ATLAS OF

PEDIATRIC DERMATOLOGY IN ASIAN SKIN

ATLAS OF PEDIATRIC DERMATOLOGY IN ASIAN SKIN

EDITORS

Mark Jean Aan Koh, MBBS
Head and Senior Consultant
Department of Dermatology
KK Women's and Children's Hospital
Singapore

Emily Yiping Gan, MBBS
Senior Consultant
Department of Dermatology
KK Women's and Children's Hospital
Singapore

Lynette Wei Yi Wee, MBBS
Consultant
Department of Dermatology
KK Women's and Children's Hospital
Singapore

Mc Graw Hill

Atlas of Pediatric Dermatology in Asian Skin

1 2 3 4 5 6 7 8 9 DSS 29 28 27 26 25 24

ISBN 978-1-264-26701-9
MHID 1-264-26701-0

This book was set in Minion Pro by KnowledgeWorks Global Ltd.
The editors were Dimana Tzvetkova and Peter J. Boyle.
The production supervisor was Richard Ruzycka.
Project management was provided by Tasneem Kauser, KnowledgeWorks Global Ltd.
The interior design was by Mary McKeon.
The cover designer was W2 Design.

Cataloging-in-publication data for this book is on file at the Library of Congress.

I dedicate this atlas to my beloved family, Evelyn, Alexandra, Isabel, Jessie, Jimmy, Melanie, Paul, Shirley, Patch, and Cosmo. Words cannot express my appreciation for your love, support, and dedication. I also dedicate this work to all my mentees; you have taught me so much more than I have taught you. May the force live on beyond our world!

We also want to express our heartfelt gratitude to our colleagues from the Department of Dermatology, KKH, and our pediatric dermatology colleagues from Singapore and the region who have contributed to this beautiful work. Finally, we want to thank our patients and their parents and caregivers, who have generously contributed their photographs and helped us learn so much more about pediatric dermatology.

Dr. Mark Jean Aan Koh

I dedicate this book to my parents, sister Nicola, husband Wee Lee, and daughters Bernadette, Caroline, and Hannah. Thank you for your patience and understanding whenever I spend time on my dermatology career. I also dedicate this to all my mentors and teachers in dermatology and pediatric dermatology, for believing in me and for giving me the opportunity to learn and practice in this field. Learning is a never-ending journey, and I am honored to have had you be a part of mine.

Dr. Emily Yiping Gan

I am deeply grateful to my mentors who have generously provided numerous opportunities, been instrumental in shaping and honing both my medical skills and personal growth, and inspired me on this educational journey, instilling the constant desire to improve and uplift others. This book is dedicated to my parents, whose unwavering support enabled my medical journey, and to my cherished family—my husband Han Feng and wonderful daughters Keira and Jamie. Your unconditional love, patience, and steadfast support have seen me through this journey.

Dr. Lynette Wei Yi Wee

Contents

Detailed Contents

Contributors

Uma Alagappan, MBBS
TDC: The Dermatology Clinic Pte Ltd
Singapore
Chapter 8

Yi Shan Ang, MBBS(Singapore), MMED(Paeds), MRCPCH(UK)
Department of Dermatology
KK Women's and Children's Hospital
Singapore
Chapter 13

Sabeera Begum, BKI, MBBS, MMED Paediatrics(UM)
Hospital Tunku Azizah
Kuala Lumpur, Malaysia
Chapter 5

Priya Bishnoi, MD Dermatology
A*STAR Skin Research Labs
Skin Research Institute of Singapore
Chapters 12 & 15

Nisha Suyien Chandran, MBBS, MMed(Int Med), MRCP(UK)
Division of Dermatology
Department of Medicine
National University Hospital
Singapore
Department of Medicine
Yong Loo Lin School of Medicine
National University of Singapore
Chapter 8

Shi Yun Chia, MBBS, MMed(Paed), MRCPCH
Department of Dermatology & General Paediatrics Service
KK Women's and Children's Hospital
Singapore
Chapters 12 & 15

Cherlyn Chin, MB BCh BAO, BSc(Hons)
Department of Dermatology
KK Women's and Children's Hospital
Singapore
Chapter 15

Jin Ho Chong, MBBS(Singapore), MRCPCH(UK), PG Dip Derm(UK), MSc Derm(UK)
Dr Chong Kids Medical & Eczema Clinic
Singapore
Chapter 2

Lynn Chua, MBBS, MMed(Paed), MRCPCH
Department of Dermatology
KK Women's and Children's Hospital
Singapore
Chapter 15

Maria Victoria C. Dizon, MD
Section Pediatric Dermatology
University of Santo Tomas Hospital
Philippines
Makati Medical Center
Philippines
Cardinal Santos Medical Center
Philippines
Chapter 6

Emily Yiping Gan, MBBS, M Med(Int Med), MRCP(UK)
Department of Dermatology
KK Women's and Children's Hospital
Singapore
Chapters 1, 7 & 14

Kathleen Mitch Uy Gomez, MD
Section of Dermatology
Cardinal Santos Medical Center
Valenzuela Medical Center
Philippines
Chapter 6

Madeline Sheun Ling Ho, MBChB(Edin), MRCP(UK), MRCP(Ireland), MSc(London)
National Skin Centre
Singapore
Chapter 3

Valerie Ho, MBBS, MMed(Paed), MRCPCH
Department of Dermatology
KK Women's and Children's Hospital
Singapore
Chapter 9

Mark Jean Aan Koh, MBBS, MRCPCH, FAMS(Dermatology), DipDermatopathology
Deparment of Dermatology
KK Women's and Children's Hospital
Singapore
Chapters 1, 10 & 13

Juin Yee Kong, MD, FAAP, FAMS
Department of Neonatology
KK Women's & Children's Hospital
Singapore
Chapter 2

Yan Ling Kong, MBBS(Singapore), PG Dip(UK), MSc(UK), FAMS
DermAlly Specialist
Skin Clinic & Surgery
Singapore
Chapter 3

Elis Lee, MBBS, MMed(Paed), MRCPCH, PG Dip Clinical Derm(UK)
Department of Dermatology
KK Women's and Children's Hospital
Singapore
Chapter 9

Hwee Chyen Lee, MBBS, MRCP(UK), FAMS(Dermatology)
Epi Dermatology & Laser Specialist Clinic
Singapore
Chapters 10 & 16

Kin Fon Leong, MBBS(UM), MRCPCH(Edin)
Women and Children Hospital
Kuala Lumpur
Chapter 4

Cheryl Jia Ling Lie, MBBS
Department of Dermatology
KK Women's and Children's Hospital
Singapore
Chapter 7

Hui Min Liew, MBChB, MRCP, FAMS(Dermatology)
HM Liew Skin and Laser Clinic
Gleneagles Medical Centre
Singapore
Chapter 2

Charmaine Lim, MBBS, FAMS(Dermatology)
Department of Dermatology
KK Women's and Children's Hospital
Singapore
Chapter 8

Pamela Ng, MBBS, MMed(Paed), MRCPCH
Department of Dermatology
KK Women's and Children's Hospital
Singapore
Chapter 9

Shanna Ng, BMedSci, MBBS
The Dermatology Practice
Singapore
Chapter 14

Amelie Seghers, MD, MSc, MRCP(UK), MRCP(Derm)
www.drameliesegher s.com
London
United Kingdom
Chapter 14

Colin Weixuan Tan, MBBS, MRCS(Edin), GDFM
Department of Dermatology
KK Women's and Children's Hospital
Singapore
Chapter 7

Jenny Tan, MBBS(UM), MRCPCH(UK)
Subang Jaya Medical Centre
Selangor, Malaysia
Chapter 4

Lucinda Tan, MBBS, MRCP, MMed(Int Med)
National Skin Centre
Singapore
Chapter 8

Maria Celi Rico-Tantianpact, MD, DPPS
Department of Pediatrics
Makati Medical Center
Philippines
Chapter 6

Yong Kwang Tay, MBBS, M Med(Int Med), MRCP, MRCP, FRCP, FRCP, FAMS
Department of Dermatology
Changi General Hospital
Singapore
Chapter 14

Suruchi Vohra, MBBS, MRCP(UK), MD(Dermatology)
King's College Hospital
Dubai
Chapter 11

Wilsie Walinsundin, MD
University of Santo Tomas Hospital
Philippines
Pediatric Dermatology Unit
East Avenue Medical Center
Philippines
Dr. Jose N. Rodriguez Memorial Hospital
Philippines
Chapter 6

Aileen Wee, MD(UPM), MRCPCH(UK)
Growell Baby & Child Specialist Clinic (Ampang)
Selangor, Malaysia
Chapter 5

Lynette Wei Yi Wee, MBBS(Singapore), MMED(Paeds), MRCPCH(UK), DIP DERM(UK)
Department of Dermatology
KK Women's and Children's Hospital
Singapore
Chapters 1, 10, & 13

Sharon Wong, MBBS, MRCPCH(UK)
Department of Dermatology & General Paediatrics Service
KK Women's and Children's Hospital,
Singapore
Chapter 11

Foreword

The skin of individuals of Asian descent spans the full range of Fitzpatrick skin pigmentation types but differs from other races, such as Caucasians, Hispanics, and Africans, in skin thickness, density and size of cutaneous appendages, and hair and nail thickness and texture. Even among Asian races, physiological differences can occur, e.g., between lighter races, such as northern Chinese, and darker races, such as East Indians. As a result, the presentation of skin disease can vary both between Asian and other races and among different Asian races.

During the last century, due to rapid globalization and ease of travel, Asians have moved to every continent, especially to the Americas, Europe, and Australia. Indeed, based on the 2020 US Census data, 19.9 million people in the United States self-identified as Asian and another 4.1 million as Asian in combination with other races. During the past two decades, numerous textbooks, atlases, and journal articles have focused on Asian populations, emphasizing the importance of understanding the skin and skin disease in this vast group of individuals. While pediatric dermatology as a field has expanded greatly since the late 20th century, there are few textbooks or atlases dedicated to pediatric dermatology in Asian children and adolescents.

The *Atlas of Pediatric Dermatology in Asian Skin* provides comprehensive and concise information on common pediatric skin conditions, as well as high-resolution photographs of dermatoses as they present in the various Asian races. Co-edited by Drs. Koh, Gan, and Wee, with chapters co-authored by colleagues from Singapore and elsewhere in the Southeast Asian and South Asian region, the atlas exemplifies the strong collaboration among pediatric dermatologists from the region, bolstered by the efforts of the Asian Society of Pediatric Dermatology (ASPD) and International Society of Pediatric Dermatology (ISPD).

I am confident that this atlas will be an excellent tool to aid in recognition and understanding of skin conditions in children and a useful resource for pediatricians, dermatologists, general practitioners, nurses, and pediatric dermatologists in daily clinical practice.

Amy S. Paller, MD
Chair, Department of Dermatology
Director, Skin Biology and Diseases Resource-Based Center

Walter J. Hamlin Professor of Dermatology
Professor of Dermatology and Pediatrics
Northwestern University
Chicago, Illinois

Preface

Our aim in compiling this atlas is to provide not only a teaching tool for the recognition and management of common (and some less common) pediatric dermatological conditions in Asian skin types, but also to provide a resource of photographs for healthcare professionals in daily practice. Our intended audience includes pediatricians, dermatologists, family practitioners, nurses, and allied health professionals who consult and manage Asian children and adolescents in their daily practice. This atlas is also intended to be a useful learning resource for medical students, trainees, residents, and fellows, especially those with an interest in pediatrics and dermatology.

We have compiled a large and extensive compendium of high-resolution clinical images of pediatric dermatological conditions presenting in Asian races, collected not only from our own pediatric dermatology practice at KK Women's & Children's Hospital in Singapore, a cosmopolitan melting-pot of Asian races, but also from our co-authors and contributors from the Southeast and South Asian regions. To enable the atlas to be an everyday working reference, we have provided up-to-date vignettes to aid in the diagnosis, investigations, and treatment of the various pediatric dermatological conditions. A small section on "pearls and practical tips" at the end of each sub-chapter adds important practice points arising from our co-authors' clinical experience. Some of these points may not be found in other publications. Chapter 16, the last chapter of the atlas, provides practical tips on performing common dermatological procedures in pediatric patients. For readers with online subscriptions to the atlas, on-demand videos of some of these procedures have been provided from our clinical practice, in addition to additional digital photographs which include less classical presentations of pediatric dermatology conditions, and rarer diagnoses. The videos may be obtained by visiting the book on AccessDermatologyDxRx.com.

We sincerely hope that you will find this atlas as useful as we have while compiling the text and photographs of the book.

Dr. Mark Jean Aan Koh
Dr. Emily Yiping Gan
Dr. Lynette Wei Yi Wee

Introduction: Development & Biology of Asian Skin

Asia is the largest continent in the world. Asians comprise more than half of the total global population, and a large proportion are regarded as having pigmented skin. Even among individuals of Asian descent, skin types can vary from Fitzpatrick skin type II or III (e.g., Chinese, Koreans, Japanese) to Fitzpatrick skin type VI (e.g., South Indians), with many races in between these two extremes. Importantly, with the increasing mobility of the world's population over the past two centuries, Asians now comprise a significant proportion of populations throughout the world and in all continents.

Apart from differences in some aspects of skin biology, the prevalence and presentation of various pediatric skin conditions in Asians can differ from Caucasian or African pediatric populations.

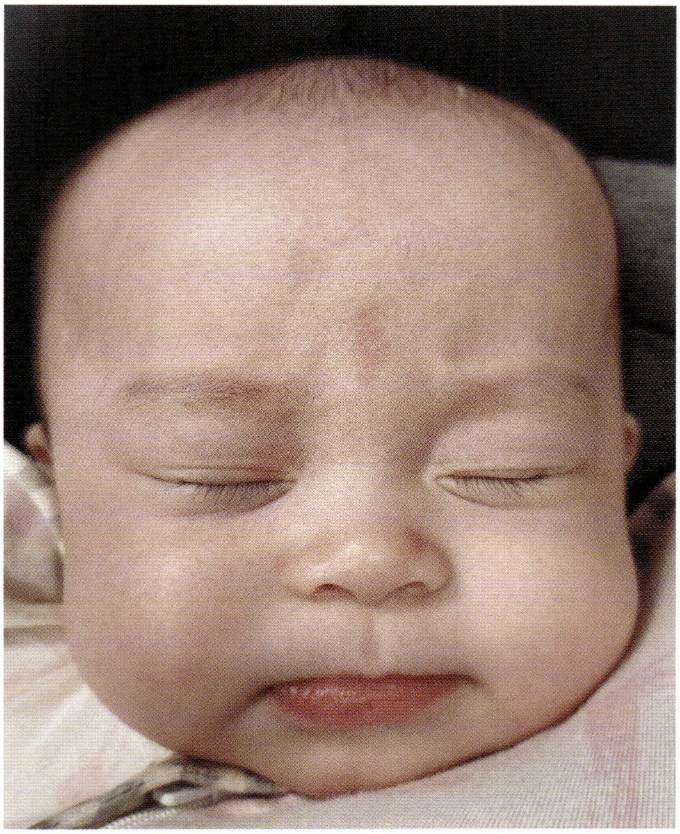

FIGURE 1-1. Chinese child with Fitzpatrick skin type II.

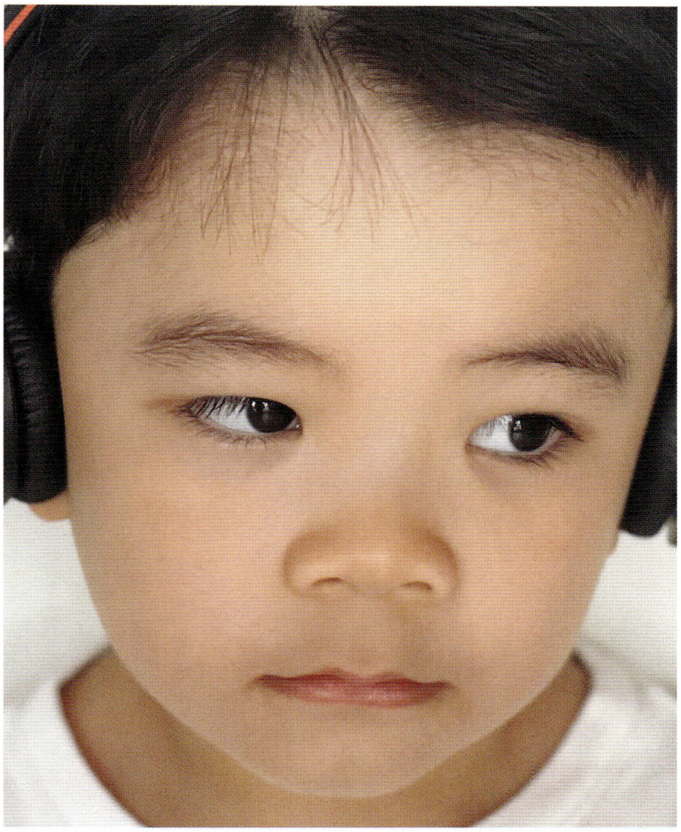

FIGURE 1-2. Chinese child with Fitzpatrick skin type III.

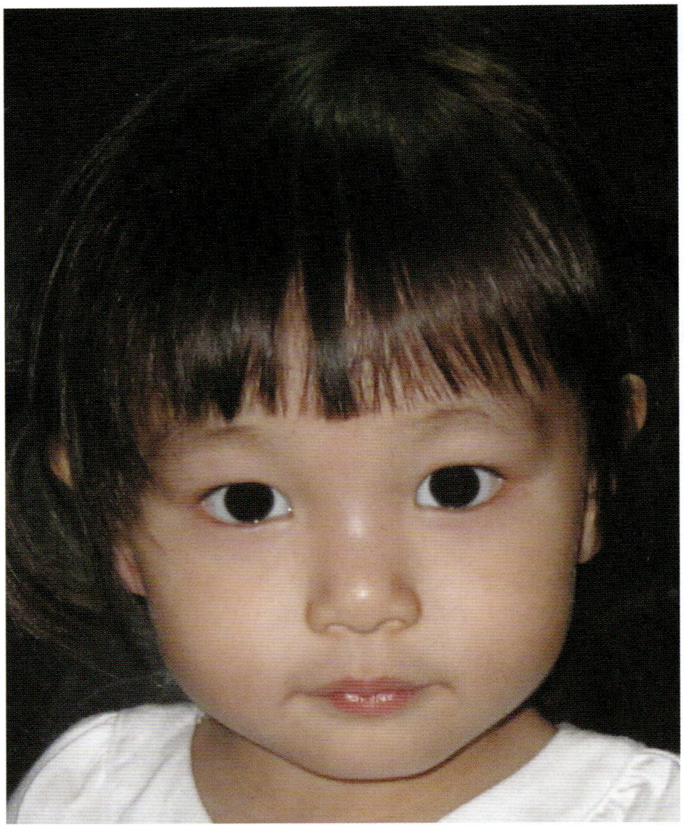

FIGURE 1-3. Chinese child with Fitzpatrick skin type IV.

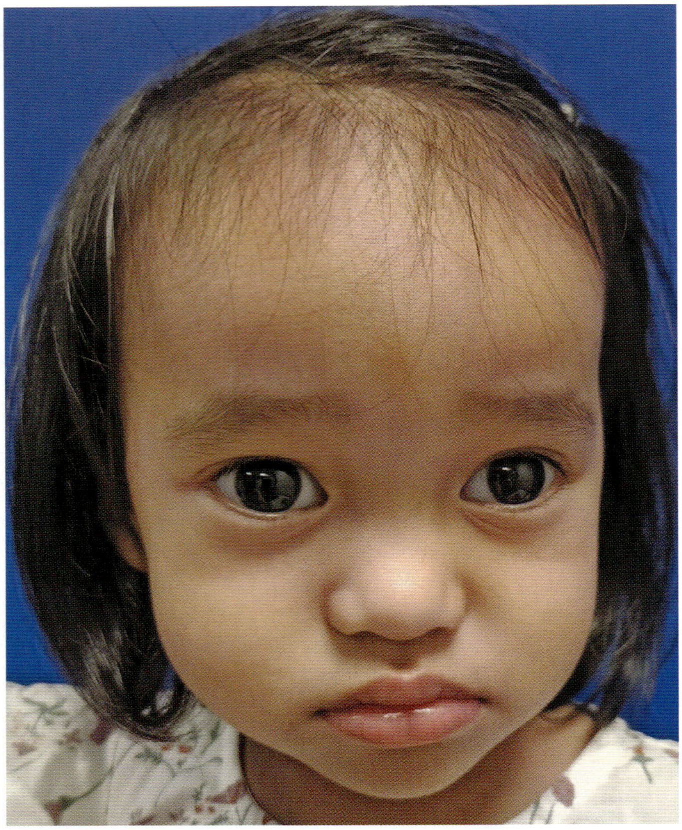

FIGURE 1-4. Malay child with Fitzpatrick skin type IV.

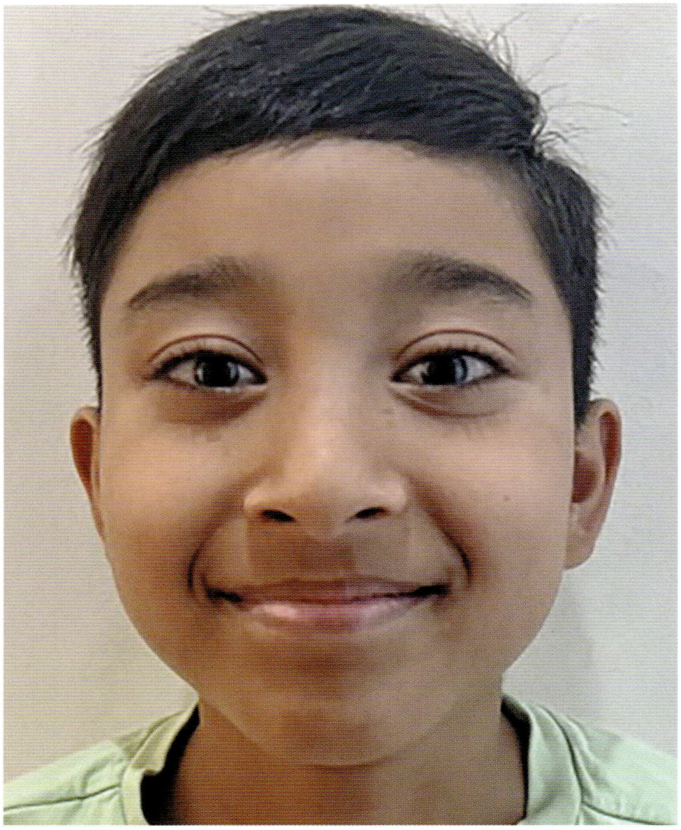

FIGURE 1-5. Indian child with Fitzpatrick skin type V.

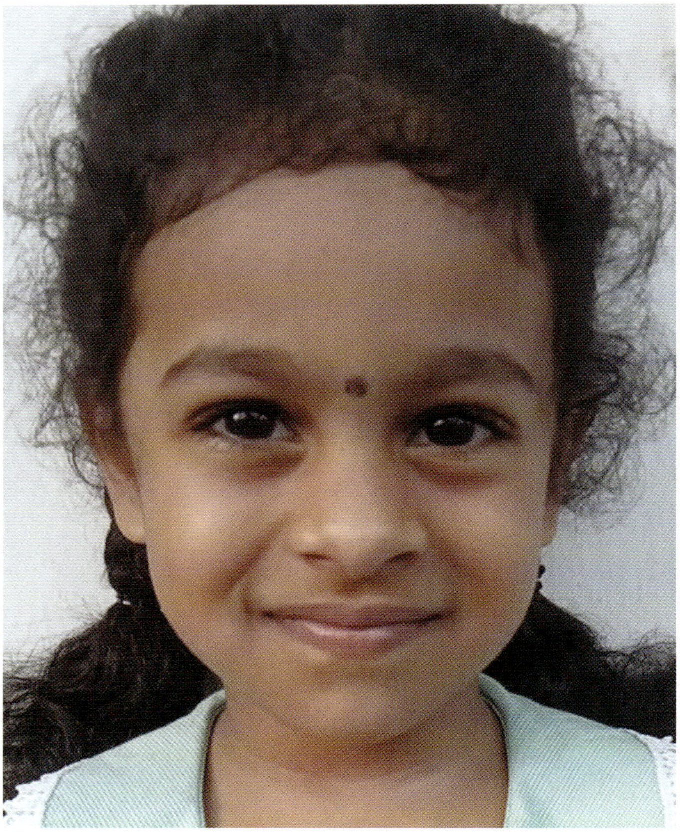

FIGURE 1-6. Indian child with Fitzpatrick skin type VI.

BIOLOGY OF PIGMENTATION IN ASIAN SKIN

- The hallmark of pigmentation of individuals with skin of color is the amount and distribution of melanin in the skin.
- Melanin is synthesized by melanocytes within melanosomes. Melanosomes are transferred to keratinocytes either as aggregated or single particles. Two forms of melanin are synthesized within melanocytes: eumelanin, which is brown-black, and pheomelanin, which is yellow-red.
- The difference in skin color between different races is due to differences in number, size, aggregation, and distribution of melanosomes in melanocytes and keratinocytes. There is no difference in absolute number of melanocytes between races.
- Due to the biology of melanin and melanosomes in Asian skin of color, pigmentary disorders are much more common compared to Caucasians. Post-inflammatory dyspigmentation, which can appear as either hypo- or hyperpigmentation, is very common in Asian children. This can worsen with increased sun exposure.
- The presentation of various dermatoses in darker Asian races can vary considerably with light Asian races and Caucasians; that is, the erythema seen in various dermatoses, such as atopic dermatitis, is poorly seen in darker skin types, with lesions appearing more hyperpigmented.

BIOLOGY OF THE EPIDERMIS AND DERMIS OF ASIAN SKIN

- The epidermis comprises four main layers, which, from the most superficial to the deepest layer, is composed of the stratum corneum, stratum granulosum, stratum spinosum, and stratum basale.
- Data on racial differences in the structure, function, and properties of the stratum corneum have been conflicting. A study found significant differences in the ceramide/cholesterol ratios between different racial groups, with Asians having the highest ratio compared to white-skinned individuals and Africans.[1]
- Although there is no proven difference in the thickness of the dermis between races, there have been differences at the cellular level, including the amount of collagen 1 and 3, fibrillin-rich microfibrils, and fibulin-5.[2]
- The dermal-epidermal junction (DEJ) is an important structure in the skin. Specific skin-associated components of the DEJ include hemidesmosomes, anchoring filaments, anchoring fibrils, type VII collagen, laminin 332, and BP180. Collagen VII has been shown to be more widely distributed in East Asian skin compared to the more discrete distribution seen in African skin, but there was no significant difference in the distribution of laminin-332 and integrin β4.[2]

BIOLOGY OF ADNEXAL STRUCTURES IN ASIAN SKIN

- Adnexal structures of the skin include hairs, sebaceous glands, and sweat glands. Certain areas of the skin are richer in the different adnexal structures. Hair is found most abundantly on the scalp, with increased hair developing over the facial, axillary, and genital regions during puberty, and in males. Sebaceous glands are found most abundantly on the face, scalp, and chest regions; eccrine glands are found throughout the skin; and apocrine glands are found in limited sites, such as the axillae, groin, and around the nipples.
- The density of hair follicle orifices on the scalp of Asians has been shown to be less than Caucasian skin but similar to African skin.[3,4] The hairs of Asians are more round or circular, with the largest cross-sectional area compared to Caucasians. Asians have been found to have the smallest follicular infundibulum volume compared to Caucasians and Africans, leading to more significant transcutaneous absorption of substances, as the follicular infundibulum serves as a reservoir for these substances applied topically.[5]
- Sebaceous glands are attached to the hair follicle by the pilosebaceous duct, and secrete sebum, which contains a mixture of squalene, cholesterol, cholesterol esters, wax esters, and triglycerides. Studies have shown conflicting results on the amount and composition of sebum in different skin types.
- There are two main types of sweat glands. Eccrine glands can be found over almost the entire body, although different regions show different densities. Apocrine sweat glands are mostly found in the intertriginous regions and become active during puberty. The effect of race on the size and function of sweat glands is less than the effect of climate.

References

1. Jungersted JM, Høgh JK, Hellgren LI, Jemec GBE, Agner T. Ethnicity and stratum corneum ceramides. Br J Dermatol 2010;163:1169–73.
2. Langton AK, Sherratt MJ, Sellers WI, Griffiths CE, Watson RE. Geographical ancestry is a key determinant of epidermal morphology and dermal composition. Br J Dermatol 2014 Aug;171(2):274–82.
3. Mangelsdorf S, Otberg N, Maibach HI, Sinkgraven R, Sterry W, Lademann J. Ethnic variation in vellus hair follicle size and distribution. Skin Pharmacol Physiol 2006;19:159–67.
4. Lee HJ, Ha SJ, Lee JH, Kim JW, Kim HO, Whiting DA. Hair counts from scalp biopsy specimens in Asians. J Am Acad Dermatol 2002;46:218–21.
5. Luther N, Darvin ME, Sterry W, Lademann J, Patzelt A. Ethnic differences in skin physiology, hair follicle morphology and follicular penetration. Skin Pharmacol Physiol 2012;25:182–91.

2

Neonatal Dermatoses

PHYSIOLOGICAL SKIN CHANGES OF THE NEWBORN

Physiological skin changes are common, benign skin manifestations that should be recognized and differentiated from more pathological skin changes. An important differentiating factor is the general clinical condition of the baby. An irritable or extremely quiet child, poor feeding or feed intolerance, and respiratory distress are possible suggestions of an unwell baby.

CUTIS MARMORATA

Most often found in neonates and young infants, **cutis marmorata is a transient skin condition** that occurs when the child is exposed to cool ambient temperature and presents with **a bluish-red marbling pattern** of the skin.

Clinical Features

- "Lace-like" mottled pattern of dusky erythema on the trunk or extremities, which is more pronounced when the skin is cooled, and fades with warmer ambient temperatures.
- The child is clinically well.
- The phenomenon is due to the simultaneous contraction and dilation of superficial blood vessels in the skin.

Differential Diagnosis

- Cutis marmorata telangiectatica congenita (CMTC)
  - This is a rare vascular malformation characterized by persistent reticular erythema or purpura that is usually localized to a specific area, especially a limb. Skin ulceration may be seen. Unlike cutis marmorata, the lesions do not lighten with warming the skin.
- Skin mottling
  - This appears quite similar to cutis marmorata but occurs in an ill child and is associated with prolonged capillary refill time.

Investigations & Treatment

- The diagnosis is made clinically and no treatment is required, except for rewarming of the infant.

Pearls & Practical Tips

- If the onset of reticulate erythema or purpura is recent and baby's general condition is poor, consider skin mottling from underlying sepsis.

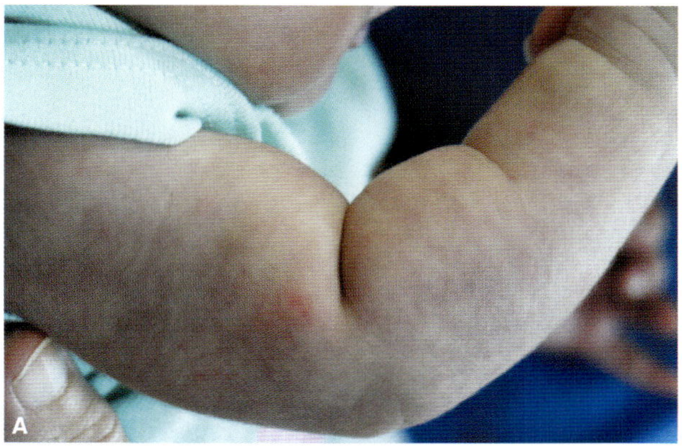

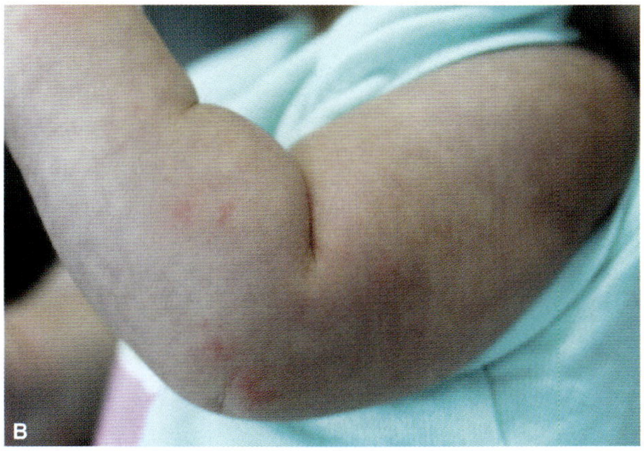

FIGURE 2-1A & 1B. Cutis marmorata on the limbs of a Chinese neonate, presenting as a bluish-red marbling pattern on the arms and legs.

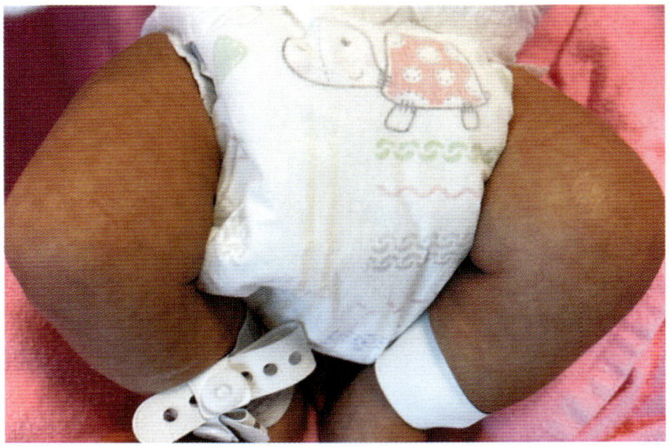

FIGURE 2-2. Cutis marmorata on the legs of a neonate.

HARLEQUIN COLOR CHANGE

Harlequin color change is a transient phenomenon present in about 10% of newborns that is characterized by sharply demarcated red color change affecting half of the body. This has been hypothesized to be due to the immature hypothalamic center that results in dilation of peripheral blood vessels.

Clinical Features

- When an affected baby is placed on one side, an erythematous flush with a sharp demarcation at the midline is seen on the dependent side, with the non-dependent side appearing pale.
- A transient phenomenon that commonly affects healthy newborns between day 2 and 5 of life and can occur as late as 3 weeks of life.

Differential Diagnosis

- Port wine stain
  - The erythema of port wine stain persists regardless of position.

Investigations & Treatment

- This is a clinical diagnosis and no treatment is required.

Pearls & Practical Tips

- Rarely, this condition may be a result of a serious underlying central nervous system disorder, especially if associated with other neurological abnormalities.

CEPHALOHEMATOMA

A cephalohematoma is a collection of blood between the skull and periosteum that occurs as a result of ruptured small blood vessels crossing the periosteum during the birth process. It is a self-resolving condition with no intracranial complications.

Clinical Features

- Cephalohematoma presents as a fluctuant swelling with or without overlying purpura or bruising, bounded by the suture lines of the skull.
- It occurs during vertex deliveries, especially with prolonged labor and instrument-assisted delivery with forceps or vacuum extractor.
- Complications include hyperbilirubinemia causing neonatal jaundice, and rarely, cellulitis.

Differential Diagnosis

- Caput succedaneum and subgaleal hematoma
  - Caput succedaneum is a soft tissue swelling with irregular borders that crosses the suture line, while a subgaleal hematoma is a fluctuant to tense scalp swelling that also crosses the suture lines.
- Cranial meningocele or encephalocele
  - These are rare meningeal outpouchings that contain cerebrospinal fluid.

Investigations & Treatment

- Diagnosis is clinical and no treatment is required, with spontaneous resolution in 7 to 10 days.

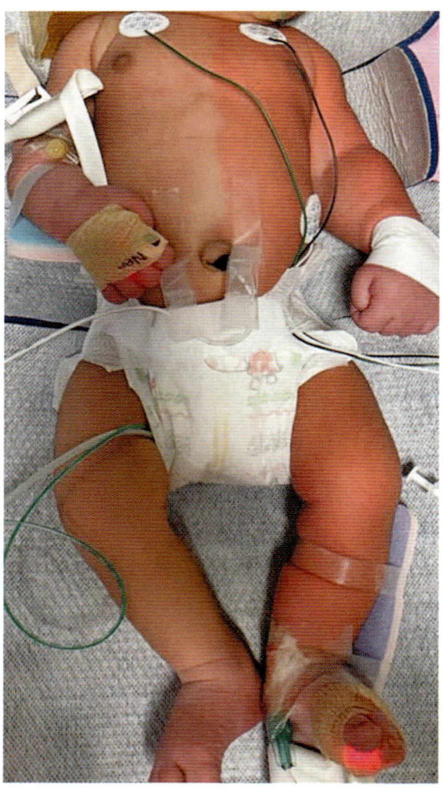

FIGURE 2-3. Harlequin color change in a neonate with hypoxic ischemic encephalopathy presenting with sharply demarcated unilateral red color with midline demarcation.

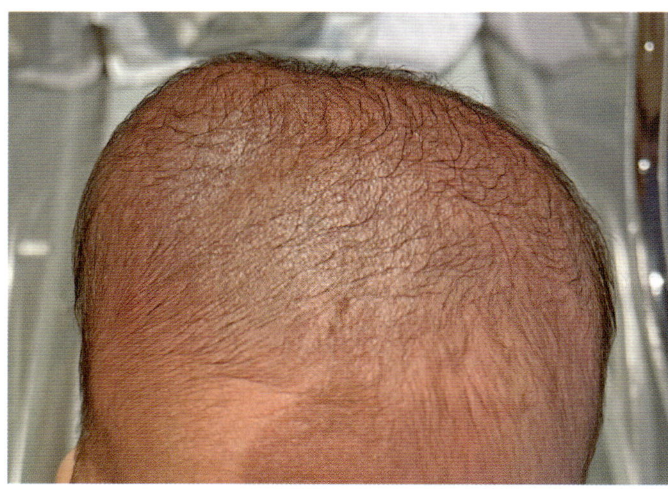

FIGURE 2-4. Cephalohematoma in a newborn presenting with a swelling on the right parietal region with overlying erythema. The swelling is bounded by the suture lines.

CAPUT SUCCEDANEUM

Caput succedaneum is a soft tissue **swelling around the** vertex of a **newborn's head**, giving rise to a **"conehead" appearance.** It occurs as a result of pressure from the uterus or vaginal wall during a vertex delivery, especially with prolonged labor and instrument-assisted delivery with forceps or vacuum extractor.

Clinical Features

- It presents as subcutaneous, extraperiosteal edema over the presenting part of the head, with the swelling crossing the suture lines.
- It feels soft without a well-defined outline.

Differential Diagnosis

- Cephalohematoma (see above)
- Cranial meningocele or encephalocele (see above)

Investigations & Treatment

- Diagnosis is clinical and no treatment is required, with resolution in a few days.

Pearls & Practical Tips

- Rare complications include bruising of the skin over the swelling with necrosis resulting in scarring, and alopecia can occur.

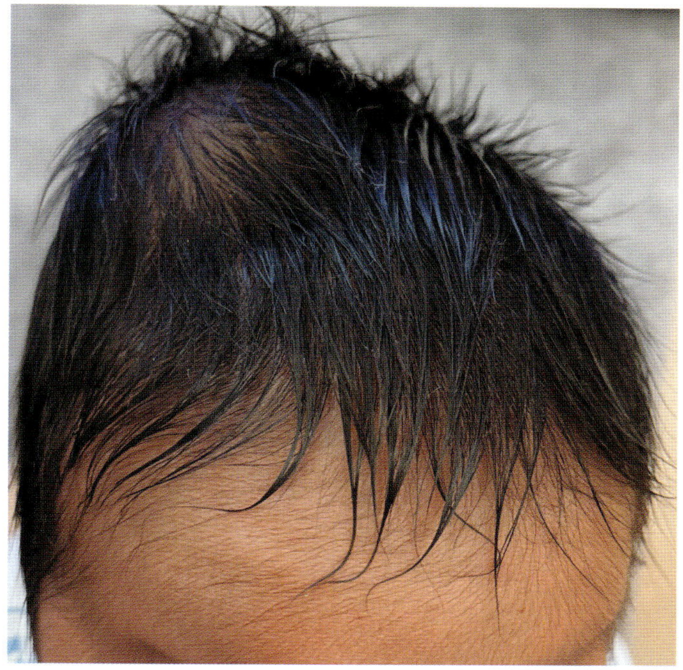

FIGURE 2-5. Caput succedaneum in a newborn, presenting as a swelling around the skull, with a "conehead" appearance.

CUTANEOUS DISORDERS OF THE NEWBORN

ERYTHEMA TOXICUM NEONATORUM

Erythema toxicum neonatorum is a very common benign cutaneous eruption in infants, appearing within 24 to 48 hours of life. Affected infants are generally well.

Clinical Features

- Usually occurs in the first 2 days of life, but onset can be as late as 2 weeks.
- Erythema toxicum presents as elevated small yellowish papules and pustules, with surrounding erythema and sometimes wheals.
- The infant is generally well, and the rash is asymptomatic.

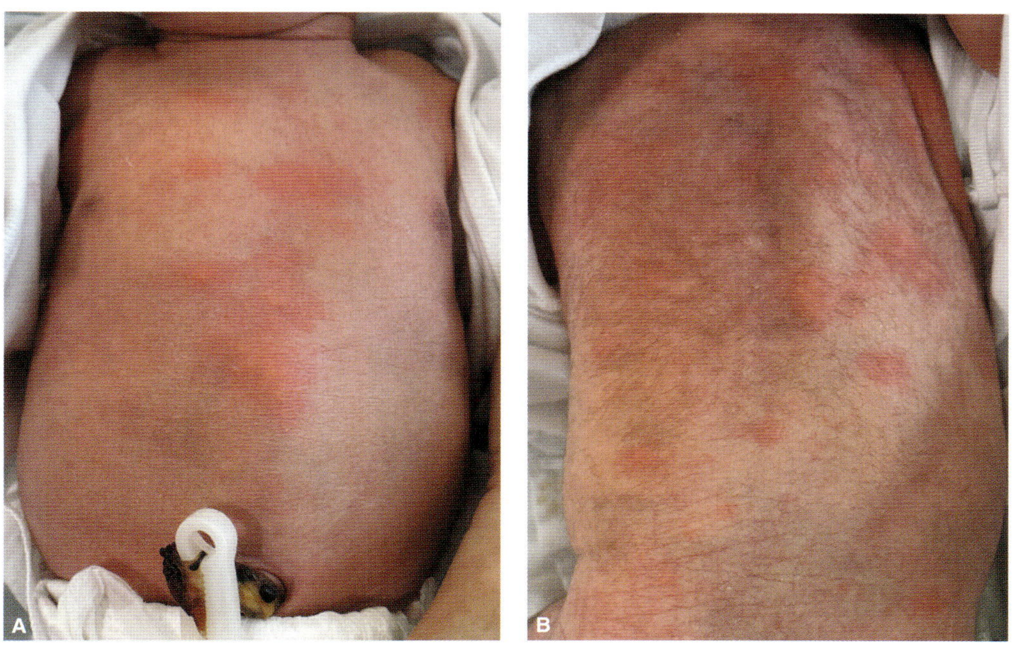

FIGURE 2-6A & 6B. Erythema toxicum neonatorum in a 3-day-old neonate, presenting with multiple blotchy erythematous patches and plaques on the trunk.

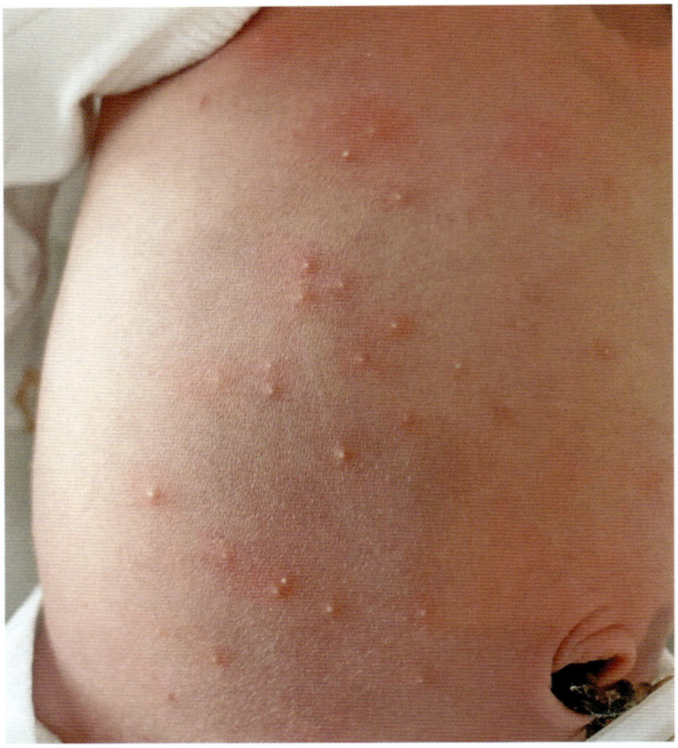

FIGURE 2-7. Erythema toxicum neonatorum in a neonate presenting with pustules and erythematous patches and plaques on the trunk.

- The trunk is most commonly affected but the rash can also affect the face and limb, with sparing of acral sites.

Differential Diagnoses

- Neonatal herpes simplex infection
  - Lesions are more vesicular rather than papulopustular. There may be a history of herpes simplex infection in the mother.
- Impetigo
  - Pustules are usually larger and more flaccid, denuding to form superficial erosions. The baby is more unwell and may be febrile.
- Congenital cutaneous candidiasis
  - Lesions are also pustular but tends to have a scalier background.

Investigations & Treatment

- The diagnosis is made clinically, and investigations are not necessary.
- Microbiological investigations may be required to exclude infections if the infant is systemically unwell.
- Spontaneous resolution of these lesions occurs within a week, and no treatment is required.

Pearls & Practical Tips

- Parents may be alarmed by the appearance of the rash, especially when extensive. Reassurance is usually sufficient as long as the child is generally well and afebrile.

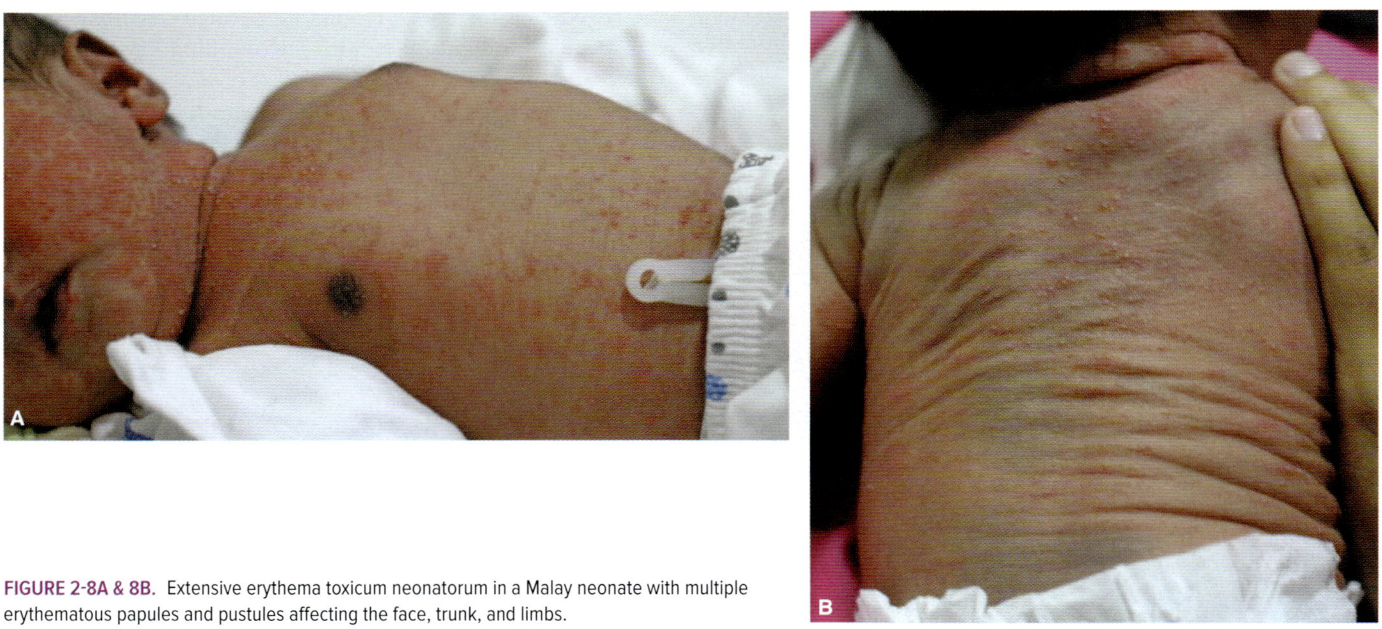

FIGURE 2-8A & 8B. Extensive erythema toxicum neonatorum in a Malay neonate with multiple erythematous papules and pustules affecting the face, trunk, and limbs.

TRANSIENT NEONATAL PUSTULAR MELANOSIS

Transient neonatal pustular melanosis is a benign idiopathic skin dermatosis most commonly affecting newborns of skin of color. It is characterized by vesicles, superficial pustules, and hyperpigmented macules.

Clinical Features

- Transient neonatal pustular melanosis presents from birth with vesicles and pustules without an erythematous base, or pigmented macules with collarette of scales.
- Most commonly affected sites include the chin, forehead, nape, lower back, and shins.
- The lesions heal after a few days, leaving hyperpigmented macules.

Differential Diagnosis

- Erythema toxicum neonatorum
  - Some consider transient neonatal pustular melanosis as a variant of erythema toxicum neonatorum occurring in skin of color.
  - Erythema toxicum neonatorum usually appears after 24 to 48 hours of life rather than from birth.
- Infantile acropustulosis
  - This has a more acral distribution.
- Neonatal herpes simplex infection
  - This presents with vesicles on an erythematous base, with subsequent crusting.
- Congenital cutaneous candidiasis
  - Lesions are also pustular but tends to have a scalier background.
- Neonatal cephalic pustulosis
  - This is a variant of neonatal acne that typically erupts on the face and scalp during the third week of life.

Investigations & Treatment

- The condition is diagnosed clinically, although a smear of the contents of a vesicle or pustule will reveal neutrophils, and occasionally, eosinophils.
- The Lesions resolve spontaneously without treatment after a few weeks to months, leaving residual hyperpigmentation.

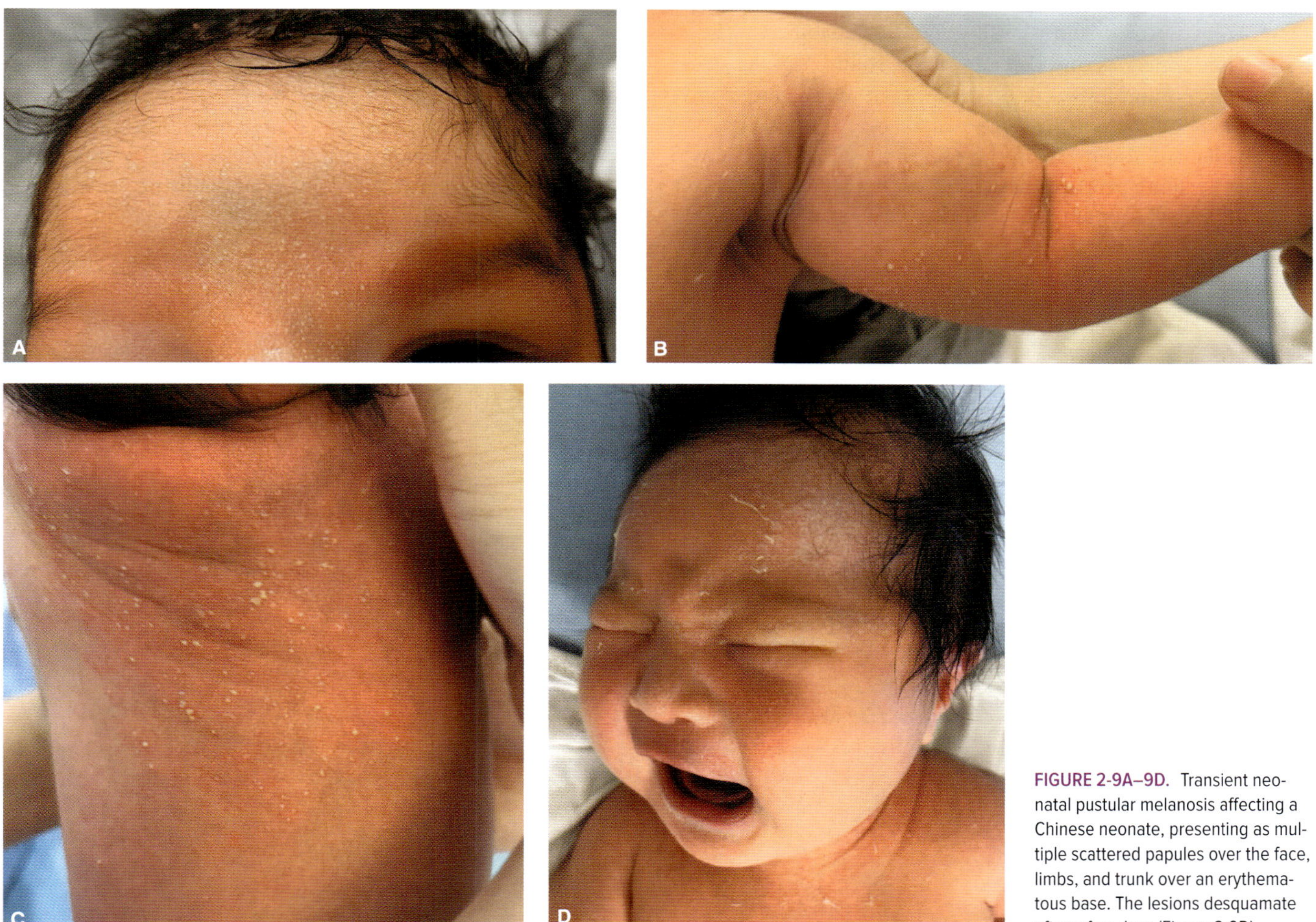

FIGURE 2-9A–9D. Transient neonatal pustular melanosis affecting a Chinese neonate, presenting as multiple scattered papules over the face, limbs, and trunk over an erythematous base. The lesions desquamate after a few days (Figure 2-9D).

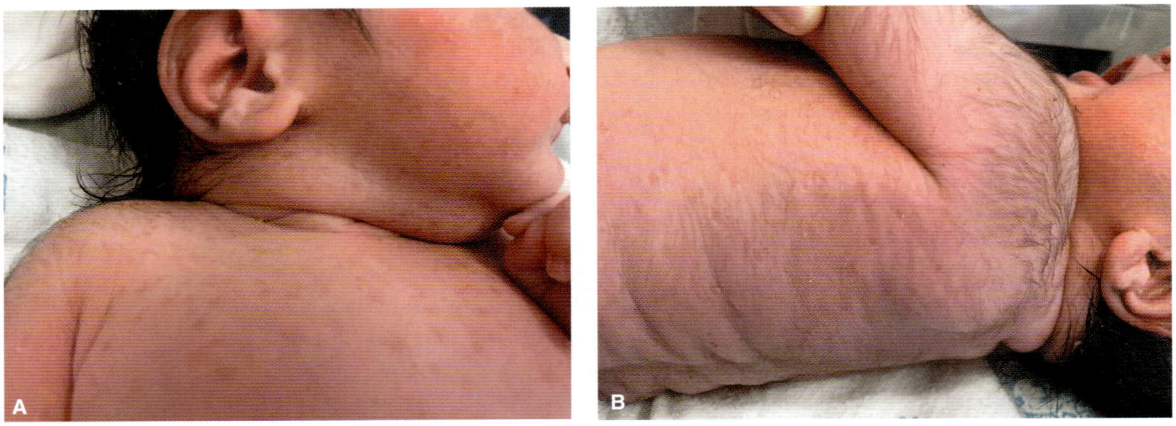

FIGURE 2-10A & 10B. Transient neonatal pustular melanosis in an Indian neonate presenting as multiple erythematous papules and pustules with desquamation. (Photograph courtesy of Dr. Kong Juin Yee, Neonatology, KK Women's & Children's Hospital.)

MILIA

Milia are common papules that occur on the face of neonates and infants. They represent small epidermal cysts with keratinaceous content.

Clinical Features

- Milia occurs in almost 50% of newborn babies.
- They appear as tiny, discrete, white, round papules.
- They commonly occur on the face but may be found anywhere on the skin surface.
- Milia can also occur in the oral mucosal and are known as Epstein's pearls if they occur on the palate and Bohn's nodules if they appear on the lingual surfaces of the alveolar ridges.

Differential Diagnoses

- Sebaceous hyperplasia
  - These appear as multiple, clustered, yellowish papules on the nose.

Investigations & Treatment

- Milia are diagnosed clinically.
- Milia usually resolves spontaneously over several months.

Pearls & Practical Tips

- If the lesion is persistent or large, it may be removed by pricking the lesion with a sterile needle or blade and expressing the contents. There is usually no scarring and does not recur.

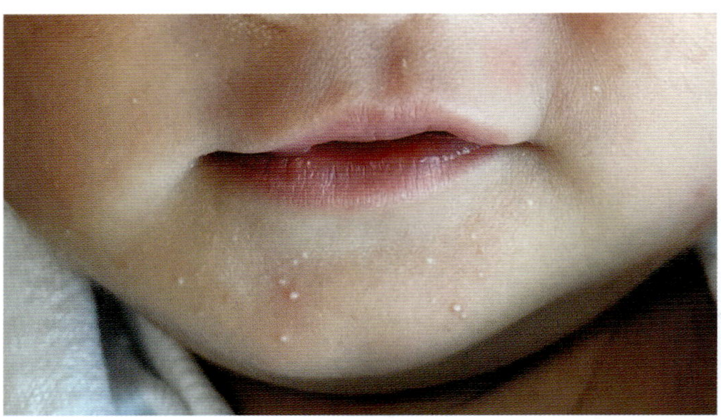

FIGURE 2-11. Multiple milia on the chin of this Chinese neonate, presenting as small, white papules.

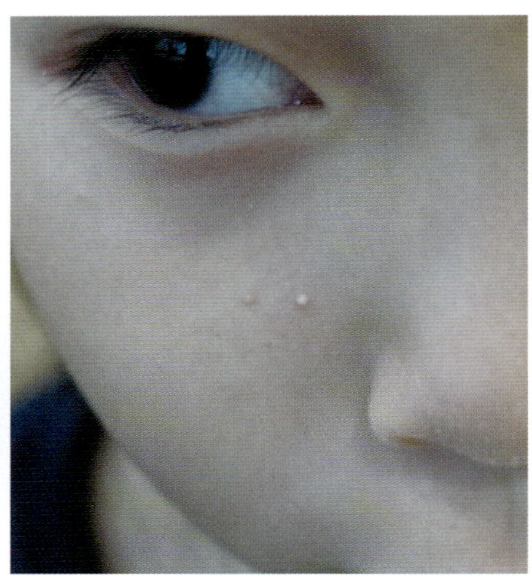

FIGURE 2-12. Milia on the cheek of an older Chinese child, with small, white, scattered papules.

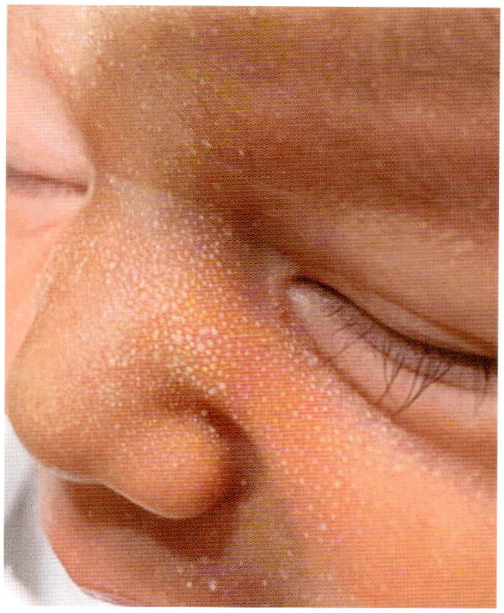

FIGURE 2-13. Sebaceous hyperplasia on the nose and medial cheek of a newborn, presenting as pinpoint, evenly spaced, white-to-yellow papules.

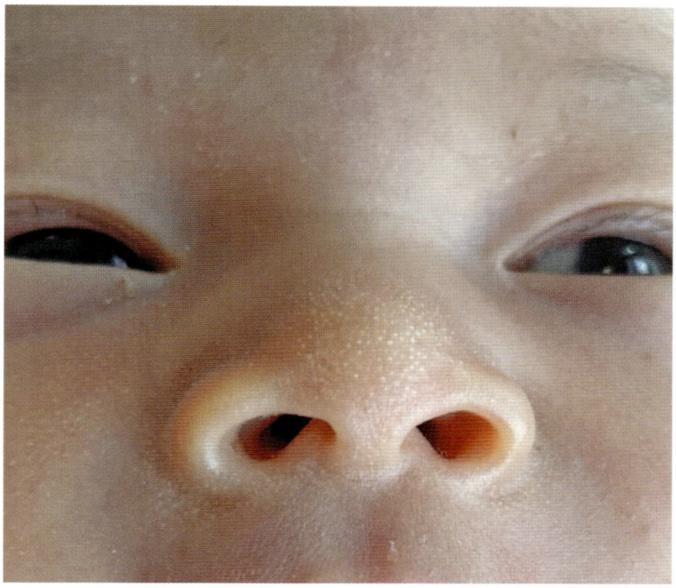

FIGURE 2-14. Sebaceous hyperplasia on the nose of a Chinese neonate.

SEBACEOUS HYPERPLASIA

Sebum secretion in a newborn is influenced by maternal hormones causing hyperplasia of the sebaceous glands.

Clinical Features

- Lesions are usually present from the first week of life.
- They appear as minute yellow papules distributed evenly around the nose and upper lip. There is no surrounding erythema.

Differential Diagnoses

- Milia
  - These present as discrete white papules; usually only one or a few are present.

Investigations & Treatment

- Diagnosis is made clinically.
- Spontaneous resolution of these lesions occurs within first few weeks of life and no treatment is required.

SUCKING BLISTERS

Sucking blisters are blisters that occur in newborns induced by vigorous sucking of the affected body part in utero. The occurrence is fairly common, and may be mistaken for other conditions, such as epidermolysis bullosa.

Clinical Features

- Sucking blisters present as 0.5- to 2-cm oval, tensed, fluid-filled blisters, which rupture to form shallow, clean erosions.
- Most commonly affected sites include the dorsal aspect of the fingers, thumb, wrist, lips, or radial aspects of the forearm. Rarely, they may appear at more distant sites, such as the toes or feet due to in-utero positioning of the baby.

Differential Diagnosis

- Bullous impetigo
  - Bullous impetigo presents with multiple small to large flaccid bullae affecting the face, trunk, and perineal region. There may be systemic symptoms, such as fever.
- Herpes neonatorum
  - Herpes presents with small, grouped vesicles with an erythematous base, and may be associated with mouth ulcers and/or conjunctivitis. The neonate may be febrile and constitutionally unwell.
- Epidermolysis bullosa
  - In epidermolysis bullosa, there will be recurrent, new blisters forming over sites of trauma. There may be a family history or parents are consanguineous.

Investigations & Treatment

- The diagnosis is made clinically and lesions spontaneously resolve rapidly and without sequelae or recurrence.

Pearls & Practical Tips

- Sucking blisters are often mistaken for other more dangerous conditions, as listed in the differential diagnoses section. The presentation, site, and morphology can provide clues to the diagnosis. Importantly, the neonate is constitutionally well.

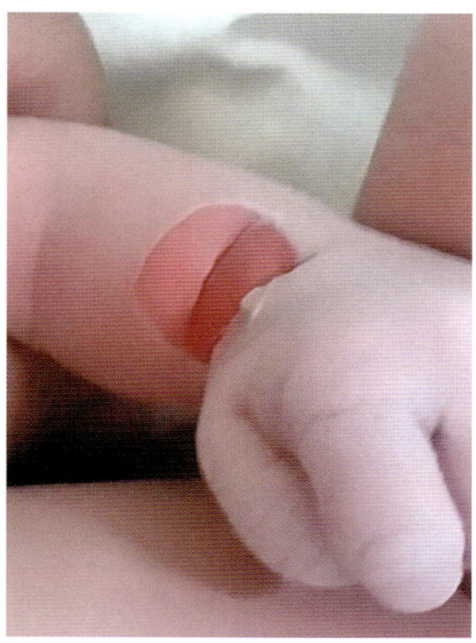

FIGURE 2-15. Superficial erosion on the left wrist of a newborn secondary to sucking blister. (Photograph courtesy of Dr. Wai Lun Tun.)

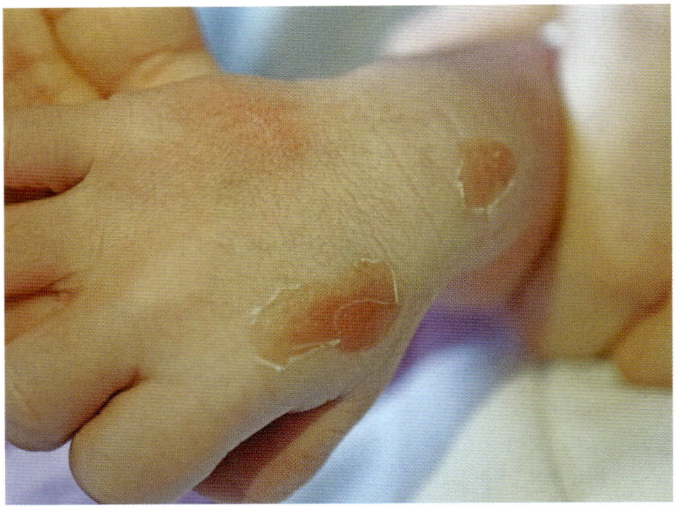

FIGURE 2-16. Two superficial erosions on the right hand dorsum of a newborn secondary to sucking blister.

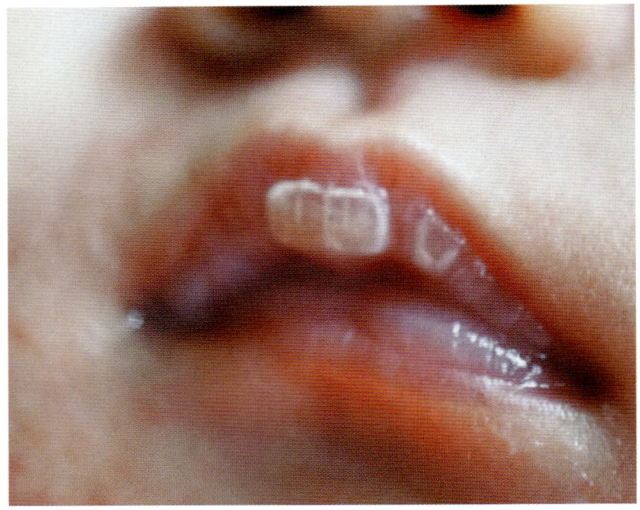

FIGURE 2-17. Sucking blister on the upper lip of young neonate.

MILIARIA

Miliaria, also known as heat rash, occurs secondary to obstruction of the eccrine ducts. It occurs commonly in infants in warm climates, especially when heavily swaddled or are febrile due to infection.

Clinical Features

- The clinical manifestations of miliaria depend on the level of obstruction of the eccrine duct. The baby is otherwise generally well.
- Miliaria crystallina appears as clear non-inflammatory vesicles and is due to sweat duct obstruction at the subcorneal or intracorneal layer of the epidermis.
- Miliaria rubra appears as erythematous papules or papulopustules and occurs due to obstruction of the eccrine ducts within the epidermis, with inflammation around the obstructed ducts. It has a predilection for occluded skin, such as the flexures and upper trunk and forehead.
- Miliaria profunda is much less common than miliaria crystallina and rubra. It presents as inflamed edematous papules and nodules and occurs secondary to obstruction of eccrine ducts at or below the dermal-epidermal junction.

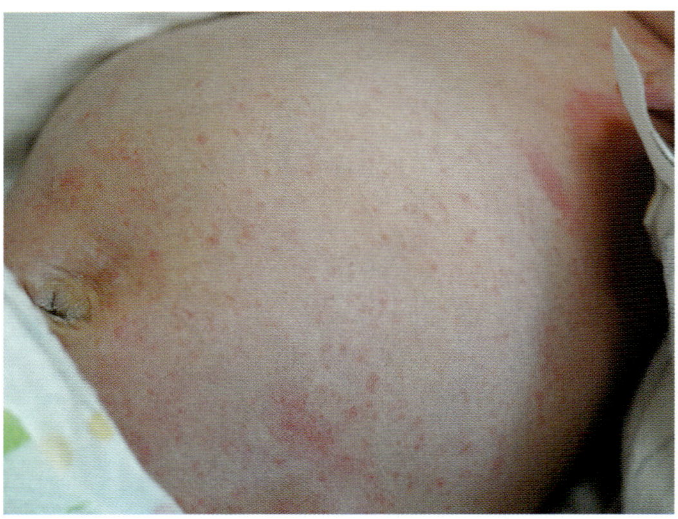

FIGURE 2-18. Miliaria rubra on the trunk of a neonate presenting as small, pinpoint, erythematous papules.

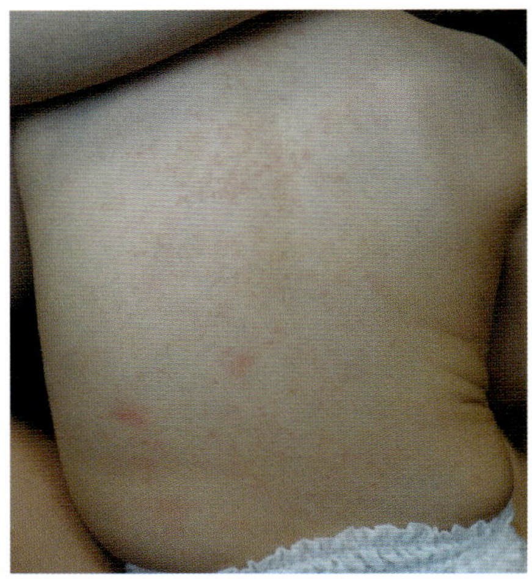

FIGURE 2-19. Miliaria on the back of a Japanese infant, with small pinpoint, erythematous papules.

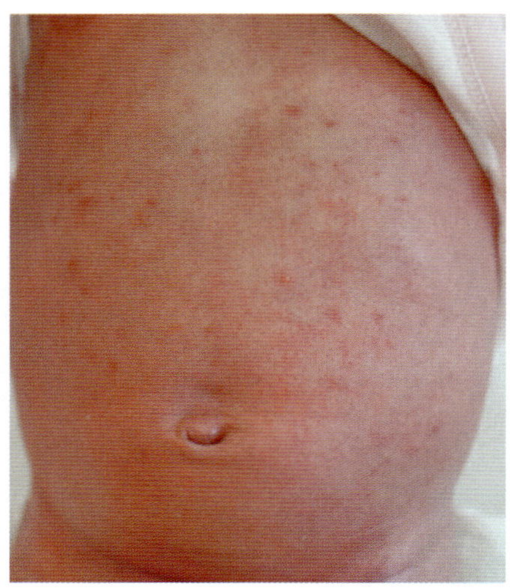

FIGURE 2-20. Miliaria rubra and miliaria pustulosa on the trunk of an infant with Netherton syndrome.

Differential Diagnoses

- Neonatal cutaneous infections
  - These include candidiasis, impetigo, herpes simplex, or varicella infections.
- Erythema toxicum neonatorum
  - This usually presents in the first few days of life, while miliaria usually presents later.

Investigations & Treatment

- Investigations are usually not required for diagnosis. If skin biopsies are performed, histological examination will show acute and/or chronic inflammation around the eccrine ducts, either in the epidermis or superficial dermis.
- Treatment includes measures to reduce body temperature, such as nursing in a cool air-conditioned room, avoiding swaddling, wearing of lightweight cotton clothing, bathing in cool or tepid water, and application of light moisturizers.
- Mild topical corticosteroids may be required for inflamed lesions, for example in miliaria rubra.
- If the newborn is febrile, examination and investigations should be undertaken to determine the source of infection and promptly treated.

Pearls & Practical Tips

- Avoid the use of heavy moisturizers, for example paraffin, in patients with miliaria, as this can exacerbate the sweat duct obstruction.

NEONATAL ACNE

Neonatal acne is one of the most common transient skin conditions in infants. It has been hypothesized to occur secondary to maternal hormonal stimulation, with concomitant inflammatory reaction to *Pityrosporum (Malassezia)* species of both *M. furfur* and *M. sympodialis*.

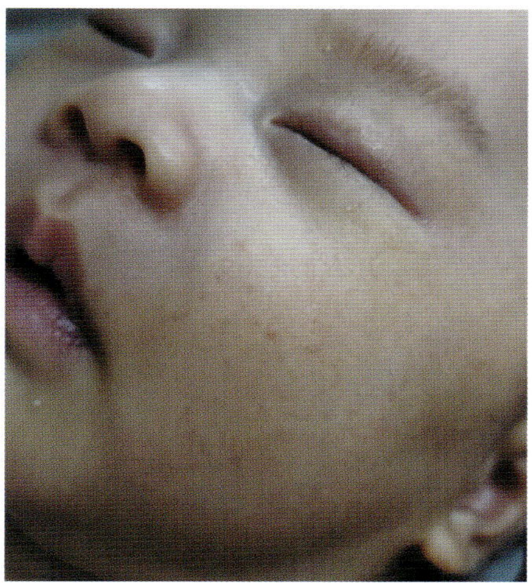

FIGURE 2-21. Mild neonatal acne on the cheeks of this Chinese infant. She also has a milia on her chin.

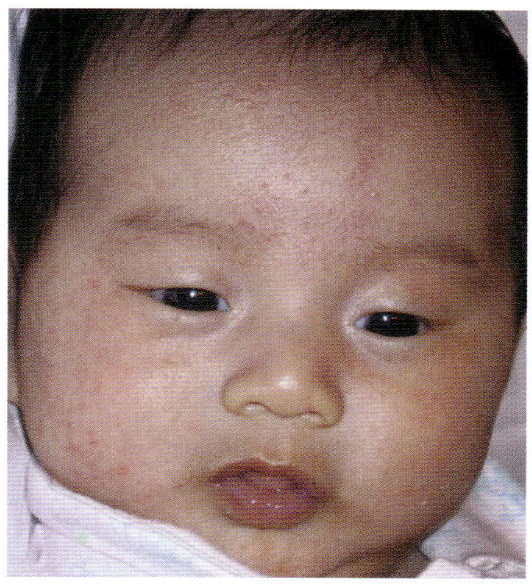

FIGURE 2-22. Mild neonatal acne with concomitant seborrheic dermatitis in a Chinese infant.

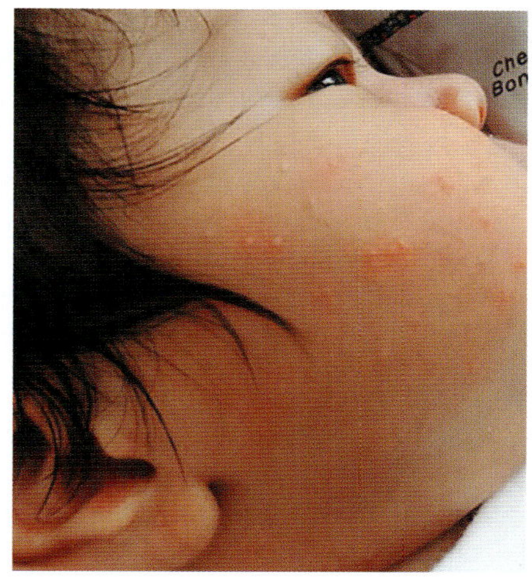

FIGURE 2-23. Mild neonatal acne on the cheeks of a Chinese neonate.

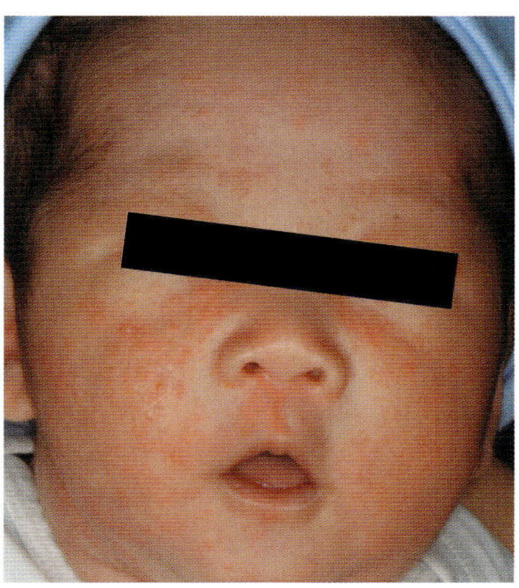

FIGURE 2-24. Neonatal acne in a Chinese baby.

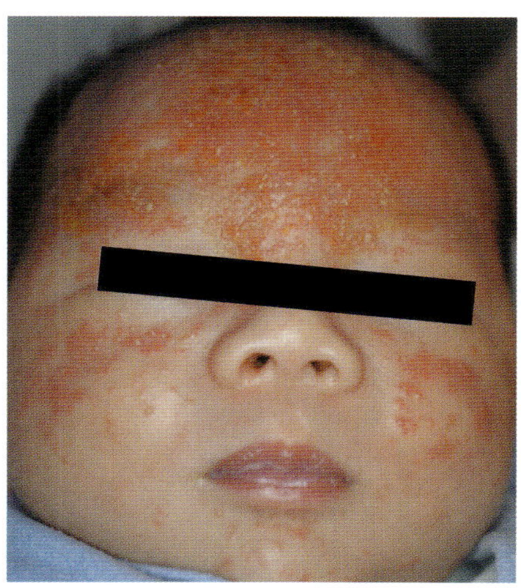

FIGURE 2-25. Neonatal acne with concomitant seborrheic dermatitis on the forehead and cheeks of a neonate, presenting with yellow, oily, scaly, papules.

Clinical Features

- Neonatal acne usually presents after the first few weeks of life.
- It presents with small, rather monomorphic papulopustules, situated on the cheeks, forehead, sometimes extending onto the scalp. Comedones, nodules, and large pustules are not seen.
- A more severe form is known as neonatal cephalic pustulosis.
- It spontaneously resolves after a few months without scarring.

Differential Diagnoses

- Milia
  - These present as single or a few small, white papules.

Investigations & Treatment

- Diagnosis is made clinically, and investigations are not necessary.
- Treatment is usually not required as it resolves spontaneously. However, in more extensive disease, topical antifungals with topical anti-inflammatory medications such as mild topical corticosteroids may be useful.

Pearls & Practical Tips

- Neonatal acne commonly occurs concomitantly with features of infantile seborrheic dermatitis, especially in babies with a family history of atopy.
- We usually treat with antifungal shampoos and mild topical corticosteroids with or without a topical antifungal.

NEVUS SIMPLEX

Nevus simplex, also called stork bite, angel's kiss, or salmon patch, is the most common type of capillary malformation, as a result of capillary dilation which are remnants of fetal blood circulation affecting infants.

Clinical Features

- Nevus simplex presents as pinkish to erythematous macules and patches, usually noticed at birth or after a few days or weeks of life.
- It occurs most commonly over the glabella, eyelids, and occiput, and less commonly on the nose and upper lip.
- Most lesions of nevus simplex over the glabella and eyelids will resolve over months to years. However, the large majority of lesions at the occiput persist.

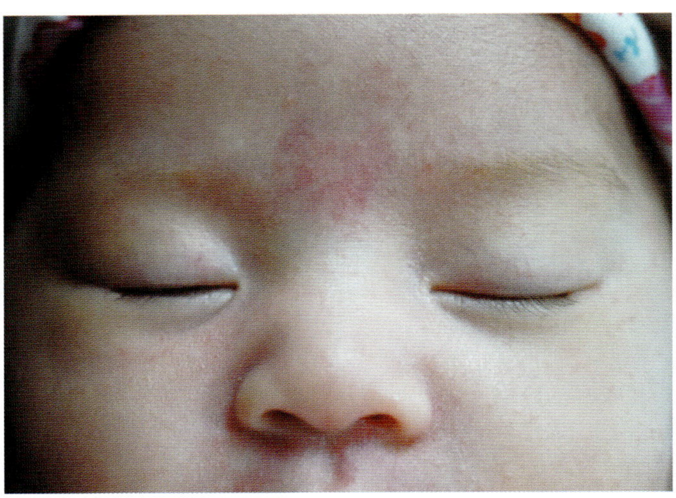

FIGURE 2-26. Nevus simplex on the glabella of a Chinese infant girl.

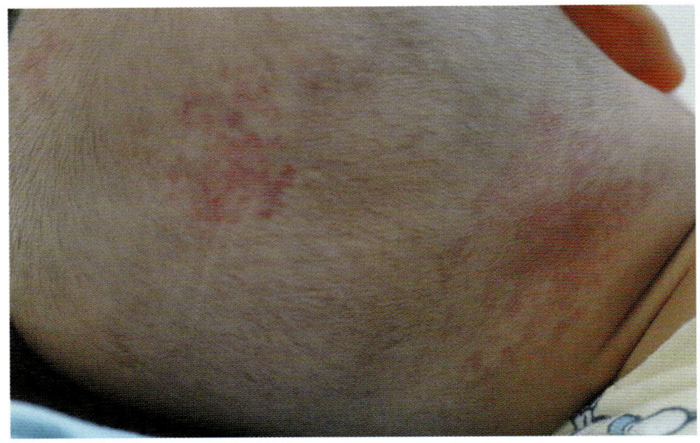

FIGURE 2-27. Nevus simplex on the nape and occipital scalp of this Chinese infant.

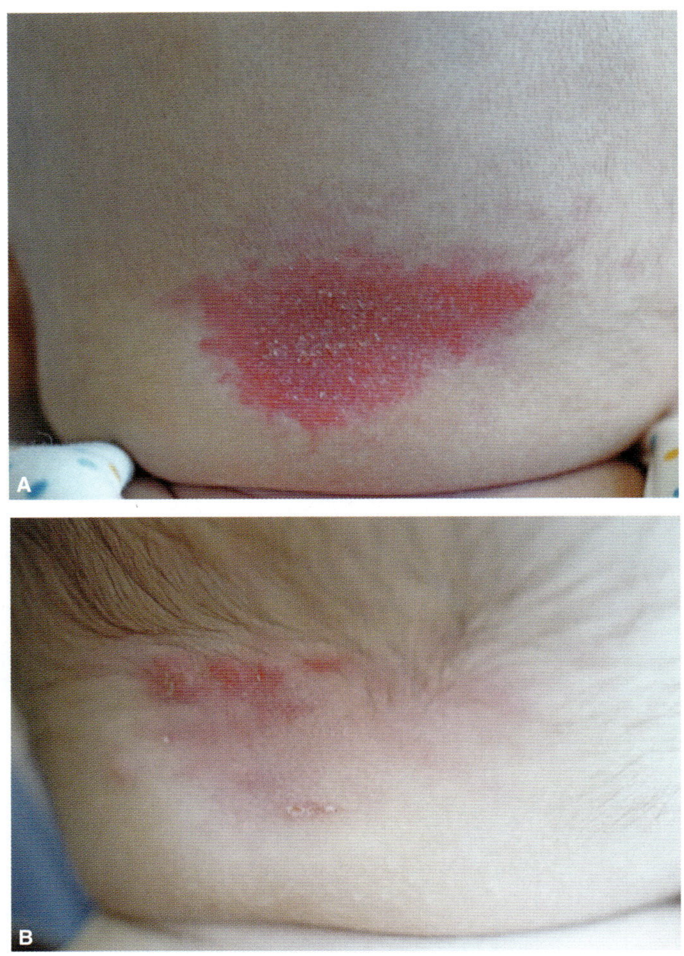

FIGURE 2-28A & 28B. Nevus simplex on the nape of this Chinese neonate with overlying eczematous changes. Figure 28B shows the same lesion 2 weeks after commencing treatment of the eczema.

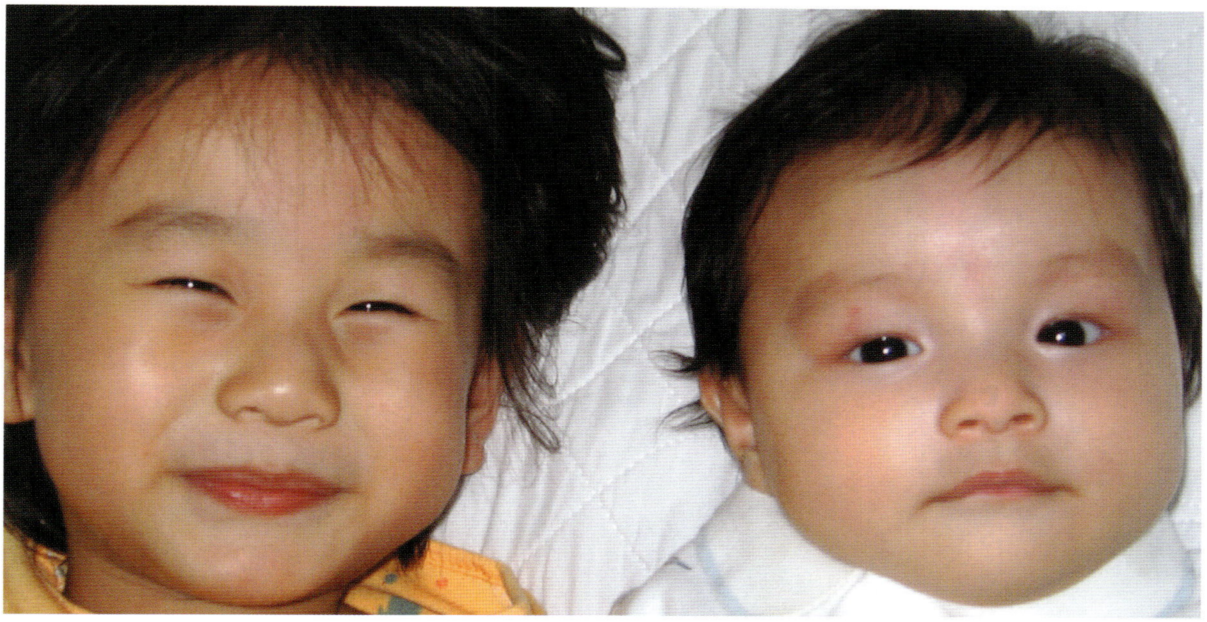

FIGURE 2-29. Nevus simplex on the glabella and forehead of both daughters of one of the co-authors (Dr. Mark Jean-Aan Koh), aged 3 years and 3 months. The younger daughter also has nevus simplex on her bilateral eyelids.

Differential Diagnoses

- Port-wine stain
  - These present with more extensive and well-demarcated, red to violaceous patches, usually asymmetrically and can darken and thicken over time.

Investigations & Treatment

- Investigation and treatment for nevus simplex is not required. Vascular lasers such as pulsed-dye lasers have been used to treat more persistent and darker lesions that are cosmetically concerning.

Pearls & Practical Tips

- Lesions of nevus simplex are usually centrally located, while port-wine stains are usually laterally located and darker, and can darken and thicken with age.
- Parents often notice that nevus simplex lesions can become more obvious with changes in weather or when the child cries.
- Eczematous changes over the nevus simplex can occur in babies with a strong family history of atopy, making the lesion appear more red.

SUBCUTANEOUS FAT NECROSIS

Subcutaneous fat necrosis (SFN) is an uncommon condition that usually occurs in full-term or post-term infants. It is usually associated with perinatal complications such as asphyxia, hypothermia, meconium aspiration, and intrapartum medications, although it can also be seen in infants without any obvious perinatal stress.

Clinical Features

- SFN presents in the first few days or weeks of life with solitary or multiple well-circumscribed, indurated, erythematous or violaceous, subcutaneous nodules or plaques, measuring from one to several centimeters.
- In some cases, the lesions may be subtle, and can only been appreciated by palpation.
- It is usually located on the trunk, thighs, buttocks, and less commonly, on the face.
- Affected infants are usually generally well and asymptomatic.
- In most cases, the lesions of SFN will regress over several months without sequelae.
- In rare cases, secondary infection or calcifications can occur.

Differential Diagnoses

- Vascular tumors or malformations
  - Vascular tumors, such as Kaposiform hemangioendothelioma and infantile hemangiomas, as well as vascular malformations, such as venous malformations, can also present with indurated, erythematous, or violaceous plaques.
  - Imaging and biopsies may be required to differentiate.
- Other causes of panniculitis
  - Subcutaneous nodules in a sick infant should raise the suspicion of other causes of panniculitis, such as sclerema neonatorum, infectious panniculitis, and nodular panniculitis.

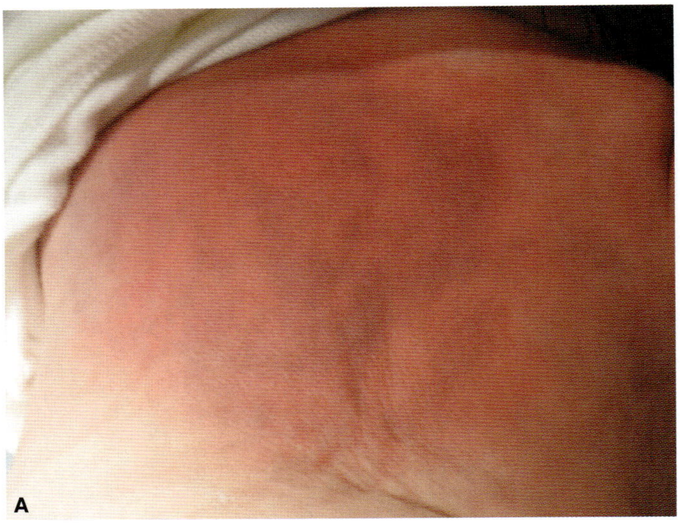

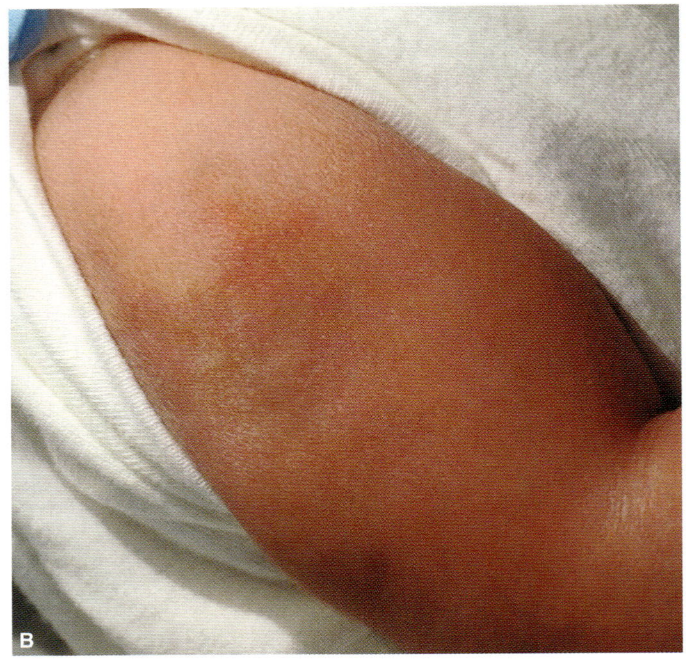

FIGURE 2-30A & 30B. Subcutaneous fat necrosis presenting as erythematous, indurated, poorly demarcated plaques on the back and arm of a neonate.

Investigations & Treatment

- SFN is often diagnosed clinically, especially in a well infant. However, if the baby is systemically unwell and the presentation is atypical, a skin biopsy should be performed to confirm the diagnosis of SFN and exclude other diagnoses.
- Histology of SFN will have features of lobular panniculitis with mixed inflammatory infiltrate, and radially arranged, needle-shaped clefts within adipocytes.
- Investigations to exclude hypercalcemia should be performed in all cases of SFN. This can occur up to 6 months after onset. Serial serum calcium levels should be performed. The risk of hypercalcemia corresponds to the severity of the perinatal stress.
- In most cases, medical intervention is not required apart from supportive measures. The lesions will resolve after a few months without sequelae.
- If hypercalcemia is present, intravenous fluids and calcium-wasting diuretics, and rarely, intravenous corticosteroid, can be given. In severe hypercalcemia, etidronate has been reported to be effective in regulating calcium levels.[1]

Reference

1. Pérez Martínez E. Treatment with bisphosphonates in severe hypercalcemia due to subcutaneous fat necrosis in an infant with hypoxicischemic encephalopathy. J Perinatol 2014;34: 492-3.

ACROPUSTULOSIS OF INFANCY

Acropustulosis of infancy is an idiopathic condition characterized by small, itchy blisters and pustules on the palms and soles of infants from a few months to 3 years of age.

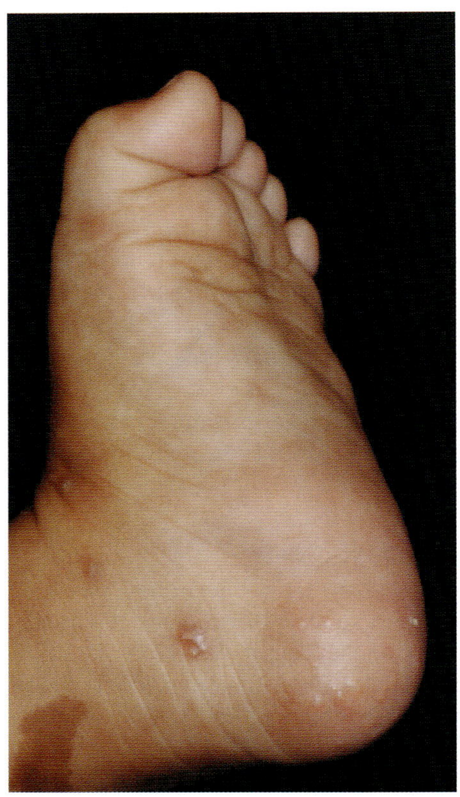

FIGURE 2-31. Pruritic papules and pustules on the feet of a 7-month-old Malay infant with acropustulosis of infancy.

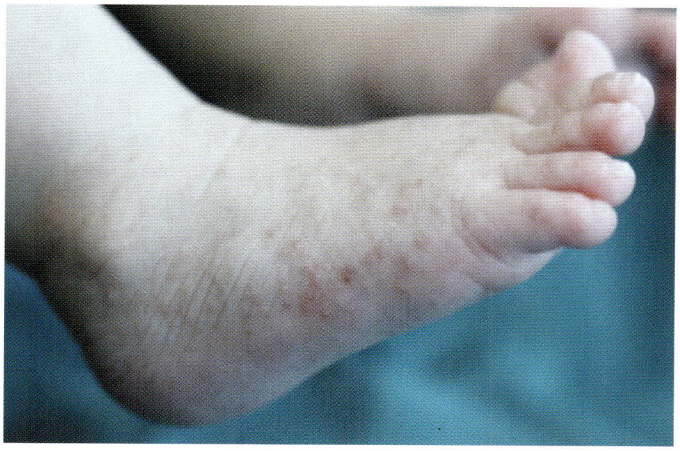

FIGURE 2-32. Acropustulosis on the feet of a 4-month-old infant with pruritic papules and pustules.

Clinical Features

- Acropustulosis presents with intensely pruritic papules and pustules, located mostly on the extremities, especially the palms and soles.
- The lesions heal with post-inflammatory hyperpigmentation.

Differential Diagnosis

- Scabies
  - The presentation of acropustulosis can be very similar to scabies. In fact, many infants with acropustulosis are invariably treated initially for scabies.
  - There may be positive contact history for scabies within the household. Burrows are commonly seen, and other common sites of involvement of scabies include the interdigital spaces, groin, axilla, and trunk.
- Eosinophilic folliculitis
  - This usually affects the scalp rather than the extremities.
- Hand, foot, and mouth disease
  - This has a more acute presentation with associated fever and pharyngeal ulcers.

Investigations & Treatment

- The diagnosis of acropustulosis is made clinically, although investigations may be performed to exclude infectious etiologies, especially for scabies.
- Treatment of acropustulosis is mainly symptomatic, with the use of topical corticosteroids and systemic antihistamines.

Pearls & Practical Tips

- Although previously postulated to occur secondary to a hypersensitivity reaction to scabies mites, this is now known to be untrue. The majority of cases of acropustulosis do not occur after scabies.
- The condition can recur up to 3 years of age.

DIAPER DERMATITIS

Diaper dermatitis, or nappy rash, is a common occurrence in infants and toddlers. It can occur due to various factors, most commonly secondary to irritant contact dermatitis from urine and feces. Other factors include seborrheic dermatitis, friction from diapers, candida infection, and bacterial infection. Rare causes of diaper rash include psoriasis, Langerhans' cell histiocytosis, and zinc deficiency. Some of these are discussed in other sections of the atlas.

IRRITANT DIAPER DERMATITIS

Irritant diaper dermatitis is the commonest cause of nappy rash and is caused by contact with urine, feces, and excessive use of wet wipes. Prolonged occlusion from diapers can lead to maceration of the stratum corneum and increased skin pH, predisposing to irritant dermatitis.

Clinical Features

- Irritant diaper dermatitis often develops after the first 3 weeks of life and peaks at about 10 months. It can be precipitated by a bout of diarrhea.
- It presents with erythema with very minimal scaling, and variable oozing.
- It most commonly occurs over the convex surfaces of the groin region—areas that are most often in contact with urine and feces, such as the inner upper thigh, lower abdomen, and buttocks. The creases are classically spared.
- Secondary infection with candida or bacteria may lead to more severe inflammation.
- Jacquet's erosive dermatitis is a severe form of irritant diaper dermatitis that presents with punched-out ulcers and erosions. This is less common now due to the use of disposable diapers. It may be more common in infants with underlying bowel disease such as short bowel syndrome.

Differential Diagnoses

- Seborrheic dermatitis
  - Seborrheic dermatitis can present in the diaper area but most commonly affects the inguinal folds. Many of these patients progress to atopic dermatitis. Other typical areas such as the scalp, face, and axilla are also commonly affected.

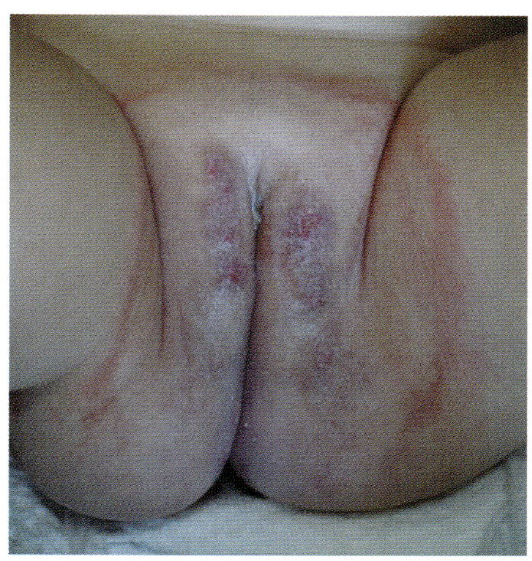

FIGURE 2-33. Irritant diaper dermatitis affecting the convex surface of the groin region of this Chinese infant. She coincidentally has frictional dermatitis from tight-fitting diapers, with linear, erythematous patches on both inner thighs and suprapubic region.

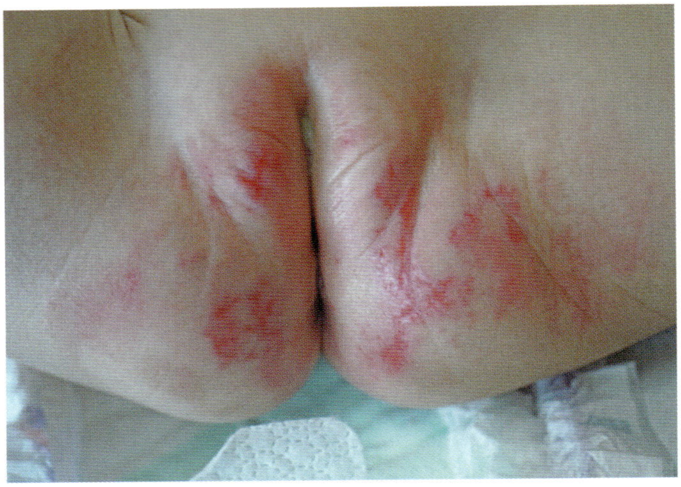

FIGURE 2-34. Irritant diaper dermatitis with erosions (Jacquet's dermatitis) affecting the convex surfaces of the groin and perianal region of this Chinese infant.

- Psoriasis
  - This is uncommon and classically presents with well demarcated, beefy erythematous patches and plaques, but lacking the silvery scales. It can be rather persistent.
- Allergic contact dermatitis
  - This is uncommon but can occur secondary to allergy to chemicals in baby wipes, for example methylchloroisothiazolinone/methylisothiazolinone (MCI/MI), and diaper dyes such as disperse blue and disperse yellow. The site of involvement may vary with the contact allergen, that is, margin of the diaper with diaper dyes, entire diaper area, with topical products or wet wipes.

Investigations & Treatment

- Investigations are usually not required for diagnosis but skin swabs for fungal microscopy and culture or bacterial culture can be done to exclude secondary infection.
- Good diaper hygiene practices such as regular change of soiled diapers, airing the perineum dry before wearing the new diaper, as well as the use of barrier creams may help to improve the condition of the skin.
- Treatment of moderate to severe cases includes mild topical corticosteroids with or without antifungals or antimicrobials, and bland moisturizers. Oral antibiotics may be required if there is secondary bacterial infection, and oral nystatin may be required for secondary candida infection.

Pearls & Practical Tips

- Frictional dermatitis from tight diapers usually presents with erythema at the creases, where the elastic bands of diapers are most in contact with the skin.
- Pull-up diapers can cause irritation of skin in contact with the elastic band areas, for example waist, lower back, and lower abdomen.
- In severe diaper dermatitis, we recommend time off diapers, especially in the day, as well as judicious use of a bland moisturizer such as white soft paraffin.

DIAPER, CONGENITAL, AND NEONATAL CANDIDIASIS

Diaper candidiasis is caused by the yeast *Candida albicans* and is common in infants. Some may have concomitant oral thrush, caused by transfer from the mother's vaginal canal. Diaper candidiasis may occur in isolation but commonly also complicates irritant diaper dermatitis. Congenital candidiasis is defined as skin lesions being present from birth to the first 6 days of life. It is acquired in utero and may be associated with preterm labor. Neonatal candidiasis is acquired during the birth process due to candida vaginal colonization, and typically presents with skin lesions after the first week of life.

Clinical Features

- Diaper candidiasis presents in two common forms. It can present as a diffuse erythematous patch extending into the perineum with scaling and satellite lesions, or as small

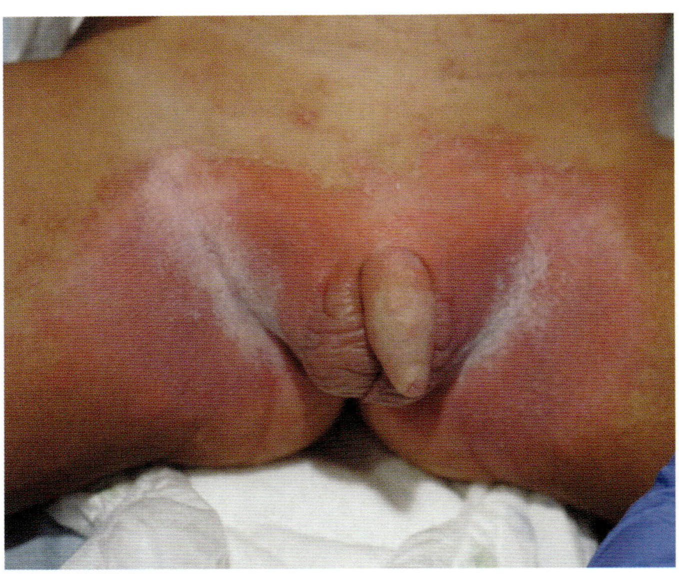

FIGURE 2-35. More severe irritant contact dermatitis affecting a Chinese male infant.

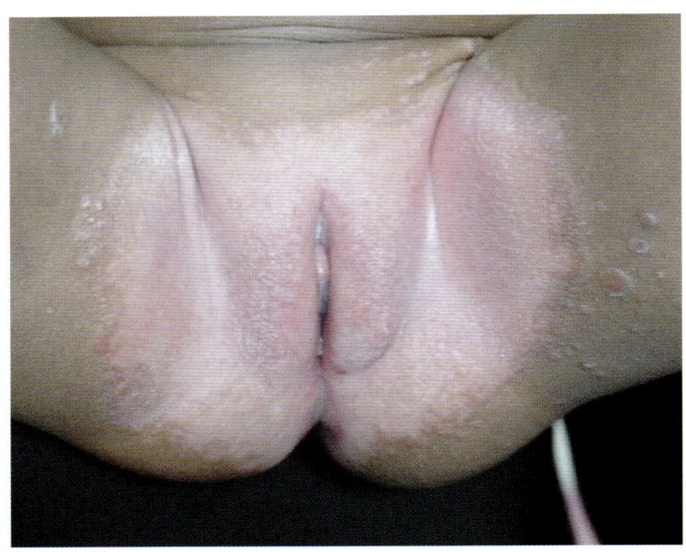

FIGURE 2-36. Diaper candidiasis in a Malay infant, presenting with confluent, scaly, pink-to-erythematous plaque with satellite papules.

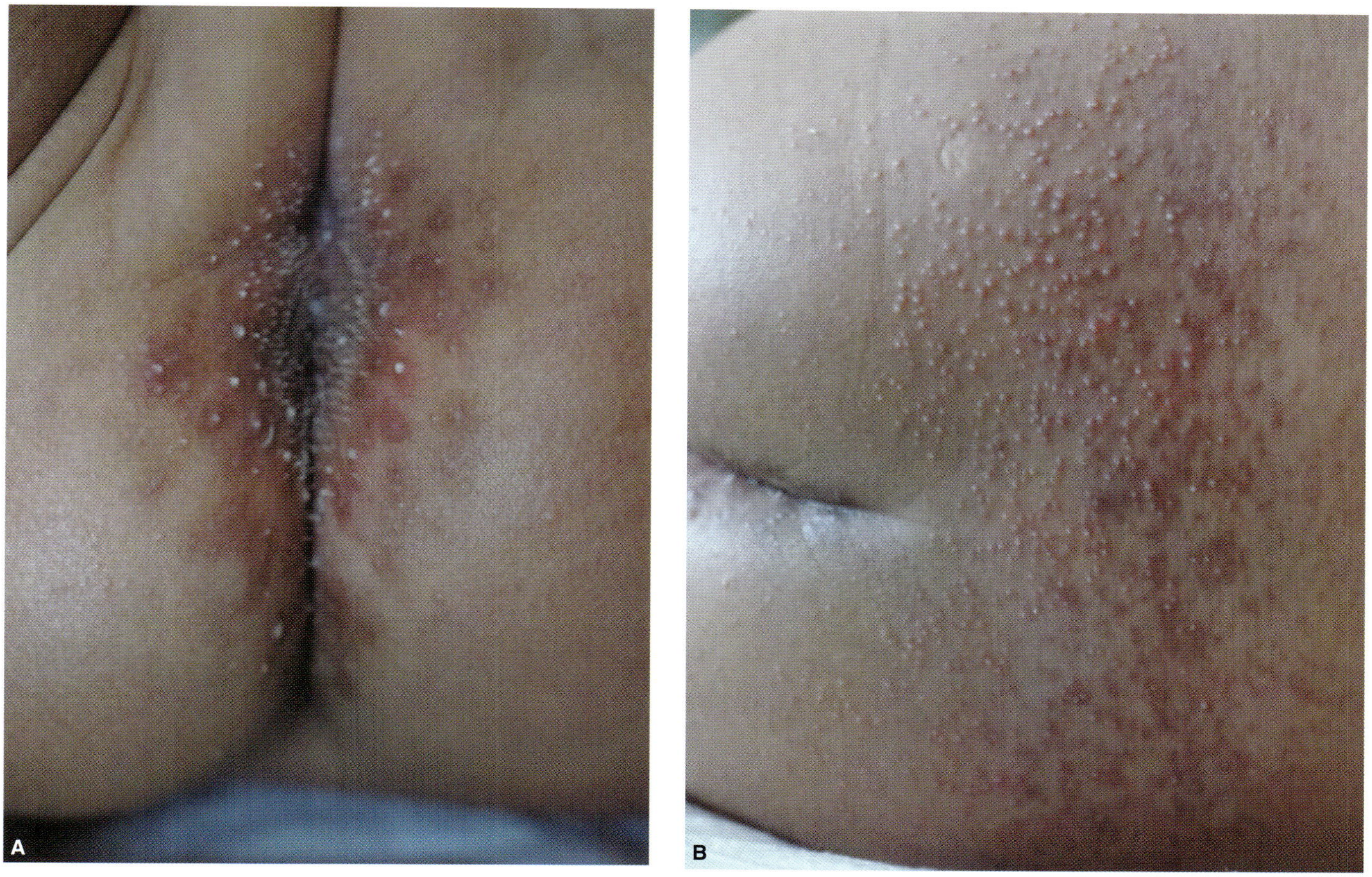

FIGURE 2-37A & 37B. Diaper candidiasis in a Chinese infant, presenting with multiple papules and pustules over the vulva and lower back region.

erythematous macules and papules with scaling and small pustules. Concomitant oral thrush may be present. Often, there are concomitant manifestations of irritant contact dermatitis.

- Neonatal cutaneous candidiasis presents with widespread multiple scaly erythematous macules, papules and pustules, neonatal erythroderma, or a diffuse scaling dermatitis. Commonly affected sites include the back, extensor surfaces of the extremities, and skin folds, with relative sparing of the diaper area. Pustules on the palms and soles may be present.
- Congenital candidiasis is benign in full-term healthy infants but could be associated with serious systemic infection in extremely low birthweight premature infants.

Differential Diagnoses

- Differential diagnoses for diaper candidiasis:
  - Irritant diaper dermatitis
    - » This often occur with diaper candidiasis. The creases are usually spared in irritant diaper dermatitis.
  - Perianal streptococcal infection
    - » This can also present with bright red erythema around the perianal skin. There may also be small pustules over the lesion.

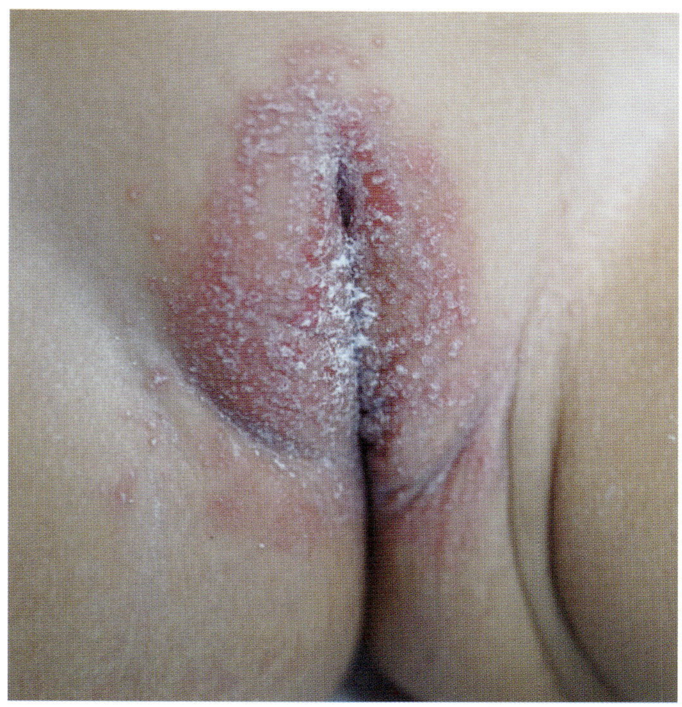

FIGURE 2-38. Diaper candidiasis in a Chinese infant, presenting as scaly erythematous plaques over the labia majora with satellite papules and pustules.

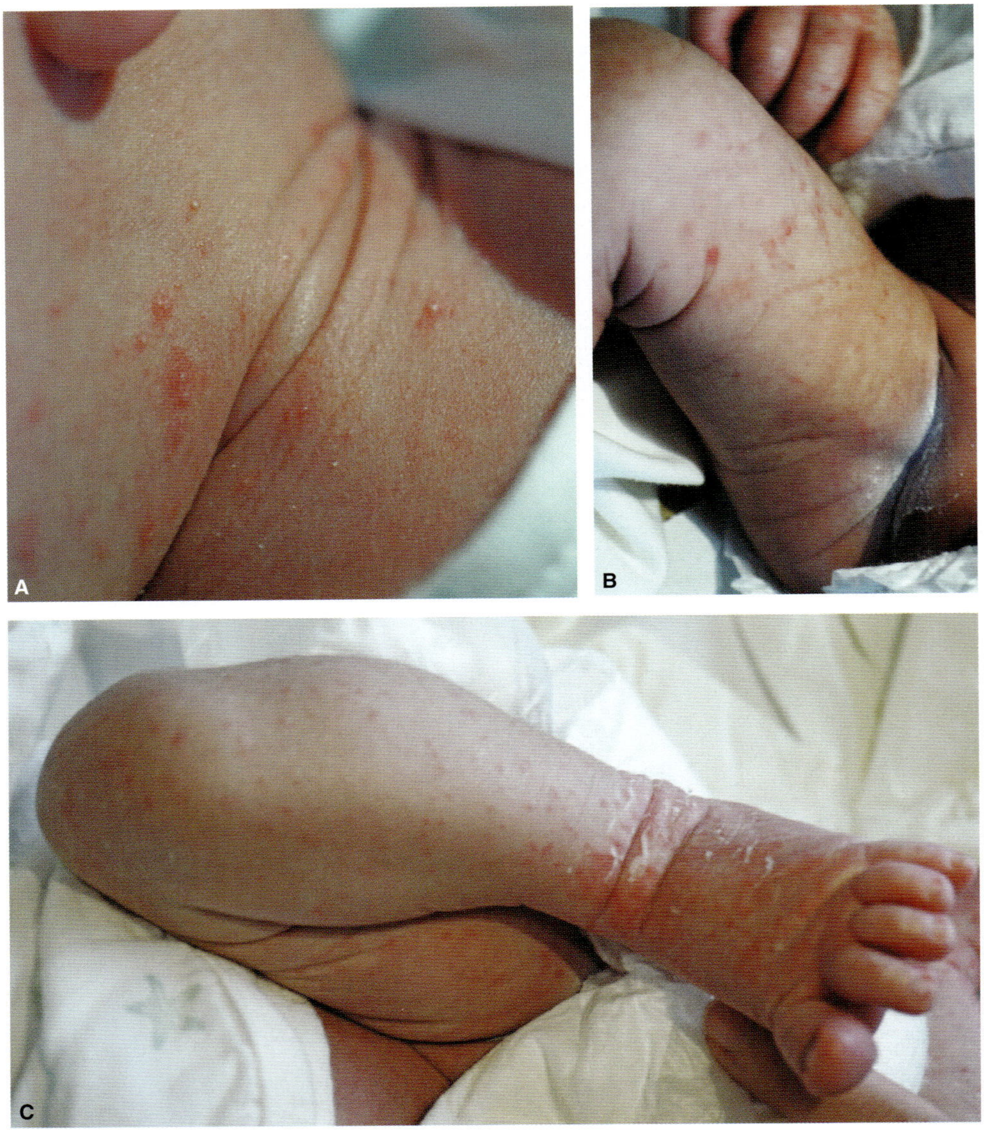

FIGURE 2-39A–39C. Neonatal candidiasis presenting in a 1-week-old neonate with erythematous papules and pustules. He had concomitant oral thrush (not shown).

  » Swab for bacterial and fungal cultures may be required to differentiate.
- Infantile seborrheic dermatitis
  » There are usually no satellite lesions or pustules seen, and other areas of seborrheic dermatitis are often present.
- Psoriasis
  » This can also present with beefy red plaques in the genital area. Satellite lesions are usually absent, and fungal microscopy and cultures are negative.

- Differential diagnoses of neonatal or congenital candidiasis include other neonatal infections such as listeria, impetigo, varicella, herpes, and syphilis, and non-infectious conditions presenting with pustular skin eruptions in newborns such as Langerhans cell histiocytosis and pustular psoriasis.

Investigations & Treatment

- Diaper candidiasis can be diagnosed clinically, but swabs for fungal microscopy and culture can help to confirm the diagnosis.
- Treatment with topical antifungals for at least 2 weeks is often sufficient. If lesions are more inflamed, addition of a mild topical corticosteroid may be helpful.
- Good diaper hygiene practices such as regular change of soiled diapers, airing the perineum dry before wearing the new diaper, as well as the use of barrier cream may help to improve the condition of the skin.
- Treatment of congenital or neonatal candidiasis is with topical and/or systemic antifungals, depending on the extent and severity of the disease.

Pearls & Practical Tips

- In more extensive cases of diaper candidiasis or cases that do not respond to topical treatment, we find the use of oral nystatin very useful.

ZINC DEFICIENCY

Zinc is an essential mineral crucial in the function of over 100 enzymes in human physiology.[1] Zinc deficiency is an uncommon cause of diaper dermatitis. It can occur in three circumstances. It most commonly occurs secondary to maternal dietary zinc deficiency. It can also occur when there is insufficient zinc in a mother's breast milk despite normal serum levels. This condition is termed transient neonatal zinc deficiency (TNZD).[2] The rarest form is acrodermatitis enteropathica (AE), which is caused by a defect of dietary zinc absorption in the baby's gut, caused by a mutation in the SLC39A4 gene, inherited as an autosomal recessive disorder.[3]

Clinical Features

- All three forms of zinc deficiency present with fairly similar features, including dermatitis, diarrhea, poor weight gain, alopecia, and irritability. Recurrent infections can also occur in more severely affected patients.

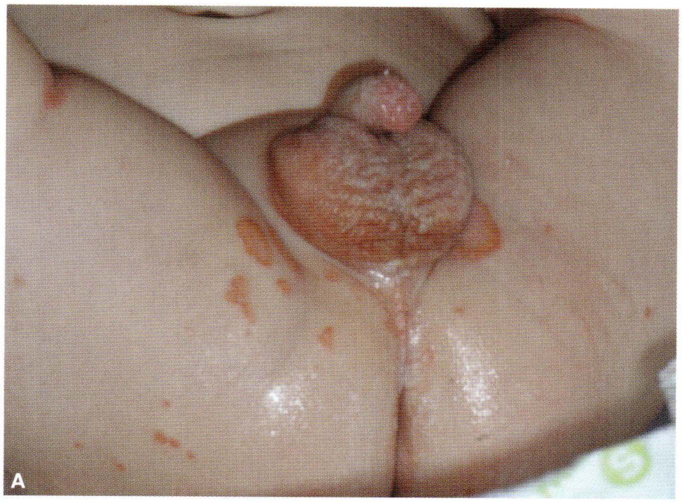

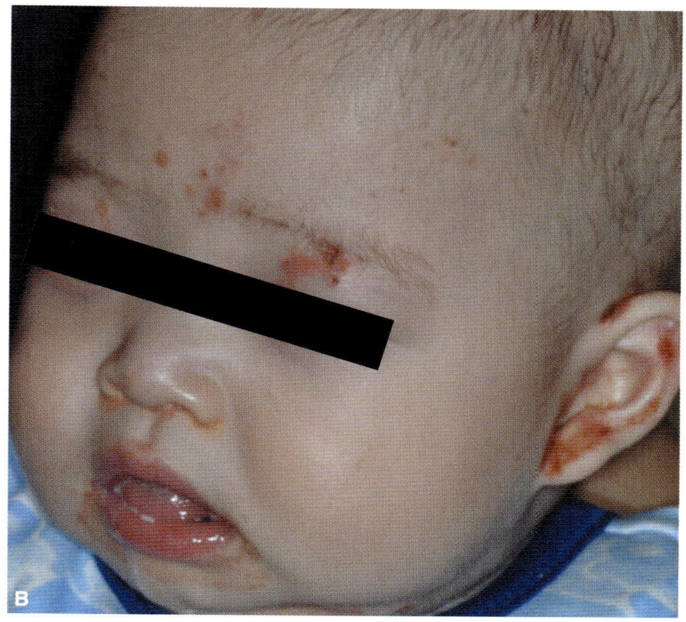

FIGURE 2-40A & 40B. TNZD in a Chinese infant presenting with erosive psoriasiform papules and plaques in the groin and periorificial region. The baby's mother was found to have a mutation in SLC30A2.

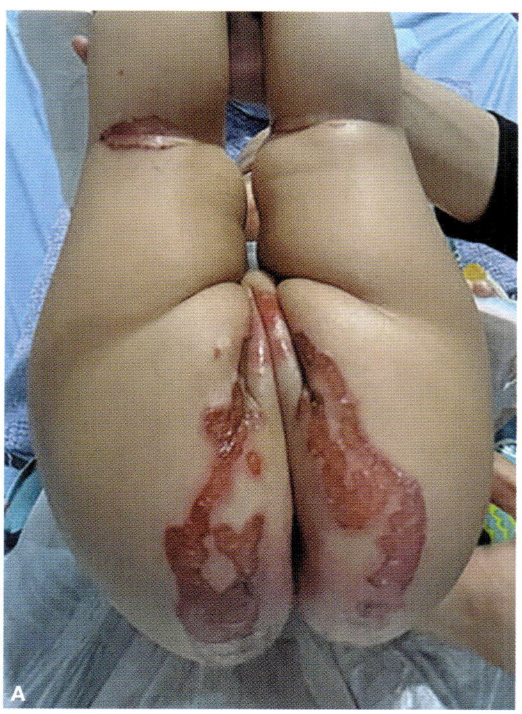

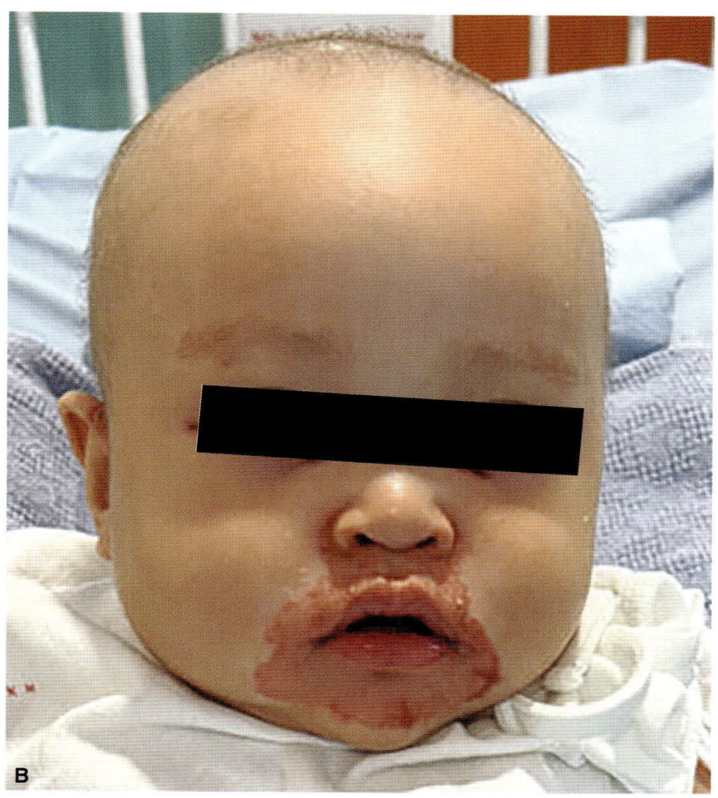

FIGURE 2-41A & 41B. Zinc deficiency in a Malay infant presenting with erosive psoriasiform plaques in the groin and periorificial regions.

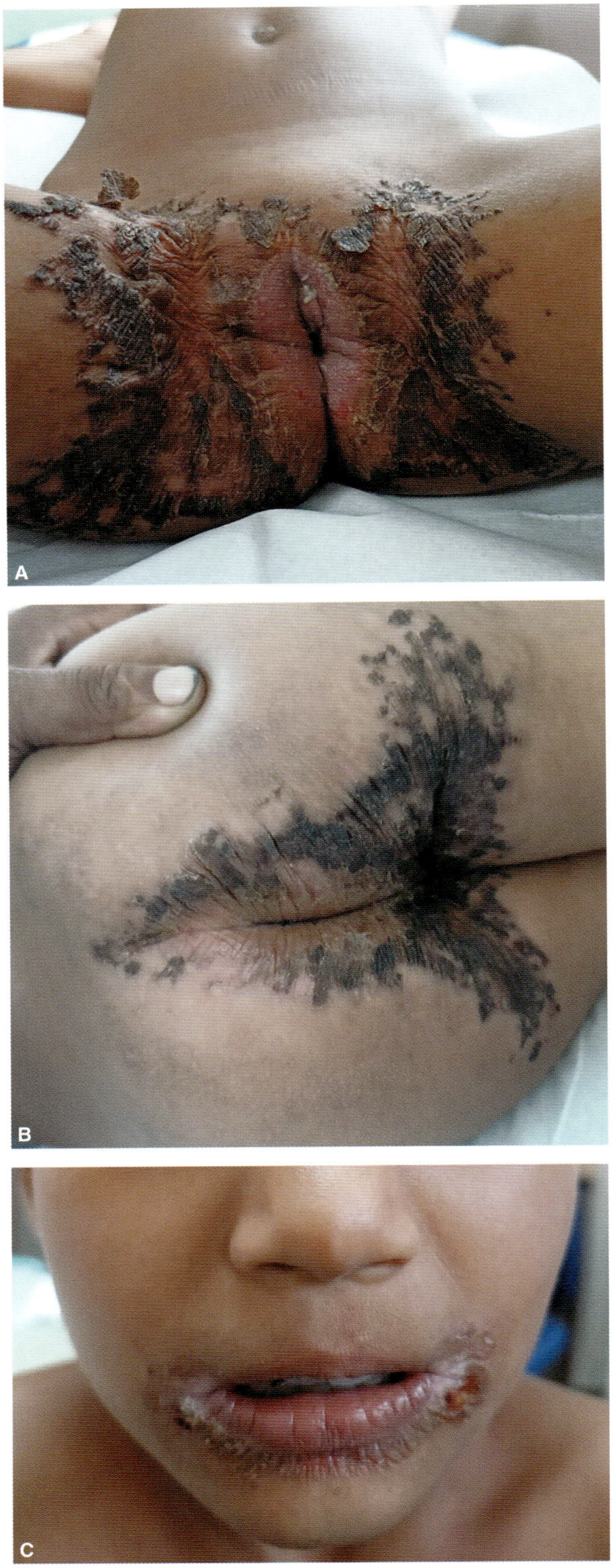

FIGURE 2-42A–42C. Acrodermatitis enteropathica in an Indian child presenting with exfoliative rash in the diaper and perioral region. (Photograph courtesy of Dr. Sandipan Dhar, Kolkata, India.)

- The rash caused by zinc deficiency can either appear as well-demarcated psoriasiform plaques or more erosive, oozy papules and plaques.
- The rash most commonly affects the periorificial areas, such as the groin, genitalia, perianal region, and around the ears, nose, mouth, and eyes. It frequently also affects acral sites such as the hands and feet.
- Zinc deficiency due to low maternal serum zinc levels can present early, within a few months of life, and more commonly in fully breast-fed infants.
- TNZD is caused by a mutation in the SLC30A2 gene in the mother of affected babies. It encodes the ZnT2 transporter that is expressed in breast ducts, leading to low zinc levels in breast milk. It commonly presents at babies at 3 to 4 months of life who are exclusively breast fed.
- AE usually presents when affected infants are weaned from breast milk to cow's milk, as the availability of zinc in breast milk is higher than in cow's milk.

Differential Diagnoses

- Other causes of zinc deficiency
  - Zinc deficiency can also occur in other circumstances, such as in premature breastfed infants with high nutritional demands, and in children with malabsorption disorders.
- Other deficiency disorders
  - These include biotin deficiency and pellagra, with deficiency in vitamin B3.
- Other causes of diaper dermatitis
  - These include irritant diaper dermatitis, psoriasis, seborrheic dermatitis, candidiasis, and Langerhans cell histiocytosis, which are described in other sections.

Investigations & Treatment

- Serum or plasma zinc levels confirm the diagnosis of zinc deficiency.
- Other blood investigations that support a diagnosis of zinc deficiency include low serum alkaline phosphatase (ALP), anemia, and leukopenia.
- Genetic testing for SLC39A4 and SLC30A2 mutations if indicated.
- Empirical treatment with oral zinc supplementation (3–5 mg/kg/day) will lead to rapid improvement in symptoms within days.
- AE will require zinc supplementation for life. Other forms of zinc deficiency may only require zinc replacement until there is adequate restoration of dietary zinc, such as TNZD.

Pearls & Practical Tips

- In babies that we diagnose with low serum zinc levels, the next step is to check mother's serum zinc levels. If this is normal, we will analyze the mother's breast milk zinc levels. If this is also normal and no other cause of zinc deficiency is apparent, we recommend performing genetic testing for AE.
- Irritability is the first symptom to resolve soon after zinc supplementation in zinc deficient infants. The resolution of rash occurs soon after.

References

1. Prasad AS. Zinc: an overview. Nutrition 1995;11(1 Suppl):93-9.
2. Küry S. Identification of SLC39A4, a gene involved in acrodermatitis enteropathica. Nat Genet 2002;31(3):239-40.
3. Liew HM, Tan CW, Ho CKM, Chee JN, Koh MJA. Transient neonatal zinc deficiency caused by a novel mutation in SLC30A2 gene. Pediatr Dermatol 2017:34:e104-e105.

CONGENITAL LUMPS AND BUMPS

Congenital lumps and bumps often present at or shortly after birth, and can occur from incomplete regression, problems during embryological migration, or incomplete tissue closure during embryological development. The diagnosis depends on the site, morphology, and associated features, and often requires additional investigations with imaging or histopathological examination.

Pearls & Practical Tips

- Minor developmental defects are usually isolated and benign but may also give a clue to possible underlying systemic associations and syndromes.

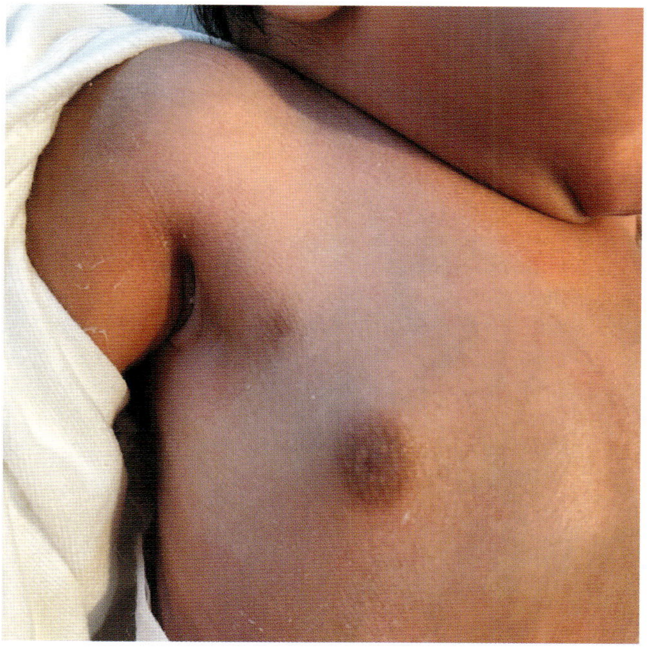

FIGURE 2-43. Supernumerary nipple on the right upper chest along the milk line between the axilla and the normal nipple.

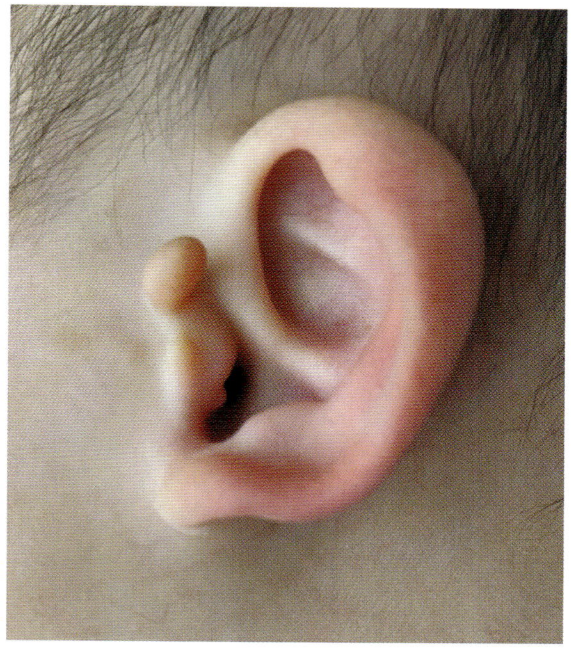

FIGURE 2-44. Accessory tragus in a Chinese infant. (Figure courtesy of A/Prof Henry Tan, Otolaryngology, KK Women's & Children's Hospital.)

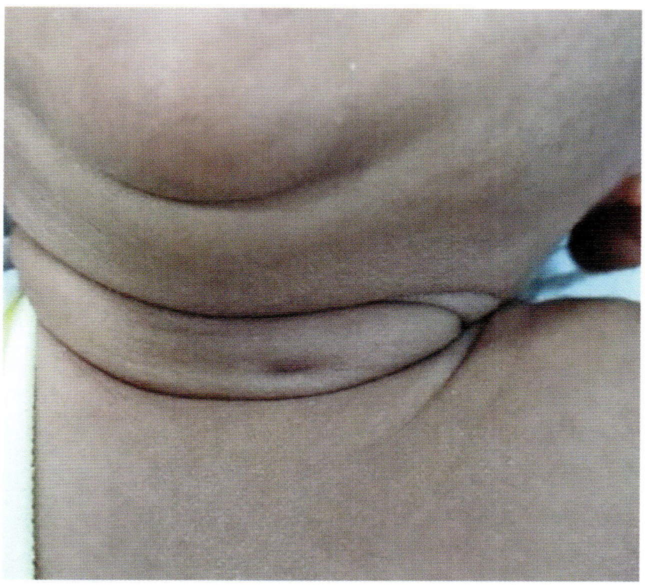

FIGURE 2-45. Branchial cleft cyst/sinus on the neck of a Chinese newborn. (Figure courtesy of Dr. Kong Juin Yee, Neonatology, KK Women's & Children's Hospital.)

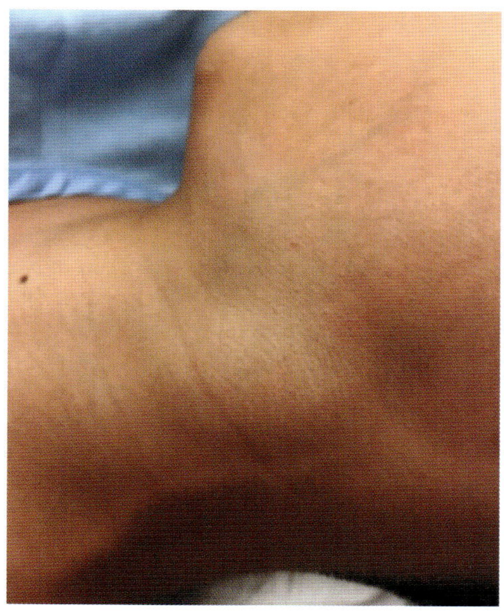

FIGURE 2-46. Branchial cleft cyst on the neck of a Chinese child, presenting as a localized swelling, skin-colored lump. (Figure courtesy of A/Prof Henry Tan, Otolaryngology, KK Women's & Children's Hospital.)

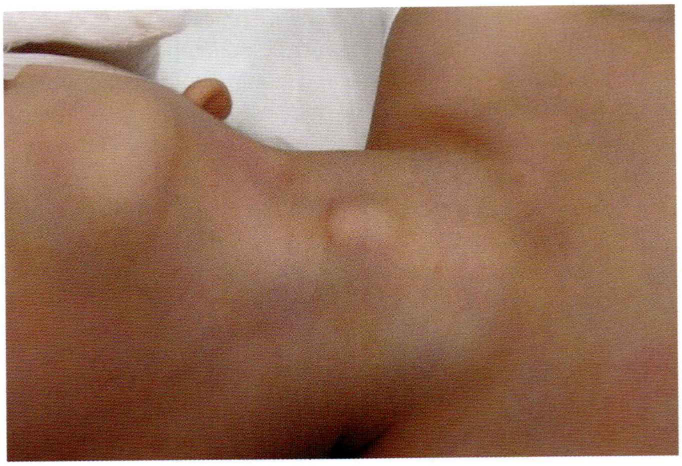

FIGURE 2-47. Thyroglossal duct cyst presenting as a skin-colored, midline lump in this Chinese boy. (Figure courtesy of A/Prof Henry Tan, Otolaryngology, KK Women's & Children's Hospital.)

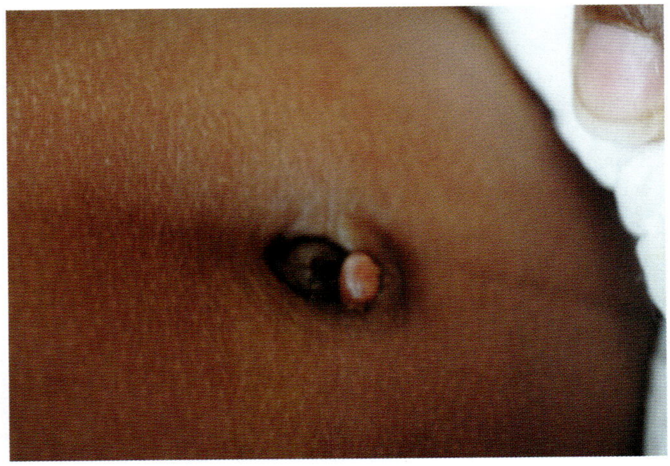

FIGURE 2-48. Umbilical granuloma in an Indian neonate.

Congenital lumps and bumps

Condition	Cause	Site	Clinical features	Differential diagnoses	Investigations and treatment	Systemic associations
Supernumerary mammary tissue	• Due to incomplete regression of the mammary ridge during embryonic development	• Along embryonic breast lines from axilla to inner thigh	• Accessory nipples and areola • Soft, brown pedunculated papules • Can occur in both males and females • May present as more than one lesion	• Congenital nevus • Dermatofibroma • Scar tissue • Lipoma • Wart	• Surgical excision may be offered for cosmesis, tenderness during puberty, or if there is discomfort from lactation	• Possible nephro-urinary malformations
Accessory tragus	• A benign congenital anomaly of the external ear derived from the first branchial arch	• Along the line from preauricular region to ipsilateral corner of mouth • Rarely on glabella or suprasternal region	• Soft, pedunculated, flesh-colored nodule • Can occasionally be covered with vellus hair	• Preauricular skin tag • Epidermal cyst • Adnexal tumor • Branchial cyst • Thyroglossal cyst	• Consider complete surgical resection	• Other developmental abnormalities of the first branchial arch • Goldenhar & Treacher-Collins syndrome, VACTERL association
Infantile myofibroma (IMF)	• A rare congenital benign mesenchymal tumor presenting in the first 2 years of life • Associated with *PDGFRB* and *NOTCH 3* mutations	• Commonly involved sites are the head and neck, trunk, and upper limbs	• Asymptomatic superficial or deep rubbery, firm to hard subcutaneous nodules • May occur as solitary disease, multicentric disease with lesions in skin, bone, and soft tissues, or generalized disease with visceral organ involvement	• Other soft tissue tumors such as congenital fibrosarcoma, neurofibromas, metastatic neuroblastoma	• Skin biopsy for histopathology • Usually resolve spontaneously in the first few years of life sometimes leaving residual skin atrophy • For generalized disease, multidisciplinary team management, chemotherapy may be required	• Generalized IMF can affect any visceral organ

(*Continued*)

Congenital lumps and bumps (Continued)

Condition	Cause	Site	Clinical features	Differential diagnoses	Investigations and treatment	Systemic associations
Branchial cleft cyst	• Due to improper closure of the branchial arches during embryonic development	• Along the lower third of the lateral aspect of neck near anterior border of sternocleidomastoid muscle • May be unilateral or bilateral	• Asymptomatic, mobile, soft cystic swellings, measuring 1–2 cm that may swell during an episode of upper respiratory infection • May drain onto skin or into pharynx • Secondary infection may occur	• Unilateral lymphadenopathy • Parotid or thyroid tumors • Thyroglossal cyst • Dermoid cyst • Neurofibroma	• Diagnosis can be made clinically • Imaging to look for underlying sinus • Surgically excised to prevent infection	NIL
Thyroglossal duct cyst	• Persistent tract formed during embryological migration of thyroid gland from base of tongue to anterior neck	• Midline of neck, or just lateral to midline	• Midline neck cyst that moves upward with tongue protrusion or swallowing • Usually asymptomatic	• Branchial clefts/sinuses • Cutaneous bronchogenic cysts • Undescended lingual thyroid gland	• Surgical excision recommended to prevent infection.	NIL
Umbilical granuloma	• Result of poor re-epithelization of the umbilicus	• Over the umbilicus after premature detachment of the cord within the first week of life	• Small, red, and friable papule • Usually asymptomatic	• Urachus and omphalomesenteric duct • Umbilical hernia	• Silver nitrate stick application	NIL

3

Atopic Dermatitis and Other Eczematous Conditions

ATOPIC DERMATITIS

Atopic dermatitis (AD), also known as atopic eczema, is a chronic skin condition that is common in infants, children, and adolescents. Itchy, dry skin is a prominent clinical feature. AD commonly presents during infancy, although it can occur at any age. A family history of atopy is often present. Potential aggravating factors include infections, dust mites, sweating, hot water baths, allergens (food, contact), irritants (harsh soaps, contact), and stress.

Clinical Features

- In infancy, the cheeks and scalp are usually affected. Older children often have flexural involvement. However, in both age groups more extensive involvement may occur.
- Eczema can present in the acute, subacute, or chronic stages. Acute eczema presents with erythematous patches, papules, plaques, with overlying crusting and oozing, and vesicles.
- The acute stage may transition into the subacute stage, which presents mainly with erythema and scaling.

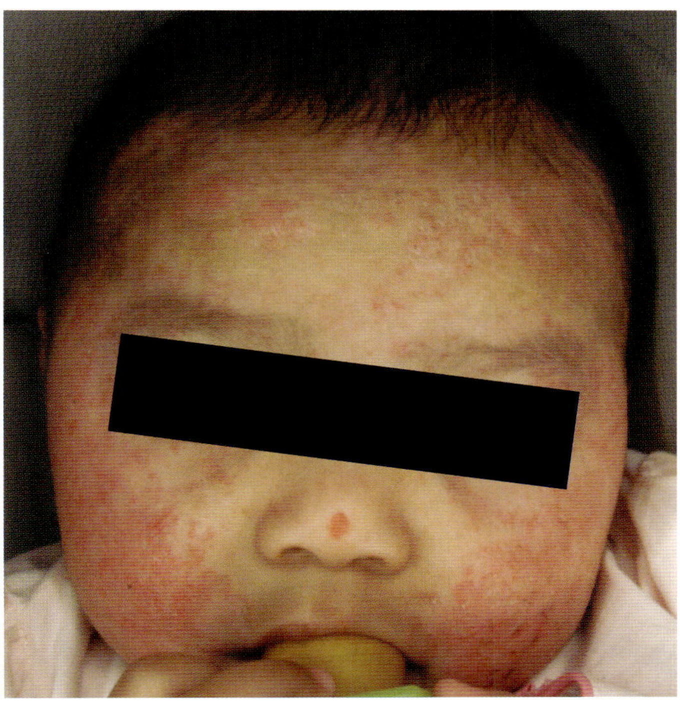

FIGURE 3-1. Infantile AD affecting the cheeks, forehead, and periorbital regions of a Malay infant.

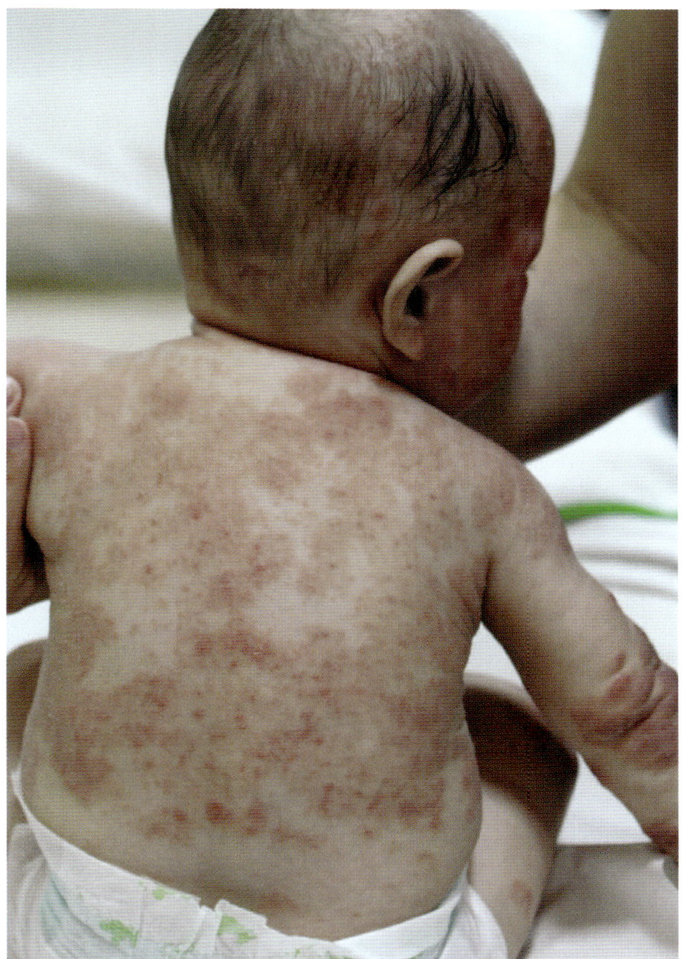

FIGURE 3-2. Extensive AD affecting the face, trunk, and limbs of a Chinese infant.

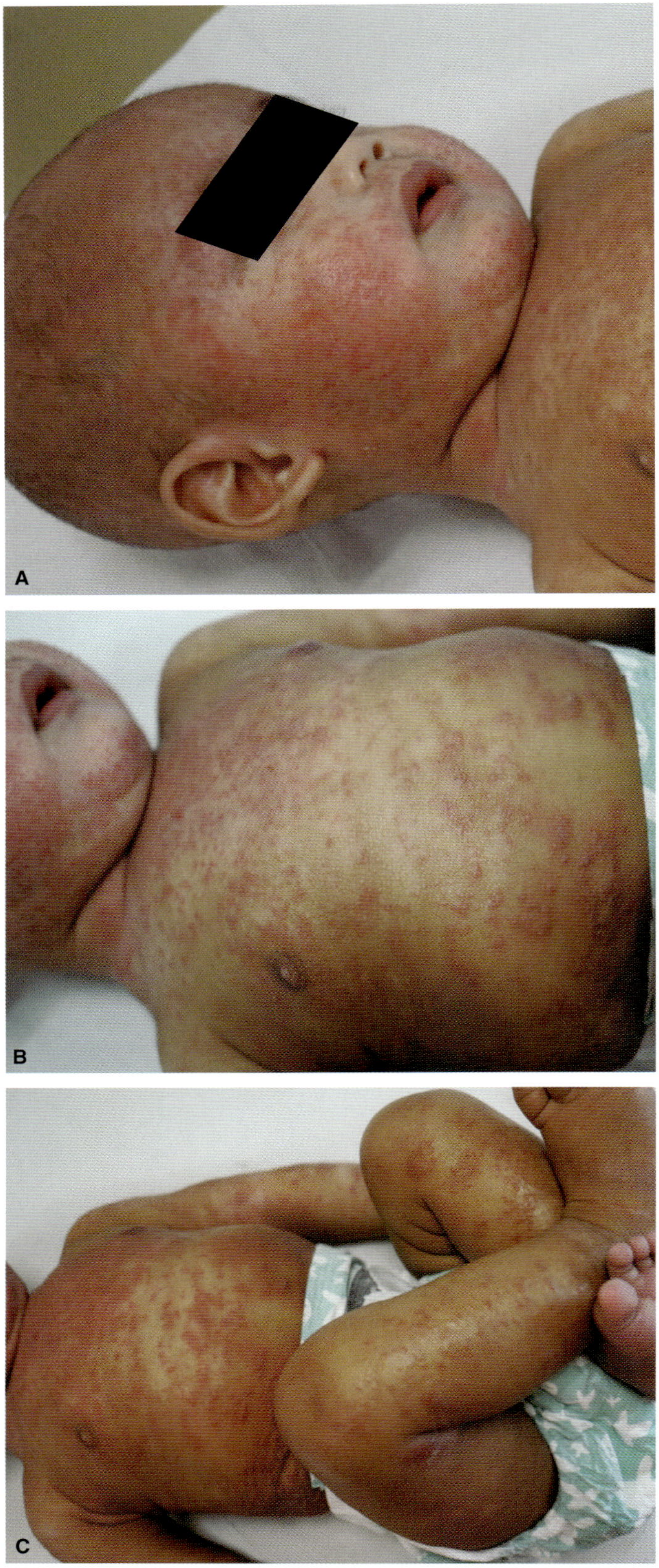

FIGURE 3-3A–3C. Extensive infantile AD in a Malay infant presenting with thick, scaly, erythematous-to-hyperpigmented papules and plaques affecting the face, trunk, and limbs.

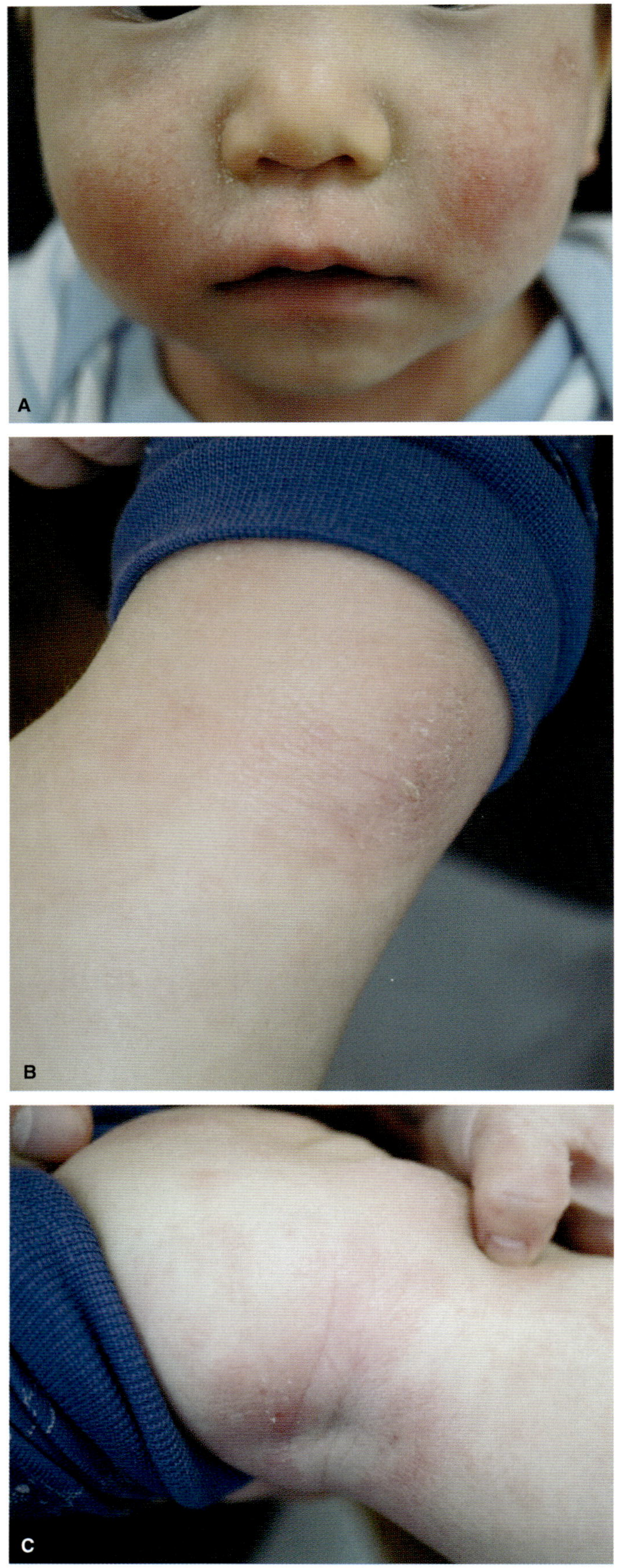

FIGURE 3-4A–4C. AD affecting the face and flexures of a Chinese toddler.

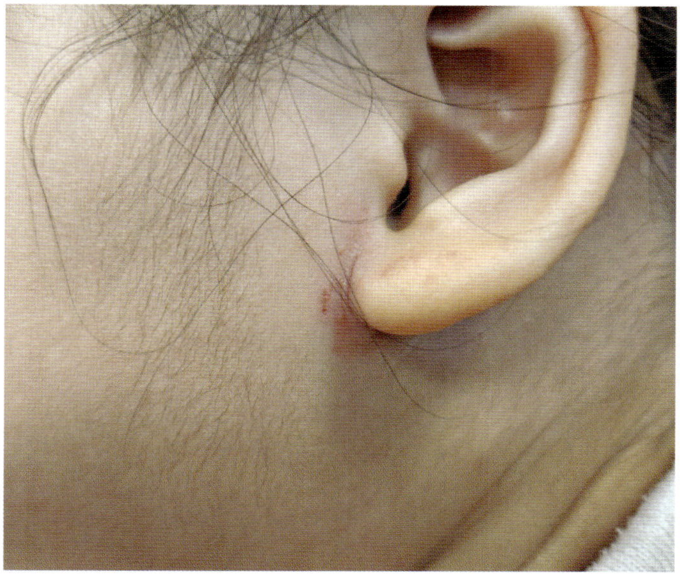

FIGURE 3-5. Involvement around the earlobe with erythema, scaling and fissuring is characteristic for younger patients with AD.

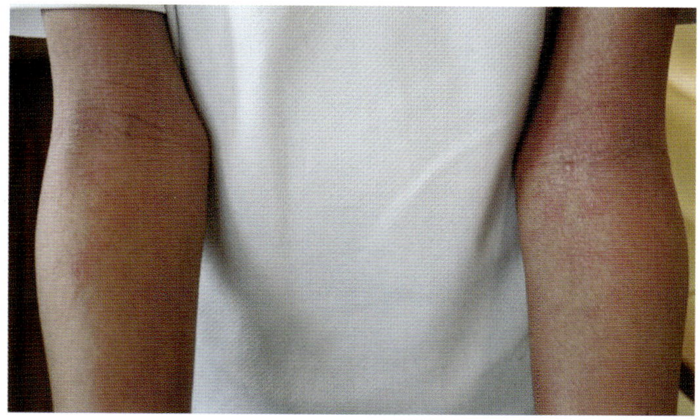

FIGURE 3-7. Scaly, lichenified plaques affecting bilateral cubital fossae of an older child with AD.

- In chronic eczema, lichenification, scaling, xerosis, and excoriations are seen. Pigmentary changes consisting of hyper-, hypo-, or depigmentation (leukoderma) may be present. Annular scaly patches and plaques may be seen, often confused with tinea.
- A rippled pattern of hyperpigmentation on the neck, called a "dirty neck" appearance, may occur in adolescence. It is postulated to be a result of both frictional melanosis and post-inflammatory hyperpigmentation.
- Follicular eczema is a subtype of AD, which can be present in all skin types but is most common in children of Asian, African American, and Hispanic descent. In this subtype, follicular prominence or perifollicular accentuation may be accompanied by pruritus, without the typical eczematous changes.
- Atopic individuals may have palmar hyperlinearity, keratosis pilaris, Dennie-Morgan lines, and white dermographism.
- Eczema herpeticum is a known complication of eczema. It should be suspected when there is rapid worsening of eczema with painful blisters or erosions. Clinically, there are punched-out erosions, small vesicles, and hemorrhagic crusts. Treatment with antivirals such as acyclovir should not be delayed.
- Impetiginized eczema occurs when there is secondary bacterial infection with *Staphylococcus aureus,* manifesting as honey-colored crusting and purulent exudates. Treatment

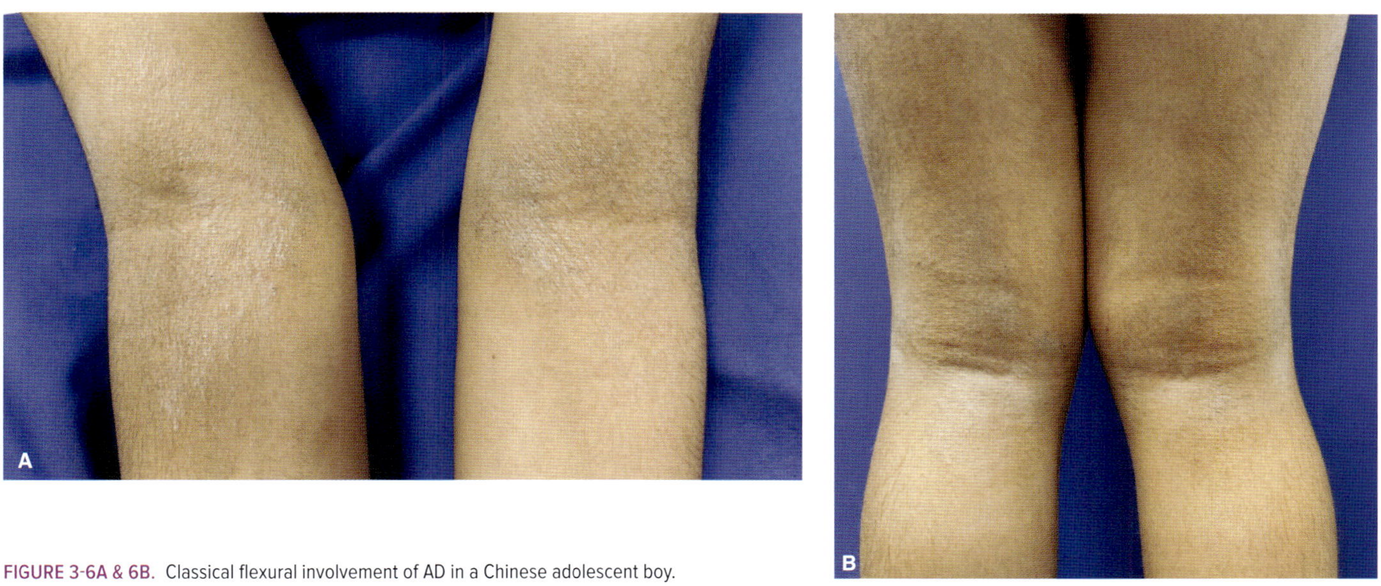

FIGURE 3-6A & 6B. Classical flexural involvement of AD in a Chinese adolescent boy.

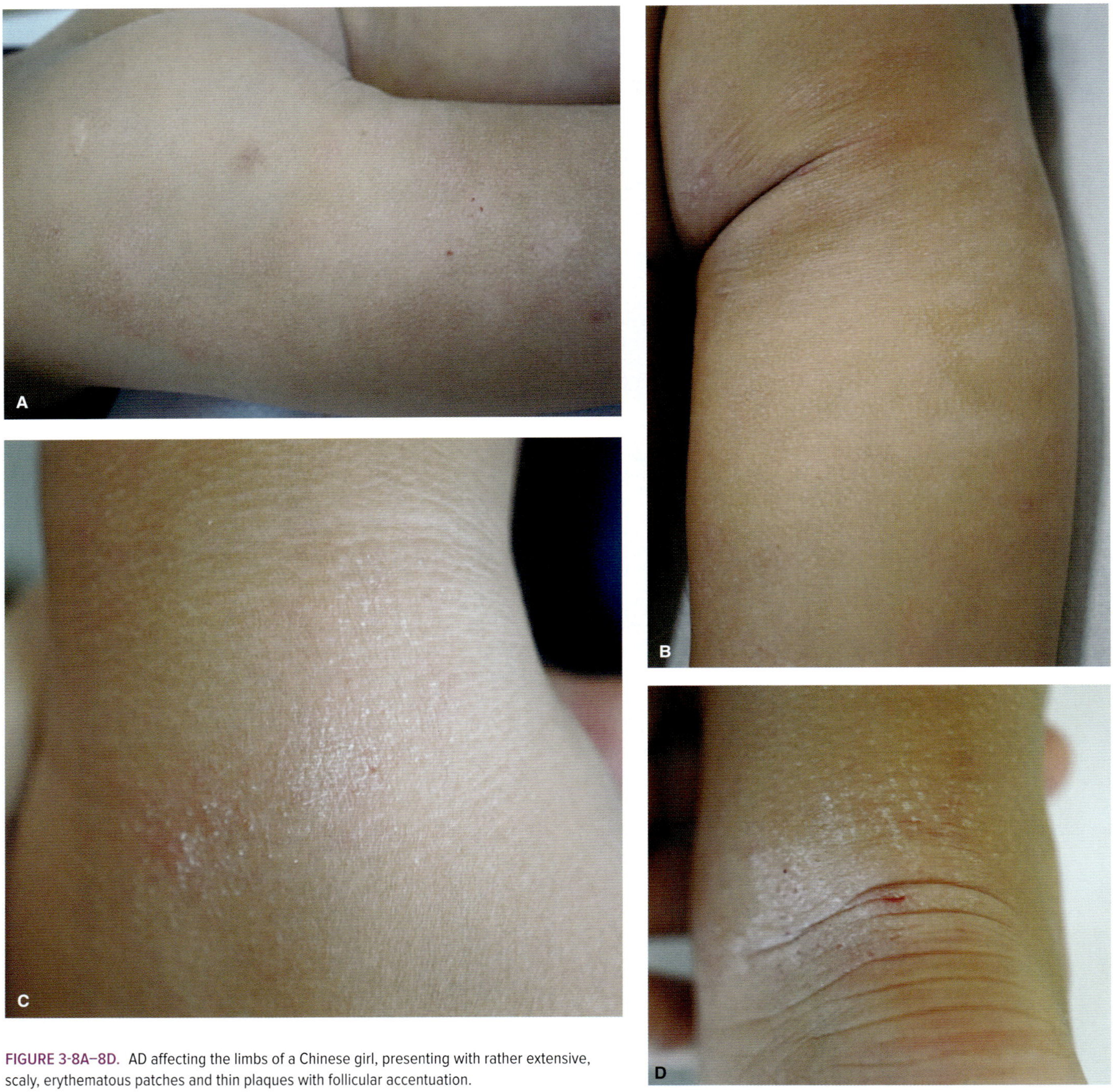

FIGURE 3-8A–8D. AD affecting the limbs of a Chinese girl, presenting with rather extensive, scaly, erythematous patches and thin plaques with follicular accentuation.

with anti-staphylococcal antibiotics such as cephalexin, cloxacillin, or amoxicillin/clavulanate is indicated. Nasal swab for *S. aureus* carriage and antiseptic body washes are useful in those who are prone to recurrent infections.

Differential Diagnosis

- Seborrheic dermatitis
  - Although the two conditions may occur at the same time, especially in infancy, seborrheic dermatitis is usually less pruritic and tends to present with greasy scales on the scalp and eyebrows.
- Contact dermatitis
  - This may also coexist with AD but the history may reveal exposure to a potential irritant or allergen on the affected site(s). A patch test is necessary to confirm allergic contact dermatitis.
- Diaper dermatitis
  - This presents with erythematous patches and plaques on the skin surfaces covered by the diaper. It is usually multifactorial in etiology, and can be secondary to irritation from urine and feces, candida and bacterial

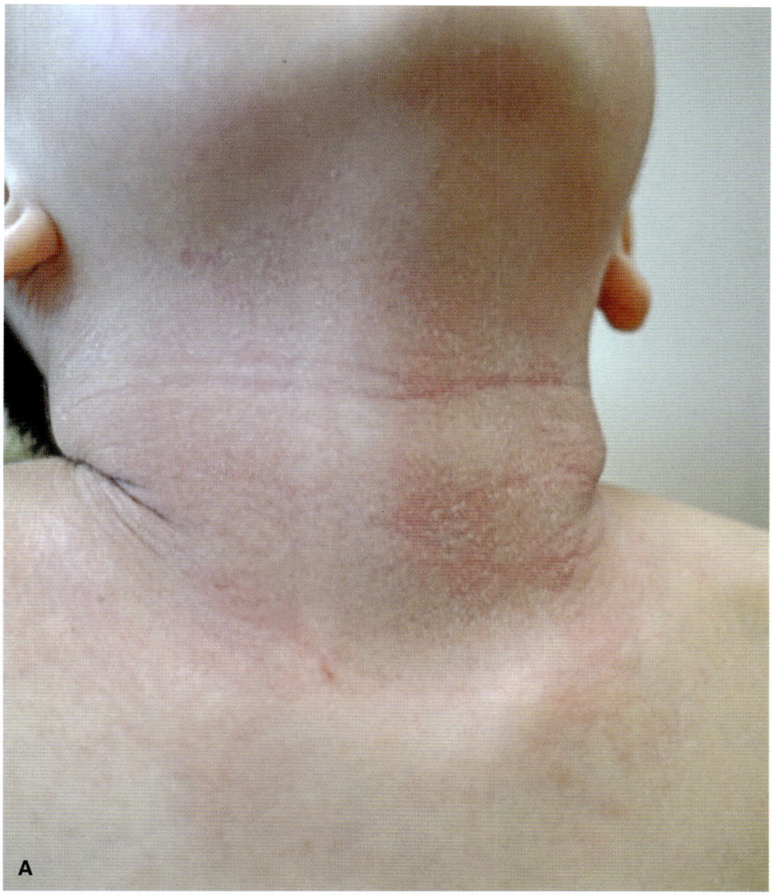

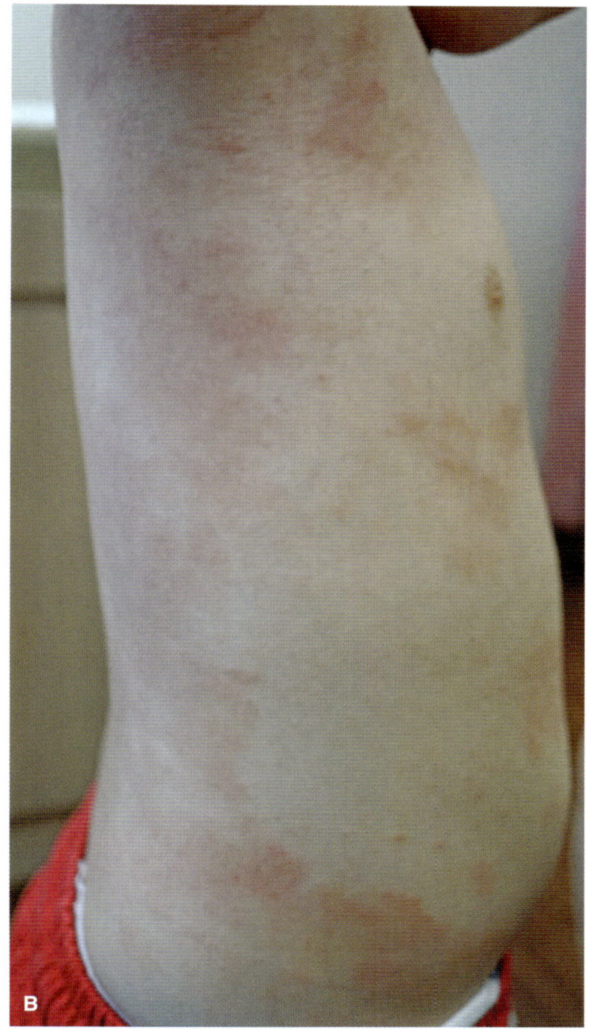

FIGURE 3-9A & 9B. AD affecting a young Chinese boy presenting with a more urticarial dermatitis phenotype. There are areas presenting with scaly, erythematous plaques and some areas with a more urticarial component.

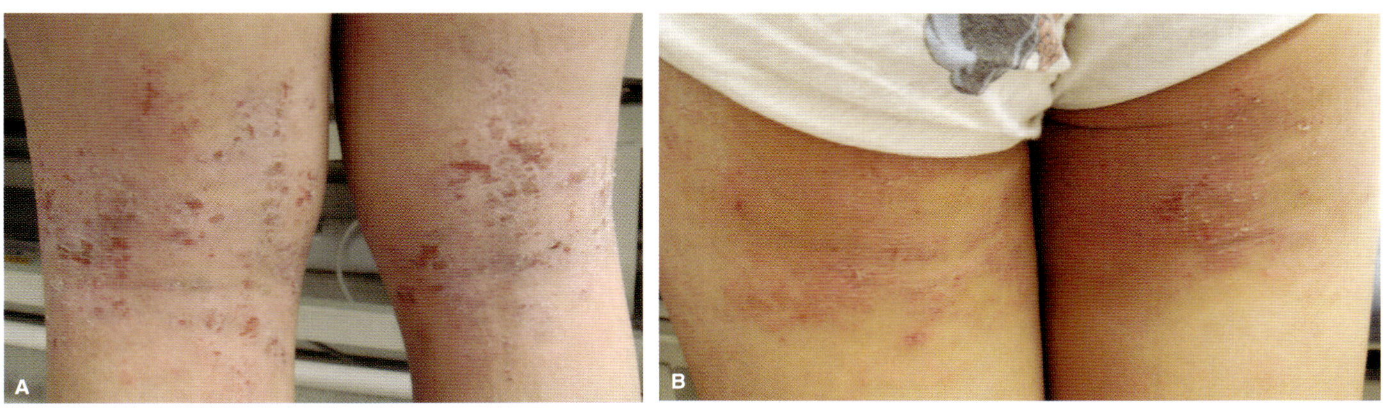

FIGURE 3-10A & 10B. Thick, scaly, excoriated and lichenified plaques affecting the popliteal fossae and posterior thighs of a Chinese child with chronic AD.

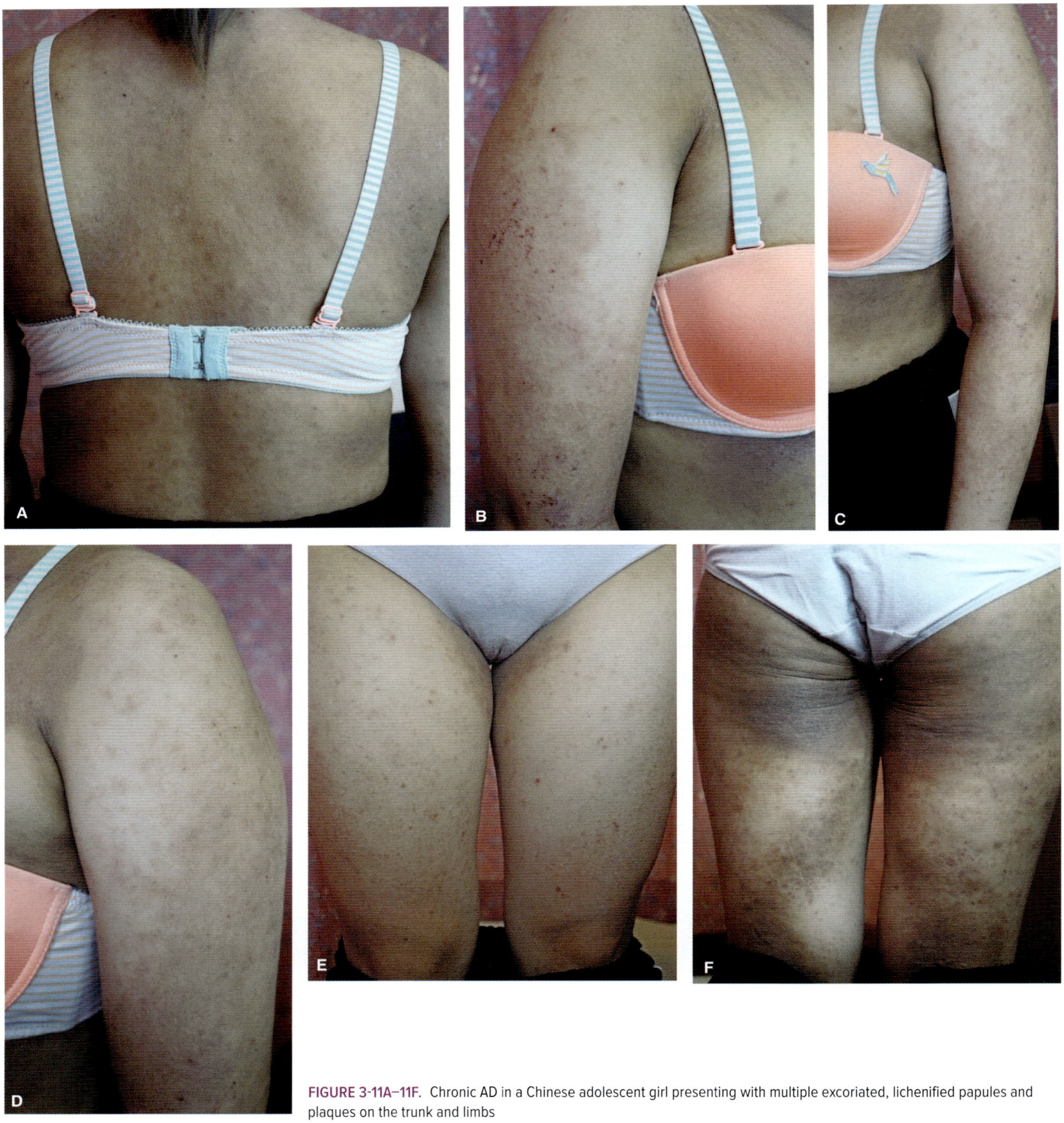

FIGURE 3-11A–11F. Chronic AD in a Chinese adolescent girl presenting with multiple excoriated, lichenified papules and plaques on the trunk and limbs

infection, and possibly contact dermatitis to wet wipes or diaper creams.

- Tinea corporis
  - This presents with annular scaly plaques. If it is inappropriately treated with topical corticosteroids, the original rash slowly expands, leading to tinea incognito. Skin scraping for fungal microscopy and culture can help to confirm the diagnosis.
- Scabies
  - This should be suspected if an infant presents with a pruritic eruption with vesiculopustules on the palms and soles, and/or nodules on the axillae and groin.

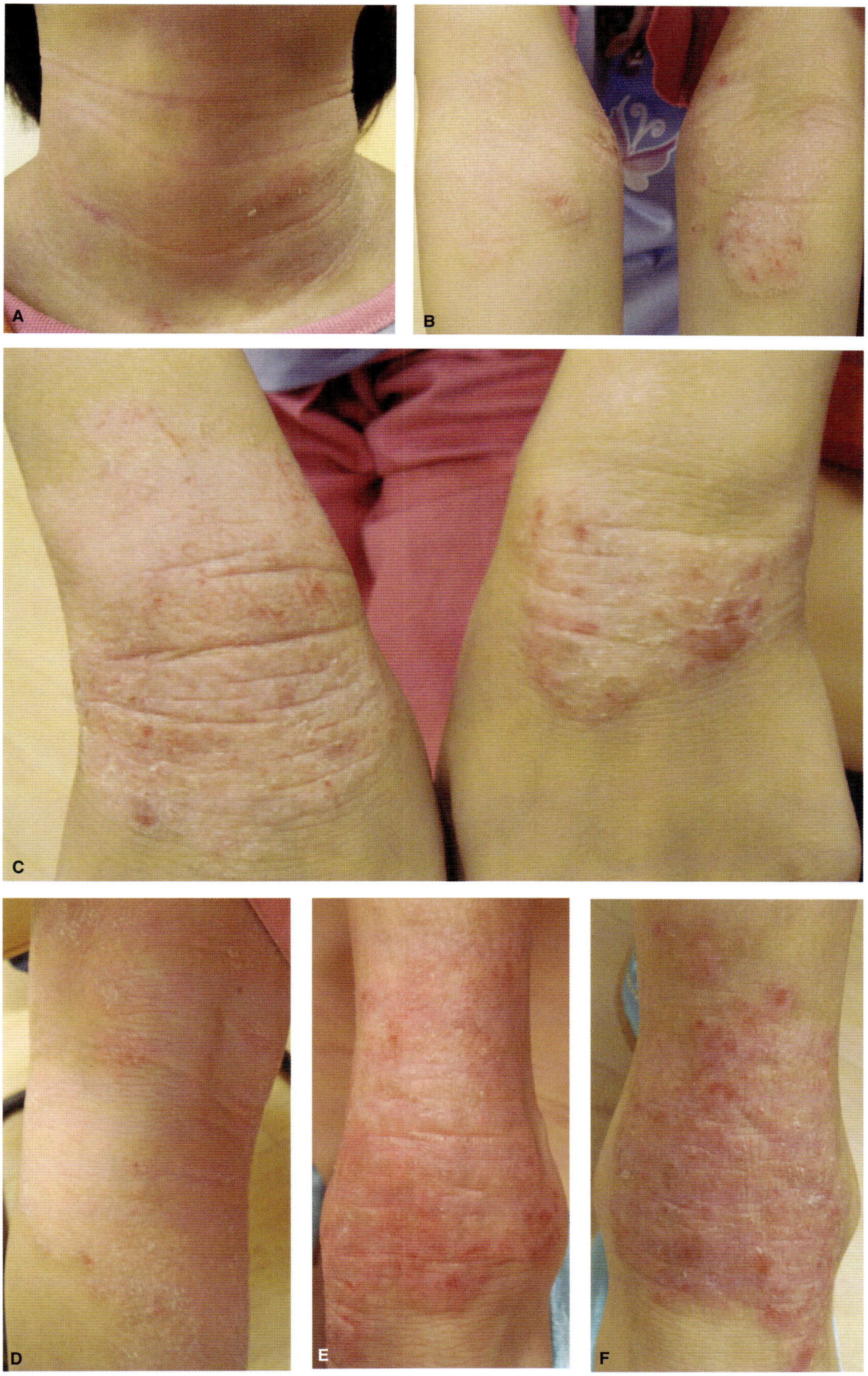

FIGURE 3-12A–12F. Erythematous, scaly and lichenified plaques on the flexor and extensor aspects of the limbs and neck in a Chinese female with moderate-to-severe AD.

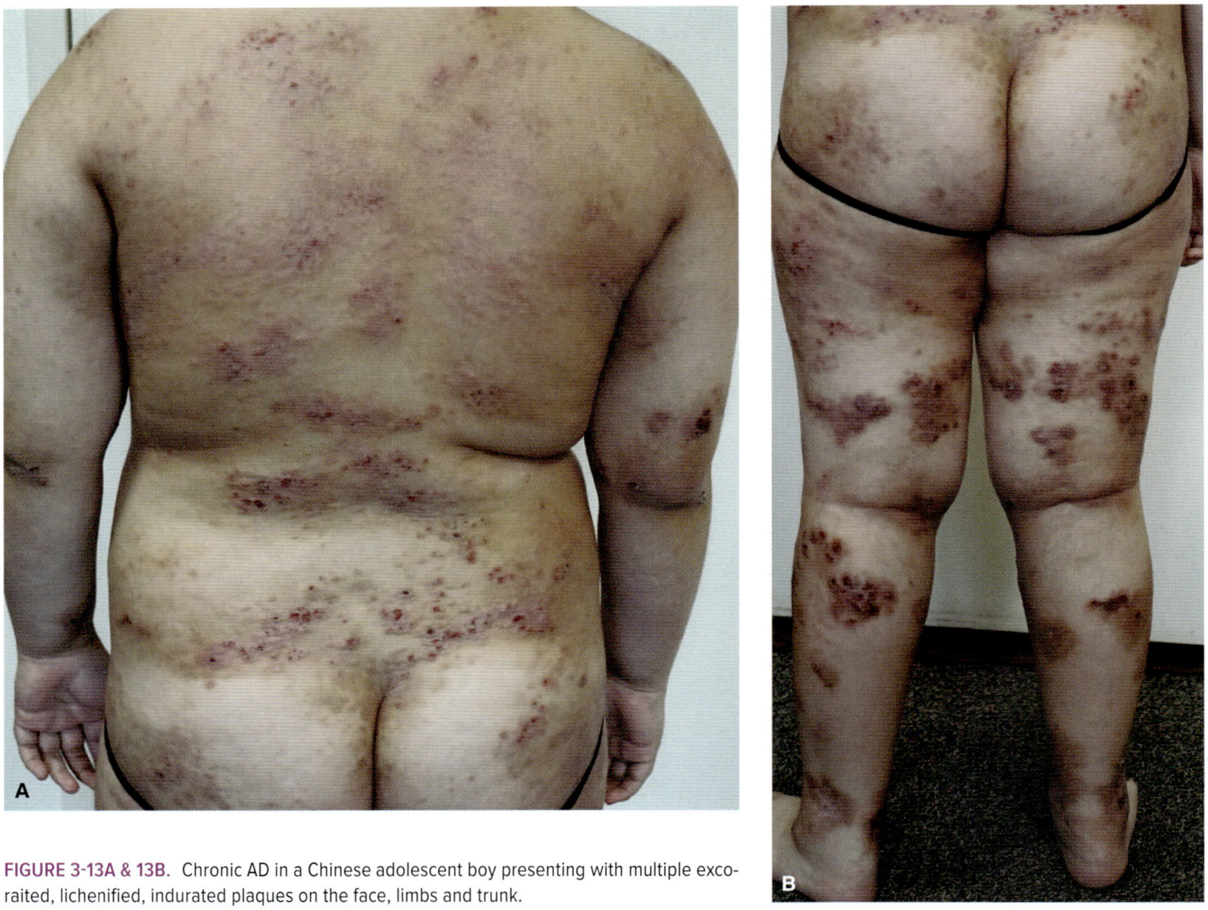

FIGURE 3-13A & 13B. Chronic AD in a Chinese adolescent boy presenting with multiple excoraited, lichenified, indurated plaques on the face, limbs and trunk.

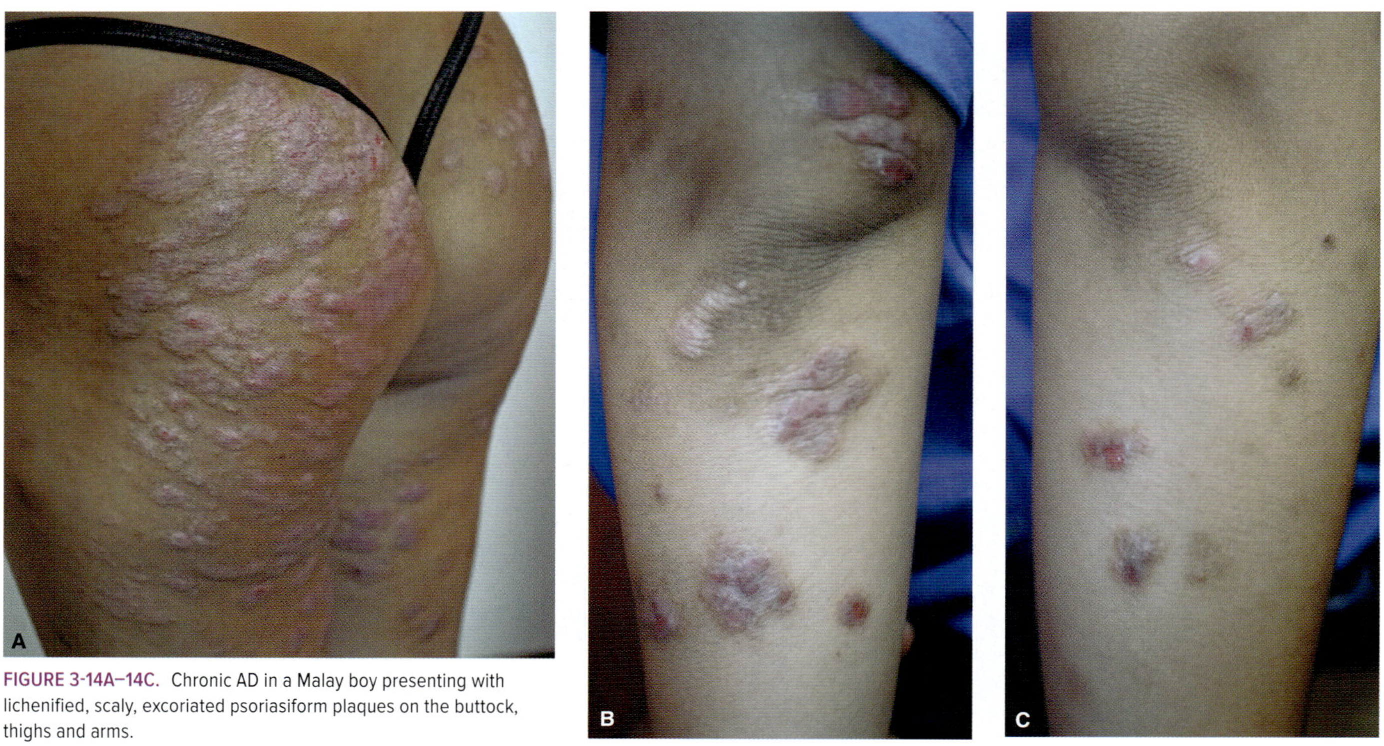

FIGURE 3-14A–14C. Chronic AD in a Malay boy presenting with lichenified, scaly, excoriated psoriasiform plaques on the buttock, thighs and arms.

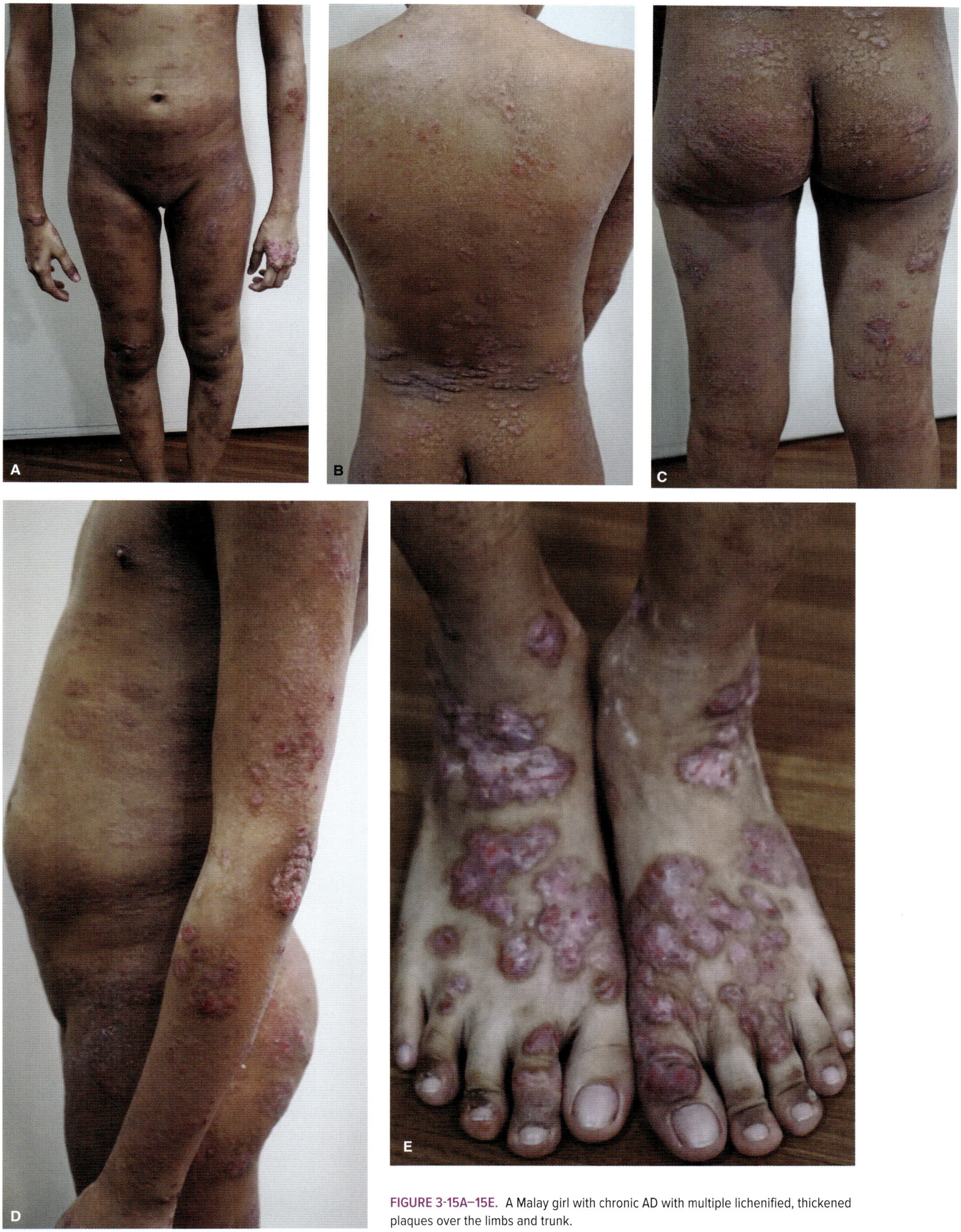

FIGURE 3-15A–15E. A Malay girl with chronic AD with multiple lichenified, thickened plaques over the limbs and trunk.

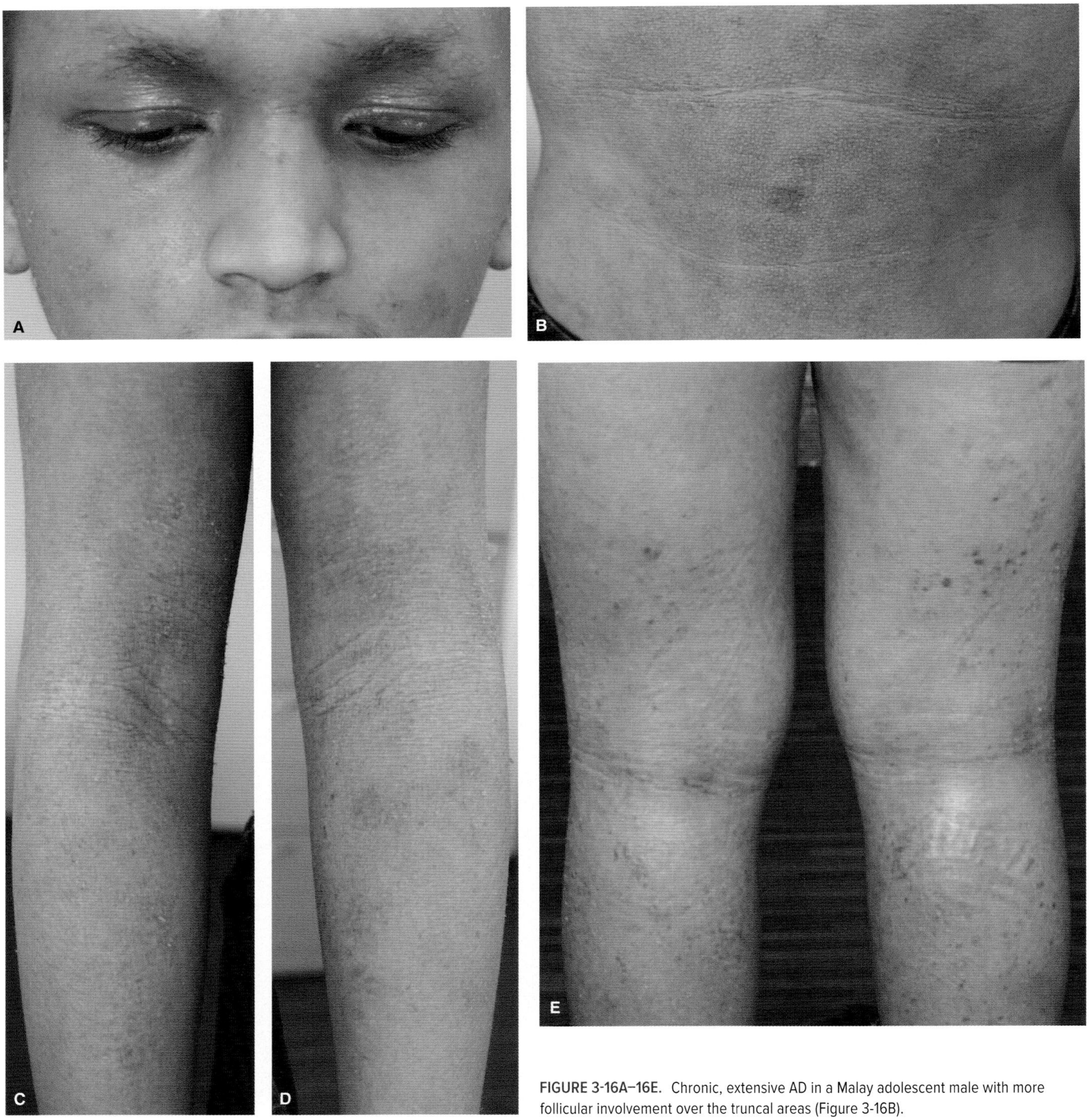

FIGURE 3-16A–16E. Chronic, extensive AD in a Malay adolescent male with more follicular involvement over the truncal areas (Figure 3-16B).

A positive contact history or a history of other family members and caregivers with recent onset of pruritic rashes is suggestive. Skin scraping for scabies mites or eggs can help to confirm the diagnosis.

- Psoriasis
  - Pediatric psoriasis is less common than AD. The most common plaque type presents with well-demarcated erythematous scaly plaques on the extensor surfaces and scalp. Facial and intertriginous areas are commonly involved in children, with predilection for the diaper area in infants. Nail changes such as pitting, distal onycholysis, ridging, and discoloration may serve as clues to the diagnosis.

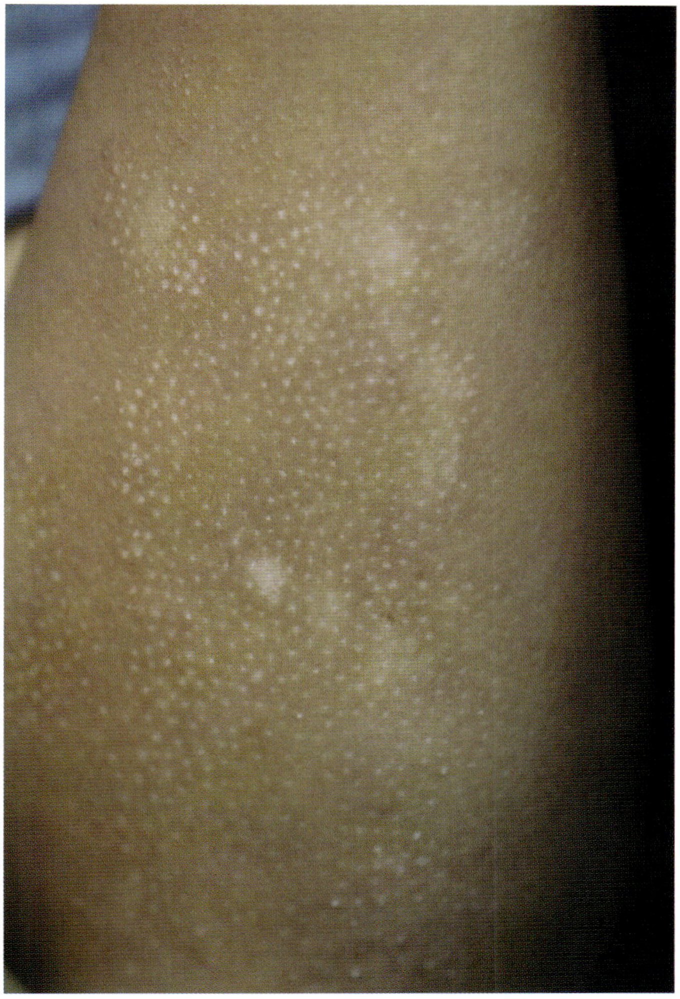

FIGURE 3-17. Follicular eczema on the arms of a darker-skinned Chinese child with AD, associated with post-inflammatory hypopigmentation.

Investigations

- Skin swab for bacterial culture in patients with infected eczema guides the choice of antibiotics.
- Skin swab for herpes simplex PCR to confirm a diagnosis of eczema herpeticum may be useful.
- Skin prick tests can be performed for environmental allergens such as house dust mite, and animal dander.
- Food allergies may worsen eczema in some individuals, especially infants and young children with severe, extensive eczema. Where testing for food allergies is indicated, skin prick test and specific IgE measurements can be done. These tests are more useful as negative predictors. A positive specific IgE result confirms sensitization but this does not necessarily mean an actual allergy exists. Correlation with a history of reaction to foods is necessary, and a double-blind oral food challenge is the gold standard for diagnosis of food allergy. As children can outgrow certain allergies such as cow's milk and egg, positive skin prick tests may be repeated.
- Patch testing may be carried out to exclude allergic contact dermatitis.

Management of Atopic Dermatitis

- Moisturizers are essential to repair the skin barrier and improve xerosis and pruritus. They are crucial for maintenance therapy. Moisturizers typically contain combinations of humectants such as glycerin, occlusives such as paraffin, and emollients such as lanolin. Newer-generation moisturizers may also contain ceramides.
- Gentle cleansers, bath oils, or soap substitutes are recommended for patients with AD. Showers should be limited in duration and frequency, and use of tepid to lukewarm water is preferred over hot water.
- Topical corticosteroids are the main anti-inflammatory medication used. The choice of potency depends on body location, age of patient, and severity of eczema.
- It is best to avoid potent topical steroids in infants, but in severe facial and flexural infantile AD, a 1- to 2-week course of a potent topical corticosteroid (avoid periorbital areas) can be effective.[1] Tapering to milder topical corticosteroids should follow as the eczema improves.[1]
- If the patient has frequent relapses of eczema, during periods of remission, proactive treatment with twice-weekly topical calcineurin inhibitors or mild topical corticosteroids can be used on the sites with frequent flares.
- Although systemic corticosteroids are sometimes used as rescue therapy for acute, severe flares, these should generally be avoided in children and adolescents.
- Topical calcineurin inhibitors (tacrolimus and pimecrolimus) are useful for areas that are more susceptible to side effects of topical corticosteroids, such as the face (especially the periorbital region), neck, groin, and flexural areas. There is no link between the risk of malignancy and use of calcineurin inhibitors.[2]
- Potassium permanganate diluted to a pale pink color is a useful antiseptic to dry any oozy eczematous lesions.
- Sedating antihistamines, which may help with pruritus and sleep disturbance at night, have potential side effects such as impaired concentration at school. Therefore, they should only be taken as needed.
- Non-sedating antihistamines are not as useful to treat pruritus in AD but may be useful when there is concomitant allergic rhinitis or urticaria.
- Phototherapy and systemic immunosuppressants (cyclosporine, methotrexate, azathioprine, mycophenolate mofetil) are second-line options for moderate-to-severe eczema.
- Dupilumab, the biologic targeting IL-4 and IL-13 signaling, is now used to treat moderate-to-severe AD in patients aged 6 months and older. Janus kinase (JAK) inhibitors, such as upadacitinib, have been approved for use in adolescents with moderate-to-severe AD.

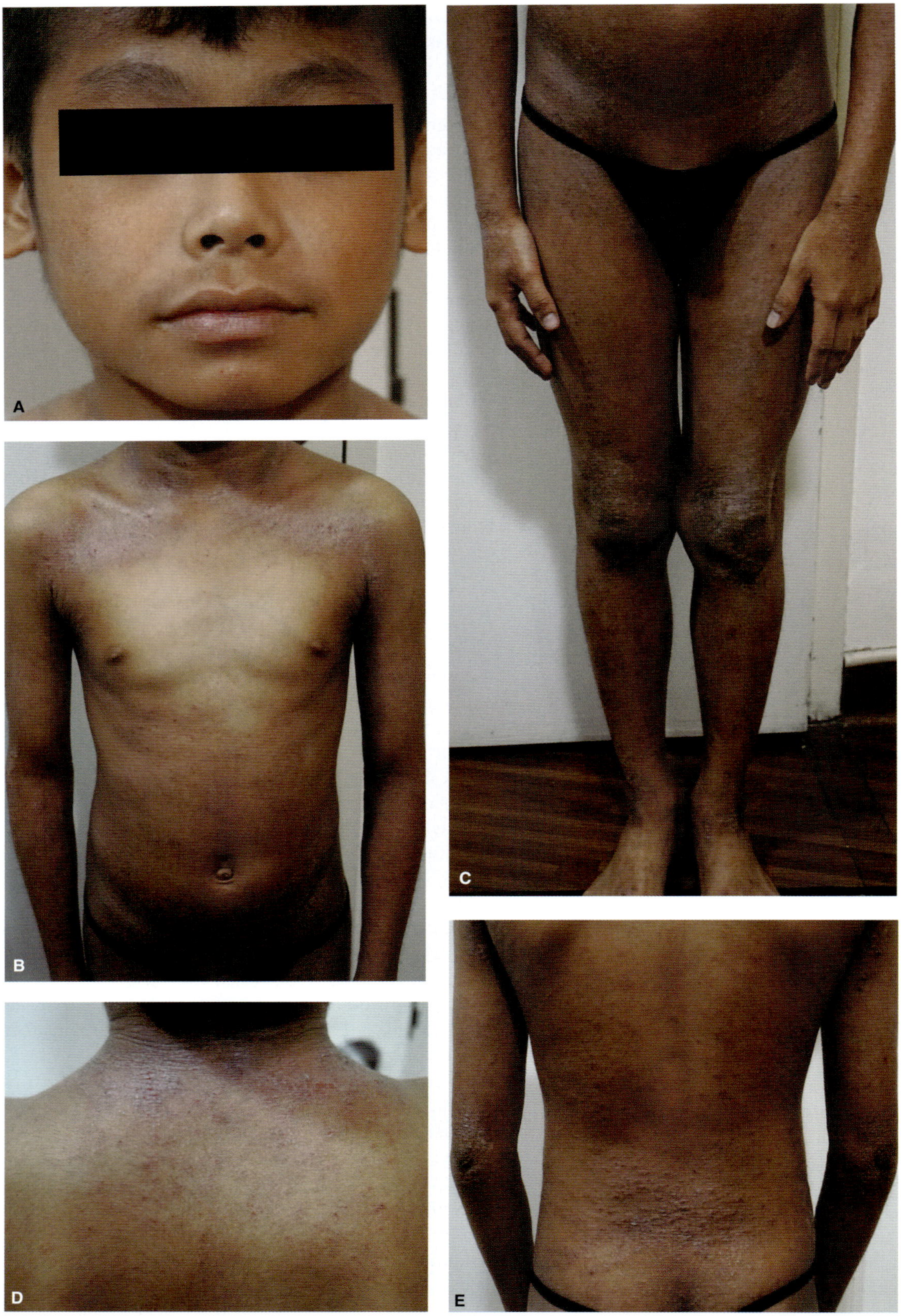

FIGURE 3-18A–18E. Moderately severe AD in a darker-skinned Malay boy with extensive, erythematous to hyperpigmentedy plaques over the face, trunk, and limbs.

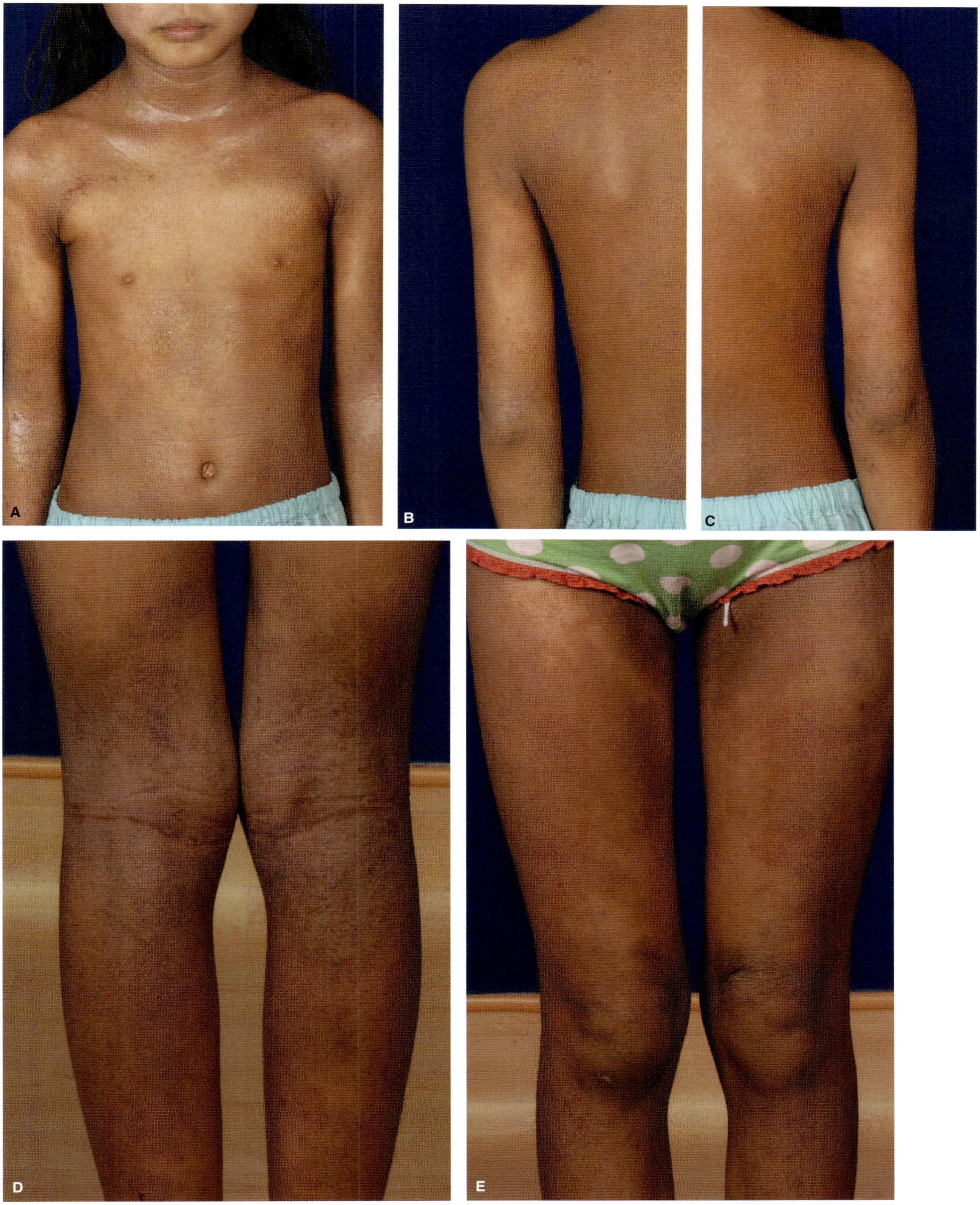

FIGURE 3-19A–19E. Extensive hyperpigmented, scaly patches and plaques affecting the face, limbs, and trunk in a Malay girl with severe AD.

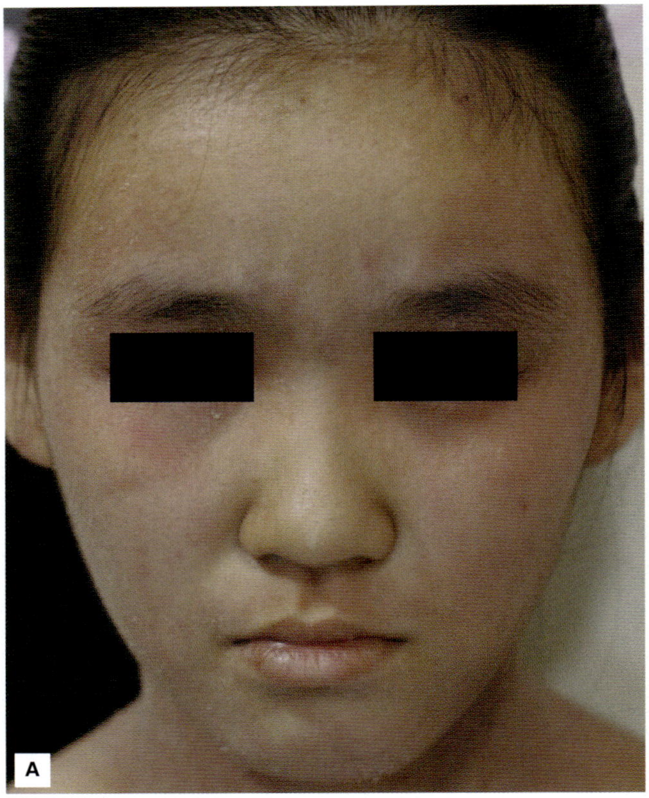

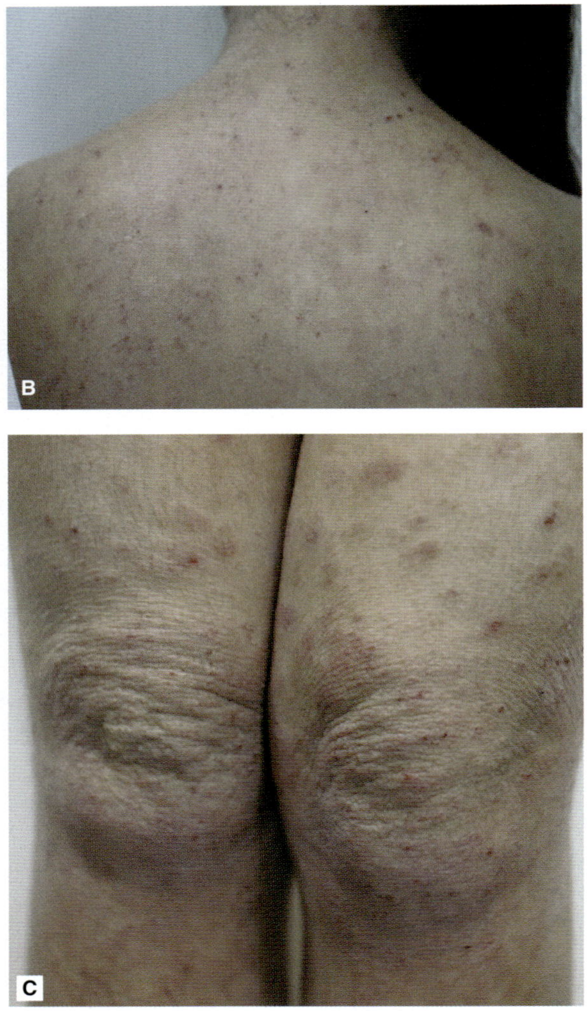

FIGURE 3-20A–20C. Extensive scaly, excoriated, erythematous plaques on the face, periorbital region and back of a Chinese adolescent girl with chronic AD. There are excoriated lichenified plaques on the knees of the same patient (Figure 3-20C).

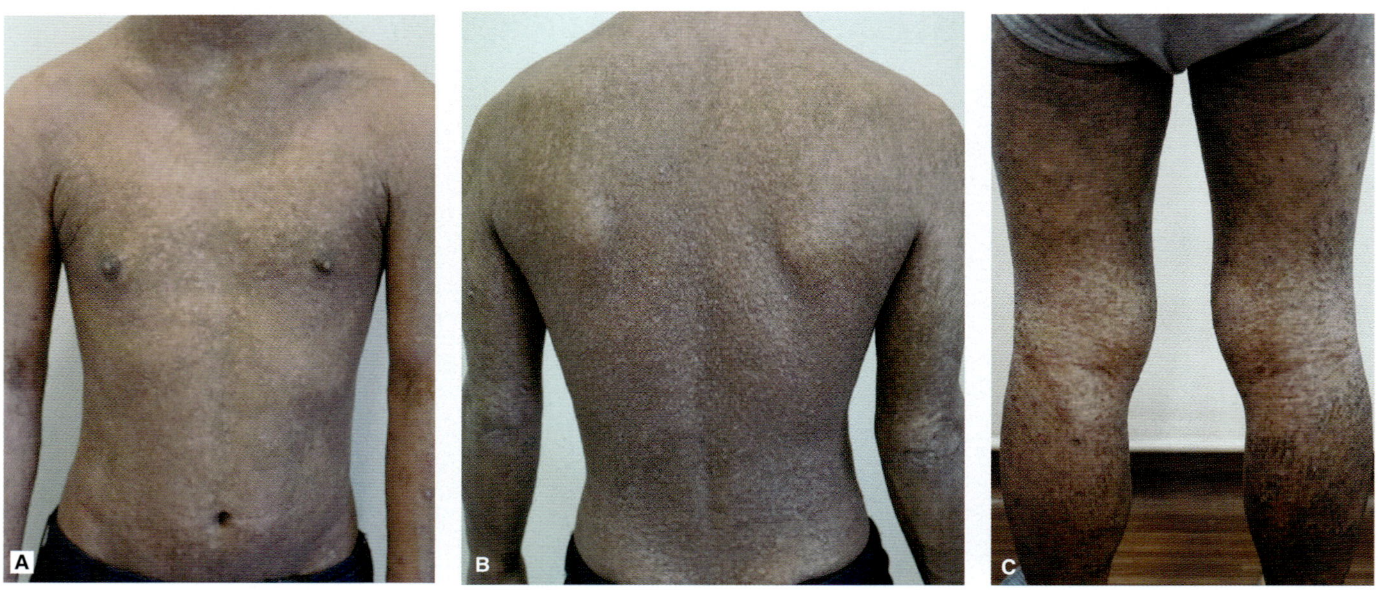

FIGURE 3-21A–21C. Severe, chronic AD in a Malay adolescent male presenting with extensive scaly, dry, excoriated plaques over his trunk, thicker lesions over his lower limbs and dyspigmentation of affected areas (Figure 3-21C).

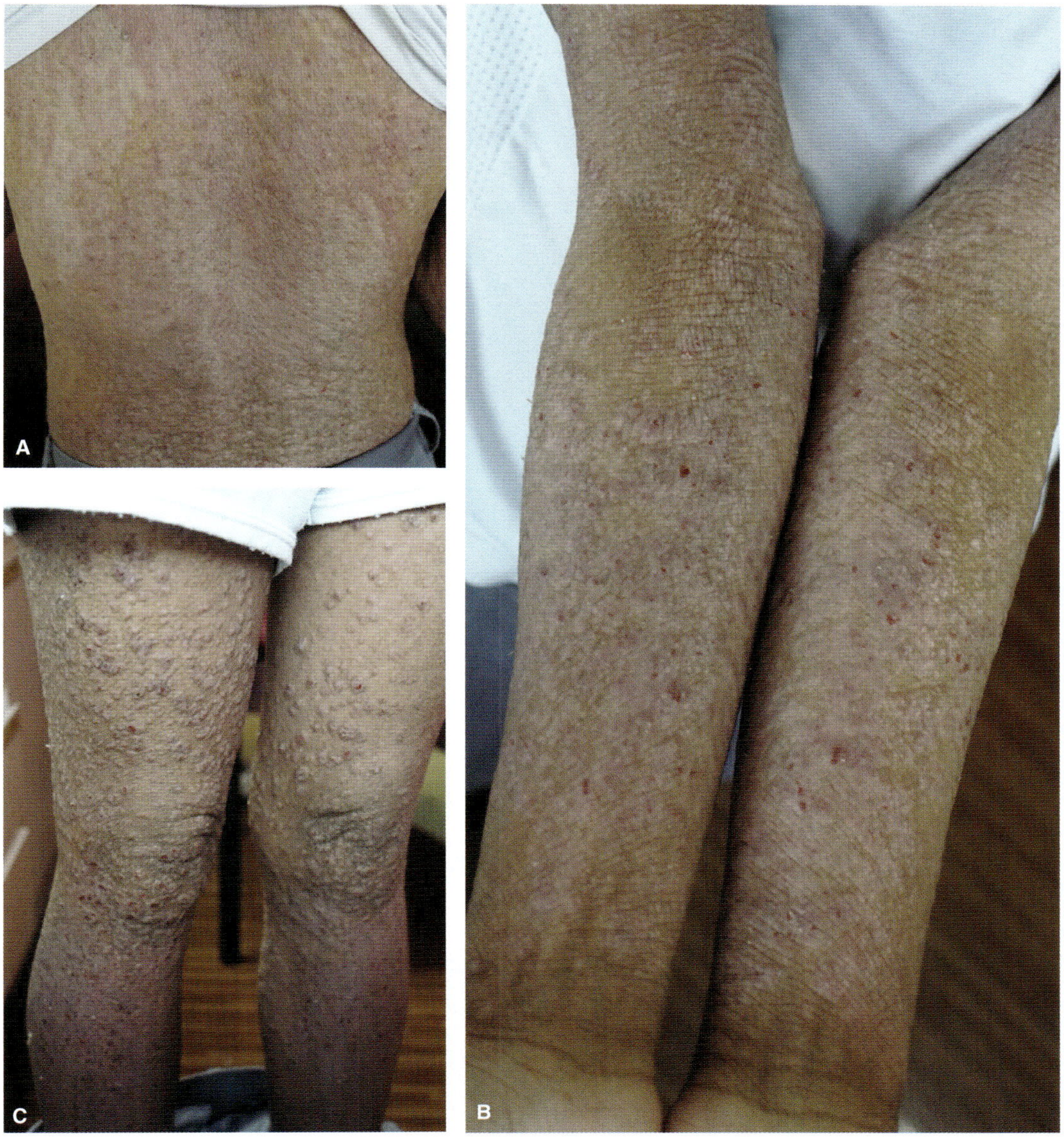

FIGURE 3-22A–22C. Severe, chronic AD in a Chinese adolescent male presenting with extensive eczematous, scaly, excoriated patches and plaques over his trunk and prurigo nodules over his limbs.

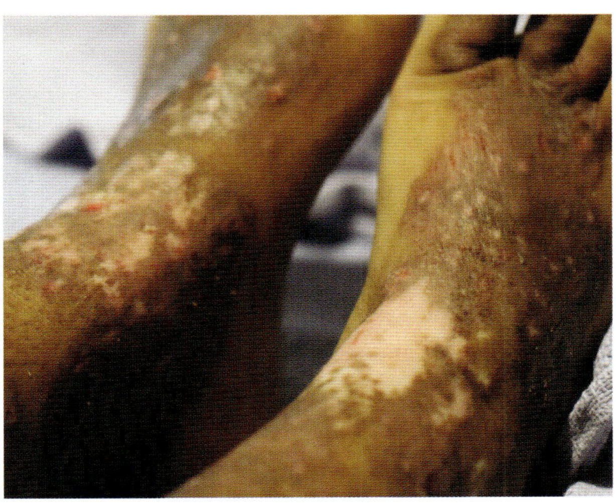

FIGURE 3-23. A darker-skinned adolescent with chronic AD, with areas of post-inflammatory leukoderma.

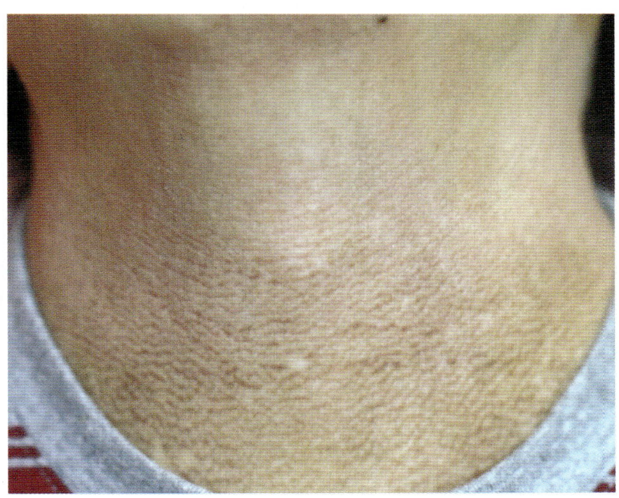

FIGURE 3-24. Rippled, hyperpigmented patches on the neck of a child with severe AD ("dirty neck").

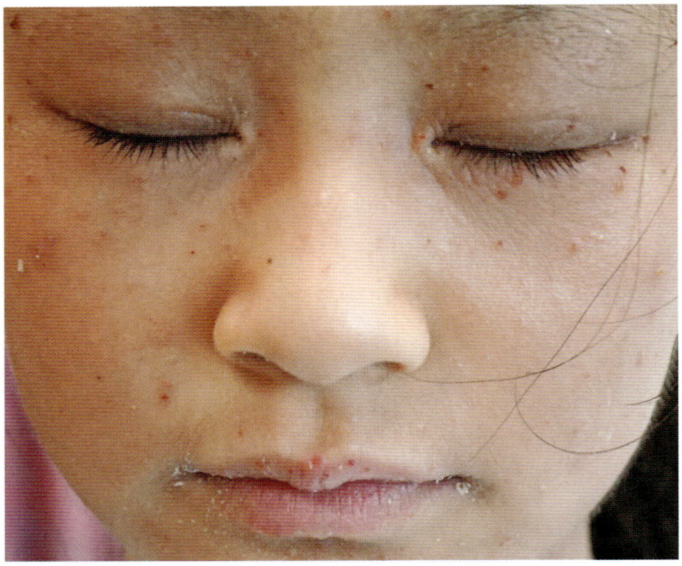

FIGURE 3-25. An adolescent with eczema herpeticum presenting with acute onset of punctate erosions on her face.

Pearls & Practical Tips

- It is important to address steroid phobia. Judicious use of topical corticosteroids avoids potential side effects such as atrophy.

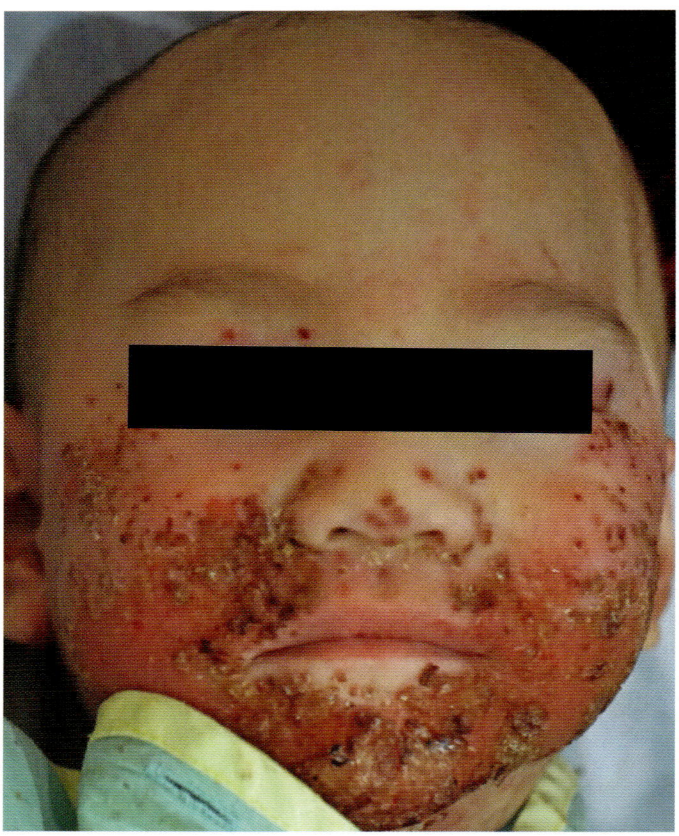

FIGURE 3-26. Vesicles and punctate, punched-out erosions with overlying honey-colored crusts on the face of a child with eczema herpeticum and secondary "impetiginization."

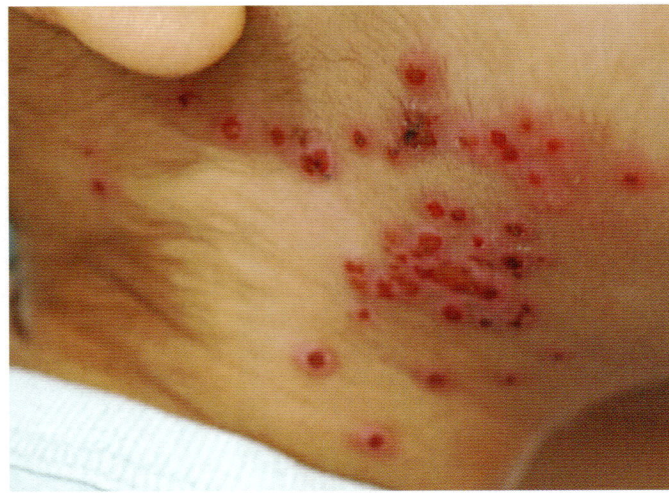

FIGURE 3-27. Punctate, crusted erosions on an erythematous base in a child with eczema herpeticum.

- Patient and caregiver education increases compliance with application of topicals.
- Simple practical tips such as avoiding long, hot showers and moisturizing after swimming are helpful for the patient.
- Wet wraps are a safe and inexpensive method of increasing efficacy of topicals if tolerated and done correctly.
- AD can cause significant psychosocial problems, which should be addressed.

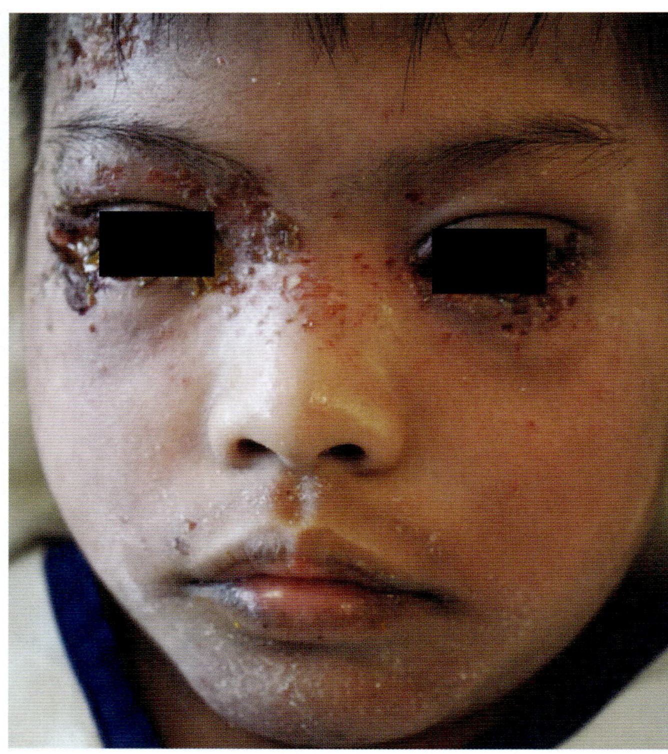

FIGURE 3-28. A Malay boy with eczema herpeticum and secondary bacterial infection affecting his face and eyelids.

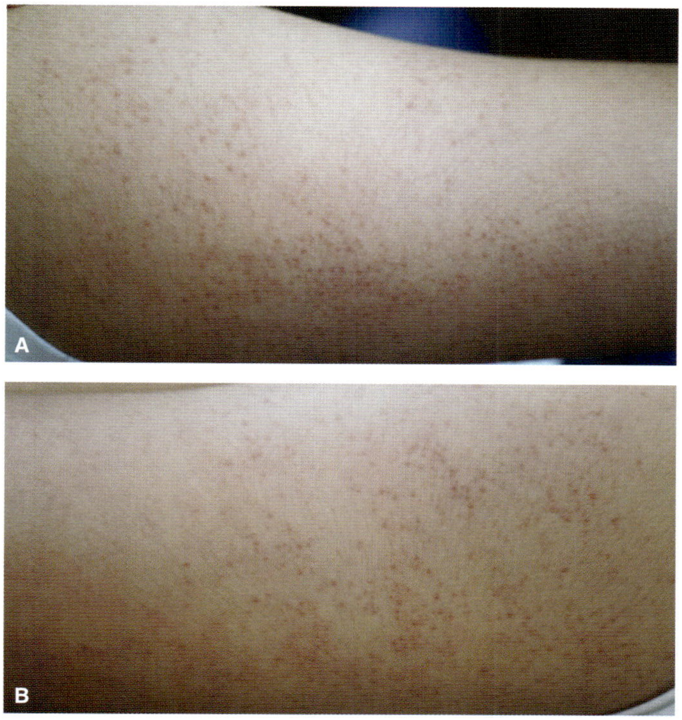

FIGURE 3-29A & 29B. An adolescent Chinese girl with keratosis pilaris, associated with atopic dermatitis, presenting with mildly erythematous-to-hyperpigmented follicular papules on the outer arms.

References

1. Tay YK, Chan YC, Chandran NS, et al. Guidelines for the management of atopic dermatitis in Singapore. Ann Acad Med Singap 2016 Oct;45(10):439-50.
2. Siegfried EC, Jaworski JC, Kaiser JD, et al. Systematic review of published trials: long-term safety of topical corticosteroids and topical calcineurin inhibitors in pediatric patients with atopic dermatitis. BMC Pediatr 2016 Jun 7;16:75.

SEBORRHEIC DERMATITIS

Seborrheic dermatitis is a common inflammatory skin condition most prominent on sebum-rich skin of the scalp and face. The infantile form of seborrheic dermatitis usually starts in early infancy and resolves within the first year of life. Seborrheic dermatitis can also occur in adolescence and adulthood. Infants with seborrheic dermatitis, who have a strong family history of atopy, commonly evolve to develop more classical features of atopic dermatitis as they get older.

Clinical Features

- Seborrheic dermatitis typically presents as pink to erythematous patches with thick, greasy, white-to-yellowish scales.
- Commonly affected sites include the scalp, face (especially the eyebrows and nasolabial folds), and posterior auricular, nuchal, axillary, and inguinal folds. In adolescents, it characteristically involves the scalp, post-auricular areas, eyebrows, nasolabial folds, and anterior chest.
- Some babies with Fitzpatrick types IV to VI skin tone present with hypopigmented scaly macules and patches in the eyebrow region, neck, upper back, and chest, without a significant preceding erythematous rash.
- Pityriasis amiantacea is a reaction pattern that can occur in patients with atopic dermatitis or seborrheic dermatitis. It presents with thick silvery or yellowish scales on the scalp accompanied by tufts of matted, bound-down hair.

Differential Diagnoses

- Atopic dermatitis
  - Many infants with seborrheic dermatitis may eventually develop clinical features of atopic dermatitis, especially if there is a strong family history of atopy. Atopic dermatitis is classically more itchy than seborrheic dermatitis.
- Psoriasis
  - Psoriasis is rare in infancy and presents with more persistent well-demarcated erythematous plaques, with thicker whitish scales.
- Tinea capitis
  - Tinea capitis may occur in prepubertal children and is uncommon in infants. Presentation can range from localized erythematous scaly patches, usually with accompanying alopecia, to boggy alopecic plaques called favus or kerion. The diagnosis should be confirmed by Wood's lamp examination, fungal

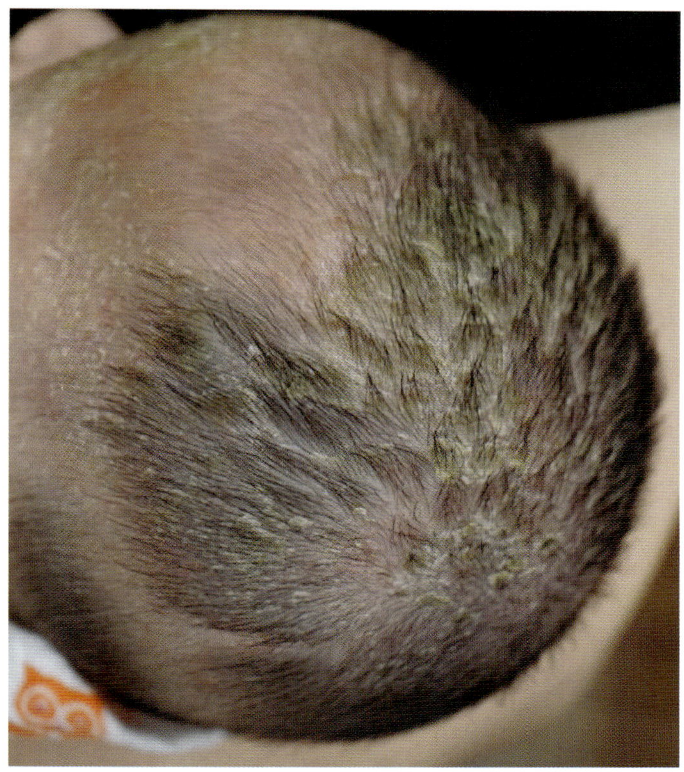

FIGURE 3-30. Thick, yellow, matted scales on the scalp of an infant with seborrheic dermatitis.

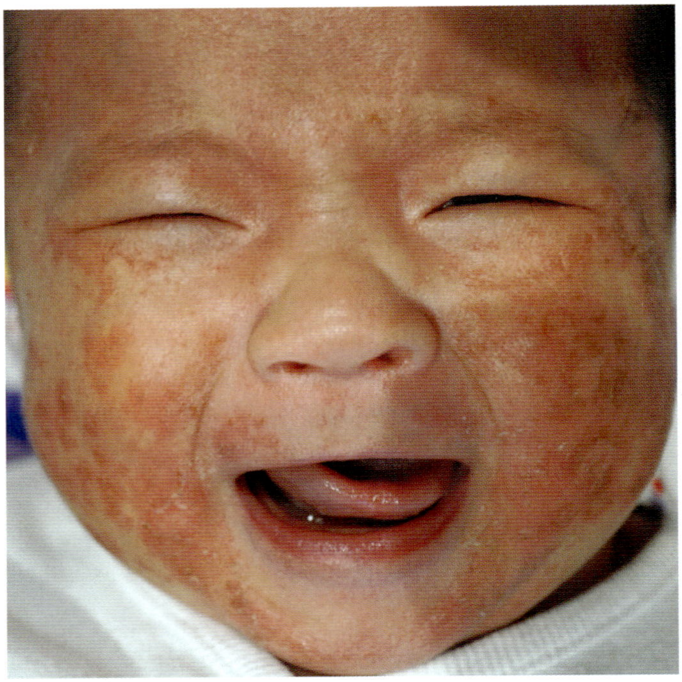

FIGURE 3-31. Patchy erythema with greasy, yellow scaling on the face of an infant with seborrheic dermatitis.

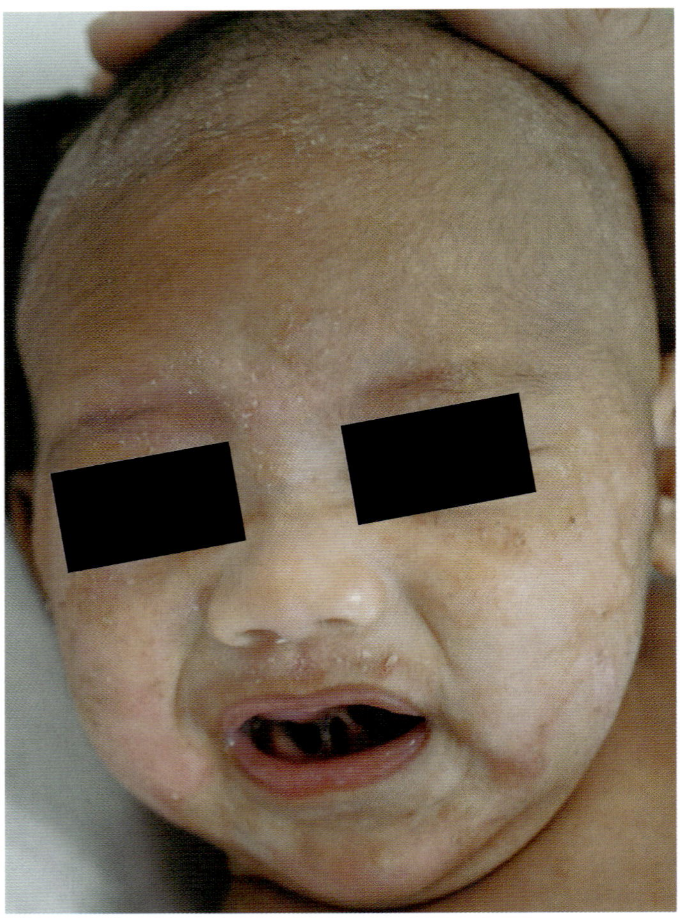

FIGURE 3-32. Scaly, erythematous, poorly demarcated patches and plaques on the face and scalp of a darker-skinned infant with seborrheic dermatitis.

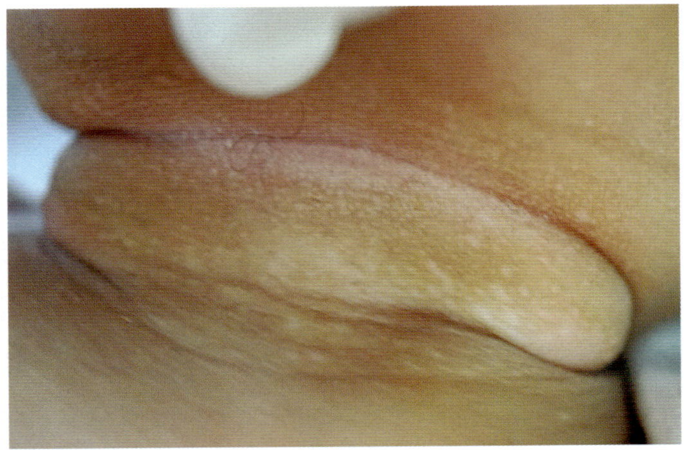

FIGURE 3-33. Mildly erythematous patches with post-inflammatory hypopigmentation on the neck of an infant with seborrheic dermatitis.

microscopy, and culture. A history of contact with animals, especially cats, should prompt suspicion for tinea capitis.

- Langerhans cell histiocytosis
  - Langerhans cell histiocytosis (LCH) can present with rashes in a similar distribution to seborrheic dermatitis. Morphological features that are more in keeping with LCH are brownish erythematous, hemorrhagic, or purpuric macules, papules, or plaques. Surface ulceration is also more commonly seen, especially at intertriginous sites. The diagnosis is confirmed by skin biopsy.

Investigations & Treatment

- Investigations are not usually required for seborrheic dermatitis.
- Oils such as olive oil and baby oil can be applied to the greasy scales on the scalp 30 to 60 minutes before bathing. This facilitates the easy removal of scales.

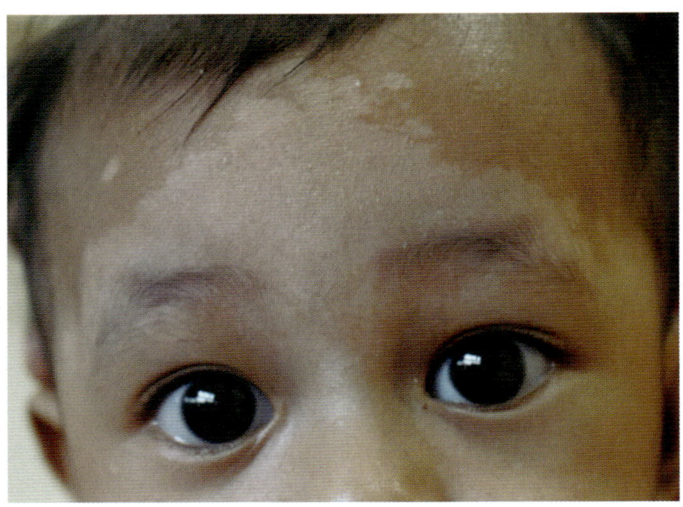

FIGURE 3-34. Post-inflammatory hypopigmentation on the forehead of a darker-skinned infant with seborrheic dermatitis. Mild scaling is still visible.

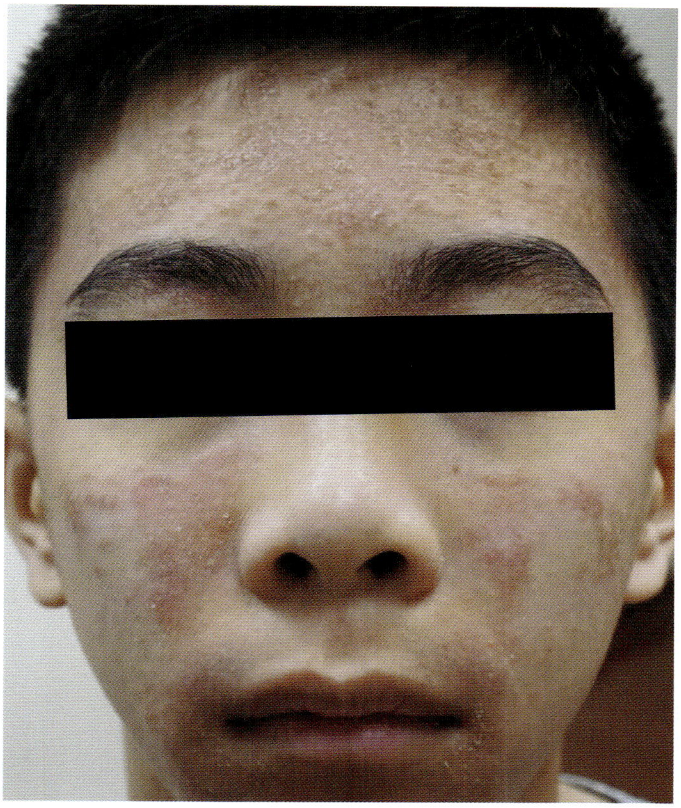

FIGURE 3-35. Patchy, erythematous papules and plaques with fine greasy yellow scales in an adolescent with seborrheic dermatitis.

- Use of an azole shampoo (e.g., ketoconazole shampoo), followed by application of a low-potency topical corticosteroid or azole cream, and moisturizers may be useful for more extensive or severe cases.
- In adolescents, application of a calcineurin inhibitor (e.g., pimecrolimus, tacrolimus) may also be useful to reduce inflammation on the face.

Pearls & Practical Tips

- As this condition is self-limiting in infancy, management can be conservative, with skin care and education of the parents and caregivers.
- Post-inflammatory dyspigmentation, usually hypopigmentation, may occur, especially in darker-skinned infants. Parents should be advised that resolution may take a few months. No treatment is necessary.

PRURIGO NODULARIS

Prurigo nodularis is a chronic pruritic skin disorder presenting with papulonodules secondary to long-term, repetitive scratching and picking of the skin, which is often habitual. It can occur in isolation or may occur in association with other dermatoses, such as atopic dermatitis or papular urticaria.

Clinical Features

- Patients present with excoriated, scaly, hyperkeratotic dome-shaped papulonodules that may be skin colored, erythematous, and hyper- or hypopigmented.
- The extensor surfaces of the limbs, upper back, and buttocks are commonly affected. There is usually sparing of the upper central back, as this area is typically difficult to reach ("butterfly sign").
- Features of other itchy dermatoses may be present, such as atopic dermatitis, insect bite reactions, or papular urticaria.

Differential Diagnoses

- Perforating diseases
  - This group of diseases may be inherited or acquired, and include conditions like reactive perforating collagenosis and acquired perforating dermatosis. Skin biopsies may be required to exclude this diagnosis.

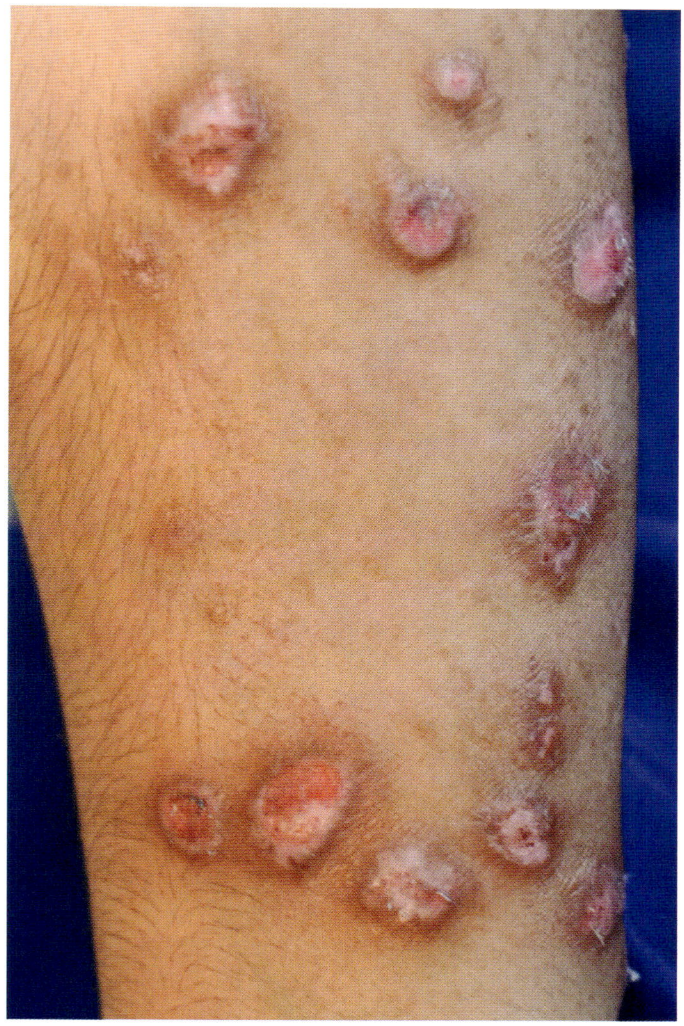

FIGURE 3-36. Multiple excoriated, thickened, prurigo nodules on the arm of an adolescent.

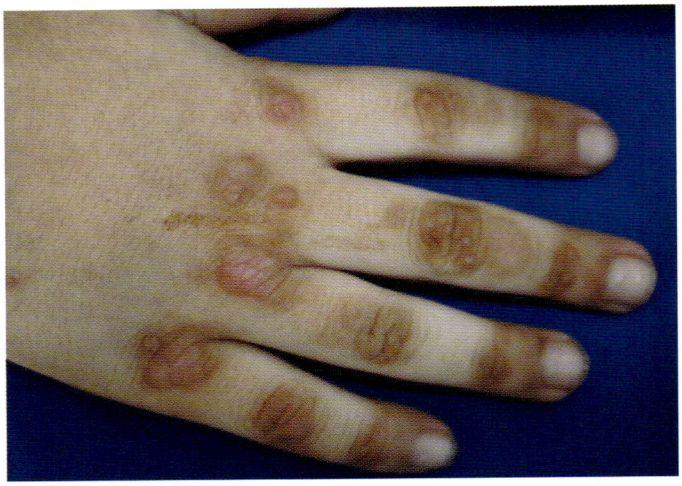

FIGURE 3-37. Multiple pink-to-hyperpigmented papulonodules on the dorsum of the fingers in a young boy with severe prurigo nodularis and concomitant AD.

- Patients present with papulonodules usually with a central keratotic core which is not seen in prurigo nodularis.
- Epidermolysis bullosa pruriginosa
  - This rare genetic disorder is a subtype of dystrophic epidermolysis bullosa.
  - Clinically, patients present with blisters and erosions in infancy or early childhood that gradually progress to develop coalescent lichenoid papulonodules.
  - There is a predilection for the pre-tibial area and there may be concomitant nail changes.
  - A positive family history of the same condition may be present.
- Nodular scabies
  - Nodular scabies is a variant of scabies that occurs most commonly in infants and young children.
  - Patients present with pruritic nodules that develop as a hypersensitivity reaction to the infestation, and lesions may persist even after successful anti-scabetic treatment.
  - Unlike prurigo nodularis, nodular scabies may be accompanied by other lesions classical of scabies, like papules, burrows, and vesicles, that occur typically in the digital webspaces, genitals, and axillae. A positive contact history may also aid diagnosis of nodular scabies.

Investigations & Treatment

- Investigations are generally not required for diagnosis.
- Skin biopsy shows a dome-shaped nodule with compact hyperkeratosis and parakeratosis, epidermal hyperplasia, and vertically streaked collagen in the papillary dermis.
- Therapeutic options include potent topical corticosteroids and anti-pruritic agents such as menthol-containing formulations. Cryotherapy, intralesional corticosteroids, phototherapy with UVA and UVB, or systemic immunosuppressants like cyclosporin may also be used.

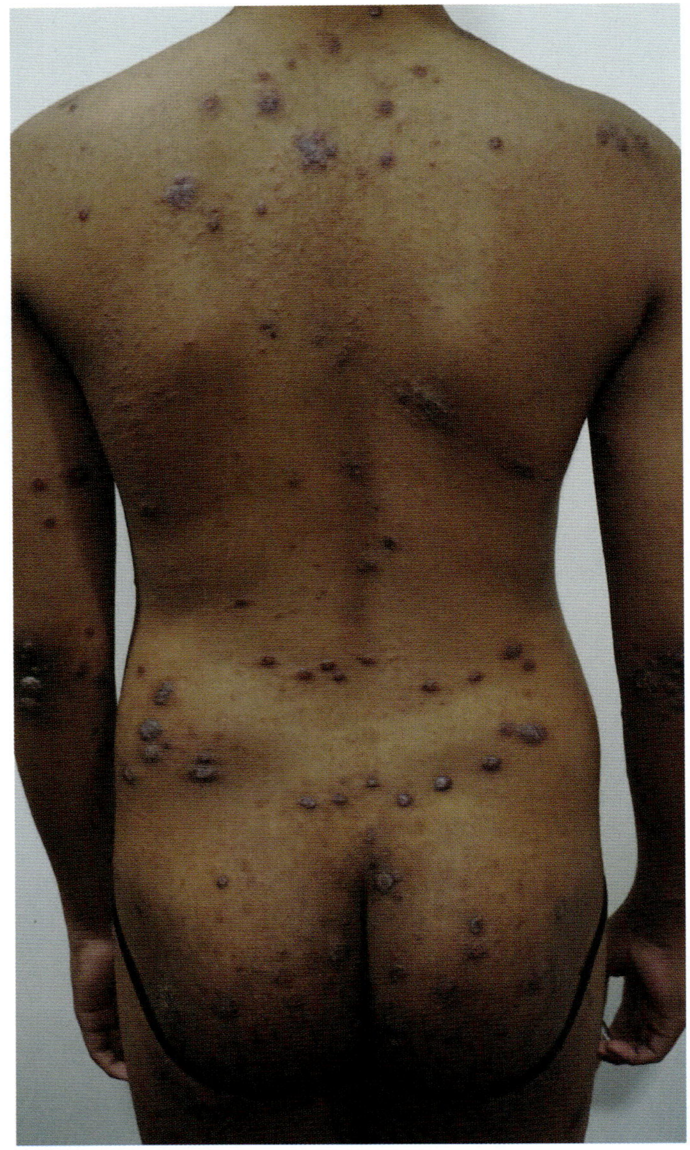

FIGURE 3-38. Extensive hyperpigmented prurigo nodules on the back, buttocks, and arms of a darker-skinned adolescent.

Pearls & Practical Tips

- Regular application of emollients, use of soap substitutes, and avoidance of rough clothing are important adjunctive general measures when managing prurigo nodularis.
- Actinic prurigo is a condition predominantly affecting children and should be considered if the lesions affect mainly sun-exposed sites.
- The scratching and picking of lesions can be habitual in some patients with prurigo nodularis and oftern reported to be worsening during times of stress. Therefore, co-management with a psychologist may be required to reduce the habitual picking.

LICHEN SIMPLEX CHRONICUS

Lichen simplex chronicus (LSC) refers to a well-demarcated area of skin thickening resulting from repeated, habitual trauma of the skin, for example by rubbing or scratching. Although it can occur in isolation, it more commonly occurs in patients with underlying atopic dermatitis or other types of eczema.

Clinical Features

- LSC can occur at any age but is more common in older children or adolescents.
- It is most commonly seen in patients with pre-existing pruritic skin conditions such as atopic dermatitis or psoriasis, but may also occur in those with systemic disorders causing generalized pruritus.
- Presents as a well-circumscribed area of thickened skin that may be skin colored, hyper- or hypopigmented. There are often overlying scales or occasionally scabs. The skin lines are accentuated over the area (lichenification).

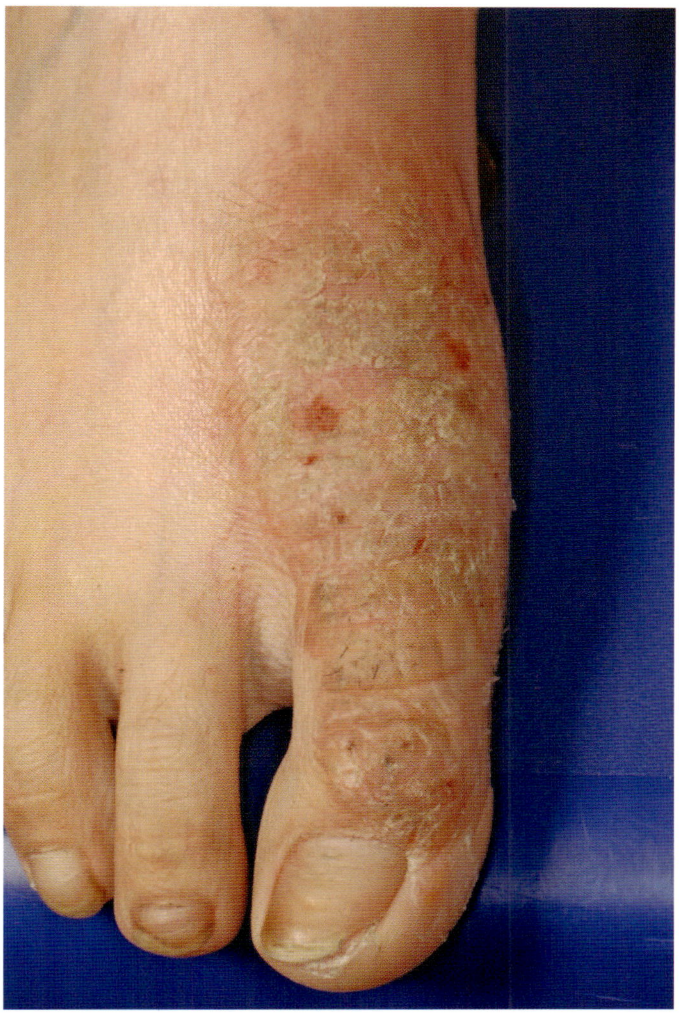

FIGURE 3-39. LSC on the forefoot and big toe of a Chinese boy showing a well-circumscribed, scaly, lichenified plaque.

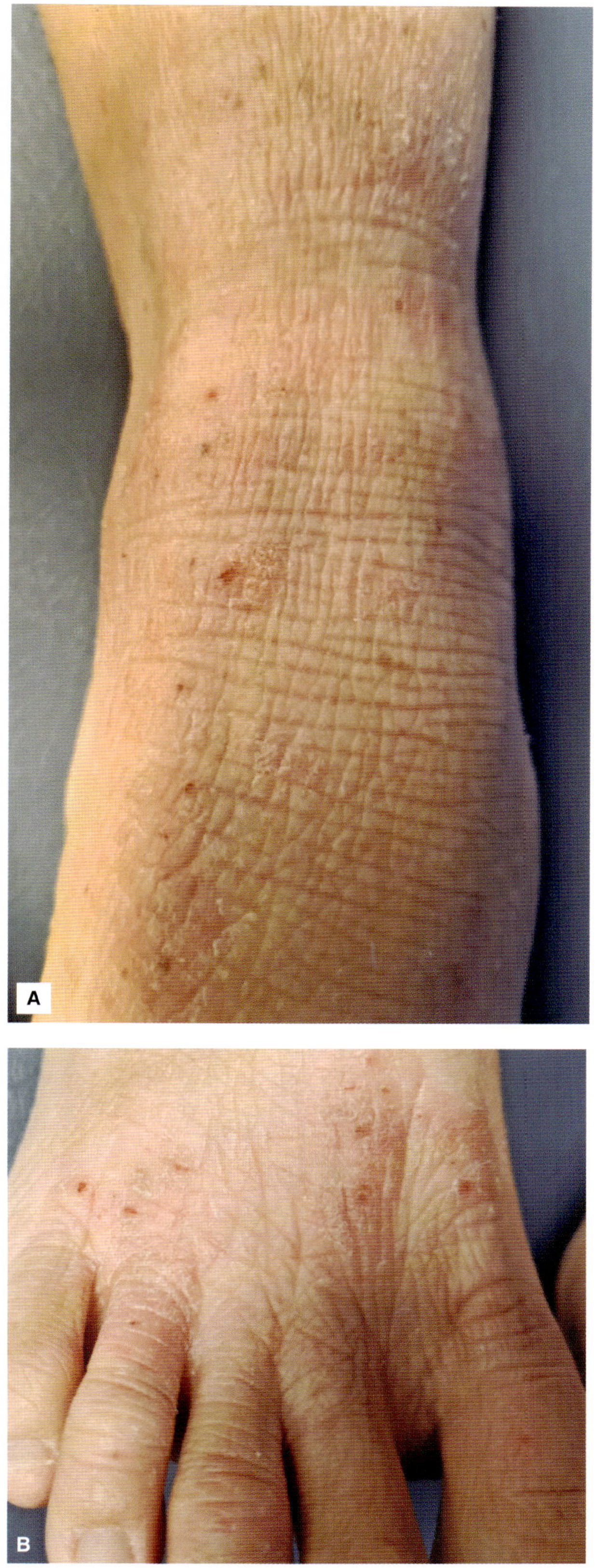

FIGURE 3-40A & 40B. LSC on the ankle and forefoot of a Chinese adolescent, presenting as a well-circumscribed, scaly, lichenified plaque.

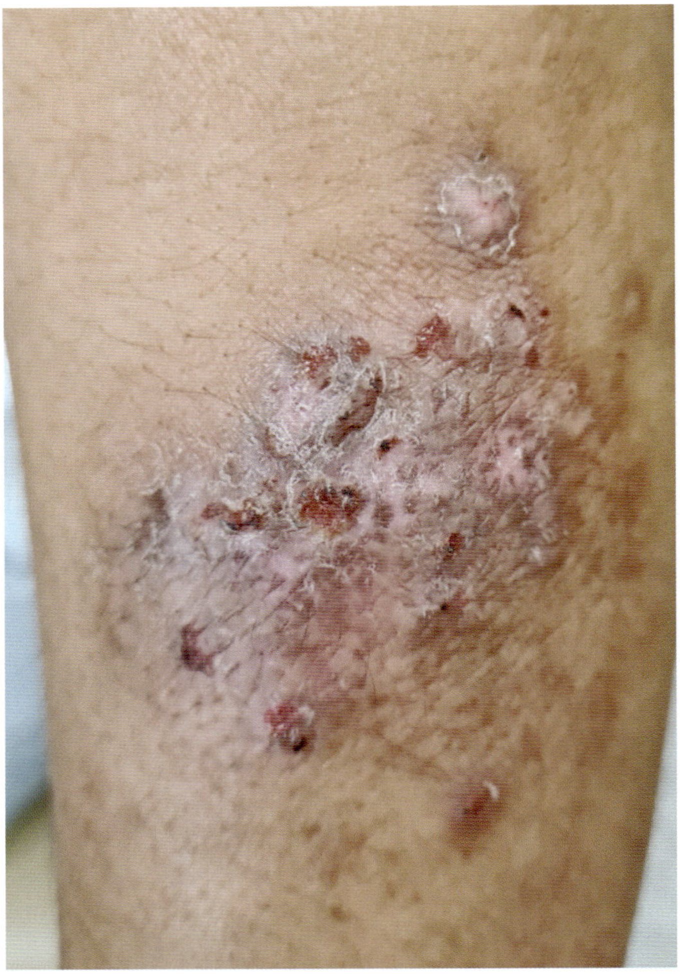

FIGURE 3-41. A Chinese child with chronic AD and LSC on the extensor elbows, manifesting as a fairly well-demarcated, thick, scaly excoriated plaque with dyspigmentation.

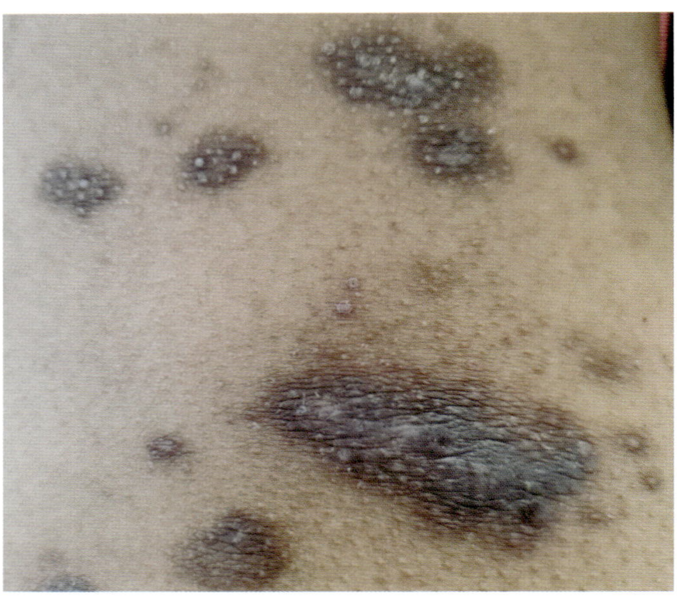

FIGURE 3-42. An Asian child with chronic eczema presenting with hyperpigmented plaques of LSC together with a follicular type of eczema.

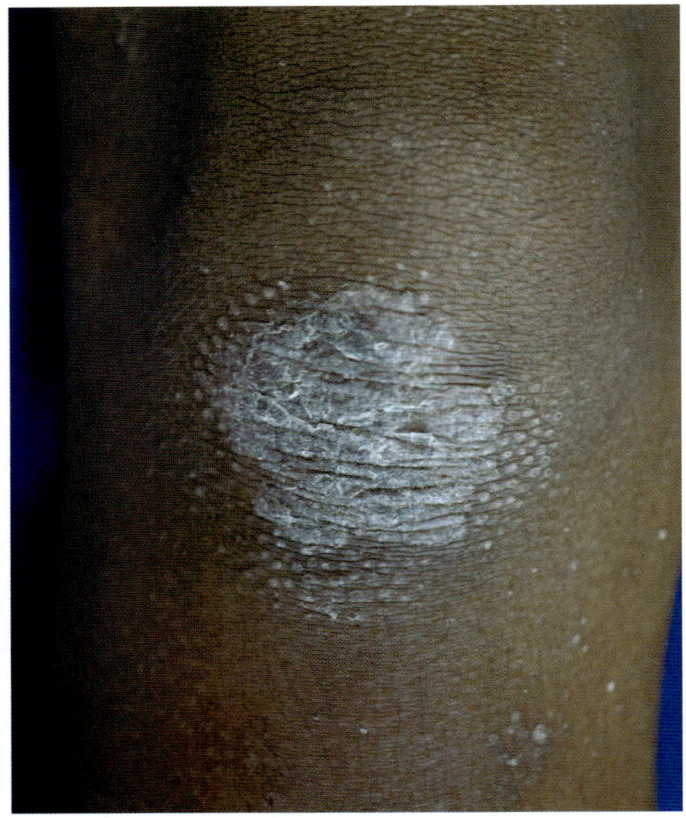

FIGURE 3-43. LSC presenting as a well-circumscribed, thick, scaly plaque on the anterior knee of an Indian child. There is follicular type of eczema seen around the plaque of LSC.

- Lesions are usually intensely pruritic.
- Commonly affected sites include body parts accessible to scratching, including the extensor surfaces of the limbs, ankles, posterior neck, and the anogenital region.

Differential Diagnoses

- Chronic plaque psoriasis
  - Chronic plaque psoriasis presents with well-defined erythematous scaly plaques on extensor surfaces.
  - Unlike LSC, the plaques tend to be symmetrically distributed and the scales are silvery-white in color. There may also be associated nail changes and joint involvement.
- Discoid eczema
  - This is a subtype of eczema that may occur in older children and adolescents, although younger children may also be affected.
  - Clinically, discoid eczema presents with coin-shaped, scaly, erythematous plaques, usually on the limbs, which may occasionally be weepy and exudative.
- Chronic atypical mycobacterial and deep fungal infections
  - Very rarely, atypical mycobacterial infections (e.g., fish-tank granuloma) and deep fungal infections (e.g., chromoblastomycosis, mycetoma) can present as localized, lichenified, scaly plaques. If there is a history

of exposure, especially in the absence of eczema elsewhere, biopsies for histology, and mycobacterial and fungal cultures should be performed to exclude these infections.

Investigations & Treatment

- Investigations are not required for diagnosis.
- If performed, skin biopsy will show compact hyperkeratosis with parakeratosis, irregular psoriasiform hyperplasia of the epidermis, and vertically streaked collagen in the papillary dermis.
- Disruption of the itch-scratch cycle is the cornerstone of the management of LSC.
- Pharmacological treatment options include potent topical corticosteroids and anti-pruritic agents such as menthol-containing formulations. Cryotherapy and intralesional corticosteroids are also effective therapeutic options, although these are more painful and may not be suitable for younger children.

Pearls & Practical Tips

- Underlying psychosocial stressors may precipitate the itch-scratch cycle and should be addressed.
- Topicals may be applied under occlusion to improve absorption and also to prevent patients from further traumatizing the lesions.

DISCOID ECZEMA

Discoid eczema, also known as nummular eczema, is a fairly common, chronic relapsing condition characterized by itchy coin-shaped eczematous plaques. It is usually super-infected with *Staphylococcus aureus.*

Clinical Features

- Discoid eczema can occur at any age, although it is more common in older children and adolescents.
- It presents with intensely pruritic, round, coin-shaped erythematous plaques, which may be oozy and studded with scales or pustules.
- Lesions are typically exudative and crusted in the acute phase and evolve to be dry, scaly, and lichenified in chronic disease. Concomitant skin xerosis is usually present. In patients with skin of color, discoid eczema may present with hyperpigmented scaly or oozy plaques.
- The limbs, especially the legs, are usually affected, although the involvement may be more generalized in more severely affected patients.
- Triggers for discoid eczema include insect bites, contact dermatitis, and skin infections, for example molluscum in children.
- The condition tends to be more persistent and treatment resistant than atopic dermatitis.

Differential Diagnosis

- Tinea corporis
  - Discoid eczema may be mistaken for tinea corporis, where the skin lesions appear annular and scaly. Skin scraping for fungal microscopy or fungal culture confirms the diagnosis.

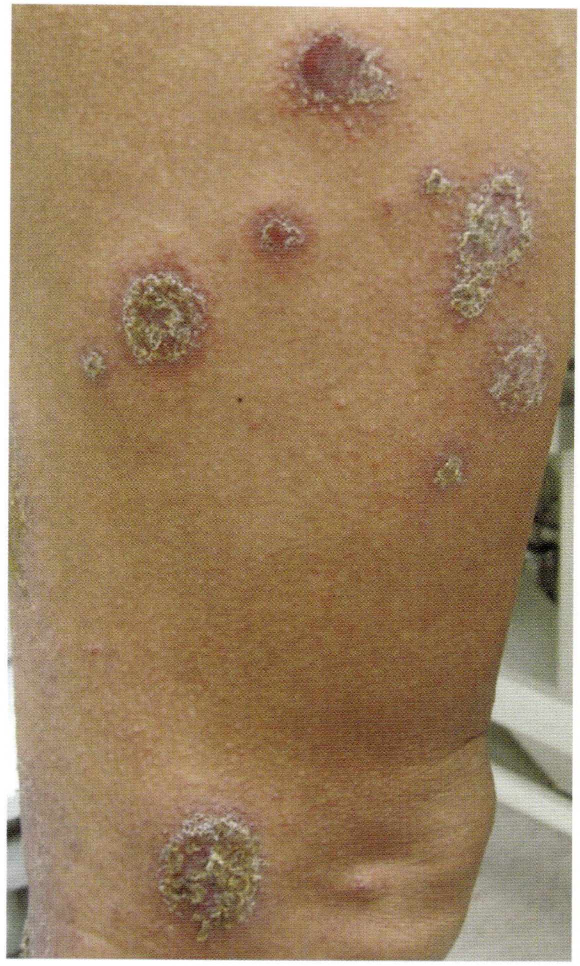

FIGURE 3-44. Discoid eczema in a Chinese child presenting as rather well-demarcated, round-to-ovoid plaques with overlying yellow scaling.

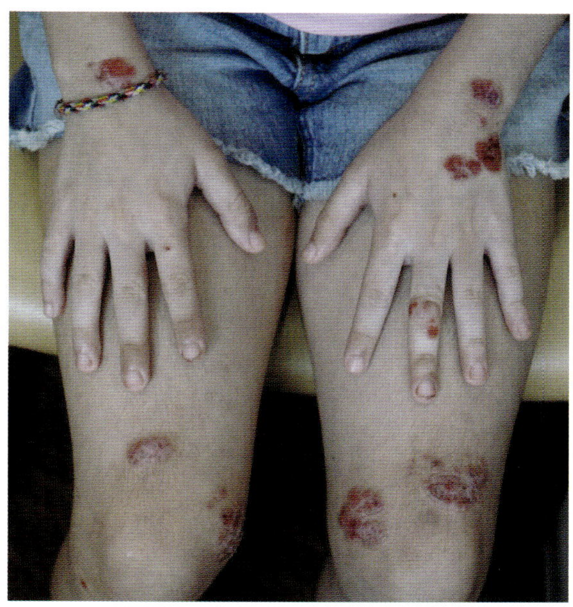

FIGURE 3-45. Thick, excoriated, scaly, discoid eczema plaques on the dorsum of the wrists, fingers, and on the thighs of a Chinese girl.

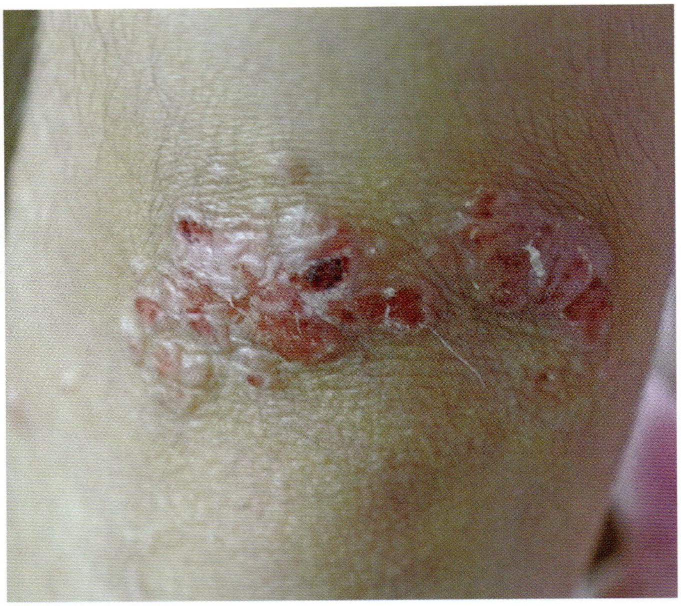

FIGURE 3-46. Excoriated, scaly and thick discoid plaques on the extensor aspect of the elbow of a Chinese child with discoid eczema.

- Plaque psoriasis
  - This presents with well-demarcated erythematous scaly plaques, typically on the extensor surfaces and the scalp. Concomitant nail changes or joint involvement may be present.
- Allergic contact dermatitis
  - Lesions may be indistinguishable from discoid eczema.
  - Patch testing should be offered if the clinical history and examination are suggestive.

Investigations & Treatment

- Discoid eczema is usually diagnosed clinically.
- For exudative and crusted lesions, a skin swab may be performed for bacterial culture.
- If the clinical history and examination suggest possible allergic contact dermatitis, patch testing may be required.
- High-potency topical corticosteroids are used to treat this condition. A combination of topical steroid with topical antibiotic may be useful in more oozy lesions.
- Topical calcineurin inhibitors, such as tacrolimus ointment or pimecrolimus cream, are alternative therapeutic options and can be given for maintenance or proactive treatment.
- Potassium permanganate soaks and compresses are useful for exudative lesions.
- Mild soap-free cleansers and moisturizers should also be used.
- Oral antibiotics to cover for *S. aureus* infection (e.g., cephalexin or cloxacillin) may be required if clinically infected.
- In severe disease, a short course of oral corticosteroids may be needed.
- In refractory disease, narrow-band UVB phototherapy, ciclosporin, azathioprine, methotrexate, and dupilumab are possible treatment options.

Pearls & Practical Tips

- Discoid eczema often occurs on a background of atopic dermatitis or other atopic conditions. However, it can also occur without a history of other eczemas.
- This condition tends to be chronic, with relapses and remissions.
- If left untreated, chronic scratching of discoid eczema may lead to formation of prurigo nodules.

HAND AND FEET ECZEMA

Hand eczema can occur in patients of all ages, with onset often in childhood. It arises due to a combination of factors including underlying atopic dermatitis as well as irritant or allergic contact dermatitis. A third of patients with atopic hand eczema also have feet eczema.

Clinical Features

- Features of hand and feet eczema include palmar hyperlinearity, scaly erythematous plaques, hyperkeratosis, edema, fissures, and erosions.
- Pompholyx, also known as dyshidrotic eczema, is a subset of hand and feet eczema. Patients present with very itchy vesicles on the palms and soles, especially on the lateral aspects of the digits.
- Juvenile plantar dermatosis is a characteristic condition common in young children with atopic diathesis. Clinically, patients present with symmetrical, shiny, glazed fissured plaques on the soles and plantar surfaces of the toes, especially the forefoot and big toes. Hyperhidrosis, as well as, irritation from friction, sweating and synthetic footwear may aggravate the condition.

Differential Diagnoses

- Palmoplantar psoriasis
  - This presents with well-demarcated, erythematous, and scaly plaques. Small pinpoint pustules may often be seen.
  - Presence of psoriatic plaques elsewhere on the skin, synovitis, and psoriatic nail changes are features that would allow differentiation from hand and feet eczema.
- Tinea pedis/tinea manuum
  - This presents with erythematous, scaly, and more demarcated powdery patches and plaques. Interdigital spaces are often affected.
  - The rash may have an annular appearance, and there may be concurrent onychomycosis.
- Scabies
  - Interdigital scaling often occurs in scabies. Close inspection may reveal burrows in the webspaces.
  - A positive contact history, a history of family members with new-onset pruritus, and the presence of burrows, papules, and tracks in the interdigital webspaces, axillae, groins, inter- and inframammary areas raise suspicion for scabies infestation.

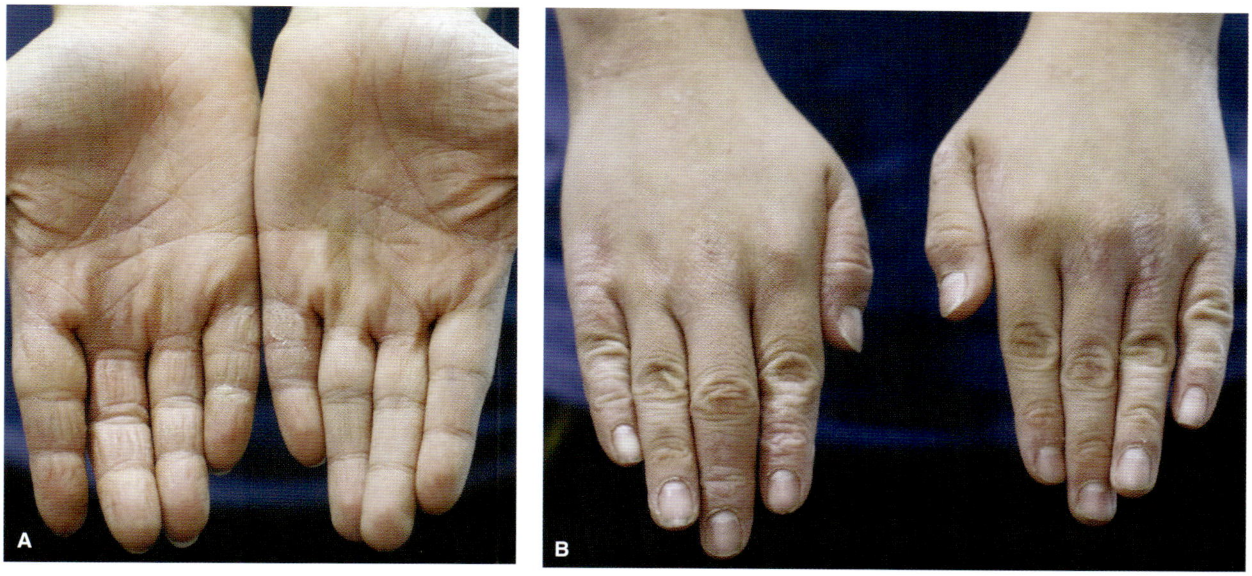

FIGURE 3-47A & 47B. Mild hand eczema presenting with scaling on the palms of an older Chinese child. Patient in Figure 3-47A with hand eczema also affecting the dorsum of the hands.

Investigations & Treatment

- The diagnosis of hand and foot eczema is usually made clinically.
- If there is concern about differential diagnoses, investigations such as skin scrapes to exclude tinea pedis and scabies as well as a patch test to exclude allergic contact dermatitis can be carried out.
- General measures include wearing waterproof gloves (extending to mid-forearm) for wet work, using soap substitutes for handwashing, generous, frequent application of moisturizers, and conscious avoidance of known allergens and irritants. Other measures include reducing the frequency of handwashing and minimizing the use of hand sanitizers.
- Because the hands and feet have a thicker stratum corneum, percutaneous absorption of topical medications is reduced and hence higher potency topical steroids may be needed. The patient can step down to a milder topical steroid or switch to topical calcineurin inhibitors (tacrolimus ointment) when the condition is better. The latter can also be used for preventive or maintenance (proactive) treatment.
- For patients with severe or recalcitrant and chronic disease, phototherapy or systemic medications like immunosuppressants (ciclosporin, azathioprine, and methotrexate) may be considered.

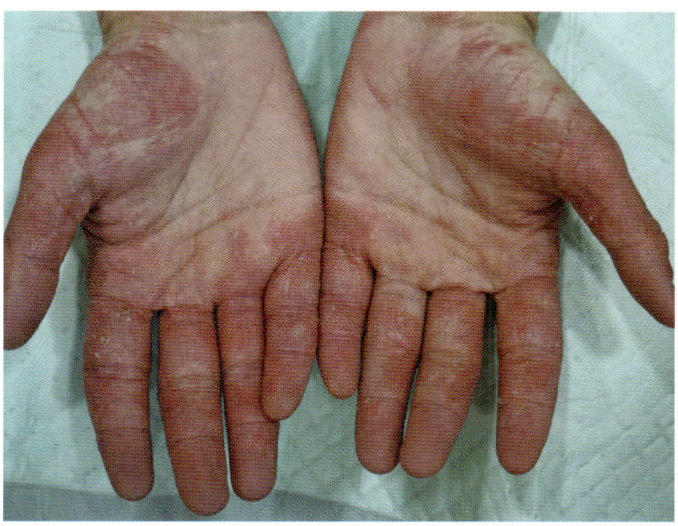

FIGURE 3-48. More severe hand eczema presenting with erythema and scaling on the palms and palmar aspect of the fingers of a Chinese adolescent with underlying AD.

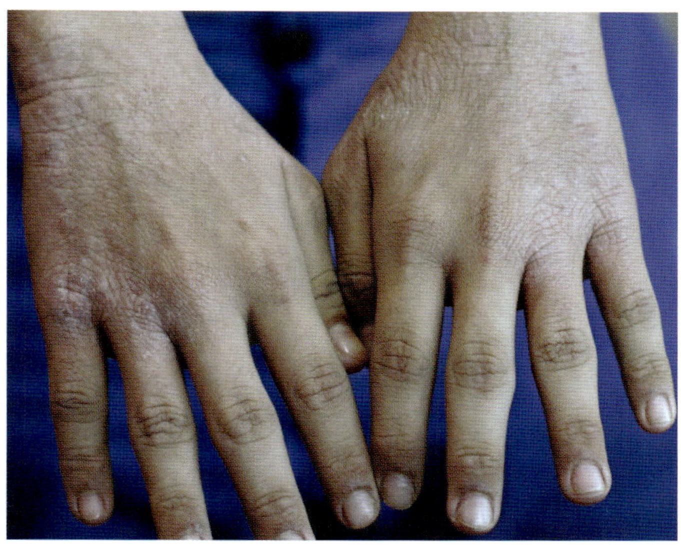

FIGURE 3-49. Chronic hand eczema in a darker-skinned adolescent with underlying AD, presenting as lichenified, dry, hyperpigmented to erythematous plaques.

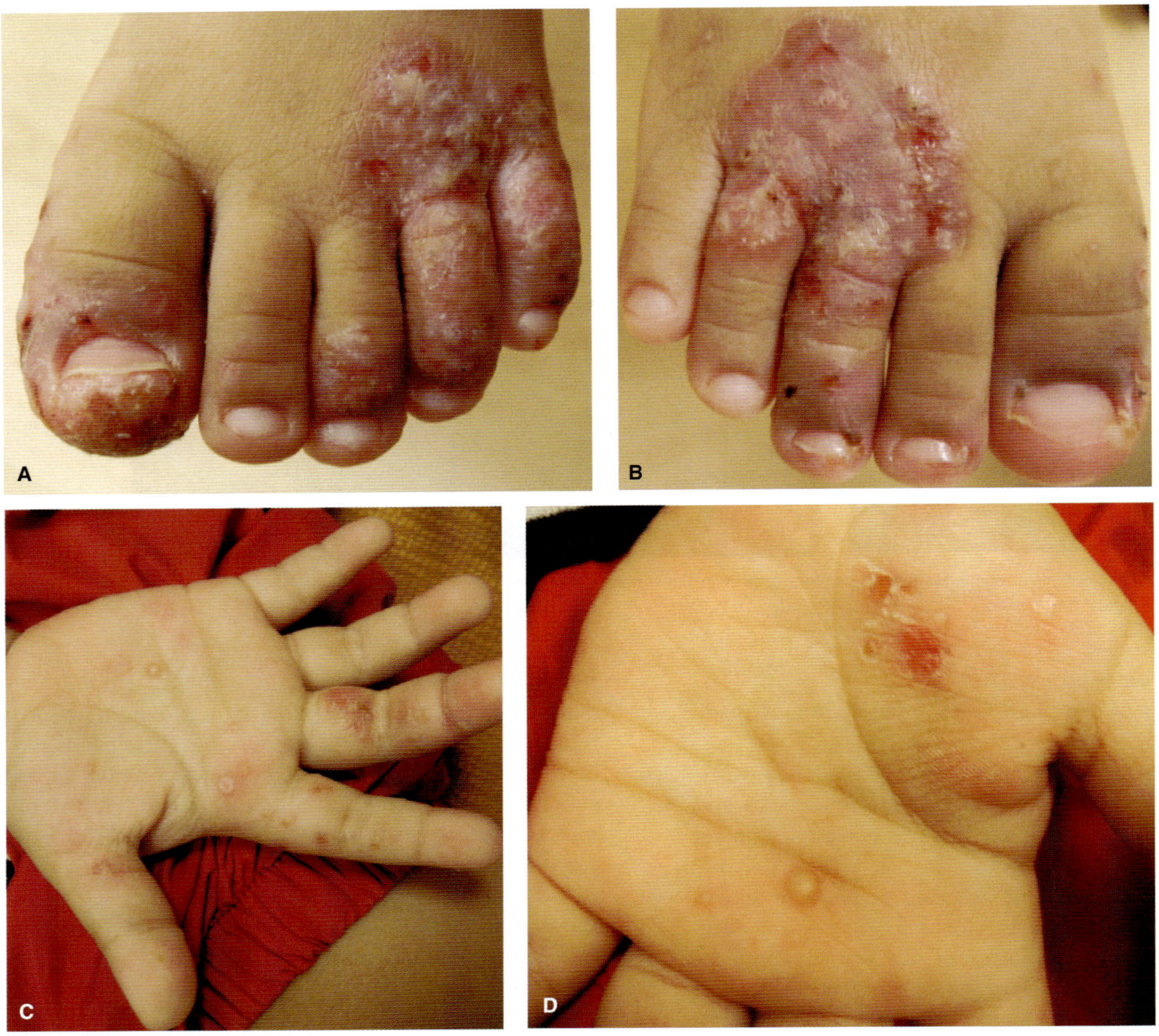

FIGURE 3-50A–50D. Secondarily infected hand and feet eczema in a Chinese child, presenting with oozy, erythematous plaques with formation of blisters and pustules.

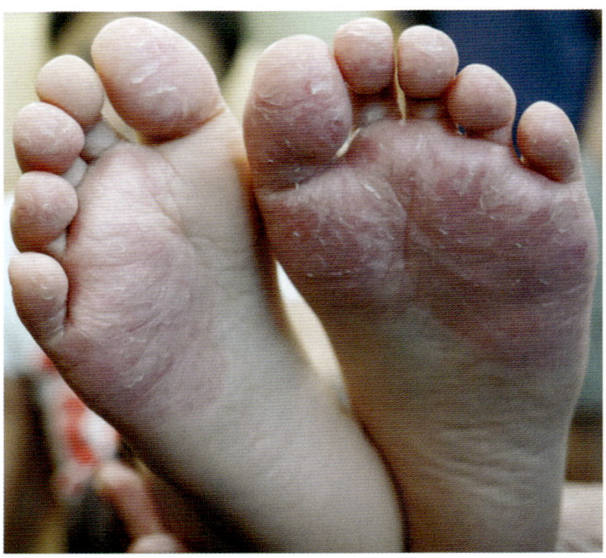

FIGURE 3-51. Classical presentation of juvenile plantar dermatosis on the toes and forefoot of bilateral feet with well-demarcated scaling and erythema.

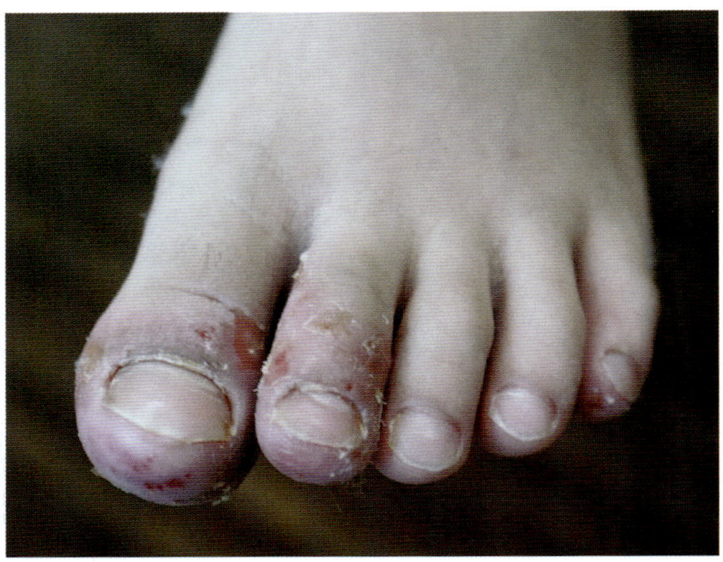

FIGURE 3-52. Juvenile plantar dermatosis affecting the toes of a young Chinese girl.

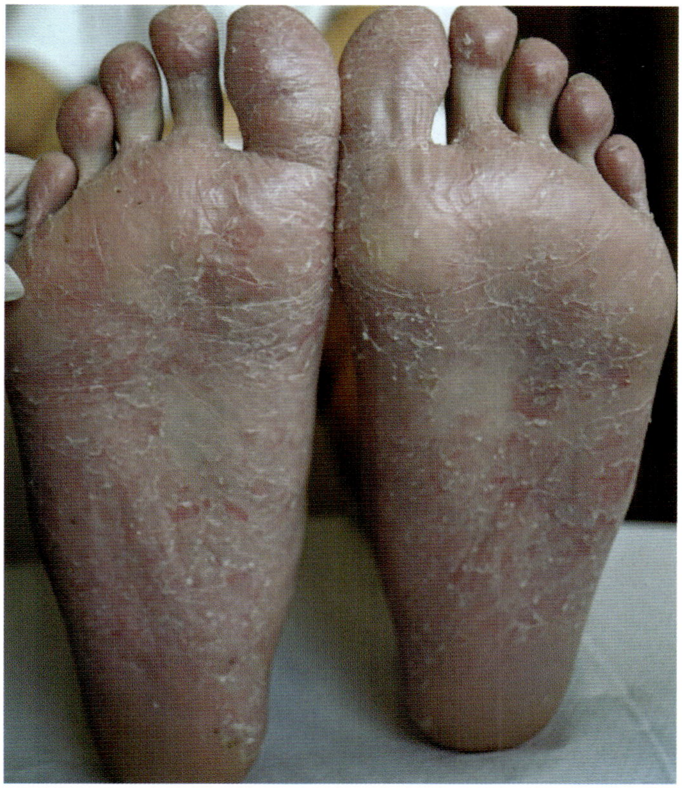

FIGURE 3-53. Severe juvenile plantar dermatoses in a young child presenting with diffuse scaling and erythema of the entire feet bilaterally.

- Juvenile plantar dermatosis is a self-limiting condition and usually resolves by adolescence. Avoidance of synthetic and occlusive footwear, as well as frequent use of moisturizers, are key to treatment. Like atopic hand and feet eczema, mid-to-high potency topical steroids may be used during flares.

Pearls & Practical Tips

- Fungal infection should be excluded in patients presenting with unilateral hand or foot involvement, or if there is involvement of both feet and one hand (two feet-one hand syndrome).
- If lesions also affect the webspaces, consider concomitant irritant contact dermatitis.
- Hyperhidrosis often aggravates any underlying hand and feet eczema. If this is significant, it should be treated.
- Due to the COVID-19 pandemic, children are often required to wash their hands or use hand sanitizers frequently, especially at school. A soap-free cleanser rather than an alcohol-based sanitizer is recommended. Sanitizers formulated with moisturizers are also preferred. Care should also be taken to dry the hands thoroughly after washing, paying special attention to the webspaces, and this should be followed by generous application of moisturizers.

CONTACT DERMATITIS

Contact dermatitis can be broadly divided into two subgroups: allergic contact dermatitis (ACD) and irritant contact dermatitis (ICD). ACD results from a type IV delayed hypersensitivity reaction to an allergen applied topically, whereas ICD is not immunologically mediated.

Clinical Features

- Contact dermatitis usually presents with a pruritic, well-demarcated, eczematous eruption, which may be acute, subacute, or chronic. In the acute stage, the rash appears as weepy, erythematous papules, and plaques, often with vesicles and bullae. In the subacute and chronic stages, hyperkeratotic, dry, fissured and lichenified plaques predominate.
- Rashes secondary to ACD may extend beyond sites in contact with the allergen due to autosensitization, whereas ICD usually occurs at the sites of contact with irritants.
- Toilet-seat dermatitis has been more commonly reported in Asian countries recently, associated with more stringent hygiene practices in the region. Previously reported to be an ACD to wooden toilet seats with varnish, lacquers, and paints more recently, the use of harsh detergents on toilet seats has been implicated to cause ICD. Eczematous plaques involving the buttocks and upper posterior thighs in a distribution corresponding to the configuration of a toilet seat is classical. It is more common in toddlers and young children who have just weaned from diapers and may need to use the toilet more frequently, although it may also be seen in adolescents and adults. Patients often have underlying atopic dermatitis.
- The higher prevalence of ACD in patients with AD may be attributed to the defective epidermal barrier, which in turn leads to higher risk of contact sensitization. In addition, children with AD are inherently exposed to more topical medicaments.
- Table 3-1 illustrates the more common allergens responsible for contact dermatitis in the pediatric population, and their sources.

TABLE 3-1. Common allergens and possible sources.

Class	Allergen	Examples of possible sources
Metals	Nickel	Costume jewelry, cosmetics, musical instruments, electronic devices like cellphones and tablets
	Cobalt	Costume jewelry, cosmetics
Fragrances	Myroxylon pereirae (balsam of Peru) and fragrance mixes I & II	Scented candles, essential oils, cosmetics, perfumes
Preservatives	Methylisothiazolinone and methylchloroisothiazolinone (MI/MCI)	Wet wipes, homemade "slime," shampoos/soaps, sunscreen
Topical medicaments	Neomycin and Bacitracin	Topical antibiotics

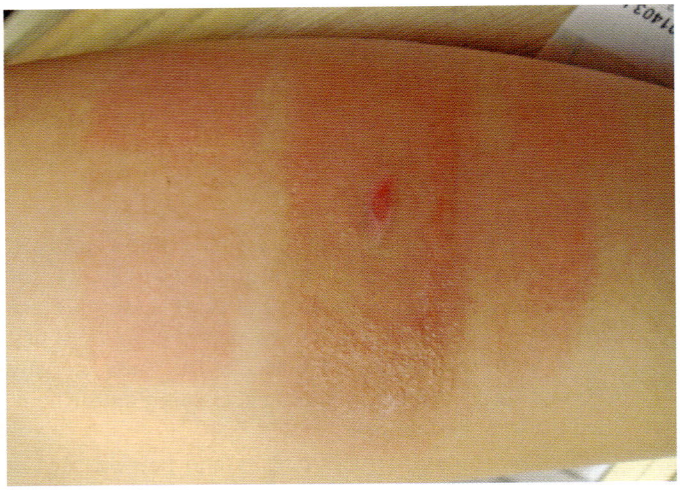

FIGURE 3-54. Acute contact dermatitis to medicated plasters (bandaids) presenting as well-demarcated, erythematous plaques on the arm of a Chinese adolescent.

Differential Diagnoses

- Atopic dermatitis
  - Atopic dermatitis also presents with eczematous rashes but tends to have a predilection for the face in infants, and for the flexures in young children. There is usually a personal or family history of atopy.
- Seborrheic dermatitis
  - Seborrheic dermatitis usually affects the eyebrows and nasolabial folds. There may be a history of atopy.
- Candidiasis
  - Diaper candidiasis is common in young children and may mimic contact dermatitis in the diaper area.
  - While both contact dermatitis and candidiasis in the diaper area may present with erythematous patches affecting the buttocks, satellite lesions/pustules are commonly seen with candidiasis.
  - There is usually sparing of the groin and buttock folds in diaper contact dermatitis but not in candidiasis.

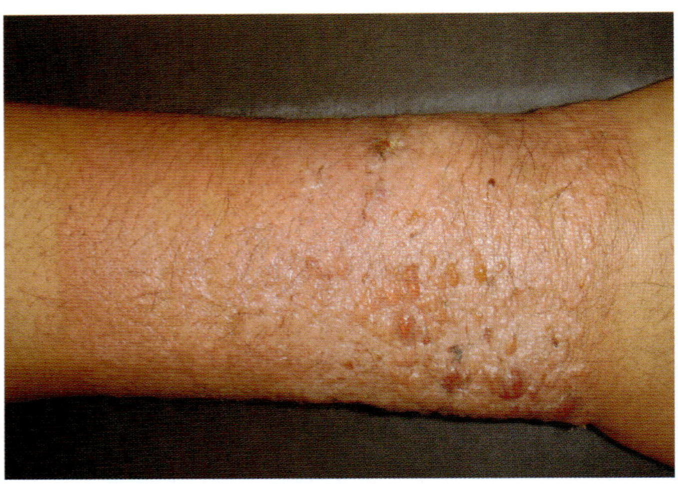

FIGURE 3-55. Acute contact dermatitis to topical traditional Chinese medications (TCM) on the arm of a Chinese adolescent, presenting as a well-demarcated, intensely erythematous plaque with small blisters.

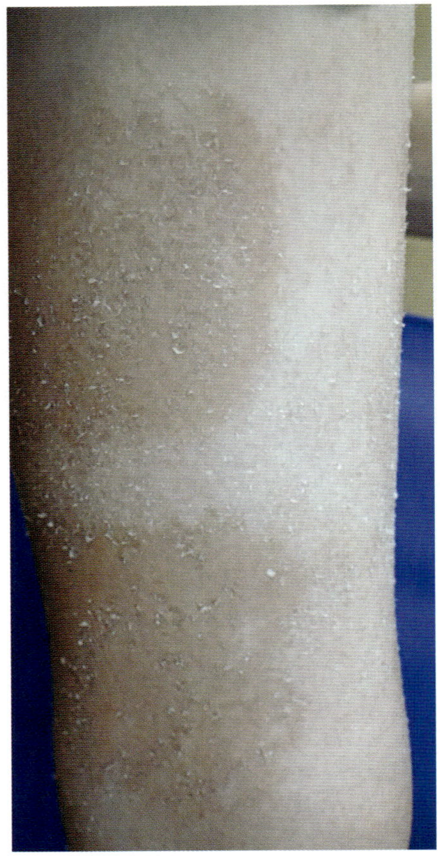

FIGURE 3-56. Well-demarcated scaly, eczematous, hyperpigmented patches on the upper thigh in a child with contact dermatitis.

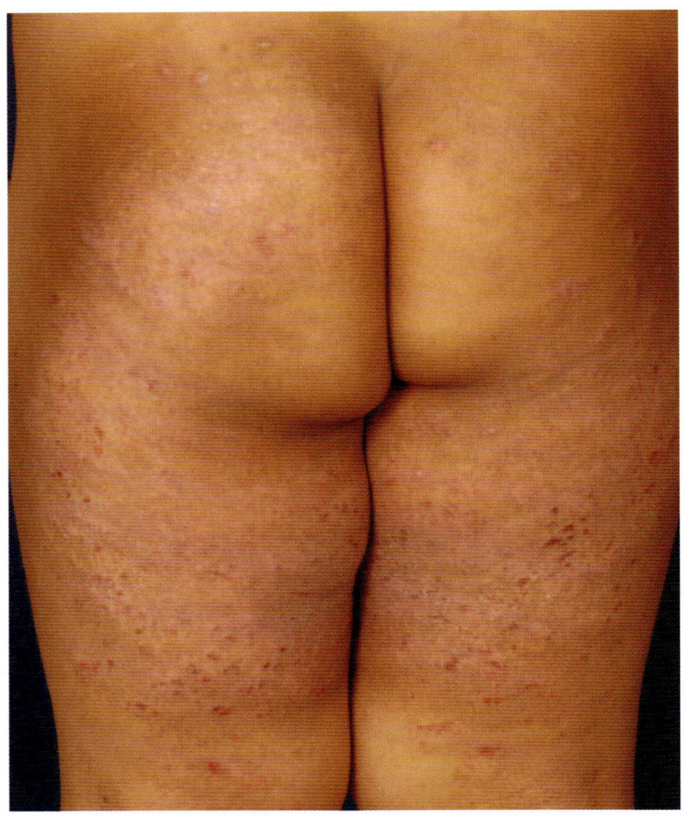

FIGURE 3-57. Toilet-seat dermatitis in a Malay child presenting as erythematous, scaly, excoriated plaques in the shape of a toilet seat on the buttocks and posterior thighs.

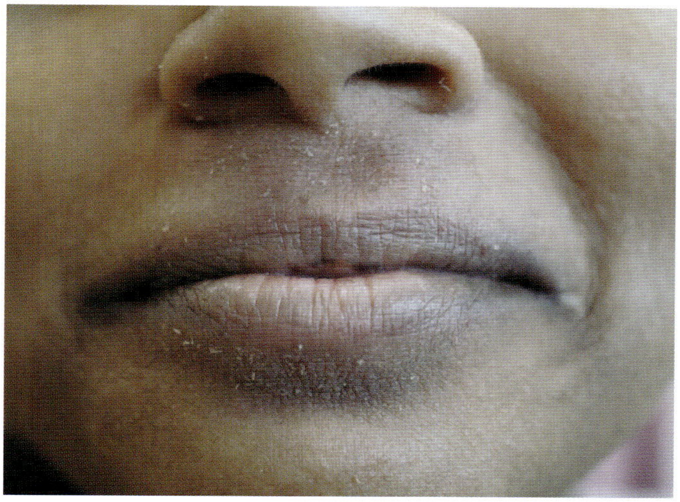

FIGURE 3-58. Irritant contact dermatitis on and surrounding the lips of this Indian adolescent female due to frequent lip licking and lip smacking—"lip-licker's dermatitis."

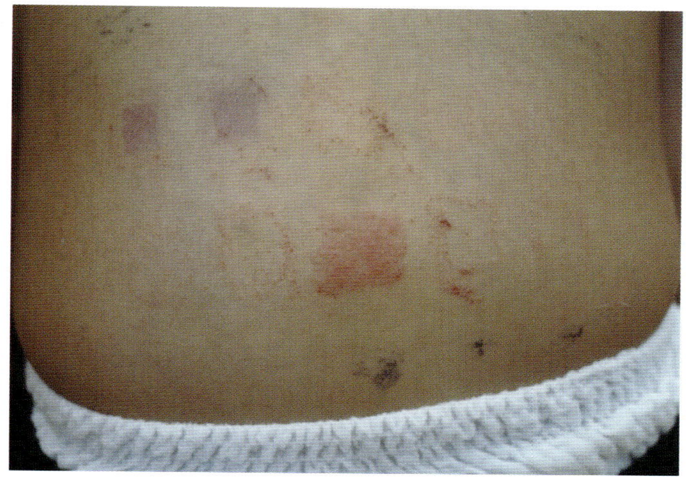

FIGURE 3-59. Positive patch test on the mid lower back of a young child, demonstrated by erythema and induration.

Investigations & Treatment

- A thorough history, including details of the child's exposure to medicaments, toys, and personal care products, should be sought. The child's hobbies and after-school activities should also be queried.
- Patch testing can be carried out to identify the culprit allergen(s) for children with ACD.
- Avoidance of irritants and allergens is important in the management of contact dermatitis.
- Application of topicals such as corticosteroids or calcineurin inhibitors (pimecrolimus, tacrolimus) can expedite resolution of the dermatitis following allergen/irritant withdrawal. Short courses of systemic corticosteroids may benefit those with extensive contact dermatitis, especially during the acute stage.

Pearls & Practical Tips

- Contact dermatitis, both ACD and ICD, are more prevalent in children and adolescents with atopic dermatitis and should be considered in patients with recalcitrant or severe disease despite appropriate treatment, or if the rashes are atypically distributed (e.g., acral sites, buttocks and thighs, eyelids, diaper area).
- For dermatoses that are steroid responsive such as atopic dermatitis or psoriasis, ACD to topical corticosteroids should be considered if patients have persistent or worsening rashes despite compliance to treatment.
- It is important to consider "consort dermatitis" in children, who may be exposed to allergens (e.g., hair dye or perfumes) through contact with their caregivers.
- It is useful for the child to bring his or her favorite toys and frequently used topical products for the dermatologist to consider patch testing to.
- Use of distraction techniques such as videos and toys reduces stress and hence improves placement of allergens during patch testing.

Papulosquamous Disorders

PITYRIASIS ROSEA

Pityriasis rosea is an acute, benign, self-limiting papulosquamous disorder that can affect all age groups, especially children, adolescents, and young adults. The exact etiology is unknown but has been postulated to be a viral-induced condition due to the presence of prodromal symptoms, seasonal variation, and clustering in communities. Reactivation of latent human herpesvirus-6 and 7 infections has been reported.

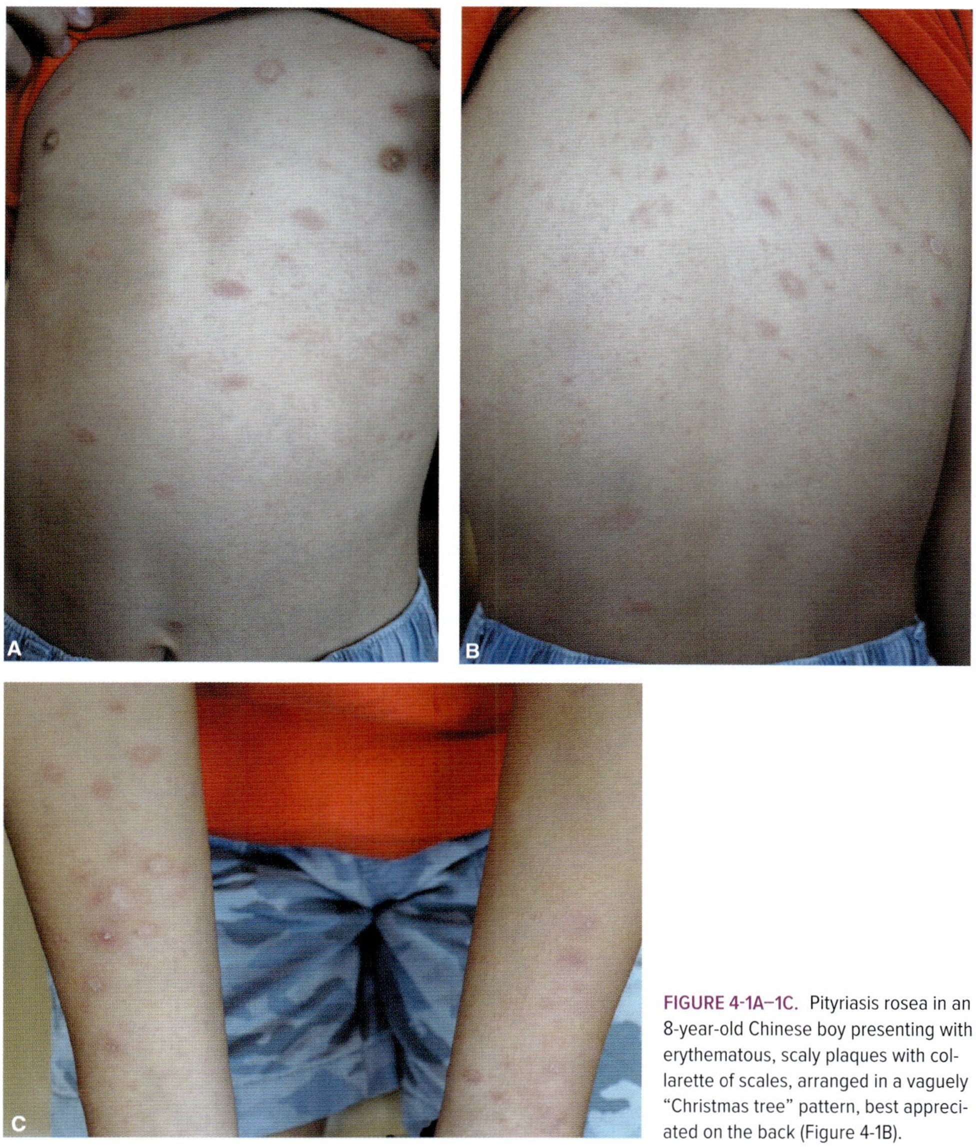

FIGURE 4-1A–1C. Pityriasis rosea in an 8-year-old Chinese boy presenting with erythematous, scaly plaques with collarette of scales, arranged in a vaguely "Christmas tree" pattern, best appreciated on the back (Figure 4-1B).

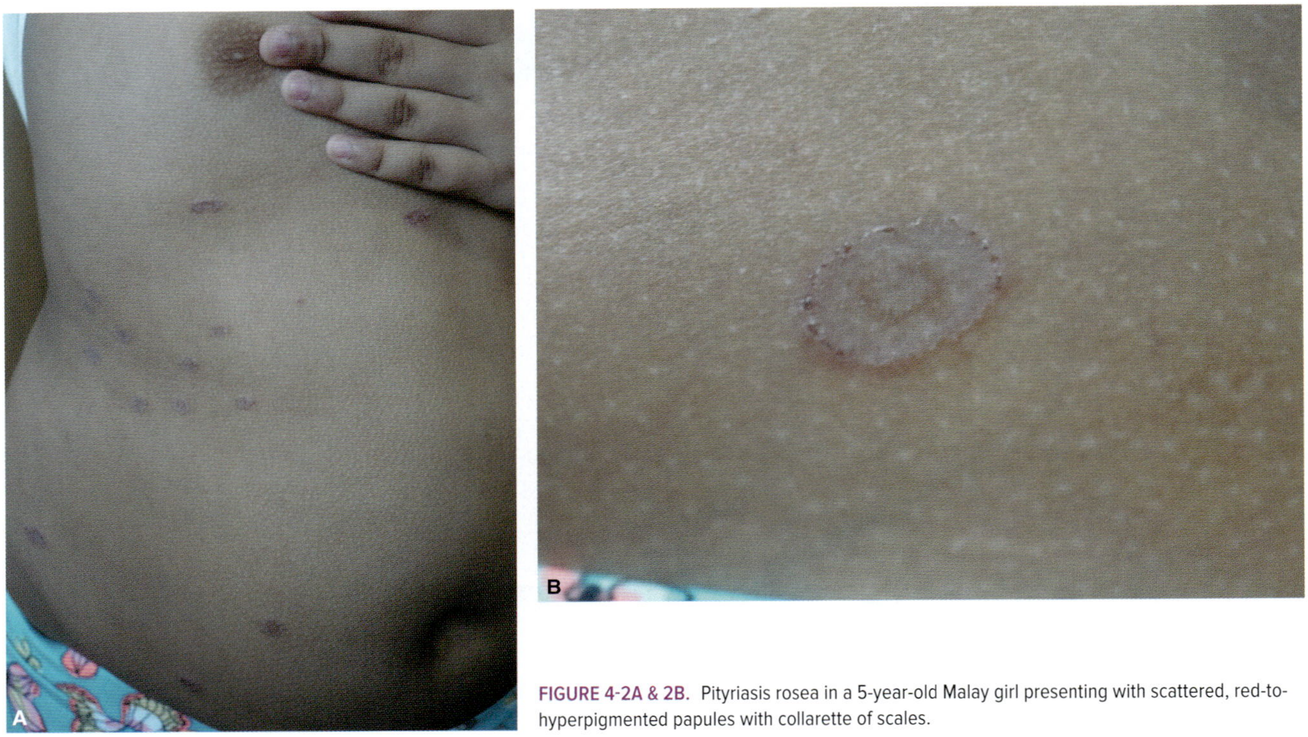

FIGURE 4-2A & 2B. Pityriasis rosea in a 5-year-old Malay girl presenting with scattered, red-to-hyperpigmented papules with collarette of scales.

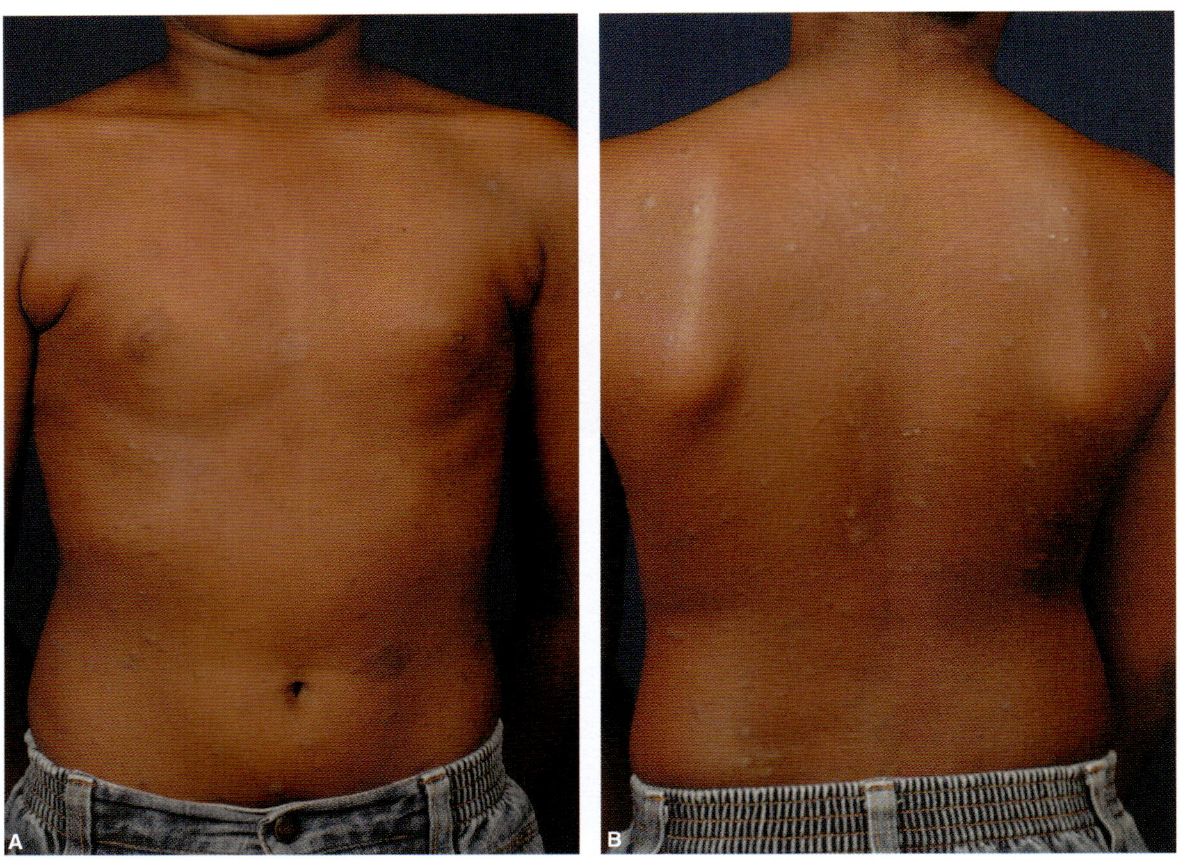

FIGURE 4-3A & 3B. Pityriasis rosea in a 10-year-old Indian boy, presenting with scaly, hypopigmented and hyperpigmented macules over his trunk in a "Christmas-tree" pattern.

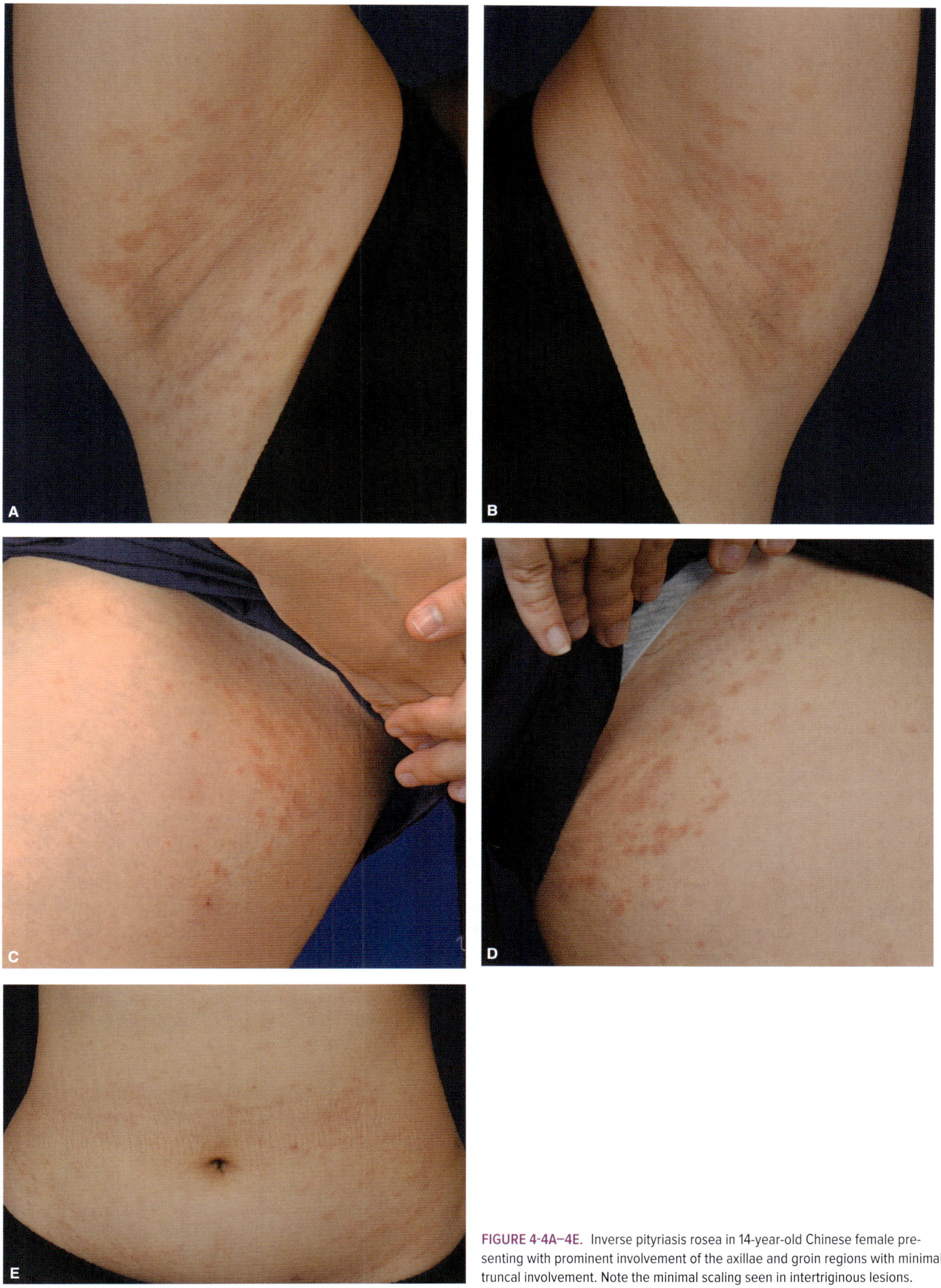

FIGURE 4-4A–4E. Inverse pityriasis rosea in 14-year-old Chinese female presenting with prominent involvement of the axillae and groin regions with minimal truncal involvement. Note the minimal scaling seen in intertriginous lesions.

Clinical Features

- Pityriasis rosea is characterized by an acute onset of a generalized eruption consisting of round to ovoid papules, patches, and plaques, with a collarette of scales (pityriasiform scaling), appearing in crops over a few days. Pruritus is variable, occurring in about 25% of cases.
- The acute eruption is often preceded by a solitary, well-defined scaly plaque termed the *herald patch*. There may sometimes be a prodrome of fever, sore throat, gastrointestinal symptoms, and arthralgia.
- The lesions often run parallel to the lines of skin cleavage, leading to a "Christmas tree" pattern, especially on the posterior trunk. There is less involvement of the face, scalp, and distal extremities. The palms and soles are classically spared.
- Spontaneous resolution typically occurs within 6 weeks, but may be as long as 5 months, often leaving behind post-inflammatory hypo- or hyperpigmentation that may persist for months, especially in dark-skinned individuals.
- Atypical presentations, representing about 20% of cases, that have been described include vesicular, follicular, erythema multiforme-like, urticarial, or purpuric, and occur on acral areas or intertriginous areas (inversus), and may be relapsing in nature.

Differential Diagnosis

- Tinea corporis
  - The annular scaly rash of the herald patch and the annular configuration of the generalized eruption can resemble tinea corporis. The lesions of tinea corporis tend to be larger plaques.
  - In doubtful cases, skin scrapings from the scaly areas can be sent for fungal microscopy and culture.
- Pityriasis lichenoides
  - Pityriasis lichenoides can also present with multiple reddish-brown papules, sometimes with annular scaling. Some lesions have a hemorrhagic central crust, which is not seen in pityriasis rosea. The course of pityriasis lichenoides is also more chronic than pityriasis rosea.
  - In doubtful cases, skin biopsies will differentiate between the two conditions.
- Nummular/discoid eczema
  - The lesions of discoid eczema are often more oozy, with yellowish scales, as compared to pityriasis rosea. The limbs are also more often affected. There are often other features of atopic dermatitis or other atopic diathesis. The time course is more chronic, with a waxing and waning course.
- Guttate psoriasis
  - The lesions of guttate psoriasis are more pink, and the scaling is more diffuse over the entire lesion, as compared to the peripheral scaling of pityriasis rosea. The Auspitz sign is also positive.
- Secondary syphilis
  - The lesions and time course of secondary syphilis can resemble pityriasis rosea, but the palms and soles are often involved. There may be a positive sexual contact history or history of preceding chancre.
  - In doubtful cases, non-treponemal and treponemal tests should be performed.

Investigations & Treatment

- Diagnosis is usually made clinically.
- If performed, skin biopsy will show a spongiotic pattern. However, this is not fully diagnostic and clinical correlation is required.
- Treatment is usually unnecessary due to the benign and self-limited nature of the condition.
- If lesions are pruritic, moisturizers, topical corticosteroids, and topical antipruritics such as menthol-containing formulations and oral antihistamines may be helpful.
- Exposure to sunlight or ultraviolet light may hasten resolution of lesions.
- A 2-week course of oral erythromycin has also been reported to hasten resolution.

Pearls & Practical Tips

- In dark-skinned patients, the papules can sometimes appear gray, dark brown, violaceous, or black.
- The herald patch is often misdiagnosed as discoid eczema or tinea.
- Secondary syphilis has to be excluded serologically if there is involvement of the palms and soles. It may be difficult to obtain an accurate sexual history from adolescents.

Bibliography

1. Litchman G, Nair PA, Le JK. Pityriasis Rosea. In: StatPearls. Treasure Island (FL): StatPearls Publishing; 2020 Jan.

PSORIASIS

Psoriasis is a common chronic immune-mediated inflammatory disease that primarily affects the skin and joints. Psoriasis is now considered a systemic inflammatory condition, that has associations with obesity, metabolic syndrome, and psychological conditions. It is caused by a complex and dynamic interaction between the immune system, psoriasis-associated susceptibility loci, autoantigens, and environmental factors. Approximately a third of psoriasis begins in childhood, and 2% below 2 years of age. There is a slight female preponderance. Known triggers include streptococcal pharyngitis, diaper candidiasis, and viral illnesses. Psoriasis in children is associated with increased pruritus compared to adults, and lesions are relatively thinner and less scaly.

Clinical Features

- Based on morphology, pattern, and distribution, childhood psoriasis is classified into several subtypes, including plaque psoriasis, guttate psoriasis, pustular psoriasis, diaper-area psoriasis, and other variants.
- The lesions of psoriasis are characterized by well-demarcated, mildly pruritic erythematous or salmon-pink plaques, covered with silvery-white scales. Removal of scales results in fine punctate bleeding points (Auspitz sign).

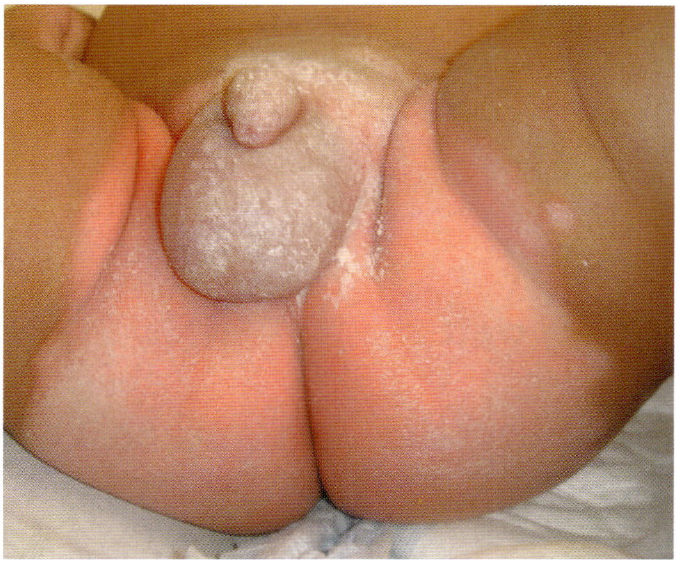

FIGURE 4-5. Infantile psoriasis in a Malay infant presenting with well-demarcated, pink, scaly plaques over the face, neck, and groin region.

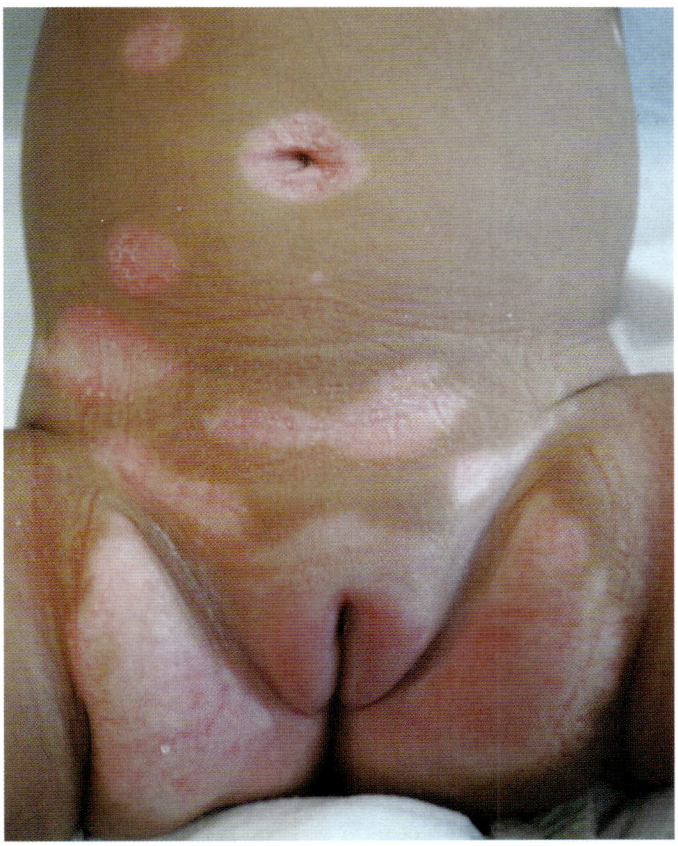

FIGURE 4-6. Infantile psoriasis in a Malay female infant with pink plaques over the intertriginous and umbilical areas.

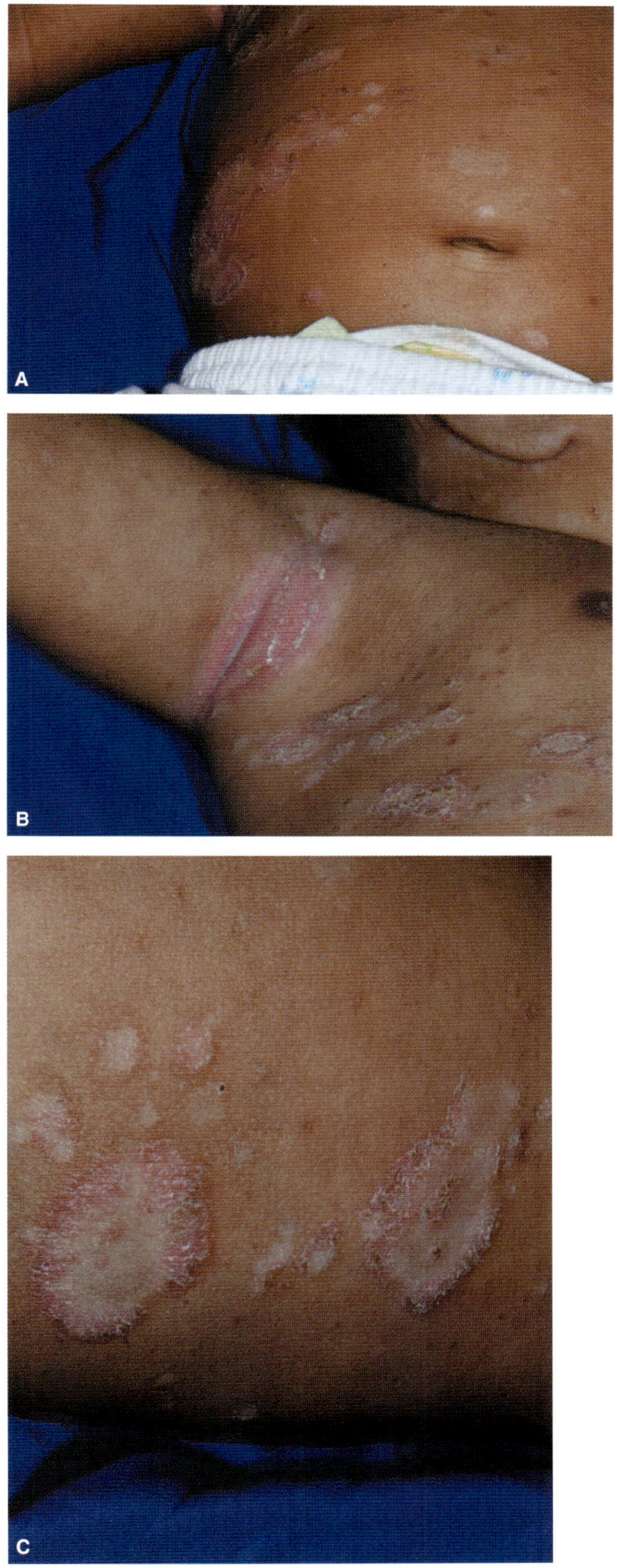

FIGURE 4-7A–7C. Extensive infantile psoriasis in a 6-month-old Indian child, presenting with widespread well-demarcated, scaly, erythematous plaques, some with annular configuration. The lesions in the axillae often lack the scaling seen at other sites.

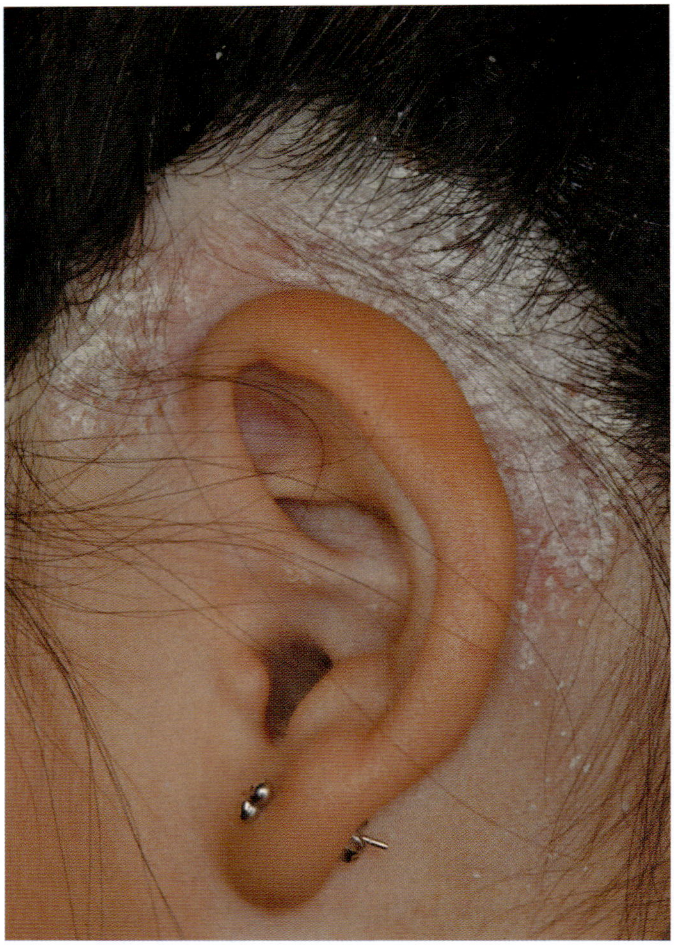

FIGURE 4-8. Scalp psoriasis in a 9-year-old Chinese girl, presenting with well-demarcated pink plaques on the hairline with thick, white scales.

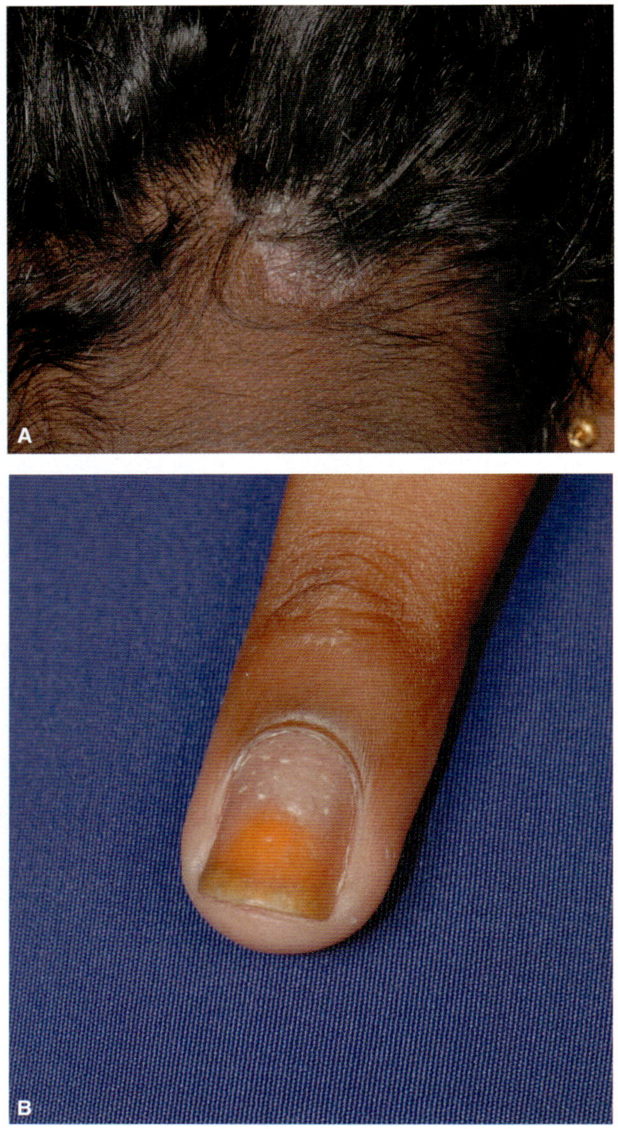

FIGURE 4-9A & 9B. Limited plaque psoriasis affecting the hairline of this 10-year-old Indian girl. She also has pitting and transverse ridging of her nails. The orange discoloration of the nail is due to application of henna.

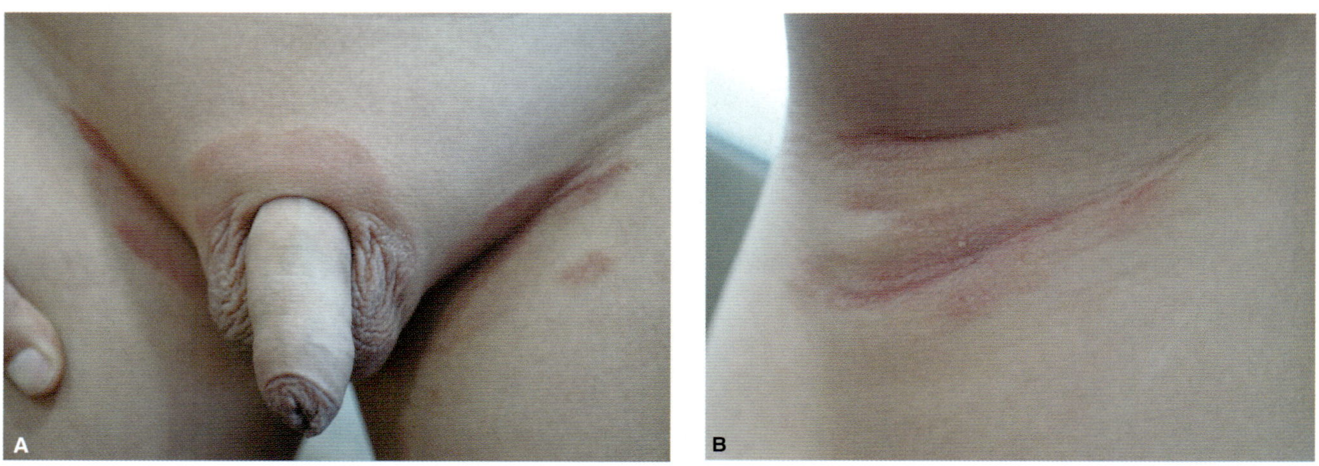

FIGURE 4-10A & 10B. "Inverse psoriasis" in an 8-year-old Chinese boy with well-demarcated pink plaques on the groin and axillae. Note the lack of scale in these lesions due to the constant maceration in these areas.

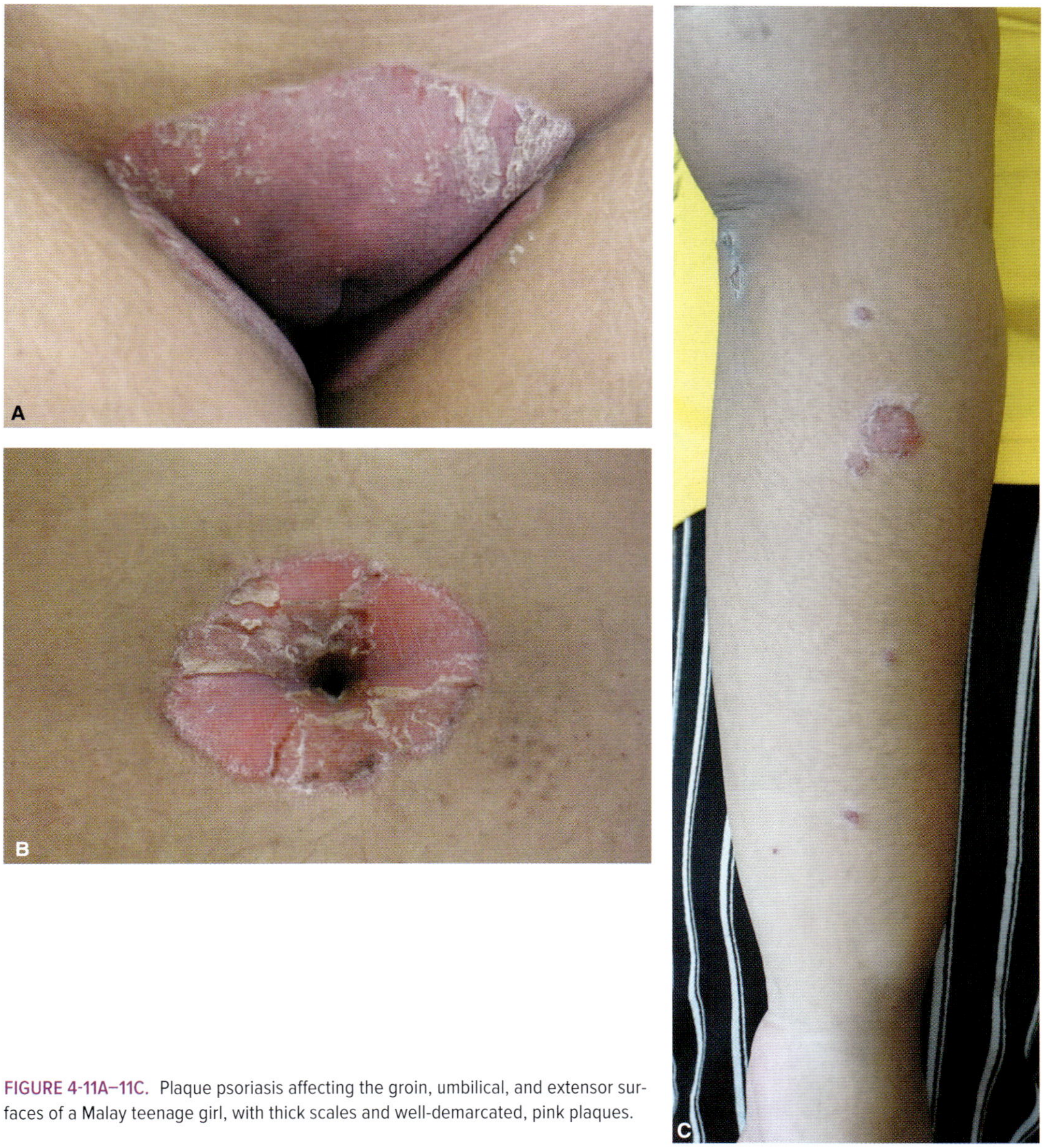

FIGURE 4-11A–11C. Plaque psoriasis affecting the groin, umbilical, and extensor surfaces of a Malay teenage girl, with thick scales and well-demarcated, pink plaques.

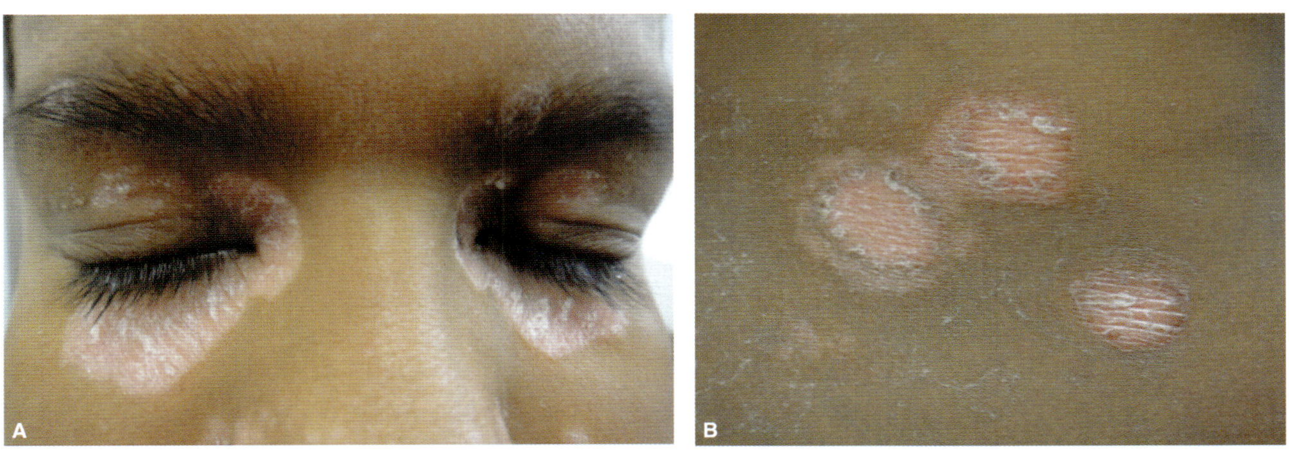

FIGURE 4-12A & 12B. Plaque psoriasis on the face and trunk of an adolescent Indian male.

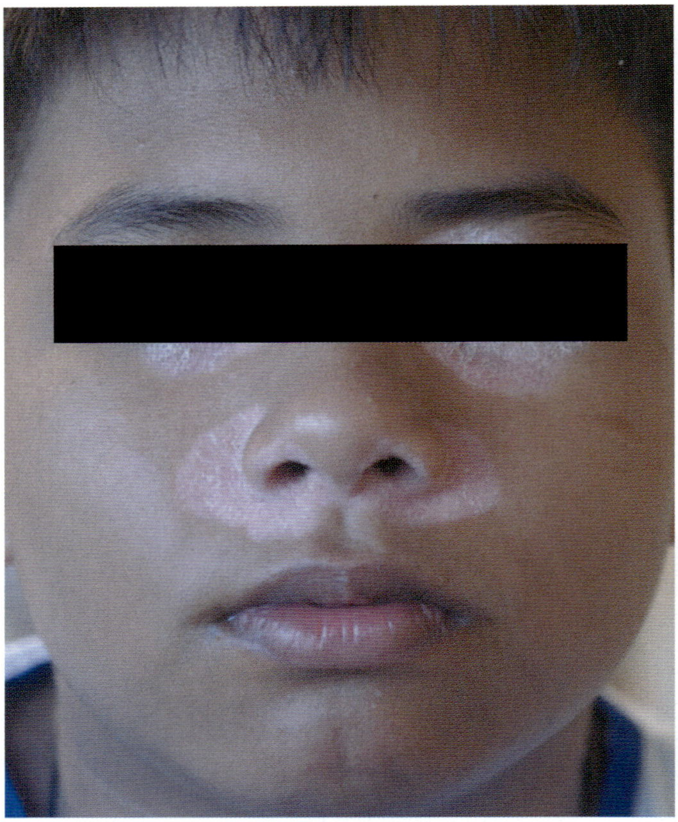

FIGURE 4-13. Plaque psoriasis on the face of a 14-year-old Eurasian boy with predominantly facial involvement.

- Nail involvement is common, and pitting is the most frequent feature. Other characteristics include onycholysis, oil-spots, brownish discoloration, subungual hyperkeratosis, and onychodystrophy. These changes can precede, coincide with, or develop after skin psoriasis.
- Plaque psoriasis
  - This is the most common variant, with childhood-onset disease arising at a mean age of 7 to 10 years.
  - Lesions are distributed symmetrically with a predilection for the scalp, eyelids, hairline, extensor surfaces of the elbows and knees, and lumbosacral and anogenital regions. The course is chronic and recurrent.
- Guttate psoriasis
  - This commonly presents acutely, 1 to 3 weeks after a streptococcal infection or viral upper respiratory tract infection.
  - It is characterized by raindrop-like (guttate) papules and small plaques distributed symmetrically over the trunk and proximal extremities, occasionally involving the face, scalp, and distal extremities.
  - Some spontaneously resolve after a few months, leaving post-inflammatory hypopigmentation, while some progress to plaque psoriasis.

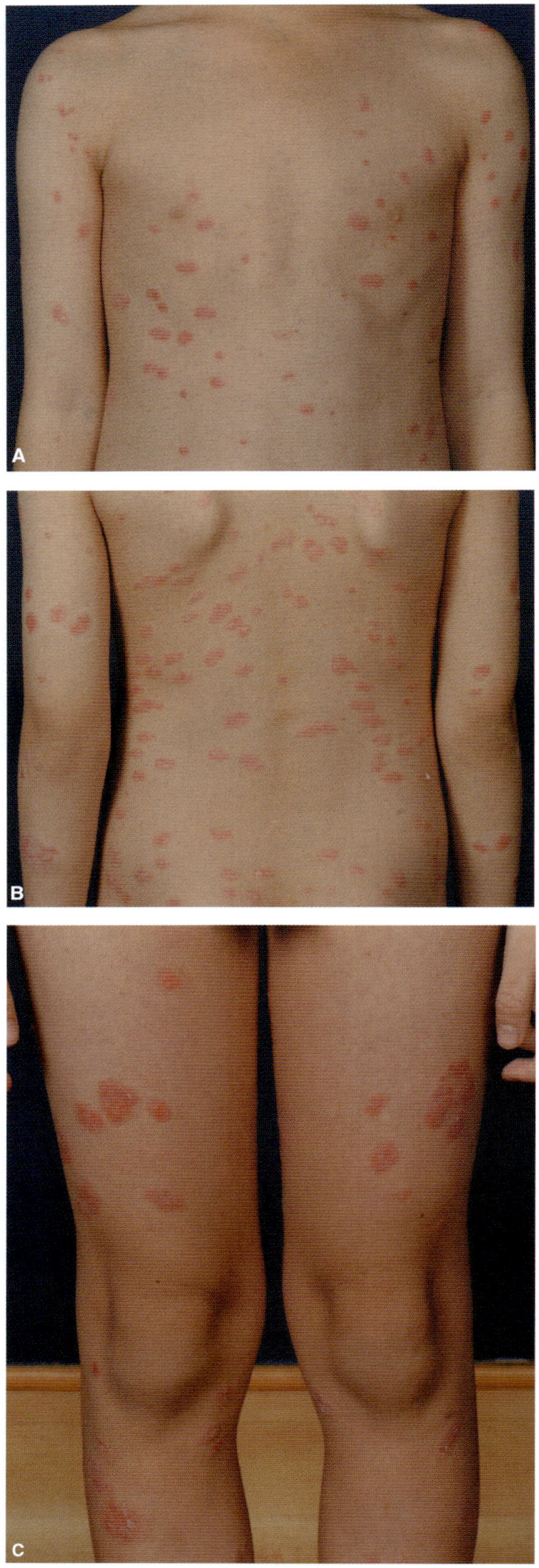

FIGURE 4-14A–14C. Guttate psoriasis affecting the trunk and limbs of a 7-year-old Chinese boy.

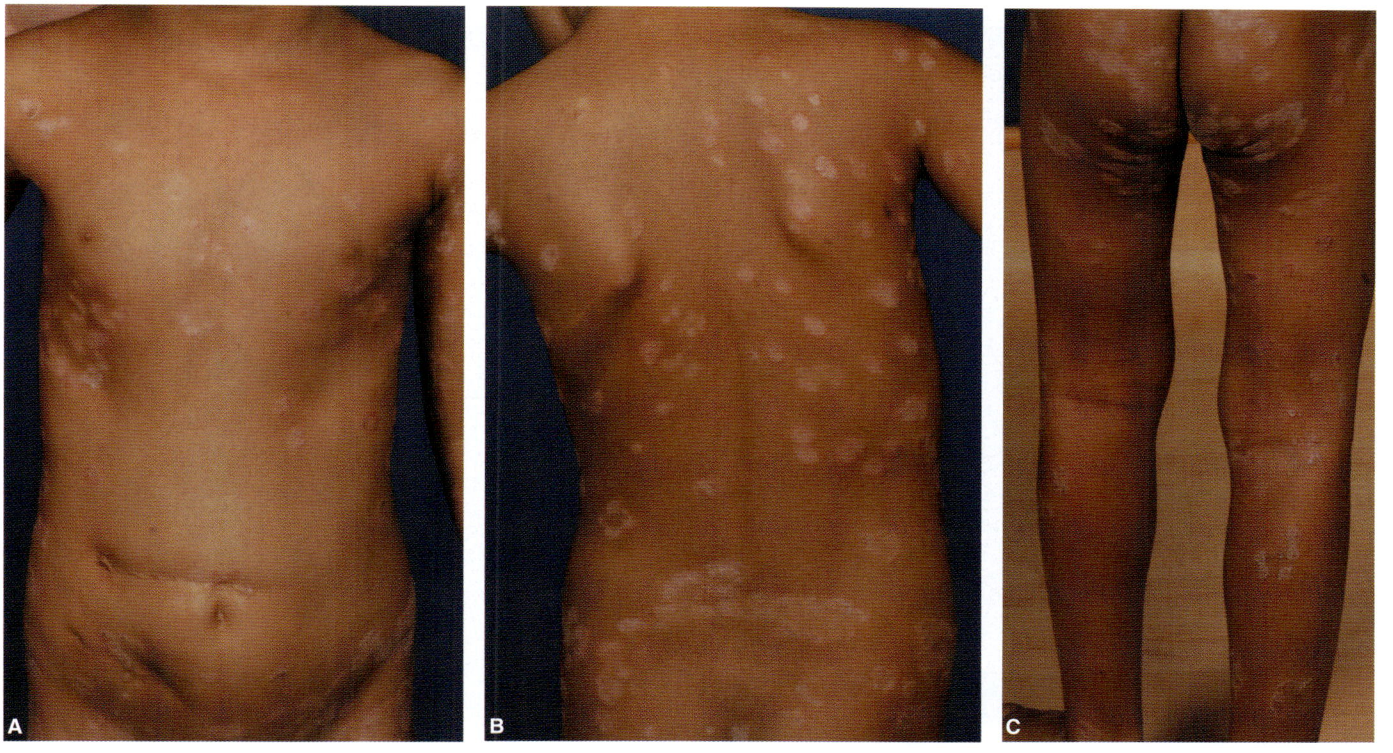

FIGURE 4-15A–15C. A 5-year-old Malay girl with both guttate and plaque psoriasis, with residual post-inflammatory hypopigmentation.

- Pustular psoriasis
  - This can occur in three forms: generalized pustular psoriasis (von Zumbusch) (GPP), palmoplantar pustulosis, where the hands and feet are involved, and acropustulosis (Hallopeau), where the nails and distal digits are involved.
  - Up to half of children with pustular psoriasis manifest during infancy. There may be a prior history of plaque psoriasis.
  - Lesions begin as superficial, non-follicular, pinpoint to slightly larger pustules that coalesce into lakes of pus. The pustules rapidly rupture, leaving a scaly rim with well-demarcated erythematous borders.
  - The lesions are often painful and can have associated systemic symptoms, such as fever and malaise, with elevated inflammatory markers, leukocytosis, and neutrophilia.
  - The clinical course is highly variable, with intermittent flares and partial or complete remission in between flares.
- Diaper-area psoriasis
  - Also known as "napkin psoriasis," this occurs in infancy or early childhood, and is characterized by well-demarcated, pink-to-erythematous plaques affecting the diaper area and inguinal folds. The lesions are not scaly due to the occlusion and subsequent maceration beneath the diapers.

Differential Diagnoses

- Atopic dermatitis/eczema
  - The lesions of eczema can sometimes resemble psoriasis, giving rise to the term "psoriasiform dermatitis." However, lesions of eczema are usually less well-demarcated, with more irregular, yellow, and crusted scaling.
  - Eczema tends to affect the flexures compared to the extensor involvement of psoriasis, and scalp involvement in eczema is more diffuse, while psoriasis tends to "hug" the hairline.
  - The lesions of discoid eczema can resemble guttate psoriasis but are usually more erythematous or hyperpigmented.
  - Itch is worse in eczema compared to psoriasis.
- Tinea
  - The characteristic annular rim with erythema and scaling, with central hyperpigmentation differentiates tinea from psoriasis, where the scaling is more diffusely distributed over the lesion.
- Pityriasis rubra pilaris (PRP)
  - Some consider PRP on a spectrum with psoriasis. Lesions of PRP have a more orange-red hue, compared to the pink and red plaques of psoriasis. Nail changes are less often seen in PRP.

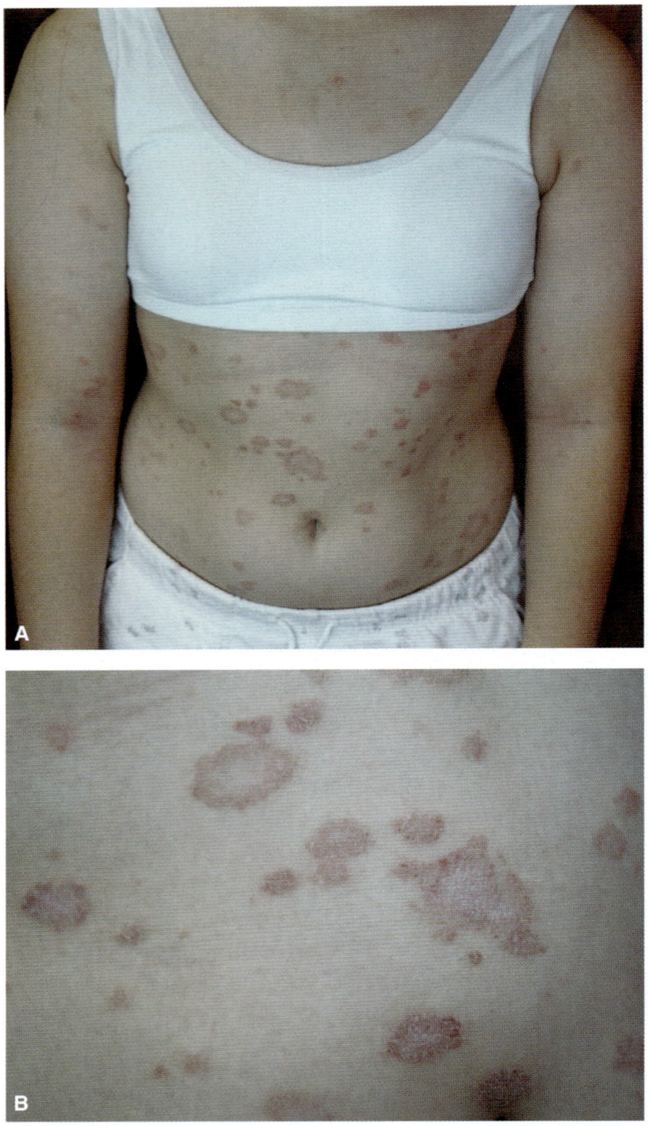

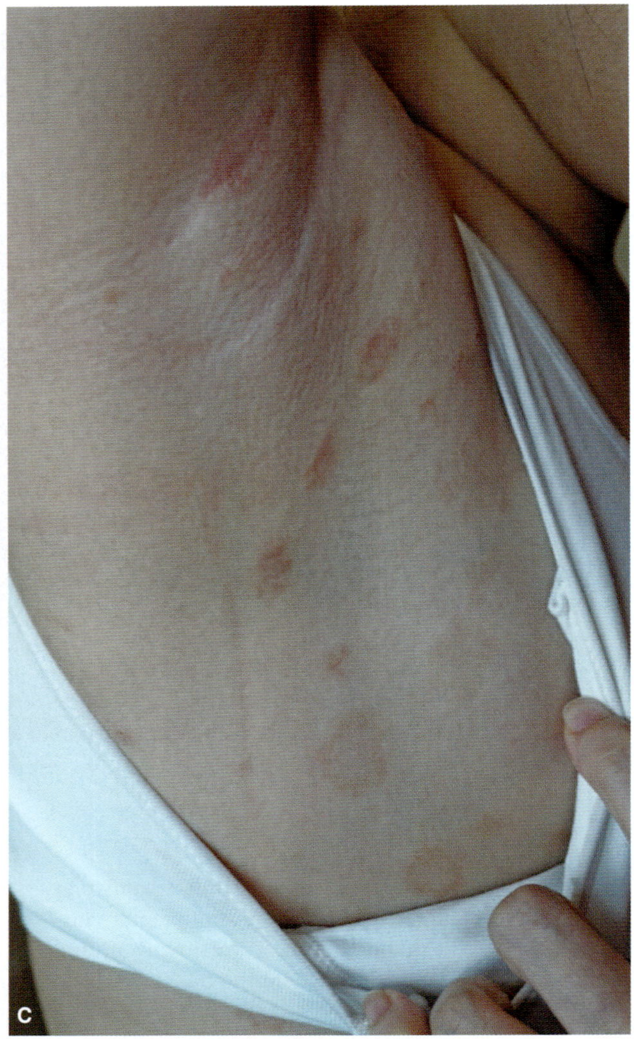

FIGURE 4-16A–16C. Guttate psoriasis in a 9-year-old Chinese girl with round, scaly plaques, with some having a more annular configuration. This presentation may be mistaken for pityriasis rosea.

- Pityriasis rosea
  - A differential for guttate psoriasis, the "pityriasiform" peripheral collarette scaling differentiates it from the diffuse scaling of psoriasis. A herald patch may be present before onset of the generalized rash distribution.
- Pityriasis lichenoides chronica (PLC)
  - A differential for guttate psoriasis, the lesions in PLC are characterized by "pityriasiform" peripheral collarette scaling. Concomitant lesions of pityriasis lichenoides et varioliformis acuta may also be present with the central hemorrhagic crust.
- Secondary syphilis
  - This is a differential of psoriasis especially in adolescents, especially if there is palm and sole involvement.
- Acute generalized exanthematous pustulosis (AGEP)
  - A differential of GPP, the onset is more abrupt and generally resolves in 2 weeks. There is often a history of an acute infection or drug ingestion.

Investigations & Treatment

- Diagnosis is usually made clinically. Skin biopsies may be required in atypical cases.
- Typical histological features of psoriasis are confluent parakeratosis, neutrophils in the stratum corneum and epidermis (microabscesses of Munro and Kogoj), hypogranulosis, regular acanthosis of the epidermis, and suprapapillary thinning of the epidermis.
- Treatment of psoriasis involves a stepladder approach depending on the age, severity of disease, subjective symptoms, and the effect on quality of life.
- Topical treatments include moisturizers, corticosteroids, coal tar preparations, salicylic acid, calcineurin inhibitors, and vitamin D analogues.
- Phototherapy may be used for more extensive disease, with narrowband ultraviolet B (nbUVB), as the preferred modality.

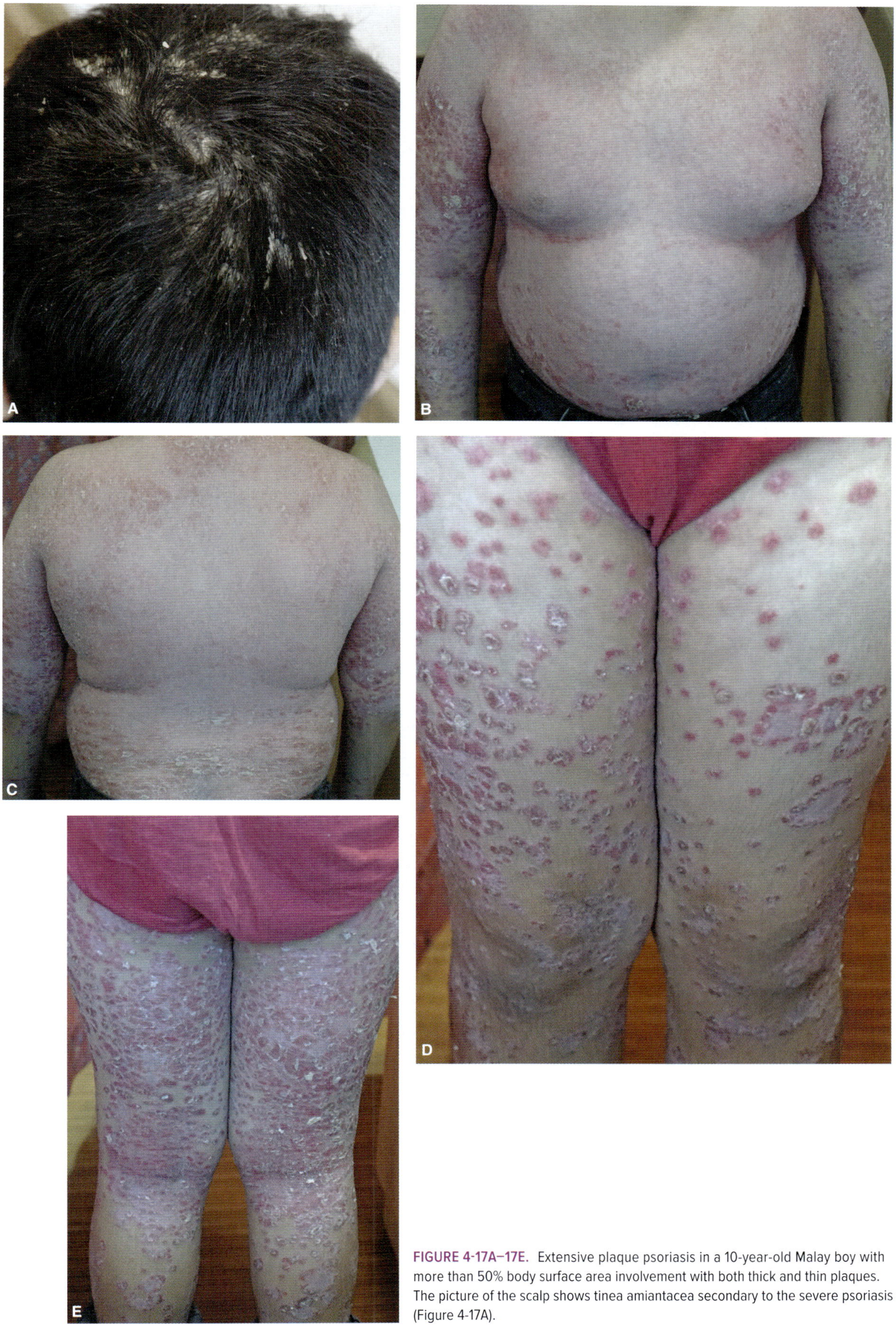

FIGURE 4-17A–17E. Extensive plaque psoriasis in a 10-year-old Malay boy with more than 50% body surface area involvement with both thick and thin plaques. The picture of the scalp shows tinea amiantacea secondary to the severe psoriasis (Figure 4-17A).

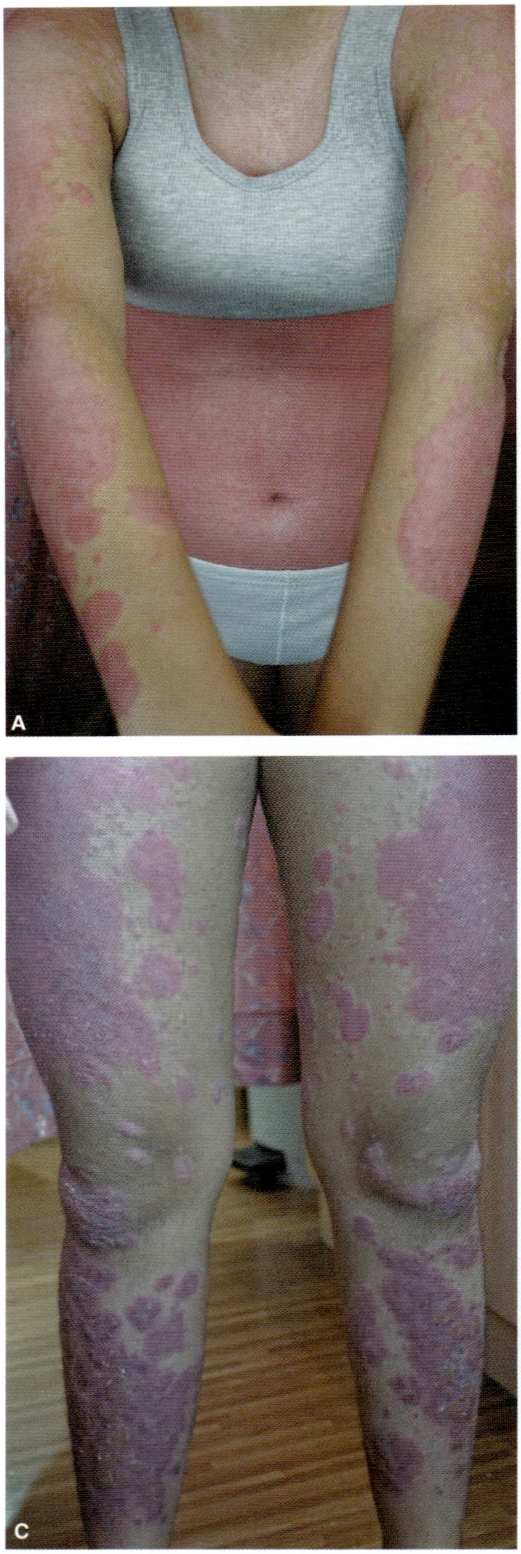

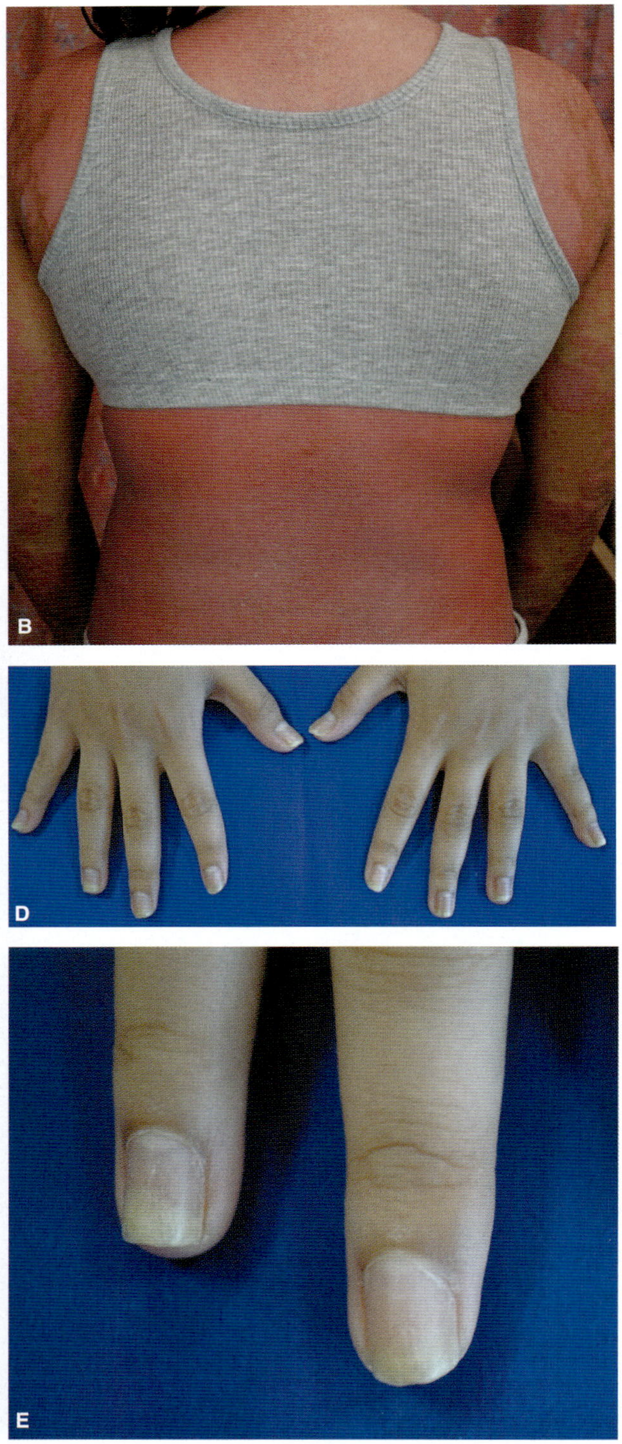

FIGURE 4-18A–18E. Extensive plaque psoriasis mainly affecting the trunk and limbs of this 15-year-old Malay girl, with concomitant and psoriatic nail changes (Figures 4-18D & 18E).

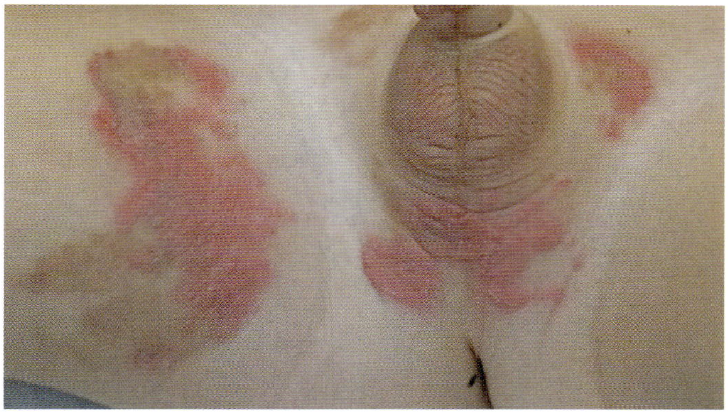

FIGURE 4-19. Annular pustular psoriasis on the thigh and groin area of a 3-year-old Chinese boy. Small pustules may be seen at the periphery of the plaques. There is significant post-inflammatory hyperpigmentation.

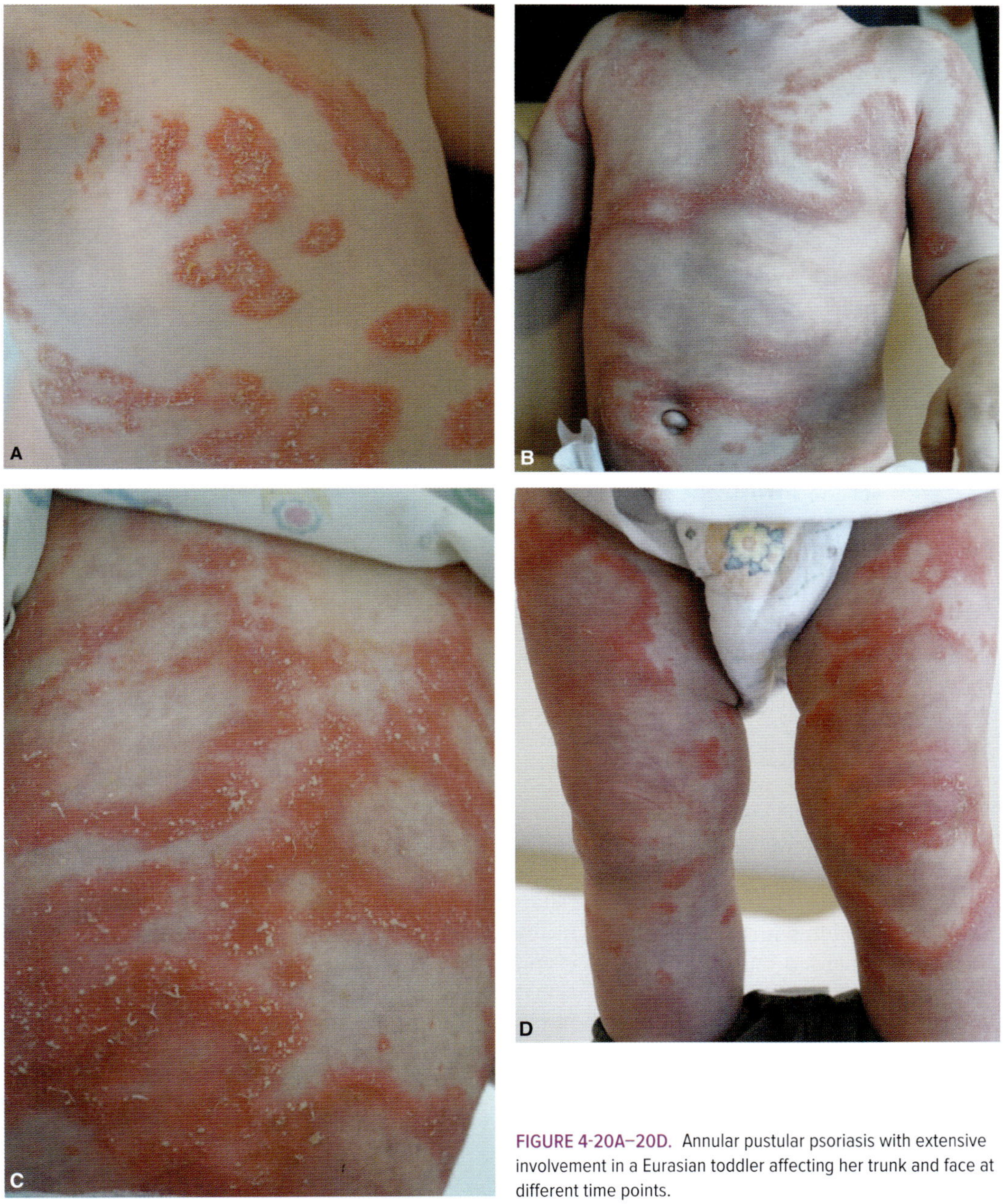

FIGURE 4-20A–20D. Annular pustular psoriasis with extensive involvement in a Eurasian toddler affecting her trunk and face at different time points.

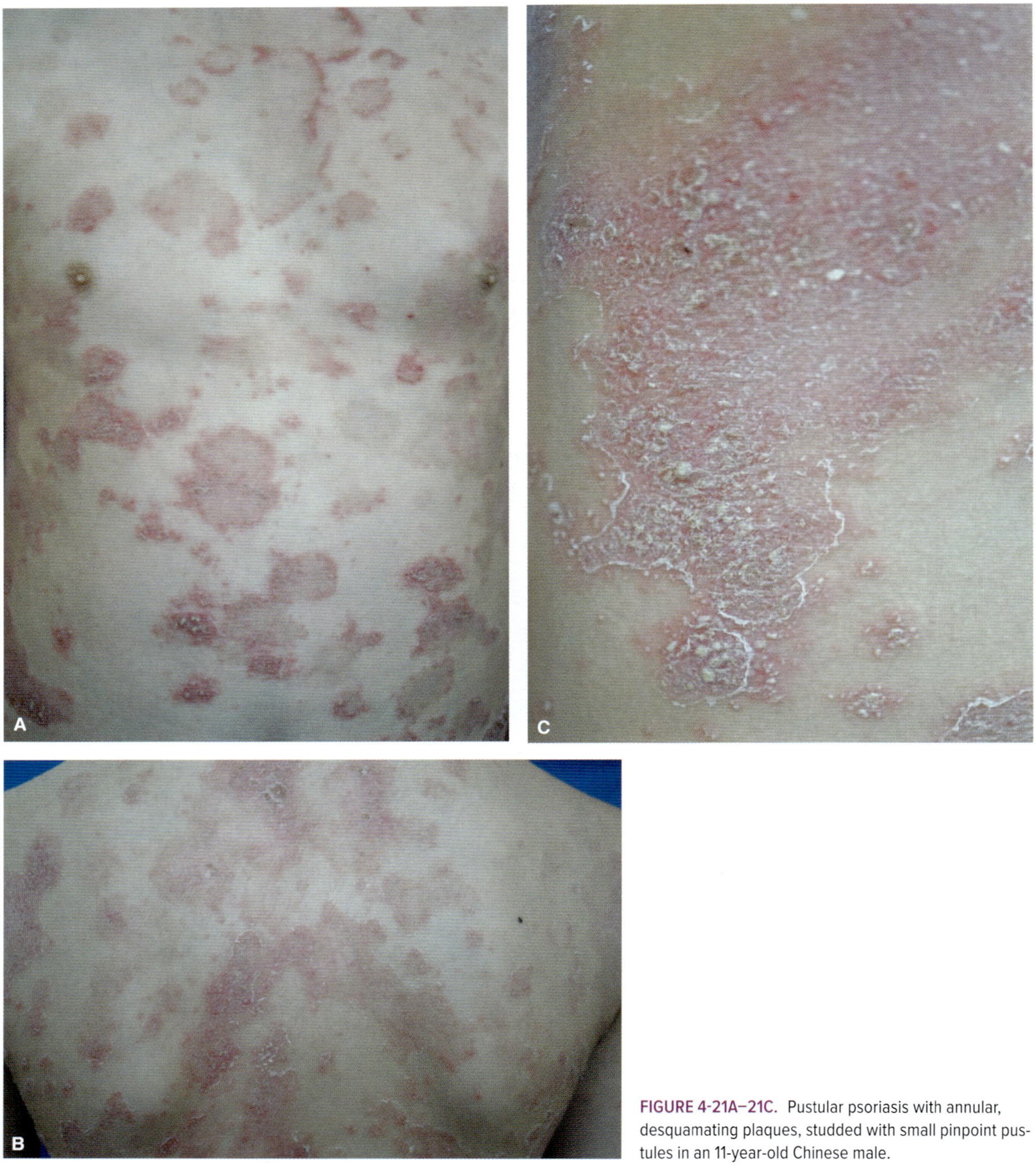

FIGURE 4-21A–21C. Pustular psoriasis with annular, desquamating plaques, studded with small pinpoint pustules in an 11-year-old Chinese male.

- Systemic treatments include acitretin, methotrexate, and cyclosporin. Acitretin and methotrexate may be combined with phototherapy.
- Biologics that have been approved in children include the tumor necrosis factor antagonists etanercept and adalimumab, ustekinumab (IL-12/23 inhibitor), and IL-17 inhibitors, secukinumab and ixekizumab.

Pearls & Practical Tips

- Actively monitor for early signs and symptoms of psoriatic arthritis, with prompt referral to a pediatric rheumatologist for assessment and management. Radiological changes can occur late.
- Consider diaper psoriasis in infants with persistent diaper rashes that do not response to conventional therapy.

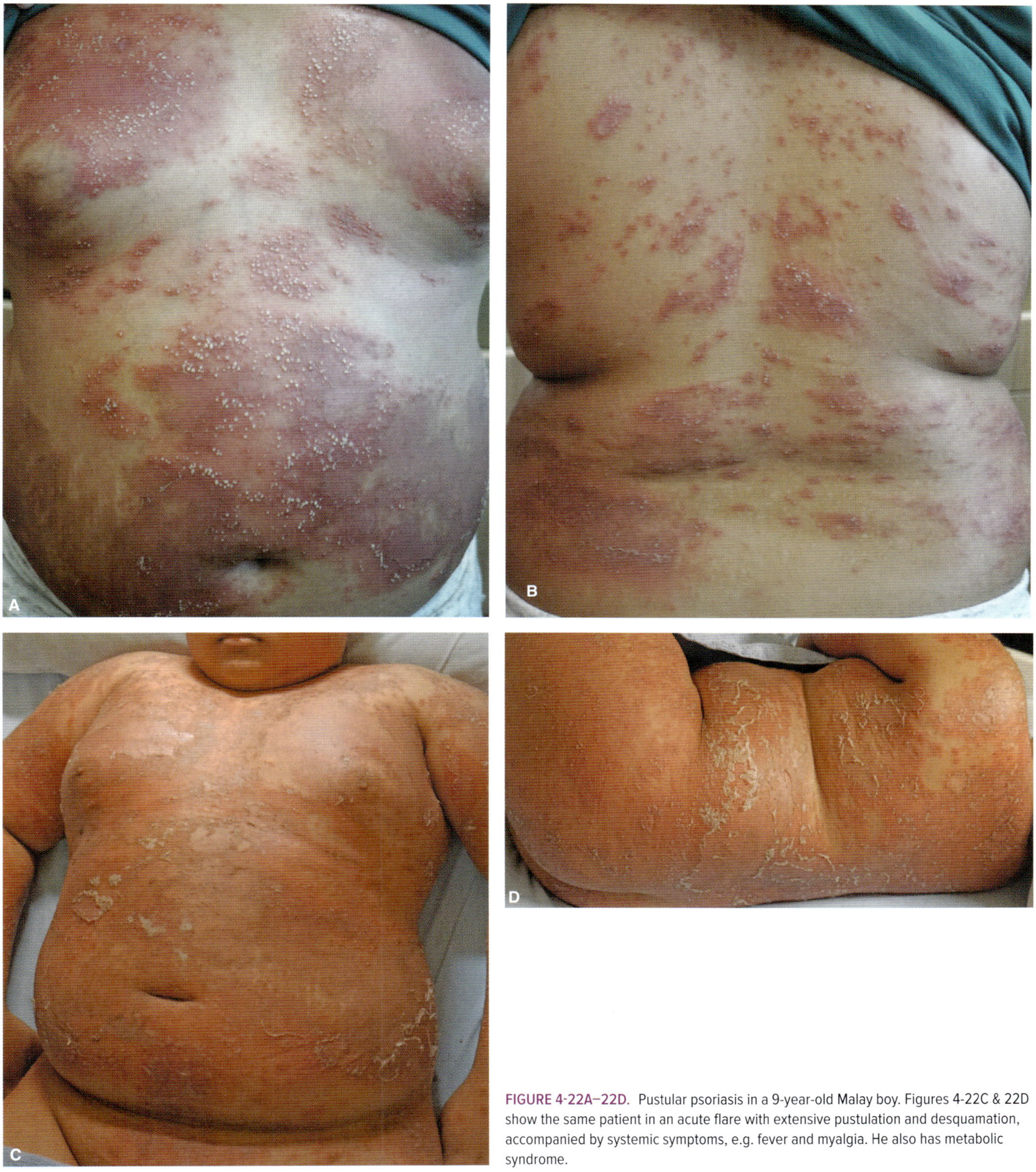

FIGURE 4-22A–22D. Pustular psoriasis in a 9-year-old Malay boy. Figures 4-22C & 22D show the same patient in an acute flare with extensive pustulation and desquamation, accompanied by systemic symptoms, e.g. fever and myalgia. He also has metabolic syndrome.

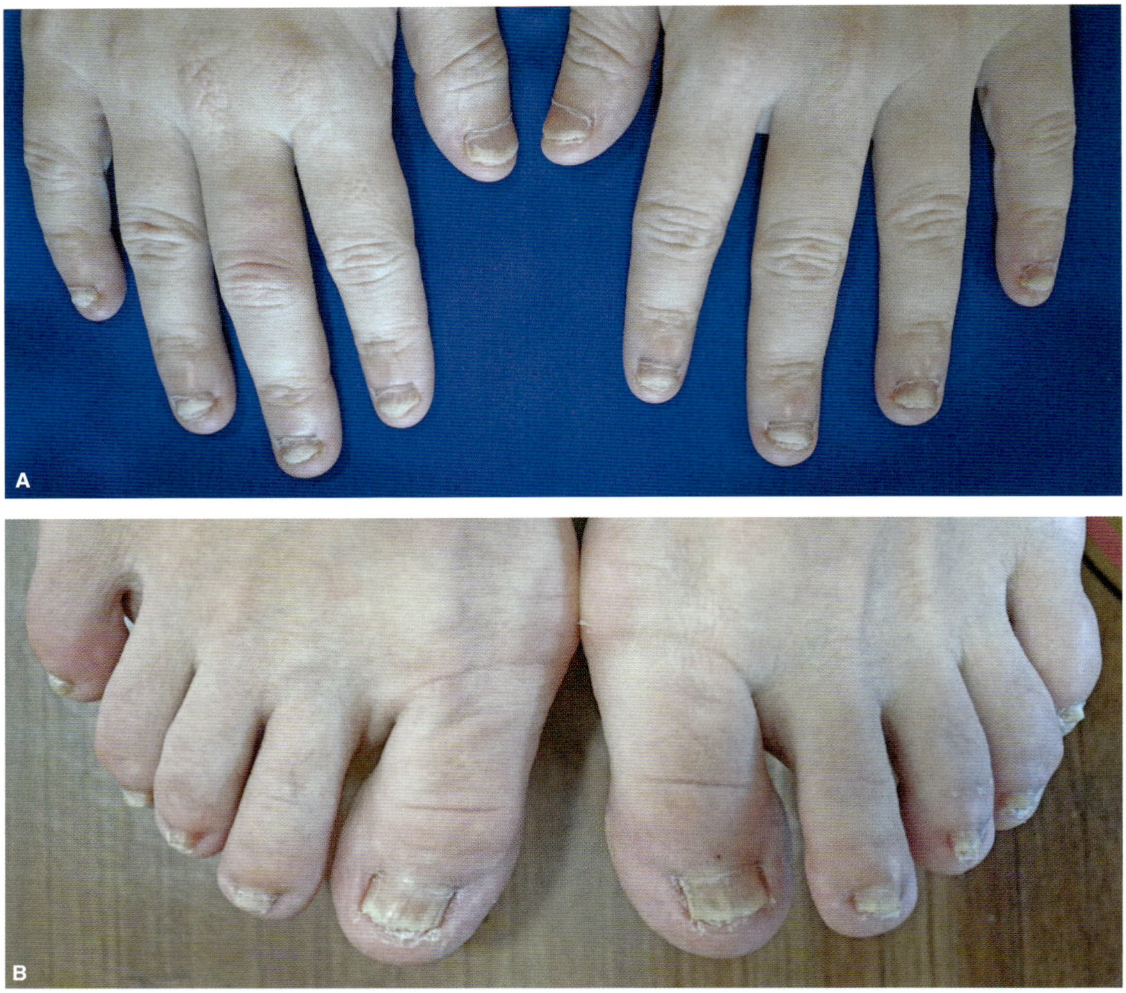

FIGURE 4-23A & 23B. Nail psoriasis with mild paronychia affecting almost all the nails of this 6-year-old Chinese boy.

- Combination topical treatments are recommended. However, regimens that are too confusing can lead to poor compliance.
- Pustular psoriasis often responds faster to treatment with acitretin compared to chronic plaque psoriasis. A short course of oral corticosteroids, started concomitantly with acitretin or ciclosporin, is useful to rapidly reduce the symptoms of GPP.
- There is increasing evidence that childhood psoriasis is associated with other systemic comorbidities including obesity, hypertension, and psychological disorders. Early education and screening of comorbidities are important in the care of pediatric patients with psoriasis.

Bibliography

1. Tangtatco JAA, Lara-Corrales I. Update in the management of pediatric psoriasis. Curr Opin Pediatr 2017;29(4):434-42.
2. Moustou AE, Kakourou T, Masouri S, Alexopoulos A, Sachlas A, Antoniou C. Childhood and adolescent psoriasis in Greece: a retrospective analysis of 842 patients. Int J Dermatol 2014;53(12):1447-53.

PITYRIASIS RUBRA PILARIS

Pityriasis rubra pilaris (PRP) is a rare papulosquamous, inflammatory dermatosis of unknown etiology, with clinical and pathological overlap with psoriasis. Activating mutations in CARD14 gene has recently been shown to be associated with some cases of childhood PRP.

Clinical Features

- Griffith's classification of PRP is shown in Table 4-1. In Asian children, type IV PRP is the most common. However, overlap between the subtypes is also common.

TABLE 4-1. Griffiths classification of pityriasis rubra pilaris.

Type I	Classic adult
Type II	Atypical adult
Type III	Classic juvenile
Type IV	Circumscribed juvenile
Type V	Atypical juvenile
Type VI	HIV-associated

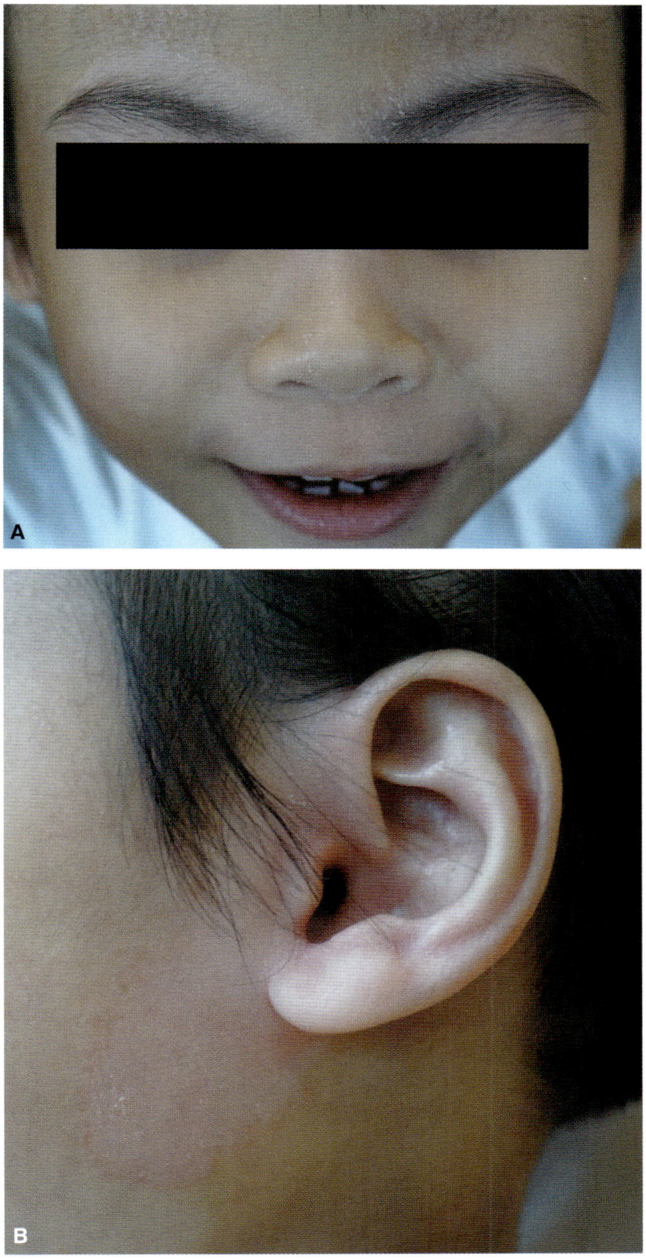

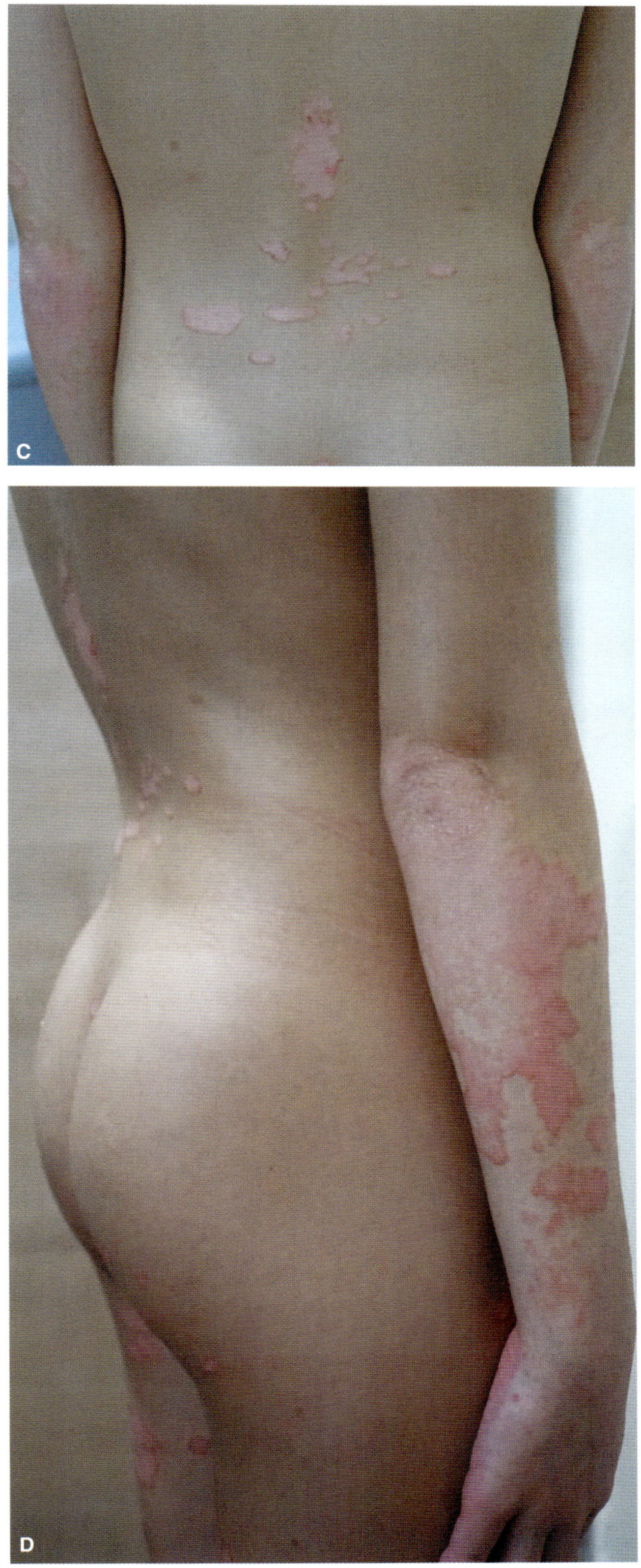

FIGURE 4-24A–24I. Classic juvenile PRP in a 7-year-old Chinese girl with well-circumscribed, psoriasiform plaques with pink-orange hue, located mostly on the extensor surfaces, associated with palmoplantar keratoderma.

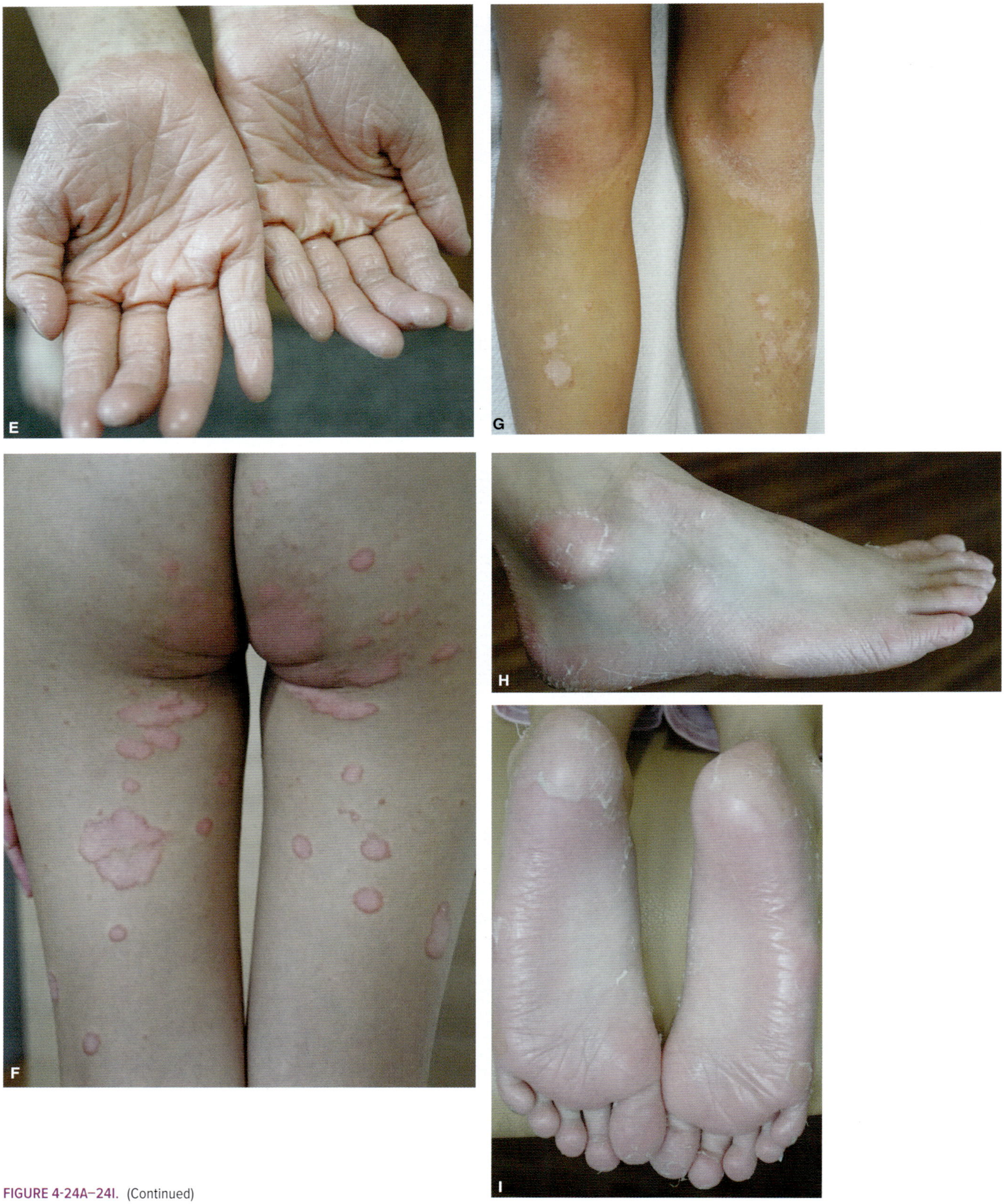

FIGURE 4-24A–24I. (Continued)

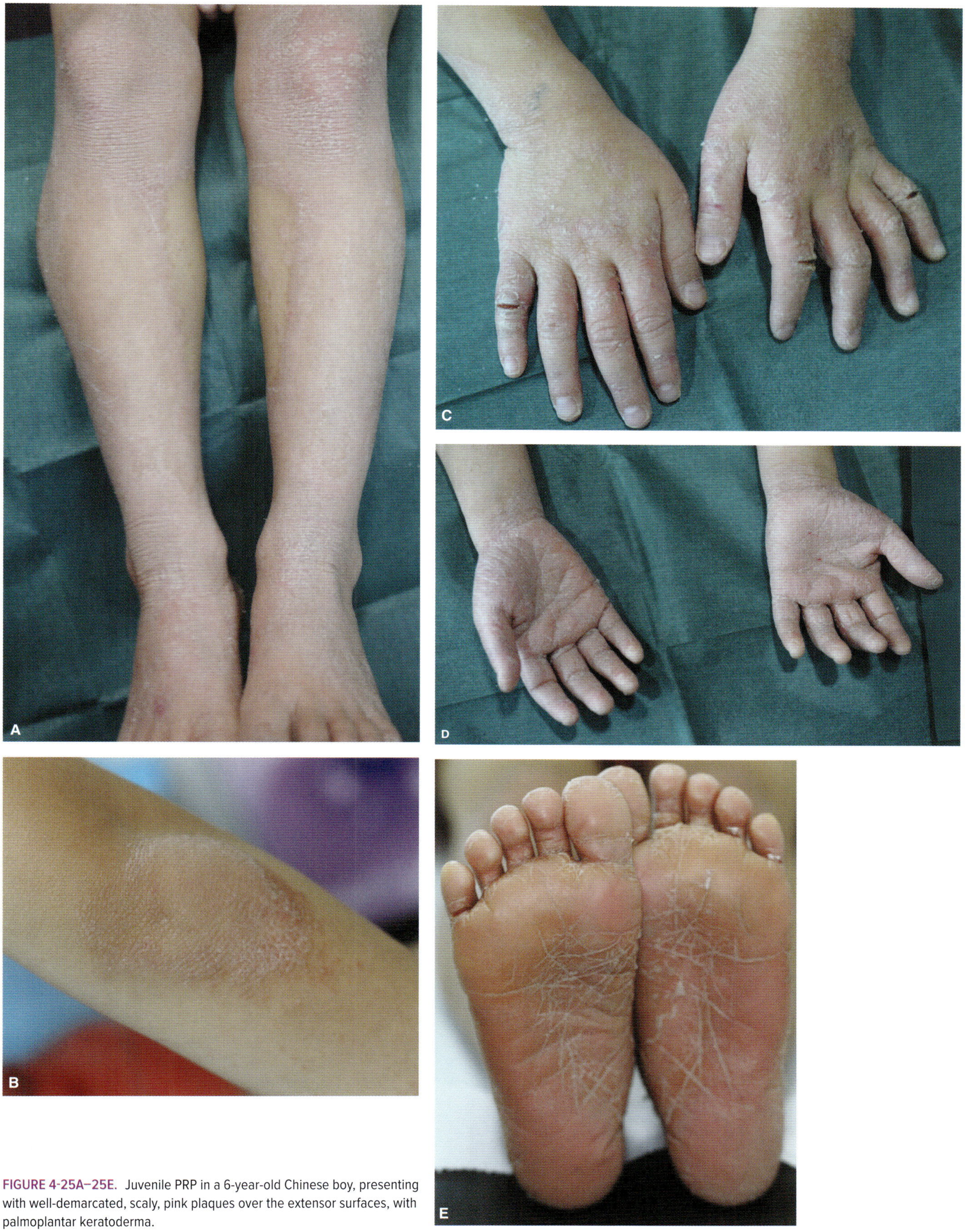

FIGURE 4-25A–25E. Juvenile PRP in a 6-year-old Chinese boy, presenting with well-demarcated, scaly, pink plaques over the extensor surfaces, with palmoplantar keratoderma.

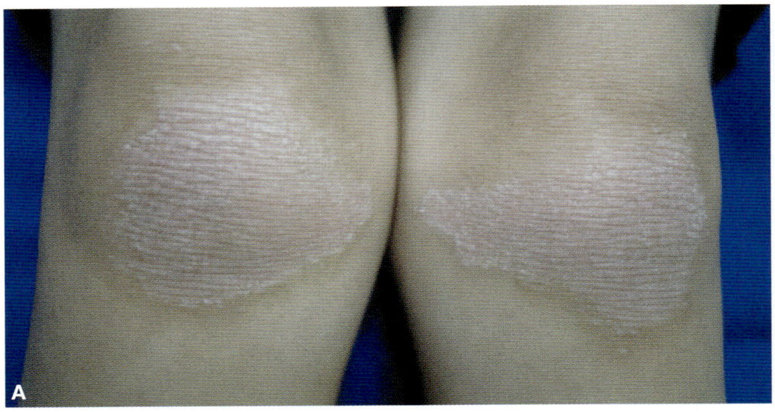

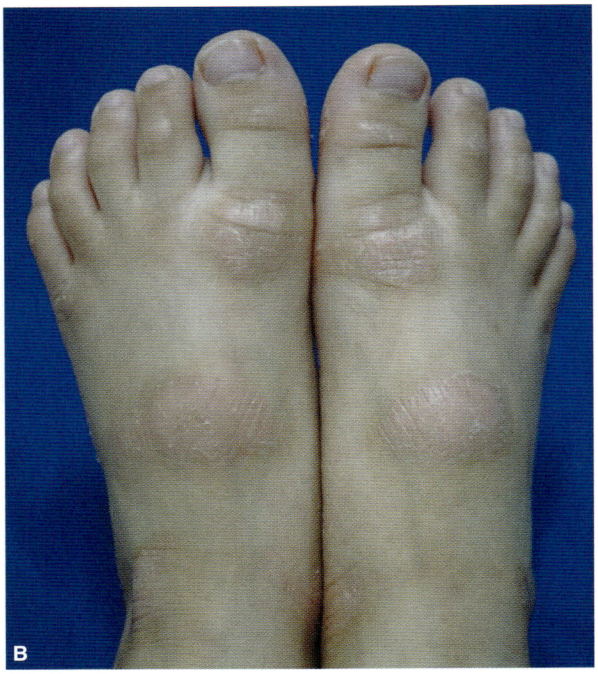

FIGURE 4-26A & 26B. Circumscribed juvenile PRP in a 4-year-old Chinese boy, presenting with well-demarcated, pink-orange, scaly plaques on the extensor surfaces.

- Time of onset for juvenile forms of PRP is usually before puberty. Familial type V PRP usually presents from birth or in the first few years of life.
- PRP is characterized by follicular papules with perifollicular erythema and a central keratotic plug that coalesce into large red to orange-red, well-demarcated, scaly plaques with distinctive islands of sparing.
- Lesions are bilateral and symmetrically affect the elbows, knees, ankles, and Achilles tendon. The plaques can progress to become more extensive, sometimes to generalized erythroderma.
- In some variants of PRP, orange-red, waxy keratoderma of the palms and soles with well-defined borders can be seen.
- Nails can be thickened, with onycholysis, transverse striations, and subungual debris.
- Itch is variable, and patients are generally well, although rarely, rapidly progressive erythroderma may be associated with systemic symptoms of fever, malaise, and chills.
- The clinical course of PRP is variable, with disease often lasting several years. The long-term outcomes for most pediatric patients do not correlate with the extent of involvement. Persistence of familial disease is the rule.

Differential Diagnosis

- Psoriasis
  - There can be considerable clinical and histological overlap between psoriasis and PRP. However, psoriasis appears more pink or red compared to the orange hue of PRP.
- Seborrheic dermatitis
  - Seborrheic dermatitis typically affects the "seborrheic" areas, such as the forehead, cheeks, upper chest, axillae, and groin.
- Atopic dermatitis (AD) and lichen simplex chronicus
  - The lesions of AD are usually not as well-demarcated as PRP. There is often overlying scale-crusting. AD tends to affect flexural areas as compared to the extensor involvement of PRP.
  - Circumscribed PRP can appear similar to lichen simplex chronicus. However, the sites of involvement are different.
- Hereditary palmoplantar keratoderma (PPK)
  - Hereditary PPK usually only affects the palms and soles, unlike in PRP where the involvement is more widespread.

Investigations & Treatment

- Diagnosis can be made clinically based on the cardinal features of follicular-based keratotic papules with perifollicular erythema, diffuse red-orange scaly plaques with islands of sparing, and bilateral waxy palmoplantar keratoderma.
- A skin biopsy may be required to support a diagnosis of PRP, although there is considerable overlap with the histological features of psoriasis.
- Topical treatments may be used for milder disease, including emollients, corticosteroids, calcineurin inhibitors, tazarotene, and keratolytic agents such as urea, salicylic acid, and alpha-hydroxy acid (AHA).
- For more extensive disease, systemic retinoids, such as acitretin or isotretinoin, methotrexate, cyclosporine, or azathioprine, can be considered.
- Some patients may respond to narrowband ultraviolet B (nbUVB) phototherapy.
- Biologics may be used for recalcitrant PRP, including etanercept, infliximab, ustekinumab, and secukinumab.

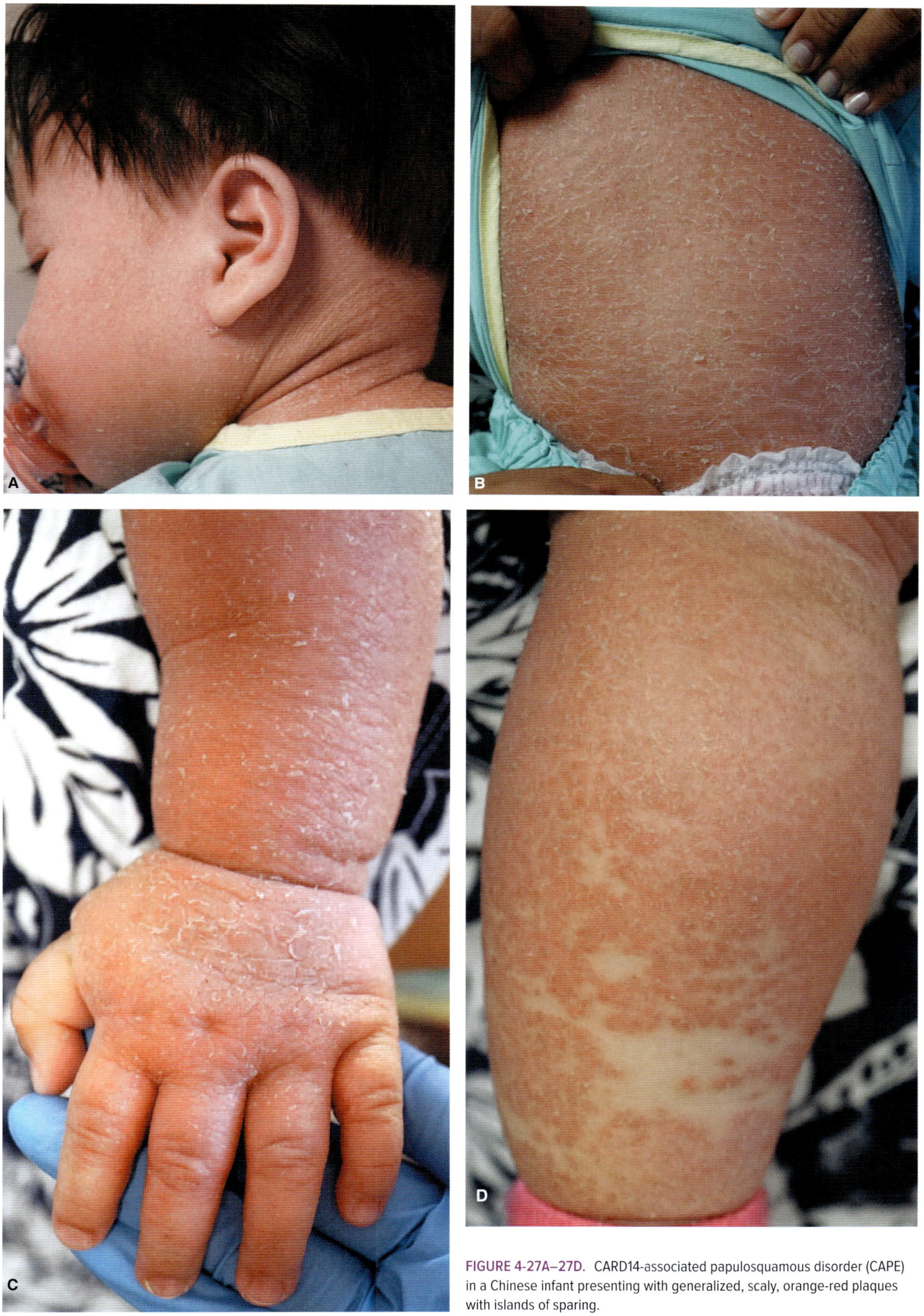

FIGURE 4-27A–27D. CARD14-associated papulosquamous disorder (CAPE) in a Chinese infant presenting with generalized, scaly, orange-red plaques with islands of sparing.

Pearls & Practical Tips

- The cephalocaudal pattern of progression of PRP lesions is classical but may not always be present.
- CARD14-associated papulosquamous eruption (CAPE) is a more recently described dermatosis that has overlapping features of psoriasis and PRP. It commonly presents in early childhood and exhibits extensive involvement, including the face. It has been reported to be unresponsive to classical treatments for PRP, with most reported patients requiring biologics for better response.

Bibliography

1. Chao-Chun Yang MD, et al. Juvenile pityriasis rubra pilaris: Report of 28 cases in Taiwan. J Am Acad Dermatol 2008;59(6):943-48.
2. Eastham AB. Pityriasis rubra pilaris. JAMA Dermatol 2019 Mar 1;155(3):404.
3. Wong GHZ, Chia SY, Wei H, Rafi'ee K, Koh MJA, Tan EC. CARD14-associated papulosquamous eruption (CAPE) in a toddler responding to treatment with acitretin. Pediatr Dermatol 2021;38(4):970-72

PITYRIASIS LICHENOIDES

Pityriasis lichenoides is uncommon, and represents a spectrum of a chronic, waxing and waning, papulosquamous disorder that manifests in three clinical forms: pityriasis lichenoides et varioliformis acuta (PLEVA), pityriasis lichenoides chronica (PLC) and the more severe Mucha-Habermann disease. It is common to observe features of both PLEVA and PLC in the same patient.

Clinical Features

- The mean age of onset of pityriasis lichenoides in the pediatric age group is between 5 and 10 years, although it can occur at any age.
- Lesions of PLEVA appear as multiple, non-pruritic, 2- to 3-mm, oval or round, reddish-brown macules and papules that progress to become vesicular, necrotic, crusted, and occasionally purpuric lesions. The lesions may be itchy or occasionally painful. They usually resolve without scarring, although atrophic scarring may occasionally be seen.
- Patients with predominantly PLEVA lesions often have a more abrupt onset of the rash, sometimes associated with fever and other constitutional symptoms.
- Lesions of PLC appear as multiple pink to reddish-brown papules with centrally adherent scales (mica scales) that resolve with hypo- or hyperpigmentation, without scarring.
- In dark-skinned patients, it is not uncommon that the eruption primarily presents as extensive hypopigmented macules and patches only. However, on close inspection, mild scaling and erythema may be appreciated.
- The lesions are often asymptomatic, although some patients may complain of mild itch.
- Patients with predominantly PLEVA lesions have a more waxing and waning course, while patients with predominantly PLC lesions have a more chronic course. However, there is substantial overlap, and the eruption can last for years.
- In both forms, lesions may involve the entire body including the trunk, proximal thighs, and upper arms. They are also more pronounced over the flexural surfaces. The face, scalp, mucous membranes, palms, and soles are often spared.

Differential Diagnosis

The duration and polymorphous nature of the eruption help to distinguish pityriasis lichenoides from other inflammatory skin disorders. Differential diagnosis of PLEVA include the following.

- Chickenpox has similar polymorphous eruptions similar to PLEVA but is usually more pruritic. It dries up within a week to 10 days. A varicella-zoster PCR from the vesicular fluid will be positive.
- Impetigo is a superficial skin infection characterized by the painful, mild pruritic yellowish crusts, which may sometimes be bullous. Fever is uncommon.
- Arthropod bites have variable presentation depending on the type of arthropod involved, including mosquitoes, fleas, bed bugs, and spiders. They can be itchy and painful, and are typically self-limited.
- Vesicular pityriasis rosea usually appears as a generalized eruption of vesicles or a rosette of vesicles with a preceding "herald patch."
- Vasculitis typically presents with palpable purpura in dependent areas and may be associated with petechiae, ulcers, hemorrhagic vesicles, and bullae. May be associated with positive autoimmune markers in the serum.
- Scabies are characterized by superficial burrows, extreme pruritus, blisters, and pustules, typically over the palms and soles and the webs of fingers and toes. There is usually a history of similarly pruritic rashes in a household member.

Differential diagnosis of PLC includes the following.

- Hypopigmented mycosis fungoides present with multiple variably sized hypopigmented macules and patches, most commonly affecting the sun-covered sites, such as the buttocks, trunk, and abdomen. Fine scales or subtle atrophy may sometimes be appreciated within these lesions.
- Guttate psoriasis is characterized by diffuse thick, white scales on an erythematous rash with positive Auspitz sign.
- Lichen planus typically has the pathognomonic feature of small, delicate white streaks that form a network on the surface of papules, called Wickham's striae.
- Pityriasis rosea usually starts as a herald patch followed by secondary papules with collarette scales affecting the back in a fir tree distribution.
- Secondary syphilis usually has non-pruritic erythematous papules with central scaly plaque lesions affecting the palms and soles.

Investigations

- Diagnosis can be made clinically. When diagnosis remains in doubt, skin biopsy will often confirm the diagnosis. An accurate description of the morphology and chronicity of the biopsied lesion is essential for better clinicopathological correlation.

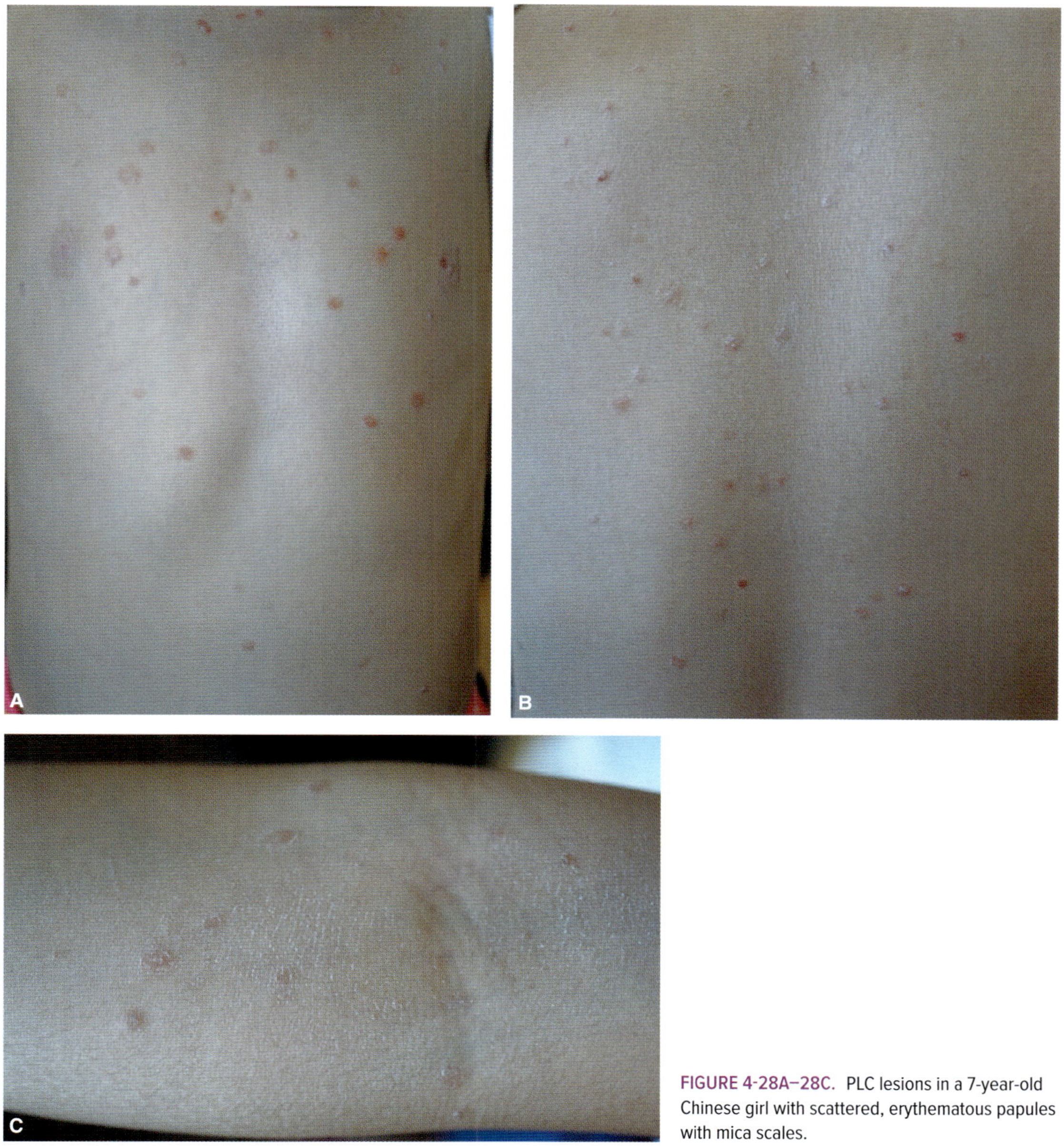

FIGURE 4-28A–28C. PLC lesions in a 7-year-old Chinese girl with scattered, erythematous papules with mica scales.

Treatment

- Topical corticosteroids as monotherapy are rarely effective except for controlling pruritus.
- Up to two-thirds of children show a partial or full response to systemic antibiotics such as erythromycin, azithromycin, doxycycline, and tetracycline. A 1- to 2-month trial is justified, especially for the acute form. Doxycycline and tetracycline are contraindicated in children younger than 8 years of age.
- Narrow-band ultraviolet B (nbUVB) is indicated as an effective second-line therapy.
- Third-line therapies such as oral methotrexate and cyclosporine are reserved for severe PLEVA.

Pearls & Practical Tips

- Pityriasis lichenoides is often not considered as the first diagnosis, especially when patients present early.
- Pityriasis lichenoides generally follows a benign course; however, long-term follow-up is recommended due to rare reports of progression to cutaneous T-cell lymphoma (CTCL).
- PLC and hypopigmented mycosis fungoides should be considered in all dark-skinned children with extensive hypopigmented macules and patches.

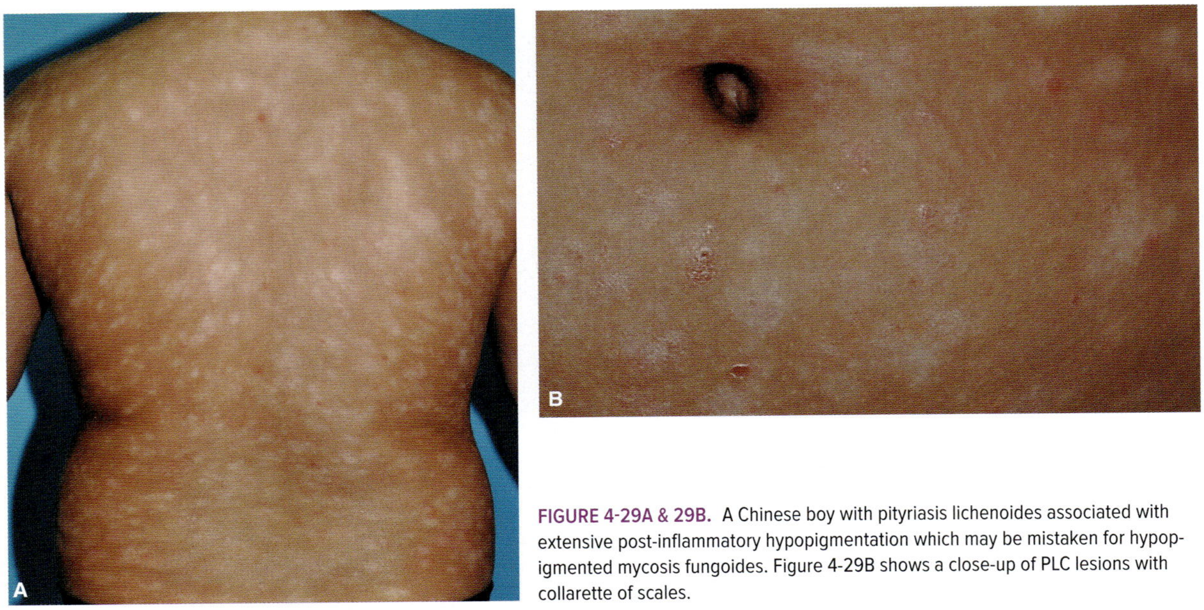

FIGURE 4-29A & 29B. A Chinese boy with pityriasis lichenoides associated with extensive post-inflammatory hypopigmentation which may be mistaken for hypopigmented mycosis fungoides. Figure 4-29B shows a close-up of PLC lesions with collarette of scales.

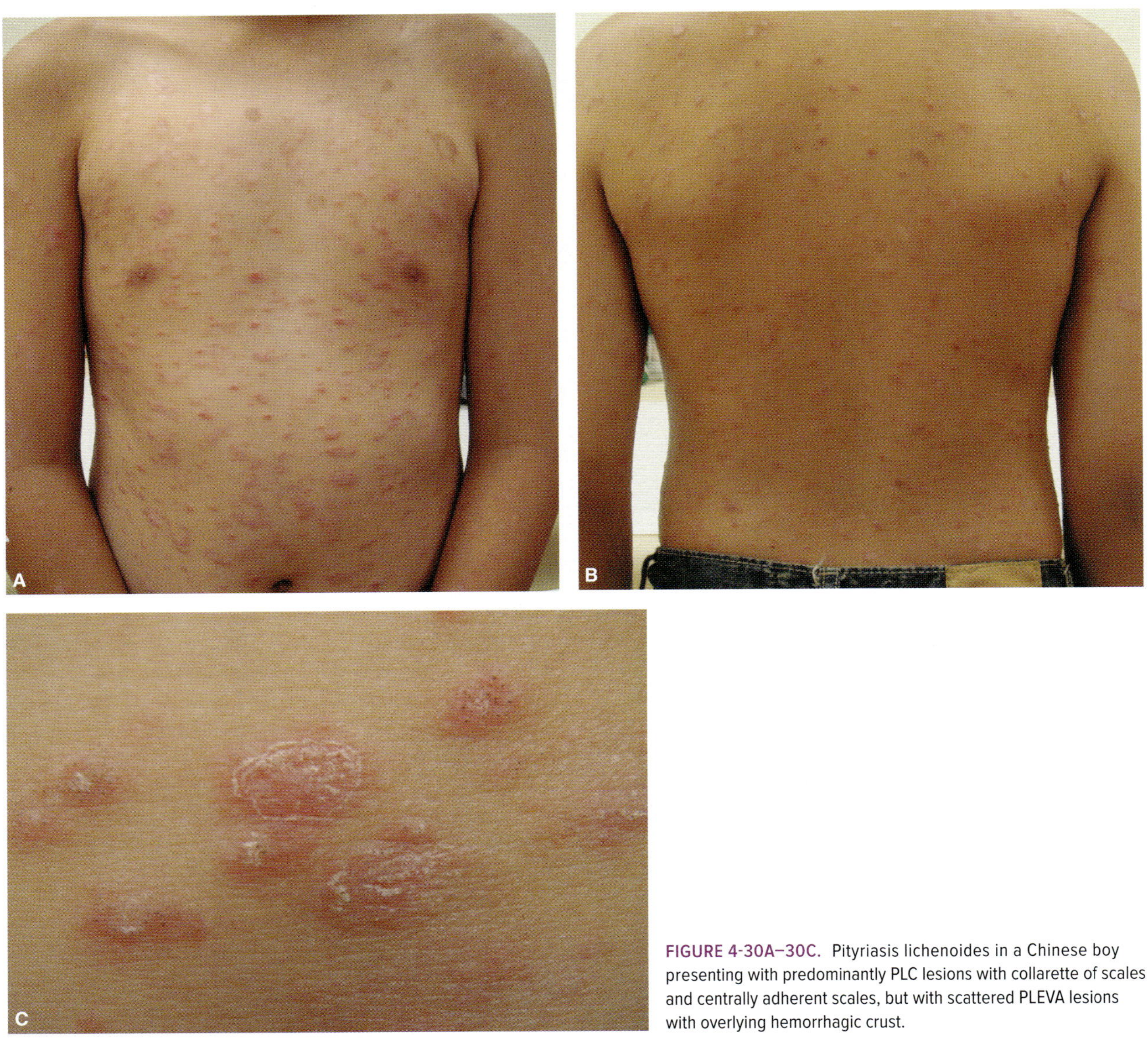

FIGURE 4-30A–30C. Pityriasis lichenoides in a Chinese boy presenting with predominantly PLC lesions with collarette of scales and centrally adherent scales, but with scattered PLEVA lesions with overlying hemorrhagic crust.

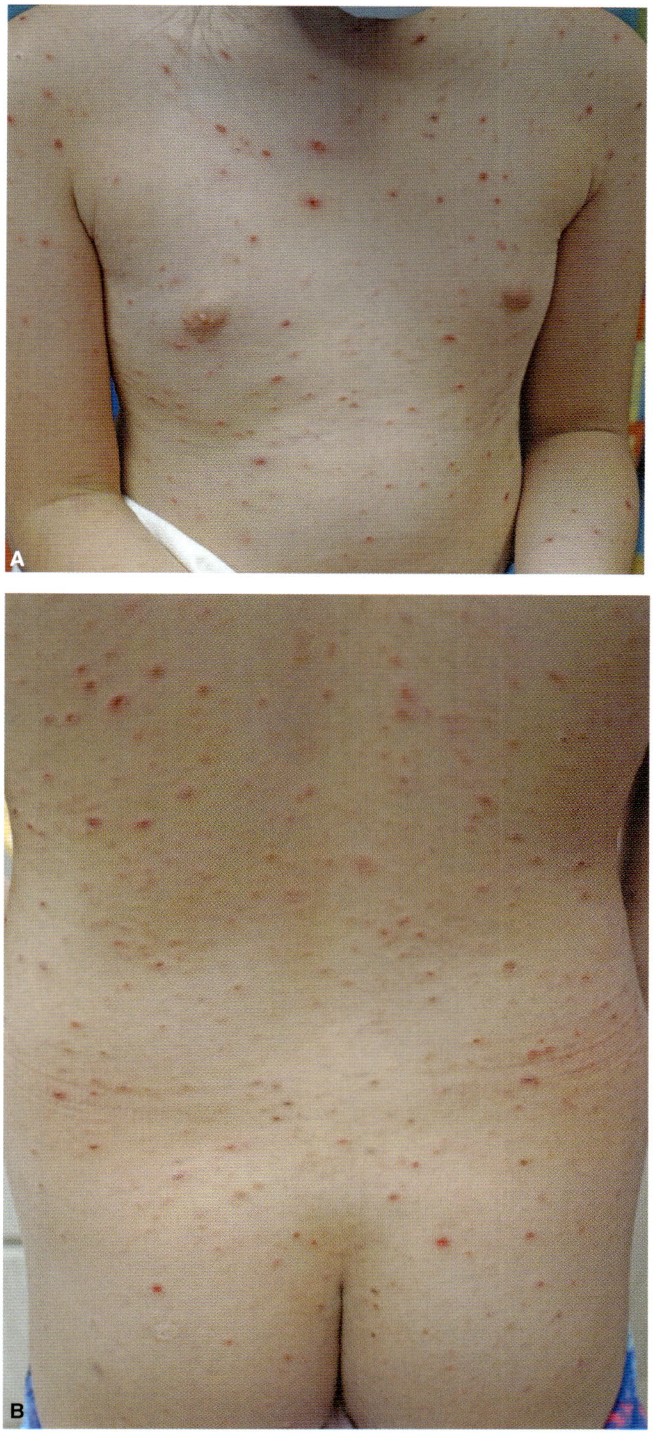

FIGURE 4-31A & 31B. Predominantly PLEVA lesions in this Chinese girl with pityriasis lichenoides.

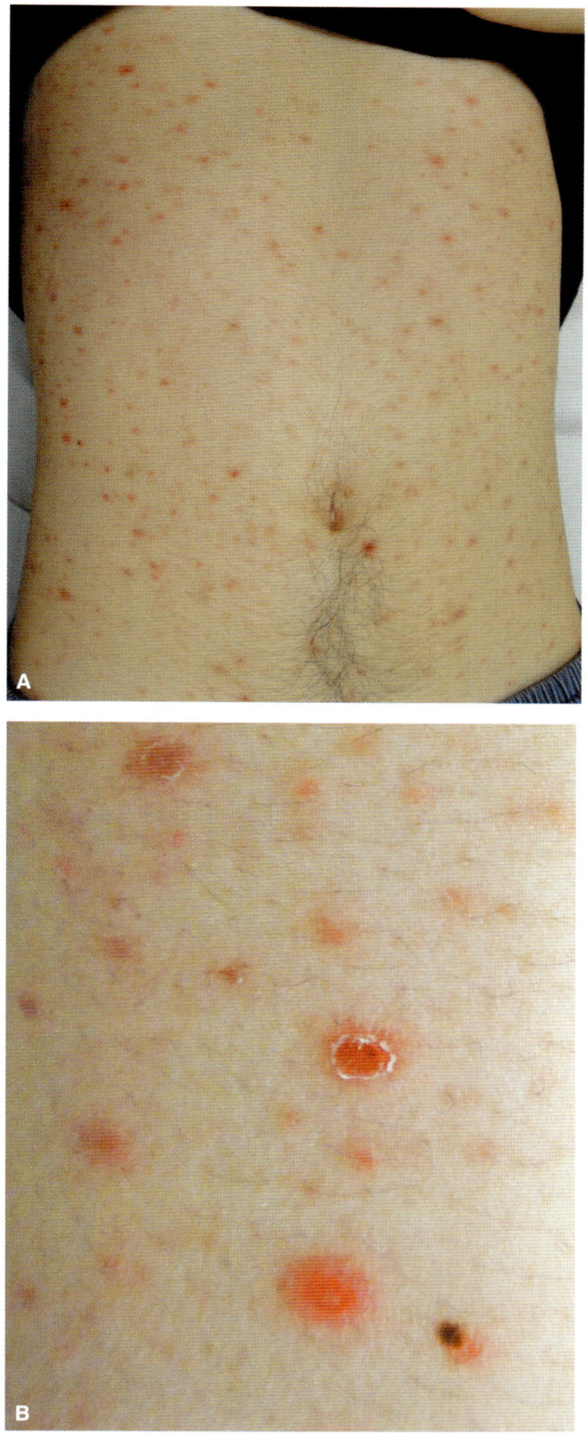

FIGURE 4-32A & 32B. Pityriasis lichenoides in a teenage Chinese male with both PLC and PLEVA lesions. Figure 4-32B shows a close-up of a PLEVA lesion with a hemorrhagic central crust and collarette of scales.

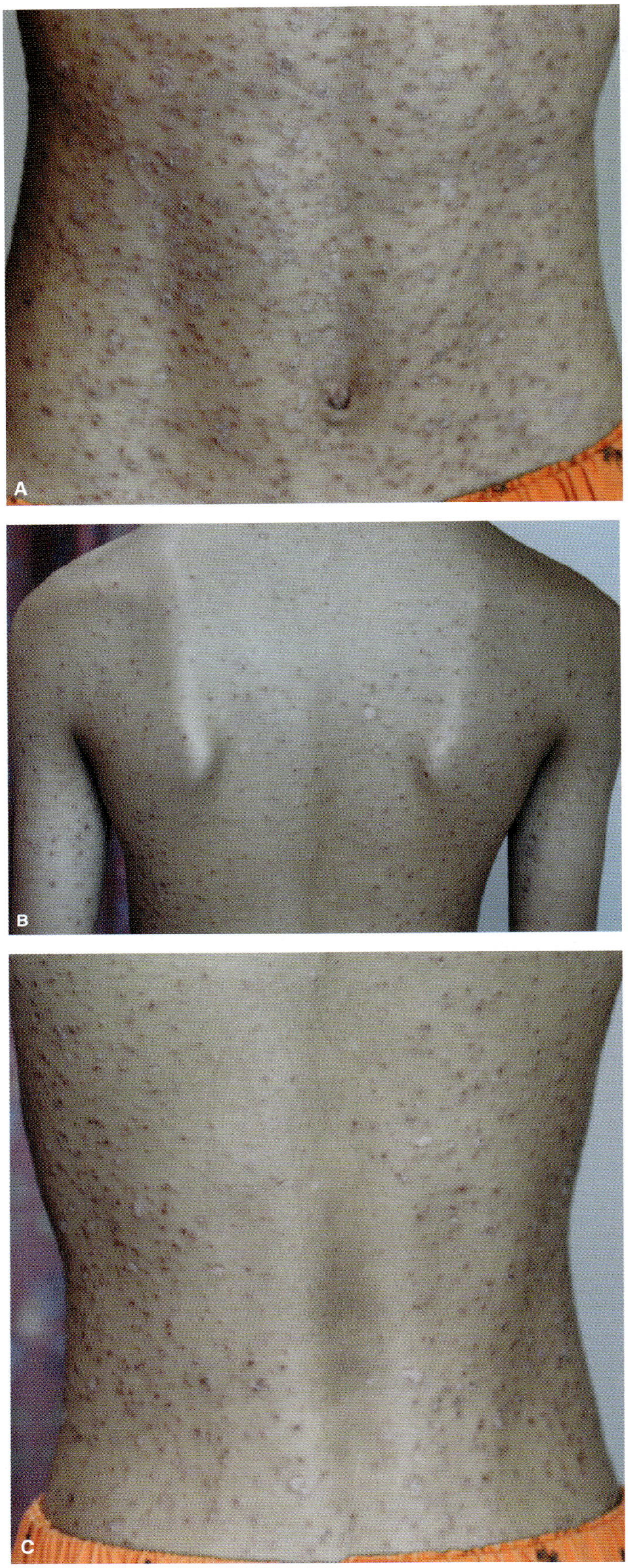

FIGURE 4-33A–33C. Extensive PLEVA in a 14-year-old Chinese boy with multiple scaly, necrotic papules scattered across his trunk.

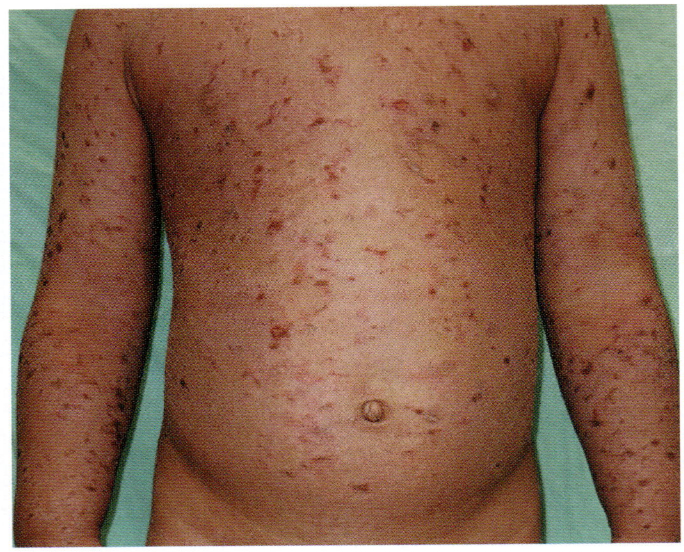

FIGURE 4-34. Extensive pityriasis lichenoides in this Malaysian child with both PLEVA and PLC lesions. There are confluent areas of hemorrhagic scabbing seen.

Bibliography

1. Gelmetti C, Rigoni C, Alessi E et al. Pityriasis lichenoides in children: a long-term follow-up of eighty-nine cases. J Am Acad Dermatol 1990;23:473-78.
2. Koh WL, Koh MJA, Tay YK. Pityriasis lichenoides in an Asian population. Int J Dermatol 2013;52:1495-99
3. Geller L et al. Pityriasis lichenoides in childhood: review of clinical presentation and treatment options. Ped Dermatol 2015;32(5):579-92.

LICHEN PLANUS

Lichen planus (LP) is a chronic inflammatory dermatosis that is uncommon in childhood. The mean age of childhood LP ranges from 7 to 11.8 years. There is a predilection for Indians compared to other Asian races. The pathophysiology of LP is unknown, although there is growing evidence that it is due to a T cell–mediated autoimmune response against unknown proteins in the skin and mucosa membranes. Some antigens postulated to trigger LP in children are hepatitis C or human herpesvirus 7 infection; vaccinations, including hepatitis B, MMR (measles, mumps, rubella), and polio vaccines; and dental amalgam fillings.

Clinical Features

- LP is characterized by symmetrically distributed polygonal, violaceous, flat-topped papules and plaques. Small, delicate white streaks that form a network on the surface, called Wickham's striae, best appreciated on dermoscopy, is pathognomonic.
- Common sites of involvement are the legs, wrists, and lower back. It rarely involves the face, palms, and soles.
- Koebner phenomenon leads to linearly oriented lesions, especially at sites of minor trauma.
- Eruptive lesions can result in widespread involvement of small hyperpigmented macules or papules.

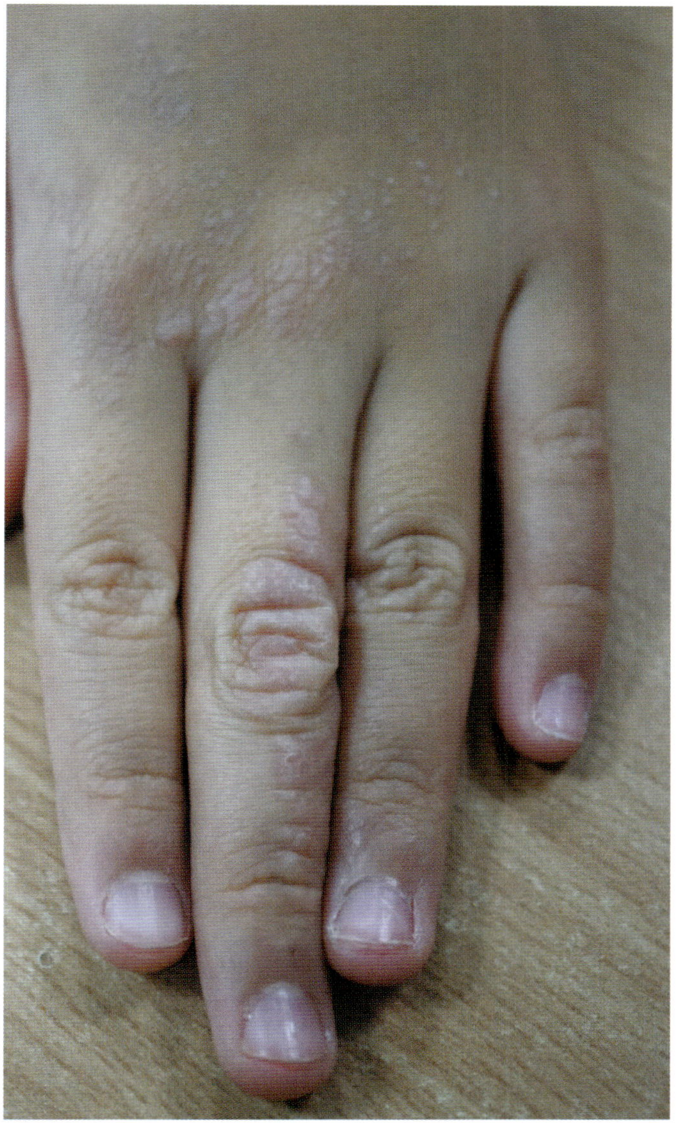

FIGURE 4-35. Localized LP on the hand of a 7-year-old Chinese boy, presenting as flat-topped, pink-to-violaceous papules and plaques with overlying mild scaling.

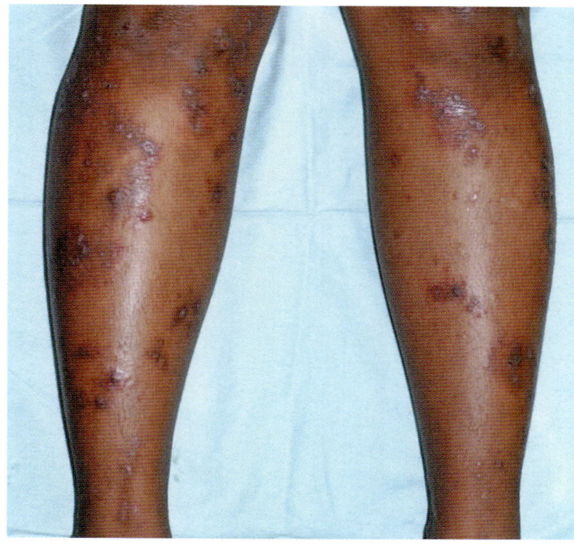

FIGURE 4-36. LP on the legs of a darker-skinned child with violaceous and hyperpigmented papules and plaques with overlying scale.

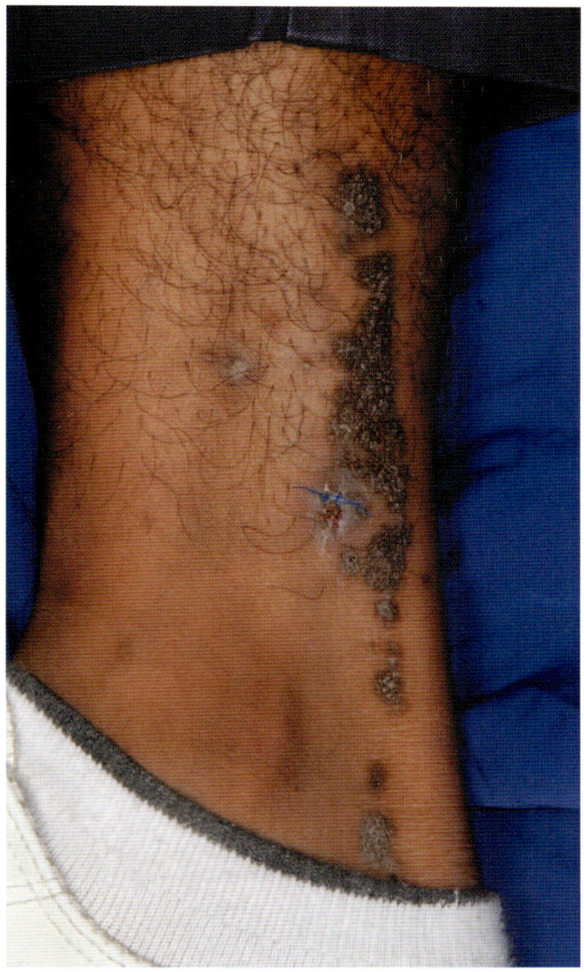

FIGURE 4-37. Linear LP on the calf and ankle of a 16-year-old Indian male, presenting as a violaceous-to-hyperpigmented linear plaque with overlying Wickham's striae.

- In true linear LP, lesions follow lines of Blaschko.
- LP pigmentosus is usually seen in Indians and darker-skinned individuals. They usually present with macular lesions, over sun-exposed sites. Some consider erythema dyschromicum perstans (Ashy's dermatosis) and idiopathic eruptive macular pigmentation (IEMP) as variants of LP pigmentosus.
- Other less common morphologic variants of LP include hypertrophic, atrophic, actinic, bullous, and pigmented lesions.
- Mucosal involvement can present in various forms, with the reticular form, presenting as lacy whitish streaks on the buccal mucosa, the most common. Erosive, papular, atrophic, and bullous subtypes are rare.

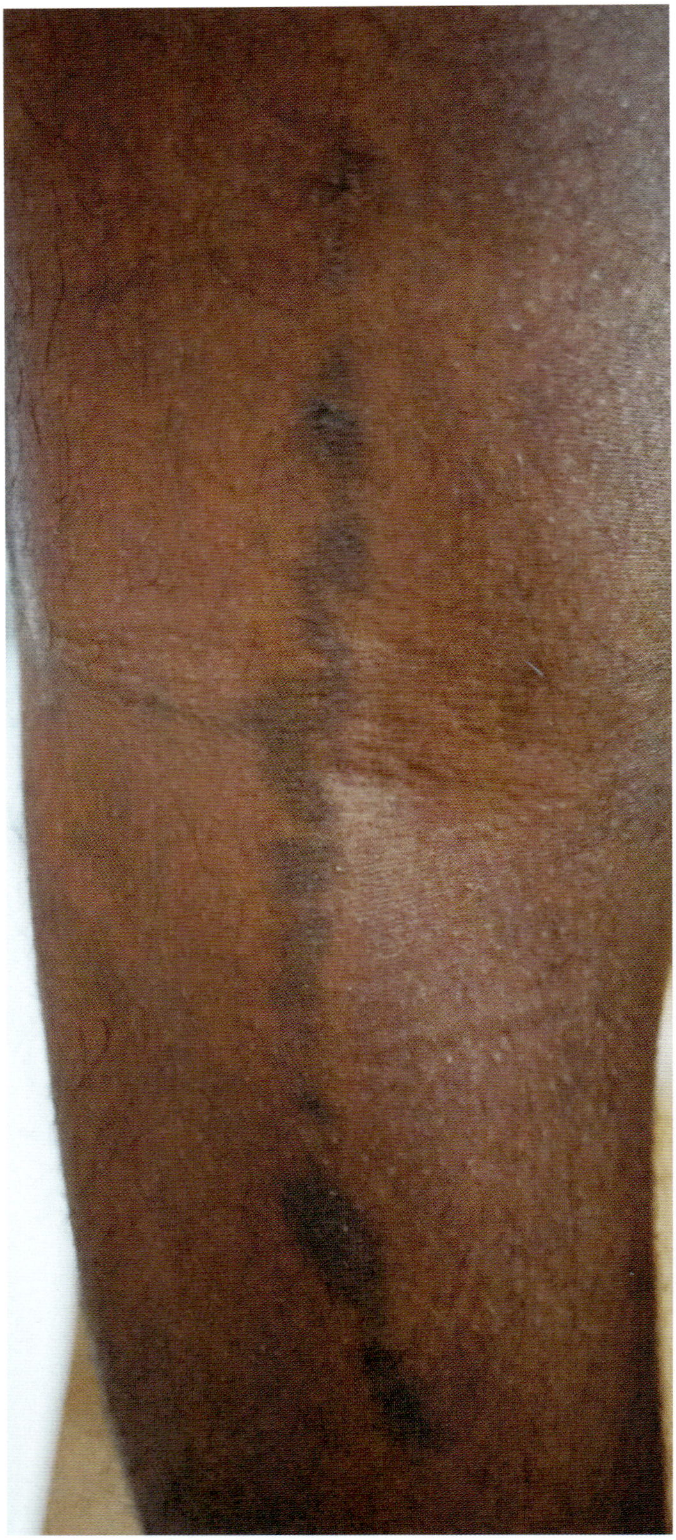

FIGURE 4-38. Linear LP on the calf of a 15-year-old Indian male, presenting as a hyperpigmented, linear plaque with mild surface scaling.

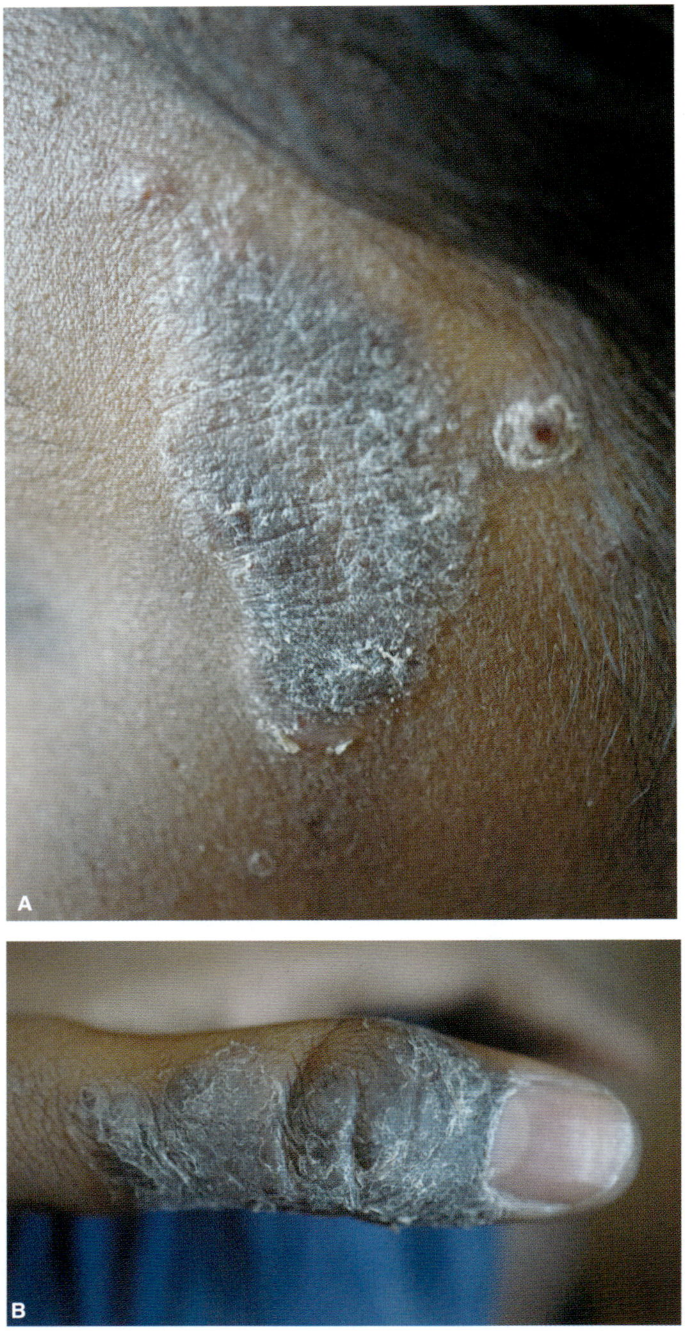

FIGURE 4-39A & 39B. Hypertrophic LP on the face and finger of a 12-year-old Indian girl, with a thickened, hyperpigmented plaque with overlying Wickham's striae.

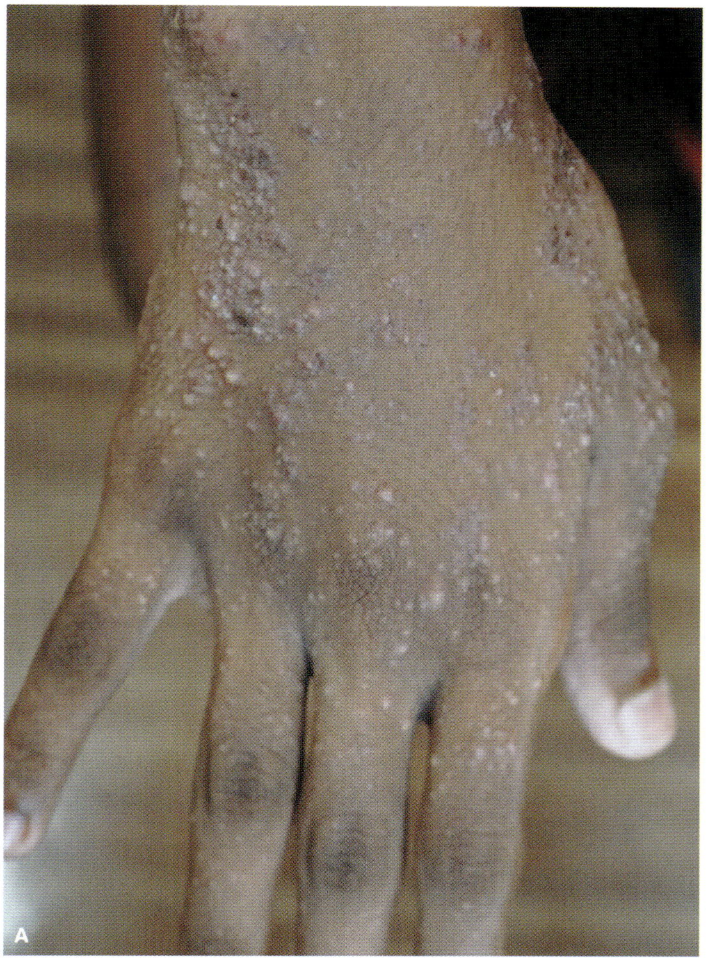

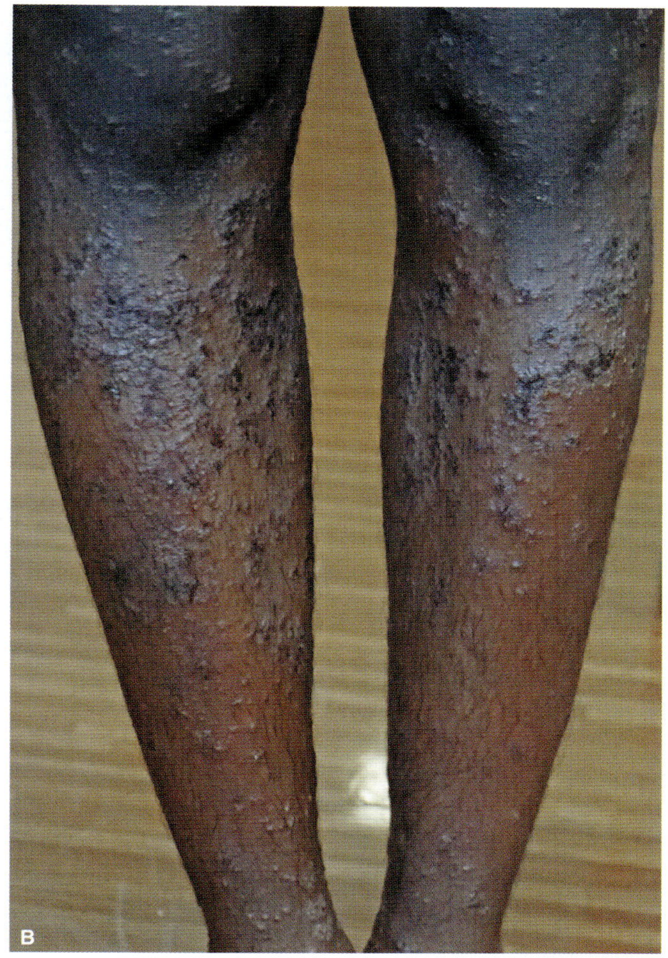

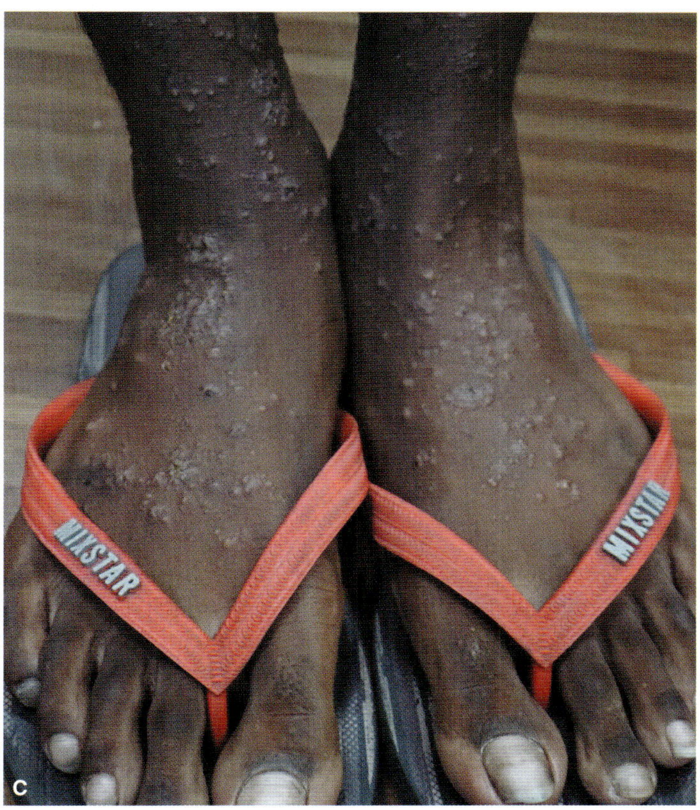

FIGURE 4-40A–40C. "Actinic" LP on the sun-exposed sites of a 14-year-old Indian male, presenting as scaly, violaceous papules and plaques over the extensor surfaces of the arms, hands, legs, and feet.

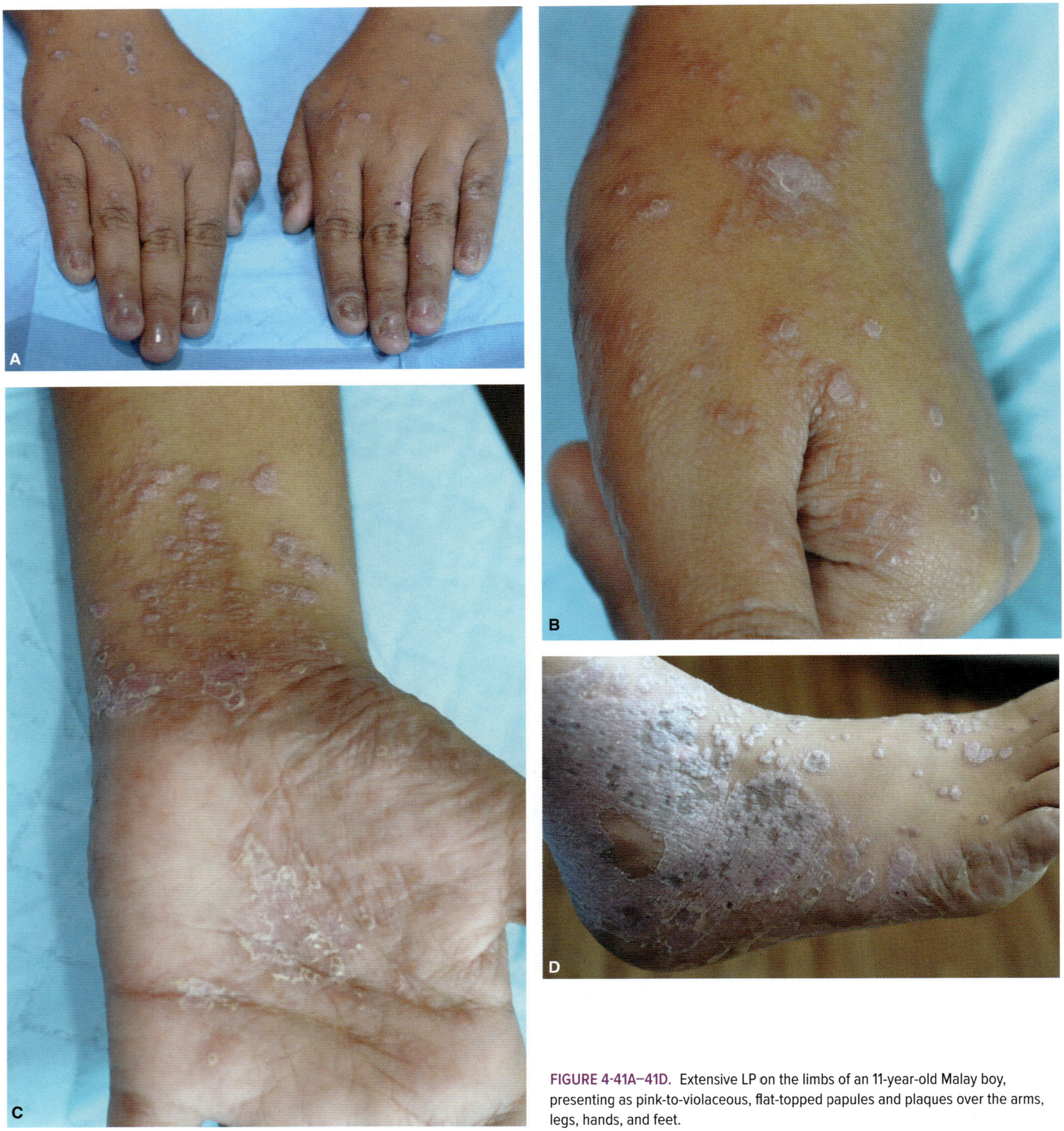

FIGURE 4-41A–41D. Extensive LP on the limbs of an 11-year-old Malay boy, presenting as pink-to-violaceous, flat-topped papules and plaques over the arms, legs, hands, and feet.

- Nail involvement can also occur in children. Pterygium formation is classical, but a late sign, and leads to permanent nail scarring. Longitudinal fissuring and ridging of the nail plate, brittleness, and onycholysis may also be seen.
- Scalp involvement leading to scarring alopecia, termed *lichen planopilaris*, is extremely uncommon in children.
- LP in children is usually a self-limiting disease and resolves after months to a few years. Lesions fade to become post-inflammatory hyperpigmentation that tends to be more persistent in darker-skinned children.

Differential Diagnosis

- Lichen simplex chronicus (LSC)
  - LSC can often mimic LP lesions. However, they are less violaceous, with more yellowish scaling. A biopsy may be required to differentiate the two conditions.

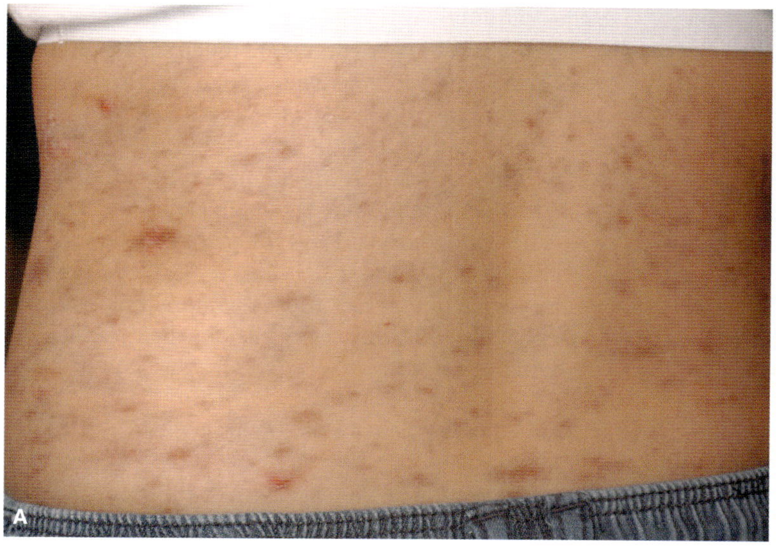

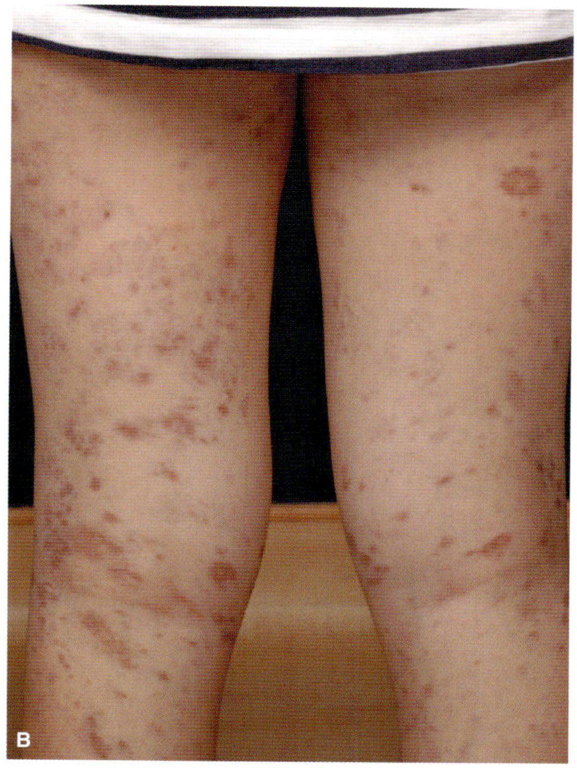

FIGURE 4-42A & 42B. Eruptive extensive LP on the trunk and limbs of a 13-year-old Chinese girl.

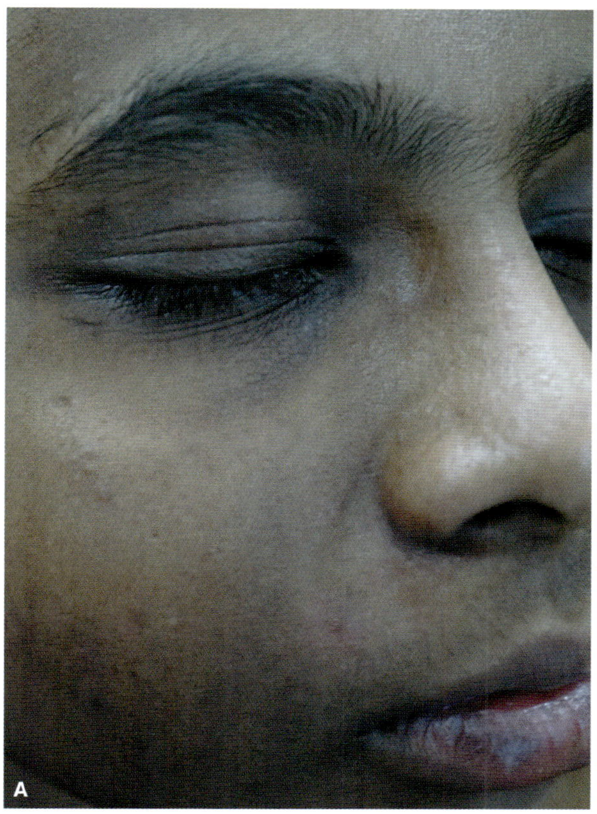

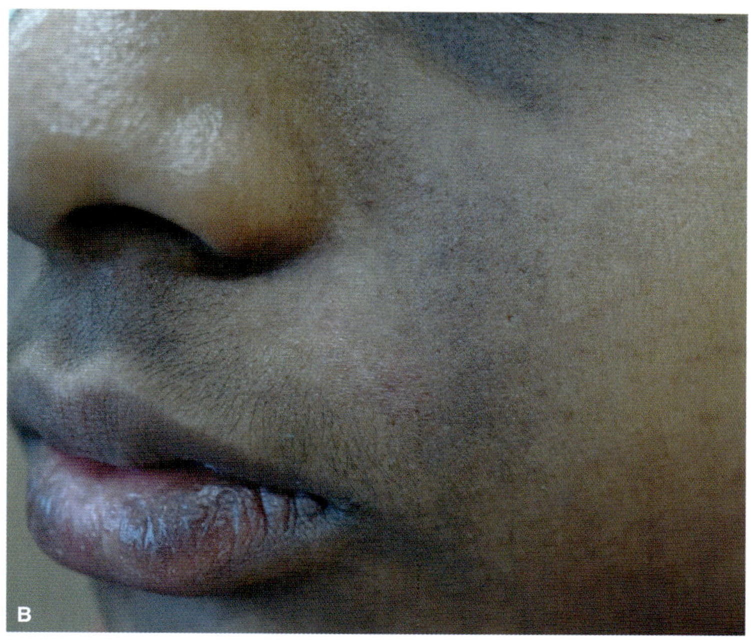

FIGURE 4-43A & 43B. Lichen planus pigmentosus on the forehead, cheeks and periorbital region of this 13-year-old Indian boy, presenting as poorly demarcated, hyperpigmented patches.

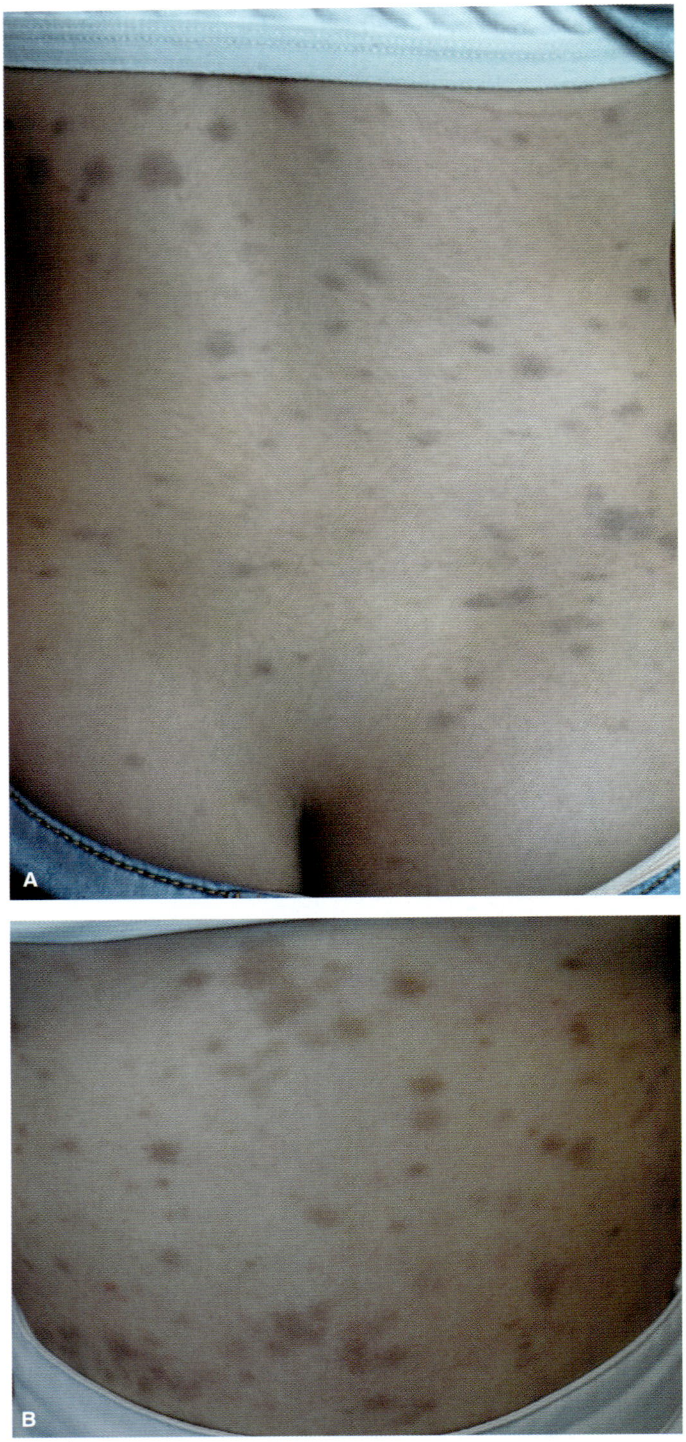

FIGURE 4-44A & 44B. Erythema dyschromicum perstans, or Ashy dermatosis, considered a variant of lichen planus pigmentosus, in a 14-year-old Chinese girl with progressively increasing numbers of dark grey-brown macules and patches on her trunk and proximal limbs.

- Lichen nitidus
  - The lesions of lichen nitidus are much smaller and less violaceous or hyperpigmented compared to lesions of LP. Lesions are also usually less pruritic.
- Lichen striatus
  - This can mimic linear LP, although the color of lichen striatus is more pink or hypopigmented as compared to linear LP, which is classically more violaceous.
- Psoriasis
  - The plaque of psoriasis is usually more pink or red as compared to the violaceous hue of lichen planus. The scaling of psoriasis is also more diffuse compared to LP.
- Discoid lupus erythematosus (DLE)
  - This presents with red to purple scaly plaques over sun-exposed areas, especially over the face. There is usually hyper- and hypopigmentation.
  - There are some cases of overlap between DLE and LP, even on biopsy. Direct immunofluorescence may be helpful in such cases.

Investigations & Treatment

- Diagnosis is usually clinical, although skin biopsy is commonly performed to confirm the diagnosis.
- Histopathology will show a lichenoid band of lymphocytes and histiocytes at the dermal epidermal junction, accompanied by basal vacuolar alteration and necrotic keratinocytes. There is also hyperkeratosis, hypergranulosis, and "saw-tooth" epidermal hyperplasia.
- Combination of potent topical corticosteroids with topical tacrolimus can be used for limited LP. A tapering course of systemic corticosteroids over 2 to 6 weeks can be added in extensive or eruptive cases.
- In more extensive and recalcitrant cases, other treatment options include phototherapy, oral antimalarials, acitretin, methotrexate, and dapsone.

Pearls & Practical Tips

- Drug-induced lichenoid eruption is rare in children but can resemble LP clinically. A detailed drug history and skin biopsy showing parakeratosis, necrotic keratinocytes at different levels of the epidermis, and eosinophils in the dermal infiltrate are clues to the diagnosis of drug-induced lichenoid eruption. There is often a long latency period of a few months to a year after introduction of the inciting drug.

Bibliography

1. Lee SH, Law GTWM, Nanu NM, Tey KE, Choon SE. Clinical profile of 128 patients with lichen planus seen in Hospital Sultanah Aminah Johor Bharu. MJD 2018;41:15-20.
2. Pandhi D, Singal A, Bhattacharya S. Lichen planus in childhood: a series of 316 patients. Paediatr Dermatol 2014;31(1):59-67.

LICHEN NITIDUS

Lichen nitidus is a fairly common benign chronic inflammatory skin eruption that occurs more commonly in children and adolescents compared to adults. It affects both genders equally. The etiology of this condition is unknown. Although most cases of lichen nitidus occur in isolation, it is known to be associated with atopic eczema, lichen planus, and Down syndrome.

Clinical Features

- Lichen nitidus is characterized by multiple discrete, nonfollicular, shiny, skin-colored 1- to 2-mm papules, which can be evenly or randomly spaced. The lesions are usually asymptomatic, although some children may complain of mild itch.
- Linear lesions along lines of trauma occur as a result of Koebner phenomenon, a hallmark of this disorder.
- Lesions are primarily located on the forearms, abdomen, and genitalia, but rarely can be more generalized.
- Most lesions resolve spontaneously after several months to a few years, usually without scarring, but post-inflammatory hypopigmentation can persist for months in children with skin of color.

Differential Diagnosis

- Lichen planus
  - Lesions of lichen planus are usually larger, more violaceous, and with overlying Wickham's striae. They are also more pruritic.
  - Both lichen planus and lichen nitidus can occur in the same patient.
- Flat warts/verruca plana
  - Flat warts are usually larger, and browner in color. Tiny dotted hemorrhagic vessels may be seen on dermoscopy.
- Follicular eczema or lichen spinulosus
  - Lesions of follicular eczema or lichen spinulosus appear more evenly spaced as they occur around the hair follicles, as compared to more random spacing in lesions of lichen nitidus. There may be other signs of atopy.

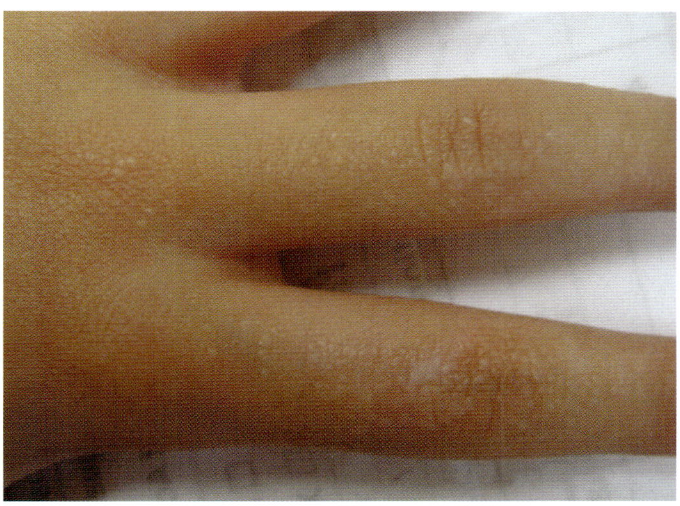

FIGURE 4-45. Lichen nitidus on the hand and finger of a Chinese boy, presenting with small, discrete, flat-topped papules, with some coalescence of the lesions.

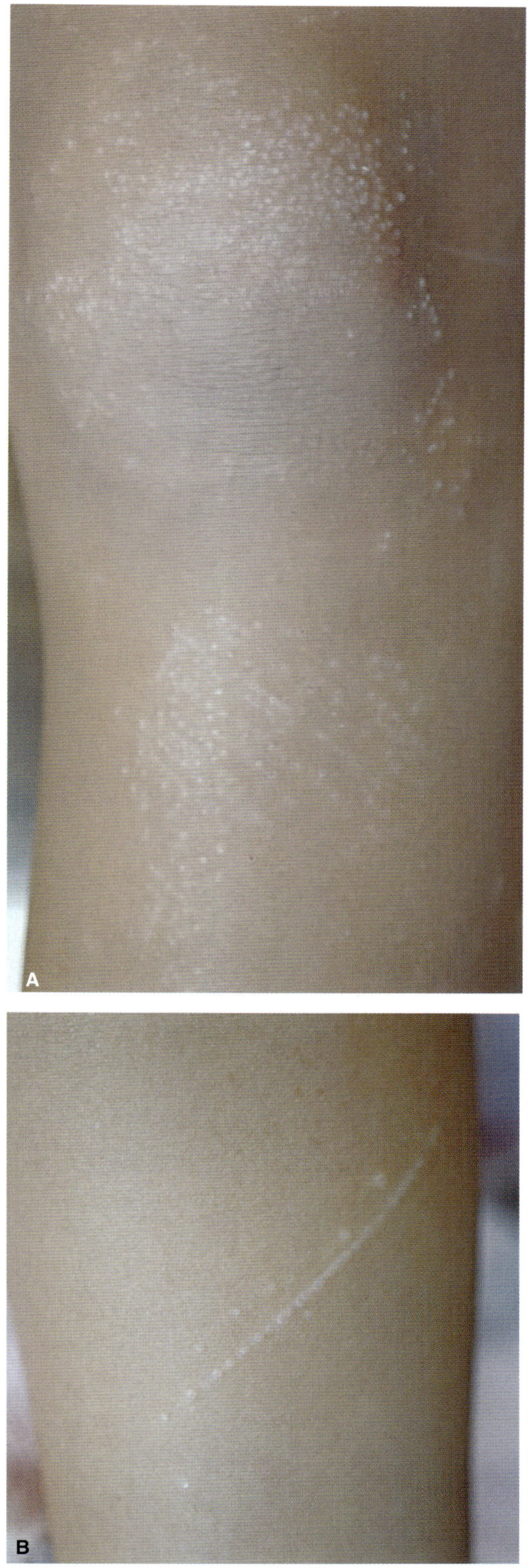

FIGURE 4-46A & 46B. Lichen nitidus on the legs of a 9-year-old Chinese girl, with randomly placed, pinpoint hypopigmented papules. Figure 4-46B shows Koebnerization with a linear lesion.

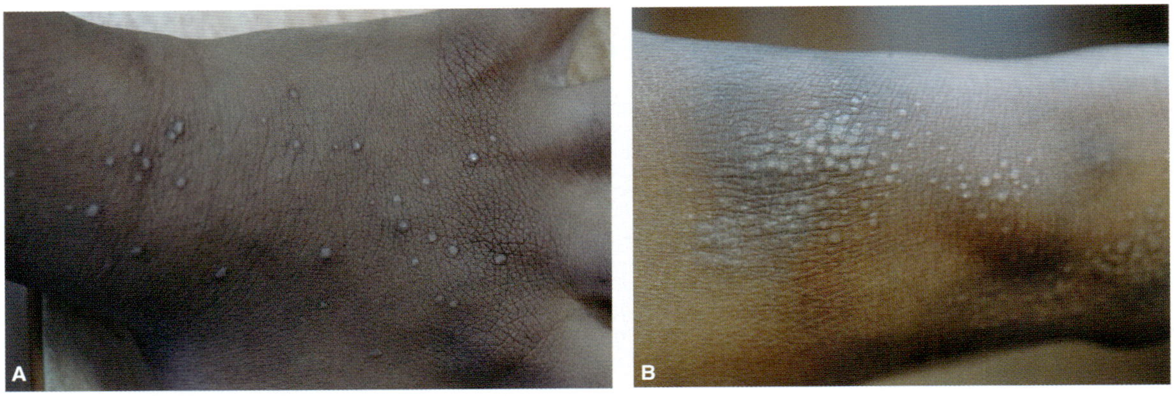

FIGURE 4-47A & 47B. Widespread lichen nitidus in a 5-year-old Indian girl, with discrete, flat-topped, hypopigmented papules on the hands and feet.

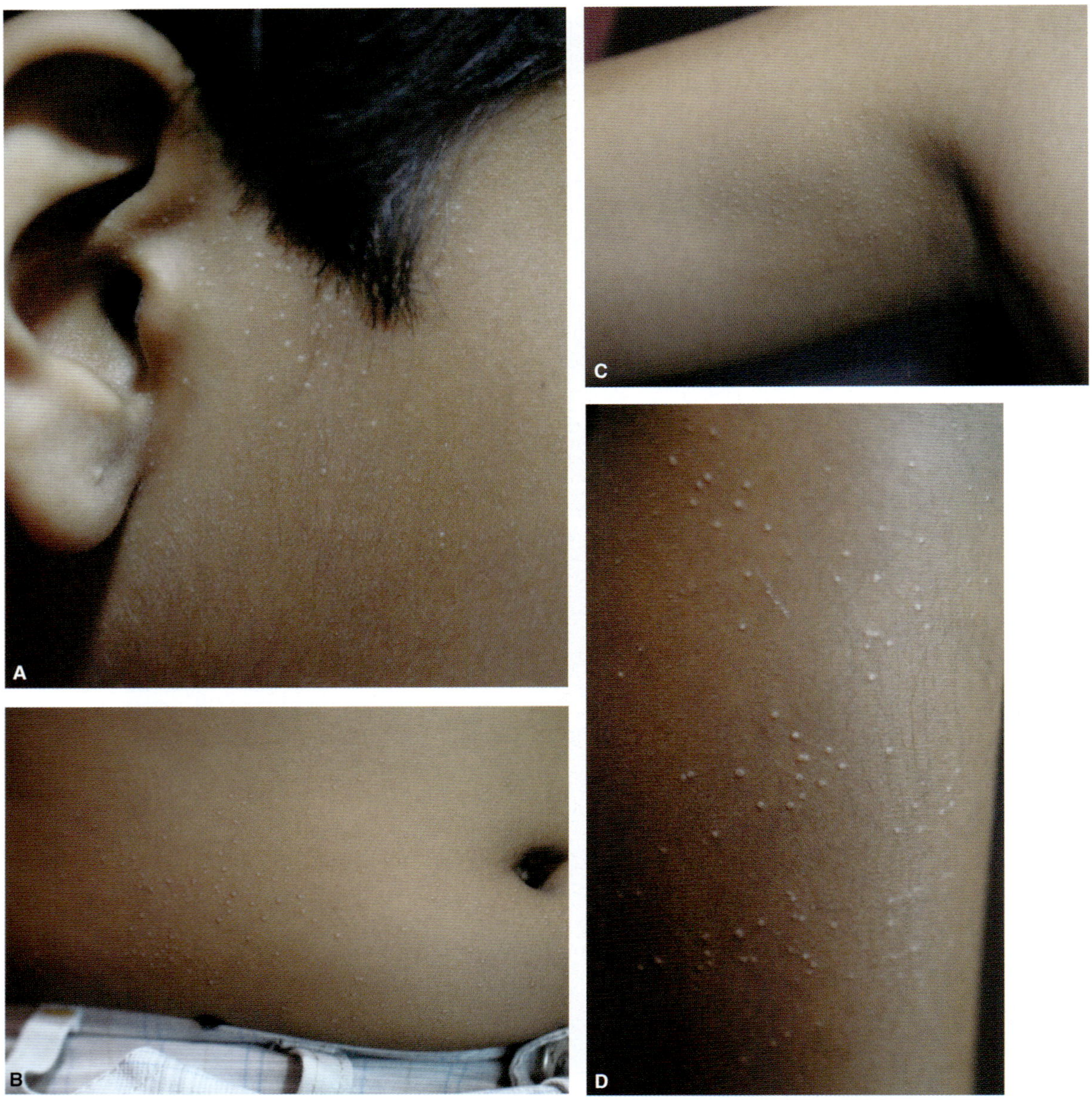

FIGURE 4-48A–48D. Widespread lichen nitidus in a 10-year-old Indian boy with Koebner's phenomenon demonstrated in Figure 4-48D, with linear lesions induced by scratching.

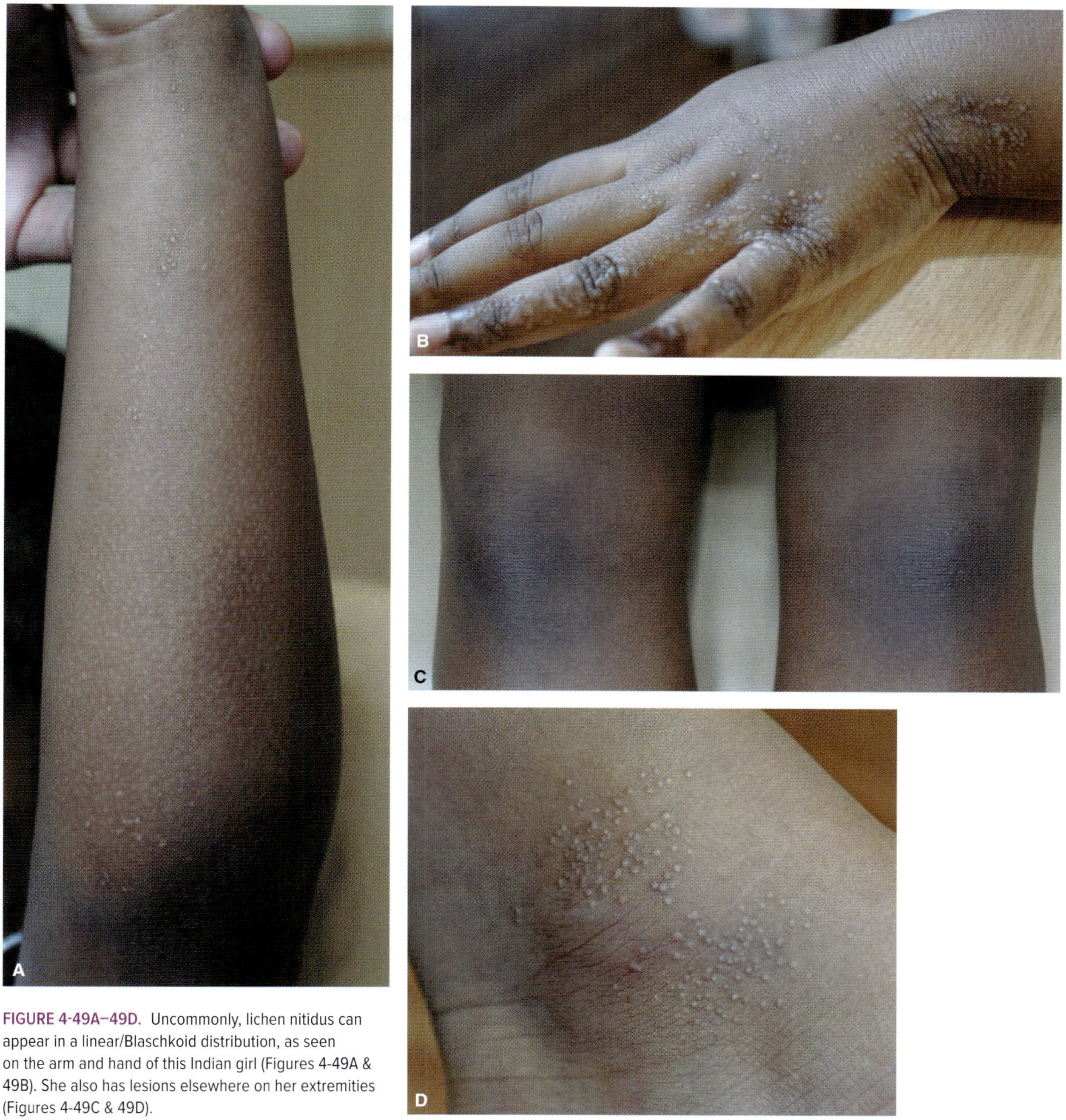

FIGURE 4-49A–49D. Uncommonly, lichen nitidus can appear in a linear/Blaschkoid distribution, as seen on the arm and hand of this Indian girl (Figures 4-49A & 49B). She also has lesions elsewhere on her extremities (Figures 4-49C & 49D).

- Keratosis pilaris
  - These appear as erythematous, skin-colored or light brown papules, typically over the outer aspects of bilateral upper arms, thighs, buttocks, and sides of the cheeks.

Investigations & Treatment

- Diagnosis is usually made clinically.
- Skin biopsies, if performed, show distinctive histological features of a lichenoid inflammatory infiltrate of lymphocytes, histiocytes, and occasionally giant cells, spanning 3 to 4 rete pegs, encircled by acanthosis of the surrounding epidermal rete ridges, resembling a hand clutching a ball.
- The condition is mostly self-limiting, and no active treatment is needed.
- Topical corticosteroids, topical calcineurin inhibitors, oral antihistamines, or narrow-band UVB therapy should be reserved for more symptomatic patients—those with a more prolonged clinical course, or with cosmetically disturbing or extensive lesions.

Pearls & Practical Tips

- To differentiate between lichen nitidus and lichen spinulosus, observe the spacing between individual lesions. In lichen spinulosus, this spacing is rather regular due to the regular spacing between hair follicles on the skin. However, as lichen nitidus affects the interfollicular epidermis, the spacing between lesions is more random.

- A lichen nitidus variant of polymorphous light eruption can be seen in children of Asian descent. Consider this if lesions are more prominent on sun-exposed sites.
- The appearance of these lesions can be quite distressing, especially to parents. As such, constant reassurance is important.

Bibliography

1. Chu J, Lam JM. Lichen nitidus. CMAJ 2014;186(18):E688.

LICHEN STRIATUS

Lichen striatus is an uncommon, self-limiting, inflammatory dermatosis in children. It has been reported in all races and appears to be more common in girls. Although the exact etiology is unknown, the distinct pattern of lichen striatus along the lines of Blaschko suggests its relation to cutaneous mosaicism, a result of postzygotic mutations that produce abnormal keratinocyte clones during early embryogenesis. These aberrant clones may remain silent until a triggering event causes immunologic intolerance and initiates an immune reaction.

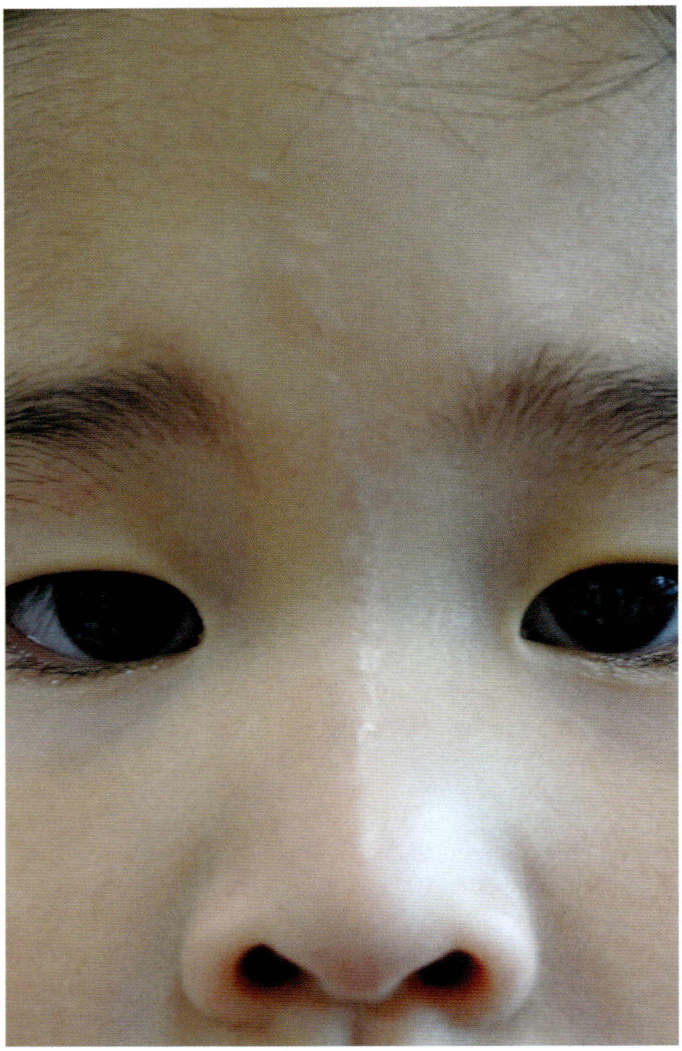

FIGURE 4-50. Lichen striatus on the forehead and nose of this 5-year-old Chinese girl presenting as a linear, pink-to-hypopigmented streak with a few erythematous papules.

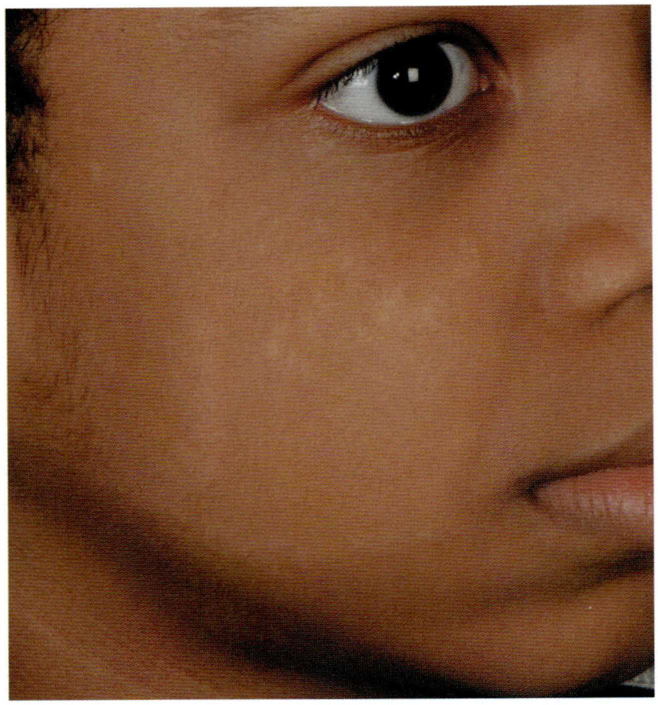

FIGURE 4-51. Lichen striatus on the right cheek of a 10-year-old Indian boy in a classical facial Blaschkoid distribution.

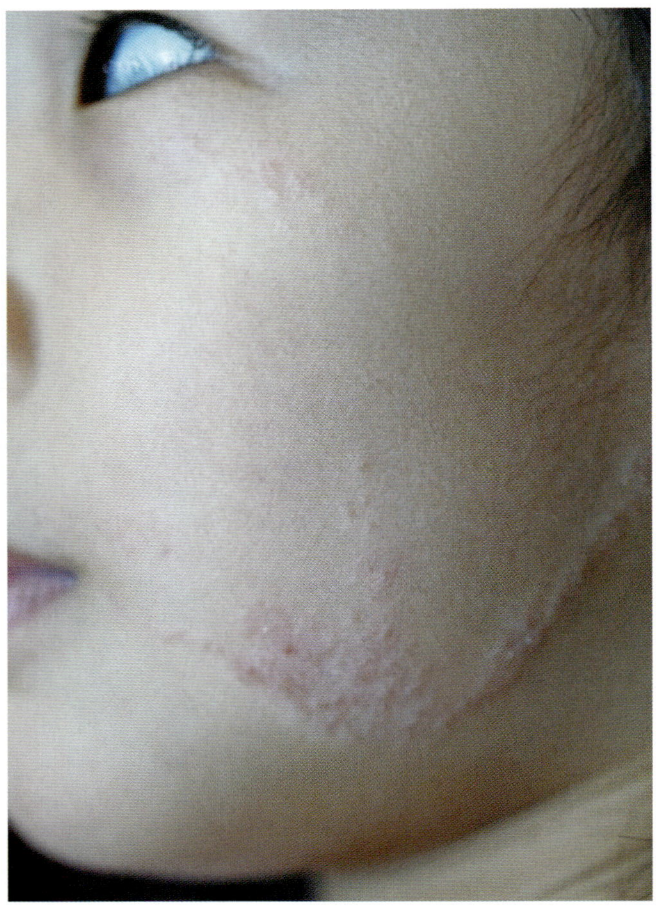

FIGURE 4-52. Lichen striatus on the left cheek of a 5-year-old Chinese girl, with more inflamed lesions.

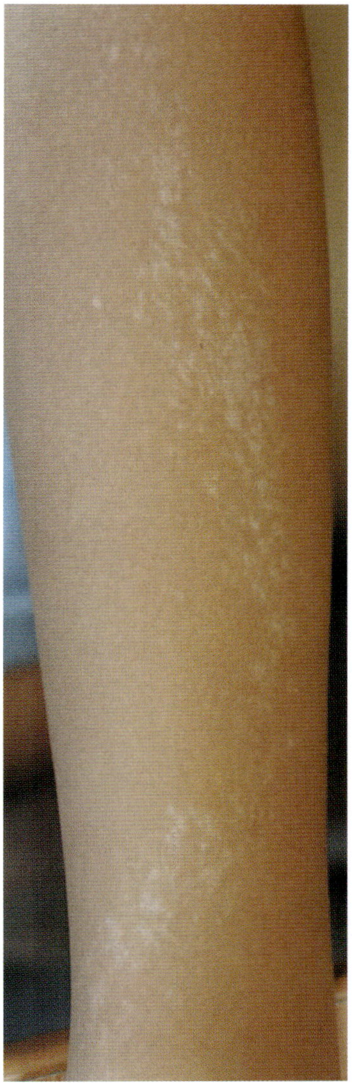

FIGURE 4-53. Lichen striatus presenting as a hypopigmented, linear patch on the forearm of a 5-year-old boy.

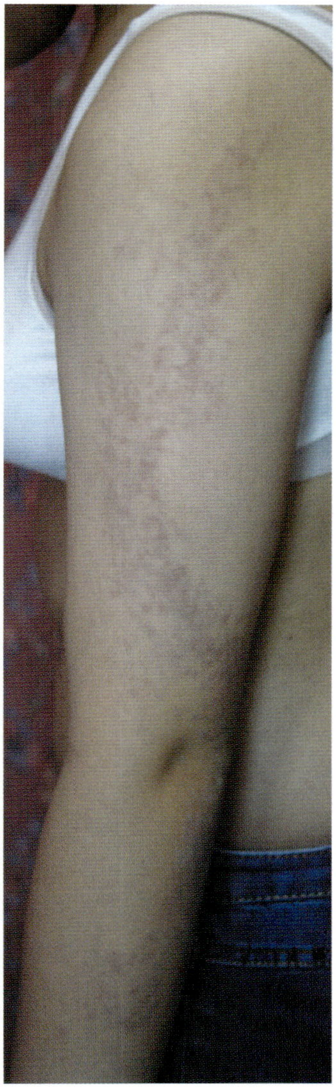

FIGURE 4-54. Lichen striatus on the arm of a 13-year-old Malay girl, presenting as an erythematous-to-violaceous, linear, Blaschkoid plaque.

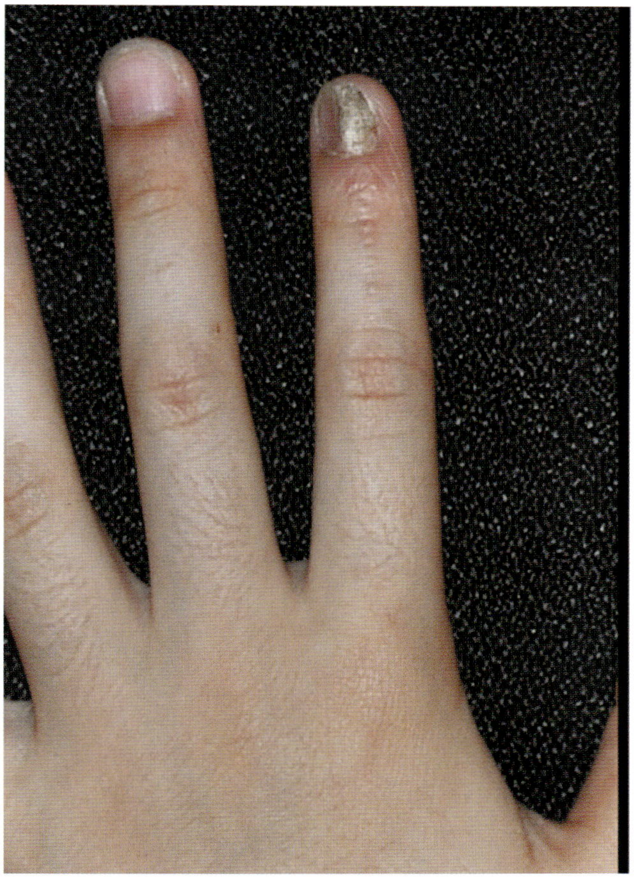

FIGURE 4-55. Lichen striatus on the dorsum of the hand extending onto the index finger with associated nail dystrophy.

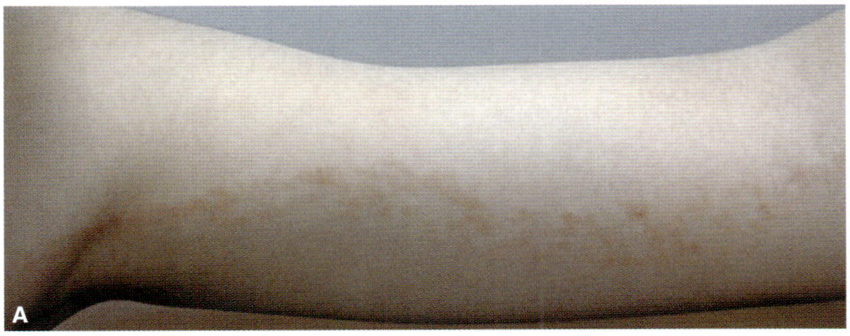

FIGURE 4-56A & 56B. Extensive lichen striatus affecting the left arm and chest of this young Chinese boy.

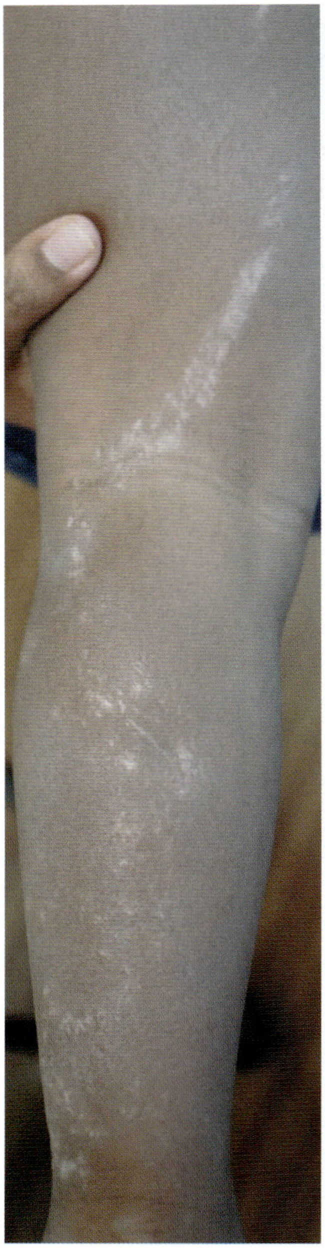

FIGURE 4-57. Lichen striatus on the arm and forearm of a 3-year-old Indian child. The hypopigmentation is very stark on the darker skin type.

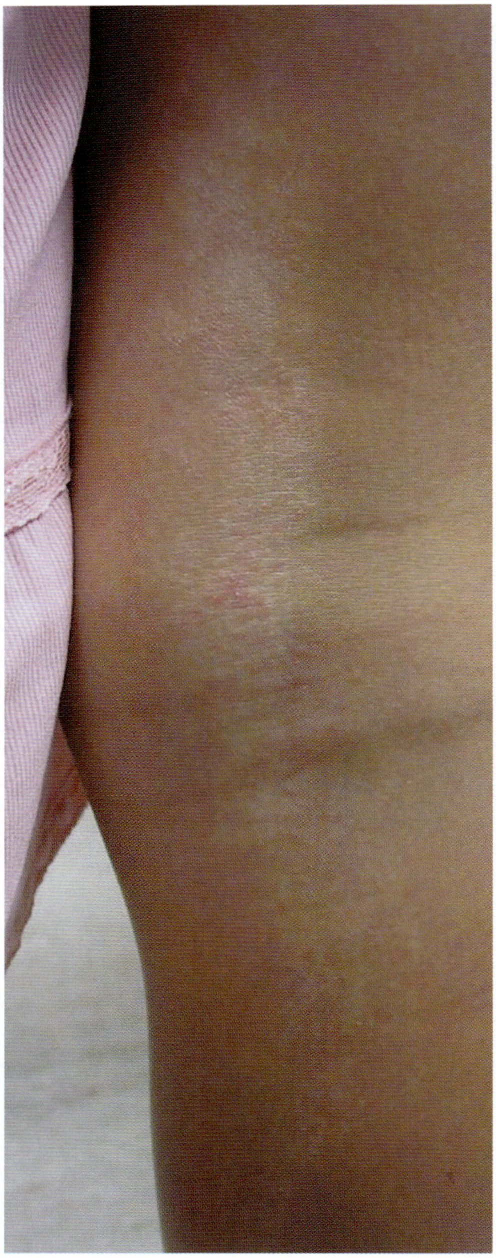

FIGURE 4-58. Lichen striatus on the posterior thigh and calf on a young Chinese girl, presenting with a pink, slightly scaly, linear plaque.

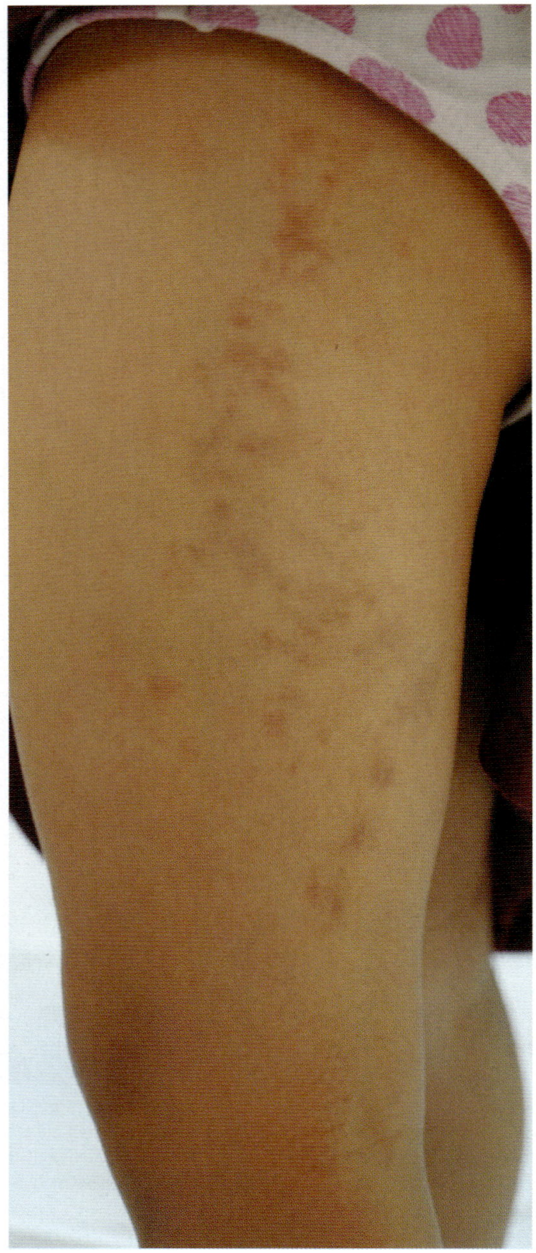

FIGURE 4-59. Hyperpigmented form of lichen striatus on the thigh of a 5-year-old Chinese girl. In this case, the lesions also do not form a continuous straight line but appear patchier.

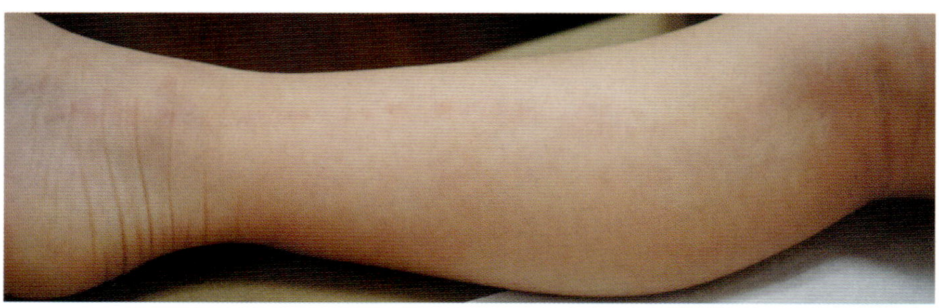

FIGURE 4-60. Lichen striatus on the calf and ankle of a 2-year-old Chinese girl.

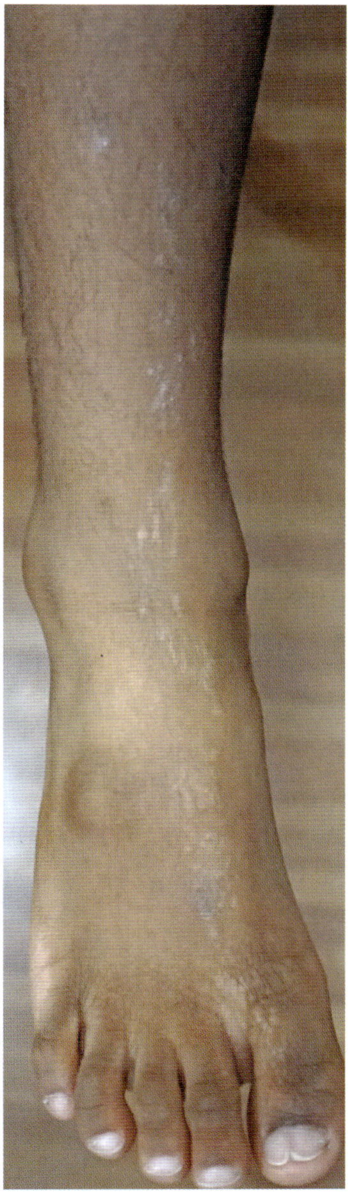

FIGURE 4-61. Lichen striatus on the shin and dorsum of the foot, extending onto the big toe of this 5-year-old Indian boy. Note the mild nail involvement with nicking of the distal nail plate.

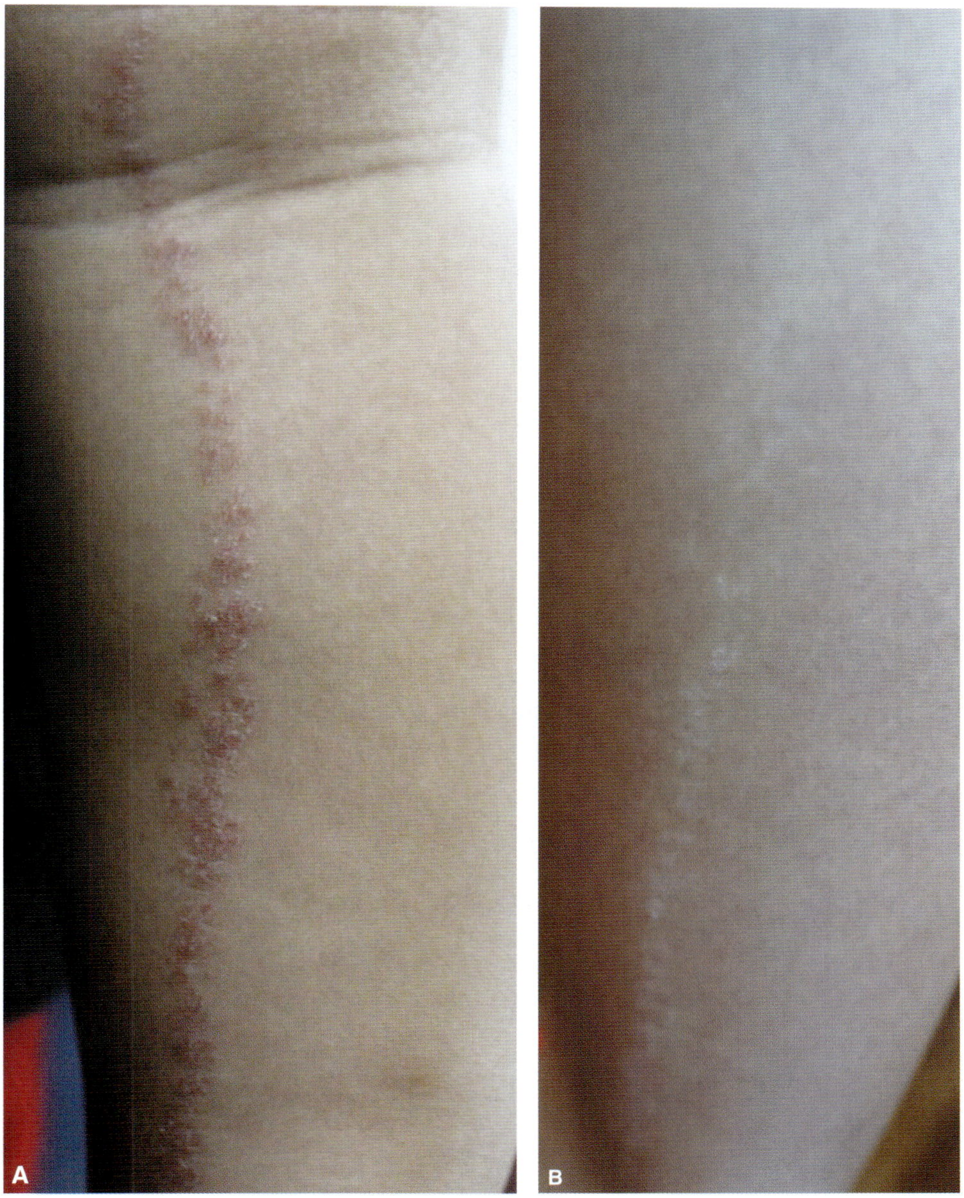

FIGURE 4-62A & 62B. Lichen striatus on the back of the calf of a 1-year-old child, presenting as a pink, flat-topped, slightly scaly, linear plaque. Figure 62B shows the same child at 5 years of age, with the same lesion appearing hypopigmented and flat.

Clinical Features

- Lichen striatus primarily affects children between 5 and 15 years of age.
- It is usually asymptomatic but may be mildly pruritic, especially in children with underlying atopic dermatitis.
- Clinically, it is characterized by small discrete pink flat-topped papules which can be smooth or scaly, that coalesce over a few weeks to form a slightly scaly, irregular band in a linear or blaschkoid pattern, usually 2 mm to 2 cm in width. The color can range from pink to red, skin-colored, or hypopigmented in dark-skinned individuals.
- It usually starts on a proximal limb and extends distally in a continuous or interrupted pattern. The length can vary from only a few centimeters to, occasionally, the entire length of the limb.
- Spontaneous resolution occurs within 6 to 12 months. However, post-inflammatory hypo- or hyperpigmentation may persist for several months, or sometimes years.
- Nails may be affected and become thick, ridged, and split or fall off.

Differential Diagnosis

- Inflammatory linear verrucous epidermal nevus (ILVEN)
  - Lesions of ILVEN can appear in the same age group as lichen striatus. The lesions are more verrucous and inflamed and persist longer than lichen striatus. Pruritus is also more prominent.
- Linear lichen planus (LP)
  - The lesions of LP are more pruritic, violaceous, with overlying Wickham striae. Other lesions of LP may or may not be present elsewhere.
- Lichen nitidus
  - Lichen nitidus appears as multiple asymptomatic, discrete, non-follicular, shiny skin-colored papules. Sometimes lesions appear in a linear configuration due to Koebner phenomenon.
- Linear psoriasis
  - This is characterized by well-demarcated erythematous plaques covered with silvery-white scales distributed in a linear manner. Other classical lesions of psoriasis may or may not be present elsewhere.
- Linear porokeratosis
  - This is rare in childhood and is characterized by small hyperpigmented erythematous, sometimes atrophic plaques with raised borders, arranged in a linear pattern.

Investigations & Treatment

- The diagnosis is usually made clinically.
- If performed, a skin biopsy will show interface and lichenoid dermatitis with a superficial and often deep inflammatory infiltrate in the dermis.
- As the condition is self-limiting and asymptomatic, treatment is usually not necessary apart from reassurance.
- If pruritus is present, topical corticosteroids or topical calcineurin inhibitors, with moisturizers will be helpful.

Pearls & Practical Tips

- Higher vigilance is needed to identify facial, neck, and truncal lichen striatus due to the complexity of Blaschkoid lines in these areas. On the face, they take on an hourglass-like pattern, converging on the nasal root and intersecting at an angle of almost 90 degrees. There is a spiral pattern on the scalp, a V-shaped pattern on the upper spine, an S-shaped pattern on the abdomen, and a U-shaped pattern on each side of the chest.
- Current treatment options will not change the natural history of lichen striatus, and parents have to be informed of this, especially if the child is seen early in the disease course.
- Lichen striatus can occur concomitantly with lichen nitidus or lichen planus in rare patients.

Bibliography

1. Charifa A, Jamil RT, Ramphul K. Lichen Striatus. Treasure Island (FL): StatPearls Publishing; 2020 Jan.

5

Acneiform Disorders

ACNE

Acne vulgaris is one of the most common dermatologic complaints in adolescents of all skin types. Although acne is not a unique condition in Asian children and adolescents, special considerations apply when treating this group. Delayed or suboptimal treatment of acne can lead to cosmetically significant complications.

Clinical Features

- The clinical features of acne appear relatively similar in all skin types. However, in patients of darker skin color, redness caused by inflammation may be masked.
- Although more common in adolescents, acne can occur at all ages. However, presentation in younger age groups is less common.
- Neonatal acne
  - See Chapter 2 (Neonatal dermatoses)
- Infantile acne
  - An uncommon condition, infantile acne begins between 3 and 6 months of age due to elevated levels of androgens produced by immature adrenal glands in girls, and immature adrenal glands and testes in boys.
  - Improvement of acne is seen when androgen levels fall by 1 to 2 years of age.
- Mid-childhood acne
  - Rare, and defined as acne occurring in children 1 to 7 years of age.
  - Evaluation for endocrine abnormalities and precocious puberty is essential.
- Preadolescent acne
  - Defined as acne occurring during preadolescent ages of 7 to 11 years.
  - Early acne presents as comedones predominantly in the T-zone, with occasional inflammatory papules.
  - Polycystic ovarian syndrome (PCOS) needs to be excluded if acne in this age group is severe or is recalcitrant to treatment.
- Adolescent acne
  - Classic acne lesions occur as open (blackheads) and closed (whiteheads) comedones, inflammatory papules, and pustules. Cysts and nodules may be seen with more severe disease.
  - The forehead is often the earliest site affected, followed by the cheeks, nose, and jawline.
  - Truncal acne is also common and appears on the upper chest and back.
  - Atrophic scars are common, especially after more severe acne. Hypertrophic scars and keloids are less common, but can occur especially over the jawline, shoulders, upper chest, and back.

Differential Diagnoses

- Periorificial dermatitis
  - Periorificial dermatitis is characterized by small, grouped, erythematous papules in a perioral, perinasal, or periorbital distribution.

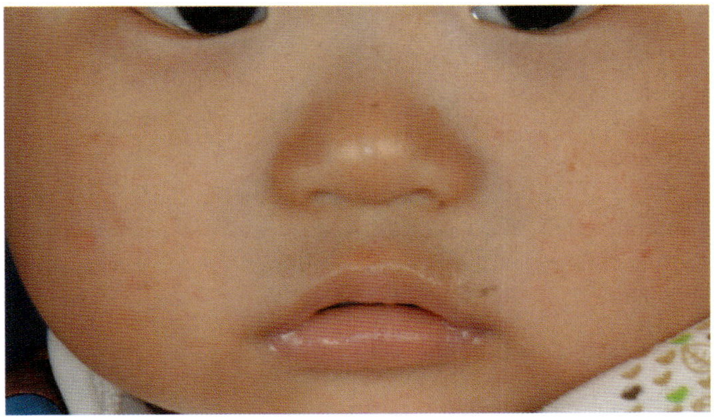

FIGURE 5-1. Mild infantile acne presenting mainly with closed comedones in a Chinese male infant. He had no other signs of hyperandrogenism, and hormonal evaluation was normal.

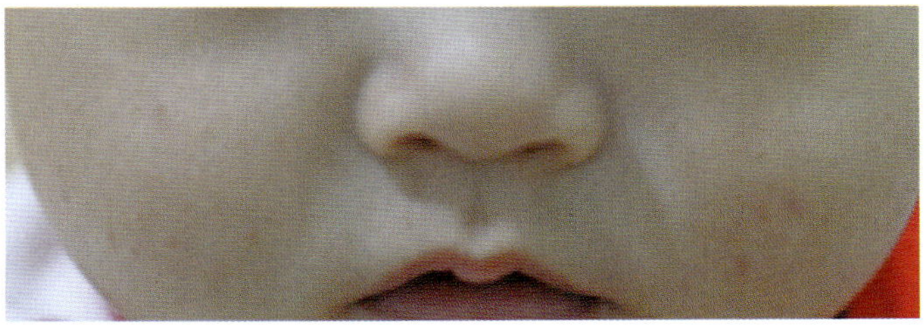

FIGURE 5-2. Chinese male infant with infantile acne presenting with comedones on the cheeks.

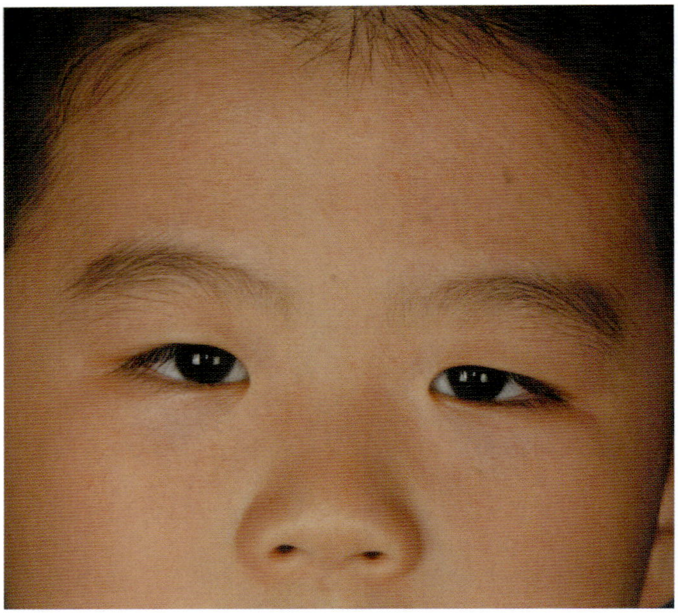

FIGURE 5-3. Mild childhood acne in a 7-year-old Chinese boy, with comedones mostly on the forehead and cheeks. There were no other signs of puberty in the child.

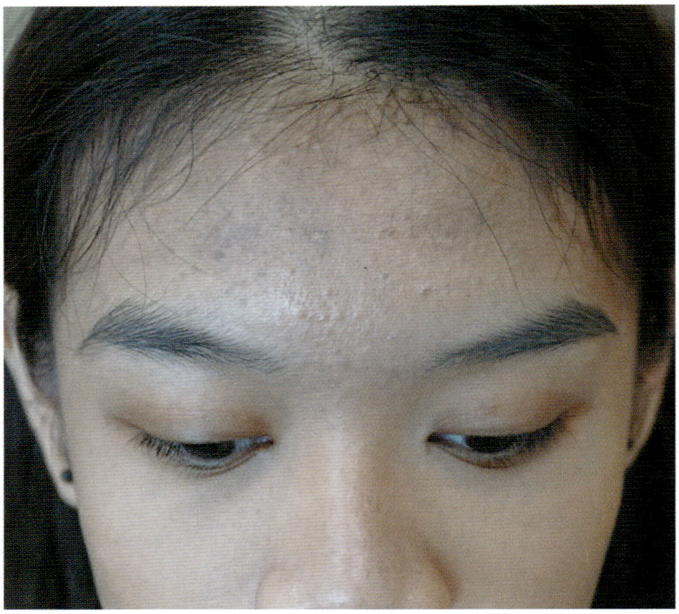

FIGURE 5-4. Comedones, both open and closed, on the forehead and nose of a 15-year-old Malay female.

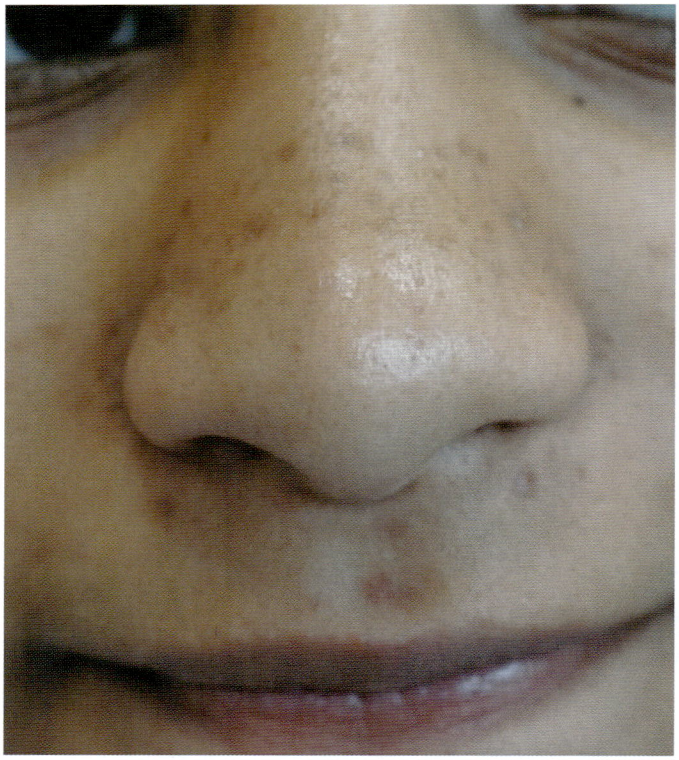

FIGURE 5-5. Open and closed comedones on the nose of an Indian teenager, with residual post-inflammatory hyperpigmentation.

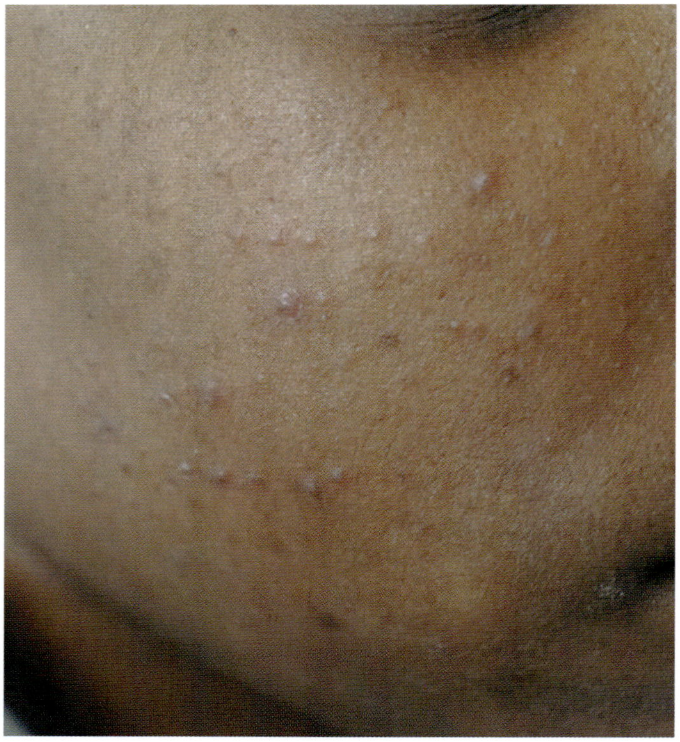

FIGURE 5-6. Predominantly comedonal acne with a few small papules on the cheek of this Indian male.

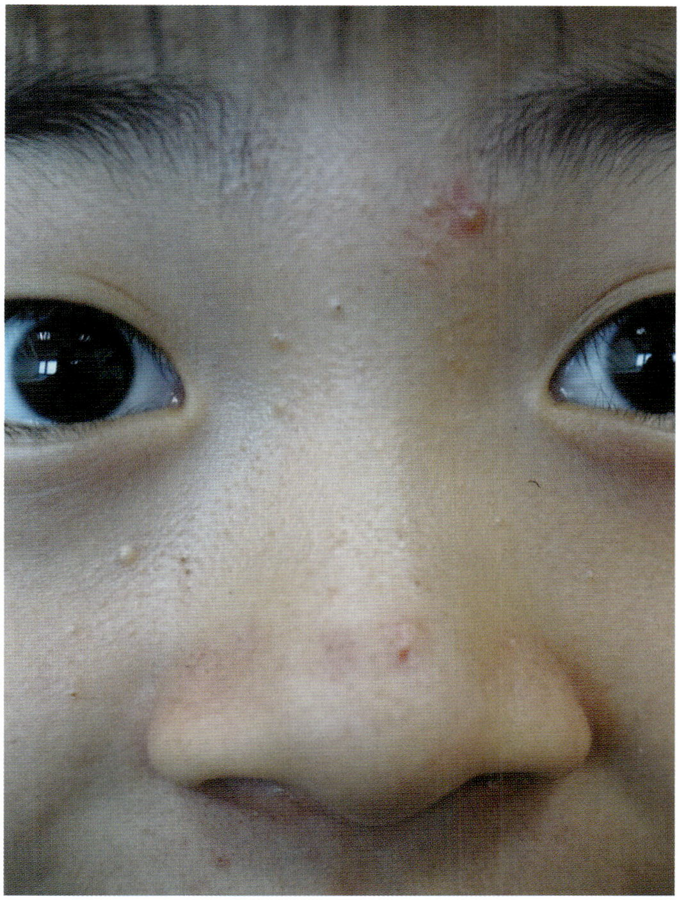

FIGURE 5-7. Several open and closed comedones, with few inflammatory papules on the face of a 9-year-old Chinese child.

- Unlike acne, the papules seen in periorificial dermatitis tend to appear more monomorphic, and comedones are not seen.
- Rosacea
  - Rosacea is rare in children and appears as erythema, telangiectasias, and papules or pustules on the central face.
  - Acne vulgaris is distinguished from acne rosacea by the presence of comedones and the absence of telangiectasias.
- Seborrheic dermatitis
  - Seborrheic dermatitis is another common condition that often has its onset in adolescence. Some patients may present concomitantly with acne and seborrheic dermatitis.
  - It presents with erythematous patches and plaques with overlying yellowish scaling. It commonly occurs over the eyebrows and nasolabial folds.

Investigations & Treatment

- Acne is a clinical diagnosis, and no investigations are necessary unless if other diagnoses need to be excluded.
- If underlying hyperandrogenism is suspected, an endocrine evaluation is essential.

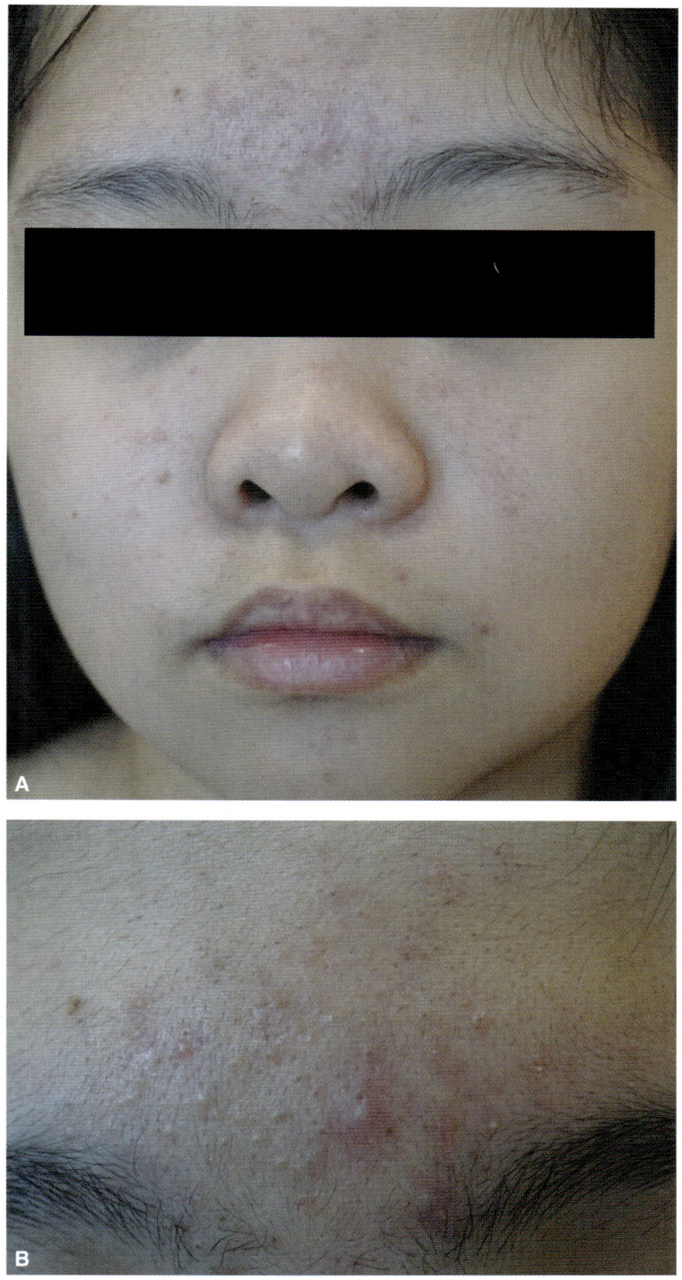

FIGURE 5-8A & 8B. Mild-to-moderate inflammatory acne on the face and cheeks of a Chinese adolescent female, with open and closed comedones, and several, small papules.

- Treatment should be customized according to severity and without inducing excessive irritation and other side effects.
- Treatment of acne should optimally be instituted early, to prevent scarring and dyspigmentation. After successful control, maintenance therapy is important to prevent or minimize recurrence. For most patients, acne will improve or resolve in the late teenage years or in early twenties.

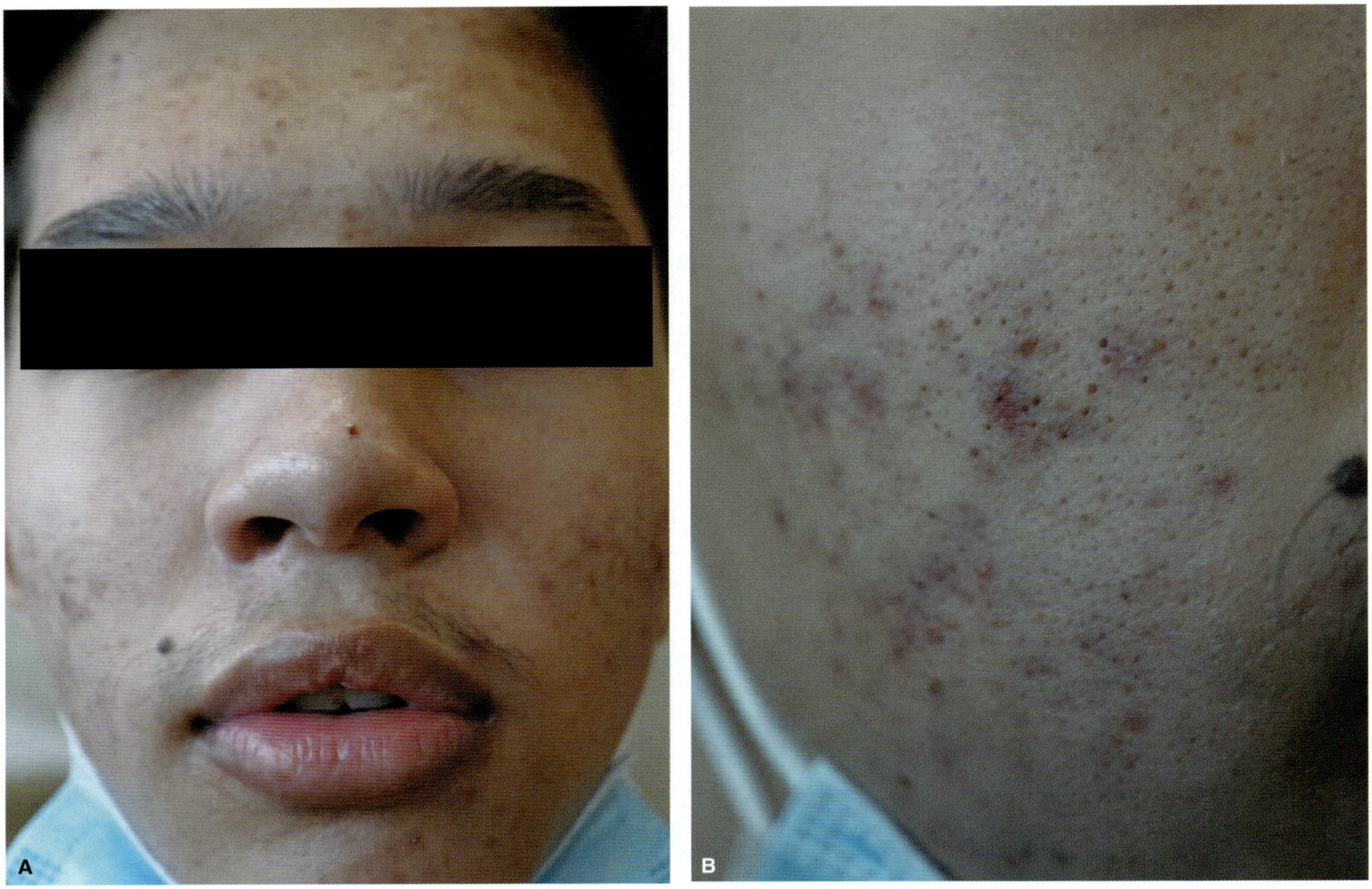

FIGURE 5-9A & 9B. Moderate inflammatory acne with erythematous papules and multiple open comedones on the cheeks of a darker-skinned Chinese adolescent male.

- Non-pharmacologic treatment
  - Gentle skin cleansing twice daily using oil-free moisturizers.
  - Avoidance of greasy emollients, hair styling products, and comedogenic cosmetic products over affected areas.
- Topical therapies
  - **Benzoyl peroxide (BPO)** is an effective bactericidal, keratolytic, and anti-inflammatory agent, and is effective in reducing inflammatory and non-inflammatory lesions. Its use has not been associated with the development of bacterial resistance. Various concentrations are available (e.g., 2.5%, 5%, and 10%). Start with the lowest concentration and titrate to higher concentrations according to clinical response. Adverse effects include erythema, dryness, flaking, and burning, but these are usually mild and transient.
  - **Topical retinoids** are synthetic derivatives of vitamin A (retinol). They have anticomedogenic, comedolytic, and anti-inflammatory properties. Retinoids reduce and prevent the development of micro-comedones and clear existing comedones. Retinoids should be applied to all acne-prone areas, even without the presence of active lesions. Common topical retinoids include tretinoin, adapalene, isotretinoin, and tazarotene. Common side effects include burning, stinging, dryness, and scaling. Retinoids should be avoided in pregnant females or those planning pregnancy.
  - **Topical antibiotics**, including topical clindamycin and erythromycin, are effective in treating mild-to-moderate inflammatory acne. However, topical antibiotics as monotherapy should be avoided, to prevent bacterial resistance.
  - **Topical azelaic acid** has antimicrobial, anti-inflammatory, and comedolytic effects. Side effects are mild and transient, which include pruritus, burning, stinging, and tingling.
  - **Topical salicylic acid** is a keratolytic agent that has antimicrobial and comedolytic properties and is effective for mild-to-moderate acne. Side effects include pruritus, tingling, desquamation, and erythema.
  - **Topical fixed combinations** (preparations with topical benzoyl peroxide, retinoids, or antibiotics) are more effective than any agent alone. There is also better compliance, as these are recommended for once-daily use. However, there is a higher risk of irritant reactions. Available combinations include clindamycin/BPO, adapalene/BPO, erythromycin/BPO, and clindamycin/tretinoin.

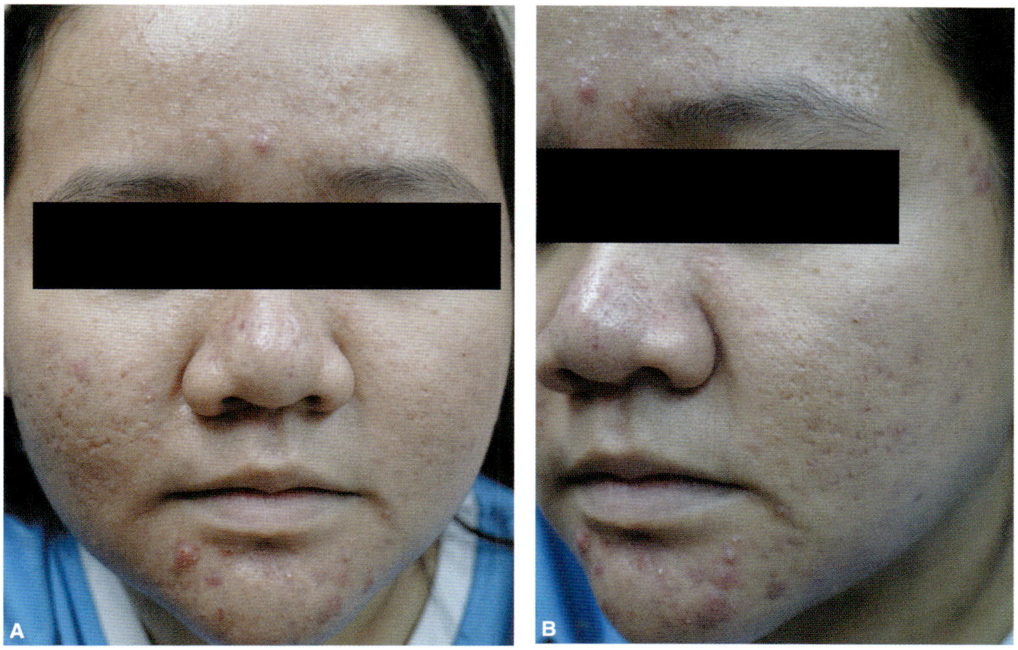

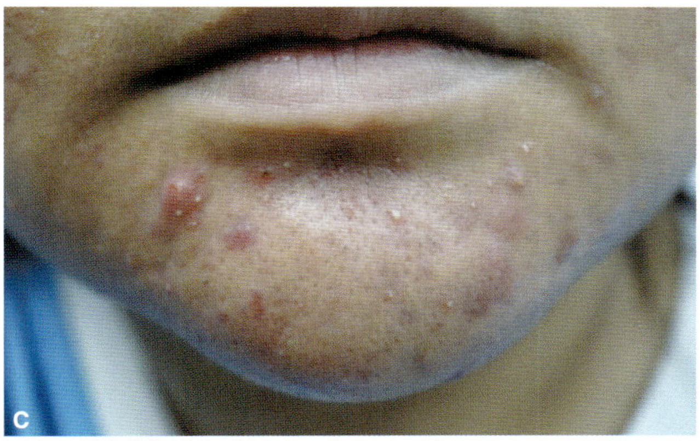

FIGURE 5-10A–10C. Severe inflammatory acne with scarring. There are multiple comedones, pustules, papules, and scattered nodules with multiple ice-pick scars, especially over the cheeks and chin area.

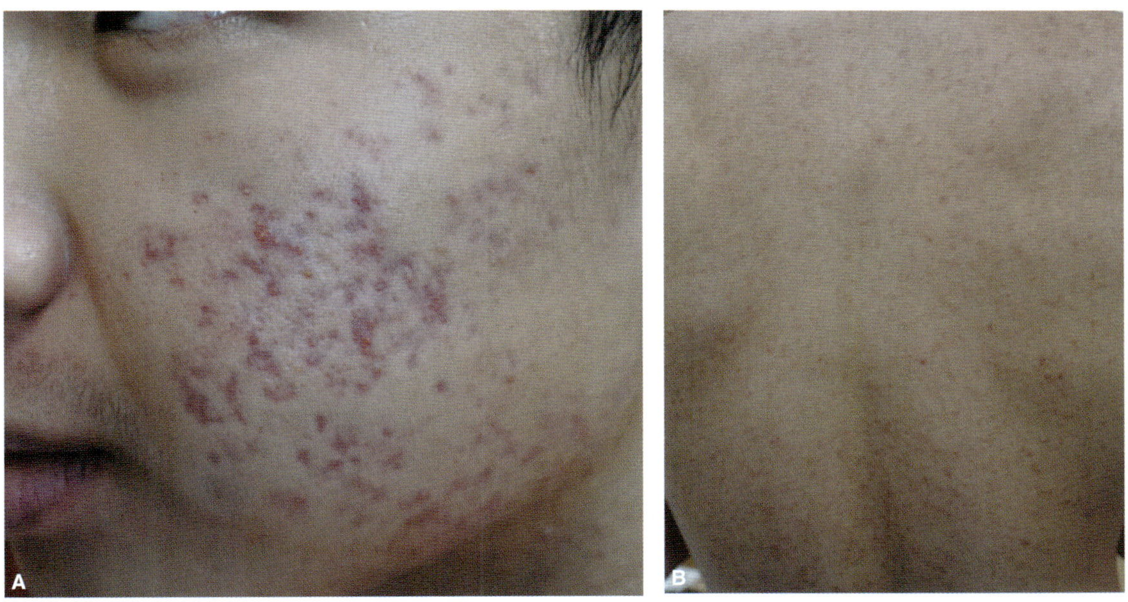

FIGURE 5-11A & 11B. Severe inflammatory acne with red atrophic scars on the cheeks of this Malay teenage boy. There is concomitant truncal acne with post-inflammatory hyperpigmentation (Figure 5-10B).

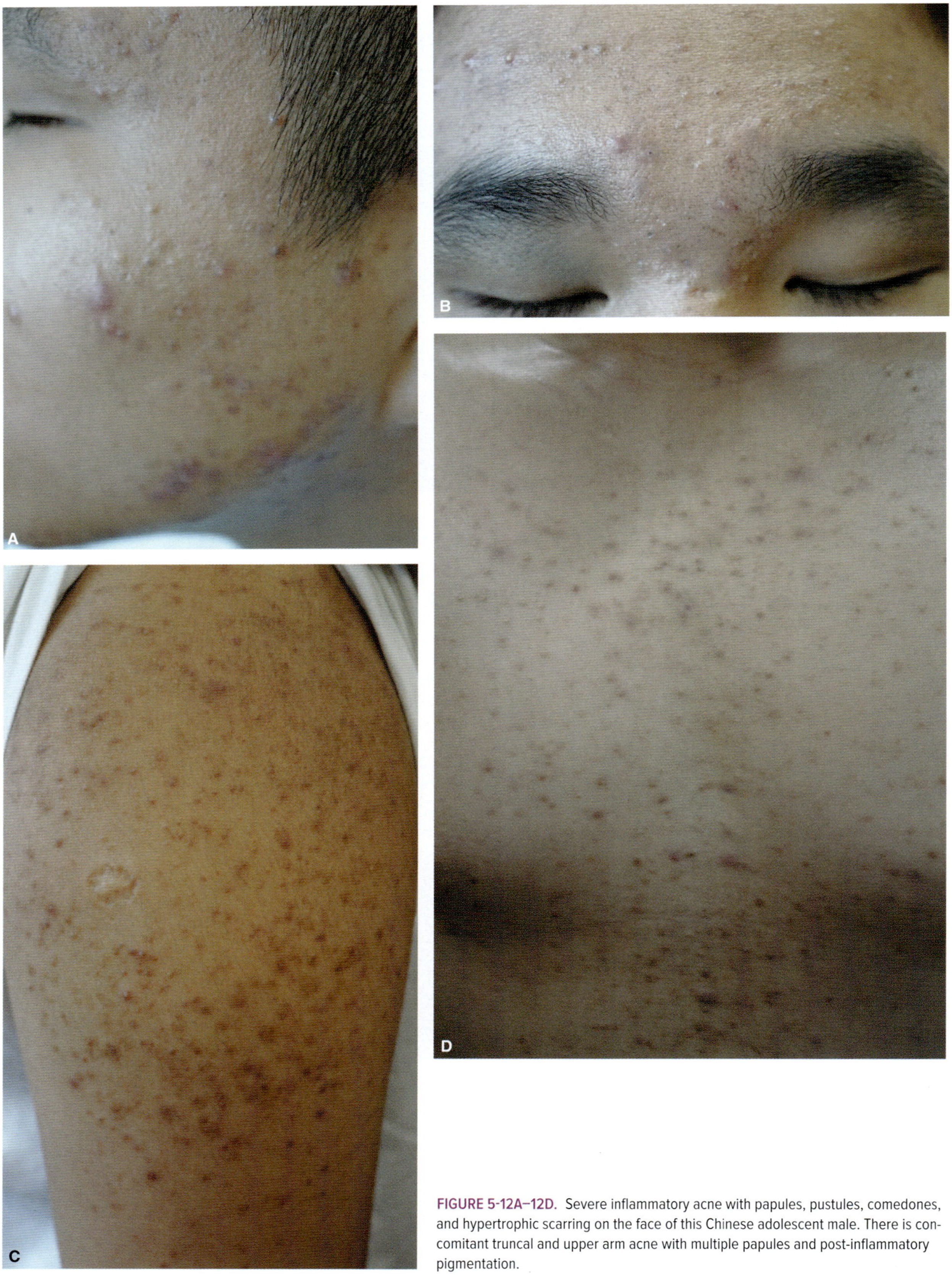

FIGURE 5-12A–12D. Severe inflammatory acne with papules, pustules, comedones, and hypertrophic scarring on the face of this Chinese adolescent male. There is concomitant truncal and upper arm acne with multiple papules and post-inflammatory pigmentation.

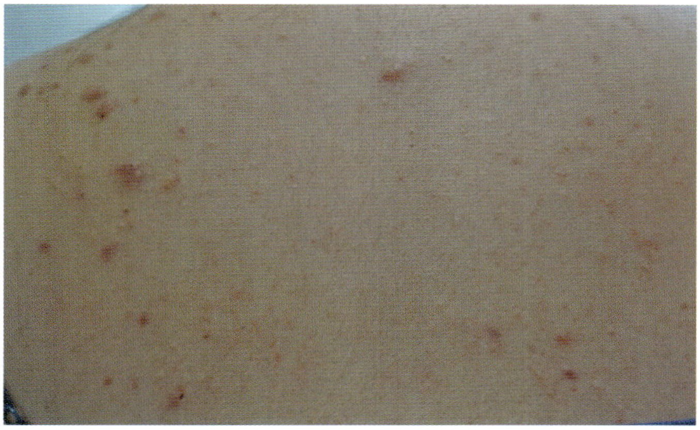

FIGURE 5-13. Back acne with inflammatory papules and nodules, in addition to comedones and hypertrophic scarring, on a Chinese adolescent female.

- Systemic treatments
  - **Oral antibiotics** are widely used for moderate-to-severe acne. Oral tetracyclines (doxycycline, tetracycline, minocycline) and macrolides (erythromycin, azithromycin) are the most commonly used. The tetracyclines are contraindicated in children less than 8 years of age. The effects of oral antibiotics take 6 to 8 weeks, and treatment is usually prolonged beyond 6 months. Prolonged use of antibiotics may be associated with bacterial resistance. Side effects are usually mild and tolerable. However, more severe side effects, such as lupus erythematosus with minocycline, have been reported and should be monitored.

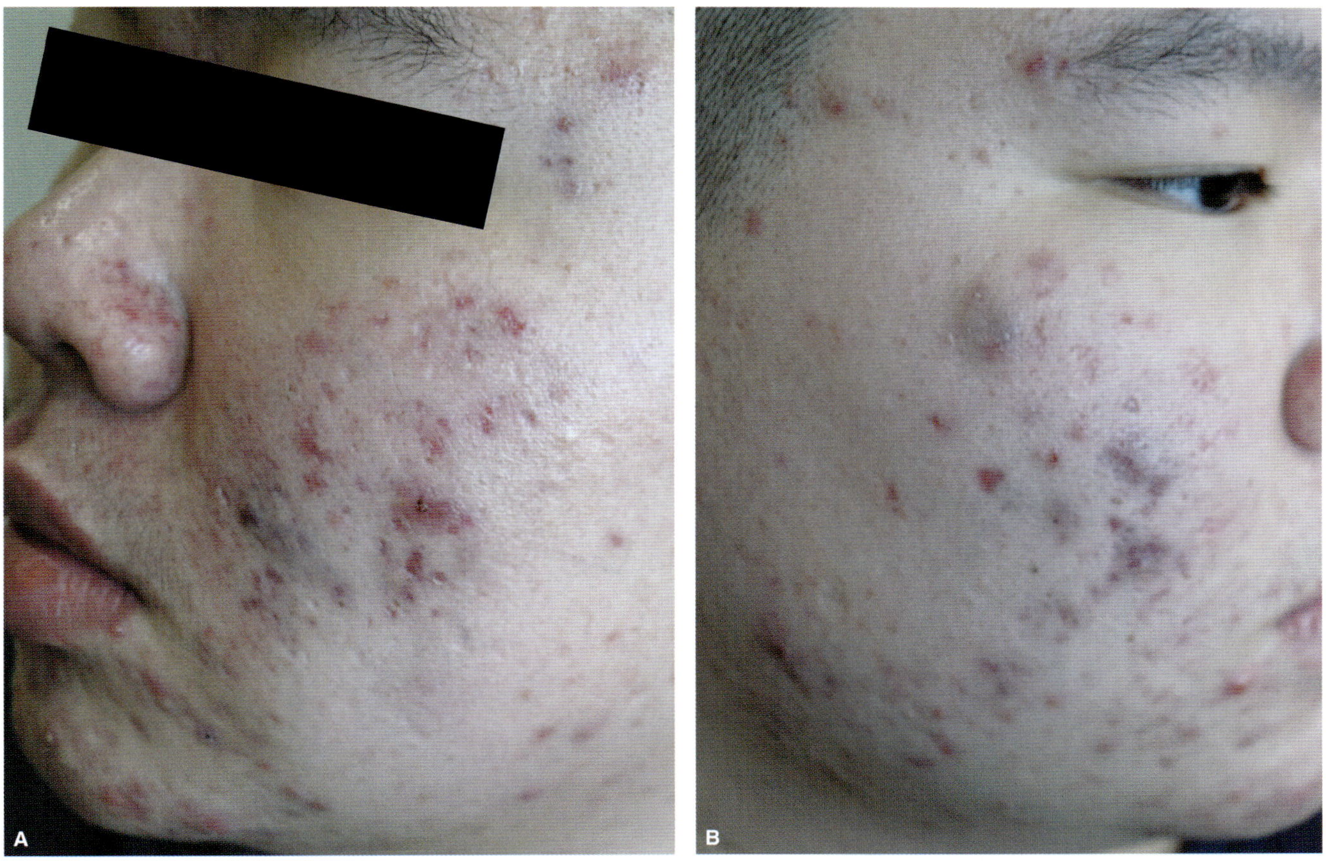

FIGURE 5-14A & 14B. Nodulocystic acne in this 16-year-old Chinese male, presenting with nodules and cysts with severe scarring and dyspigmentation.

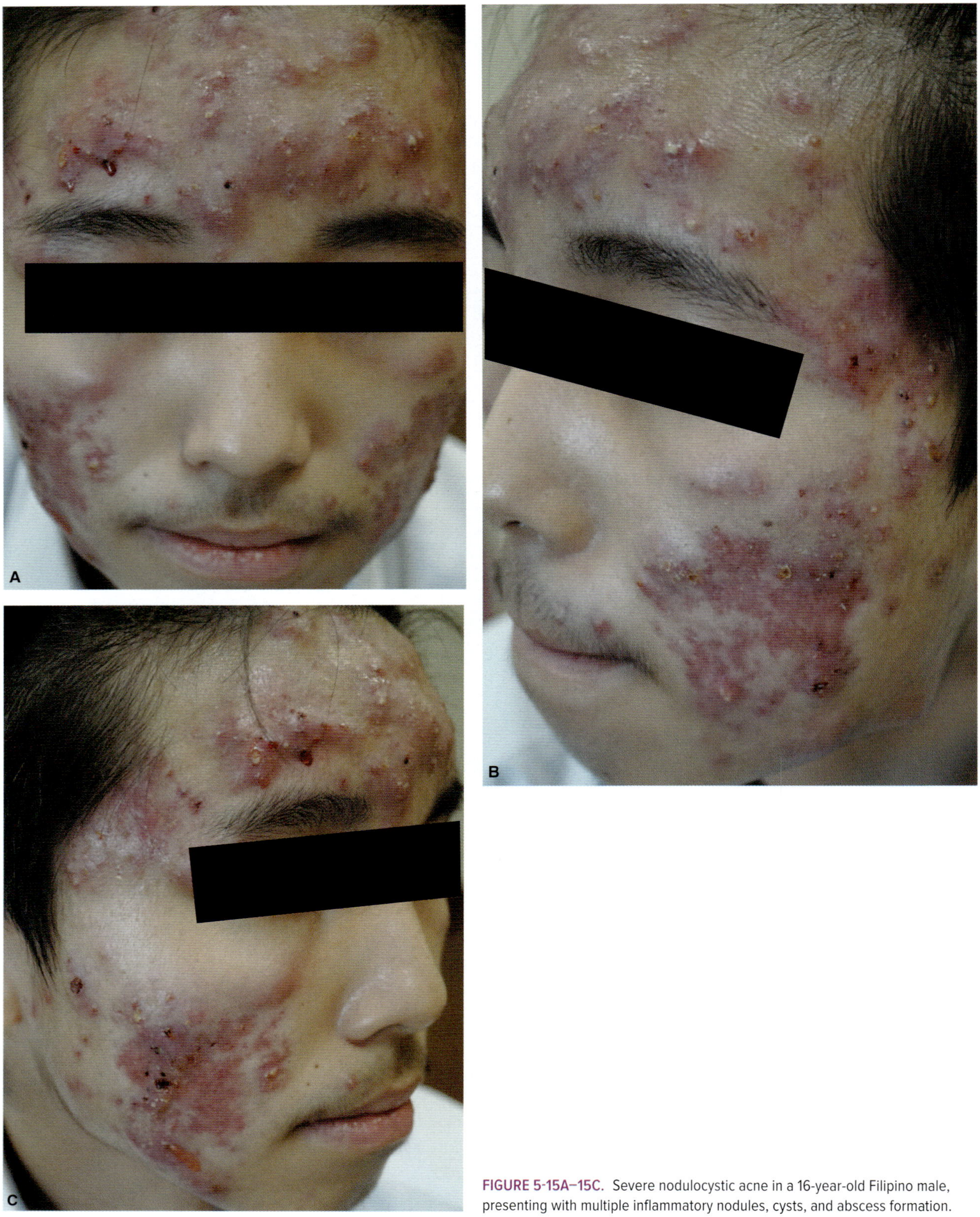

FIGURE 5-15A–15C. Severe nodulocystic acne in a 16-year-old Filipino male, presenting with multiple inflammatory nodules, cysts, and abscess formation.

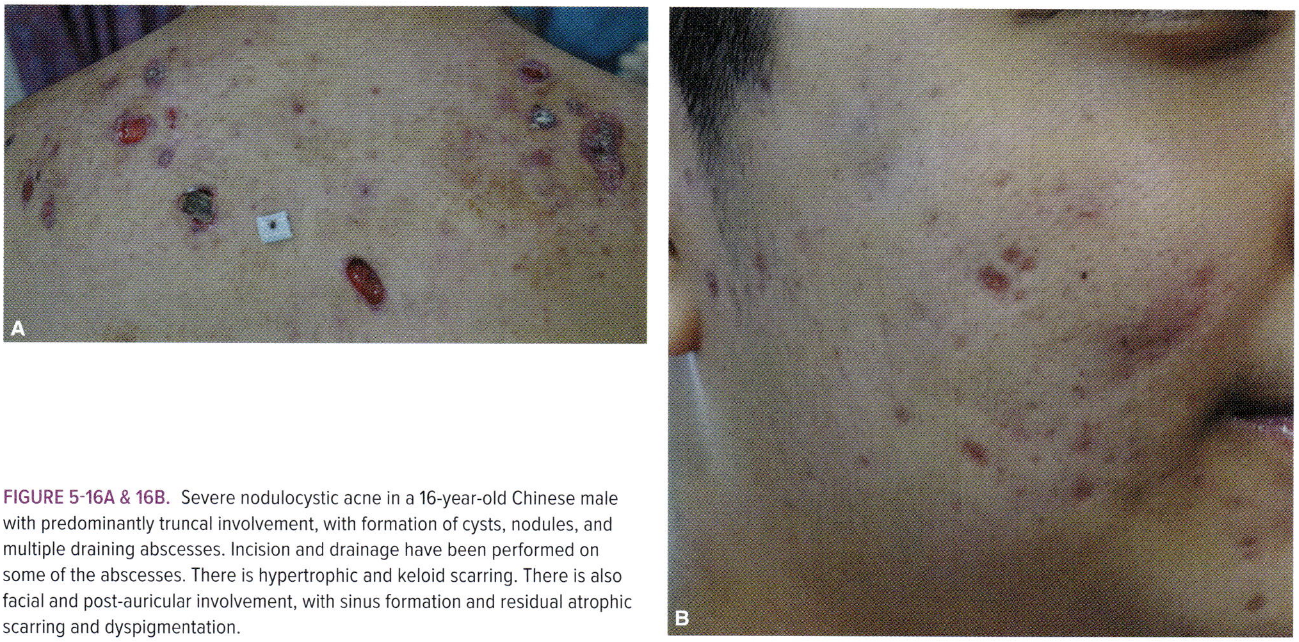

FIGURE 5-16A & 16B. Severe nodulocystic acne in a 16-year-old Chinese male with predominantly truncal involvement, with formation of cysts, nodules, and multiple draining abscesses. Incision and drainage have been performed on some of the abscesses. There is hypertrophic and keloid scarring. There is also facial and post-auricular involvement, with sinus formation and residual atrophic scarring and dyspigmentation.

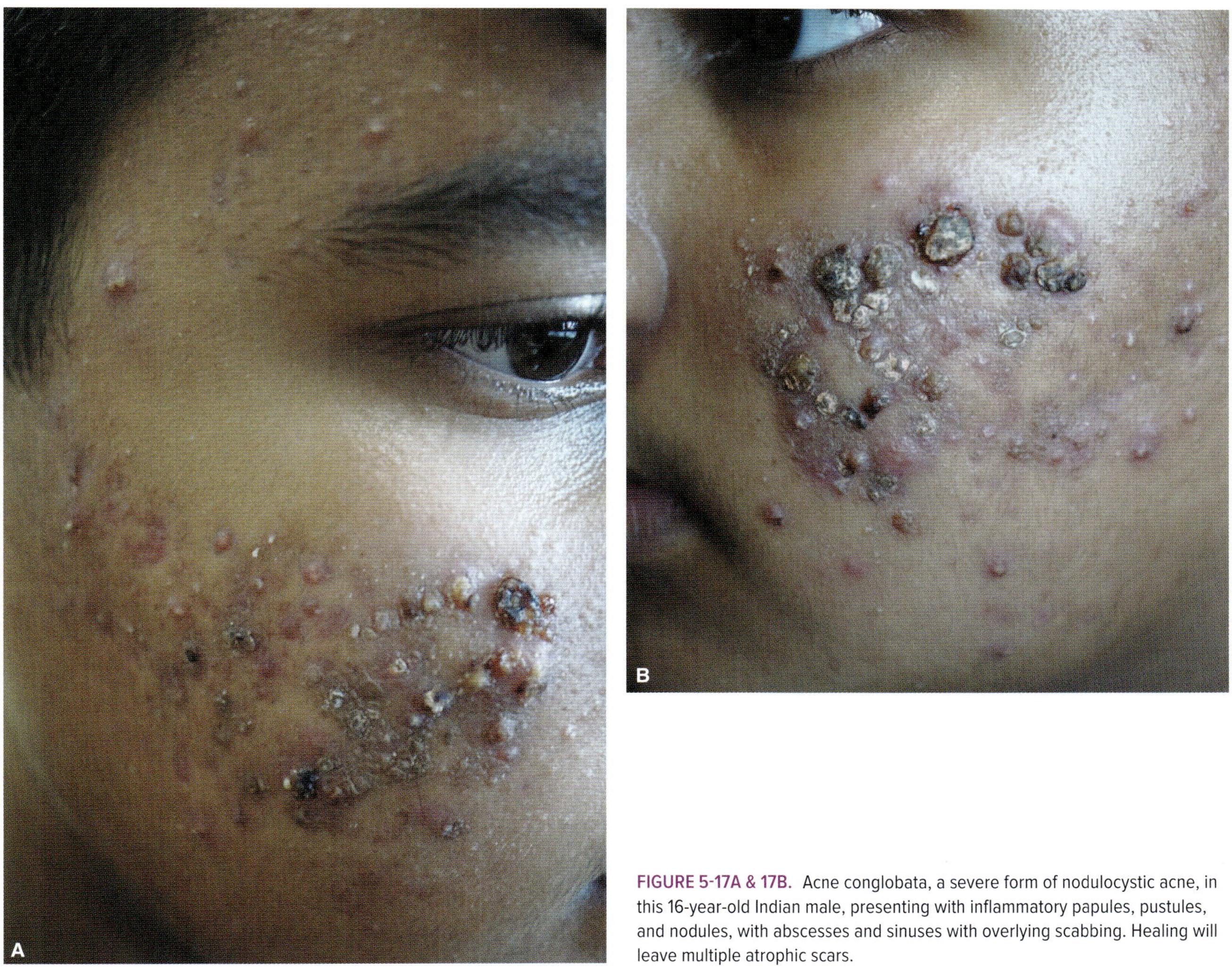

FIGURE 5-17A & 17B. Acne conglobata, a severe form of nodulocystic acne, in this 16-year-old Indian male, presenting with inflammatory papules, pustules, and nodules, with abscesses and sinuses with overlying scabbing. Healing will leave multiple atrophic scars.

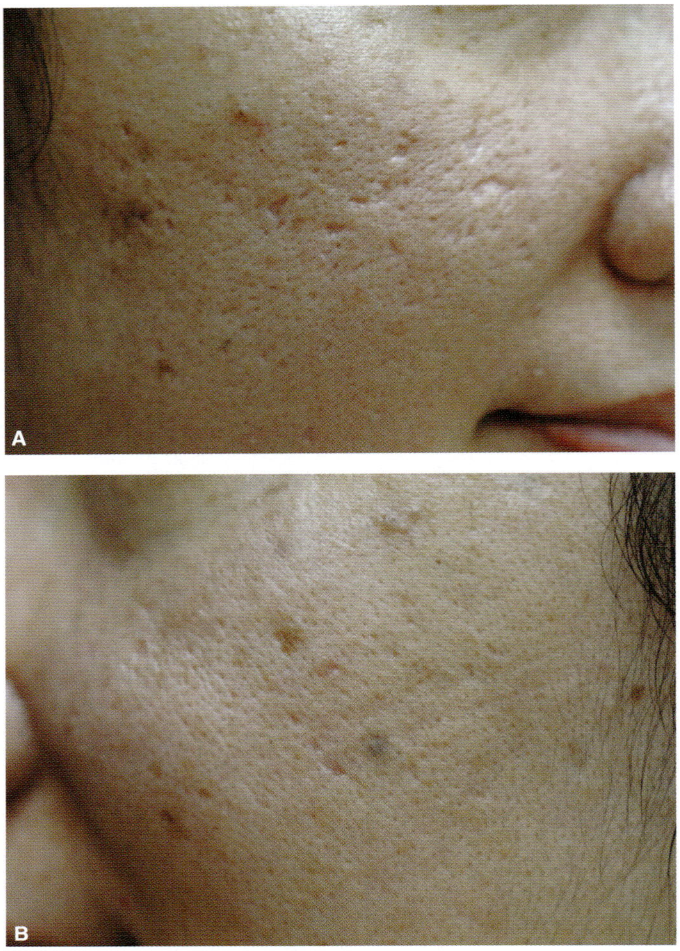

FIGURE 5-18A & 18B. Atrophic acne scars in a young adult Chinese female with previous history of severe inflammatory acne.

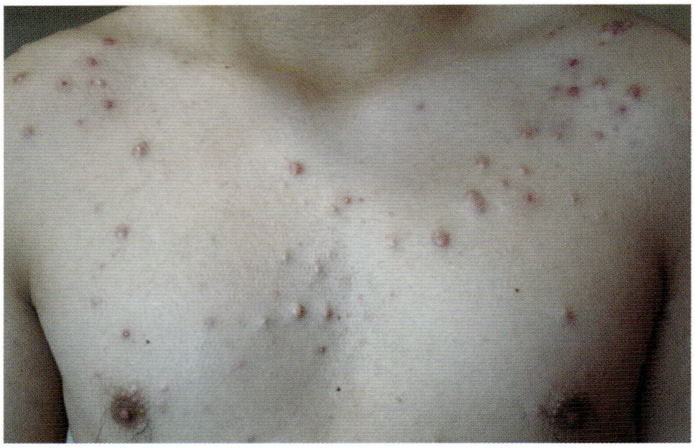

FIGURE 5-19. Multiple hypertrophic and keloid scars on the chest and shoulders of this Chinese adolescent male with nodulocystic acne with predominantly truncal involvement. He has other features of the follicular occlusion triad.

  - **Oral hormonal therapy**, in the form of combined oral contraceptives (COC) can be used as monotherapy for acne. However, their use for acne is generally avoided in the first 2 years after attaining menarche. COC may be considered for the treatment of moderate-to-severe acne in females who wish to also regulate their menstrual cycles, with inadequate response to other therapies, and acne flares associated with menstrual cycles. Common side effects include nausea, vomiting, weight gain, mood changes, and breast tenderness. There is also a risk of thromboembolic events, although this is rare in adolescents.
  - **Oral isotretinoin** is the most effective treatment for moderate-to-severe acne, especially for patients with suboptimal response to other treatments. In Asian patients, it is usually effective at a dose of 20 to 30 mg per day, although higher doses may be required in individuals not responding to these doses. Most patients require treatment for 9 to 12 months for optimal results. Common adverse effects include dose-related xerosis, especially of the lips and eyes, and myalgia. Isotretinoin is teratogenic and can cause major fetal abnormalities upon exposure.
- Adjunctive therapies that may improve acne or its complications include intralesional triamcinolone injections for cysts, nodules, and keloids; chemical peels (such as salicylic acid and glycolic acid); light-based therapies (blue light, diode laser, intense pulse light, photodynamic therapy); and lasers.

Pearls & Practical Tips

- Although acne has no major systemic complications, patients may experience adverse social and psychological effects.
- Erythema may be more difficult to appreciate in darker skin tones, and may appear as post-inflammatory hyperpigmentation. Palpation for induration or tenderness may help to signify active acne lesions.
- Post-inflammatory hyperpigmentation is more common in pigmented skin. This may be worsened with increased sun exposure and manipulation of acne.
- Most acne treatments require at least 1 to 2 months for effective response. Oral isotretinoin works the fastest, with effects within 1 to 2 weeks.
- An acute flare may occur in the first 1 to 2 weeks on starting treatment with oral isotretinoin. In these cases, a tailing course of oral corticosteroids may be required.
- Maintenance treatment with topical therapies, such as tretinoin cream, should be continued for some time—typically for a few years—after resolution is achieved.

Bibliography

1. Silverberg NB, Duran-McKinster C, Yong-Kwang T. Pediatric Skin of Color. 2015. Chapter 38:341-62.
2. Thiboutot D, Zaenglein AL. Pathogenesis, clinical manifestations and diagnosis of acne vulgaris. UpToDate Nov 12, 2019.
3. Graber E. Treatment of acne vulgaris. UpToDate Jul 28, 2020.

HIDRADENITIS SUPPURATIVA

Hidradenitis suppurativa, also known as acne inversa, is a chronic inflammatory skin condition that is more common in adults but may have its onset in adolescence. It is a chronic follicular occlusive disease that involves the follicular portion of folliculopilosebaceous unit.

Clinical Features

- Rarely seen in prepubertal children, the onset of hidradenitis suppurativa is usually in adolescence.
- Clinical manifestations can vary, ranging from comedones, recurrent inflamed nodules and abscesses, to draining sinus tracts and hypertrophic scarring.
- Primary sites of involvement are the intertriginous skin areas of the axilla, groin, perianal, and inframammary regions.
- The associated pain, malodor, drainage, and disfigurement can lead to profound psychosocial impairment.

Differential Diagnoses

- Follicular pyodermas (folliculitis, furuncles, carbuncles)
  - Follicular pyodermas are transient lesions that usually respond to appropriate antibiotic, whereas hidradenitis suppurativa typically exhibits a chronic and recurrent course. Moreover, follicular pyodermas do not cause the persistent sinus tracts, comedones, and hypertrophic scarring seen in hidradenitis suppurativa.
- Acne vulgaris
  - Severe acne vulgaris, especially the nodulocystic acne, can be associated with hidradenitis suppurativa and be part of the follicular occlusion tetrad, which also includes dissecting cellulitis of the scalp and pilonidal sinus.
  - Acne primarily affects the face, upper chest, and back, in contrast to hidradenitis suppurativa, which primarily affects the intertriginous areas.
- Pilonidal sinus
  - Pilonidal sinus is characterized by a cavity, pit, or sinus in the area of the natal cleft that may be associated with purulent or mucoid discharge. The condition can be chronic or recurrent.

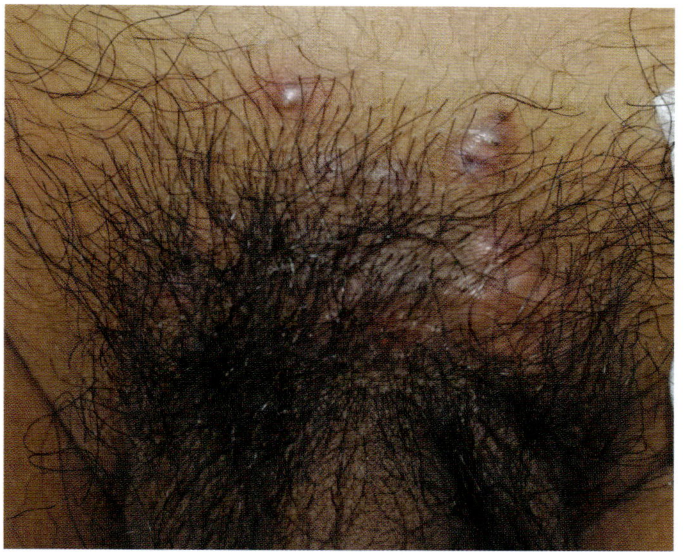

FIGURE 5-21. Early hidradenitis suppurativa on the groin area of a Chinese adolescent male, presenting as papules, pustules, and nodules.

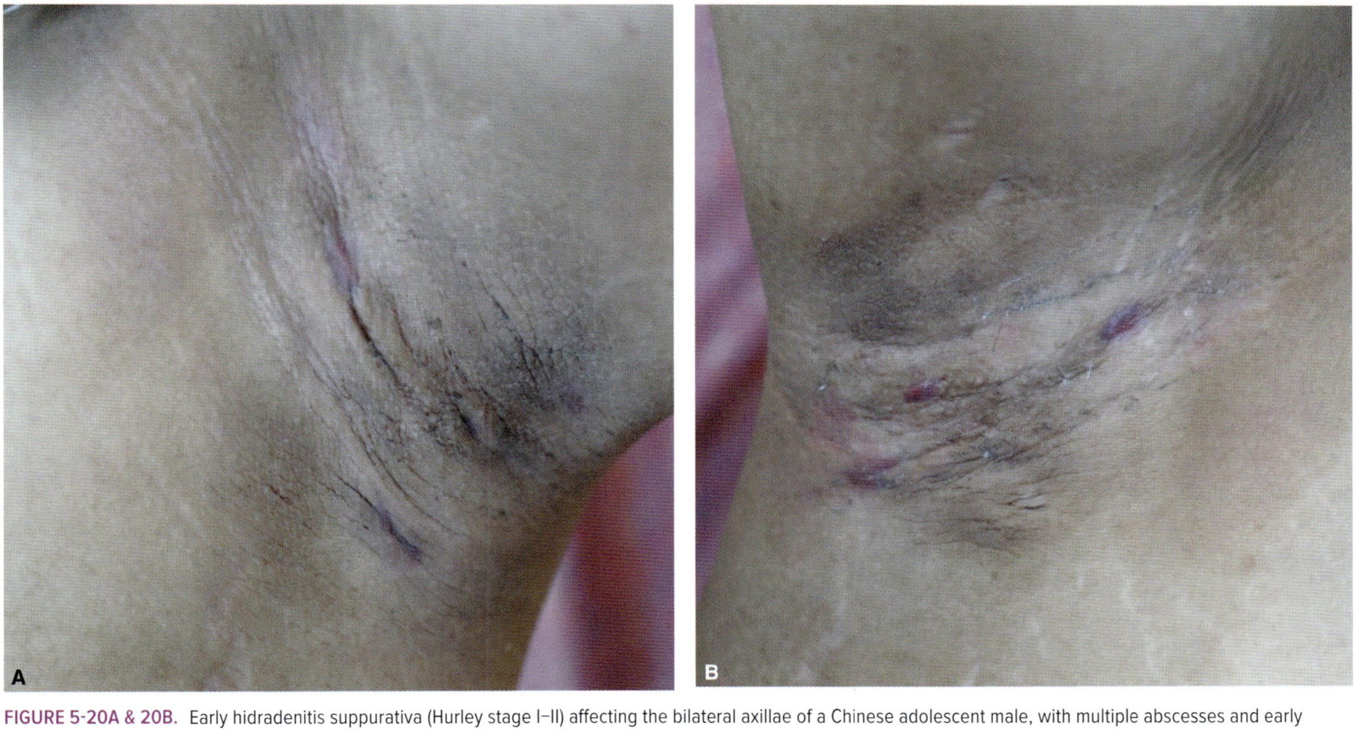

FIGURE 5-20A & 20B. Early hidradenitis suppurativa (Hurley stage I–II) affecting the bilateral axillae of a Chinese adolescent male, with multiple abscesses and early scarring.

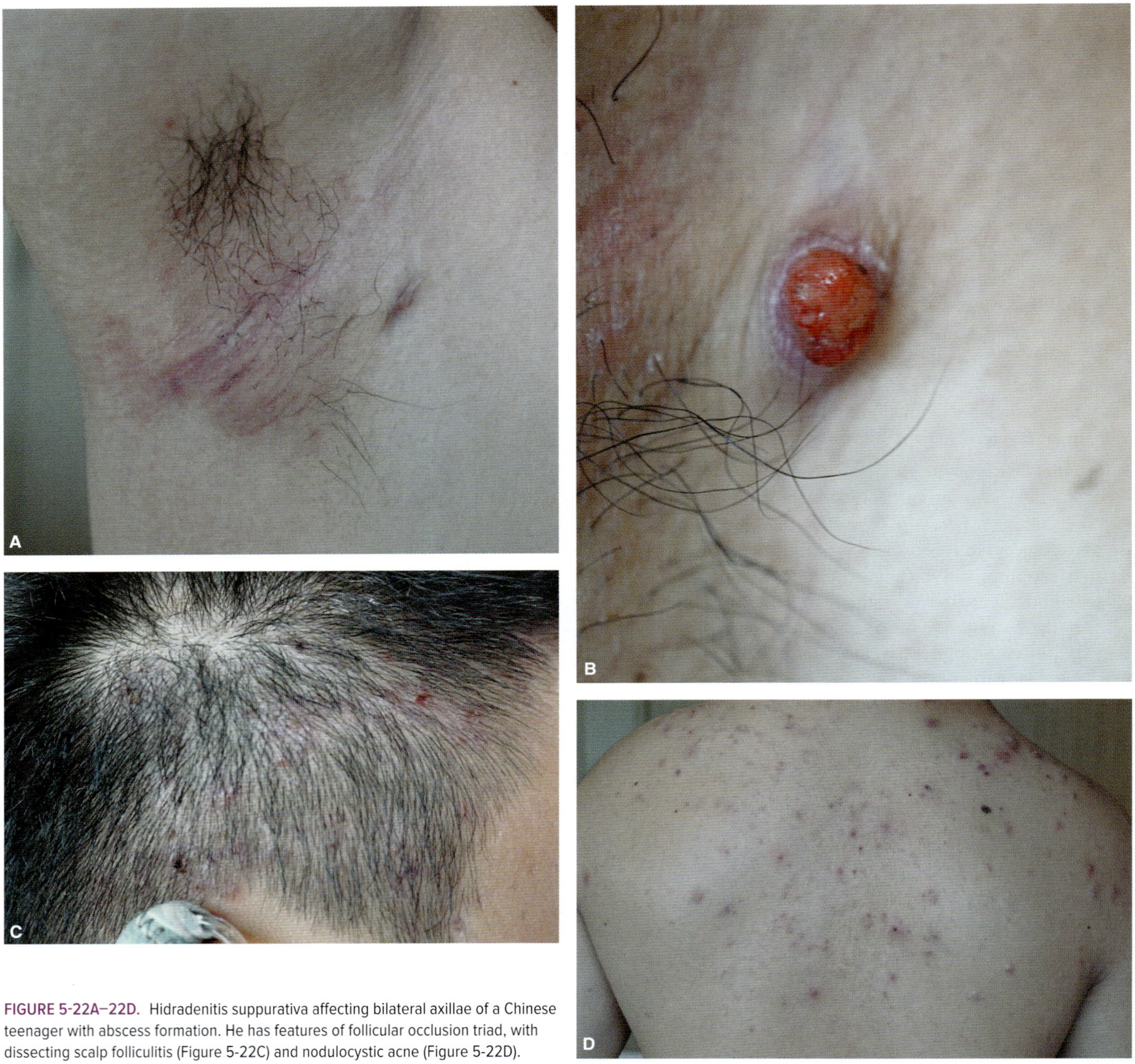

FIGURE 5-22A–22D. Hidradenitis suppurativa affecting bilateral axillae of a Chinese teenager with abscess formation. He has features of follicular occlusion triad, with dissecting scalp folliculitis (Figure 5-22C) and nodulocystic acne (Figure 5-22D).

Investigations & Treatment

- Diagnosis is mainly clinical.
- Bacterial cultures are not routinely performed but may help exclude secondary bacterial infection if required to aid antibiotic choice.
- Skin biopsies may be helpful if the diagnosis is in doubt.
- The Hurley classification system is used to stage the disease and guide management:
  - Stage I: Single/multiple abscesses without sinus tracts/scarring
  - Stage II: Abscess recurrence with sinus tracts and scarring; widely separated lesions
  - Stage III: Diffuse skin involvement with multiple sinus tracts and widespread abscess formation
- Response to treatment is determined by reduction in the severity and frequency of lesions, improvement in symptoms, and quality of life.
- Treatment includes modification of lifestyle, and topical and systemic modalities.

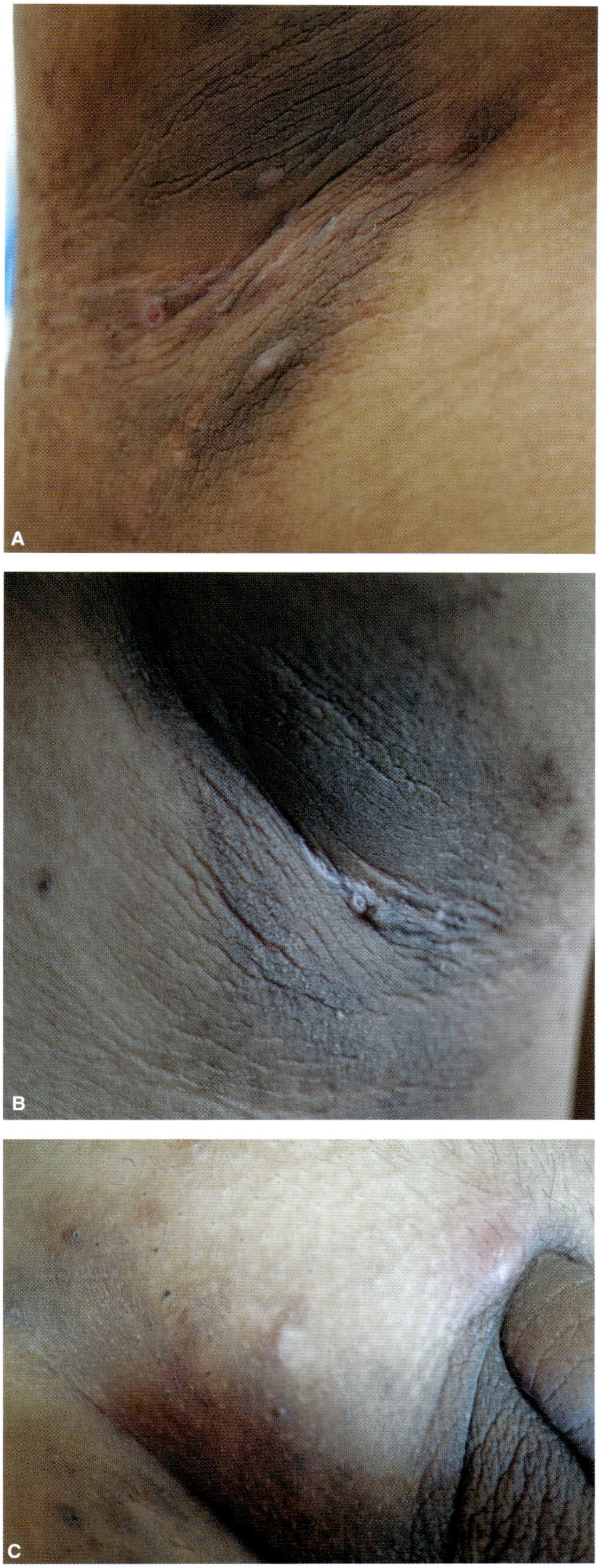

FIGURE 5-23A–23C. Hidradenitis suppurativa affecting bilateral axillae and groin on an obese Indian adolescent, with features of comedones, papules, abscesses, and scarring. There is concomitant acanthosis nigricans affecting bilateral axillae, with thickened, velvety, hyperpigmented skin.

- Advice on **modification of lifestyle** includes wearing of loose-fitting clothing, weight loss if overweight or obese, cessation of smoking, and assessment for associated diabetes mellitus and psychological issues, for example, depression.
- **Topical treatments** include topical antibiotics (e.g., clindamycin or erythromycin) and anti-septic washes (e.g., chlorhexidine or benzoyl peroxide washes). These may suffice in mild disease and can be adjunctive treatment for moderate or severe disease.
- **Oral antibiotics** may be more useful for their immunomodulatory rather than antimicrobial effects in the treatment of hidradenitis suppurativa. Examples include oral tetracycline and doxycycline. Treatment can be prolonged.
- **Oral isotretinoin and acitretin** have been used with variable outcomes. These are contraindicated in pregnant patients and women who are planning for pregnancy.
- **Hormonal therapies** may be considered in female patients with flare-ups associated with menstrual cycles. These include oral contraceptives and/or spironolactone.
- **Biologics**, especially the tumor necrosis factor inhibitors (e.g., adalimumab and infliximab) and IL-17 inhibitors (e.g., secukinumab) have shown benefit in the treatment of more severe disease or in patients not responding to other systemic treatments. Anakinra, an interleukin-1 receptor antagonist, has also been found to be effective for moderate-to-severe disease.
- Other treatments that may be useful include intralesional corticosteroid injections, such as triamcinolone and metformin.

- Surgical treatments
  - The goal of surgical procedures in the treatment of hidradenitis suppurativa is to control inflammation by removing the diseased folliculopilosebaceous unit, sinus tracts, and associated debris to prevent further progression and scarring.
  - Local procedures include punch debridement, unroofing/deroofing, skin-tissue sparing excision with electrosurgical peeling, and laser excision.

Pearls & Practical Tips

- Poorly controlled moderate and severe hidradenitis suppurativa and its long-term complications, such as scarring, has been shown to impact quality of life and lead to severe psychosocial impairment, especially if treatment is suboptimal.
- A combination of treatments, including medical and surgical treatments, may be required for optimal results.

Bibliography

1. Wipperman J, Bragg DA, Litzner B. Hidradenitis suppurativa: rapid evidence review. AAFP 2019;100(9):562-9.
2. Ingram JR. Hidradenitis Suppurativa: Pathogenesis, Clinical Features and Diagnosis and Management. UpToDate Sep 2020.

PERIORIFICIAL DERMATITIS

Periorificial dermatitis, also known as perioral dermatitis, is an uncommon acneiform eruption that occurs most commonly in children and adult women. It may be associated with the use of systemic, topical, intra-nasal or inhaled corticosteroids.

Clinical Features

- In the pediatric population, periorificial dermatitis more frequently affects prepubescent children.
- It presents with monomorphous grouped papules, papulovesicles, or papulopustules, with or without mild overlying scale. Comedones are not seen. The lesions are rarely symptomatic.
- Lesions range from pink to red to flesh colored, and may be associated with hypo- or hyperpigmentation, particularly in dark-skinned patients.
- Most commonly affects the perioral region, sparing a narrow zone around the vermilion border of the lip. Perinasal or periorbital sites are less commonly involved.
- Childhood granulomatous periorificial dermatitis is considered a clinical variant of periorificial dermatitis, and is characterized by yellow-brown or erythematous papules without pustules.

Differential Diagnoses

- **Lip-licker's dermatitis**
  - This is common in children and results from excessive lip-licking, which is most often a habit or tic.
  - It presents with more eczematous lesions with scaly, erythematous plaques that affect the lips and often extend onto the perioral skin.
- **Acne vulgaris**
  - Acne vulgaris affects pubertal patients more commonly than prepubescent children.

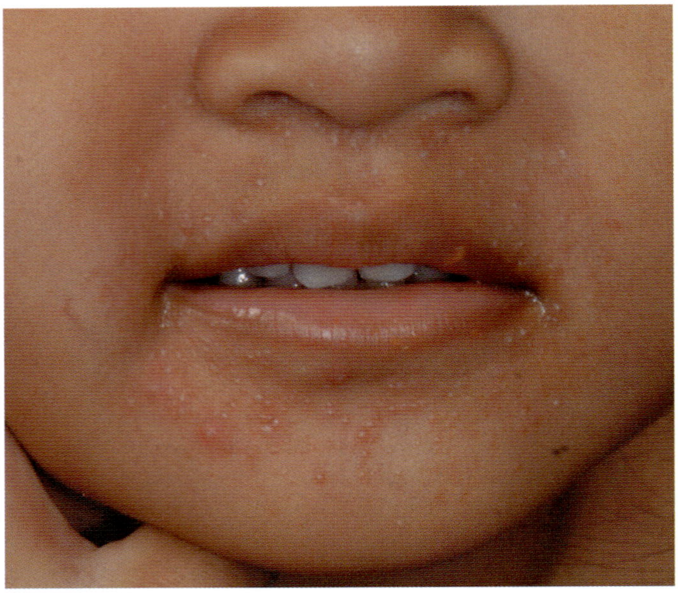

FIGURE 5-24. Periorificial dermatitis in a young Chinese girl presenting with multiple papules and few pustules around the perioral region.

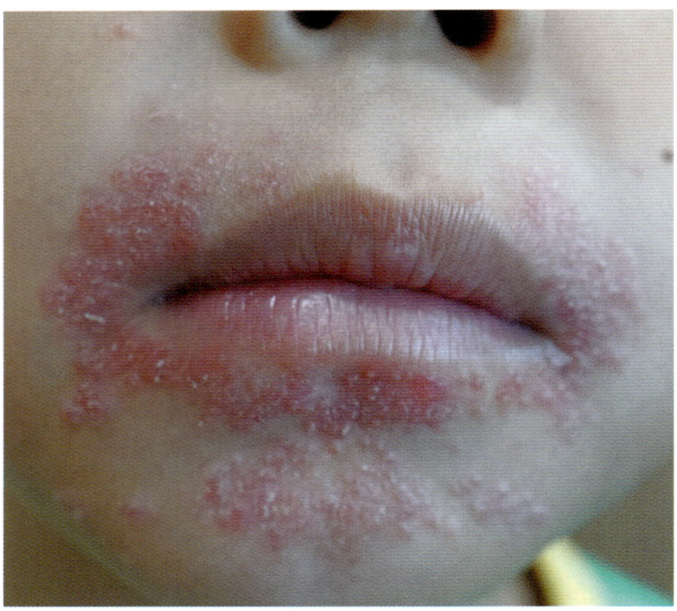

FIGURE 5-25. Periorificial dermatitis presenting as multiple, monomorphic, erythematous papules with mild overlying scaling around the mouth, in a young Chinese boy.

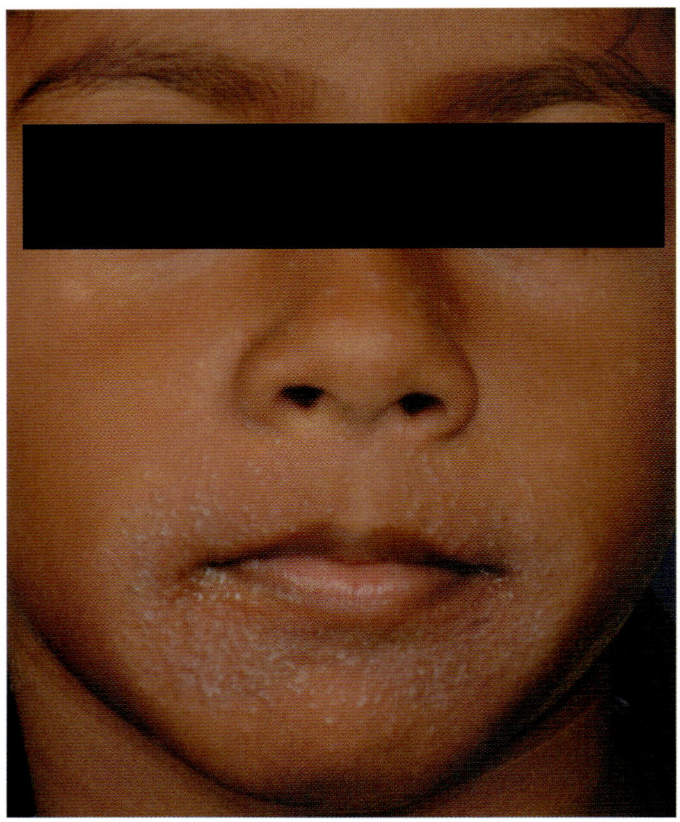

FIGURE 5-26. Periorificial dermatitis predominantly affecting the perioral, nasal, and periorbital region in a 5-year-old Indian boy, presenting with monomorphic skin-colored to hypopigmented papules.

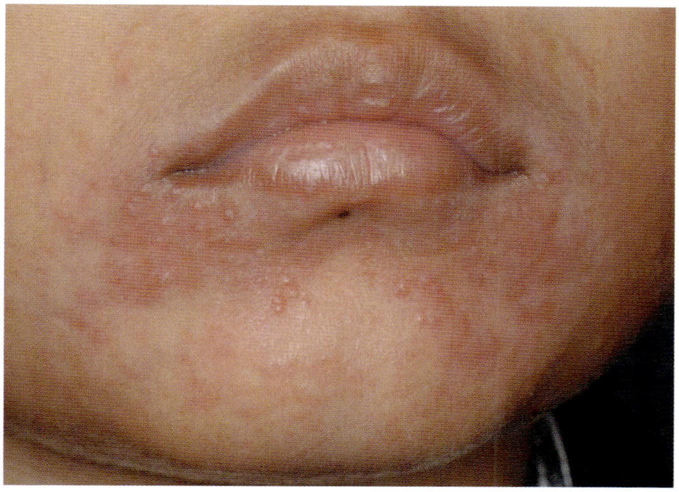

FIGURE 5-27. Close-up of periorificial dermatitis around the mouth of a 5-year-old Indian male.

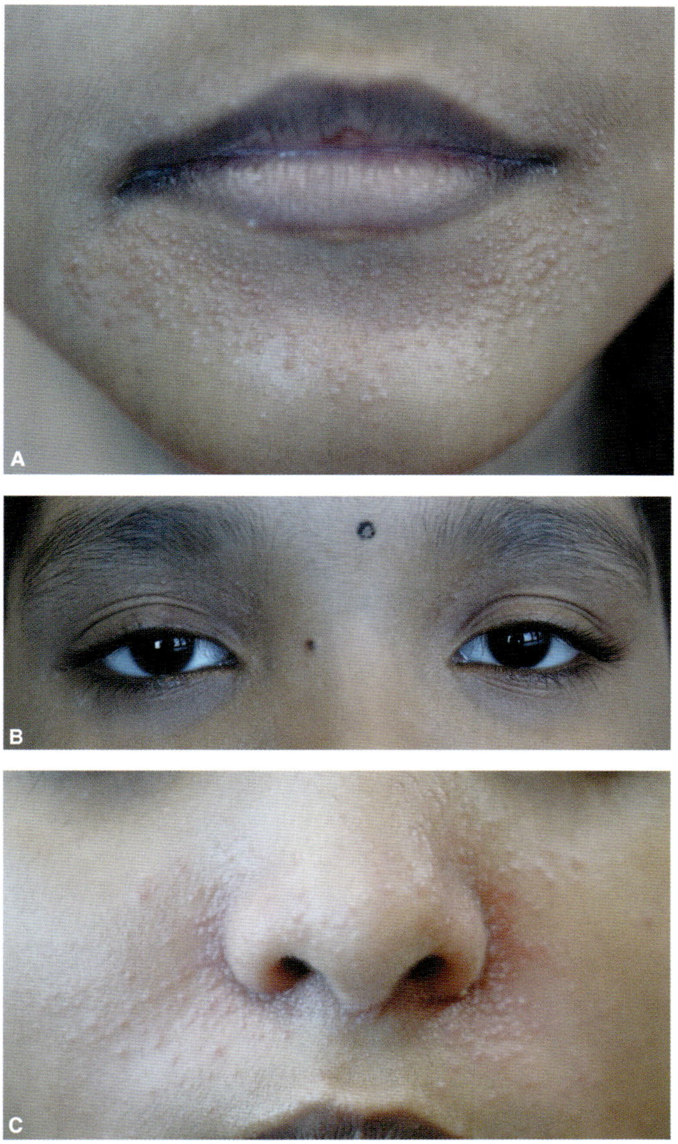

FIGURE 5-28A–28C. Periorificial dermatitis affecting the perioral and perinasal regions in an 11-year-old Indian girl. There are scattered papules around the eyes.

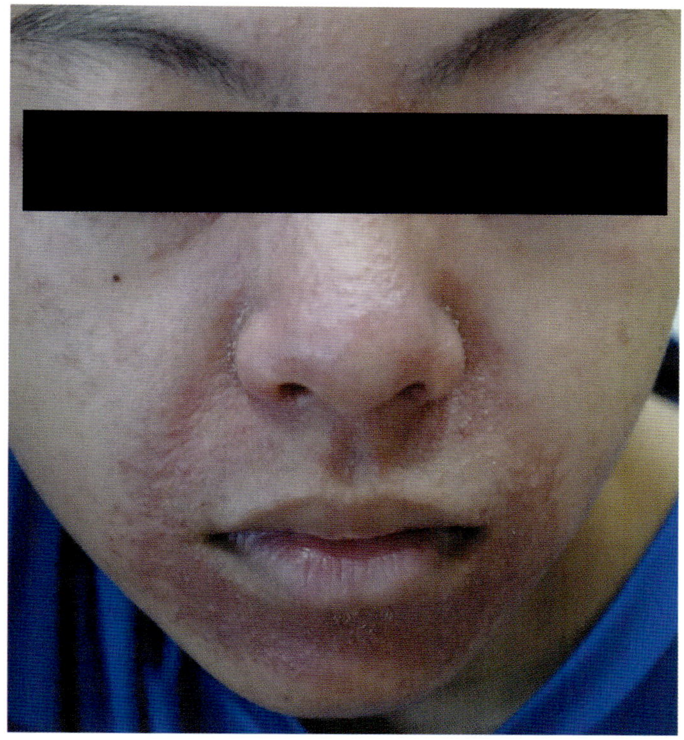

FIGURE 5-29. Extensive periorificial dermatitis in a 14-year-old Chinese male, with involvement around the eyes, nose, and mouth. Note that unlike acne vulgaris, there are no comedones.

  - It manifests as closed and open comedones and inflammatory papules or pustules, which are not commonly seen in periorificial dermatitis.
  - Unlike acne vulgaris, scarring is uncommon in periorificial dermatitis.
- **Seborrheic dermatitis**
  - Seborrheic dermatitis more commonly affects pubertal patients compared to prepubertal children.
  - It also commonly affects the perinasal area but also affects other sites, such as the scalp, eyebrows, and chest.
  - It presents with erythematous papules, patches, and plaques with overlying greasy, yellowish scales. In contrast to periorificial dermatitis, small papules are not a typical feature of seborrheic dermatitis.

Investigations & Treatment

- Diagnosis is usually made on clinical grounds. However, biopsy may be useful if the clinical diagnosis is in doubt.
- The histopathologic findings may vary with the type of biopsied lesion, and include parakeratosis, epidermal spongiosis and mild acanthosis, and perifollicular and perivascular lymphocytic infiltrates. Epithelioid granulomas may sometimes be seen.
- Topical metronidazole, applied twice daily, is useful for the treatment of periorificial dermatitis and childhood granulomatous periorificial dermatitis. Other topical antibiotics such as clindamycin and erythromycin may also be used.

- Oral erythromycin (30–50 mg/kg/day, every 6–12 hours) may be effective for children not responding to topical treatments. Other systemic antibiotics, such as tetracycline, doxycycline, or minocycline, may also be used; however, these are contraindicated in children less than 8 years of age. Treatment is usually for at least 4 to 8 weeks, and may be longer for some patients.
- In recalcitrant cases, oral isotretinoin may be used.
- Topical calcineurin inhibitors and azelaic acid may also be used as adjunctive or second-line treatment.

Pearls & Practical Tips

- Although the condition improves with the use of topical corticosteroids, it will recur quickly upon cessation.
- Prognosis is good, and the lesions commonly resolve without scarring, although dyspigmentation is common in Asian children and may last for several months.

Bibliography

1. Silverberg, NB, Duran-McKinster C, Yong Kwan T. Pediatric Skin of Color. 2015. Chapter 39:363-7.
2. Reichenberg J. Perioral (periorificial) dermatitis. UpToDate Sept 2020.

6

Cutaneous Infections

VIRAL INFECTIONS

CUTANEOUS HERPES SIMPLEX VIRUS INFECTIONS

Herpes labialis and herpes gingivostomatitis are most often caused by herpes simplex virus (HSV) type 1, and less commonly by HSV type 2. Most infections are, however, asymptomatic. Symptomatic infections can range from mild to severe, leading to dehydration and rarely, systemic manifestations. Genital herpes, most often caused by HSV type 2, is rare in children. It is most often acquired sexually. Herpetic whitlow, most often caused by HSV type 1, causes blistering on the fingers.

Clinical Features

- Herpes labialis and gingivostomatitis is the most common primary manifestation of primary HSV infection in children, usually 1 to 5 years of age.
- Initial lesions present as small vesicles that can be seen on the lips and perioral area, gingiva, hard and soft palates, tongue, buccal mucosa, and less often on the pharynx.
- Vesicles progress to develop shallow ulcers with an exudative yellowish base and surrounding erythema. Lesions may also coalesce.
- Associated symptoms vary and include malaise and fever. Tender cervical lymphadenopathy, halitosis, and drooling occur later.
- Oral lesions may persist for 2 to 3 weeks.
- Recurrence of herpes labialis may be observed in some patients (cold sores), usually within the first 2 years of initial infection.
- Patients with a history of atopic dermatitis may develop localized or widespread herpetiform lesions, known as eczema herpeticum.
- Genital herpes presents as painful, grouped, small blisters over an erythematous base, and can occur on the labia majora or minora in girls, on the penile shaft in boys, and less commonly around the anal verge. Sexual transmission has to be strongly considered in all minors presenting with confirmed genital herpes.

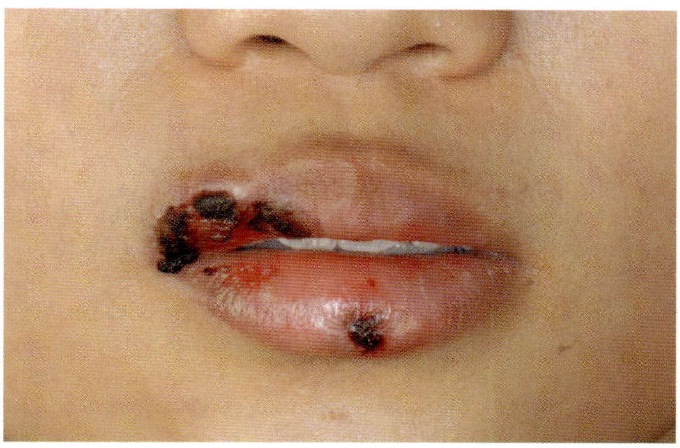

FIGURE 6-1. "Cold sores" on the lips of an adolescent girl with hemorrhagic crusting and grouped erosions.

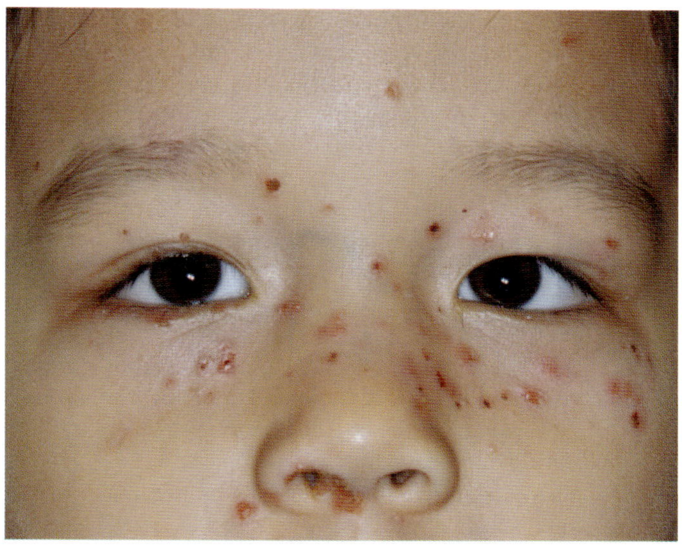

FIGURE 6-2. Eczema herpeticum in a young Nepalese boy with a background of atopic dermatitis, presenting with acute onset of small blisters and erosions on the face.

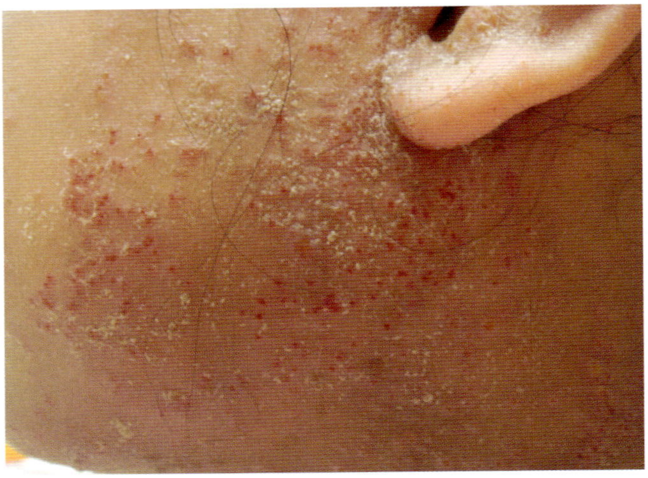

FIGURE 6-3. Eczema herpeticum in a young Chinese girl with a history of atopic dermatitis. There are multiple punctate erosions with crusting and erythema on the neck and face.

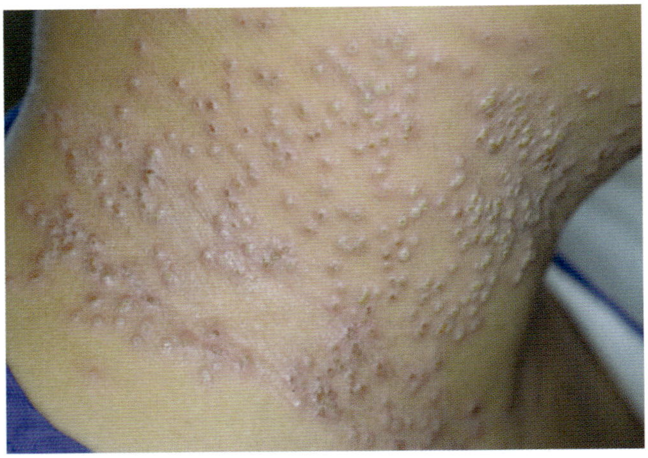

FIGURE 6-4. Eczema herpeticum in a Chinese adolescent presenting as acute onset of multiple vesicles and blisters on an erythematous base.

- Herpetic whitlow presents as painful blisters anywhere on the hand, but is most often seen on the pulp or lateral aspect of the fingers.

Differential Diagnoses

- Aphthous ulcers
  - Usually do not present with associated systemic symptoms.
  - Usually present as solitary oral ulcers; it is rare for concurrent multiple oral ulcers, and lesions do not coalesce.
  - Aphthous ulcers can also occur on the genital region, especially in girls. Also known as "Lipschutz ulcers," they commonly occur after a non-specific viral infection. Genital herpes has to always be excluded.
- Herpangina/Hand-foot-mouth disease (HFMD)
  - Often presents with fever, sore throat, malaise.
  - Ulcers are generally pinpoint in appearance and are seen on the soft palate, tonsils, uvula, and back of the throat. Lips, oral mucosa, and tongue are usually spared.
  - In HFMD, there are concomitant erythematous and purpuric macules and papules on the acral areas and buttocks.
- Impetigo
  - Presents with honey-colored crusted erosions or pustules. Lesions can affect any area of skin but are most common on the face (perinasal, perioral) and groin.
  - Does not affect the buccal mucosa, palate, or pharynx.
- Blistering distal dactylitis
  - This is a differential diagnosis for herpetic whitlow and is typically caused by Group A beta-hemolytic streptococcus.
  - Lesions present as large, tense blisters filled with seropurulent material on an erythematous base, and localized usually to the anterior fat pad of the affected finger.

Investigations & Treatment

- Diagnosis of HSV infection is most often clinical.
- Investigations, if required, include viral PCR, viral isolation, or viral culture with swab specimens obtained from fresh vesicular fluid or the base of lesions. HSV serology can also be performed but is often not able to differentiate between acute or recurrent infection.
- Mild, uncomplicated cases can often be treated supportively alone, including antipyretics, analgesics, and adequate hydration.
- Topical antiviral therapy can be considered in mild cases (e.g., topical acyclovir).
- For complicated or more severe cases, systemic treatments include:
  - Acyclovir
    - » PO 40 to 80 mg/kg/day Q 6 to 8 for 5 to 10 days (max 1 g/24 hr)
    - » IV 15 mg/kg/day Q 8 for 5 to 7 days
- Secondary bacterial infection may develop for which topical or oral antibiotics may be required.

Pearls & Practical Tips

- The ulcers from HSV gingivostomatitis most frequently affect the anterior portion of the mouth (e.g., lips, anterior tongue, anterior gingiva). The ulcers from HFMD most frequently affect the posterior portion of the mouth (e.g., pharynx, tonsils, uvula).
- Recurrent HSV infections are unusual in children and can occur in both immunocompromised and immunocompetent patients. If recurrences are frequent and symptomatic, episodic treatment with topical or oral acyclovir, or prophylactic treatment with oral acyclovir for a minimum of 6 months, may be beneficial.
- Exposure to ultraviolet light during acute HSV infections may trigger erythema multiforme or Stevens-Johnson syndrome.

Bibliography

1. Hughes H, Kahl L. The Harriet Lane Handbook. 21st ed. Philadelphia, PA: Elsevier; 2018.
2. Irvine AD, Hoeger PH, Yan AC. Harper's Textbook of Pediatric Dermatology. 3rd ed. Wiley-Blackwell; 2011.

VARICELLA ZOSTER INFECTION

Varicella or chickenpox is primary infection caused by varicella-zoster virus (VZV) and is highly contagious, transmitted via airborne droplets or by direct contact with active lesions. It most commonly affects young children but can also occur in adolescents and adults. With the more widespread use of VZV vaccine, the incidence of primary varicella has decreased over the last decade. Zoster, also known as shingles, is caused by secondary reactivation of VZV. More common in older individuals, it can also affect children and adolescents. It can rarely occur in children who have been immunized with varicella vaccine.

Clinical Features

- The incubation period for varicella is approximately 2 weeks, with a range of 10 to 21 days after exposure. Prodromal symptoms include fever, malaise, myalgia, and anorexia, and often precede the onset of rash.
- The classical rash is intensely pruritic, presenting initially as erythematous papules which evolve to non-umbilicated, oval vesicles on an erythematous base ("dewdrops on a rose petal"). The vesicular fluid evolves from clear to cloudy, followed by ulceration and crusting prior to healing and resolution.
- New crops develop every 3 to 4 days and affect all skin surfaces, including the mucous membranes. The highest concentration of lesions is seen on the trunk, leading to a centripetal distribution. Lesions are classically at different stages and become crusted by one week. Atrophic scarring can occur after resolution.
- Zoster is caused by reactivation of latent VZV in the dorsal root ganglion and spreads along the corresponding cutaneous nerve to the overlying skin or dermatome.
- Symptoms initially present as mild-to-intense localized pain and tenderness, and may be accompanied by fever and malaise.

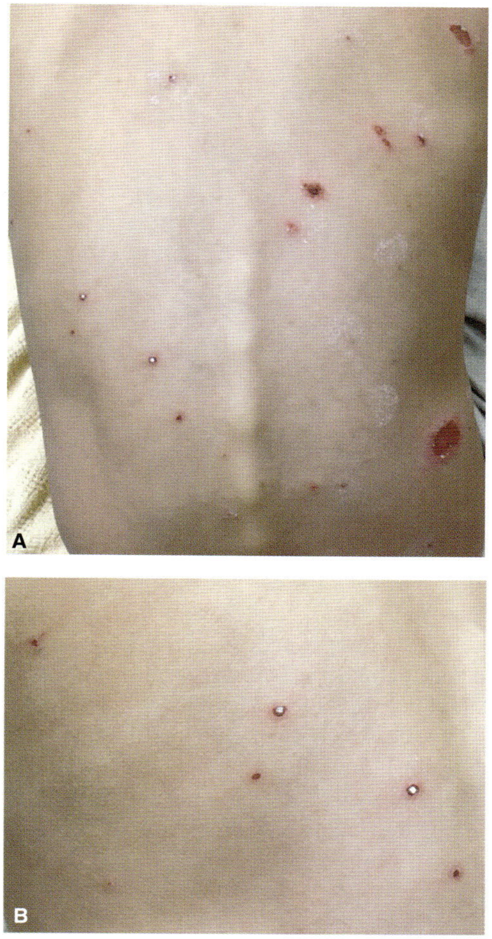

FIGURE 6-6A & 6B. Varicella in a Chinese adolescent male presenting with multiple polymorphic papules, vesicles, and erosions with surface scabbing. There is secondary impetiginization of some of the lesions.

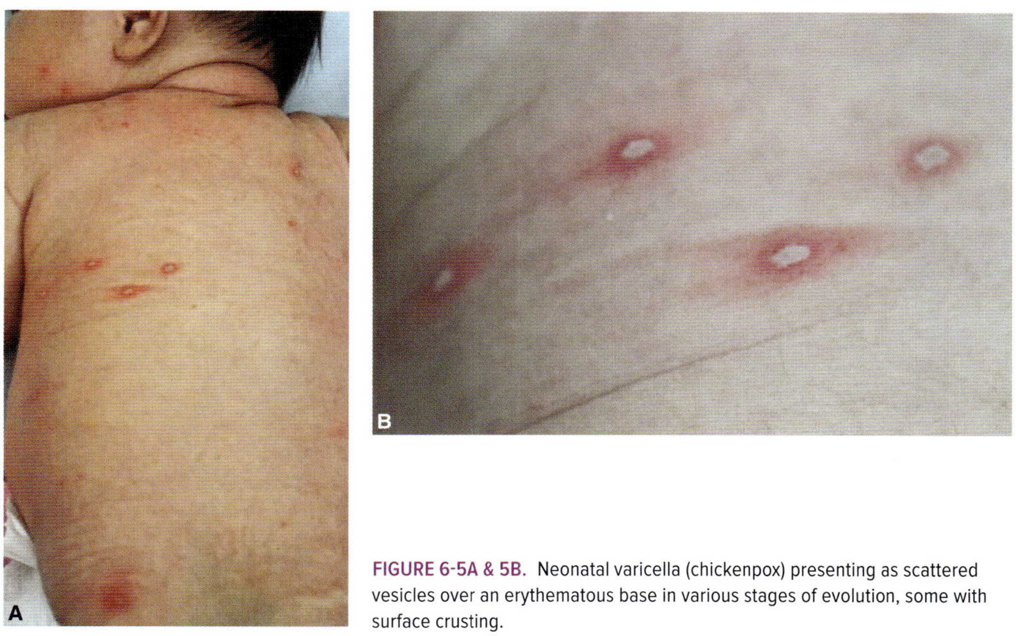

FIGURE 6-5A & 5B. Neonatal varicella (chickenpox) presenting as scattered vesicles over an erythematous base in various stages of evolution, some with surface crusting.

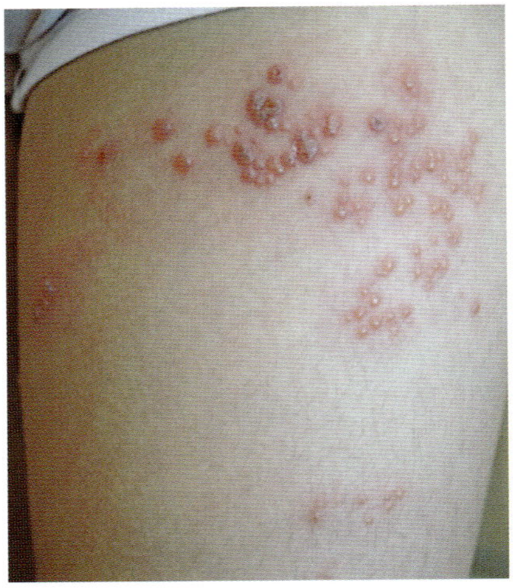

FIGURE 6-7. Zoster presenting as grouped vesicles over an erythematous base in a dermatomal distribution on the thigh of a Chinese girl.

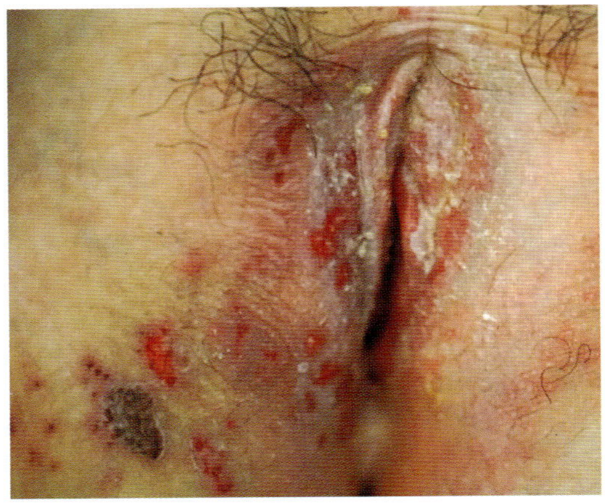

FIGURE 6-8. Zoster affecting the groin and genitalia of an adolescent Chinese girl, presenting with blisters and erosions in a dermatomal distribution.

- After a few days, an erythematous patch or plaque develops, followed by eruption of papules and vesicles, localized along the dermatome. Lesions are usually unilateral, with accompanying lymphadenopathy. Over 7 to 14 days, several crops of vesicles may appear, followed by crusting and eventual healing.
- In children, cervical or sacral dermatomes are more likely involved, as compared to lower thoracic and upper lumbar dermatomes in adults.

Differential Diagnoses

Varicella/Chickenpox

- Herpes simplex infection and eczema herpeticum
  - Can also present as vesicular eruptions but are mostly localized to certain areas (perioral, eyes, digits, genitals) and rarely have a generalized distribution.
  - Lesions are mostly clustered or grouped rather than disseminated, and are generally in the same stage of infection.
  - Lesions can be localized or widespread in eczema herpeticum, and can be confused with varicella. Lesions are more monomorphic compared to lesions in various stages seen in varicella.
- Hand, foot, and mouth disease
  - Viral infection caused by Coxsackievirus A that may also present with fever and rash, but lesions are usually vesiculopustular or vesiculopapular, and are mostly limited to the oropharynx, hands, and feet.
- Scabies
  - Caused by infestation by the *Sarcoptes scabiei* mite, lesions present as intensely pruritic papules and vesicles on the palms, soles, axillae, and trunk. The onset of lesions occurs over weeks and months. Other family members may similarly be affected.

Zoster

- Contact dermatitis
  - May also present as a localized area of erythema, swelling, and eruption of vesicles. Lesions are usually pruritic but can be painful if there is severe blistering.
  - Although a history of contact with an irritant or allergen is often present, some patients may not be able to recall a contactant. Lesions occur on the area of direct contact with the causative agent, but rarely can spread to other areas.
- Bullous impetigo
  - A bacterial infection that presents with superficial vesicles that rapidly enlarge to form flaccid bullae. Lesions eventually rupture and form yellow crusting.
  - A pathognomonic finding is a "collarette" of scale surrounding the blister roof at the periphery of ruptured lesions.
  - Lesions are more common on the face and intertriginous areas.

Investigations & Treatment

- Diagnosis is mainly clinical, but if confirmation is necessary, varicella PCR from a lesion is the current diagnostic method of choice. Detection of varicella-specific antigen in vesicular fluid by immunofluorescence using monoclonal antibodies or demonstration of a fourfold antibody increase of acute and convalescent sera is also diagnostic but not as sensitive as PCR.

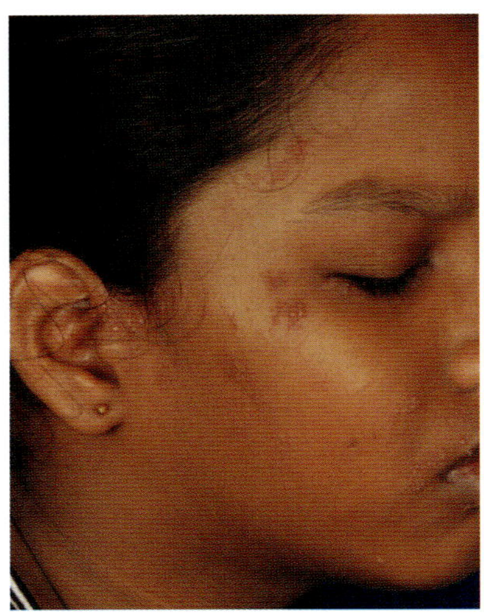

FIGURE 6-9. Zoster affecting several dermatomes on the right side of the face of an Indian girl.

- Treatment of varicella and zoster is mainly supportive, with antipyretics, topical and oral antipruritic medications, hydration, and proper hygiene.
- The need for systemic antiviral treatment for varicella depends on several factors, including patient's immune status, severity of disease, and risk or presence of complications.
- Systemic antiviral treatment for zoster accelerates cutaneous healing, hastens the resolution of pain, and reduces the risk of postherpetic neuralgia.
- The recommended dose and duration for systemic acyclovir treatment for varicella:
  - Immunocompetent
    - » Acyclovir PO (≥2 yr): 80 mg/kg/24 hr QID × 5 days (max 80 mg/kg/24 hr)
    - » Acyclovir IV (≥2 yr): 30 mg/kg/24 hr or 1500 mg/m^2/24 hr ÷ Q 8 hr × 7–10 days
  - Immunocompromised
    - » Acyclovir PO for infant and child: 20 mg/kg/dose (max 800 mg) Q6 hr × 7–10 days
    - » Acyclovir PO for adolescent: 20 mg/kg/dose (max 800 mg) 5 times daily × 7–10 days
    - » Acyclovir IV (all ages): 1500 mg/m^2/24 hr ÷ Q8 hr × 7–10 days
- The recommended dosage and duration of acyclovir for zoster:
  - Acyclovir PO 20 mg/kg/dose QID 80 mg/kg/24 hr × 5 days (max 80 mg/kg/24 hr)
  - Acyclovir IV 10 mg/kg/dose Q8H × 7–10 days

Pearls & Practical Tips

- Breakthrough varicella is infection with wild-type varicella-zoster virus occurring in a vaccinated person more than 42 days after varicella vaccination. This infection is usually mild, presenting with low-grade fever and few lesions, with a shorter disease course.
- Isolation of patients is recommended, especially for those living in contact with infants, pregnant women, and elderly and immunocompromised persons.
- Because the varicella vaccine is a live, attenuated virus, zoster can also develop in vaccine recipients, but the rate appears lower than that seen after natural infection.
- Zoster is unlikely to recur, unlike herpes simplex virus infections, which commonly recur.
- Postherpetic neuralgia, occurring after zoster, is defined as pain on the affected area persisting longer than 1 month. This is uncommon in children compared to adults.
- Urgent ophthalmological consult is required if zoster lesions affect the eyelids or tip of the nose, which corresponds to the dermatome supplied by the V1 or ophthalmic branch of cranial nerve V. Eye involvement, including keratitis and uveitis, can occur with late sequelae of glaucoma, cataracts, and corneal scarring.

Bibliography

1. Blair RJ. Varicella zoster virus. Pediatr Rev. 2019;40(7):375-7.
2. Hughes H, Kahl L. The Harriet Lane Handbook. 21st ed. Philadelphia, PA: Elsevier; 2018.
3. Chickenpox. CDC.gov. Published September 11, 2019. Accessed October 15, 2020. https://www.cdc.gov/chickenpox/hcp/index.html

OTHER VIRAL EXANTHEMS OF CHILDHOOD

Viral exanthems are very common in infants and young children, the most common of which are chickenpox (Figure 6-6A & 6B), hand-foot-mouth disease (HFMD), exanthem subitum or roseola infantum, and erythema infectiosum. Due to increased vaccinations, other exanthems, such as measles and rubella, are less common in more developed communities but may still be seen in less developed populations. Although mostly self-limiting, some of these exanthems can lead to more severe complications and increased morbidity and mortality.

Clinical Features

- Viral exanthems often present in infants and young children due to their lower immunity, but can also occur in older children or adolescents.

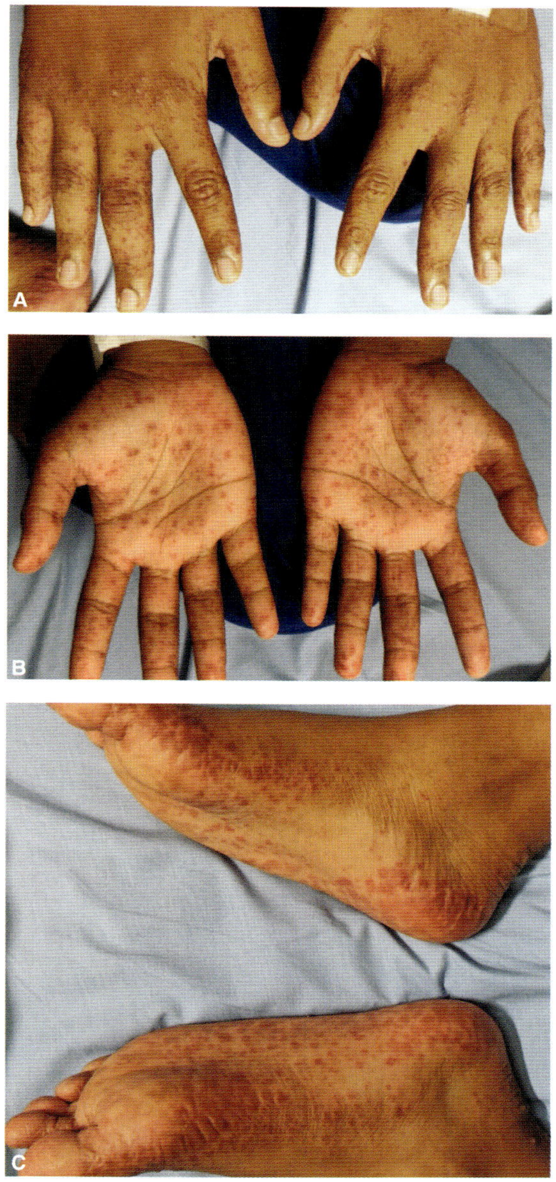

FIGURE 6-10A–10C. HFMD in a 14-year-old Malay boy, presenting with multiple violaceous macules and papules over his hands and feet. He also had oropharyngeal ulcers on the back of his throat (not shown).

TABLE 6-1. Viral exanthems of childhood.

Condition	Cause	Age at presentation	Mode of transmission	Presentation	Differential diagnoses	Investigations, treatment, sequelae, practical tips
Hand-foot-mouth disease (HFMD)	• Enterovirus (coxsackie virus A6 and A16, and enterovirus 71)	• 1–10 years	• Direct contact with oral secretions or skin lesions • Fecal-oral route	• Prodrome of fever, sore throat, dysphagia, irritability, vomiting, and diarrhea. • Oral lesions appear initially as pink to erythematous papules on the posterior tongue and palate, and pharynx, evolving into vesicles and ulcers, with difficulty feeding. • Cutaneous lesions appear as erythematous to violaceous macules and papules on palms, soles and dorsal surfaces of hands and feet, buttocks, and genitalia. Lesions vesiculate and crust before resolution in 7 to 10 days.	• Herpangina • Mucocutaneous herpes virus infection • Varicella • Gianotti-Crosti syndrome	• Enterovirus PCR or microarray • Supportive treatment; e.g., rehydration, pain relief, antipyretic • Onychomadesis is common after HFMD, especially in young children • Eczema coxsackium is HFMD occurring in a patient with atopic dermatitis and presents similar to eczema herpeticum, with concomitant features of HFMD.
Exanthem subitum/roseola infantum	• Human herpesvirus 6 or 7 (HHV6 or HHV7)	• 6 months to 3 years	• Droplets	• Abrupt onset of high fever and irritability. Fever lasts for about 3 to 5 days, with characteristic sudden eruption of widespread rash upon lysis of the fever. • The exanthem appears as rose-colored, blanching, maculopapular rash with a surrounding halo of pale skin, mainly affecting the trunk and neck, and seldomly spreads to the face and extremities. The rash fades within 1 to 3 days. • Similar lesions seen on soft palate and uvula (Nagayama spots).	• Measles • Rubella • Exanthematous drug eruption	• No confirmatory investigations • Supportive treatment including adequate hydration and fever control with antipyretics • There is an increased risk for febrile seizures, which can occur in about a third of cases
Erythema infectiosum/fifth disease	• Parvovirus B19	• School-aged children, most commonly 4–10 years	• Respiratory secretions	• Mild prodrome of low-grade fever, headache, myalgia, malaise, nausea, pharyngitis, and conjunctivitis. • Classic rash appears 7 to 10 days later, with erythema of the cheeks, giving it the "slapped cheek" appearance, with circumoral pallor. • An erythematous maculopapular rash appears on the extensors and trunk with a lacy or reticulate pattern, most common on the arms. The rash can persist for 1 to 3 weeks.	• Measles • Rubella • Scarlet fever	• Parvovirus B19 serology (IgM) or PCR • Supportive treatment, including adequate hydration and fever control • Can cause aplastic anemia in children with chronic hemolytic disorders • In utero infection may result in heart failure, hydrops fetalis, and fetal death
Measles/rubeola	• Para-myxovirus	• Most common in infants and young children	• Droplets or airborne	• Incubation ranges from 8 to 14 days. • Prodromal stage with high-grade fever, cough, coryza, and non-purulent conjunctivitis, and the appearance of pathognomonic Koplik spots (gray-white dots on the buccal mucosa opposite the lower molars) that last 12 to 24 hours. • Exanthematous stage with erythematous, macular rash during peak of fever, initially along hairline, progress in cephalocaudal manner to involve rest of body. • Recovery stage occurs when the rash fades after 4 to 5 days, with brownish discoloration and desquamation ("brawny desquamation").	• Exanthem subitum • Rubella • Erythema infectiosum • Exanthematous drug eruption	• Serologic testing for IgM antibodies • Supportive treatment with antipyretics and adequate hydration • In developing counties, the WHO has recommended administration of vitamin A, shown to improve disease outcomes in children • Prevention with two-dose series of MMR vaccine, given at 12 to 15 months and 4 to 6 years, respectively

Rubella/German measles	• Rubella virus (Togaviridae)	• Children and young adults	• Nose or pharyngeal secretions	• Prodrome of fever and malaise prior to the onset of the characteristic signs of retroauricular, posterior cervical, and posterior occipital lymphadenopathy accompanied by discrete, erythematous, maculopapular rash. • The rash has a cephalocaudal distribution, does not coalesce, and lasts for about 3 days. • Forchheimer spots (rose-colored spots on the soft palate) develop in about 20% of patients and may appear before the rash.	• Exanthem subitum • Rubeola (measles) • Scarlet fever • Infectious mononucleosis	• Serologic testing for IgM antibodies, or fourfold increase in specific IgG antibodies • Supportive treatment with antipyretics and adequate hydration • Congenital disease can lead to spontaneous abortion or premature birth and deformities; associated with infections in first trimester • Prevention by administration of a two-dose series of MMR vaccine, given at 12 to 15 months and 4 to 6 years, respectively
Dengue fever	• Dengue virus	• All age groups	• Female mosquitoes of the *Aedes* genus (esp. *Aedes aegypti*)	• Incubation period can last from 3 to 14 days (usually 4–7 days). • Sudden onset of high fever, headache, arthralgia and myalgia, nausea and vomiting. • Rash appears after a few days, initially as a flush, becoming more morbilliform after a few days, with typical islands of sparing. Petechiae are also common.	• Other viral exanthems • Chikungunya	• Leukopenia and thrombocytopenia are classical • Diagnosis by PCR, viral antigen detection (e.g., NS1), and serology • Treatment is mainly supportive
Infectious mononucleosis	• Epstein Barr virus (EBV)	• Older children, teenagers, young adults	• Oral secretions	• Clinical features include sore throat, cervical lymphadenopathy (cervical and submandibular), fever, malaise, myalgia, arthralgia, fatigue, headache. • Typical exanthem is a faint, non-pruritic generalized maculopapular rash, begins on the trunk and upper arms, then spreads to rest of the arm and face. May present as papular, morbilliform, vesicular, scarlatiniform, urticarial, petechial, or purpuric. • Although the rash is most often due to the virus itself, it can be precipitated by systemic antibiotics, most commonly amoxicillin or ampicillin. • Accompanying findings on examination include periorbital edema (especially the upper eyelids), hepatosplenomegaly, palatal petechiae, tonsillar enlargement, and genital ulcers.	• Scarlet fever • Cytomegalovirus (CMV) infection • Drug exanthem including DRESS syndrome	• A common finding is atypical lymphocytosis; other non-specific findings are neutropenia, thrombocytopenia, and elevated transaminases • Diagnosis is usually made by detecting IgM antibodies • Treatment is mainly supportive, including antipyretics, analgesia, and adequate hydration • Rest should be advised and encouraged, especially for patients with splenomegaly, and contact sports and strenuous activities should be avoided to prevent splenic rupture

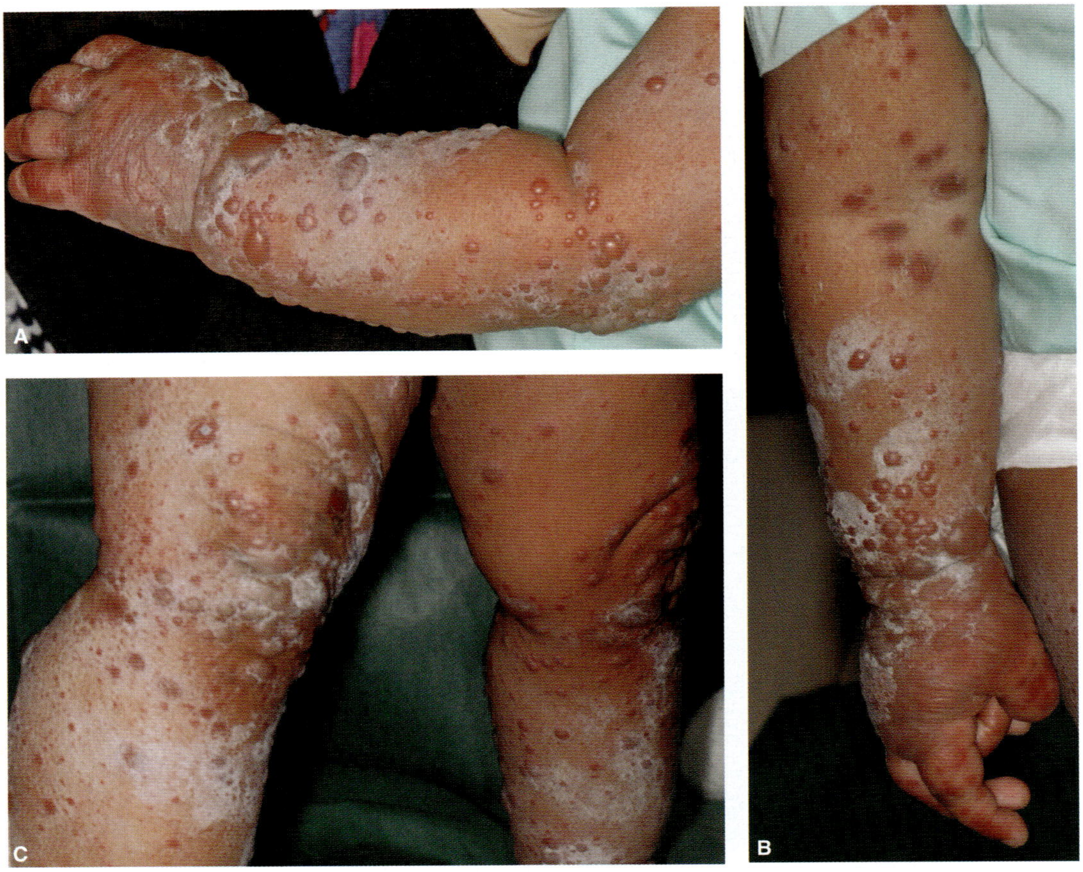

FIGURE 6-11A–11C. Bullous HFMD presenting with vesicles and papules in a Malay toddler with hand-foot-mouth disease.

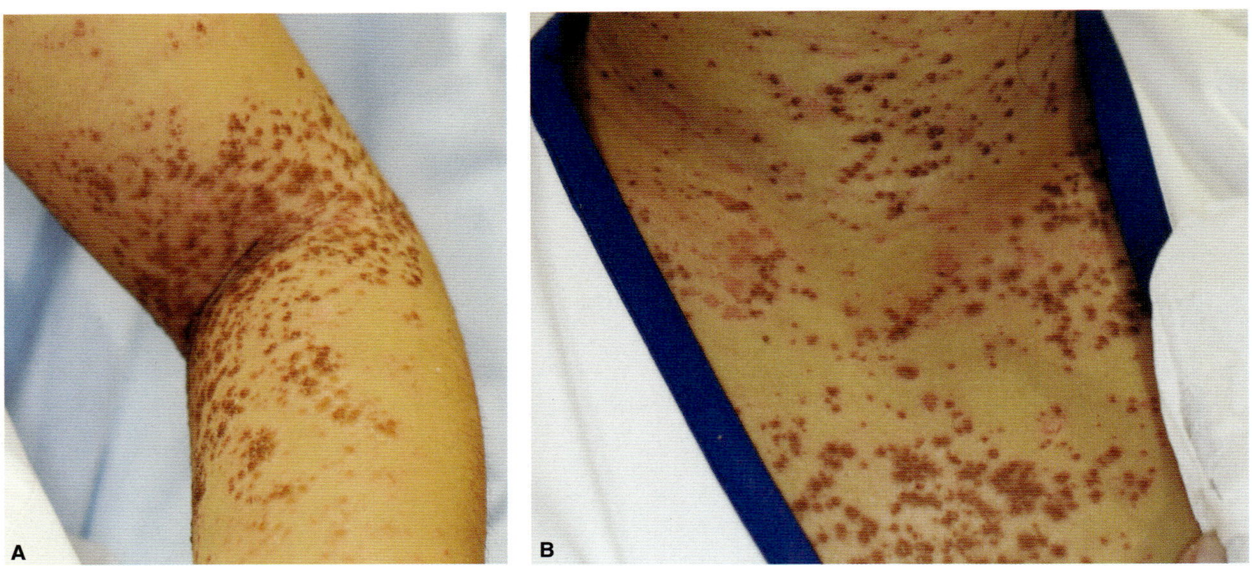

FIGURE 6-12A & 12B. Eczema coxsackium in a Chinese girl with atopic dermatitis, presenting as multiple, small, crusted or eroded papules on the flexors and chest.

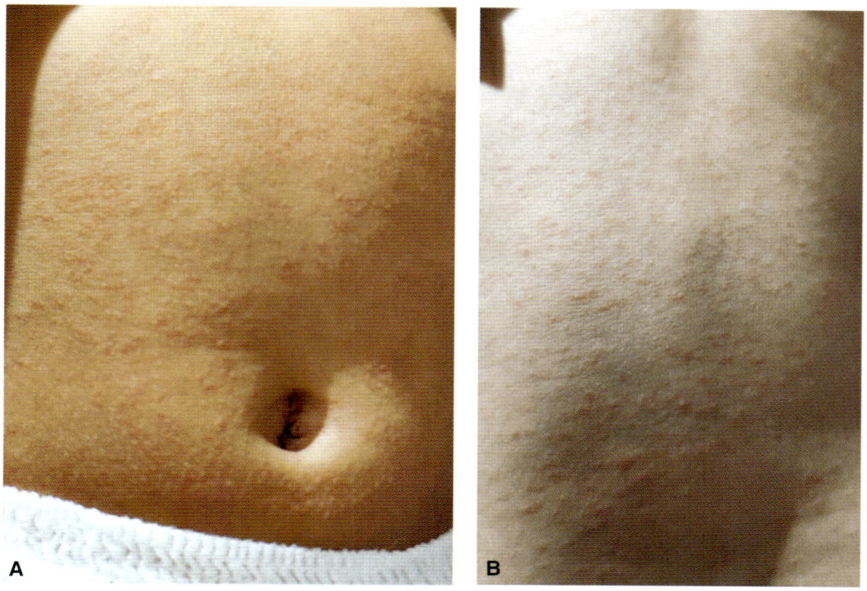

FIGURE 6-13A & 13B. Exanthem subitum in a Chinese infant, presenting with a non-specific, erythematous maculopapular rash on the trunk when the fever lysed.

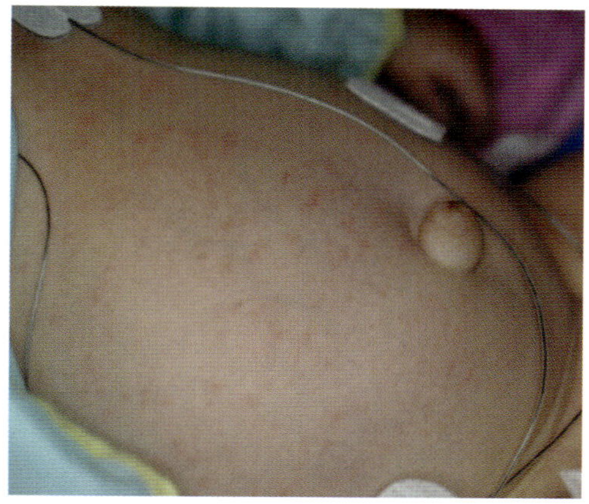

FIGURE 6-14. Exanthem subitum in a Chinese infant, presenting as blotchy, erythematous macules and papules over the trunk.

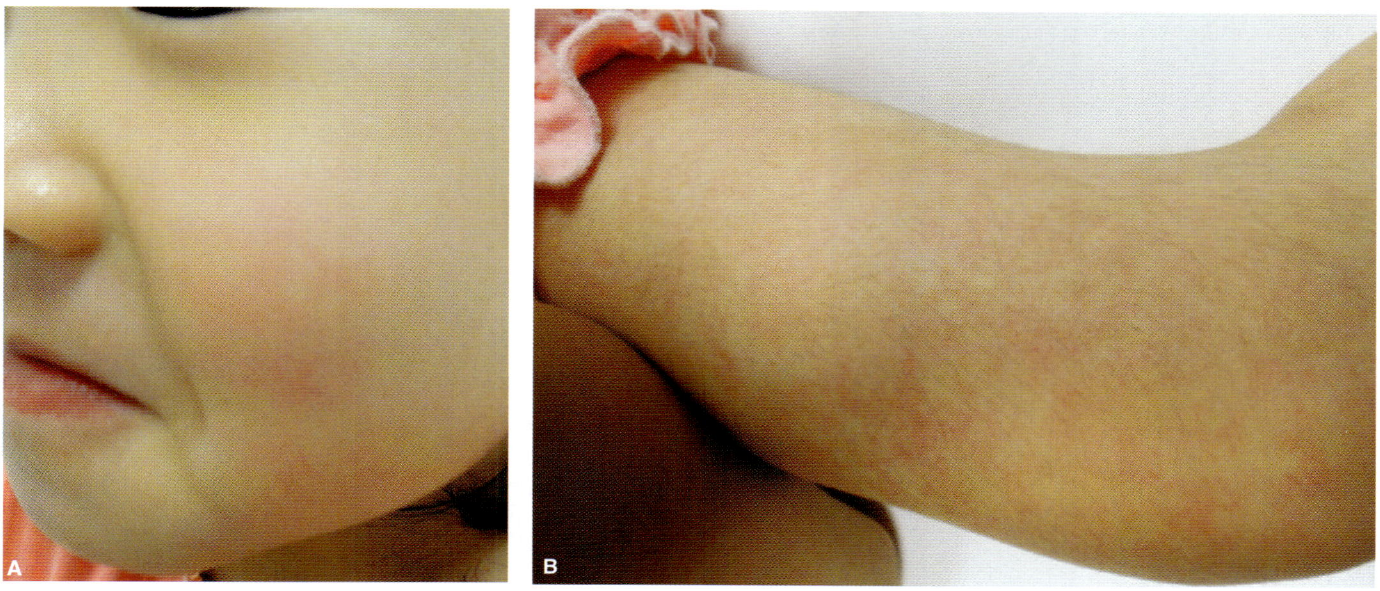

FIGURE 6-15A & 15B. Erythema infectiosum in a 6-year-old Chinese girl presenting with the classical "slapped-cheek" appearance and lacy, reticulate erythematous patches on the upper arms.

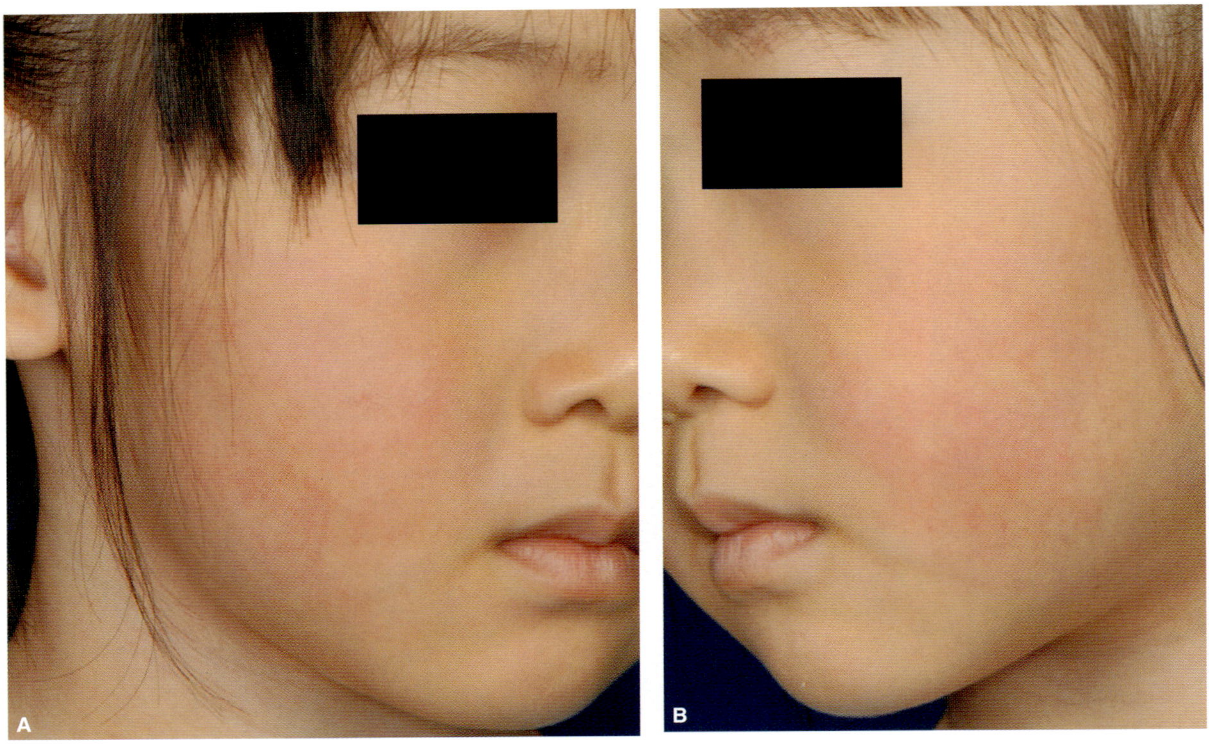

FIGURE 6-16A & 16B. A 5-year-old Chinese girl with erythema infectiosum, with classical "slapped-cheek" appearance bilaterally.

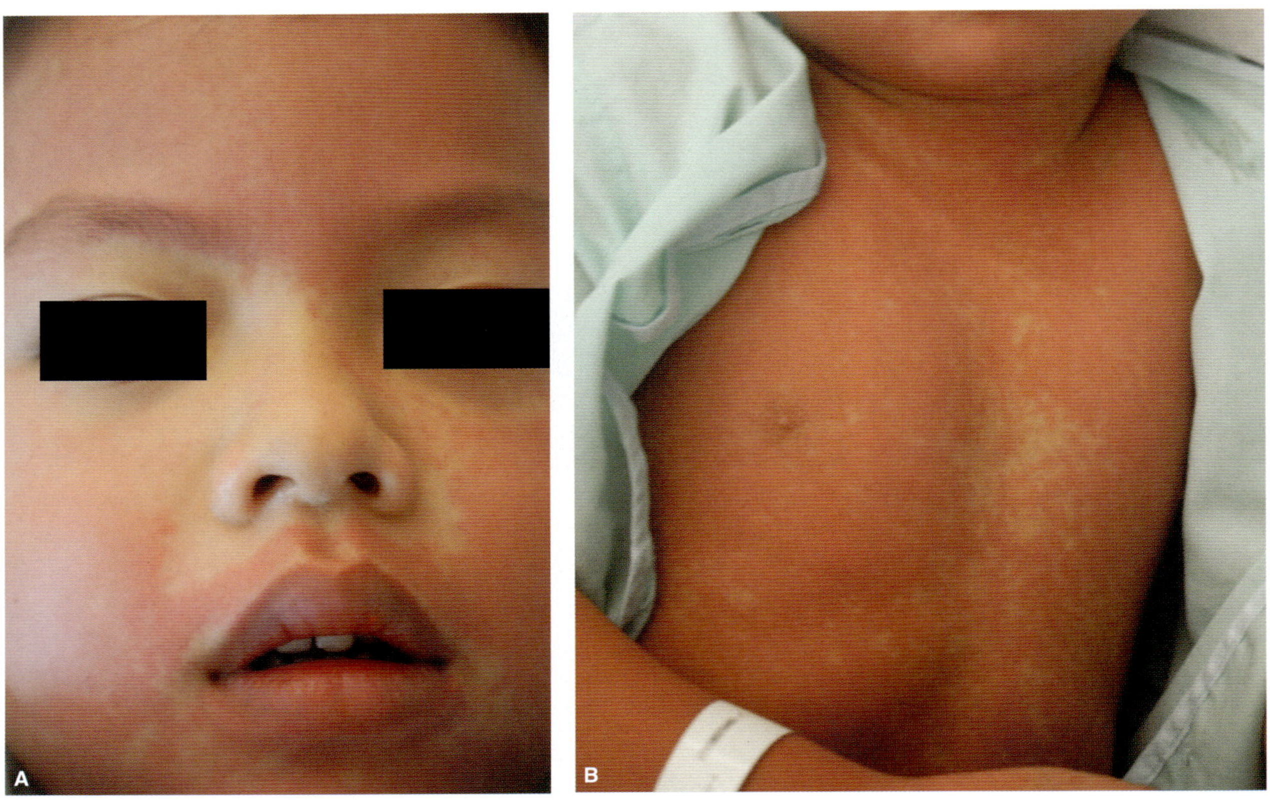

FIGURE 6-17A & 17B. A 3-year-old Chinese boy with dengue fever, presenting with fever and confluent, erythematous patches with islands of sparing.

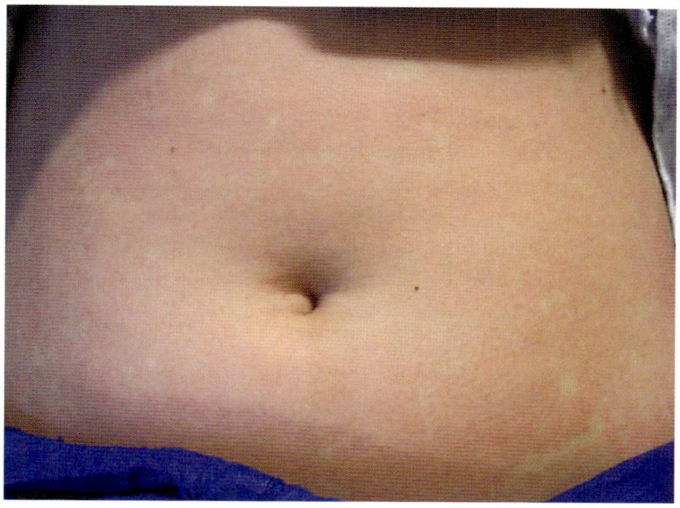

FIGURE 6-18. Dengue fever with widespread erythematous patches with islands of sparing in this Chinese boy. (Figure courtesy of Infectious Disease Service, KK Women's & Children's Hospital, Singapore.)

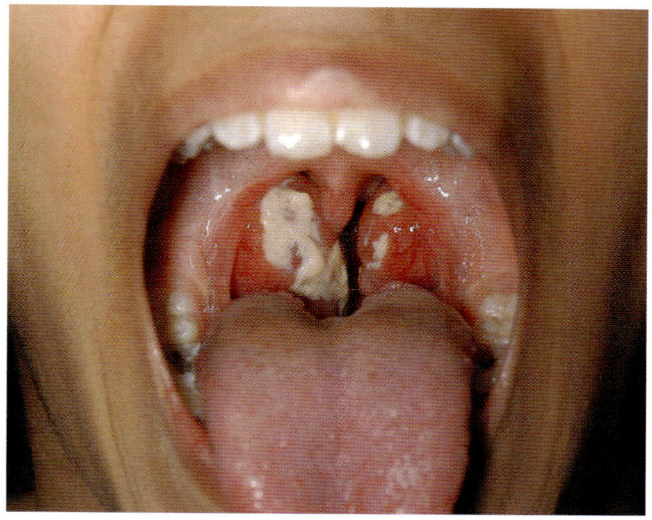

FIGURE 6-20. Infectious mononucleosis in an adolescent boy presenting with tonsillar enlargement with exudates. (Figure courtesy of Dr. Kumudhini Rajasegaran, Adolescent Medicine, KK Women's & Children's Hospital, Singapore.)

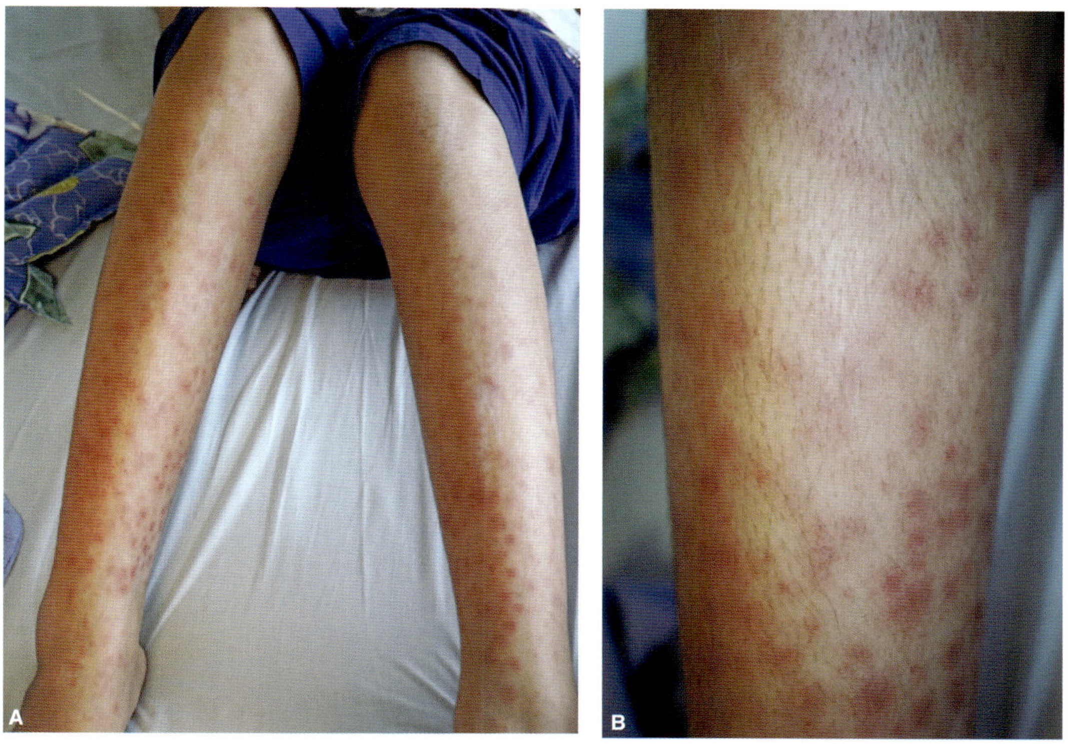

FIGURE 6-19A & 19B. Viral exanthem related to adenovirus in a 12-year-old Chinese boy, presenting as erythematous and purpuric patches over the lower legs.

- There are often preceding or concomitant systemic symptoms, such as fever, lethargy, reduced feeding, and irritability. Upper respiratory tract symptoms may also be present.
- Table 6-1 summarizes the clinical features of the common viral exanthems of childhood.

Bibliography

1. Irvine AD, Hoeger PH, Yan AC. Harper's Textbook of Pediatric Dermatology. 3rd ed. Wiley-Blackwell; 2011.
2. Marcdante K, Kliegman RM. Nelson Essentials of Pediatrics E-Book. Elsevier Health Sciences; 2014.
3. Chovel-Sella A, Ben Tov A, Lahav E et al. Incidence of rash after amoxicillin treatment in children with infectious mononucleosis. Pediatrics 2013;131(5):e1424-7.
4. World Health Organization. Immunization, Vaccines and Biologicals. World Health Organization. Published August 10, 2015. Accessed October 22, 2020. https://www.who.int/immunization/programmes_systems/interventions/vitamin_A/en/index1.html

GIANOTTI-CROSTI SYNDROME

Gianotti-Crosti syndrome, also known as papular or papulovesicular acrodermatitis of childhood, is a benign, self-limiting cutaneous response to a viral infection. It can also occur after vaccinations.

Clinical Features

- Gianotti-Crosti syndrome has been most frequently associated with hepatitis B and Epstein-Barr virus. Other etiologies include hepatitis A and C, herpesvirus 6, cytomegalovirus, coxsackievirus, adenovirus, enterovirus, echovirus, parvovirus B19, poxvirus, rotavirus, rubella, respiratory syncytial virus, polio virus, parainfluenza, and rarely, human immunodeficiency virus (HIV).[1]
- Numerous cases have also been reported following vaccinations, including DPT (diphtheria, pertussis, tetanus), polio, influenza, MMR (measles, mumps, rubella), Japanese encephalitis, and BCG (bacilli Calmette-Guerin) vaccines.[1,2]
- The condition presents as an acute eruption of monomorphic, 1- to 10-mm, flat-topped, skin-colored or pink-brown papules or papulovesicles that are non-pruritic and appear in symmetrical distribution on the extensor surfaces of the limbs, buttocks, and face. The lesions may coalesce into larger plaques over the elbows and knees. There is sparing of the flexures and mucous membranes.
- The eruption develops over a week and eventually fades in 3 to 4 weeks with mild desquamation.
- Although systemic symptoms such as low-grade fever and malaise may occur, patients are generally constitutionally well.

Differential Diagnoses

- Hand, foot, and mouth disease (HFMD)
  - HFMD is an enteroviral infection that also causes eruption of papules or papulovesicles, but involvement is usually limited to the oral mucosa, palms, and soles. Note, however, Gianotti-Crosti can be associated with HFMD, and has been reported to occur concomitantly or shortly after.
- Henoch-Schonlein purpura (HSP)
  - HSP is a small-vessel vasculitis presenting with classical symptoms of a vasculitic rash, joint pains, abdominal pains, and kidney impairment.
  - Compared to Gianotti-Crosti syndrome, the rash of HSP is more purpuric and less papular. It classically affects the shins and calves, although it can be more widespread and is often associated with joint pains, abdominal pain, and renal involvement.
- Scabies
  - Scabies can also present with widespread papules. However, compared to Gianotti-Crosti syndrome, the eruption of scabies occurs over weeks or months, is extremely pruritic, and involvement is most common over the intertriginous sites (axillae, groin), wrists, and finger webs. There is usually a positive contact history.

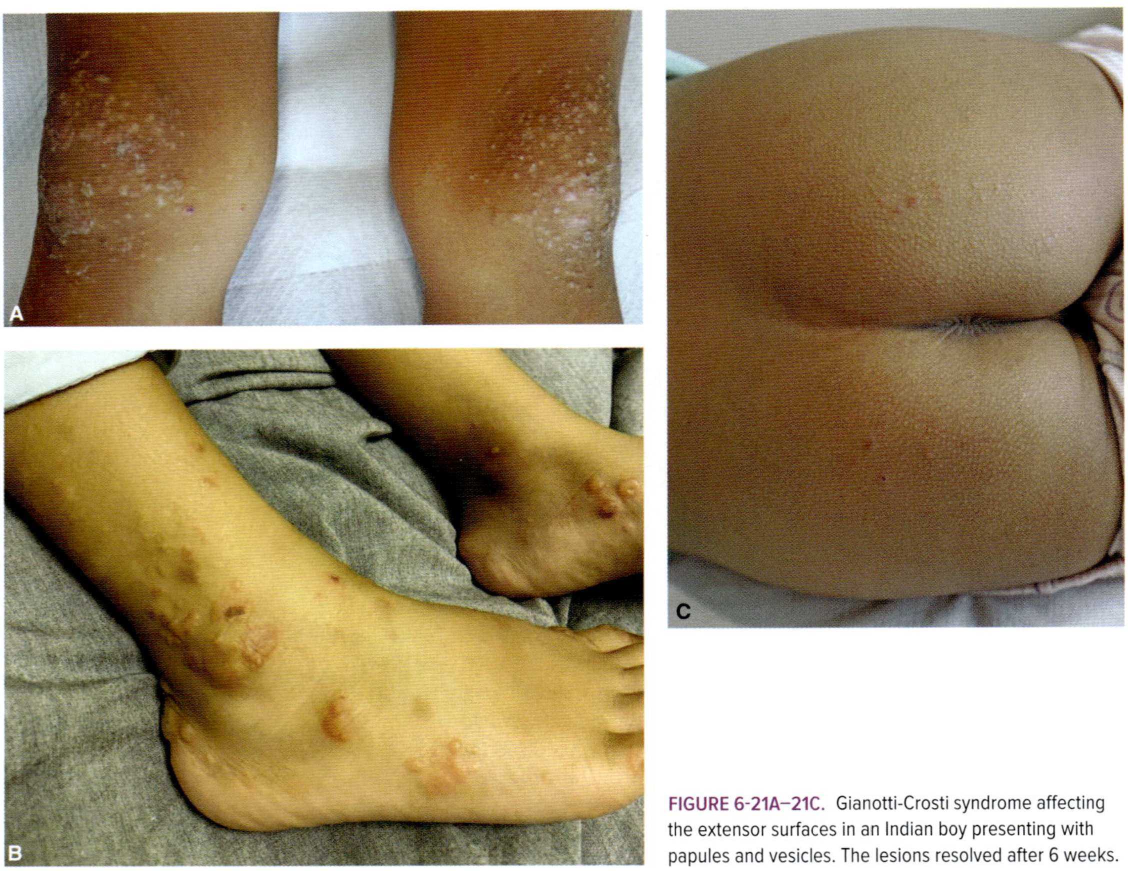

FIGURE 6-21A–21C. Gianotti-Crosti syndrome affecting the extensor surfaces in an Indian boy presenting with papules and vesicles. The lesions resolved after 6 weeks.

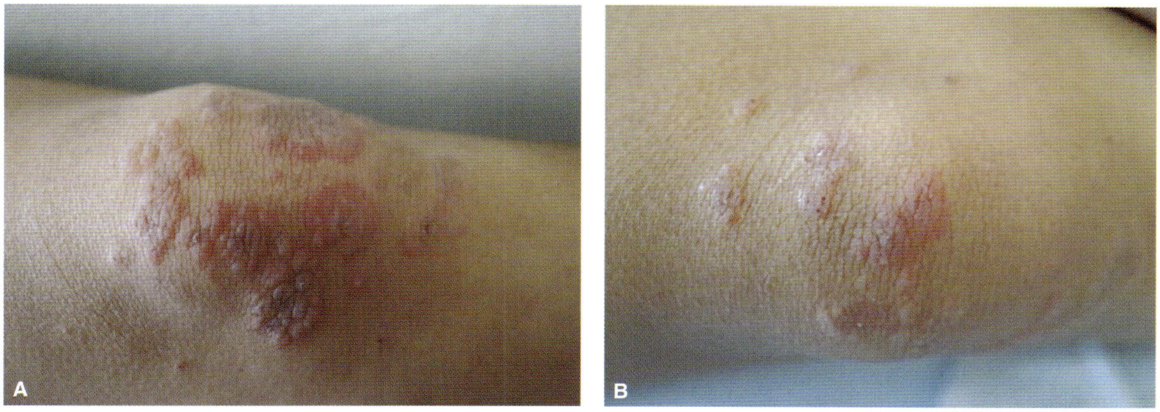

FIGURE 6-22A & 22B. Gianotti-Crosti syndrome in a Korean boy presenting with non-pruritic, pink to erythematous papules on the extensor surfaces of the elbows (not shown) and knees.

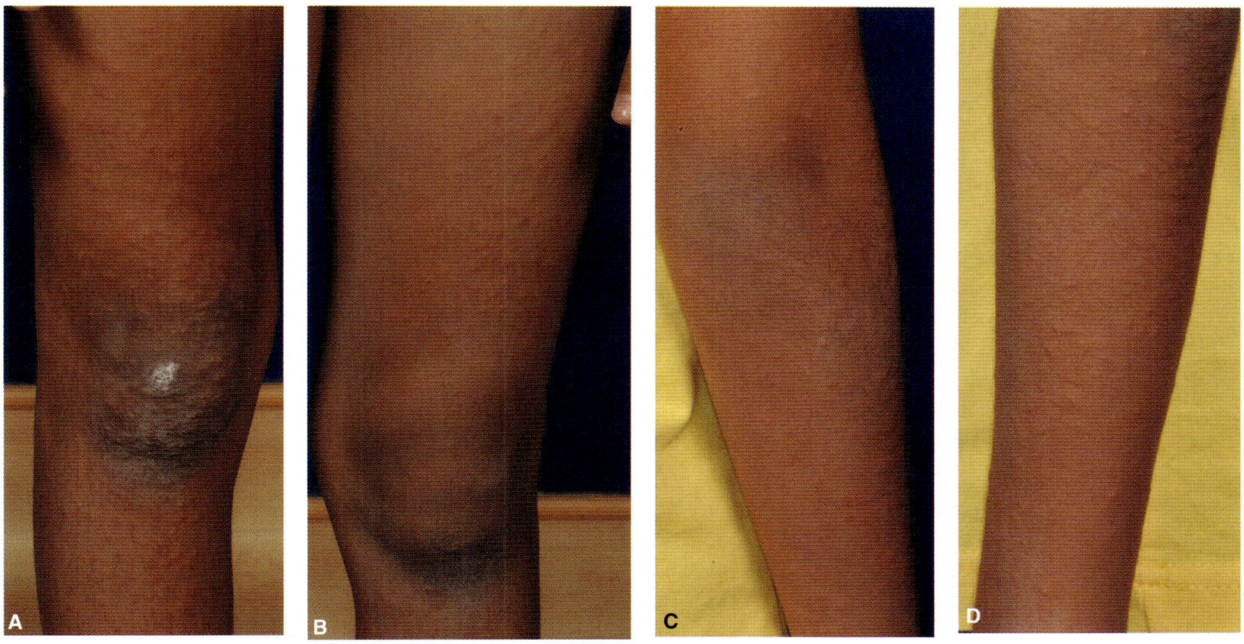

FIGURE 6-23A–23D. Gianotti-Crosti syndrome in an Indian child presenting with acute onset of non-pruritic skin-colored papules over the extensor surfaces.

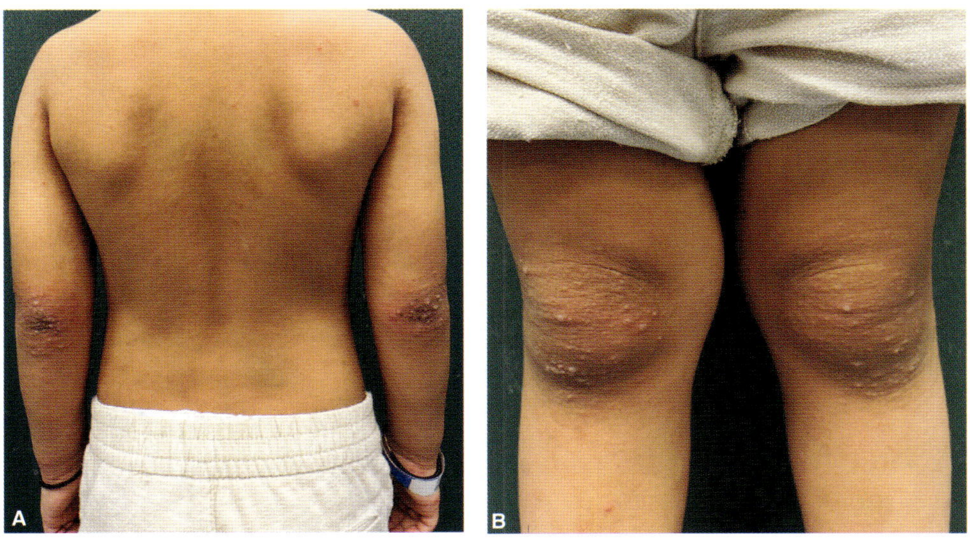

FIGURE 6-24A & 24B. Gianotti-Crosti syndrome in a young Nepalese child presenting with papules on the knees and elbows.

Investigations & Treatment

- Laboratory investigations are non-specific and non-confirmatory. Findings include leukopenia or leukocytosis with slightly elevated monocytes, and normal erythrocyte sedimentation rate.[1] Histology is non-specific.
- Treatment is mainly symptomatic and supportive. Topical corticosteroids and oral antihistamines may provide relief from pruritus.

Pearls & Practical Tips

- Gianotti-Crosti syndrome is often mistakenly diagnosed as scabies or HFMD. The duration and pattern of involvement helps to differentiate these three conditions.
- If there is no preceding illness or infection, reviewing the immunization history may be helpful.

Bibliography

1. Irvine AD, Hoeger PH, Yan AC. Harper's Textbook of Pediatric Dermatology. 3rd ed. Wiley-Blackwell; 2011.
2. Chuh AA. Diagnostic criteria for Gianotti-Crosti syndrome: a prospective case-control study for validity assessment. Cutis 2001;68(3):207-13.

VIRAL WARTS

Caused by human papillomavirus (HPV), viral warts or verrucae are common in children and adolescents. Most commonly occurring on the hands and feet, they can also occur on the face, trunk, and limbs. They may take years to self-resolve, and treatment can be prolonged. Recurrence is also common.

Clinical Features

- Warts are caused by HPV, a small, double-stranded DNA virus. It can be sexually or more commonly, non-sexually acquired, especially in children and adolescents. It is most often acquired through prolonged direct contact with another affected individual, or through fomites and autoinoculation.
- Common, flat, and plantar warts are commonly due to HPV types 1, 2, 3, 4, 7, and 10.
- Anogenital warts can occur from autoinoculation (commonly from the child's hand), inoculation from an adult during handling or diaper changes, or via vertical transmission. However, sexual abuse also needs to be considered.
- The clinical appearance varies depending on the site. The following warts are common in children and adolescents:
  - *Common warts (verruca vulgaris)*
    - » The most common type of wart in children and adolescents, most often occurring on the palms and soles.
    - » Appear as pedunculated, dome-shaped (non-acral sites) or flat-topped (acral sites), circumscribed, hyperkeratotic papules and nodules with a rough, irregular surface.
    - » Thrombosed capillaries are often seen after paring the hyperkeratotic surface. The overlying skin lines are disrupted.
  - *Flat/plane warts (verruca plana)*
    - » Common among children and young adults, and most prevalent sites are the face, neck, and dorsum of hands.
    - » Present as smooth, flesh-colored, or slightly pigmented, flat-topped brownish keratotic papules, 2 to 4 mm in size.
  - *Periungual and subungual warts*
    - » These are warts seen around or under the nails.
    - » May be painful, and treatment is challenging due to the physical obstruction by the nail.

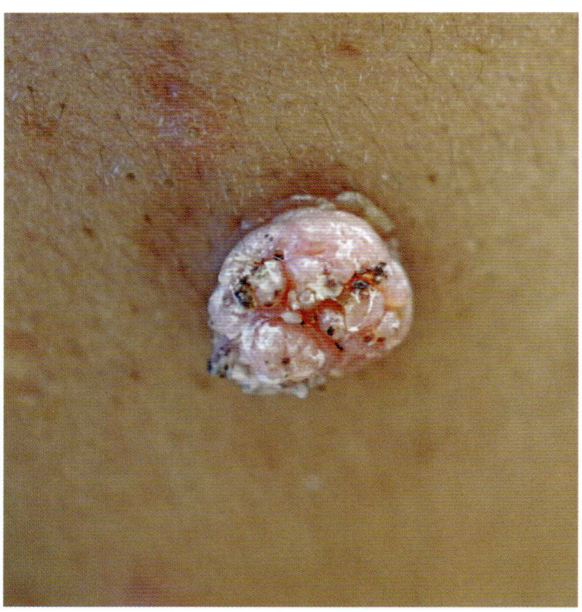

FIGURE 6-25. Viral wart on the cheek of a Malay adolescent male, presenting as a solitary, verrucous nodule.

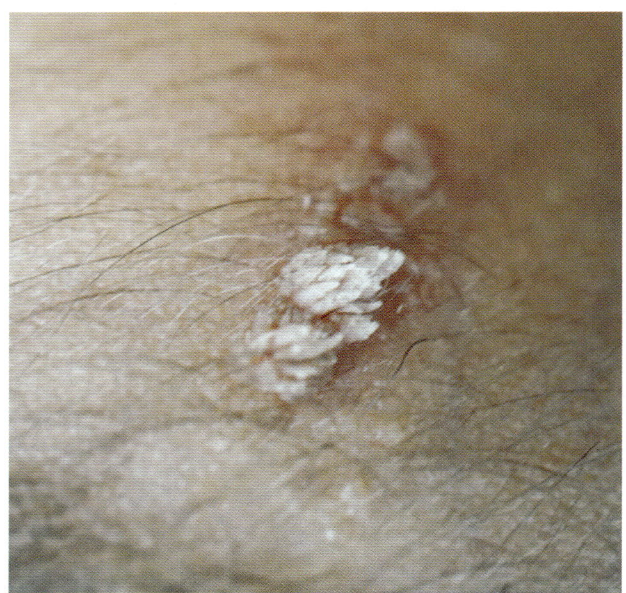

FIGURE 6-26. Filliform warts on the forehead of a young Chinese boy, presenting with keratotic finger-like projections.

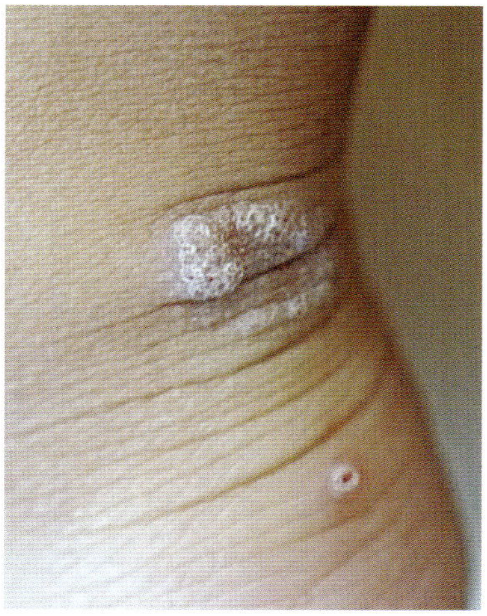
FIGURE 6-27. Warts on the back of the heel of a young Malay girl.

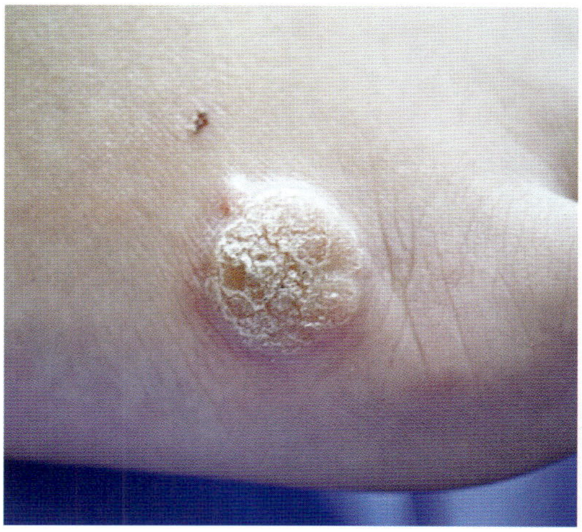
FIGURE 6-28. Large wart on the dorsum of the foot of a Chinese girl.

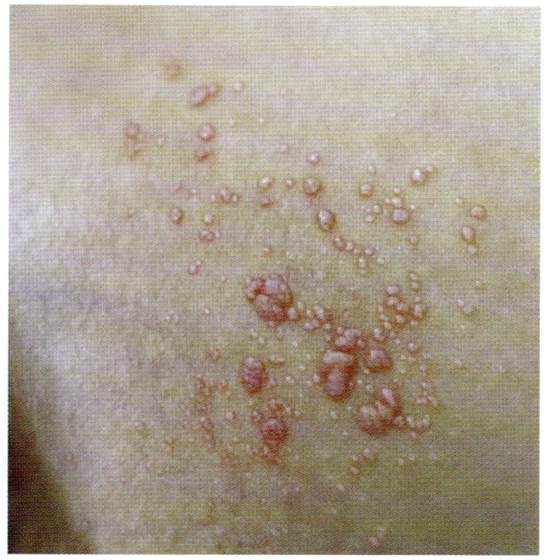
FIGURE 6-29. Multiple warts on the thigh of a Chinese adolescent girl.

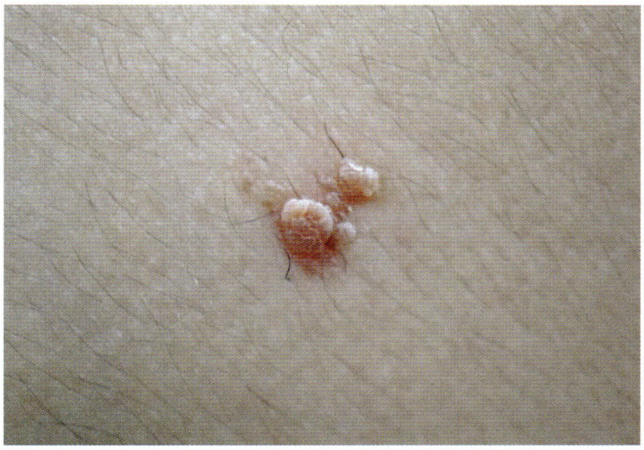
FIGURE 6-30. Viral wart on the limb.

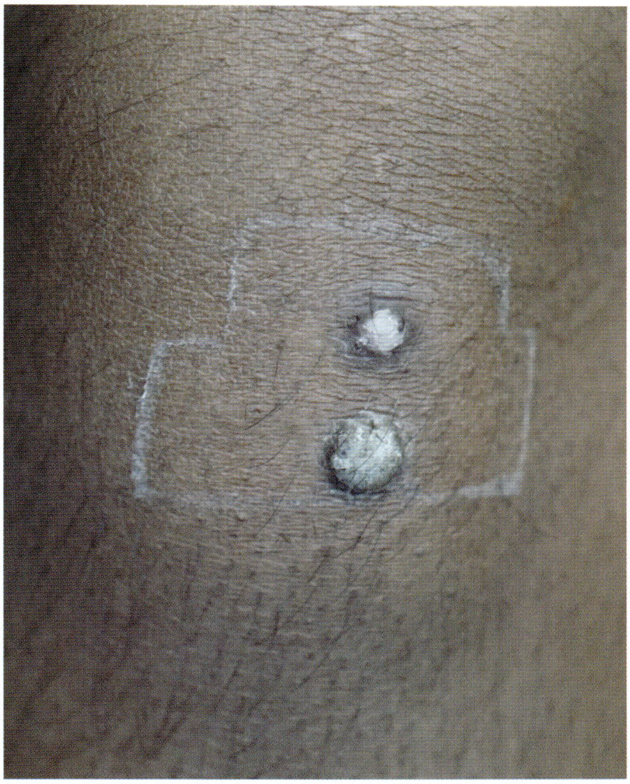
FIGURE 6-31. Warts on the knee of an Indian girl. Note the hyperkeratosis.

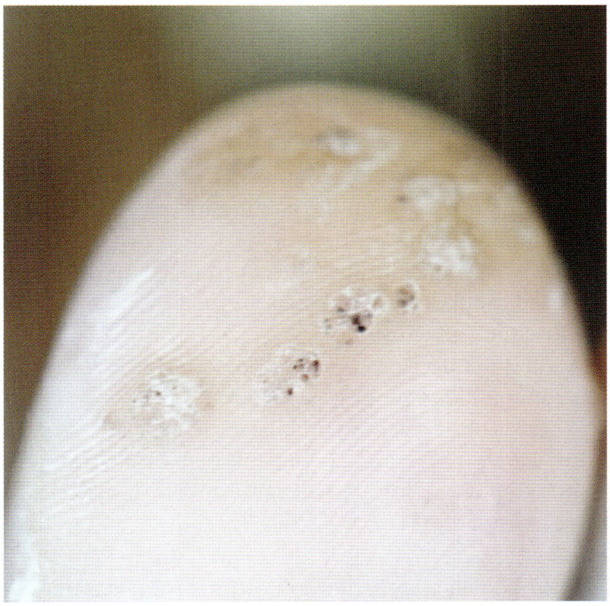
FIGURE 6-32. Multiple warts on the big toe of a young Chinese boy. Note the loss of skin lines and thrombosed capillaries.

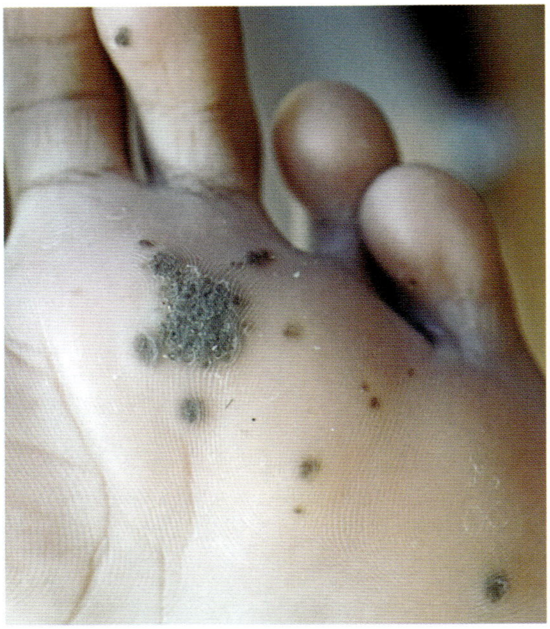

FIGURE 6-33. Multiple plantar warts in an Indian adolescent. Note the increased pigmentation seen in the warts.

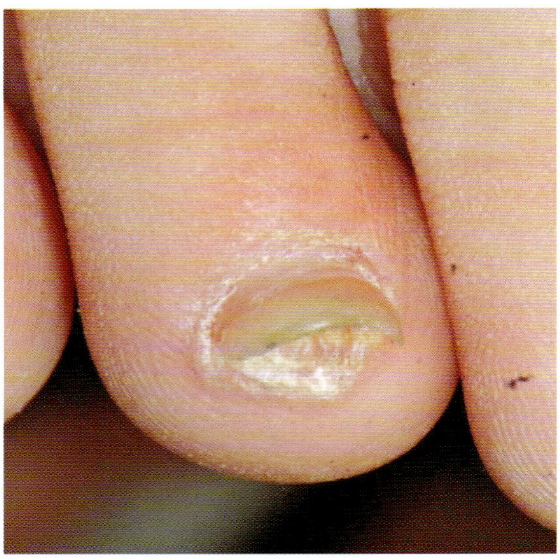

FIGURE 6-35. Subungual warts causing "tenting" of the nail plate in a young Chinese boy.

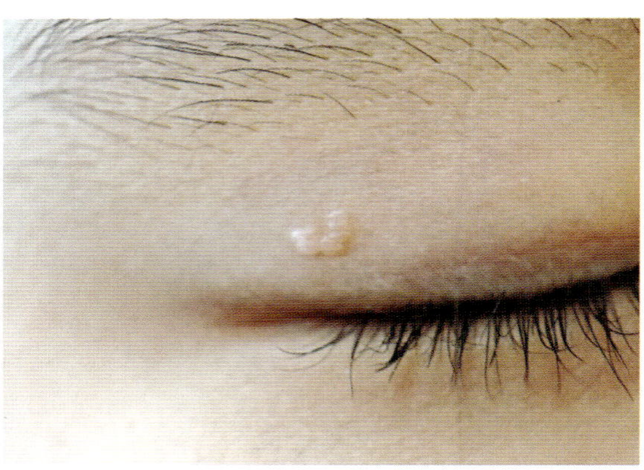

FIGURE 6-37. Plane warts on the upper eyelids of a Chinese girl.

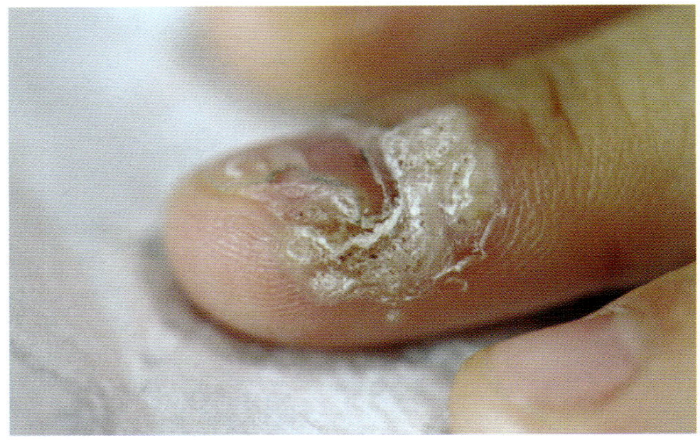

FIGURE 6-34. Periungual warts causing destruction of the nail plate in a Chinese adolescent boy.

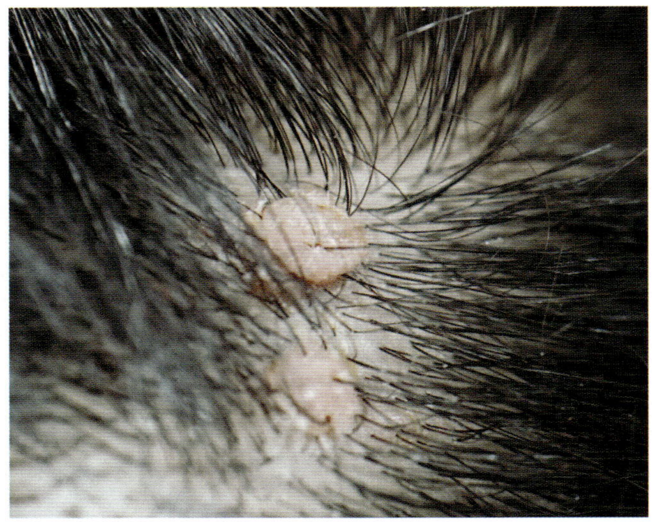

FIGURE 6-36. Viral warts on the scalp, presenting as pedunculated, verrucous papules.

Differential Diagnoses

- Callus
  - Calluses occur over pressure sites of the soles of the feet, and less often on the palms and knees, and occur bilaterally symmetrical.
  - The overlying skin lines are accentuated, and thrombosed capillaries are not seen on paring.
- Molluscum contagiosum
  - Viral skin infection caused by poxvirus that presents as skin-colored to pinkish papules.
  - There is often a central umbilication, which is not seen in warts. There are no thrombosed capillaries, and pricking of the surface will cause a whitish material to be extruded.
- Skin tags
  - Also known as acrochordon or fibroepithelial polyps, can occur anywhere, and appear as soft, pedunculated, hyperpigmented papules.

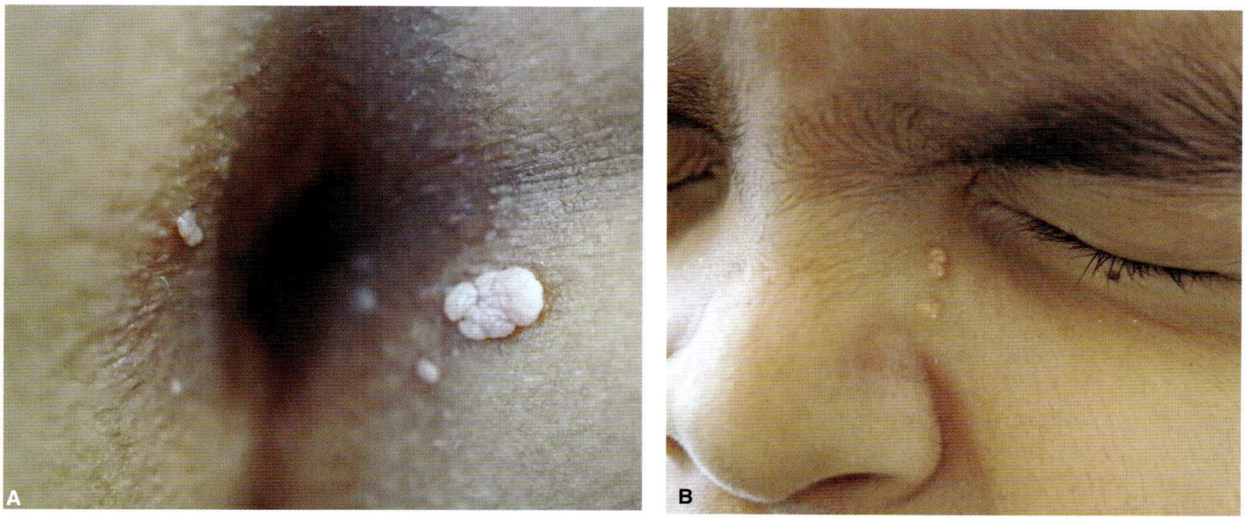

FIGURE 6-38A & 38B. Perianal warts in a Malay boy caused by autoinoculation of warts from other anatomical sites, such as the face in Figure 6-38B.

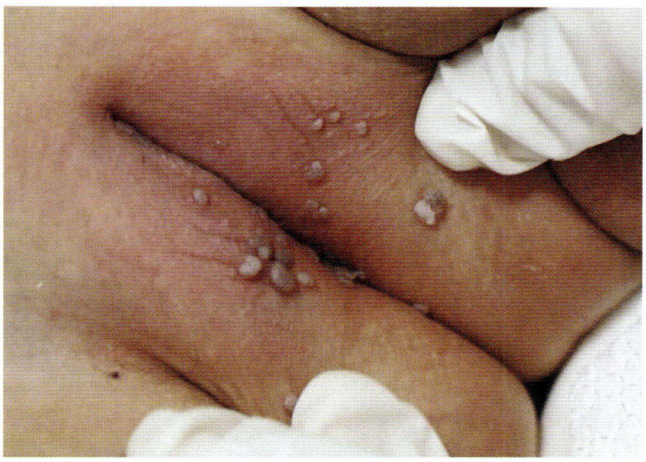

FIGURE 6-39. Multiple genital warts on the groin and vulva of a Malay infant.

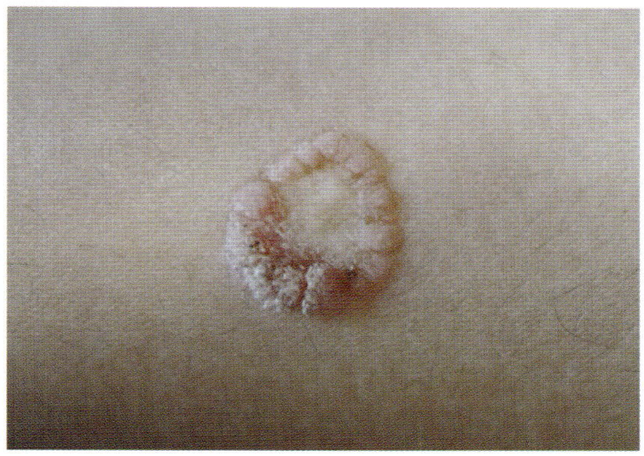

FIGURE 6-40. "Fairy-ring" warts with an annular configuration and central clearing. This can occur after cryotherapy treatment for warts.

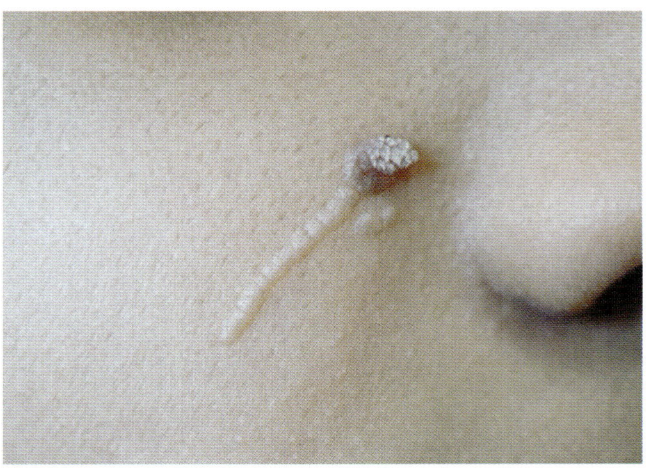

FIGURE 6-41. Koebner phenomenon is demonstrated in this Indian boy with warts on his cheek. There is a large "primary" wart and several flatter lesions seen in a line from this lesion, after self-inflicted trauma.

Investigations & Treatment

- Warts are usually diagnosed clinically. Dermoscopy may aid in diagnosis, with warts appearing as round, keratinous lesions with red or black dots on the surface representing the dilated or thrombosed capillaries.
- Various treatment options are available, based on the patient's age, number, and size and location of lesions.
- Destructive therapies include:
  - Keratolytics such as salicylic acid, are safe and effective, and can be applied at home. Efficacy is shown at about 75% after 6 to 8 weeks of use. This treatment alone is useful for young children as it is painless.
  - Imiquimod, a topical modulator, applied as home treatment, is useful for the treatment of verruca plana.

It is not as useful for highly keratinized warts, as it does not have keratolytic properties.
- Cantharidin is derived from the blister beetle *Cantharis vesicatoria*.[1] It causes epidermal cell death, acantholysis, and clinical blister formation, which can be painful. Cantharidin is applied in the physician's office every 1 to 2 weeks.
- Cryotherapy is an effective treatment in older children and adolescents, who have a higher pain threshold. Liquid nitrogen is the coldest and most effective agent used. Treatment is performed every 1 to 2 weeks. Paring the surface of the wart before cryotherapy improves the efficacy of treatment.
- Curettage and electrocautery is usually done under local anesthesia and may be required for the treatment of large, deep warts, especially on the plantar surface.
- Laser therapy is an effective mode of treatment but is mainly reserved for refractory cases since routine use is not cost-effective. Associated pain during and after the procedure makes this an option only for older children who can tolerate the discomfort. Ablative lasers (e.g., carbon dioxide laser) are most commonly used.

Pearls & Practical Tips

- The risk of recurrence after treatment is approximately 20% regardless of type of wart and treatment modality.
- In the author's experience, the use of "triple treatment" with cryotherapy every 2 weeks and application of a keratolytic, occluded overnight by duct-tape, daily between cryotherapy treatments, is especially useful in the treatment of plantar warts.
- The presence of external genital warts should always raise suspicion for sexual abuse, especially if there are no lesions elsewhere on the rest of the body. A careful and thorough social and contact history should be elicited, and a full skin examination should be performed to determine the presence of lesions at other sites. Patients should also be examined for other signs of abuse or injury.
- There are multivalent HPV vaccines currently available: a bivalent one that covers HPV 16 and 18, and a quadrivalent one that also includes HPV 6 and 11. Although these are mainly for cervical cancer prevention, there has been a decline in cases of anogenital warts since their introduction. The quadrivalent HPV vaccine has been shown to be a well-tolerated therapy for recalcitrant warts in children.[3]

Bibliography

1. Irvine AD, Hoeger PH, Yan AC. Harper's Textbook of Pediatric Dermatology. 3rd ed. Wiley-Blackwell; 2011.
2. Silverberg NB. Human papillomavirus infections in children. Curr Opin Pediatr 2004;16(4):402-9.
3. Abeck D, Fölster-Holst, R. Quadrivalent human papillomavirus vaccination: a promising treatment for recalcitrant cutaneous warts in children. Acta Dermato-Venereologica 2015;95(8):1017-9.
4. Soenjoyo KR, Chua BWB, Wee LWY, Koh MJA, Ang SB. Treatment of cutaneous viral warts in children: A review. Dermatol Ther 2020;33(6):e14034.

MOLLUSCUM CONTAGIOSUM

Molluscum contagiosum (MC) is a common cutaneous infection in children, caused by the molluscum contagiosum virus (MCV), a type of poxvirus. Mostly self-limiting, it can cause significant distress among parents and teachers.

Clinical Features

- Can occur at any age but is most common in toddlers and young children.
- Spread by direct skin-to-skin contact or through fomites. Autoinoculation can occur in affected patients, leading to formation of new lesions at other sites.
- Presents as small, pearly, skin-colored to pinkish, dome-shaped papules, sometimes with a central umbilication or depression.
- Lesions are usually asymptomatic but can occasionally be itchy.
- Although MC lesions can occur almost anywhere on the body surface, they are most common on sites subjected to more friction, such as the groin, axillae, and cubital and popliteal fossae.

Differential Diagnoses

- Viral warts
  - Viral warts tend to have a more undulating or filiform surface compared to the smooth surface of MC.
  - Tiny thrombosed blood vessels may be seen on the surface of warts, especially on paring.
  - Viral warts do not have central umbilication.
- Milia
  - Milia may look similar to MC but are whiter in color and usually occur in fewer numbers than MC.
  - They usually do not have the central umbilication.

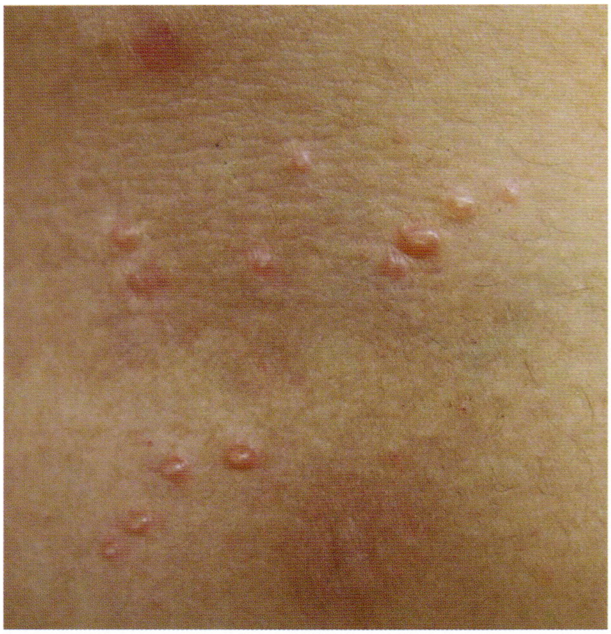

FIGURE 6-42. Molluscum contagiosum presenting as small, grouped, skin-colored, dome-shaped papules.

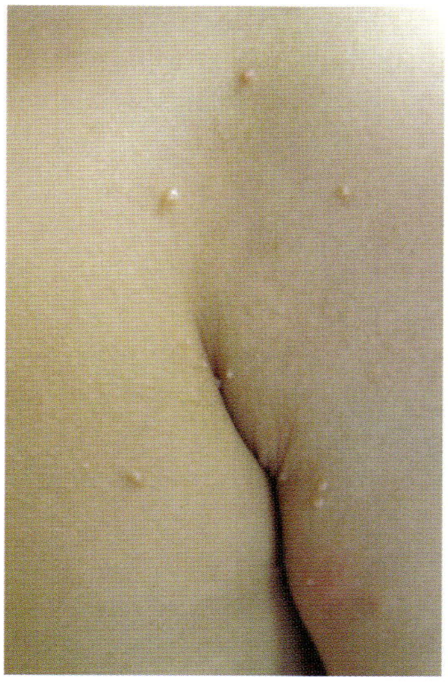

FIGURE 6-43. Multiple mollusca presenting as skin-colored, dome-shaped papules on the chest of this young Chinese child.

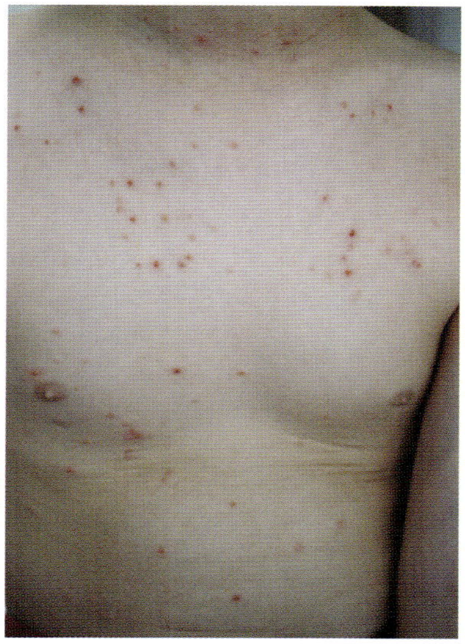

FIGURE 6-44. Extensive molluscum contagiosum on the trunk of a Korean boy. Note the surface excoriations on some of the lesions.

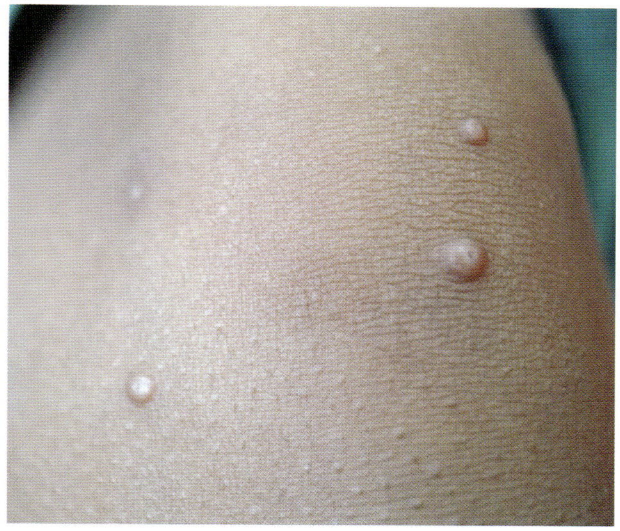

FIGURE 6-45. Several lesions of molluscum contagiosum seen on the knee of a Malay adolescent, with central umbilication.

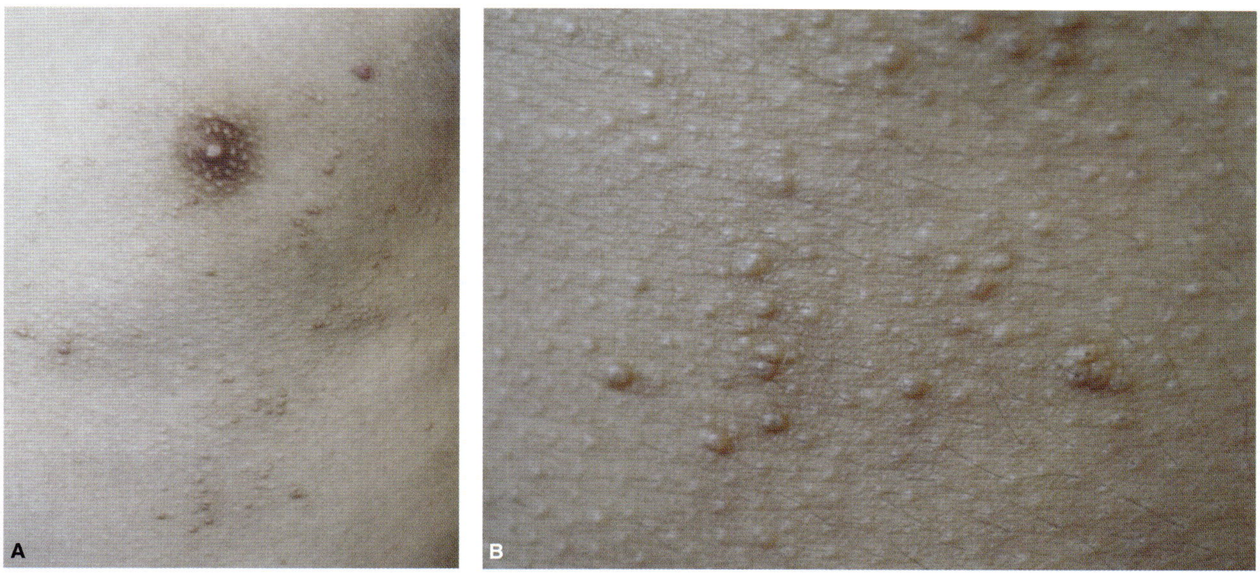

FIGURE 6-46A & 46B. Molluscum contagiosum presenting on the left chest of a Chinese adolescent with more hyperpigmented papules, some with central umbilication.

- Follicular/papular eczema
  - The distribution of follicular eczema is more evenly spaced out, following the distribution of hair follicles on the skin. They lesions also lack umbilication. Other features may be present, such as xerosis or a family/personal history of atopy.

Investigations & Treatment

- Investigations are usually not required for diagnosis.
- Skin biopsy shows a crateriform lesion with hyperplastic epidermis surrounding "molluscum bodies," which appear as eosinophilic intracytoplasmic inclusions.
- Spontaneous resolution of MC lesions can occur after 6 months to 2 years.
- Treatment may be offered if parents, caregivers, or teachers express concerns.
- Treatment options include topical therapies (imiquimod, tretinoin, cantharidin), curettage, prick and express, electrocautery, and laser ablation.[1]
- Pricking and expressing lesions of MC is a simple procedure involving extraction or evisceration of the core of the lesion with a sterile blade, edge of a glass slide, or needle. A local anesthetic cream can be applied under occlusion

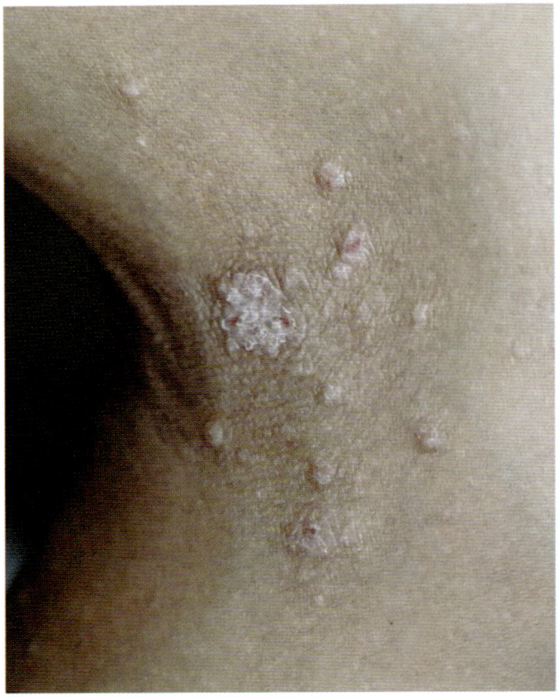

FIGURE 6-47. Molluscum contagiosum on the lateral knee of a Chinese adolescent with atopic dermatitis. Note the eczema surrounding a few of the lesions of mollusca.

prior to the procedure to minimize discomfort. After pricking the top of the lesion, the contents are expressed with gentle pressure. This can be performed on the larger lesions and can be repeated if the remaining lesions do not resolve after about 1 to 2 months.

Pearls & Practical Tips

- MC is more commonly seen and usually more extensive in children with atopic dermatitis.
- The appearance of eczematous changes around lesions of MC is a good indicator that the lesions may be resolving.
- Topical therapies need to be applied for at least 2 months to evaluate for efficacy.
- Many of the treatment options for MC can cause substantial pain and discomfort in children, and should be attempted only if other less invasive options have failed. Adequate analgesia should be applied before performing these treatments.

Reference

1. Weatherall DJ. Bone marrow transplantation for thalassemia and other inherited disorders of hemoglobin. Blood 1999;61(8):762.

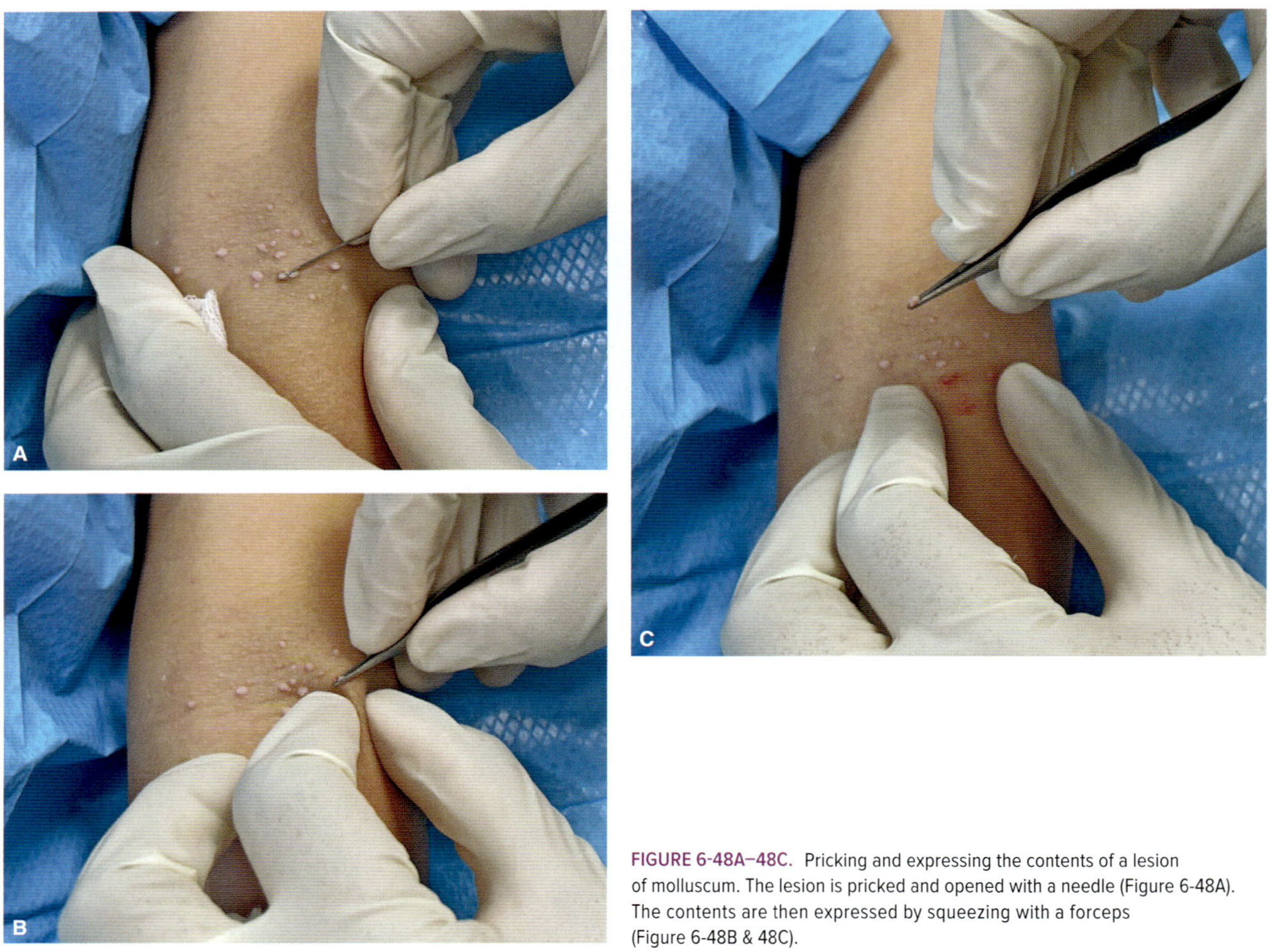

FIGURE 6-48A–48C. Pricking and expressing the contents of a lesion of molluscum. The lesion is pricked and opened with a needle (Figure 6-48A). The contents are then expressed by squeezing with a forceps (Figure 6-48B & 48C).

BACTERIAL INFECTIONS

IMPETIGO

Impetigo is a common superficial cutaneous infection in children, and less commonly in adolescents and adults. It is most commonly caused by *Staphylococcus aureus* but can also be caused by *Streptococcus*.

Clinical Features

- Impetigo is more common in lower socioeconomic areas and tropical climates. It is spread by direct contact or through fomites. It can lead to outbreaks in childcare facilities and schools.
- It is more common in patients with atopic dermatitis or other forms of eczema (e.g., discoid eczema) and other skin disorders.
- It can involve any body surface area but is most common on the face, neck, genital and buttock areas, and extremities. Lesions can progress over a few days or weeks.
- There are two forms of impetigo:
  1. Bullous impetigo is cause exclusively by *S. aureus*. Lesions present as flaccid, thin-walled bullae containing pus that rupture easily, resulting in shallow erosions with peripheral scaling.
  2. Non-bullous impetigo can be caused by *S. aureus* or group A β-hemolytic streptococci. This initially presents as a pustule or erythematous papule that forms overlying oozy, honey-crusted scaling.
- Ecthymas, caused by group A β-hemolytic streptococci or *S. aureus*, are deeper forms of impetigo and present as small, purulent, shallow ulcers with overlying thick, brown-black crusts and surrounding erythema.
- Although most children present with disease confined to the skin, complications can uncommonly occur, such as scalded skin syndrome, sepsis, osteomyelitis, septic arthritis, pneumonia, and glomerulonephritis.

Differential Diagnoses

- Infected or impetiginized eczema
  - Lesions of eczema are often infected with *S. aureus*.
  - Differentiating impetiginized eczema and impetigo is important, as treatment of impetiginized eczema requires treatment of both the infection and the underlying eczema. Look for clues of eczema, such as lichenification.
- Herpes infections
  - These also often cause bullae and may become secondarily infected with *S. aureus*. Herpetic bullae tend to be smaller and have clear discharge compared to impetigo.
  - If in doubt, microbiological investigations will be useful to differentiate, and coverage for both herpes and impetigo should be started empirically.
- Tinea
  - The progression of tinea is much slower than impetigo, progressing over weeks and sometimes months, rather than days or weeks in impetigo.
  - Does not have the same honey-crusted scaling as seen in impetigo. However, bullous lesions are also seen in tinea.
  - If in doubt of diagnosis, microbiological investigations may be useful to differentiate.
- Other bullous conditions
  - Examples include cutaneous candidiasis, bullous drug eruption, bullous erythema multiforme, and contact dermatitis. Impetiginization of these conditions can also occur commonly.
  - A thorough history, physical examination, and proper investigations will help to differentiate these conditions.

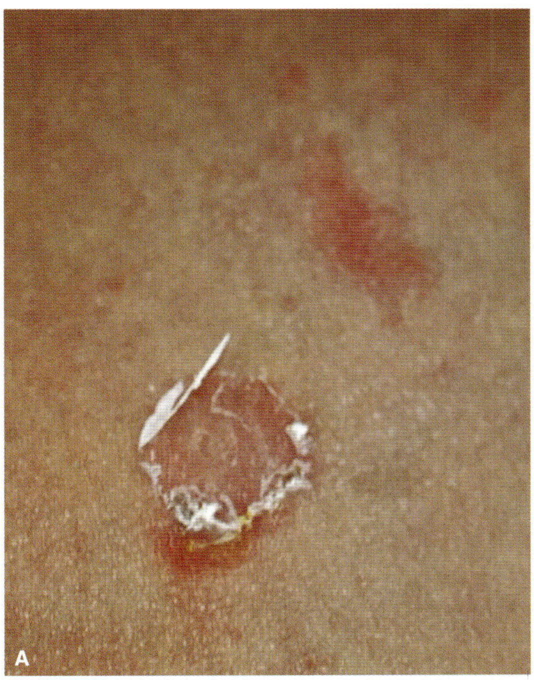

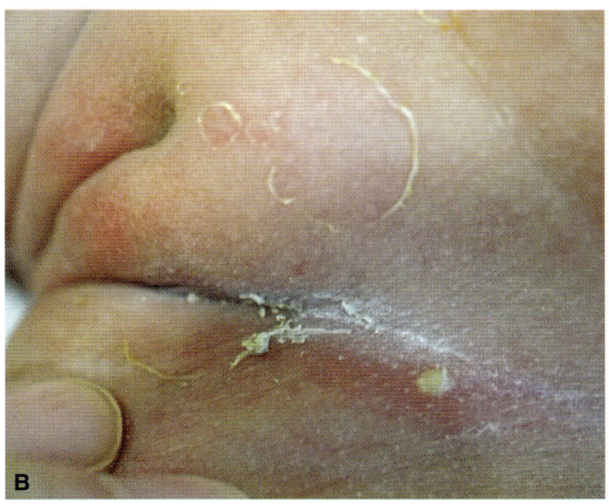

FIGURE 6-49A & 49B. Impetigo on the trunk of a young Chinese infant female neonate presenting with crusted, annular plaque, associated with lesions of localized scalded skin syndrome with circular, superficial erosions with peripheral scaling in the groin. A pustule is also seen.

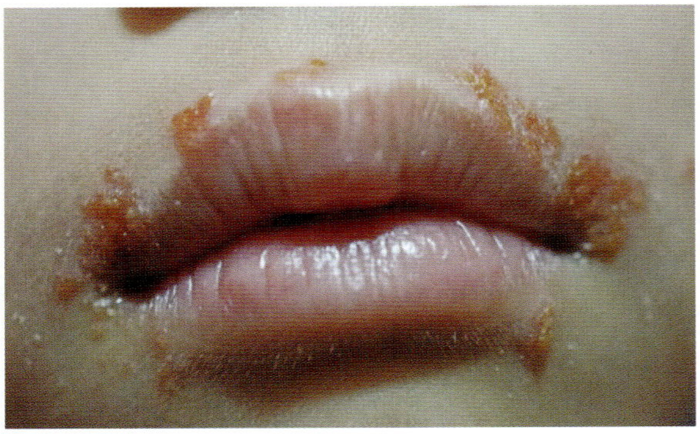

FIGURE 6-50. Bullous impetigo on the perioral region of this young Chinese boy, presenting with small pustules and vesicles, with golden-yellow crusting.

Investigations & Treatment

- Impetigo is diagnosed clinically, with microbiological investigations (e.g., Gram stain and bacterial culture) being useful adjuncts to confirm the diagnosis and aid with treatment.
- Skin biopsies are rarely performed, but if done will show subcorneal blister with acantholysis.
- Treatment of impetigo depends on the extent. In limited disease, topical antibiotics may suffice, including fusidic acid, tetracycline, and mupirocin, usually for 1 to 2 weeks until lesions resolve. In more extensive disease, systemic antibiotics will be required for 1 to 2 weeks. Most patients will respond to oral antibiotics such as cephalexin or cloxacillin. If the child is unwell, parenteral antibiotics may be required.
- Soaks with potassium permanganate or normal saline are useful adjuncts, especially in blistered or oozy lesions.

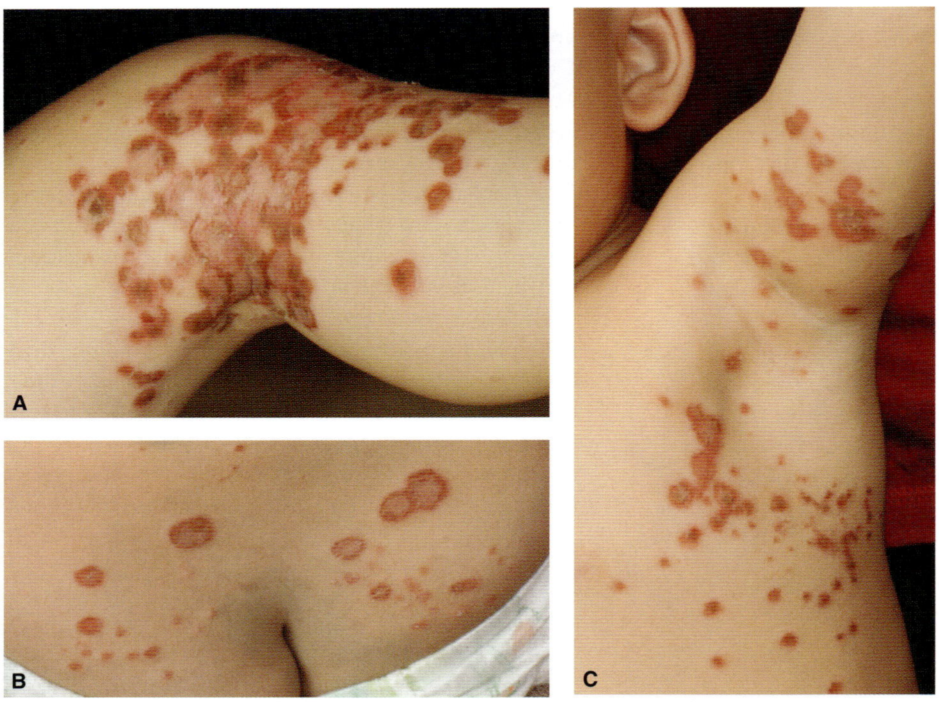

FIGURE 6-51A–51C. Widespread non-bullous impetigo affecting the legs, back, arms, and axilla in a young Chinese boy, presenting with annular, crusted papules and plaques.

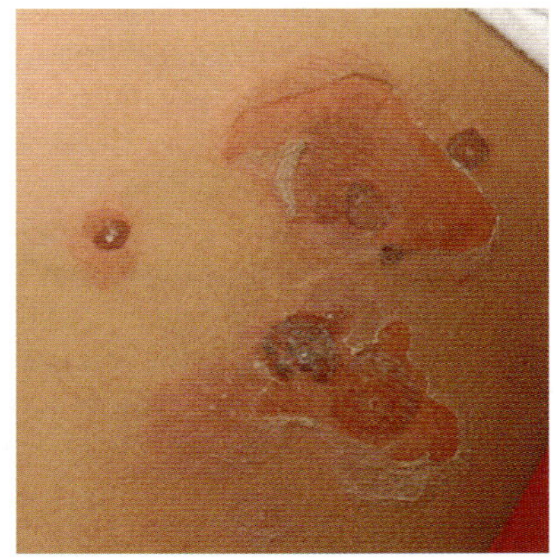

FIGURE 6-52. Bullous impetigo on the inner thigh of a young Malay girl, with flaccid blisters that break easily, leaving shallow erosions rimmed by superficial peripheral peeling.

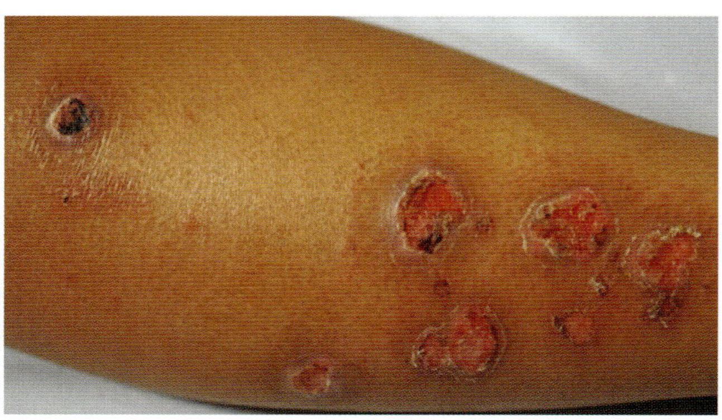

FIGURE 6-53. Lesions of impetigo on the lower calf of a young Malay girl, presenting with annular, crusted plaques. The lesion on the upper shin is consistent with ecthyma, presenting as a shallow erosion with overlying eschar.

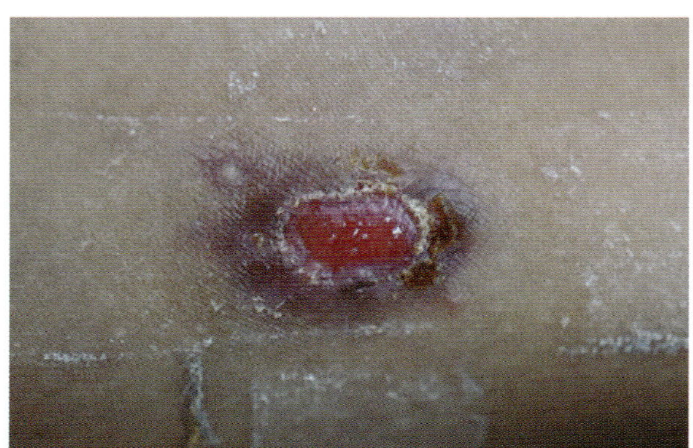

FIGURE 6-54. Ecthyma with granulation tissue seen at the base of the lesion on the leg of a teenage Chinese boy.

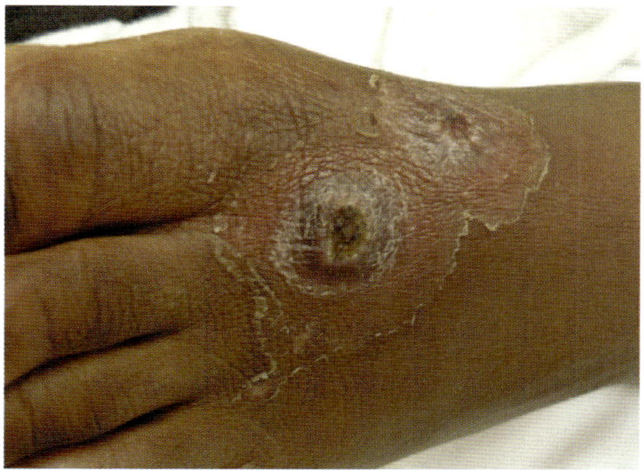

FIGURE 6-55. Ecthyma caused by group A streptococcus on the foot of this Indian boy. (Figure courtesy of Infectious Disease Service, KK Women's & Children's Hospital, Singapore.)

Pearls & Practical Tips

- The peripheral scaling is a classical sign of impetigo.
- In lesions that are extremely oozy with pus discharge, often both *S. aureus* and *Streptococcus* are isolated.
- In patients with "impetiginized" eczema, treatment should be targeted not only to the infection but also to the underlying dermatosis.
- For patients with recurrent impetigo, a nasal swab will help identify nasal carriage. Close family members should be examined for skin lesions and also undergo nasal swabs. They should also be treated if found to be carriers.
- Ecthyma gangrenosum is caused by pseudomonas bacteremia, with skin ulcers with overlying necrotic eschars. It usually occurs in patients who are critically ill and immunocompromised.

STAPHYLOCOCCAL SCALDED SKIN SYNDROME

Staphylococcal scalded skin syndrome (SSSS) is a toxin-mediated reaction secondary to *Staphylococcus aureus*. It often affects neonates, infants, and young children and is frequently preceded by localized skin infection such as impetigo. It can be potentially life-threatening if not recognized and treated early.

Clinical Features

- SSSS is associated with staphylococcal strains that produce exfoliative toxins (ETA and ETB) which target desmoglein-1, found in the intercellular desmosomes of the superficial epidermis. This leads to the loss of cohesion between the superficial keratinocytes, resulting in the classic finding of superficial blistering and exfoliation.[1]
- Commonly occurs in children less than 5 years of age. Immunocompromised individuals are also at risk for infection even until adulthood. It is postulated that the immature kidney function in younger children is unable to effectively clear the exfoliative toxins.
- There may be a preceding focus of staphylococcal infection such as impetigo or omphalitis. However, this may not be clinically obvious in many patients.
- Patients present with fever, irritability, tenderness, and diffuse, blanching erythema of the skin (hence the term scalded) that often begins around the perioral, intertriginous, or groin area. This is followed 1 to 2 days later by tissue paper–like wrinkling of the skin, and flaccid blisters that exfoliate easily, especially in areas associated with movement or pressure, including the flexures, buttocks, hands, and feet. In infants, lesions are also commonly found in the diaper area. Mucosal involvement is not seen, however, involvement of the external lip with crusting and fissuring is frequently encountered.[2]
- The superficially blistered skin peels off in sheets, leaving exposed a moist, red, and tender area. Nikolsky sign is positive (i.e., application of firm, sliding pressure creates separation of the superficial epidermis).
- Complete denudation is usually seen 5 to 7 days after onset of treatment. Healing is non-scarring, and most patients recover without complications if treatment is instituted appropriately.

Differential Diagnoses

- Stevens-Johnson syndrome (SJS)/toxic epidermal necrolysis (TEN)
  - A rare hypersensitivity reaction to drugs such as anticonvulsants, sulfonamides, beta-lactams, and nonsteroidal anti-inflammatory drugs (NSAIDs), or infections such as mycoplasma or herpes simplex virus.
  - Presentation is similar to SSSS, with initial presentation of fever, irritability, and flu-like symptoms. This is followed by an abrupt onset of tender, erythematous areas on the skin that eventually evolve to macules, purpura, targetoid lesions, and blisters that exfoliate easily.
  - In contrast to SSSS, mucous membrane involvement in SJS and TEN is prominent and severe, involving the eyes (conjunctivitis, corneal ulcerations), lips (painful cheilitis and stomatitis), pharynx, and genitalia.

Investigations & Treatment

- Diagnosis is mainly clinical, but bacterial cultures should be obtained from skin, blood, urine, or umbilical cord samples. There is leukocytosis and raised inflammatory markers such as C-reactive protein.
- The treatment should be directed toward eradication of staphylococci from the focus of infection, which involves administration of intravenous antibiotics. Patients should be treated in hospital. A penicillinase-resistant, anti-staphylococcal antibiotic such as cloxacillin or flucloxacillin is often used. Other antibiotic options include oxacillin and cephalosporins. Clindamycin is often added for its anti-toxin effect. Vancomycin is used if methicillin-resistant staphylococcal strain (MRSA) is suspected.
- Additional supportive treatments include hydration, pain management, and skin care (frequent application of emollients and non-adherent dressings), and placement in incubators for neonates.

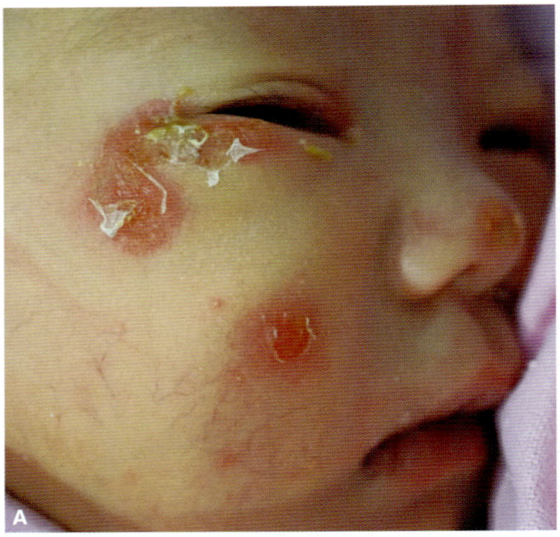
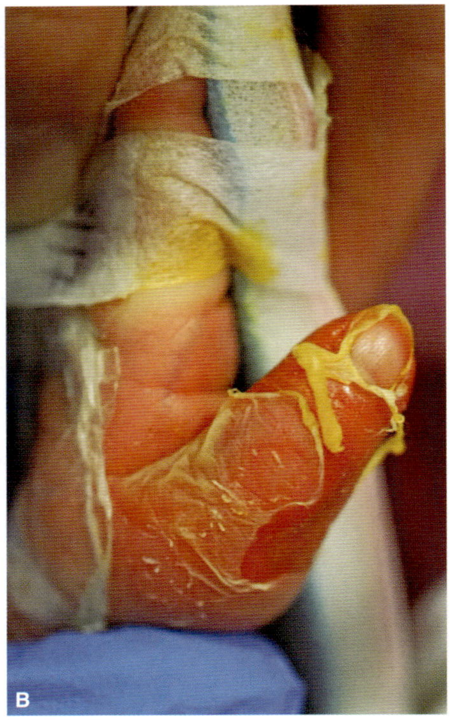

FIGURE 6-56A & 56B. Impetigo on the face of a neonate presenting with flaccid blisters and yellow-golden crusting and shallow erosions, complicated by staphylococcal scalded skin syndrome with widespread superficial skin erosion, as seen on the hand.

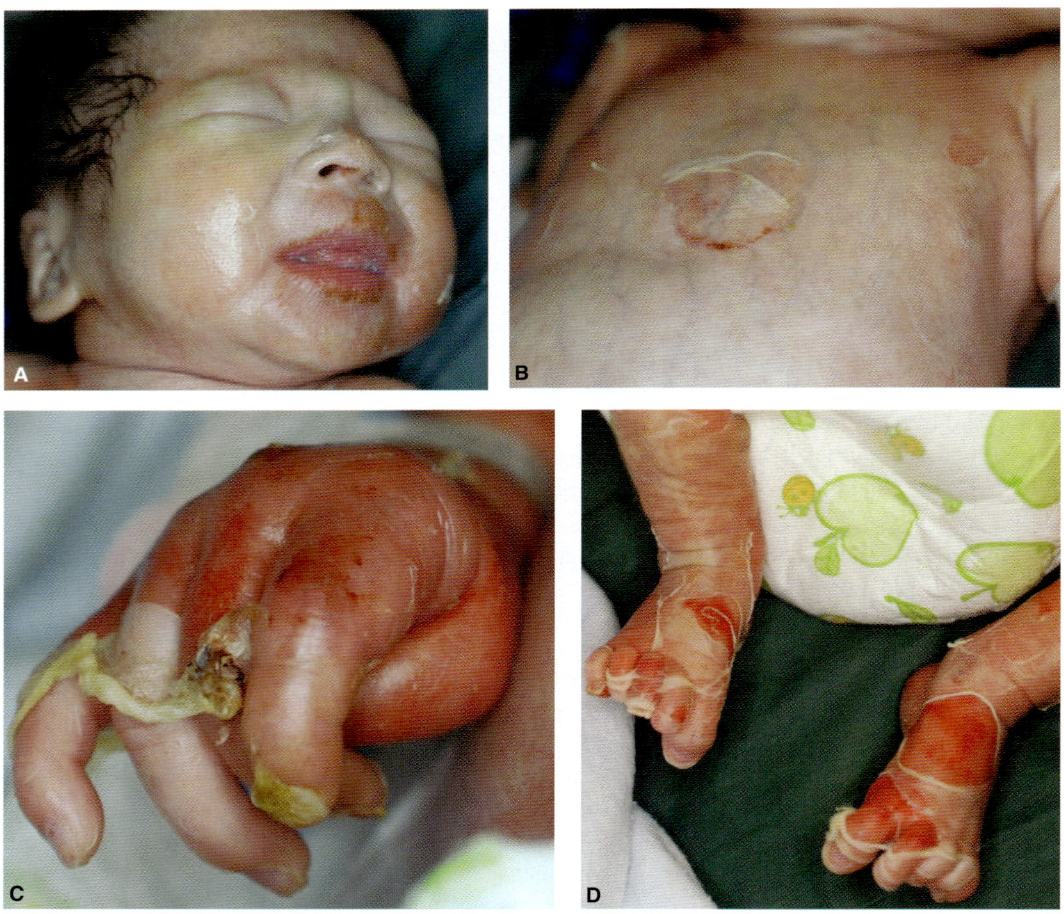

FIGURE 6-57A–57D. Staphylococcal scalded skin syndrome in an Indonesian neonate presenting with widespread superficial exfoliation of skin with underlying erythema. There is classical crusting around the perioral region (Figure 6-57A).

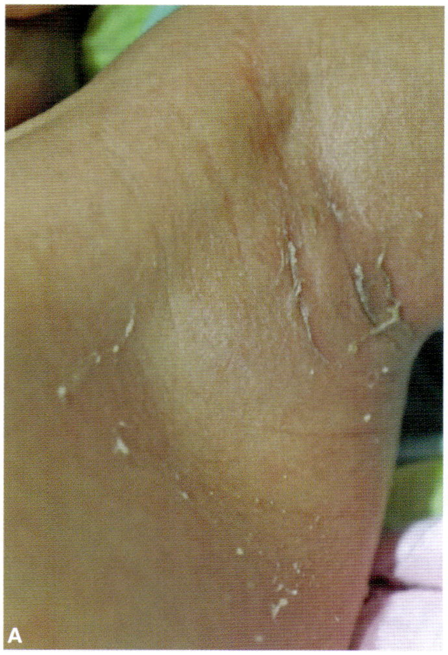
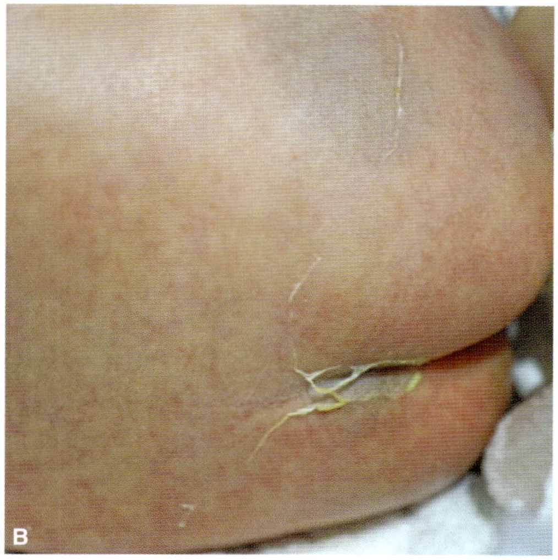

FIGURE 6-58A & 58B. Staphylococcal scalded skin syndrome with accentuation of erythema and skin denudation over the intertriginous areas in an infant.

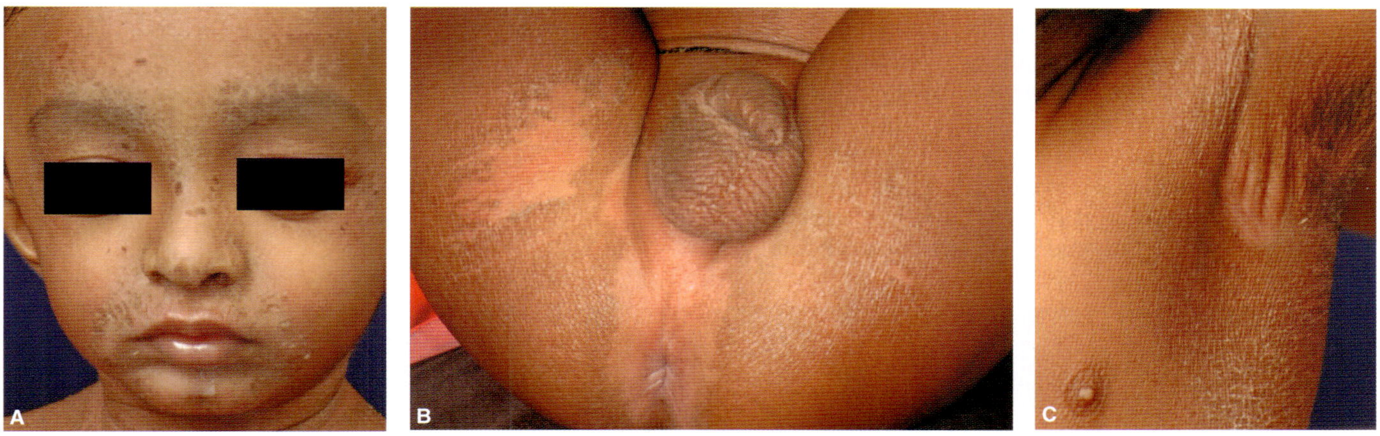

FIGURE 6-59A–59C. Staphylococcal scalded skin syndrome in a young Indian boy with impetigo on the face and superficial exfoliation and erosion, accentuated over the intertriginous regions.

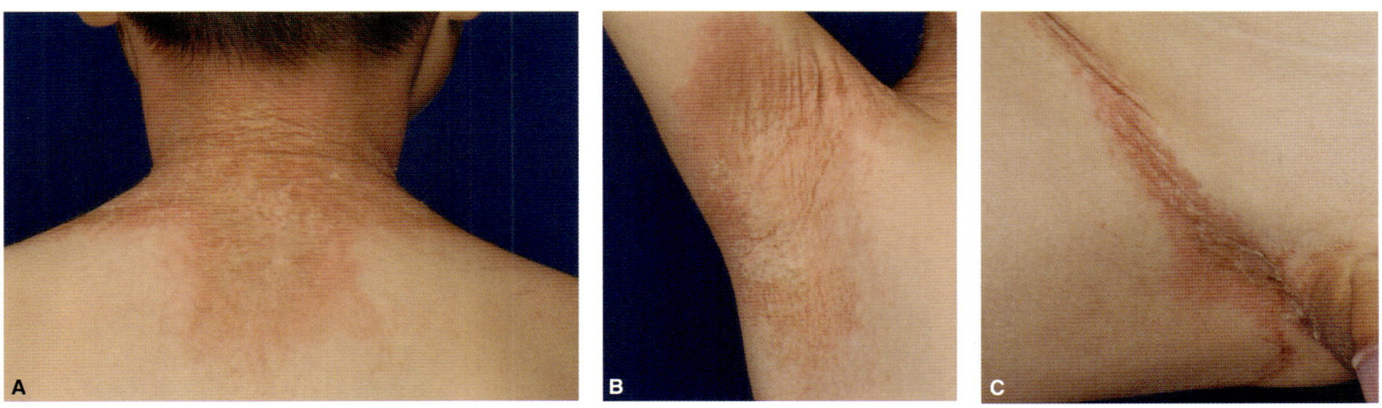

FIGURE 6-60A–60C. Staphylococcal scalded skin syndrome affecting a 5-year-old Chinese boy, mainly affecting the neck and flexures with erythema and superficial desquamation.

Pearls & Practical Tips

- The blisters seen in SSSS are sterile, hence they will not yield any growth when sampled for bacterial culture.
- The management of dehydration and electrolytes is essential, as SSSS can lead to complications and even mortality, especially in newborns and infants.
- Complications may arise if the infection is untreated, and may progress to cellulitis, pneumonia, and sepsis.
- Identification and treatment of a parent, family member, or healthcare or childcare worker colonized or infected with *S. aureus* is important to prevent recurrence. Good hygiene practices such as frequent hand washing should be encouraged at all times.

References

1. Oliveira AR, Aires S, Faria C, Santos E. Staphylococcal scalded skin syndrome. BMJ Case Rep 2013;2013:bcr2013009478
2. Irvine AD, Hoeger PH, Yan AC. Harper's Textbook of Pediatric Dermatology. 3rd ed. Wiley-Blackwell; 2011.

SCARLET FEVER & OTHER SKIN MANIFESTATIONS OF STREPTOCOCCAL INFECTION

Scarlet fever is a skin reaction caused by pyrogenic exotoxin produced by group A beta-hemolytic streptococcus. It commonly affects children, aged 1 to 10 years, and can be secondary to a cutaneous or deeper streptococcal infection or streptococcal throat infection.

Clinical Features

- The cutaneous manifestations of scarlet fever are postulated to be secondary to an enhanced delayed-type hypersensitivity reaction to streptococcal products, thereby requiring previous exposure to bacterial toxins. This explains the rarity of cases of scarlet fever in infancy, because most infants have not had previous exposure to these streptococcal toxins.[1]
- Clinical manifestations include acute onset of fever, sore throat, headache, chills, nausea, vomiting, and malaise. Physical examination findings include cervical lymphadenopathy, strawberry tongue, palatal petechiae, erythema, and edema of the pharyngotonsillar area.
- The cutaneous findings of scarlet fever classically present 12 to 48 hours after the onset of fever as erythematous patches ("boiled lobster" appearance), which then progress to become a more diffuse, finely papular, rough, sandpaper-like rash on the trunk and extremities. Minute pustules may be seen and there can be associated circumoral pallor.
- Pastia lines are linear petechial streaks seen at flexural sites, such as the antecubital fossae, axillae, and inguinal areas.
- By the sixth to seventh day of infection, the rashes start to fade, with sheets of superficial desquamation, especially on the hands and feet. This may last for 4 to 6 weeks.

Differential Diagnoses

- Viral exanthems
  - Common viral exanthems such as roseola, rubella, and measles can present with fever, lymphadenopathy, and rash. Other viral infections like Epstein-Barr virus (EBV) and cytomegalovirus (CMV) infection can also mimic scarlet fever.

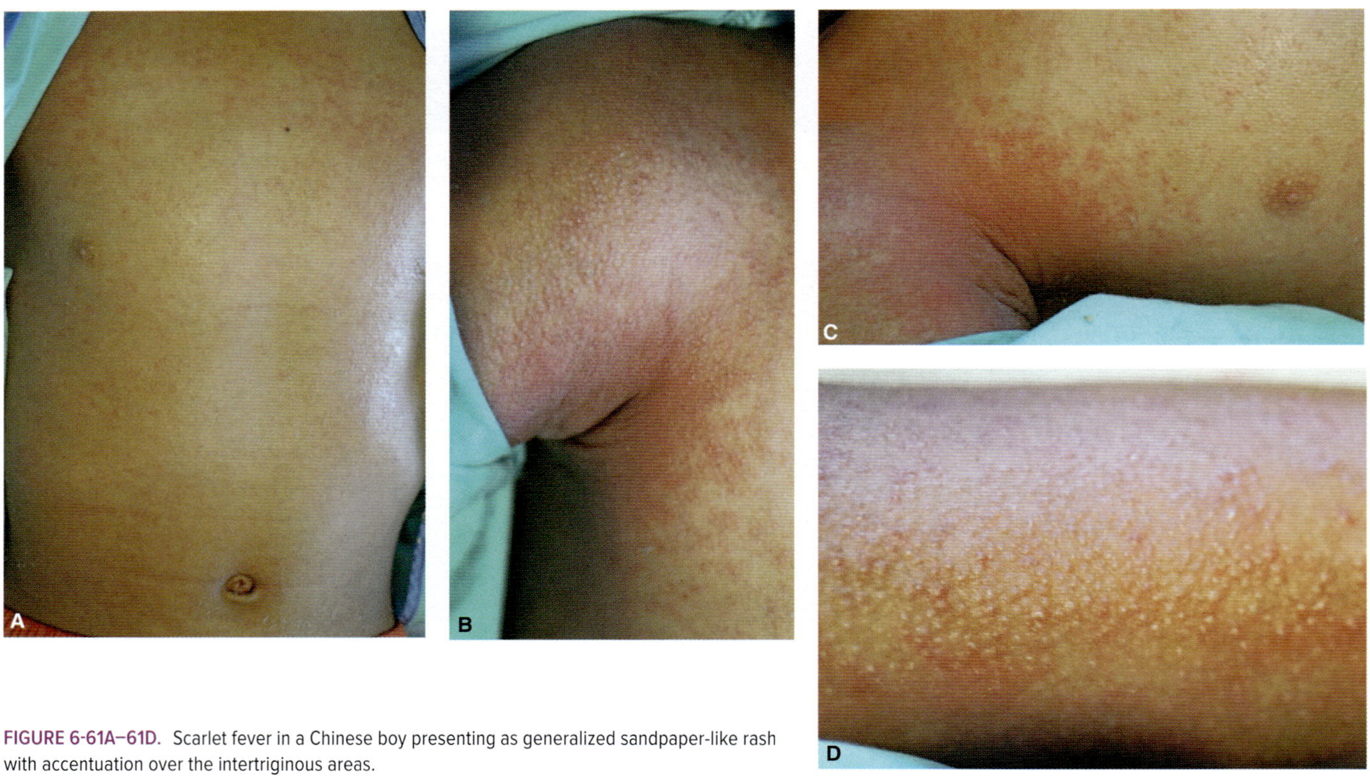

FIGURE 6-61A–61D. Scarlet fever in a Chinese boy presenting as generalized sandpaper-like rash with accentuation over the intertriginous areas.

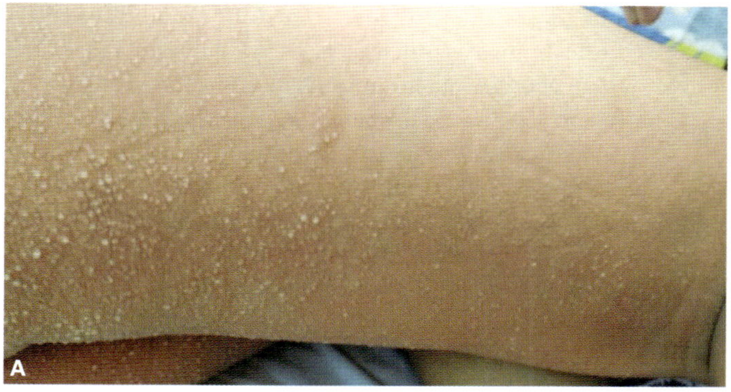

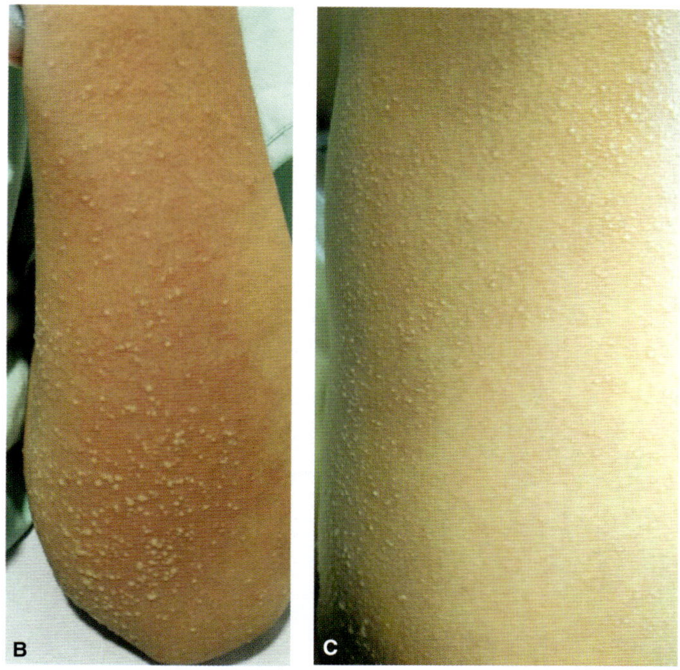

FIGURE 6-62A–62C. Scarlet fever in a Chinese child presenting with tiny erythematous papules and pustules, with a sandpaper-like consistency.

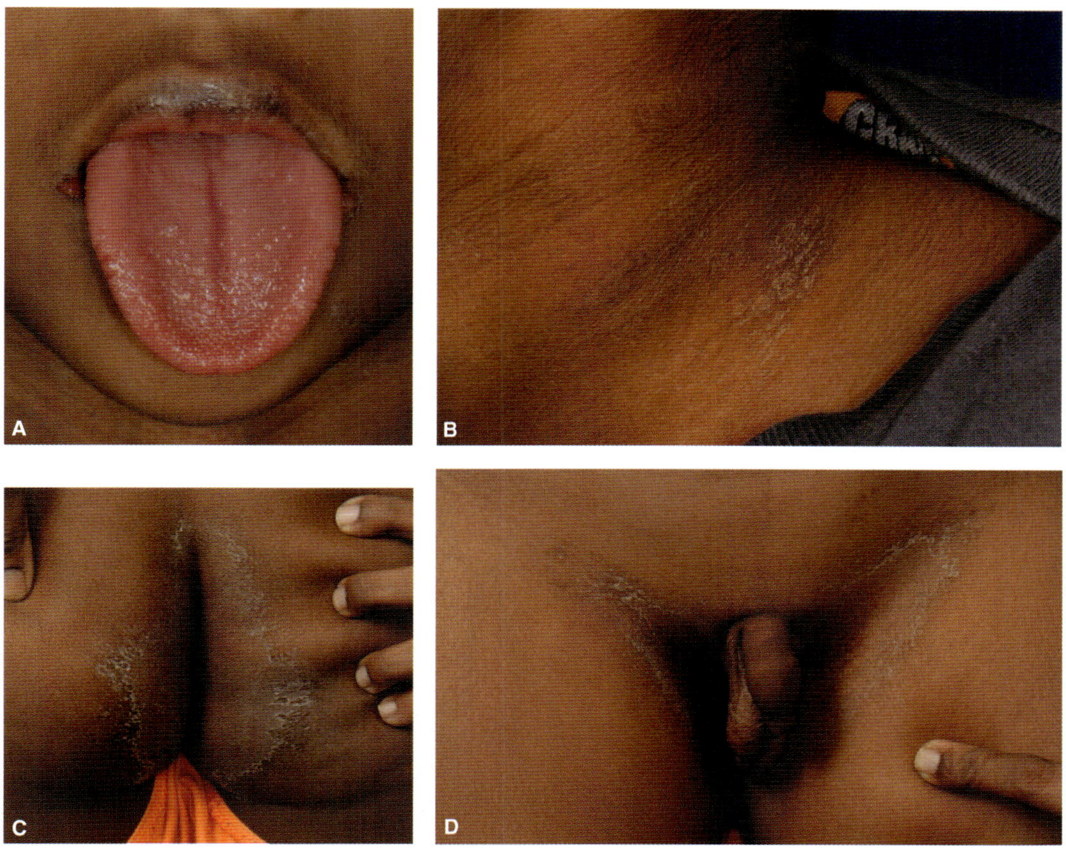

FIGURE 6-63A–63D. Scarlet fever in an Indian child presenting with strawberry tongue and exfoliative rash over the intertriginous areas.

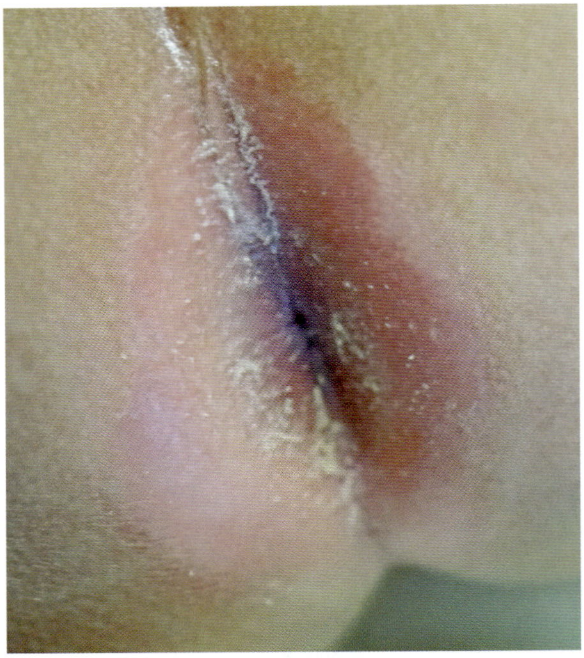

FIGURE 6-64. Perianal streptococcal dermatitis in a young Nepalese child presenting as painful and itchy, well-demarcated erythema in the perianal region.

- Kawasaki disease
  - An acute febrile illness that also presents with prolonged fever of more than 5 days, lymphadenopathies, strawberry tongue, and rash. Other cardinal signs include non-purulent conjunctivitis and edema of the hands and feet. The rash of Kawasaki varies in presentation from maculopapular to morbilliform, or target-like, as compared to the sandpaper-like rash of scarlet fever.
  - Sore throat, which is almost always seen in scarlet fever, is an uncommon finding in Kawasaki disease.

Investigations & Treatment

- Diagnosis can be made clinically but may be supported by laboratory investigations such as throat swab culture and/or antistreptolysin-O (ASO) titers. There is leukocytosis and raised inflammatory markers (e.g., C-reactive protein).
- A course of antistreptococcal antibiotic should be given to prevent subsequent post-streptococcal complications. The drug of choice is a 10-day course of penicillin or amoxicillin. Macrolides such as erythromycin and cephalosporins are alternatives to those with penicillin allergy.
- Additional supportive measures include antipyretics, pain relief, and antihistamines for control of pruritus.

Pearls & Practical Tips

- Post-streptococcal complications include rheumatic heart disease, post-streptococcal glomerulonephritis, pneumonia, osteomyelitis, and sepsis. Adequate systemic antibiotic treatment is essential to reduce the risk of these complications.
- Scarlet fever has a recurrence rate of 18%, and recent literature has shown as much as a 10-fold increase in cases due to toxin acquisition and multidrug resistance.[2]
- Perianal streptococcal infection usually affects infants and young children and is also caused by group A beta-hemolytic streptococcus. It presents as well-demarcated erythema and itch or pain around the anal region. A skin swab for culture will confirm the diagnosis, and treatment is with systemic antistreptococcal antibiotics.

References

1. Irvine AD, Hoeger PH, Yan AC. Harper's Textbook of Pediatric Dermatology. 3rd ed. Wiley-Blackwell; 2011.
2. Davies MR, Holden MT, Coupland P, et al. Emergence of scarlet fever *Streptococcus pyogenes* emm12 clones in Hong Kong is associated with toxin acquisition and multidrug resistance. Nat Genet 2015;47(1):84-7.

FOLLICULITIS, FURUNCLES, AND CARBUNCLES

These conditions occur as a result of infection or inflammation affecting hair follicles. Folliculitis signifies more superficial involvement, while furuncles and carbuncles are characterized by deeper involvement. Although less common in children than adults, they can be recurrent, whereby an underlying cause needs to be excluded.

Clinical Features

- Most commonly caused by *Staphylococcus aureus*, other common pathogens include streptococci and Gram-negative bacteria.
- Folliculitis occurs most commonly on the buttocks and upper thighs in children but can also occur on other hair-bearing sites. Lesions begin as painless, small

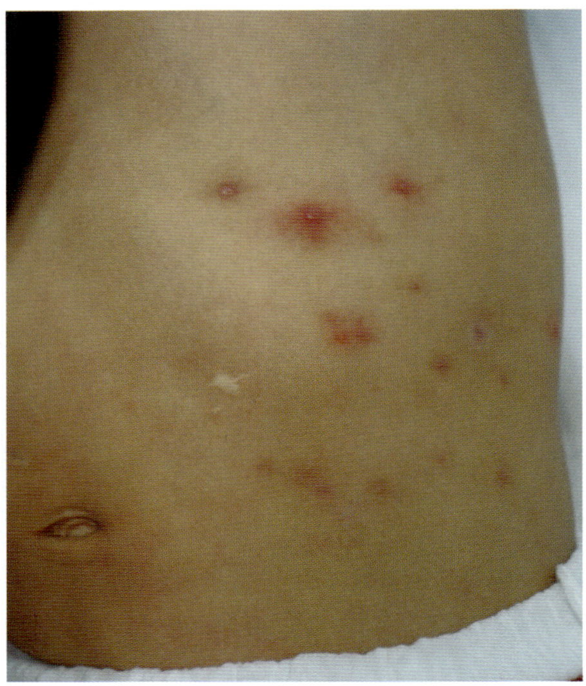

FIGURE 6-65. Folliculitis on the trunk of a Chinese toddler caused by occlusion.

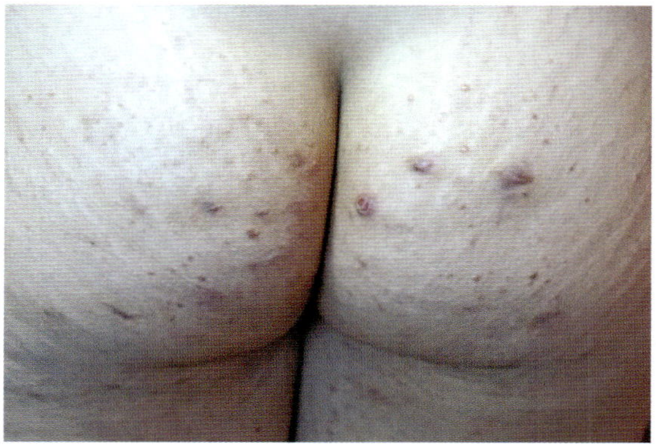

FIGURE 6-66. Chronic, recurrent folliculitis on the buttocks of an overweight adolescent female. There is a furuncle on the right inner buttock, as well as hypertrophic scarring from previous furuncles.

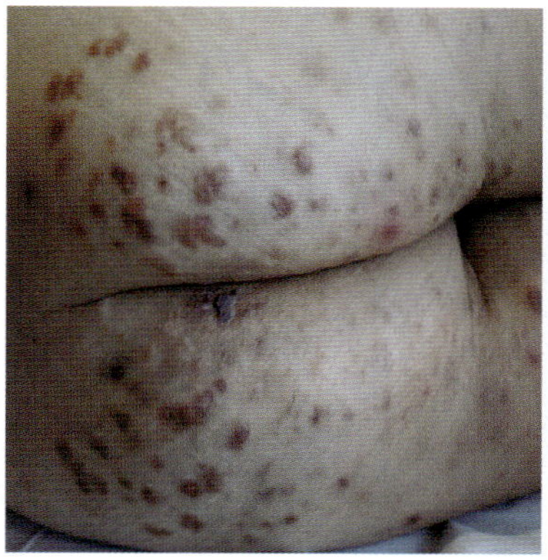

FIGURE 6-67. Severe folliculitis affecting the buttocks and groin of a teenage Chinese girl, with extensive scarring.

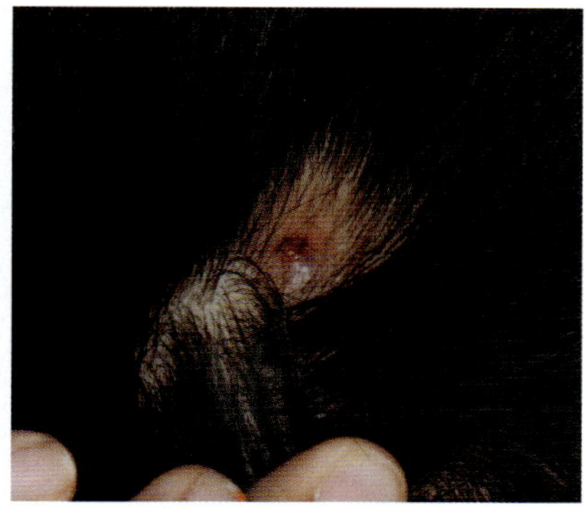

FIGURE 6-68. Scalp folliculitis presenting with a small discharging nodule with overlying and surrounding alopecia.

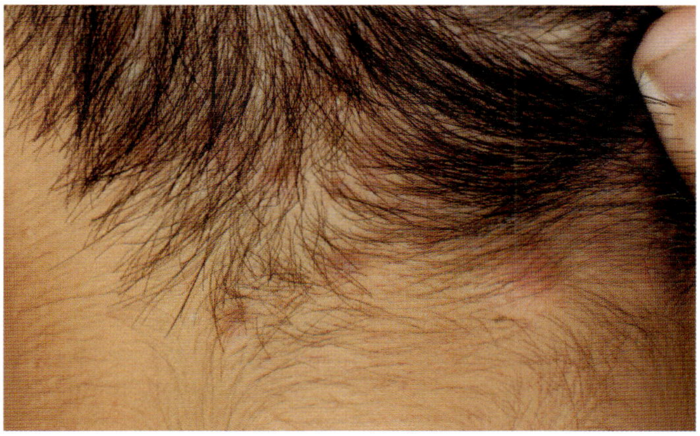

FIGURE 6-69. Scalp folliculitis presenting as recurrent erythematous papules around a hair follicle at the occipital and nape region.

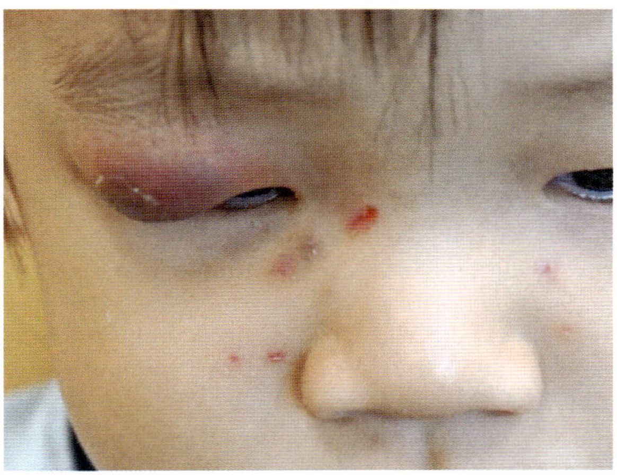

FIGURE 6-71. Right upper eyelid furuncle (abscess) in a young child. There are concomitant lesions of impetigo on his face.

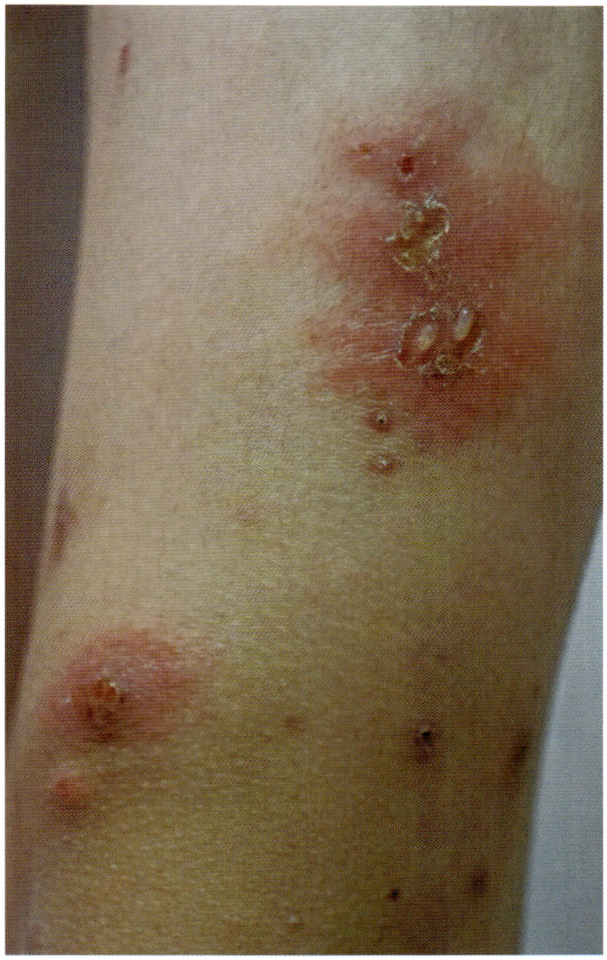

FIGURE 6-70. Folliculitis on the lower leg of a Chinese boy with formation of bigger furuncles.

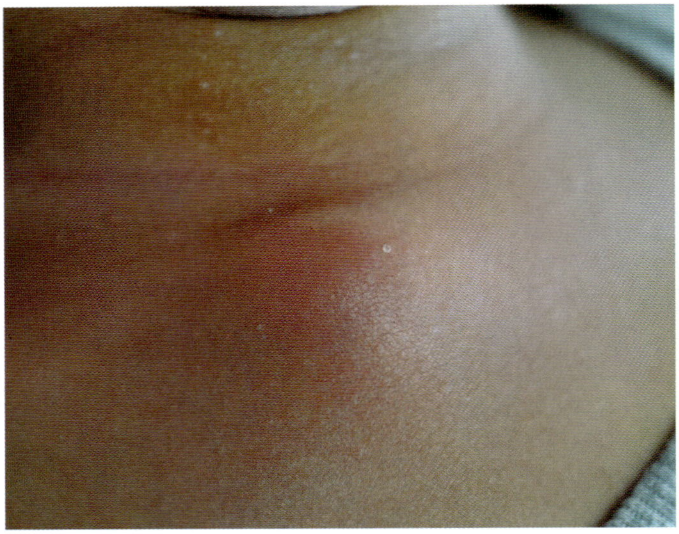

FIGURE 6-72. Abscess on the right upper chest of a young child, presenting as a fluctuant, tender erythematous nodule.

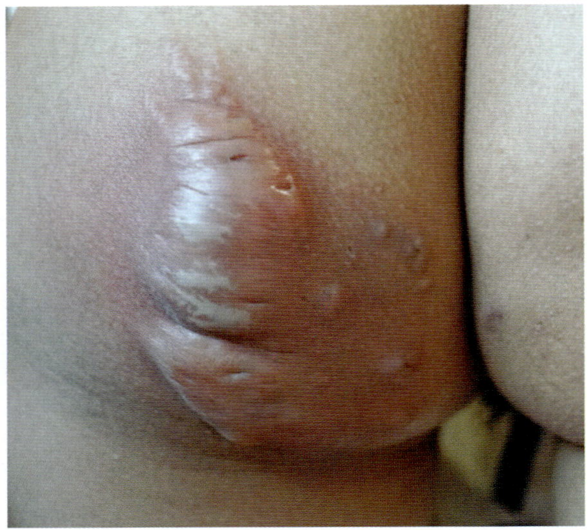

FIGURE 6-73. Carbuncle on the buttock of a teenage Chinese male with recurrent folliculitis of the buttocks with scarring.

yellowish-white papules with an erythematous rim, with a hair seen at the center of the papule. They tend to self-resolve over 1 to 2 weeks.

- Furuncles or abscesses represent deeper infections of hair follicles and are more common in adolescents and adults. They present as painful, indurated, erythematous nodules that progressively become fluctuant, and may discharge pus that can be blood tinged. Furuncles commonly occur on the back, thighs, buttocks, and intertriginous sites such as the groin and axilla.
- Carbuncles are uncommonly seen in children and adolescents. They are larger and more deep-seated and consist of interconnecting furuncles. These can drain through multiple points on the skin. Carbuncles are frequently painful and constitutional symptoms may be present, such as fever.

Differential Diagnoses

- Folliculitis
  - Impetigo can also present with pustules, but these rupture easily to leave residual golden-yellow crusts and peripheral scaling.
  - Insect bite reactions and papular urticaria can also present as grouped, acute erythematous papules. However, they are often itchy, and a central punctum may be seen. They are also not follicular based.
  - Papular or follicular eczema are more common in darker-skinned Asians and can appear as follicular-based papules. However, they are more chronic and pruritic, and other signs of atopic dermatitis or other eczemas may be seen.
  - Pseudomonal folliculitis, caused by *Pseudomonas aeruginosa*, occurs from exposure to poorly chlorinated hot tubs, swimming pools, and whirlpools. It also presents with erythematous, follicular papules, usually multiple, over the sites covered by swimming gear, such as trunk, buttocks, and thighs.
- Furuncle and carbuncle
  - Epidermal cysts and other cysts can also present with deep, rounded swellings at hair-bearing sites. However, they are usually more chronic and are not fluctuant unless secondarily infected. Epidermal cysts extrude a malodorous, whitish, keratinaceous material when ruptured.
  - Atypical mycobacterial infections are rare in children and adolescents, but may present as indurated nodules in the skin. The lesions are usually more chronic and slower growing.
  - Hidradenitis suppurativa affects most commonly the intertriginous sites, such as the axilla and groin. It also presents with discharging nodules. Comedones and hypertrophic scarring are also seen.

Investigations & Treatment

- Folliculitis, furuncles, and carbuncles are usually diagnosed clinically, although biopsies may be performed to exclude other differential diagnoses.
- Bacterial cultures may be performed to guide the choice of antibiotics, if required.
- Mild folliculitis may be treated with antiseptic washes and topical antibiotics (e.g., clindamycin, tetracycline, erythromycin, fusidic acid, or mupirocin). More extensive disease should be treated with systemic antibiotics (e.g., cephalexin, cloxacillin, or erythromycin).
- Furuncles and carbuncles are treated with systemic anti-staphylococcal antibiotics (e.g., cephalexin, cloxacillin, or erythromycin). If fluctuant, incision and drainage should also be performed.

Pearls & Practical Tips

- Folliculitis may not always be caused by an infectious agent. "Sterile" folliculitis may be caused by occlusion, friction, and shaving.

- In patients with recurrent abscesses, underlying factors need to be evaluated for and treated. These include obesity, diabetes mellitus, and rarely, immunodeficiency. Chronic carriage of *Staphylococcus aureus*, especially in the nares of patients and their family members, needs to be excluded. Twice-weekly antiseptic washes (e.g., chlorhexidine, triclosan, potassium permanganate, or sodium hypochlorite) may also be useful to prevent recurrences. However, excessive use may cause irritation.

ERYSIPELAS & CELLULITIS

Erysipelas and cellulitis are deeper cutaneous bacterial infections, with erysipelas affecting the dermal layer and cellulitis affecting the subcutaneous tissue. Both are most commonly caused by *Streptococcus* (group A β-hemolytic streptococcus) or *Staphylococcus aureus*.

Clinical Features

- Cellulitis is more common than erysipelas. However, they both can occur in the same setting, and is often preceded by trauma to the skin in children, such as insect bites or scratched eczematous skin. It occurs most commonly on the extremities, usually the legs.
- Both conditions present with erythematous, indurated, painful swelling that evolves over a few hours or days. In cellulitis, the borders are less sharply defined. In erysipelas, the borders are more demarcated, and the plaque is more red. Bullae can occur in both cellulitis and erysipelas.
- Patients usually have constitutional symptoms, such as fever and regional lymphadenopathy.
- Facial cellulitis can occur from *Haemophilus influenzae* or *Streptococcus pneumoniae*. It can arise from an odontogenic origin, and patients are more toxic.
- Periorbital cellulitis leads to erythema and swelling of periorbital tissues and can occur from trauma, conjunctivitis, or spread from paranasal sinuses. It can lead to orbital cellulitis, where children present with proptosis, ophthalmoplegia, visual problems, and appear more toxic. Complications include cavernous sinus thrombosis and brain abscess formation.

Differential Diagnoses

- Impetigo
  - Cellulitis or erysipelas can occur on the background of impetigo.
  - Impetigo presents with more surface changes (e.g., honey-yellow crusting, oozy lesions with pus discharge).
- Contact dermatitis
  - Contact dermatitis can also present with an acutely erythematous patch or plaque with overlying blisters. A history of a recent contactant will help to differentiate between cellulitis or erysipelas; however, this may often be missed.

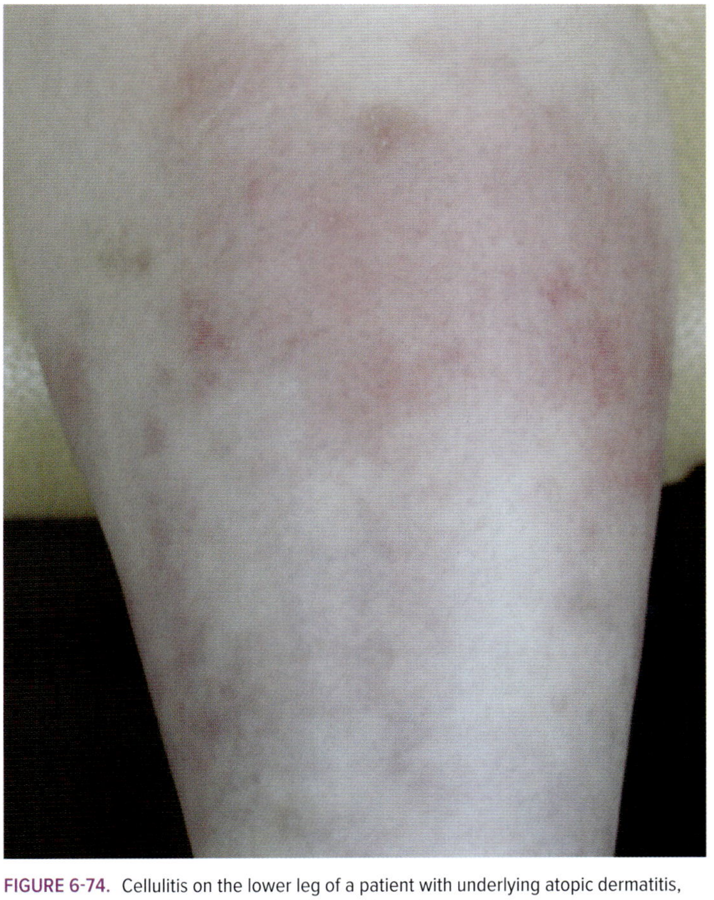

FIGURE 6-74. Cellulitis on the lower leg of a patient with underlying atopic dermatitis, presenting as a poorly demarcated pink-to-erythematous patch.

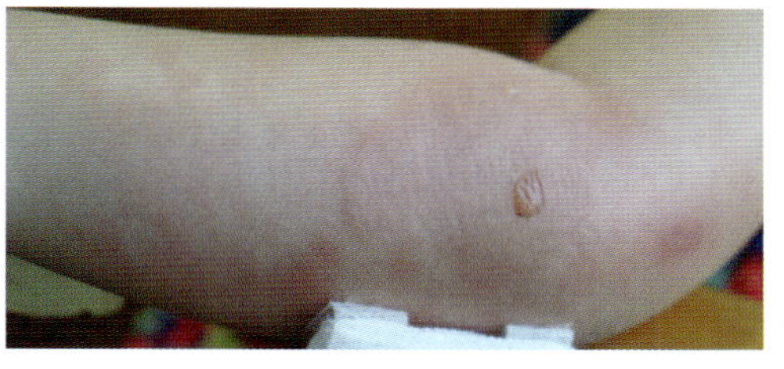

FIGURE 6-75. Cellulitis on the arm of a Chinese girl, associated with underlying arthropod bite reactions.

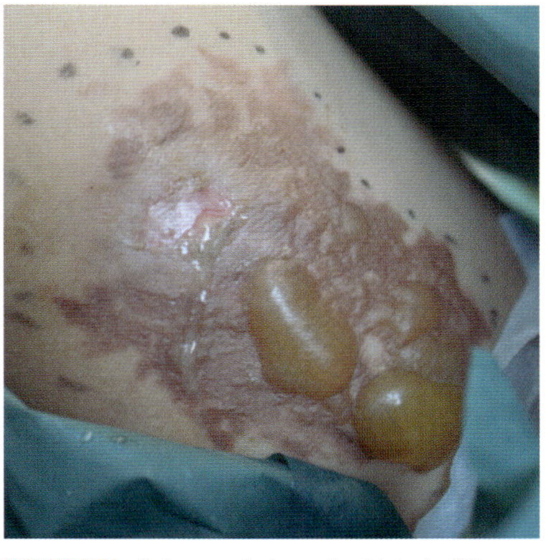

FIGURE 6-76. Bullous erysipelas on the thigh of a Chinese child presenting with well-demarcated erythematous-to-hyperpigmented plaque with well-demarcated borders and overlying tense blisters

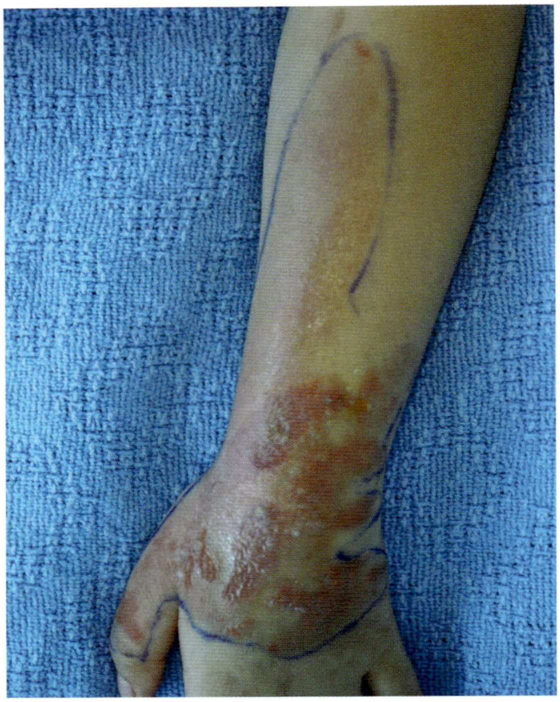

FIGURE 6-77. Bullous cellulitis on the arm of a Chinese child presenting as a erythematous plaque with localized blisters.

- Insect bite reactions
  - The surrounding skin around insect bite reactions in children can become red and indurated. This can mimic cellulitis and can be difficult to differentiate. If the child is febrile and the induration expands despite treatment with topical corticosteroids and oral antihistamines, cellulitis should be suspected and systemic antibiotics should be started.
- Necrotizing fasciitis
  - Necrotizing fasciitis can be fatal if not detected early. Early necrotizing fasciitis can mimic cellulitis.
  - Features that are more suspicious for necrotizing fasciitis include pain out of proportion to the clinical signs, hypotension, progressing erythema, fluctuance, altered mental status, hemorrhagic bullae, skin necrosis, recent surgery, and diarrhea.

Investigations & Treatment

- Cellulitis and erysipelas are diagnosed clinically. Other supporting investigation results include leukocytosis, raised C-reactive protein (CRP), and erythrocyte sedimentation rate (ESR). Blood cultures and surface cultures are often negative.
- Skin biopsies are rarely performed, but if done will show dermal or subcutaneous edema with mixed acute and chronic inflammatory infiltrate.
- Treatment of both cellulitis and erysipelas depends on the severity. In early disease without constitutional symptoms, oral antibiotics targeting both streptococcus and staphylococcus should be initiated (e.g., cephalexin or amoxicillin/clavulanic acid). If the patient is febrile or not responsive to a few days of oral antibiotics, intravenous antibiotics should be initiated (e.g., ampicillin + cloxacillin, amoxicillin/clavulanic acid, or cephazolin).
- If blisters are present, soaks with potassium permanganate or normal saline are useful adjuncts.

Pearls & Practical Tips

- In infants less than 3 months of age, group B streptococci (GBS) needs to be considered, and can be associated with invasive disease such as bacteremia or meningitis.
- Besides antibiotic treatment for the cellulitis and erysipelas, treatment for any underlying dermatoses should be initiated or continued, such as topical corticosteroids for eczema.

LEPROSY

Leprosy, or Hansen's disease, is a chronic infection caused by *Mycobacterium leprae* and affects the skin and peripheral nerves, which can lead to physical disabilities. It is a significant public health concern globally; however, with the strict implementation of multidrug therapy, its prevalence has been reduced significantly. Leprosy is an infectious disease directly transmitted from man to man via respiratory droplets. It is acquired through close contact and prolonged exposure, and only a small proportion of the population is affected.

Clinical Features

- Leprosy is transmitted via respiratory droplets and is acquired through close contact and prolonged exposure. Only a small proportion of exposed individuals develop clinically significant disease.

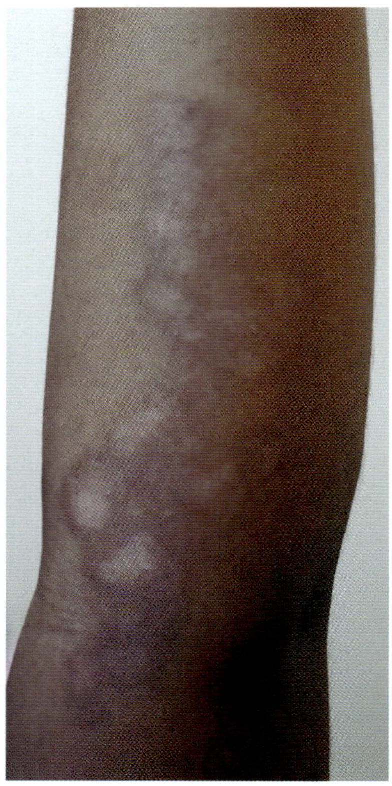

FIGURE 6-78. Leprosy in a young Indian female presenting with hypopigmented patches on her left arm with hypoesthesia. (Figure courtesy of East Avenue Medical Center Hansen's Disease Team, Dr. Jose N. Rodriguez Memorial Hospital, Manila, Philippines.)

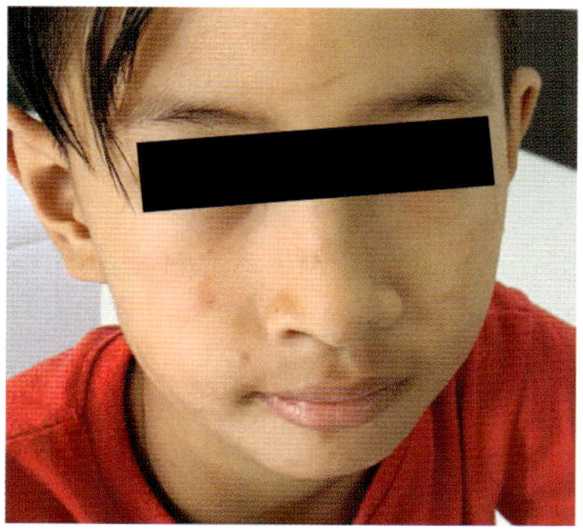

FIGURE 6-79. Leprosy in a young Filipino boy presenting with hypopigmented, hypoesthetic patches on his face with few scattered papules. (Figure courtesy of East Avenue Medical Center Hansen's Disease Team, Dr. Jose N. Rodriguez Memorial Hospital, Manila, Philippines.)

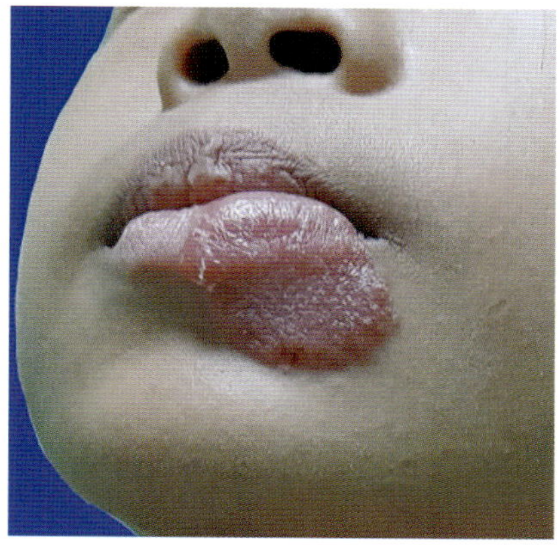

FIGURE 6-81. Tuberculoid leprosy in a Filipino child presenting as a solitary, infiltrated, hypoesthetic plaque on the face. (Figure courtesy of East Avenue Medical Center Hansen's Disease Team, Dr. Jose N. Rodriguez Memorial Hospital, Manila, Philippines.)

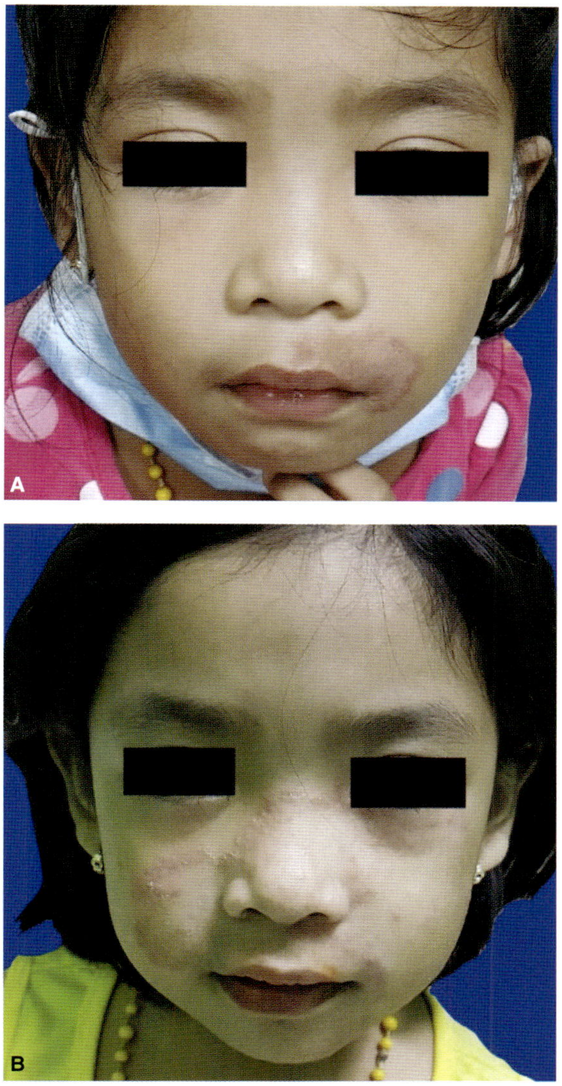

FIGURE 6-80A & 80B. Borderline tuberculoid leprosy in a young Filipino child presenting with asymmetrical, annular, mildly scaly, erythematous plaques with hypoesthesia. (Figures courtesy of East Avenue Medical Center Hansen's Disease Team, Dr. Jose N. Rodriguez Memorial Hospital, Manila, Philippines.)

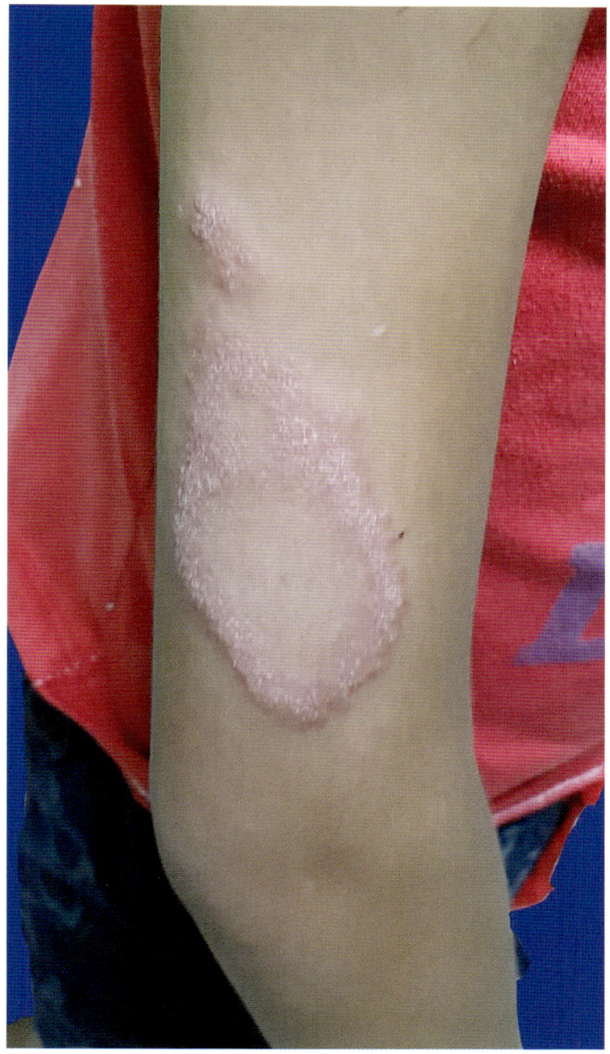

FIGURE 6-82. Tuberculoid leprosy in a Filipino child presenting as localized, annular, scaly, erythematous plaques with hypoesthesia. (Figure courtesy of East Avenue Medical Center Hansen's Disease Team, Dr. Jose N. Rodriguez Memorial Hospital, Manila, Philippines.)

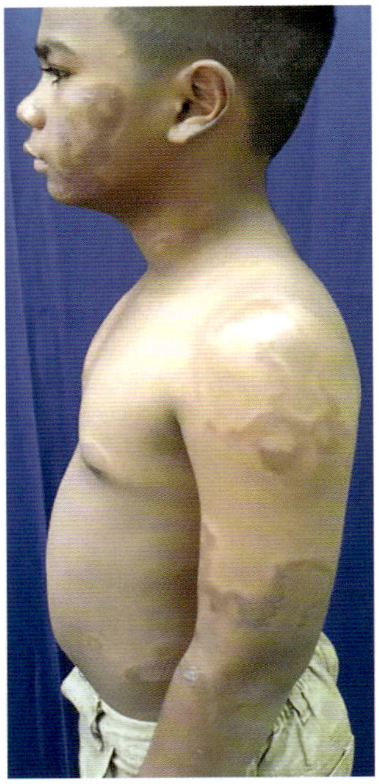

FIGURE 6-83. Borderline lepromatous leprosy in a Filipino boy presenting as widespread, annular, hyperpigmented plaques with hypoesthesia. (Figure courtesy of East Avenue Medical Center Hansen's Disease Team, Dr. Jose N. Rodriguez Memorial Hospital, Manila, Philippines.)

- An individual's immune status will determine the response to the bacilli.
- The clinical manifestations can be classified into two major ends of a spectrum: tuberculoid leprosy and lepromatous leprosy.
- Based on the Ridley-Jopling classification, there are five main types of leprosy, and all forms may be seen in children. The most prevalent type in younger children is borderline tuberculoid leprosy, while in older children the most prevalent type is borderline lepromatous leprosy, similar to the adult type.
- Children often manifest with hypopigmented macules and patches, commonly associated with hypoesthesia and decreased sweating or anhidrosis.
- Papules and plaques may also be seen in the pediatric population. However, nodules are quite rare. Many of the plaques show an annular configuration.
- Nerve enlargement is often accompanied by greater disability and impaired quality of life. Testing with the Semmes-Weinstein monofilament is necessary to quantify the sensation in macular lesions of leprosy.

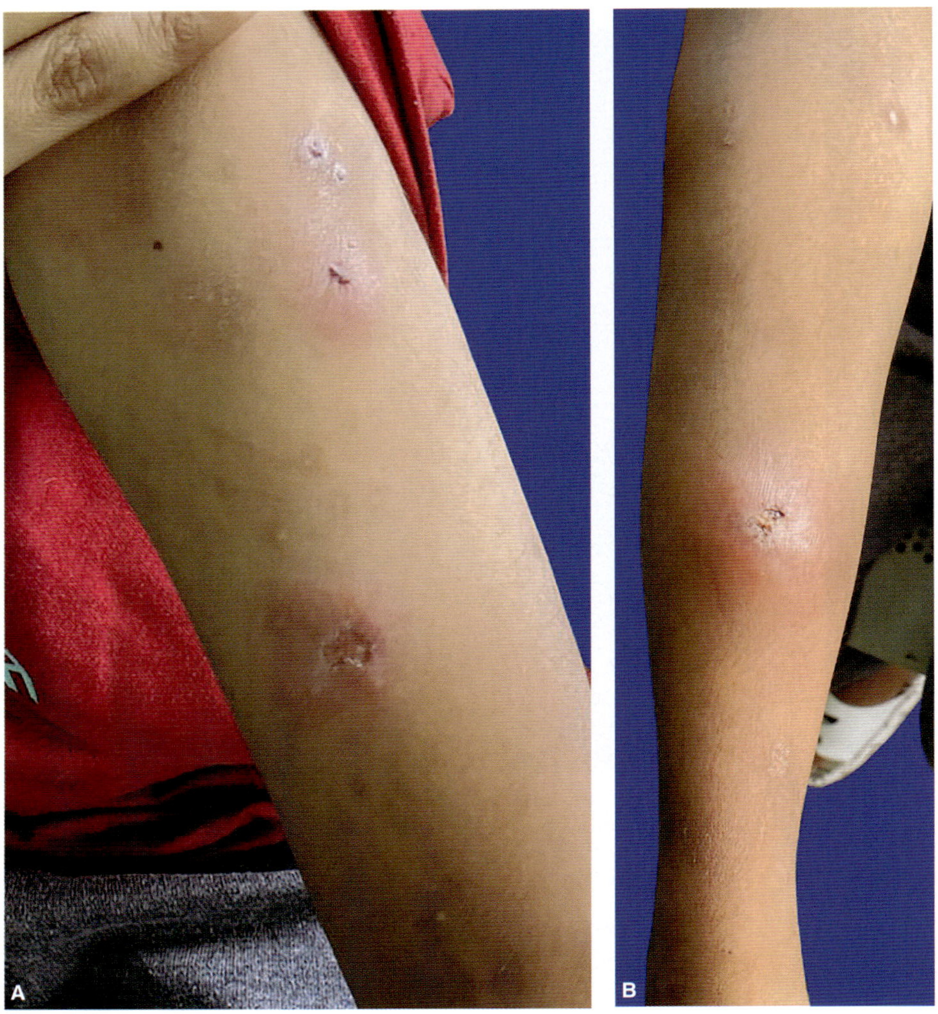

FIGURE 6-84A & 84B. Leprosy in a Filipino adolescent presenting with indurated nodules with surface ulceration. (Figures courtesy of East Avenue Medical Center Hansen's Disease Team, Dr. Jose N. Rodriguez Memorial Hospital, Manila, Philippines.)

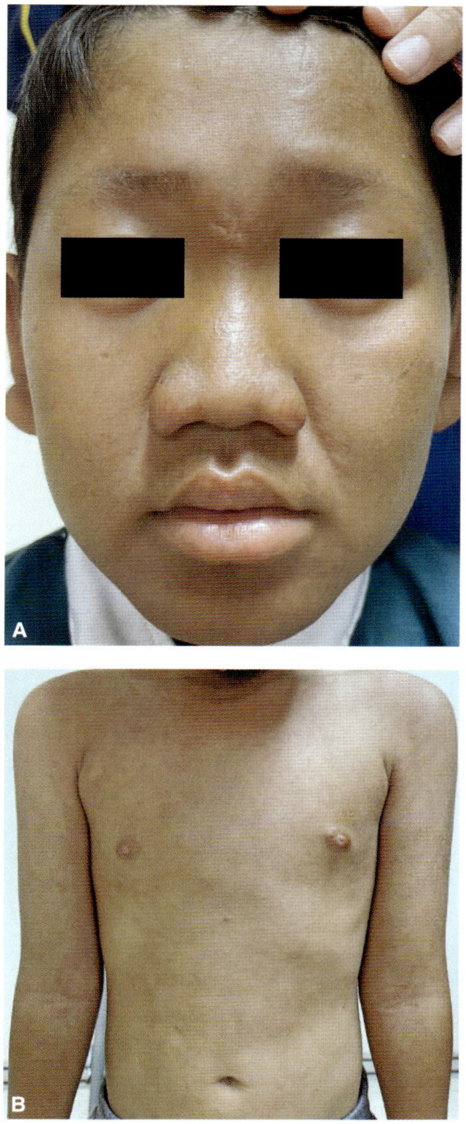

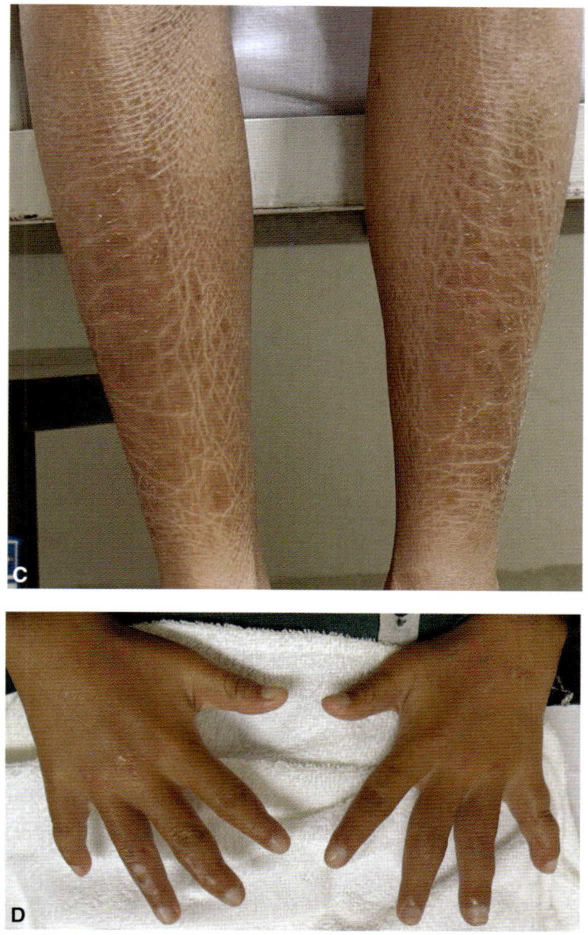

FIGURE 6-85A–85D. Lepromatous leprosy in an Indonesian adolescent boy, presenting with infiltrated plaques on his face (Figure 6-85A), hypopigmented patches and plaques on his trunk (Figure 6-85B), acquired ichthyosis on his legs (Figure 6-85C), and deformities of his hands (Figure 6-85D). (Figures courtesy of Dr. Dedianto Hidajat, SpKK, FINSDV, Faculty of Medicine University of Mataram, Indonesia.)

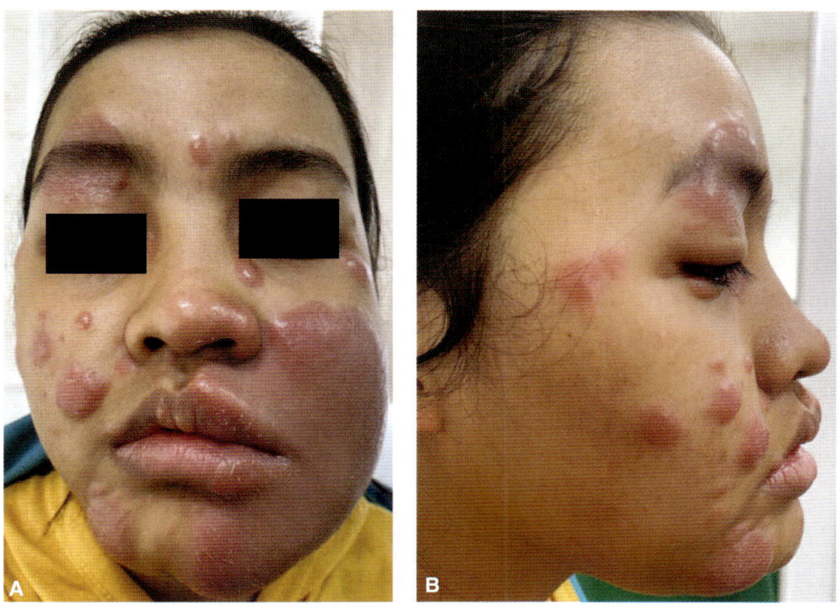

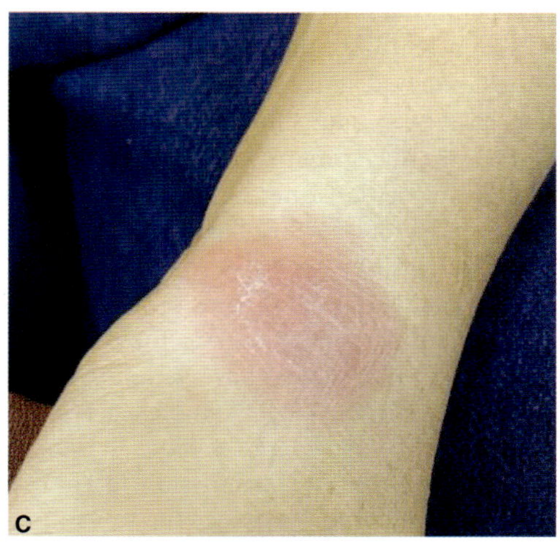

FIGURE 6-86A–86C. Type 2 lepra reaction affecting an older adolescent female from Indonesia, presenting with multiple, painful nodules on her face and limbs. (Figures courtesy of Dr. July Iriani Rahardja, Jakarta, Indonesia.)

Differential Diagnoses

- Dermatophyte infections and tinea versicolor
  - Dermatophyte infections (tinea) can also present with annular lesions but have more epidermal changes, such as scaling.
  - Tinea versicolor presents with well-demarcated hypopigmented lesions but these are usually more scaly, with no hypoesthesia.
  - Fungal microscopy and culture can be performed to diagnose tinea.
- Vitiligo
  - Hypopigmented lesions of leprosy can resemble early vitiligo. Hypoesthesia is not seen in vitiligo.
- Mycosis fungoides (MF)
  - Hypopigmented forms of MF can mimic leprosy. Hypoesthesia is not a feature of MF.
  - Biopsies can help to differentiate between the two conditions.
- Pityriasis alba and post-inflammatory hypopigmentation
  - Pityriasis alba is a common condition, presenting with hypopigmented patches mostly on the face. There is usually a history of atopy and atopic dermatitis.
  - Post-inflammatory hypopigmentation often occurs after eczema or other papulosquamous disorders. There is a history of a preceding rash before the hypopigmentation occurs.

Investigations & Treatment

- Diagnosis of leprosy is based on the classical clinical morphology supported by slit-skin smears and histopathology.
- Histopathological features depend on the clinical type. In tuberculoid and borderline tuberculoid leprosy, epithelioid noncaseating granulomas predominate, and acid-fast bacilli (AFB) are absent or rare. In borderline lepromatous and lepromatous leprosy, the infiltrate is composed of foamy macrophages, lymphocytes, and plasma cells, with numerous AFB. The Fite-Faraco stain is helpful to illustrate the acid-fast bacilli.
- Serological tests that detect antibodies produced by the host, such as anti-phenolic glycolipid-1 (PGL-1) can be used to screen for subclinical infection.
- Treatment regimens for pediatric leprosy utilize triple therapy of dapsone, rifampicin, and clofazimine for 6 months for paucibacillary, and 12 months for multibacillary disease.
- In a meta-analysis on the protective aspect of bacillus Calmette-Guérin (BCG) vaccine in the prevention of leprosy, 54.2% of studies have demonstrated more than 50% efficacy, while 20.9% of studies showed more than 75% protection against leprosy. Since familial contacts play an important role in transmission to children, BCG vaccination may partially reduce the transmission of disease.

Pearls & Practical Tips

- In highly endemic areas, patients presenting with hypopigmented lesions with hypoesthesia, biopsy, and slit-skin smears should be performed to exclude leprosy.
- It is often challenging to conduct monofilament testing in patients below 6 years; nerve ultrasound can be done instead.
- In a household with affected patients 15 years and below, active transmission within the family and community should be suspected, and contact tracing is necessary.

Bibliography

1. Irvine AD, Hoeger P, Yan AC. Harper's Textbook of Pediatric Dermatology. Chichester, West Sussex, UK: Wiley-Blackwell; 2020.
2. Dogra S, Narang T, Khullar G, et al. Childhood leprosy through the post-leprosy-elimination era: a retrospective analysis of epidemiological and clinical characteristics of disease over eleven years from a tertiary care hospital in North India. Lepr Rev 2014;85:296-310.
3. Barreto JG, de Souza Guimaraes l, Frade MA, et al. High rates of undiagnosed leprosy and subclinical infection amongst school children in the Amazon Region. Mem Inst Oswaldo Cruz 2012;107:60-7.
4. Zodpey SP. Protective efficacy of bacillus Calmette Guerin (BCG) vaccine in the prevention of leprosy: a meta analysis. Indian J Dermatol Venereol Leprol 2007;73:86-93.

CUTANEOUS TUBERCULOSIS

Tuberculosis (TB) is a communicable disease caused by *Mycobacterium tuberculosis*, an intracellular acid-fast bacillus. The disease typically affects the lungs but may involve any organ. Cutaneous involvement is relatively uncommon, affecting less than 2% of patients with TB. The global rise in HIV, use of immunosuppressive therapies, and emergence of drug-resistant strains has led to an increase in all forms of cutaneous TB. Although curable and preventable, TB remains a major public health concern, especially in developing countries.

Clinical Presentation

- Cutaneous TB is predominantly caused by *M. tuberculosis*. It may occasionally be due to *M. bovis* and its live attenuated strain, bacillus Calmette-Guérin (BCG).
- It has a worldwide distribution, occurring mostly in the tropics. Populations living in endemic areas are less susceptible to infection than if an individual has been recently exposed.
- Cutaneous TB presents with a myriad of clinical manifestations, depending on the type and extent of infection, and the status of host immunity. It can occur secondary to exogenous inoculation or endogenous spread via hematogenous, lymphatic, or contiguous spread. Tuberculids occur as a result of a hypersensitivity reaction to TB affecting another area in the body.
- Table 2 summarizes the host immunity response, clinical presentation, sites of involvement, and differential diagnoses of the various forms of cutaneous TB.

Investigations & Treatment

- Diagnosis is based on clinical manifestations, supported by host-reaction to tuberculin skin test, interferon-gamma release assays (QuantiFERON-TB Gold in tube and T-SPOT.TB tests), histopathologic analysis, and isolation of *M. tuberculosis* in culture or polymerase chain reaction.

TABLE 2. Classification, clinical features, & differential diagnoses.

Route of infection	Host immunity	Clinical disease	Presentation	Sites of predilection	Differential diagnoses
Exogenous infection (via inoculation)	Moderate to high	TB verrucosa cutis	Asymptomatic, hyperkeratotic erythematous papule or papulo-pustule with a violaceous halo, that gradually enlarges into a verrucous plaque, which may ulcerate and heal spontaneously with atrophic scarring after several years	Hands and lower extremities	Verruca, deep fungal infections, hypertrophic lichen planus, squamous cell carcinoma
	Naïve	Primary inoculation TB	Papule or erosion that appears 2 to 4 weeks after inoculation, enlarges to a painless ulcer with shallow base with granulation tissue	Face, hands, and lower extremities	Sporotrichosis, syphilis, atypical mycobacterial infections
Endogenous infection (via hematogenous, lymphatic, or contiguous spread from elsewhere in the body)	Moderate to high	Lupus vulgaris	Well-defined brownish-red plaque with smooth or hyperkeratotic surface; may have central scarring; yellow-brown color on diascopy; usually solitary but may be multiple in children	Head and neck	Discoid lupus erythematosus, sarcoidosis, leprosy, deep fungal infection, squamous cell carcinoma
		Scrofuloderma	Asymptomatic, firm, deep-seated, subcutaneous nodule which eventually becomes fluctuant and ulcerates with undermined edges; drains via sinus tracts and heals as tethered scars	Parotid, submandibular, neck, supraclavicular areas, axillae, and groin	Bacterial abscess, dimorphic fungal infections, hidradenitis suppurativa, sporotrichosis, actinomycosis
	Low	Acute miliary TB	Disseminated, minute, erythematous to violaceous macules and papules which develop central umbilication and crusting, healing with hypochromic scars; usually accompanied by fever, asthenia, and weight loss	Generalized, especially trunk	Varicella, enteroviral exanthems, pityriasis lichenoides
		Orificial TB	Friable, yellowish, or erythematous papule or nodule which develops into extremely painful, punched-out ulcers with undermined edges	Near body orifices	Aphthous ulcers, syphilis, squamous cell carcinoma, HSV, pemphigus
		Tuberculous gumma	Firm, subcutaneous nodule which may become fluctuant and ulcerate with sinus tract formation	Neck, trunk, extremities	Panniculitis, dimorphic fungal infections, hidradenitis suppurativa
Tuberculids	Unclear	Papulonecrotic tuberculid	Recurrent crops of asymptomatic, erythematous to purplish, necrotic papulonodules which heal spontaneously with atrophic scars; may be preceded by fever, asthenia, and other constitutional symptoms; may resolve spontaneously	Face, ears, extensor aspects of extremities, lower trunk, and buttocks; may become widespread	Pityriasis lichenoides, prurigo, secondary syphilis, small-vessel vasculitis
		Lichen scrofulosorum	Asymptomatic, grouped, firm, yellow-red to brown-red follicular or perifollicular papules with variable scaling; can persist for months before regressing without scarring	Trunk	Lichen nitidus, lichen planus, secondary syphilis
		Erythema induratum of Bazin	Mildly painful, dull red or bluish red subcutaneous nodules, which may ulcerate with bluish undermined borders; heals with atrophic scarring; may be recurrent	Posterior aspect of lower extremities	Erythema nodosum

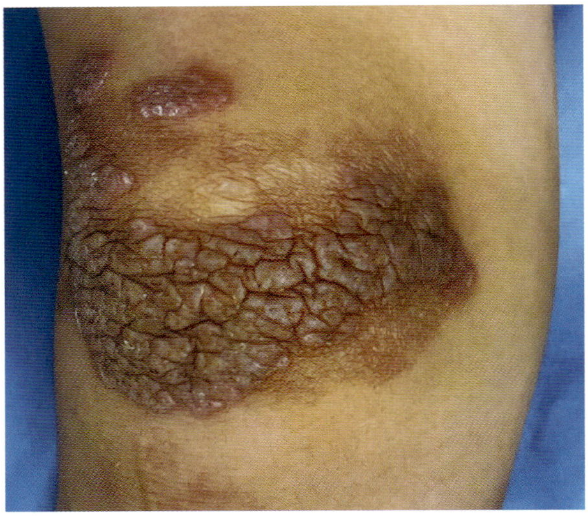

FIGURE 6-87. Tuberculosis verrucosa cutis on the knee of a 6-year-old presenting with a large, verrucous plaque. (Photo courtesy of Department of Dermatology, Ospital ng Maynila Medical Center, Manila, Philippines.)

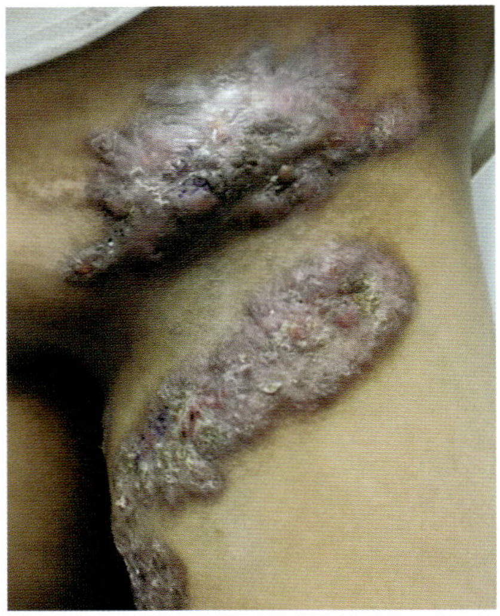

FIGURE 6-88. Tuberculosis verrucosa cutis on the abdomen and left thigh of an Indonesian child. (Photo courtesy of Dr. Deryne Anggia Paramita, Medan, Indonesia.)

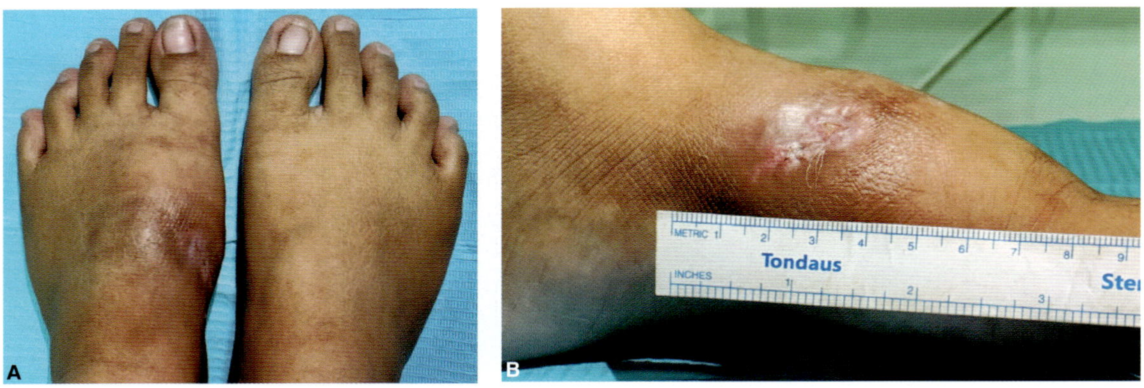

FIGURE 6-89A & 89B. Primary inoculation tuberculosis on the dorsum of the foot of a 16-year-old Filipino, presenting as a chronic, indurated, shiny plaque. (Photo courtesy of Department of Dermatology, Ospital ng Maynila Medical Center, Manila, Philippines.)

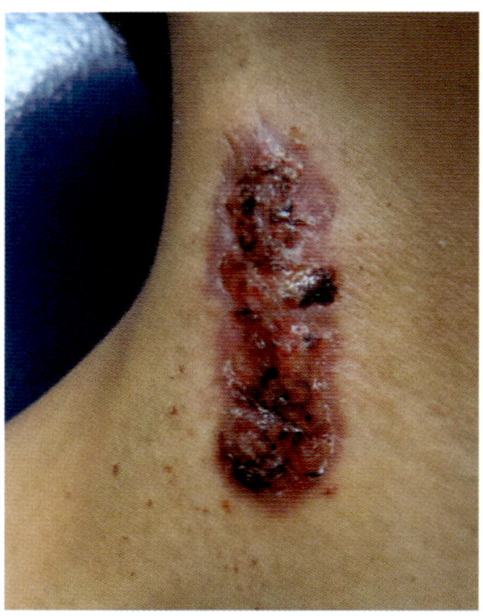

FIGURE 6-90. Scrofuloderma on the lateral aspect of the neck of a 16-year-old Filipino, presenting as a violaceous, indurated, irregular plaque. (Photo courtesy of Department of Dermatology, Ospital ng Maynila Medical Center, Manila, Philippines.)

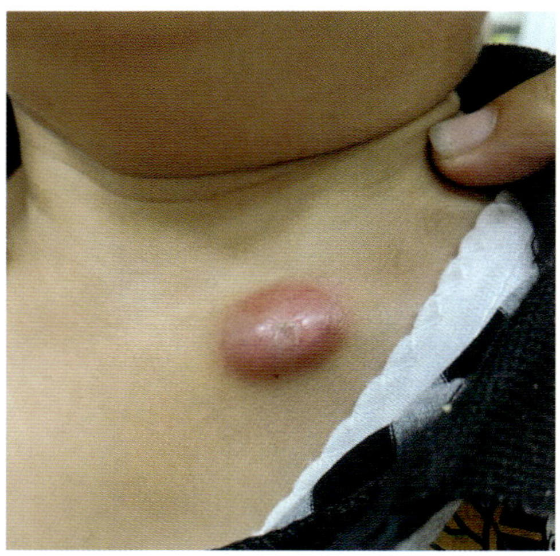

FIGURE 6-91. Scrofuloderma on the chest of an Indonesian child, presenting as an erythematous nodule with central erosion. (Photo courtesy of Dr. July Iriani Rahardja, Jakarta, Indonesia.)

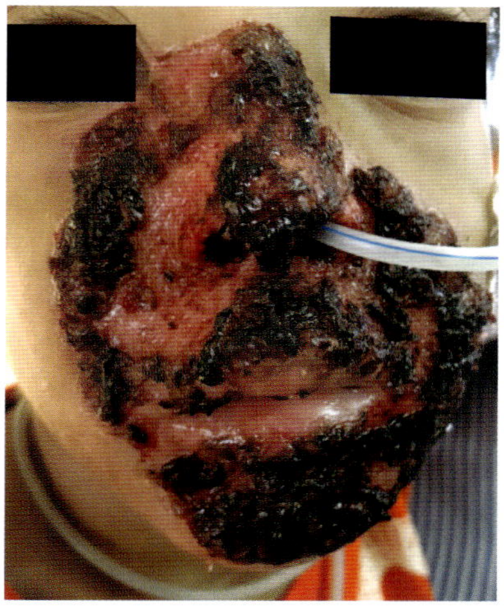

FIGURE 6-92. Lupus vulgaris presenting as a fungating mass with overlying ulceration and crusting over the face of an Indonesian boy. (Photo courtesy of Dr. Djohan Kho, Medan, Indonesia.)

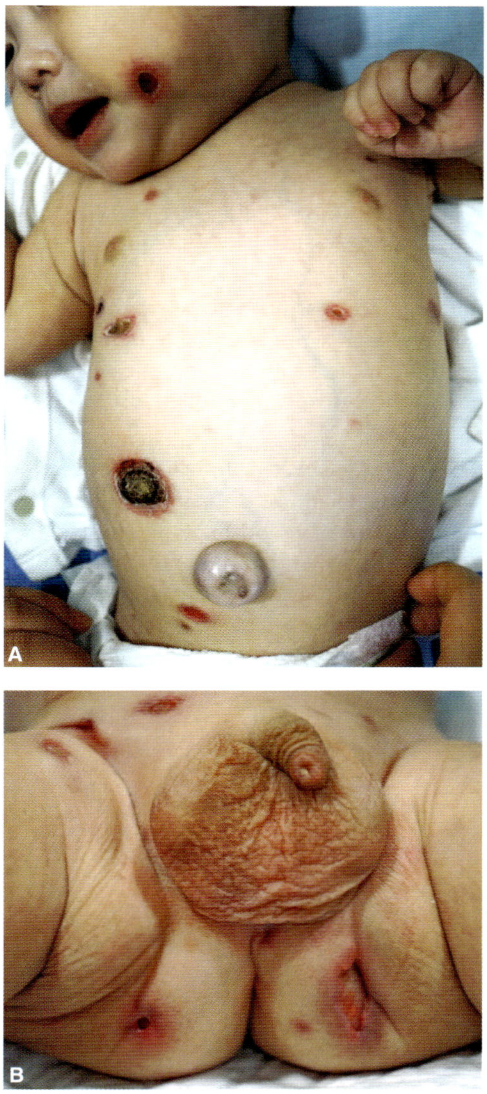

FIGURE 6-93A & 93B. Disseminated *Mycobacterium bovis* infection in a child with severe combined immunodeficiency presenting as multiple, ulcerated plaques, some with overlying eschar.

- Management of cutaneous TB is similar to that of systemic TB. For non-severe, presumed susceptible cases in children and adolescents below 16 years of age, an initial 2-month intensive phase therapy with isoniazid, rifampicin, pyrazinamide, and ethambutol followed by a 2-month maintenance therapy with isoniazid and rifampicin is currently recommended.
- Fixed-dose combinations of anti-TB drugs are available to facilitate increased adherence to medications.
- For severely malnourished and HIV-positive children on antiretroviral therapy, prophylactic supplementation of pyridoxine (10–25 mg/day) with isoniazid is recommended.
- Limited cutaneous infections such as tuberculosis verrucosa cutis, primary inoculation TB, and localized forms of lupus vulgaris with no evidence of internal TB may be treated with isoniazid alone for up to 12 months. Treatment should be extended for at least 2 months after complete involution of lesions.
- Surgical intervention may be used as adjuvant therapy in cases of scrofuloderma, tuberculosis verrucosa cutis, and small lesions of lupus vulgaris.

Pearls & Practical Tips

- The clinical presentation of cutaneous TB is myriad and includes inflammatory papules, verrucous plaques, suppurative nodules, chronic ulcers, among other lesions. For patients with chronic, non-healing skin lesions who live in endemic regions, suspicion should be high for cutaneous or atypical mycobacteria infection.
- Treatment can be curative, except for patients with severe immunosuppression.
- The most efficient way to prevent cutaneous TB is early recognition of infectious cases and appropriate therapy until complete cure. Other modalities include BCG vaccination in children and treatment of latent TB cases which can lead to development of active disease.
- Patients who do not respond to first-line treatment should be managed with other medications. Never add a single drug to a failing regimen.
- For cases with underlying systemic TB, appropriate contact investigation and treatment, whenever applicable, of household and close contacts must be done.

Bibliography

1. World Health Organization. Global Tuberculosis Report 2021. Geneva (CH): World Health organization; 2021. Available from: https://www.who.int/teams/global-tuberculosis-programme/tb-reports/global-tuberculosis-report-2021. Accessed 14 Nov 2021.
2. Santos JB, Figueiredo AR, Ferraz CE, Oliveira MH, Silva PG, Medeiros VL. Cutaneous tuberculosis: epidemiologic, etiopathogenic and clinical aspects - part I. An Bras Dermatol 2014;89(2):219-28.
3. Dias MF, Filho FB, Quaresma MV, Nascimento LV, Nery JA, Azulay DR. Update on cutaneous tuberculosis. An Bras Dermatol 2014;89(6):925-38.
4. World Health Organization. Guidance for national tuberculosis programmes on the management of tuberculosis in children. Geneva (CH): World Health Organization; 2014. Available from https://www.who.int/publications/i/item/9789241548748. Accessed 14 November 2021.

5. World Health Organization. Rapid communication on updated guidance on the management of tuberculosis in children and adolescents. Geneva (CH): World Health Organization; 2021. Available from https://apps.who.int/iris/handle/10665/344382. Accessed 21 November 2021.
6. Handog EB, Gabriel TG, Pineda RT. Management of cutaneous tuberculosis. Dermatol Ther 2008;21(3):154-61.
7. Sethuraman G, Ramesh V. Cutaneous tuberculosis in children. Pediatr Dermatol 2013;30(1):7-16.

CUTANEOUS NON-TUBERCULOUS MYCOBACTERIAL INFECTIONS

Non-tuberculous mycobacteria (NTM), or atypical mycobacteria, refers to mycobacteria other than *M. tuberculosis* complex and *M. leprae*. Although found ubiquitously in the environment, overt disease is uncommon due to the relatively low virulence of NTM. Prevalent NTM species differ geographically, with *M. avium* complex and the rapid growers *M. abscesses* and *M. fortuitum* more frequently implicated in cases from Asia.

Clinical Features

- Cutaneous NTM infection is far more common in adults compared to the pediatric population.
- Disease presentation may be localized or disseminated, depending on the causative species, route of exposure, and host immunity.
- Localized cutaneous infection mostly arises via direct inoculation following trauma, cosmetic and surgical procedures, or exposure to contaminated water.
- Cutaneous NTM may take months to become clinically apparent and present with a variety of non-specific lesions such as pustules, plaques, nodules, ulcers, and draining sinuses, especially in immunocompromised hosts. Only *M. marinum* and *M. ulcerans* produce more characteristic clinical features.
- Often referred to as "fish-tank granuloma," cutaneous *M. marinum* infection presents as a solitary, bluish-red, scaly nodule or pustule which can form hyperkeratotic crusts or suppuration. Multiple lesions follow a lymphocutaneous or "sporotrichoid" spread. There may be exposure to marine fish or other aquatic organisms.
- Cutaneous *M. ulcerans* infection presents as a solitary, asymptomatic, firm subcutaneous nodule which progresses after a month into a fluctuant ulcer with undermined edges and a deep necrotic base. There is a lack of regional lymphadenopathy and inflammatory response. It may either heal as depressed scars or spread extensively with scarring and deformity.
- Disseminated lesions or involvement of underlying structures may occur in immunocompromised hosts.

Differential Diagnoses

- Lichen simplex chronicus (LSC)
  - Lesions of LSC can often be mistaken for cutaneous NTM infection. LSC often occurs in patients with a background of atopy or AD, and there is a chronic history of scratching.
- Pyogenic bacterial infections
  - These are far more common and include folliculitis, ecthyma, and furuncles. The presentation is more acute, and specimen cultures will confirm the diagnosis.
- Other opportunistic infections
  - Due to the variable presentation of NTM, other opportunistic infections can present fairly similarly, with chronic, non-healing, scaly plaques or ulcers. These include cutaneous melioidosis, cutaneous tuberculosis, deep fungal infections, and actinomycoses.
  - Histology and tissue specimens for bacterial, mycobacterial, and fungal cultures should always be performed if a cutaneous opportunistic infection is suspected.

Investigations & Treatment

- Cutaneous NTM can be suspected clinically, but isolation of mycobacteria in tissue culture is the gold standard for diagnosis. However, depending on the type of mycobacteria, specific requirements and long incubation periods may be required, which can delay treatment.

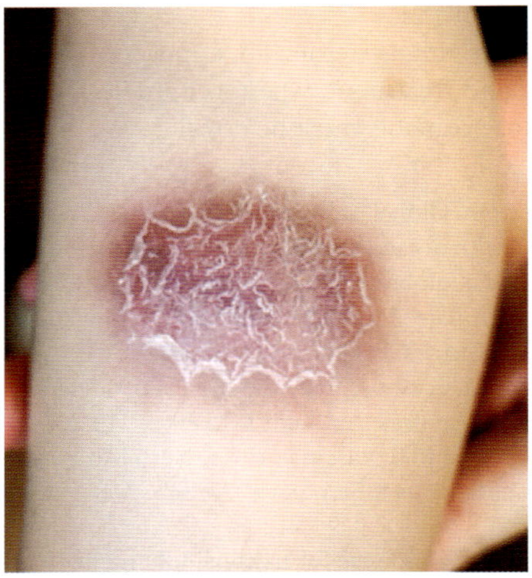

FIGURE 6-94. Solitary asymptomatic chronic erythematous scaly plaque on the leg of a child caused by *Mycobacterium abscessus*.

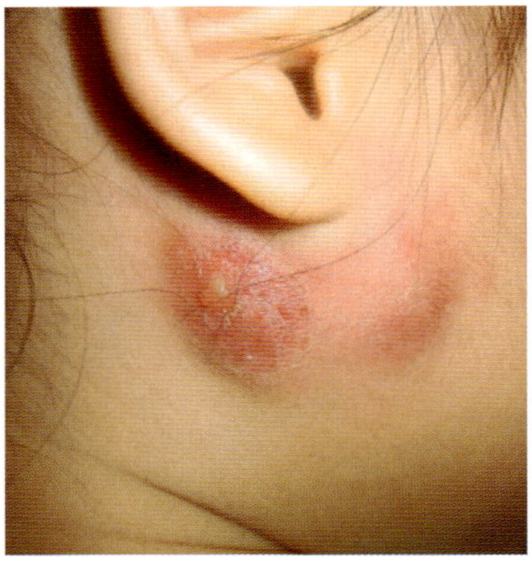

FIGURE 6-95. NTM infection of a cervical lymph node with overlying skin changes in a Chinese girl. (Photo courtesy of Infectious Disease Service, KK Women's & Children's Hospital, Singapore.)

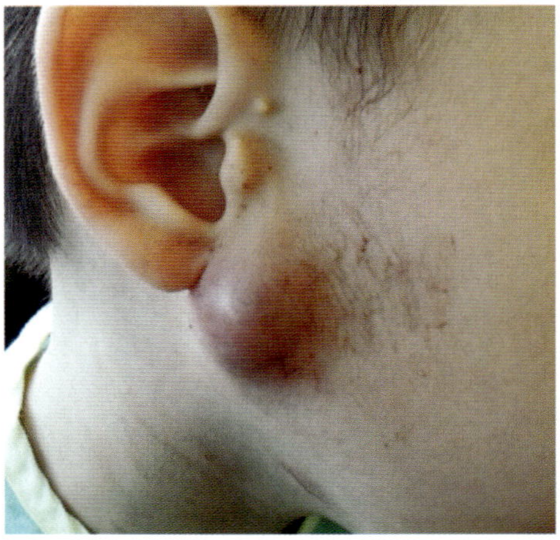

FIGURE 6-96. NTM infection of a cervical lymph node with overlying violaceous discoloration in a Chinese boy. (Photo courtesy of Infectious Disease Service, KK Women's & Children's Hospital, Singapore.)

- Histopathologic analysis is supportive but does not distinguish the mycobacterial species. Findings include chronic inflammation, suppuration, abscess, and granuloma formation, with or without caseation. Presence of acid-fast bacilli is variable, depending on the degree of host tissue reaction.
- Evolving techniques which provide rapid and more accurate identification of NTM include polymerase chain reaction assays, nucleic acid probes, and gene sequencing.
- NTMs are less responsive to standard antituberculous drugs. Multidrug regimen with chemotherapeutic agents for at least 3 to 6 months is recommended.
- Clarithromycin has been reported to be the best single empiric option in cases where immediate treatment is necessary. Additional antibiotics include rifampicin, ethambutol, and minocycline. Treatment should be in conjunction with a pediatric infectious disease expert.
- Surgical management can be used in some cases to expedite recovery and limit sequelae.

Pearls & Practical Tips

- Always consider NTM infection in patients with persistent cutaneous lesions that fail to improve despite appropriate antibiotic therapy, especially those occurring at sites of prior trauma or procedures.
- Monotherapy should be avoided to prevent acquired bacterial resistance. Treatment should be based on antimicrobial susceptibility findings. The use of combined antibiotics, with or without adjunctive surgical excision, is currently recommended.

Bibliography

1. Sharma SK, Upadhyay V. Epidemiology, diagnosis & treatment of non-tuberculous mycobacterial diseases. Indian J Med Res 2020;152(3):185-226.
2. Ford TJ, Silcock RA, Holland SM. Overview of nontuberculous mycobacterial disease in children. J Paediatr Child Health 2021;57(1):15-18.
3. Nogueira LB, Garcia CN, Costa MSCD, Moraes MB, Kurizky PS, Gomes CM. Non-tuberculous cutaneous mycobacterioses. An Bras Dermatol 2021;96(5):527-38.
4. Chung J, Ince D, Ford BA, Wanat KA. Cutaneous infections due to nontuberculosis mycobacterium: recognition and management. Am J Clin Dermatol 2018;19(6):867-78.

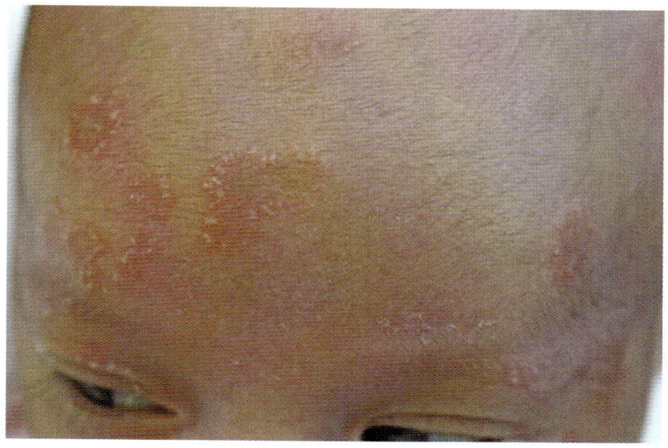

FIGURE 6-97. Tinea faciei in a young Malay infant presenting with scaly, annular, erythematous plaques on her forehead.

FUNGAL INFECTIONS

DERMATOPHYTE INFECTIONS

Dermatophytes are a common cause of superficial cutaneous infections, especially in tropical humid climates but also in temperate regions. Although uncommon in children, they are fairly common in adolescents, especially those with poor hygiene practices, and in overweight individuals. Dermatophyte infection can occur on the skin (tinea faciei, tinea corporis, tinea cruris, tinea manuum, tinea pedis), nails (tinea unguum), hair and scalp (tinea capitis). Tinea capitis is the only dermatophyte infection that occurs more commonly in children than adults.

Clinical Features

- Tinea is caused by three dermatophyte genera, namely *Trichophyton*, *Microsporum*, and *Epidermophyton*.
- Transmission of dermatophyte infection is usually indirect, occurring through the infected skin scales, hair, or nails shed from infected human or animal hosts. Contaminated combs and hairbrushes can be the source of infection in tinea capitis, while clothing, towels, and bed linens are also possible sources of infection.
- Clinical presentation is dependent on the site of infection.
- Tinea capitis (scalp/hair)
  - Most commonly caused by *Microsporum canis*, this can be acquired from infected animals, especially cats.
  - Slowly extending circular or ovoid patches with alopecia, mild erythema, and scaling. Infected hairs break off at the surface of the scalp, giving a "black-dot" characteristic.
  - Kerion and favus are inflammatory forms of tinea capitis and present as solitary or several lesions with induration, erythema, and overlying pustules or scales. Delayed treatment can cause permanent scarring alopecia.
  - On dermoscopy, the presence of comma-shaped, zigzag-shaped, cockscrew-like, and "morse-code" hairs are indicative of tinea capitis.
  - Wood's lamp examination is useful, especially in cases of infection with *Microsporum canis*, where lesions appear with light green fluorescence.

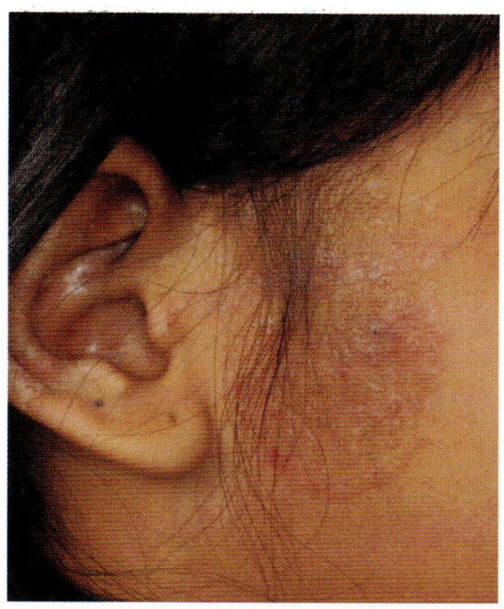

FIGURE 6-98. Tinea faciei in a Malay child with annular, scaly, erythematous plaques in an asymmetrical distribution.

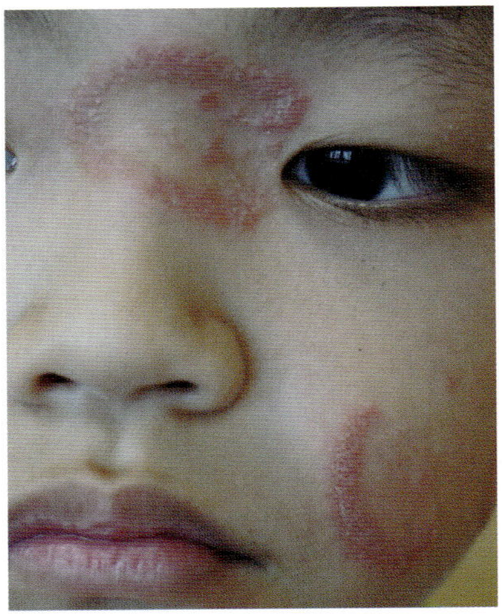

FIGURE 6-99. Tinea faciei on the face of a Chinese boy presenting with annular, scaly, erythematous plaques asymmetrically.

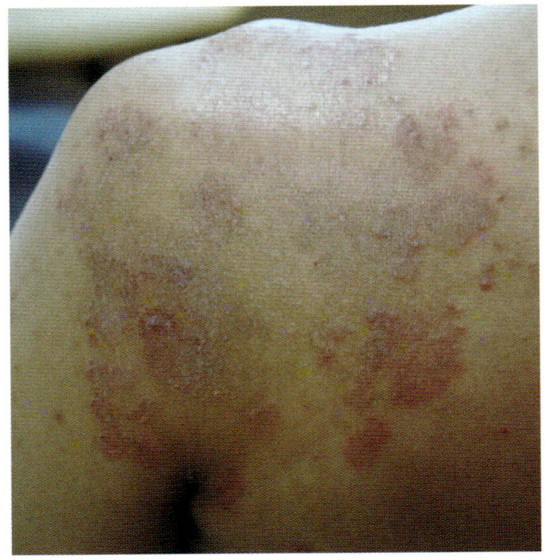

FIGURE 6-100. Tinea corporis on the left shoulder and back of a Nepalese adolescent male, presenting with annular, scaly, erythematous plaques.

- Tinea faciei (face) and tinea corporis (body)
  - Lesions in these areas appear as skin-colored to erythematous, circular plaques with distinct raised, scaly borders and hyperpigmented central areas, in a classical annular configuration.
- Tinea cruris
  - Erythematous and scaly lesions extending symmetrically from the groin down the inner surface of the thighs with a marginated, raised, scaly edge. Pustules may sometimes be seen. The lesions are often itchy.
- Tinea pedis (feet) and tinea manuum (hands)
  - Tinea pedis is more common in adolescents who wear closed footwear in hot, humid environments for prolonged periods. Tinea manuum is very uncommon in children and adolescents and can occur due to autoinoculation from tinea at other sites.
  - Tinea pedis usually arises from the interdigital spaces, especially between the fourth and fifth toes, and spreads in a circular pattern.
  - The lesions are usually itchy and can appear as small, clear vesicles that rupture to become erythematous patches or plaques with a scaly annular edge. Chronic lesions can appear diffusely scaly and can affect the heels, sides, and dorsa of the feet.
  - Lesions of tinea manuum classically appear annular with a scaly, raised, and erythematous leading edge.
- Tinea unguum
  - This is extremely uncommon in children and adolescents, and if present usually signifies autoinoculation from other sites of tinea involvement.

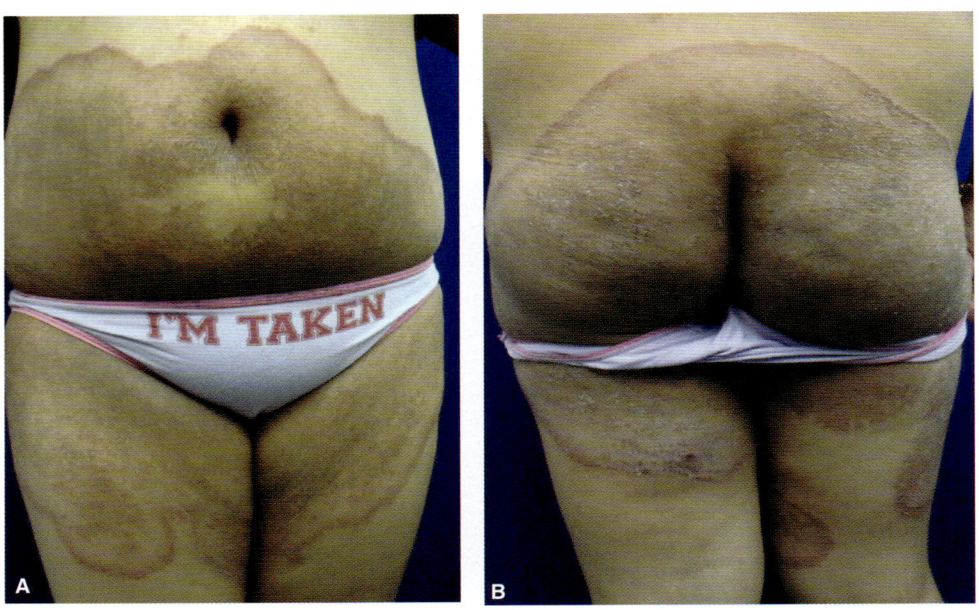

FIGURE 6-101A & 101B. Tinea corporis and cruris on the abdomen, groin, buttocks, and upper thighs of a Filipino adolescent female who is overweight. Note the annular borders with central hyperpigmentation.

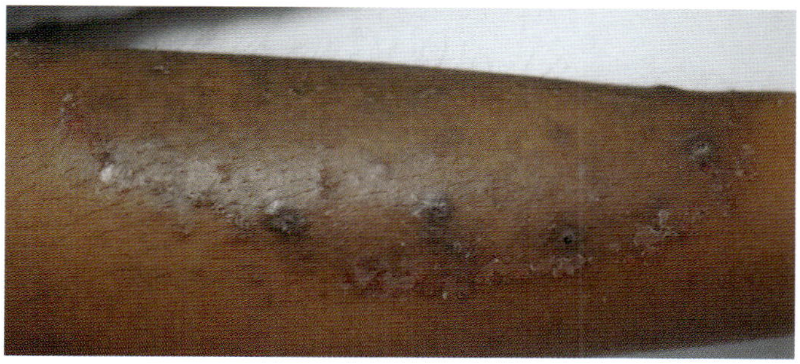

FIGURE 6-102. Tinea on the shin of a young Indian boy with features of Majocchi's granuloma with involvement of the hair follicle.

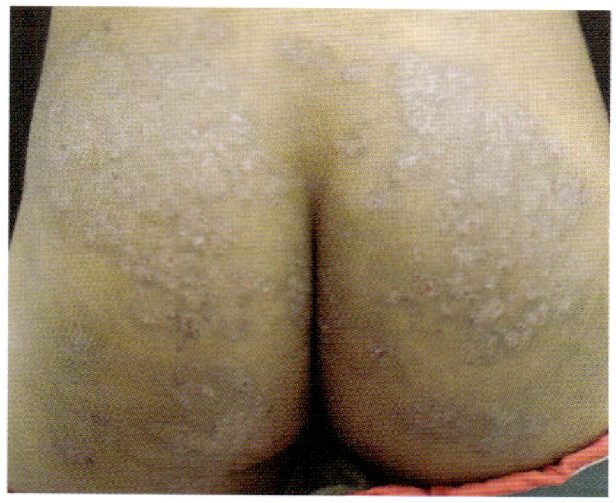

FIGURE 6-103. Tinea incognito on the buttocks of a Malay adolescent. Note that the usual annular configuration is attenuated, and the rash can be misdiagnosed as buttock eczema.

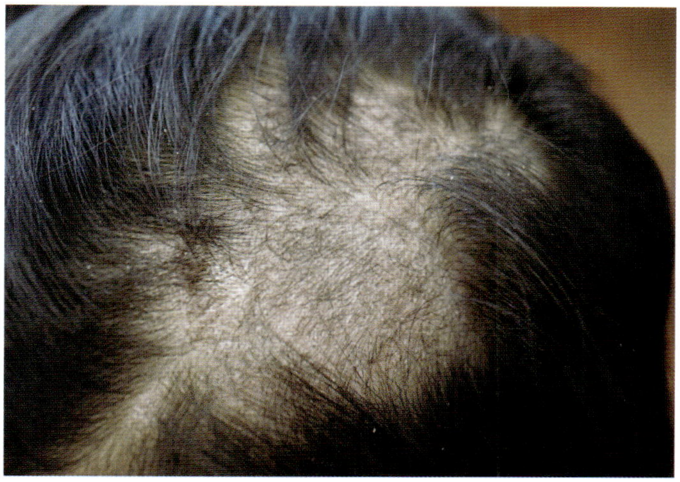

FIGURE 6-104. Tinea capitis affecting a large area of the scalp in a young Malay girl, presenting with alopecia, scaling, and mild erythema of the scalp.

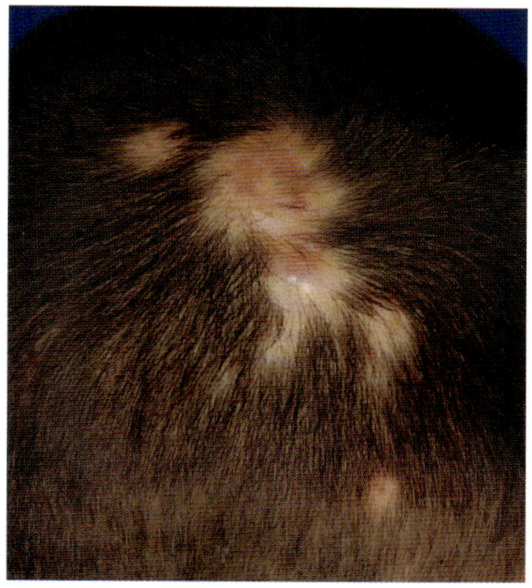

FIGURE 6-105. Tinea capitis in a Chinese boy, presenting with alopecia with erythema and mild induration of the underlying skin.

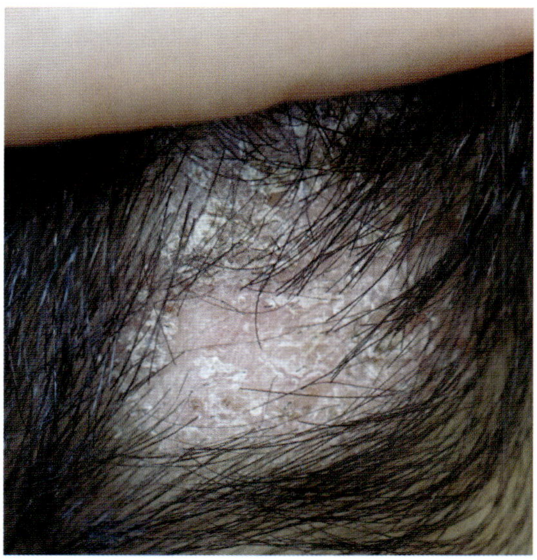

FIGURE 6-106. Inflammatory tinea capitis in a Chinese boy, presenting with erythema, scaling, scabbing, and localized hair loss.

- Invasion commences at the distal end and side of the nail and spreads proximally up the nail. The nail plate becomes friable and thickened.

Differential Diagnoses

- Tinea capitis
  - Scalp eczema, scalp psoriasis, and seborrheic dermatitis can all present as scaly patches on the scalp. Hair loss in these conditions is unusual unless manipulated by the patient. The rest of the skin should be examined for classical features of these dermatoses. Dermoscopy and Wood's lamp examination are also useful in making the distinction.
  - Alopecia areata and trichotillomania can present with localized hair loss in children and adolescents. In alopecia areata, lesions are commonly entirely devoid of hair and not scaly, whereas in lesions of tinea capitis, small, broken hairs are usually found with scaling of the scalp. In trichotillomania, short, broken hairs may also be found. However, the distribution is usually more bizarre, and hair pull test is negative. Wood's lamp examination may be useful to exclude tinea capitis. Scalp biopsy may be required in difficult cases.

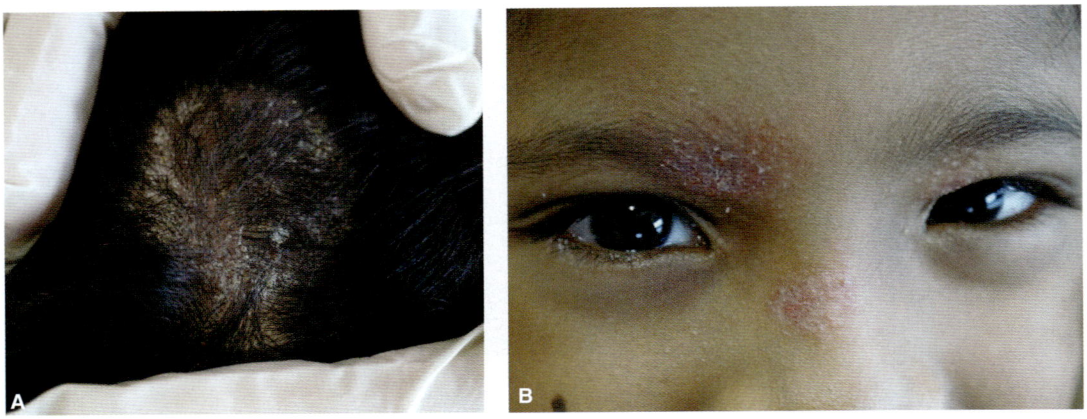

FIGURE 6-107A & 107B. Inflammatory tinea capitis with favus formation in a young Indian male. There is concomitant tinea faciei.

- Tinea faciei
  - Atopic dermatitis (AD) can present as annular lesions, especially in infants and young children. Presence of other atopic features and classical lesions of AD should be sought.
  - Seborrheic dermatitis usually affects the T-zone of the face, including the eyebrows and nasolabial folds. Other features of atopy may also be present.
  - Lupus erythematosus (LE) can occur in the neonatal period or in childhood and adolescence. Neonatal LE can also present with an annular rash, usually in the first few weeks or months of life. Subacute lesions of LE in children and adolescents can present as annular, psoriasiform eruptions, especially in sun-exposed sites. Other features of LE, especially systemic LE, have to be elucidated from the history and clinical examination. Laboratory investigations and skin biopsy can differentiate from tinea.
- Tinea corporis
  - AD, psoriasis, or psoriasiform dermatitis can present as demarcated, pink to erythematous papules and plaques with thick adherent scales, uncommonly in an annular configuration. Classical involvement of these dermatoses and family history should be sought. Fungal microscopy and cultures should be performed to exclude tinea infection.
  - Pityriasis rosea often presents as an annular, ovoid, salmon-colored patch or plaques with distinctive collarette of scales (herald patch). This then erupts into a more widespread rash, with some patches or plaques having annular configurations. The eruption is usually self-limiting, even without treatment.
  - Mycosis fungoides (MF), a form of cutaneous T-cell lymphoma, can present with annular patches and plaques, although the hypopigmented form is more common in Asian children and adolescents.

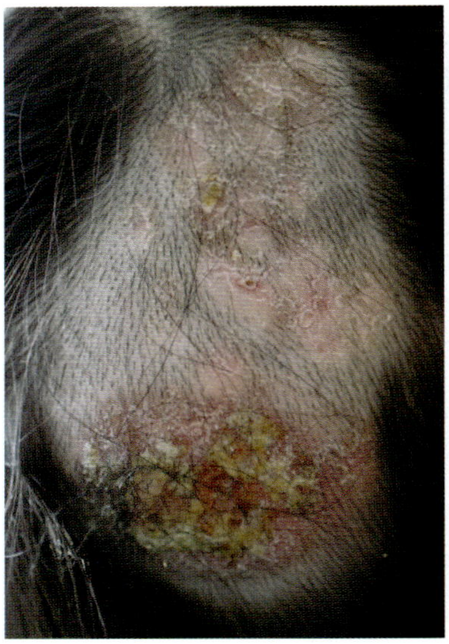

FIGURE 6-108. A Chinese girl presenting with inflammatory tinea capitis/favus.

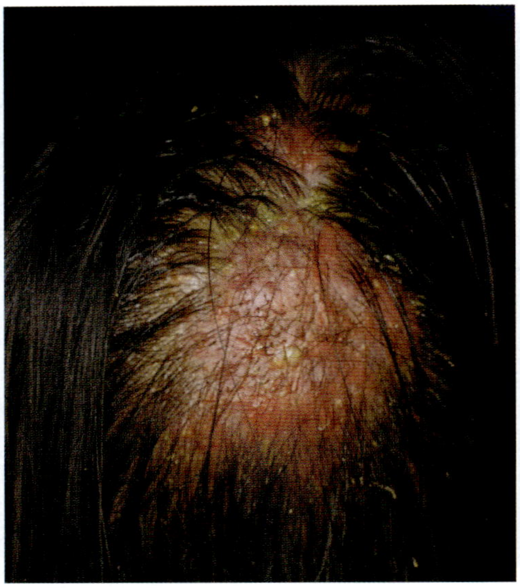

FIGURE 6-109. A young Malay girl with a kerion presenting as a red, boggy plaque with alopecia.

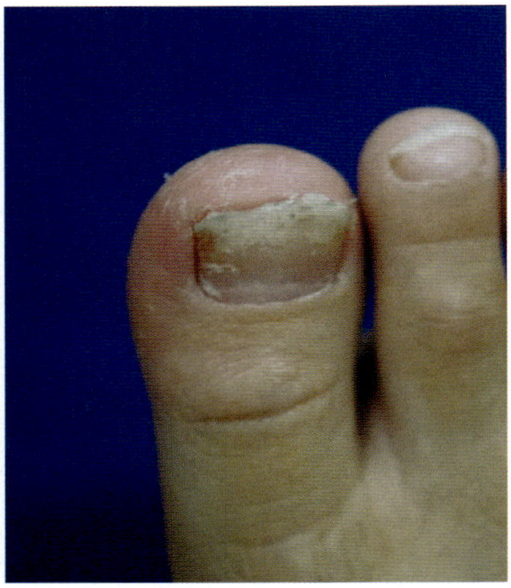

FIGURE 6-110. A rare case of tinea unguum of the big toenail in an older Chinese child, presenting with whitish discoloration of the distal nail plate with subungual debris.

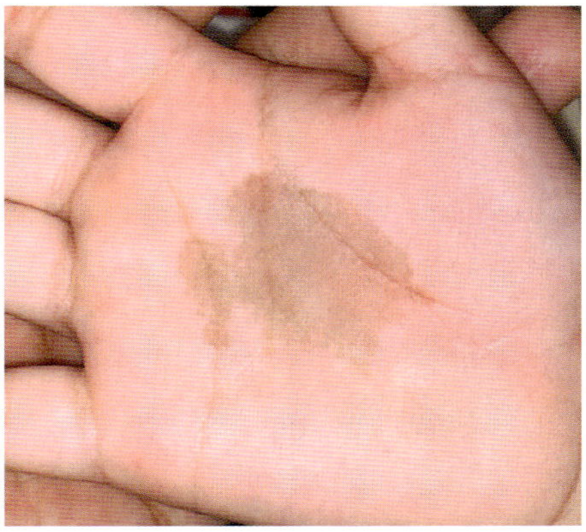

FIGURE 6-111. A rare case of tinea nigra on the palm of a young Chinese girl, caused by a mould, *Hortaea werneckii,* which is usually found in soil.

Skin biopsies, sometimes multiple, may be required to exclude MF, especially if there is poor response to treatment with antifungal agents and fungal investigations return negative.

- Tinea cruris
  - Inverse psoriasis can present as pink-to-red patches and occurs at flexural sites such as axilla and inframammary, inguinal, and gluteal folds.
  - Diaper dermatitis commonly affects children 3 to 15 months of age and occurs secondary to irritation from urine and feces. Tinea cruris is rare at this age.
  - Intertrigo is characterized by erythematous patches and plaques on body flexures such as behind the ears, folds of the neck, axillae, under a protruding abdomen, groin, between the buttocks, and in the finger and toe webs. Infection with candida or other yeast is often present.
- Tinea pedis and tinea manuum
  - Dyshidrotic eczema or hand and foot dermatitis can present as recurrent crops of deep-seated blisters on the palms and soles. They cause intense itch or a burning sensation. The blister roof peels off and the skin appears red and oozy, with painful fissures. Secondary bacterial infection is common. Dyshidrotic eczema usually affects bilaterally, whereas tinea is usually unilateral. Fungal microscopy and cultures may be required to differentiate.
  - Contact dermatitis affecting the hands and feet can present as itchy, erythematous, scaly papules, patches, and plaques. It is important to obtain a history of contactants, although this is often difficult to illicit. Patch testing may be required to exclude allergic contact dermatitis.

Investigations & Treatment

- Confirmation of dermatophyte infection is through demonstration of fungal elements in specimens from infected skin, hair, or nails using 20% to 30% potassium hydroxide on a microscope slide, or by fungal cultures from these specimens. Although microscopic examination yields faster results than fungal cultures, which may take a few weeks to more than a month, the sensitivity of microscopy is lower.
- Molecular diagnosis utilizing internal transcribed spacer region of the ribosomal DNA is recommended as the gold standard for the identification of atypical or difficult dermatophytic isolates.[1]
- Treatment of dermatophyte infections depends on the site and extent of involvement. For infections affecting non-hair-bearing sites, such as tinea corporis or tinea cruris, topical antifungal agents can be used, including topical miconazole, clotrimazole, ketoconazole, sertaconazole, isoconazole, and terbinafine. Compliance needs to be emphasized, and we usually recommend application until lesions have resolved and to continue for 2 weeks thereafter. Personal hygiene needs to be emphasized, especially in patients with recurrent infections.
- Treatment of tinea capitis, especially the inflammatory forms, requires the use of oral antifungal agents such as griseofulvin, itraconazole, or terbinafine. Extensive involvement of non-hair-bearing sites as well as more limited disease not responding to topical treatments may also be considered for oral treatment. Griseofulvin is the most widely studied systemic antifungal agent in children, especially for the treatment of tinea capitis. Treatment is prolonged for months, and both clinical improvement as well as microbiological test-of-cure should be relied upon to decide on total duration of treatment.

Pearls & Practical Tips

- The classical annular configuration of tinea corporis, faciei, and cruris may be obscured with the use of topical corticosteroids (tinea incognito).
- In children and adolescents referred to exclude nail fungal infection, nail involvement due to psoriasis or eczema or 20-nail dystrophy need to be considered, as these are far more common.
- If dermatophyte infection is strongly suspected, we usually recommend performing both fungal microscopy and culture for confirmation.
- Addition of topical keratolytic agents on thick areas of the body like the feet and hands can be beneficial in the treatment of superficial fungal infection.

Reference

1. Normand AC, Packeu A, Cassagne C, Hendrickx M, Ranque S, Piarroux R. Nucleotide sequence database comparison for routine dermatophyte identification by internal transcribed spacer 2 genetic region DNA barcoding. J Clin Microbiol 2018;25;56(5):e00046-18.

PITYROSPORUM (MALASSEZIA) INFECTIONS

Tinea or pityriasis versicolor, and pityrosporum folliculitis, caused by a *Malassezia* yeasts, are some of the most common cutaneous fungal infections, especially in adolescents and young adults in hot and humid climates. Poor hygiene practices can lead to repeated infections.

Clinical Features

- Tinea versicolor
  - Represents superficial epidermal infection by *Malassezia* yeasts.

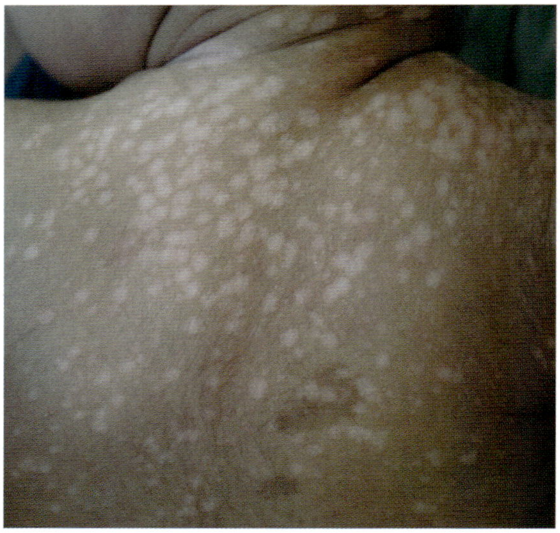

FIGURE 6-112. Tinea versicolor on the upper back of a young Malay infant presenting with well-demarcated hypopigmented patches with mild overlying erythema and scaling.

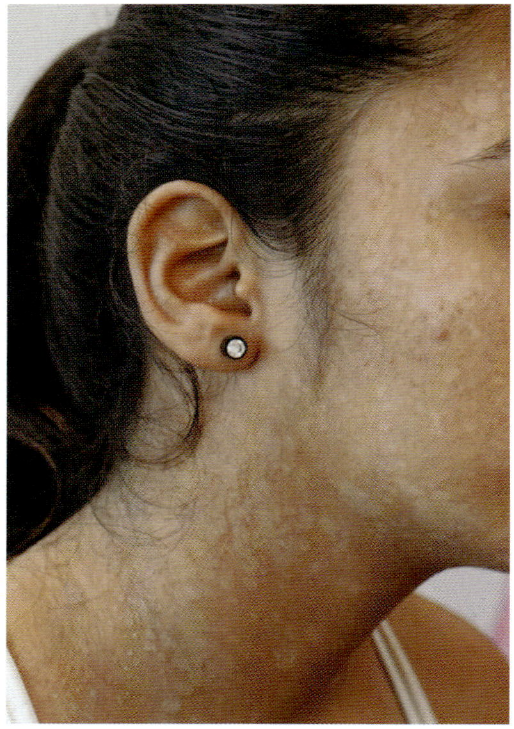

FIGURE 6-113. Tinea versicolor in an Indian adolescent girl presenting with well-demarcated, pink, coalescing, scaly patches and plaques over the axillae, as well as more hypopigmented, scaly patches on the face and neck.

  - It presents most commonly with well-demarcated hypopigmented, pink or hyperpigmented macules and patches, with overlying fine scales. The lesions may be itchy or asymptomatic.
  - The most common sites of involvement are the upper chest, shoulders, and back. However, in more extensive cases, the lesions may also involve the lower face, neck, arms, abdomen, and lower back.
- Pityrosporum folliculitis
  - Represents infection of the pilosebaceous follicles by *Malassezia* yeasts.
  - It occurs most commonly in teenagers who are pubertal, especially in hot, humid climates or when involved in prolonged physical activities. It can also occur after a course of systemic corticosteroids or less commonly, systemic antibiotics.
  - It presents with small, dome-shaped, erythematous, monomorphic papules, most commonly affecting the chest, upper back, and shoulders. Although usually asymptomatic, some patients may complain of mild itch.

Differential Diagnoses

- Tinea versicolor
  - Pityriasis alba occurs most commonly in children and less commonly in adolescents. Patients usually have associated atopic dermatitis or other atopic conditions.

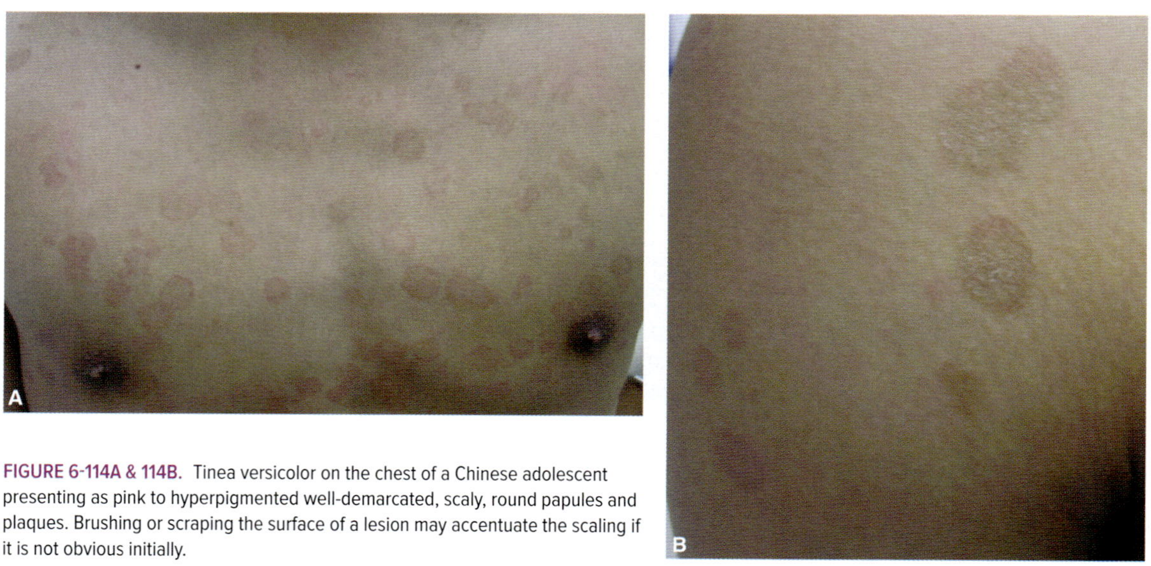

FIGURE 6-114A & 114B. Tinea versicolor on the chest of a Chinese adolescent presenting as pink to hyperpigmented well-demarcated, scaly, round papules and plaques. Brushing or scraping the surface of a lesion may accentuate the scaling if it is not obvious initially.

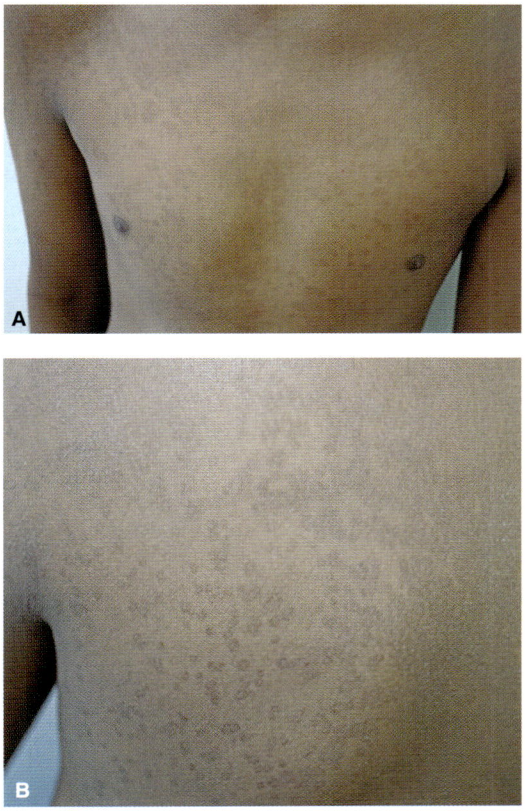

FIGURE 6-115A & 115B. Hyperpigmented form of tinea versicolor in a Malay adolescent male with well-demarcated, hyperpigmented, scaly papules.

It is characterized by non-pruritic, hypopigmented-to-pink patches with fine flaky scales. It occurs most commonly on the cheeks, and lesions are less well-demarcated compared to tinea versicolor.

- Mycosis fungoides is the most common type of cutaneous T-cell lymphoma, which is often misdiagnosed as other dermatoses. In Asian children, it commonly presents as hypopigmented macules and patches. However, it most commonly affects the sun-covered sites, especially the buttocks and trunk, although if more extensive can also affect the face.
- Tuberculoid leprosy, or Hansen's disease, a chronic skin and peripheral nerve infection caused by *Mycobacterium leprae*, can present as large, hypopigmented patches, especially in children from endemic areas. There is decreased sensation and sweating over the affected areas.

• Pityrosporum folliculitis
  - Acne vulgaris can present on the trunk and chest and is often co-existent with pityrosporum folliculitis. Acne presents with polymorphic lesions, including open and closed comedones, papules, pustules, nodules, and cysts, and lesions often also affect the face.
  - Steroid-induced acne is also postulated to be related to pityrosporum, and the treatment is similar.
  - Folliculitis caused by bacteria, including *Staphylococcus* and *Pseudomonas* infection. Staphylococcal folliculitis usually presents as one or a few grouped lesions and can occur anywhere on the body. Compared to pityrosporum folliculitis, lesions are usually larger and contain pus. Pseudomonas folliculitis can occur from exposure to contaminated water from hot tubs, swimming pools, and bathtubs. Lesions can be numerous and appear as erythematous follicular papules, mostly over the covered areas of the trunk. The history is usually shorter compared to pityrosporum folliculitis, and there is usually an exposure to a source of the pseudomonas.

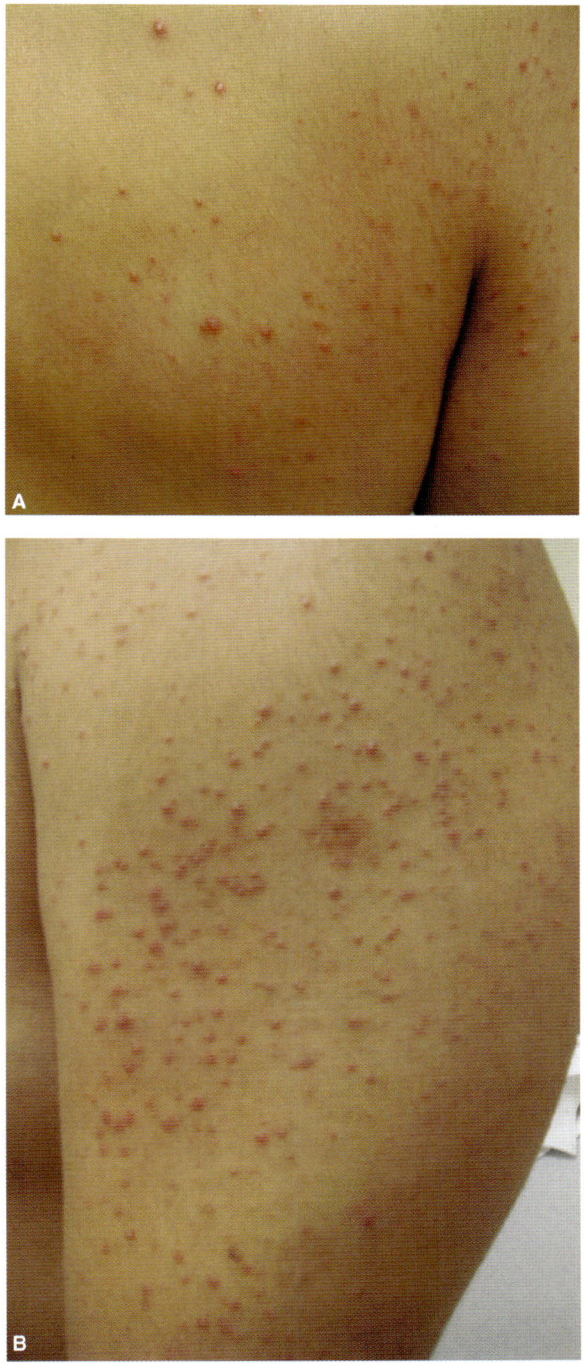

FIGURE 6-116A & 116B. Extensive pityrosporum folliculitis on the back, shoulder, and upper arm of an adolescent Chinese male presenting as multiple, dome-shaped, monomorphic, bright-red papules.

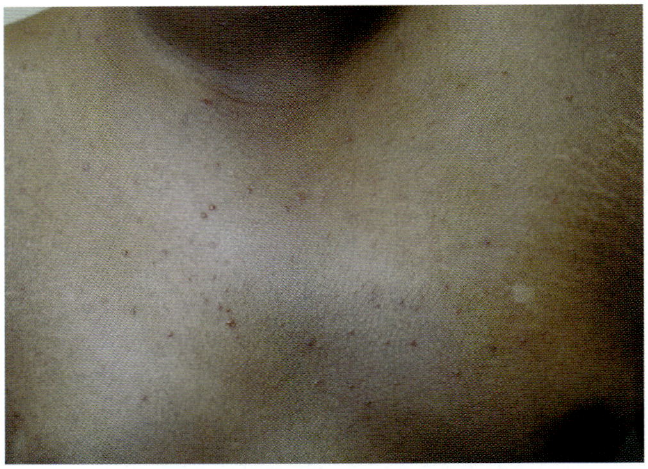

FIGURE 6-117. Pityrosporum folliculitis on chest of an Indian adolescent male presenting with monomorphic, discrete, dome-shaped, hyperpigmented papules. Note the color is brown rather than red in darker-skinned patients.

Investigations & Treatment

- Diagnosis of tinea versicolor and pityrosporum folliculitis is usually clinical. Microscopy examination of scrapings of the scales of tinea versicolor or by pricking a papule of pityrosporum folliculitis, treated with potassium hydroxide (KOH) may show the classical "spaghetti-and-meatballs" configuration of the fungus. However, the fungus is difficult to culture and this is not routinely done for diagnosis.
- Treatment of tinea versicolor is usually with topical azoles, such as miconazole, clotrimazole, ketoconazole, sertaconazole, or isoconazole. We also commonly prescribe an antifungal shampoo, such as ketoconazole or selenium sulfide shampoo, to be applied and left on for 5 to 10 minutes before rinsing off. For patients with extensive involvement, oral azoles may be required, such as itraconazole or fluconazole.
- Treatment of pityrosporum folliculitis is usually with oral azoles such as itraconazole or fluconazole. We usually also prescribe adjunctive treatment with topical antifungal agents, similar to the treatment of tinea versicolor as outlined above.

Pearls & Practical Tips

- Children with pityriasis alba are often misdiagnosed with tinea versicolor. Tinea versicolor is uncommon in childhood and usually occurs in adolescents. The latter affects mostly the trunk, compared to pityriasis alba which usually affects the face. Lesions of pityriasis alba are less well demarcated than tinea versicolor.
- It is important to exclude mycosis fungoides in Asian children and adolescents who present with hypopigmented patches. Always examine sun-covered areas of the skin to look for these lesions. Skin biopsies are required for definitive diagnosis.
- Pityrosporum folliculitis can occur after a course of systemic corticosteroids, such as prednisolone or methylprednisolone. This most often occurs in teenagers.

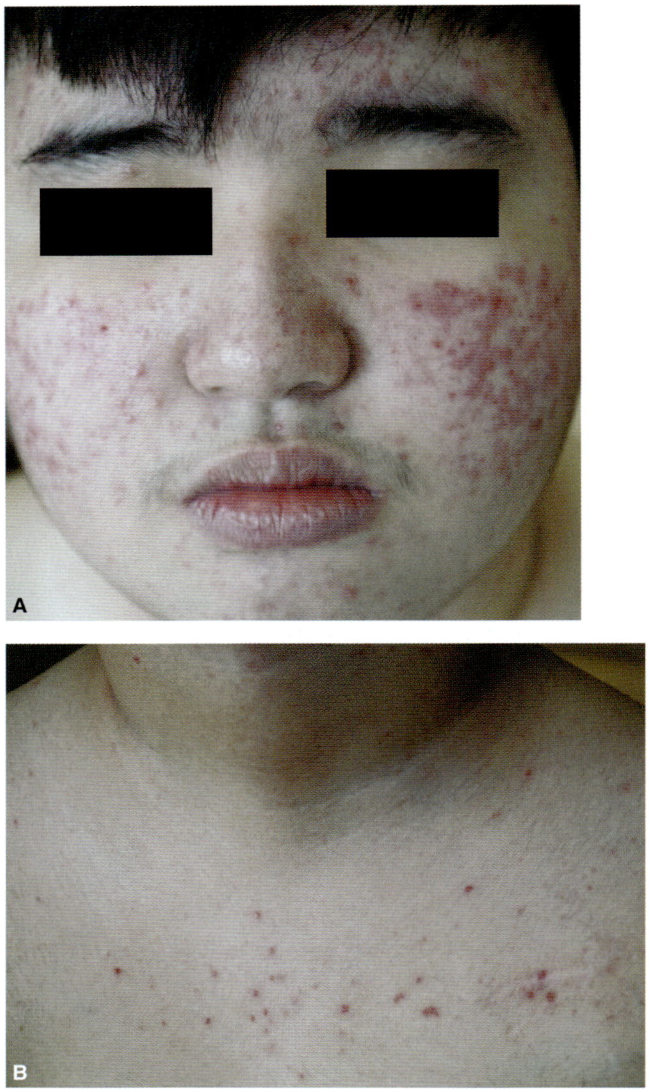

FIGURE 6-118A & 118B. Extensive pityrosporum folliculitis on the face, chest and back of a Chinese adolescent male on treatment with trametinib (MEK inhibitor) and systemic corticosteroids for underlying brain tumor. He has concomitant facial and mild truncal acne.

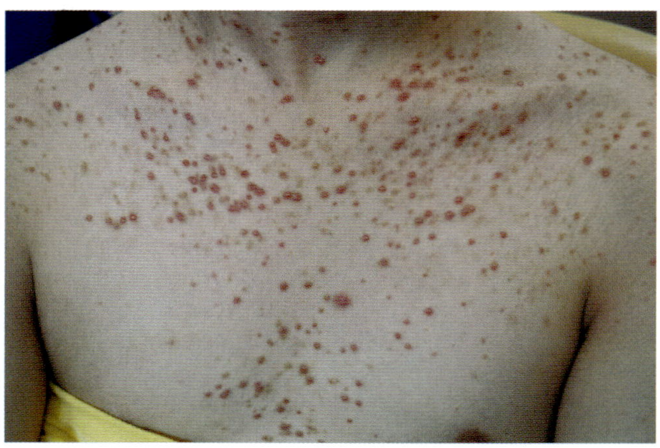

FIGURE 6-119. Extensive pityrosporum folliculitis in a Chinese adolescent male.

- Emphasizing the importance of personal hygiene is important to prevent recurrence of both tinea versicolor and pityrosporum folliculitis. Twice-weekly use of an antifungal shampoo such as ketoconazole or selenium sulfide shampoo, leaving it on for 5 to 10 minutes before rinsing off, may also help to prevent recurrences.

PARASITIC INFECTIONS

SCABIES

Scabies is a contagious skin infestation caused by the *Sarcoptes scabiei* mite. It affects all age groups and is seen worldwide. The infestation causes severe pruritus, especially at night, with the cutaneous eruption postulated to be due to a hypersensitivity response to the mites and their products in the skin.

Clinical Features

- Scabies is spread through prolonged direct contact with a carrier, and it can also sometimes be spread by fomites.
- There is an incubation period of a few weeks to 2 months.
- The clinical manifestation is variable between individuals, although children are usually more symptomatic than adults.
- Commonly affected sites include the finger and toe webs, wrists, genitalia, axillae, umbilicus, and breast areolae. In infants, involvement of the palms and soles is common, and the head and neck region can also be involved.
- Patients present with progressive, severe itch, more pronounced at night, occurring at the same time as the eruption, which manifests as erythematous papules and nodules with excoriations, secondary eczematous, or impetiginous changes. Rarely, vesicles or bullous lesions may occur.
- Burrows may also be seen, especially in the finger webs and wrists. Dermoscopy may aid in identifying these burrows. The typical burrow is a serpiginous tract that measures 1 cm in length.

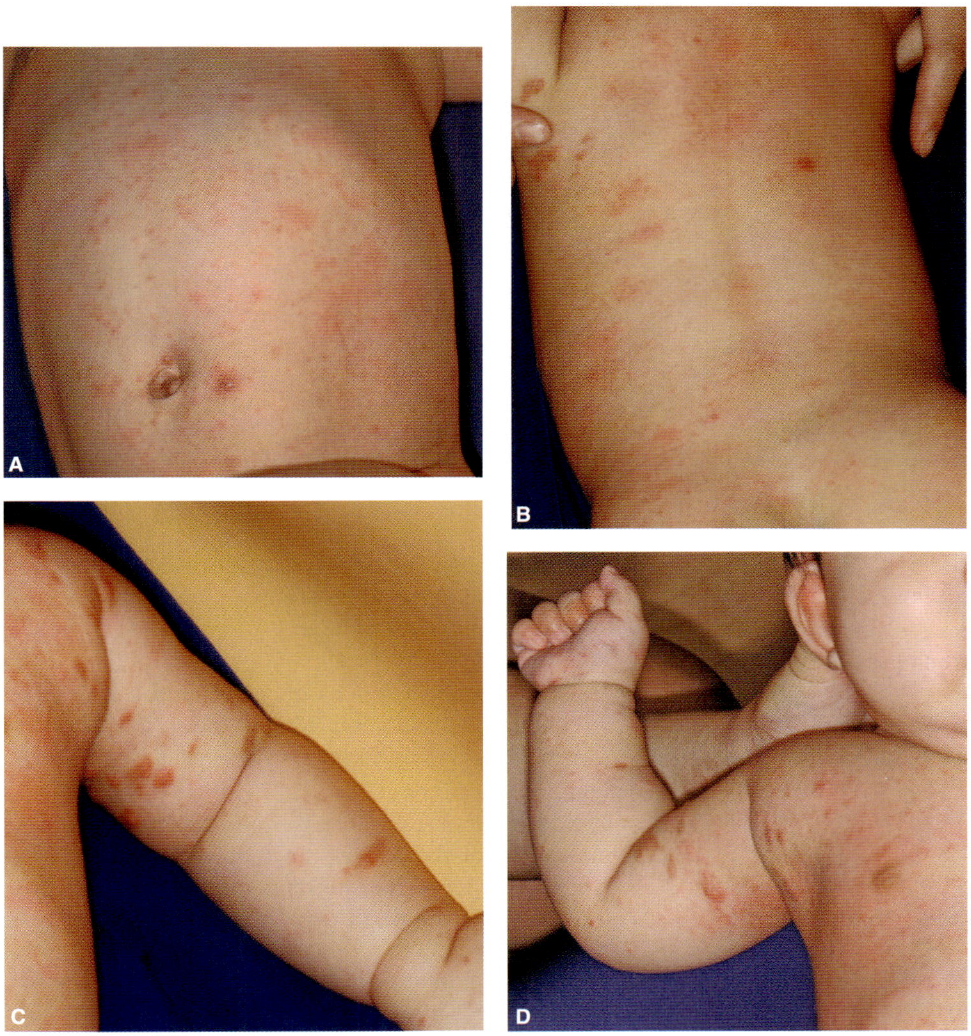

FIGURE 6-120A–120D. Scabies in a Chinese infant presenting with multiple erythematous-to-brown, pruritic papules and nodules with secondary urticaria.

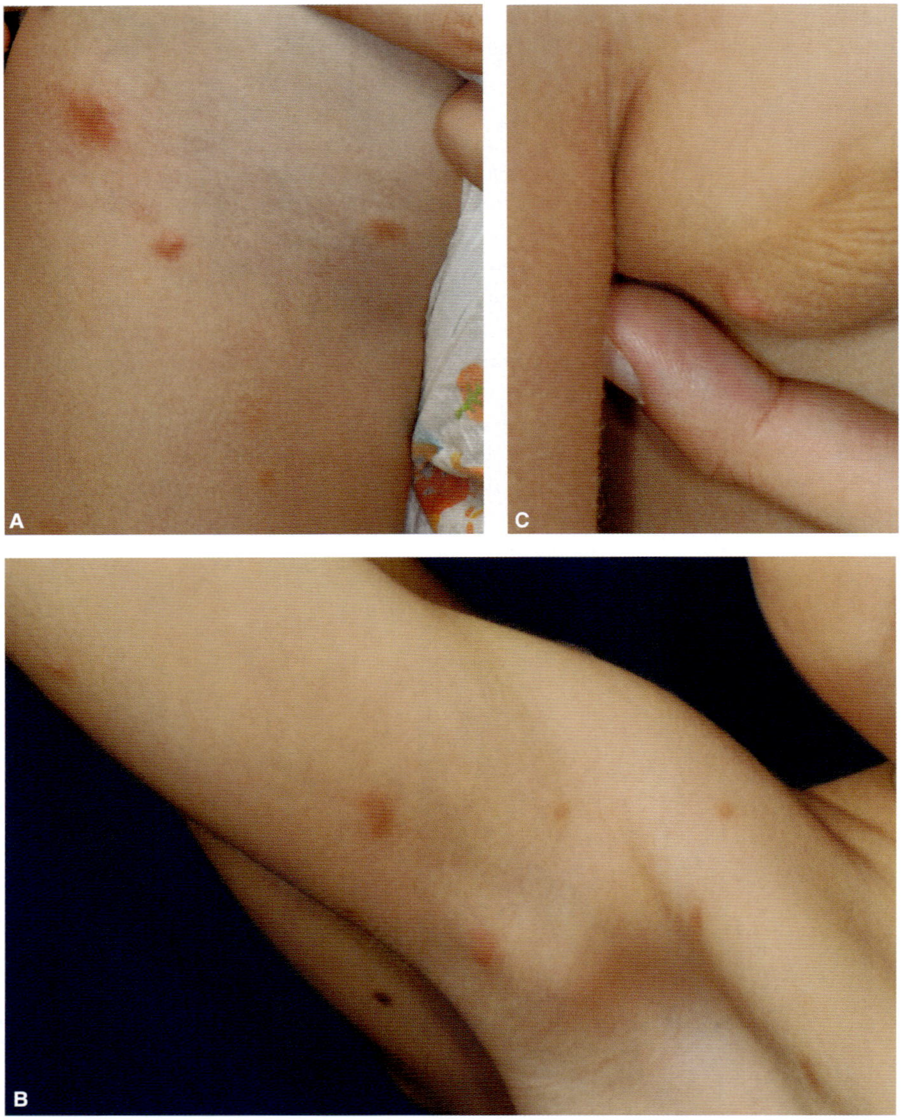

FIGURE 6-121A–121C. Multiple pruritic, red-brown papules on the thigh, axilla, and scrotum of a Chinese toddler with scabies.

Differential Diagnoses

- Atopic dermatitis (AD) or other eczemas
  - Eczematous changes may be seen secondary to scabies, especially in patients with a strong personal or family history of atopy.
  - AD may also be a differential diagnosis of scabietic eruptions. However, the lesions of AD occur at characteristic sites, such as the neck and flexural areas, and often appear as patches and plaques with scaly and oozy surface changes.
  - Prurigo nodularis often presents with nodules, but the lesions are more long-standing, and distribution is usually on exposed sites of the skin.
- Papular urticaria or insect bite reactions
  - Papular urticaria represents a hypersensitivity reaction to insect bites, such as mosquitoes or sandflies.
  - Symptoms occur more acutely over days, compared to scabies, and lesions are characterized by itchy clusters of red papules and wheals with occasional blisters. The lesions usually occur on exposed sites of the skin, such as the arms, legs, and face.
- Infantile acropustulosis
  - Vesiculopustular lesions on palms and soles can be confused with infantile acropustulosis, and the presence of larger blisters may suggest bullous disorders.

Investigations & Treatment

- The diagnosis of scabies can be confirmed by microscopic illustration of the scabies mites or eggs. Although the specificity is 100%, the sensitivity may be low and dependent on the technique of the skin scraping. Scraping can be done with a number 15 scalpel and facilitated by application of small amount of saline or mineral oil on the area to be sampled. Scrapings from the ends of burrows have the highest yield.
- A quantitative polymerase chain reaction (PCR) assay detecting the *cytochrome c oxidase subunit 1* (*cox1*) gene

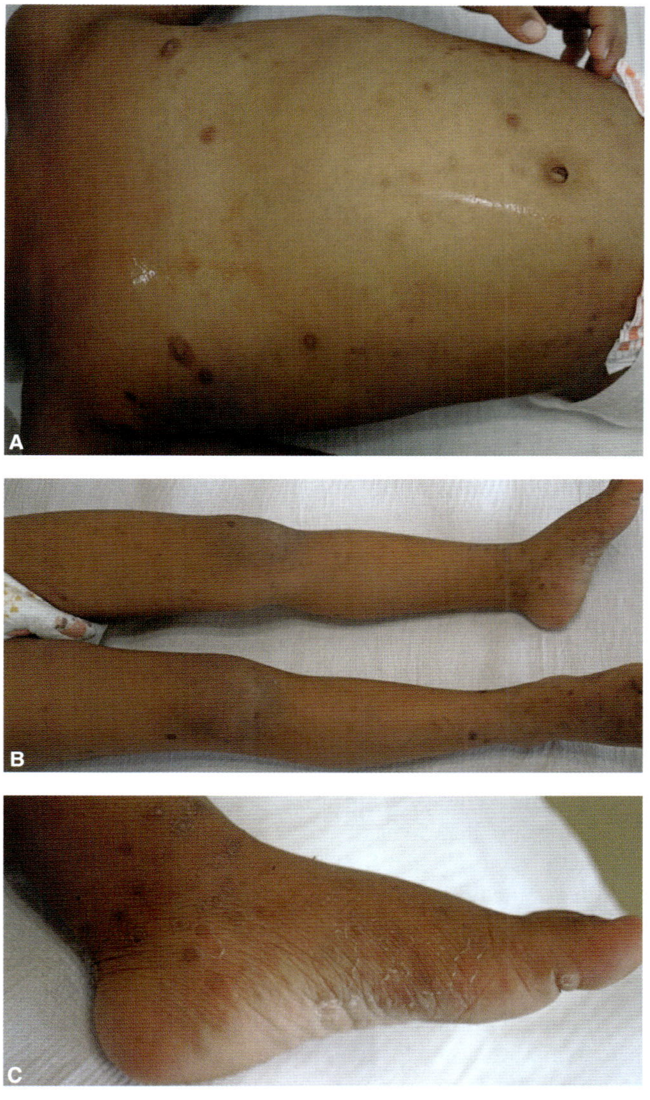

FIGURE 6-122A–122C. A young Malay child with scabies with multiple, excoriated, hyperpigmented, slightly scaly papules on the trunk, limbs, and feet.

of *S. scabiei* from skin scrapings has been shown to have good sensitivity and specificity.

- Treatment involves elimination of mites, alleviation of symptoms, and treatment of secondary infections if present.
- Topical scabicides such as malathion, permethrin, lindane, sulfur, and crotamiton may be used to treat scabies. Their availability depends on approval by each country's drug authorities. Examples of treatment regimens are found in the table below.
- Oral ivermectin is an antihelminthic that has proven efficacy for the treatment of human scabies.
- Oral or topical antibiotics may be required for treatment of secondary bacterial infection of the scabietic lesions.
- After completing treatment with anti-scabietic medications, topical corticosteroids, moisturizers, and oral antihistamines can be prescribed for treatment of post-scabietic itch. These may be required for weeks to months after treatment.

Pearls & Practical Tips

- It is imperative to treat all other household contacts at the same time, as well as the disinfestation of fomites such as bed linens, and car seat coverings, by warm washing. Recurrences are common if contacts are not treated appropriately.
- The symptoms of scabies may persist for up to several weeks or months after the eradication of the mites, and this may be prolonged in patients with atopic dermatitis.
- The reappearance of burrows is an indication of active reinfestation, and patients as well as household contacts should be retreated.

Bibliography

1. Bae M, Kim JY, Jung J, Cha HH, Jeon N-Y, Lee H-J, et al. Diagnostic value of the molecular detection of Sarcoptes scabiei from a skin scraping in patients with suspected scabies. PLoS Negl Trop Dis 2020;14(4):e0008229.

Treatment guidelines for scabies.

Medication	Dose/application	Frequency	Comments
Malathion	1 application, leave on for 24 hours	2 applications, 1 week apart	• Safe for >1 year of age • Apply to all skin surfaces from neck down
Permethrin	1 application, leave on for 8 hours	2 applications, 1 week apart	• Safe for use at all ages • For <1 year of age, apply to all skin surfaces including scalp, face, and neck • For >1 year of age, apply from neck down
Ivermectin (oral)	15–24 kg: 3 mg 25–35 kg: 6 mg 36–50 kg: 9 mg 51–65 kg: 12 mg 66–79 kg: 15 mg ≥80 kg: 200 mcg/kg single dose, repeat dose in 7 days	Single dose, repeat dose in 7 days	Limited literature available on the safety of ivermectin in children less than 5 years of age and less than 15 kg

PEDICULOSIS/LICE INFESTATIONS

Pediculosis infestation in humans is a significant health concern, as it affects children and adolescents worldwide in all communities. It is spread by close contact with an affected person. There are three types of lice infestation: pediculosis capitis (head louse), pediculosis corporis (body louse), and pediculosis pubis (crab or pubic louse). Pediculosis capitis is the most common louse infestation seen in children and adolescents.

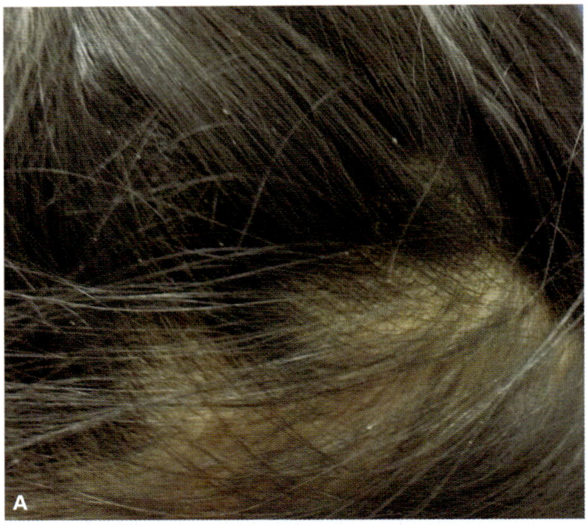

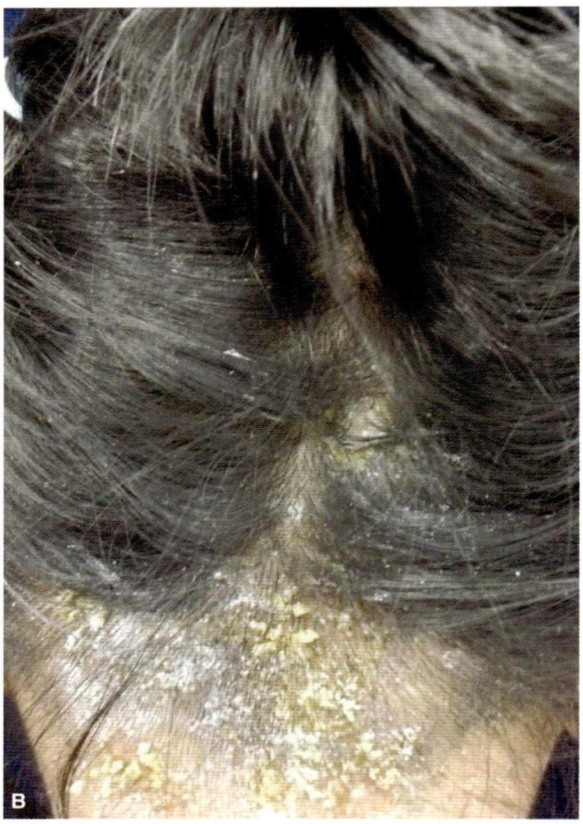

FIGURE 6-123A & 123B. Head lice can be seen by the naked eye on this Filipino girl with pediculosis capitis. There are secondary eczematous lesions on the nape.

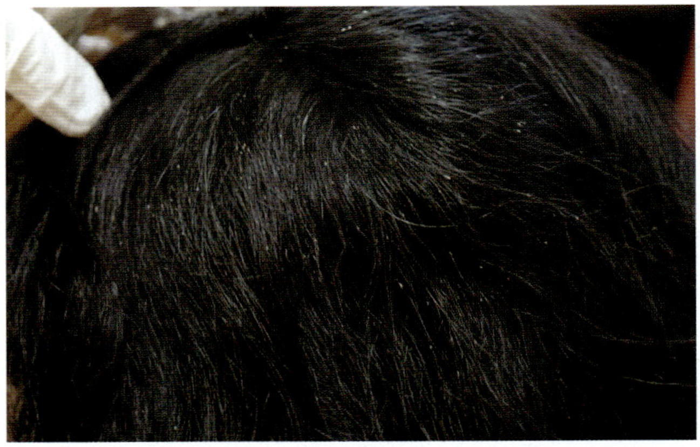

FIGURE 6-124. Pediculosis capitis presenting with white nodes on hair shafts. There is usually intense itching of the scalp.

Clinical Features

- In children and adolescents, the scalp is the most commonly affected body part.
- The patient is initially asymptomatic until 2 to 6 weeks after infestation, when sensitization occurs.
- Pruritus can be severe, and occurs due to hypersensitivity reaction to louse antigens injected either from the louse saliva or fecal matter onto the skin. There can be accompanying lymphadenopathy.
- Persistent itching may give rise to excoriations, papules, scaling, and hemorrhagic crusts on the scalp. Eczematous reactions with lichenification can occur on the nape and sides of the neck.
- Lice may be seen along hair shafts, which are better visualized using a dermatoscope.
- Nits are seen firmly attached to the hair shaft and are most commonly found at the occipital and temporal regions. Nits found closer to the scalp are more commonly viable, whereas nits found on the distal hair parts represent empty or nonviable egg cases.

Differential Diagnoses

- Pityriasis capitis (dandruff)
  - Dandruff can be caused by scalp conditions such as scalp eczema, seborrheic dermatitis, and psoriasis.
  - Other areas of the skin should be examined for presence of these common dermatoses, such as flexures for

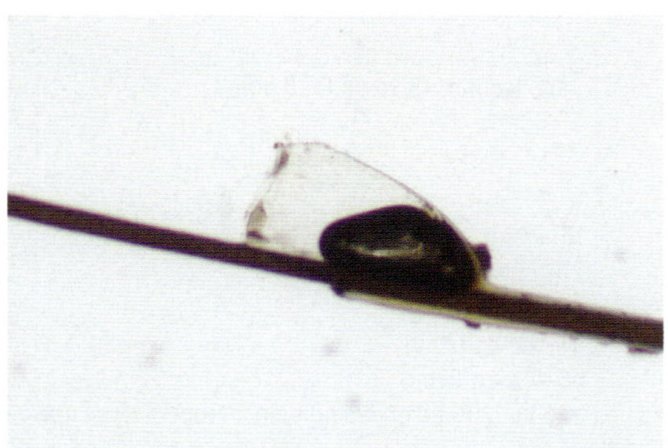

FIGURE 6-125. A hair louse nit as seen under the microscope.

atopic dermatitis, extensors and nails for psoriasis, and "T"-zone for seborrheic dermatitis.
  - It is also common to find eczematous lesions on the scalp, nape, and neck in patients with head lice.
- Hair casts
  - Hair casts, or pseudonits, are commonly found on the scalp of children and may be mistaken for hair lice.
  - They are postulated to result from failure of the inner root sheath to disintegrate before the hair emerges from the skin surface.
  - Unlike nits, hair casts can be easily dislodged from the hair shaft. Itch is also not prominent in these patients.
- White piedra
  - White piedra is caused by a fungus, *Trichosporon beigelii*.
  - It usually presents as numerous asymptomatic, discrete, soft nodules attached to the hair shaft.
  - Microscopic visualization of potassium hydroxide (KOH 10%) wet mounts of affected hairs may show the septate hyphae.

Investigations & Treatment

- Diagnosis is mainly by identifying the lice and nits by clinical examination and dermoscopy. The use of a fine-toothed comb is especially useful for the direct visualization of live head lice.
- Nits on direct microscopy appear as oval, translucent masses attached to the side of a hair shaft.
- Treatment is directed to the elimination of the adult lice and the mechanical removal of nits. This may be achieved by wet combing or hot hair treatment.[1] The hair is washed using an ordinary shampoo. A conditioner is then applied, and the hair is straightened and detangled using a wide-toothed comb. A fine-toothed "head lice detection" comb is then run though the hairs carefully. After each stroke, the comb is checked for lice, which are removed by wiping or rinsing the comb. The conditioner is rinsed out thereafter. This should be repeated every 2 days until no more lice are found.
- Topical therapies include malathion, permethrin, carbaryl, lindane, benzyl alcohol, ivermectin, and spinosad.
- Systemic treatment includes oral ivermectin, albendazole, levamisole, and cotrimoxazole.

Pearls & Practical Tips

- In eliminating live nits, application of petrolatum-based sulfur ointment on the hair and then covering it with a plastic shower cap for 8 to 12 hours is helpful.
- Apart from the use of conditioners, the application of mineral oil or essential oils can aid in the mechanical removal of nits.
- It is important to treat all household and school contacts of patients with head lice to prevent reinfestation.

Reference

1. Hill N, Moor G, Cameron MM, et al. Single blind, randomised, comparative study of the Bug Buster kit and over the counter pediculicide treatments against head lice in the United Kingdom. BMJ 2005;331(7513):384-7.

ARTHROPOD BITES AND PAPULAR URTICARIA

Arthropod bites and papular urticaria are very common in children and adolescents. Although mostly an acute reaction, symptoms can be chronic and persistent, especially in younger children. Both conditions are postulated to be a hypersensitivity reaction to the bites of various arthropods, with the most common being mosquitoes, sand flies, fleas, and bedbugs. Papular urticaria is thought to be caused by a hematogenously disseminated antigen deposited by an arthropod bite in a patient who is sensitive. The lesions can occur away from the actual bites.

Clinical Features

- Arthropod bites and papular urticaria can occur in all age groups, although it is far more common in children compared to adults, especially papular urticaria.
- Lesions appear as urticated, indurated, erythematous-to-violaceous papules or nodules, ranging from 0.2 to 2.5 cm in diameter. A central punctum or scab is often present. Itch is variable but can be severe.

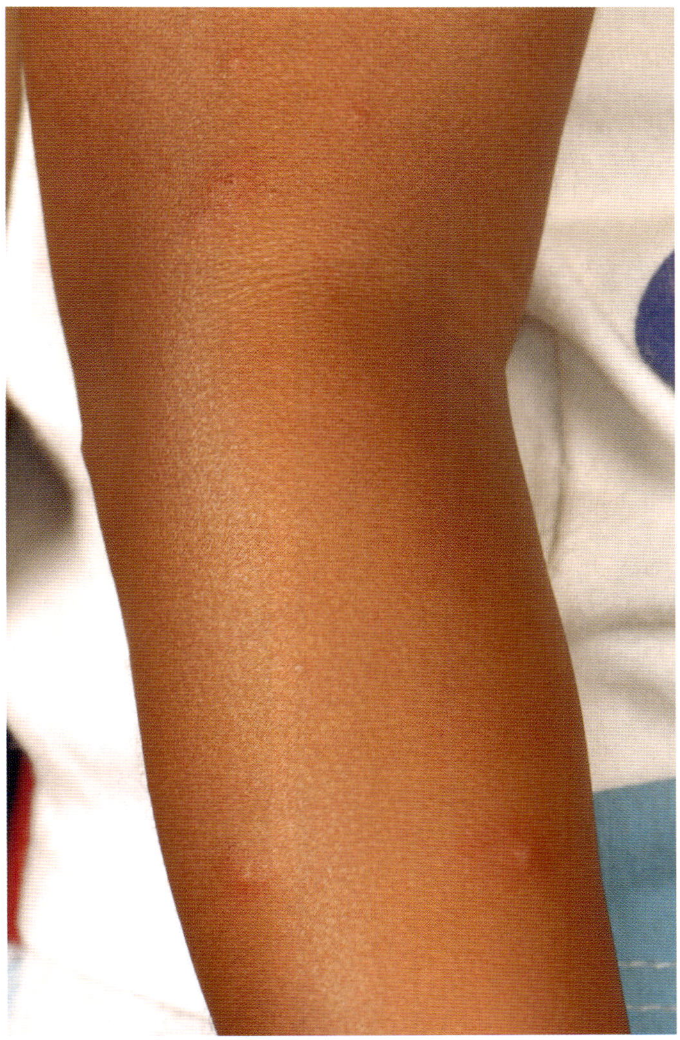

FIGURE 6-126. Mosquito bites on the arms of a young Malay child, presenting with pruritic, erythematous, indurated wheals with central punctum.

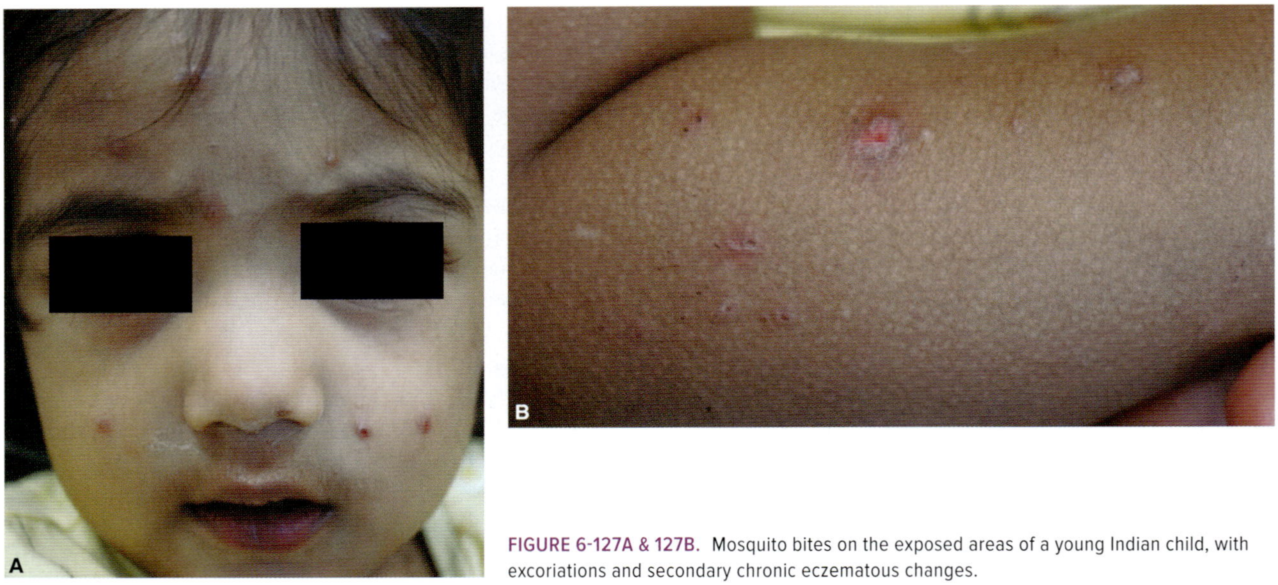

FIGURE 6-127A & 127B. Mosquito bites on the exposed areas of a young Indian child, with excoriations and secondary chronic eczematous changes.

- Blisters are also common, either over normal skin or with underlying erythema. Cellulitis can occur, especially after scratching.
- Lesions may occur singly or more often, in crops or clusters, and often occur on the uncovered areas of the skin, especially the lower legs, arms, and face. Lesions along the waistline are also fairly common.
- Lesions usually resolve after a few days or weeks, often with post-inflammatory hyper- or hypopigmentation.

Differential Diagnosis

- Urticaria
  - This is another common condition in children. Lesions appear as larger wheals compared to arthropod bites, with each wheal lasting for less than 24 to 48 hours.

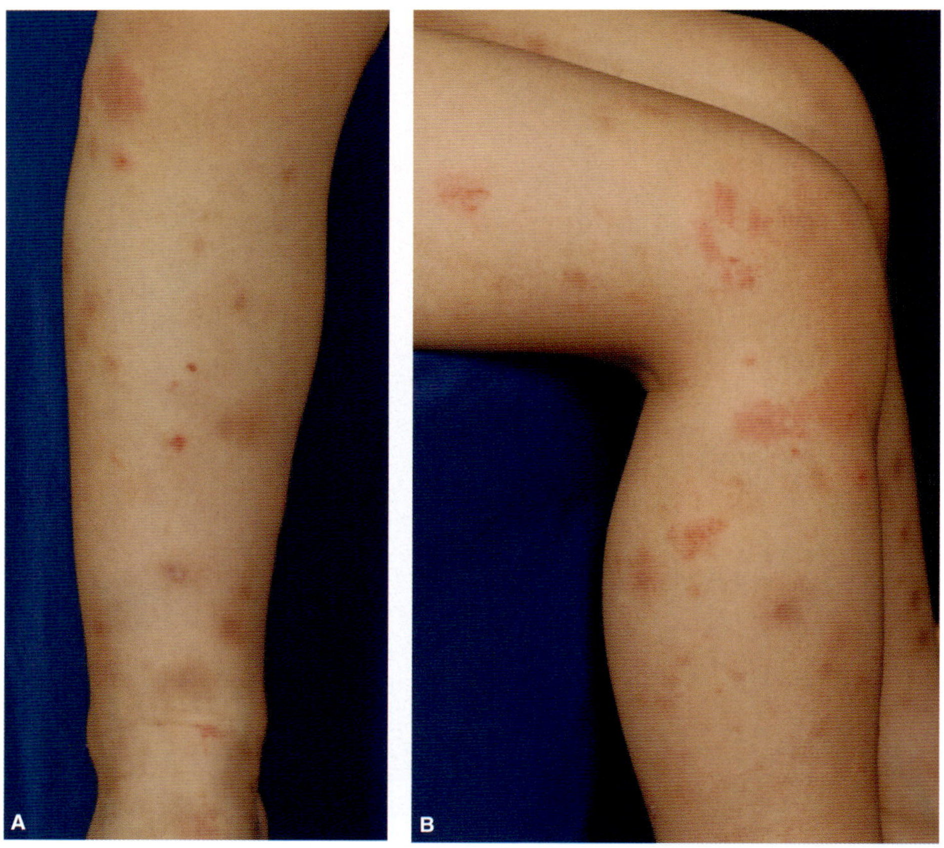

FIGURE 6-128A & 128B. Classical presentation of insect bite reactions in a Chinese girl, with erythematous papules, wheals, and hyperpigmented macules on the exposed sites of the legs.

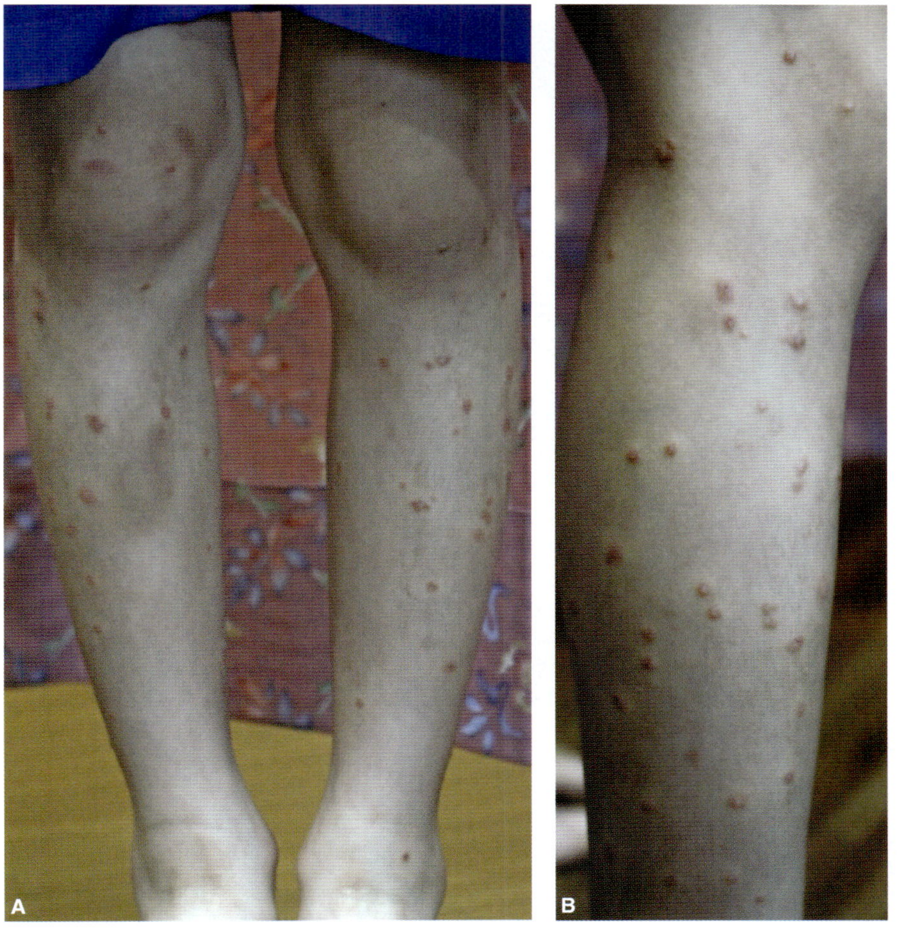

FIGURE 6-129A & 129B. Extensive chronic sandfly bites on the legs of a Chinese boy, presenting as pruritic, red to hyperpigmented, firm papules.

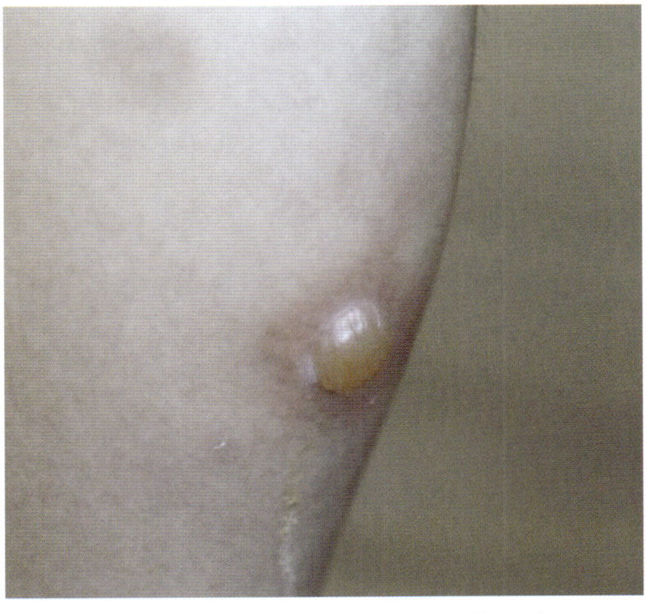

FIGURE 6-130. Bullous insect bite reaction on the calf of a Chinese boy.

- Scabies
  - The lesions of scabies are also extremely pruritic and appear papular but scabies often also affects covered sites, such as the genitalia, axillae, and trunk. The finger and toe webs are also often affected, and burrows may be present.
- Atopic dermatitis (AD)
  - Arthropod bites are often eczematized in AD patients and can trigger lesions of AD at more classical sites, such as the flexures.
  - Patients with AD are also more prone to arthropod bite reactions.
- Pityriasis lichenoides
  - Lesions of pityriasis lichenoides can present with small papular lesions with central scabbing. However, it is less itchy and more extensive than arthropod bites or papular urticaria, often affecting the trunk in addition to the limbs.
- Panniculitis
  - Panniculitis of various causes can also present with nodular lesions, especially over the legs. Lesions are usually painful rather than itchy, and last longer than arthropod bite reactions.

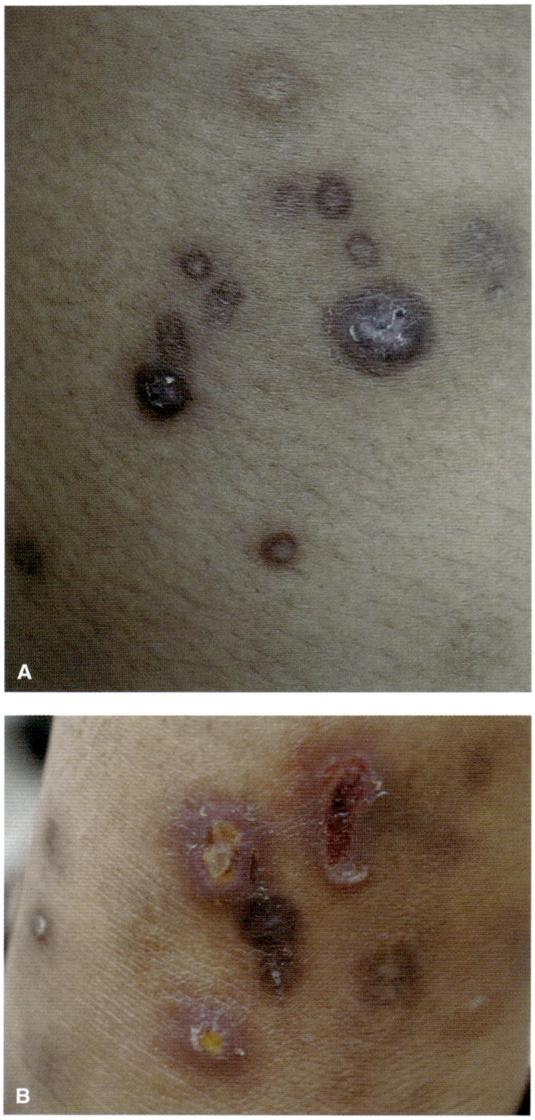

FIGURE 6-131A & 131B. Persistent arthropod bite reaction in a darker-skinned Malay girl, with dyspigmentation and formation of prurigo nodules.

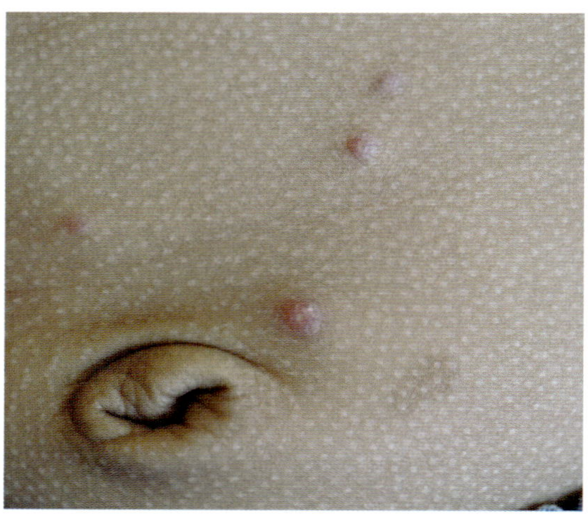

FIGURE 6-132. Papular urticaria on the abdomen of a Chinese child, presenting as itchy erythematous papules in a "linear" distribution.

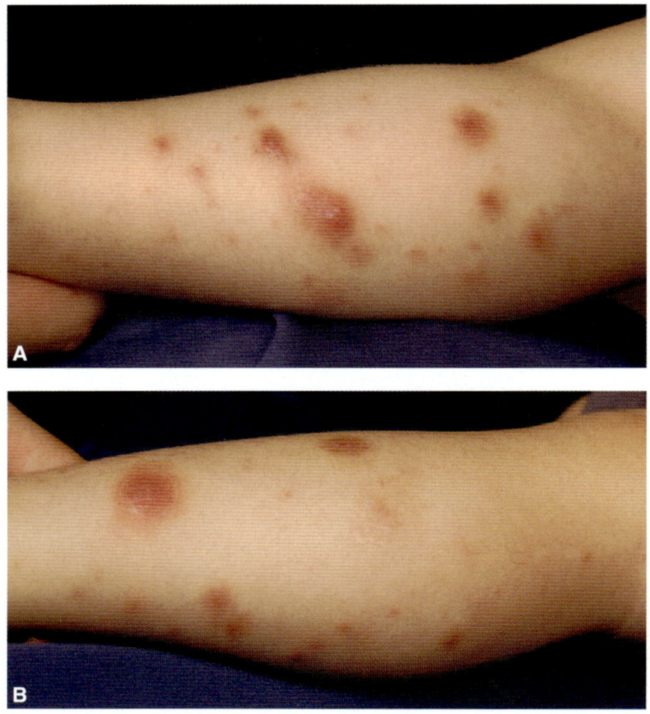

FIGURE 6-133A & 133B. Exaggerated insect bite reactions with papular urticaria on the lower limbs of a Chinese boy, with secondary infection and early abscess formation.

Investigations & Treatment

- Arthropod bites and papular urticaria are usually diagnosed clinically. A punch biopsy may be required in atypical cases.
- Histology is classical, with a superficial and deep perivascular and peri-adnexal mixed inflammatory infiltrate that includes eosinophils.
- Treatment of arthropod bites and papular urticaria is with potent topical corticosteroids and oral antihistamines. Treatment is continued until the lesions have resolved. If there is secondary infection, systemic antibiotics may be required.

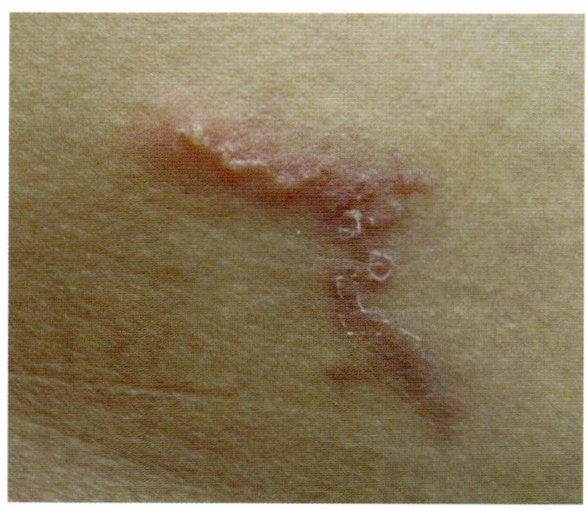

FIGURE 6-134. Cutaneous larva migrans, caused by larvae of hookworm, presenting as a serpiginous, erythematous track.

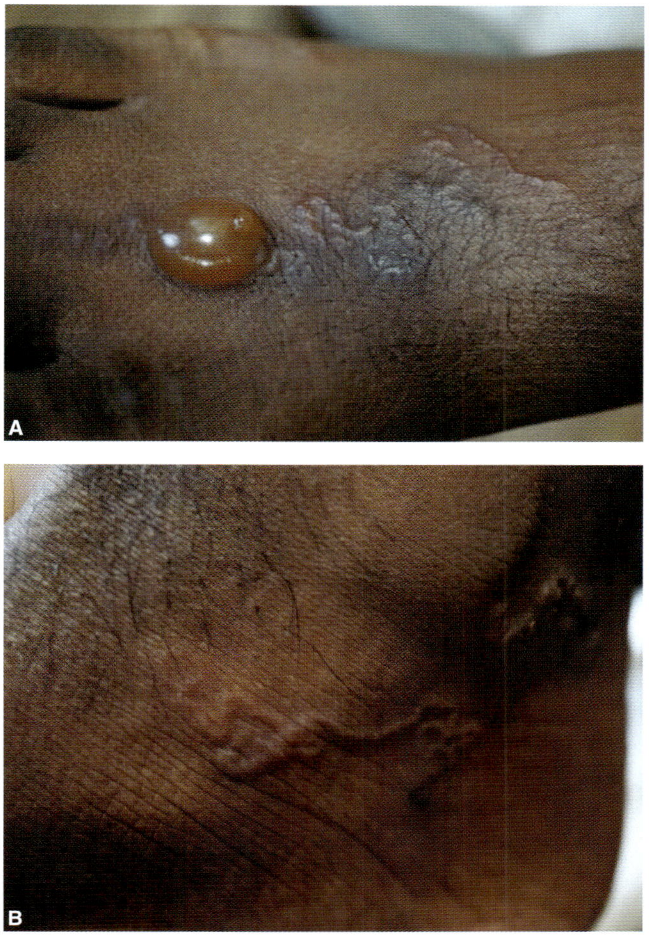

FIGURE 6-135A & 135B. Cutaneous larva migrans occurring in an Indian boy as a serpiginous track with blister formation.

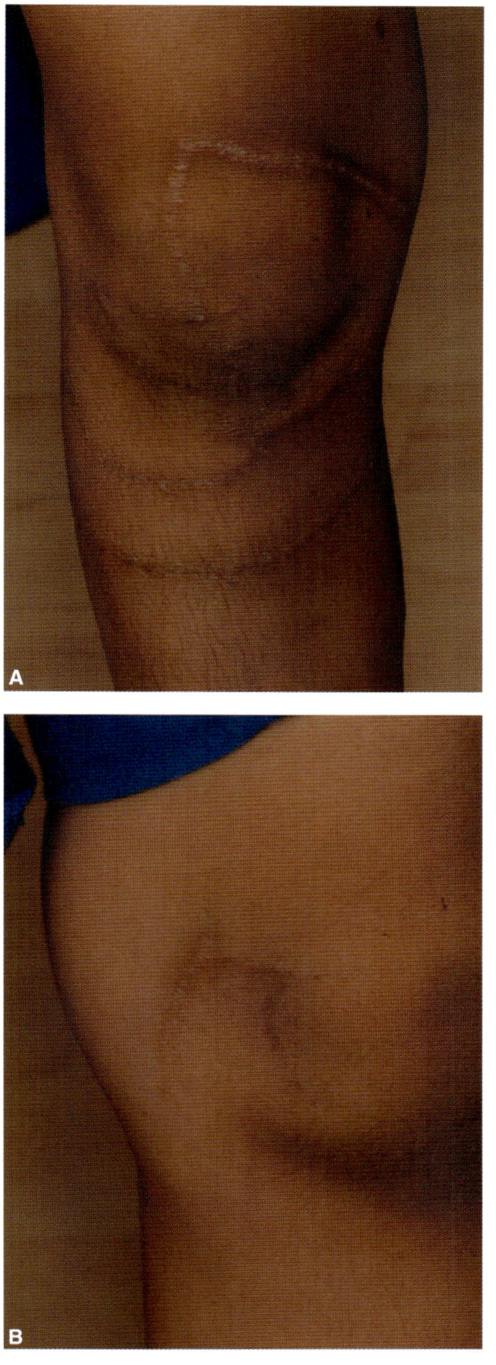

FIGURE 6-136A & 136B. Classical presentation of reaction to jellyfish sting on the legs of an Indian boy who went swimming in the sea. There are bizarre linear, scaly, hyperpigmented plaques over the exposed sites.

- Prevention of further arthropod bites is essential to prevent recurrence, especially in patients with papular urticaria. Preventive measures include avoiding outdoor activities at dawn and dusk, use of insect repellants and mosquito "patches," and use of covering clothing, including long pants and long-sleeved shirts, socks, and closed shoes.
- Hyperpigmentation of previous lesions will usually fade over months to years, but using sunscreen on a regular daily basis can help them go away faster.

Pearls & Practical Tips

- Parents and caregivers often do not give a history of arthropod bites. Careful history taking will often reveal the source of the arthropod bites, such as a visit to a park or beach. Convincing caregivers of the causative etiology is often the most difficult part of management.
- Lesions caused by flying insects, such as mosquitoes and sandflies, often appear on exposed sites, such as the lower legs, arms, and face. Lesions caused by crawling insects, such as bedbugs, often occur over covered sites, such as the trunk.
- Sandfly bites can last for many months compared to mosquito bites, which usually last for 1 to 2 weeks.
- The classically described "breakfast, lunch, and dinner" distribution is typical of papular urticaria (Figure 6-132).

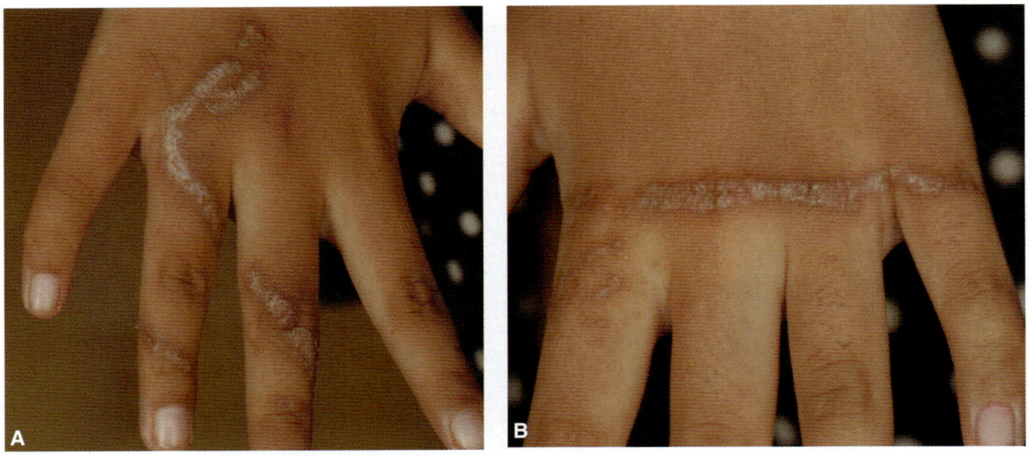

FIGURE 6-137A & 137B. Reaction to jellyfish sting in an Indian girl who went swimming in the sea. There are hyperpigmented, scaly, linear plaques on both hands.

7

Disorders of Pigmentation

PITYRIASIS ALBA

Pityriasis alba is a common skin disorder in Asian children and is thought to represent a mild form of dermatitis presenting with hypopigmentation. There is usually a background history of atopy in the patient or a family history of atopy, especially atopic dermatitis.

Clinical Features

- Pityriasis alba occurs most commonly in childhood but may also occur in adolescence. It affects both males and females equally.
- Lesions are usually not or only mildly itchy.
- On examination, there are poorly demarcated, hypopigmented, sometimes slightly scaly patches on both cheeks and other areas of the face. There may be mild patchy erythema.
- Other areas of the skin may exhibit classical lesions of atopic dermatitis or other eczemas.

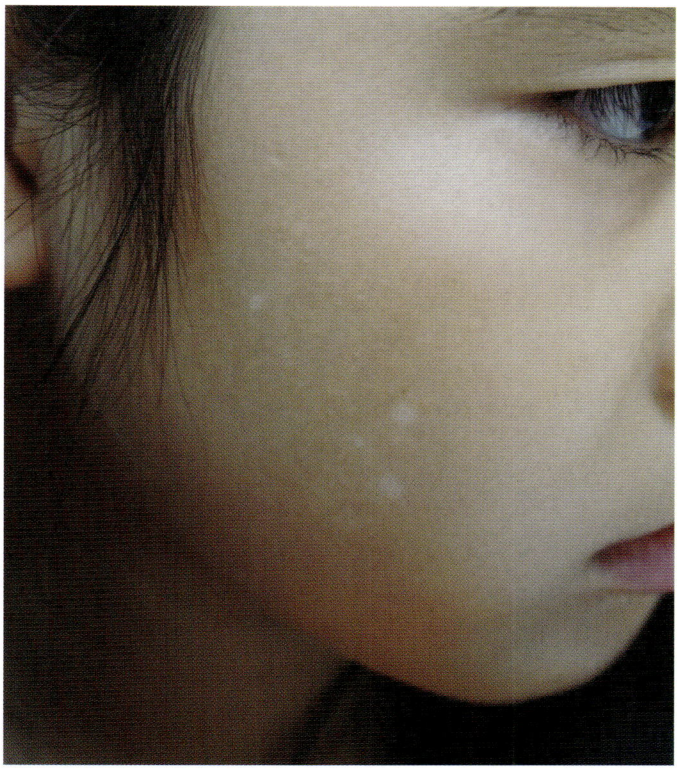

FIGURE 7-1. Pityriasis alba on the cheek of a Chinese girl, presenting with more well-demarcated, small, hypopigmented macules.

Differential Diagnoses

- Tinea versicolor
  - This usually presents in older children, adolescents, and adults, and affects primarily the upper trunk and back but may spread to the face and upper arms. Lesions appear more demarcated than in pityriasis alba.
  - In addition to hypopigmented lesions, hyperpigmented or pink lesions may also be present.
- Vitiligo
  - Vitiligo is less common than pityriasis alba. Lesions are depigmented rather than hypopigmented. No scaling is seen, and the borders are more demarcated than in pityriasis alba.
  - Lesions of vitiligo fluoresce brightly with a Wood's lamp, unlike pityriasis alba.
- Mycosis fungoides (MF)
  - MF is a primary cutaneous T-cell lymphoma and is rare in children. However, the hypopigmented form of MF is more common in Asian children and has a predilection for sun-covered sites, such as the buttocks. Facial involvement can occur in more extensive disease.
- Nevus depigmentosus
  - This usually presents in the first 2 years of life, and is unilateral and non-symmetrical. The borders are better demarcated compared to pityriasis alba, and lesions are non-progressive.

Investigations & Treatment

- No investigations are usually required for diagnosis. Fungal microscopy may sometimes be required to exclude tinea versicolor.
- Pityriasis alba can be treated conservatively, especially if asymptomatic and the child and parents are not bothered cosmetically.
- If required, it can be treated with application of light moisturizers, topical low-potency corticosteroids (e.g., hydrocortisone 1% cream or desonide 0.05% cream), or topical calcineurin inhibitors (e.g., pimecrolimus 1% cream or tacrolimus 0.03% ointment) until repigmentation is achieved.
- Application of sunscreens with at least SPF 30 when under the sun, especially when swimming, is recommended to prevent worsening or recurrence.

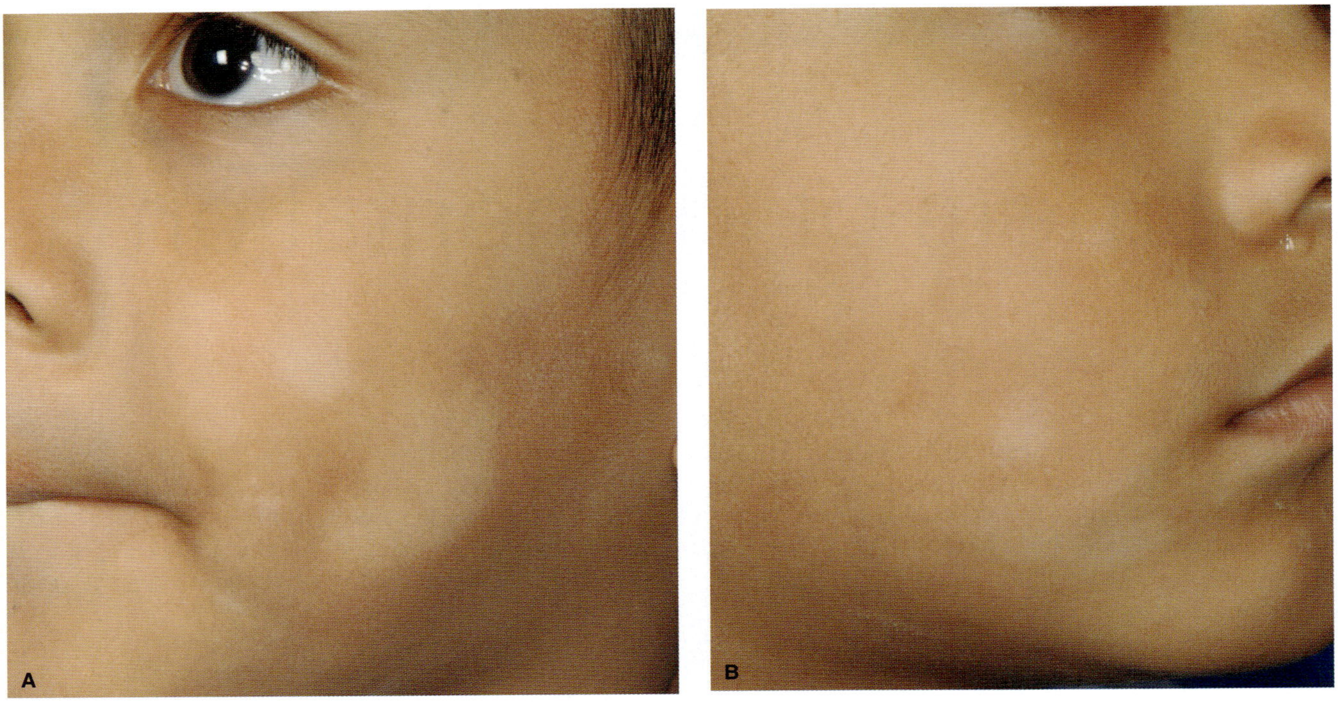

FIGURE 7-2A & 2B. Pityriasis alba on the cheeks of a Malay boy, presenting with patchy hypopigmentation.

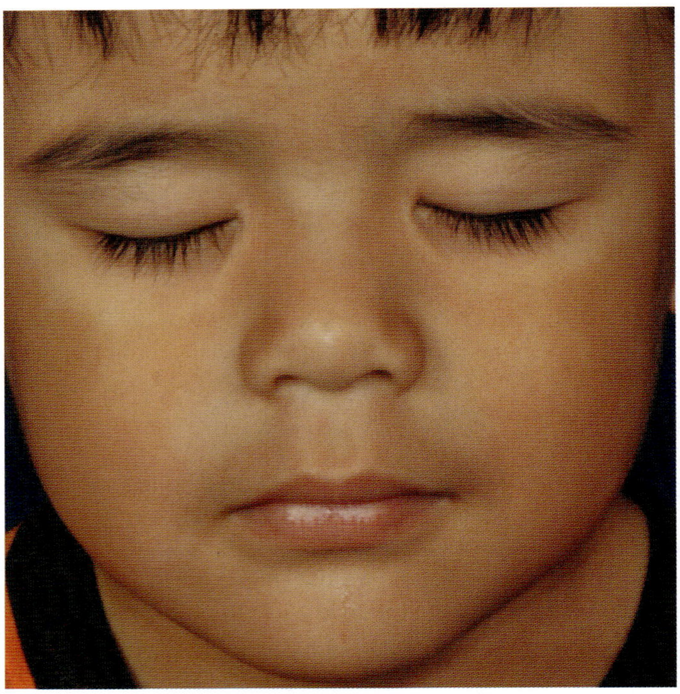

FIGURE 7-3. Pityriasis alba on the cheeks and perinasal area of a young Malay boy. The hypopigmentation in the periorbital region is secondary to prolonged wearing of swim goggles while swimming in the day.

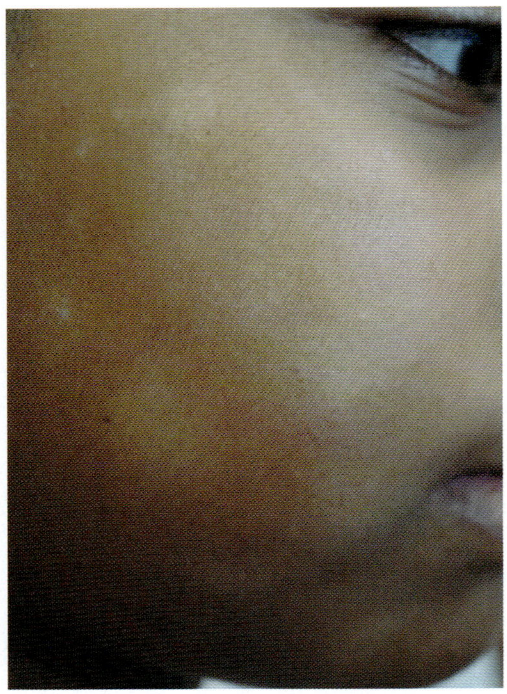

FIGURE 7-4. Pityriasis alba on the cheeks of an Indian boy, with patchy, slightly scaly, hypopigmentation.

Pearls & Practical Tips

- A recent history of increased sun exposure such as regular swimming lessons often precedes the onset of pityriasis alba.
- If the patient has concurrent atopic dermatitis, hypopigmented patches may also be apparent on other sites of the body. This is usually termed post-inflammatory hypopigmentation.
- Patients with pityriasis alba are often mistakenly treated for fungal infection.
- It is important to examine all skin surfaces in patients presenting with pityriasis alba to exclude MF. In doubtful cases, skin biopsies should be performed from sun-covered sites.

VITILIGO

Vitiligo has a worldwide prevalence of 0.5% to 2%, with studies showing no difference between pediatric and adult populations. Almost half of cases of vitiligo begin before the age of 20 years, and one-quarter occur before the age of 10 years. Compared to adult-onset vitiligo, vitiligo in children exhibits certain different clinical characteristics.

Clinical Features

- Vitiligo presents with depigmented macules and patches, either in a generalized distribution (non-segmental vitiligo) or in a localized area (focal or segmental vitiligo).
- Non-segmental vitiligo is the most common subtype of vitiligo seen in children. Segmental vitiligo, although less common than the non-segmental variant, has a higher prevalence in children compared to adults.
- In children, the head and neck are the most common sites of onset of vitiligo. Other frequently affected areas are the perineum, buttocks, and perianal region.
- Depigmented skin patches may be accompanied by depigmented hair shafts (leukotrichia/poliosis). A distinct subtype, follicular vitiligo, occurs when the initial depigmentation affects mostly the hair with or without skin involvement.
- Koebnerization can occur in patients with vitiligo, with depigmentation appearing after friction or injury to the skin, as evidenced by the frequent involvement of the diaper area in toddlers.
- The halo phenomenon can occur around nevi in children with vitiligo, especially in patients with generalized vitiligo.
- Wood's lamp examination reveals fluorescence and accentuation of the depigmented macules and patches.
- Repigmentation of vitiligo occurs in several well-described patterns, including perifollicular, diffuse, marginal, mixed, and medium spotted.
- A positive family history of vitiligo and autoimmune disease occurs more frequently in children with vitiligo. There is an increased risk of other autoimmune disease occurring in children with vitiligo.
- Childhood vitiligo can be associated with significant psychological morbidity and impairment of quality of life in both the patient and family.

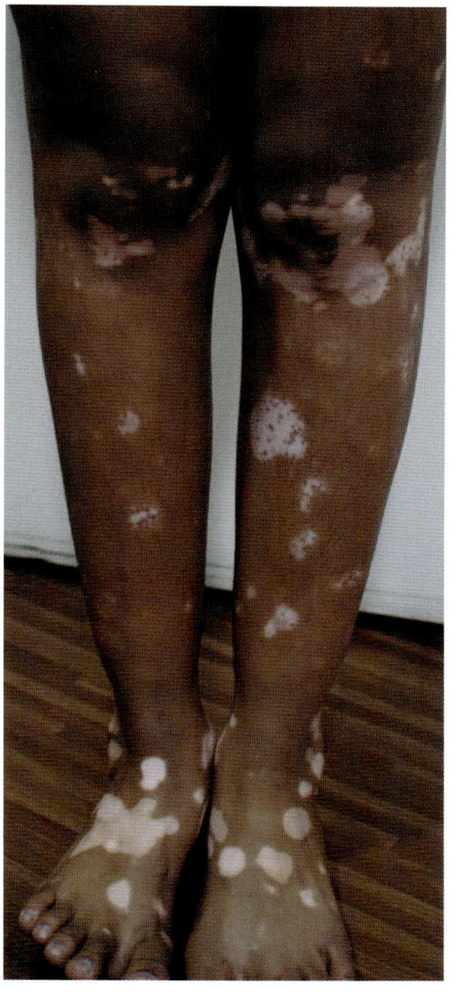

FIGURE 7-5. Non-segmental vitiligo on the lower limbs of a Malay child, presenting with multiple well-demarcated, depigmented patches. Perifollicular repigmentation is seen on some of the patches.

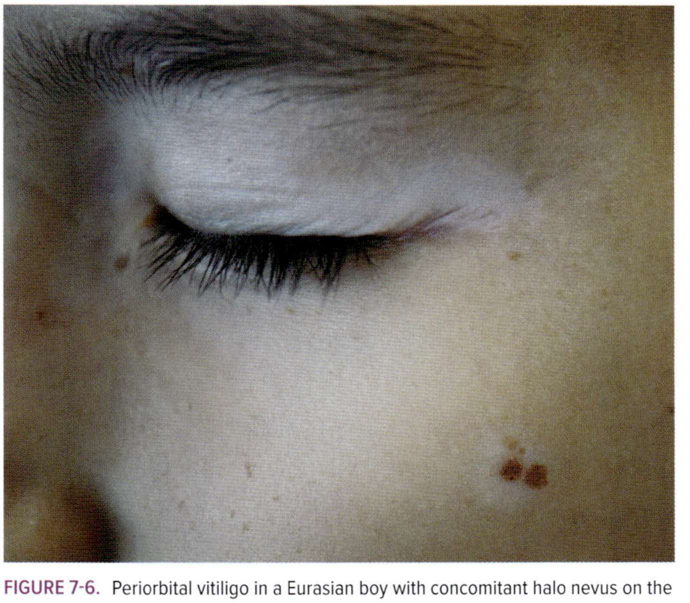

FIGURE 7-6. Periorbital vitiligo in a Eurasian boy with concomitant halo nevus on the left cheek. As the child is quite fair, the demarcation with normal skin is not as stark.

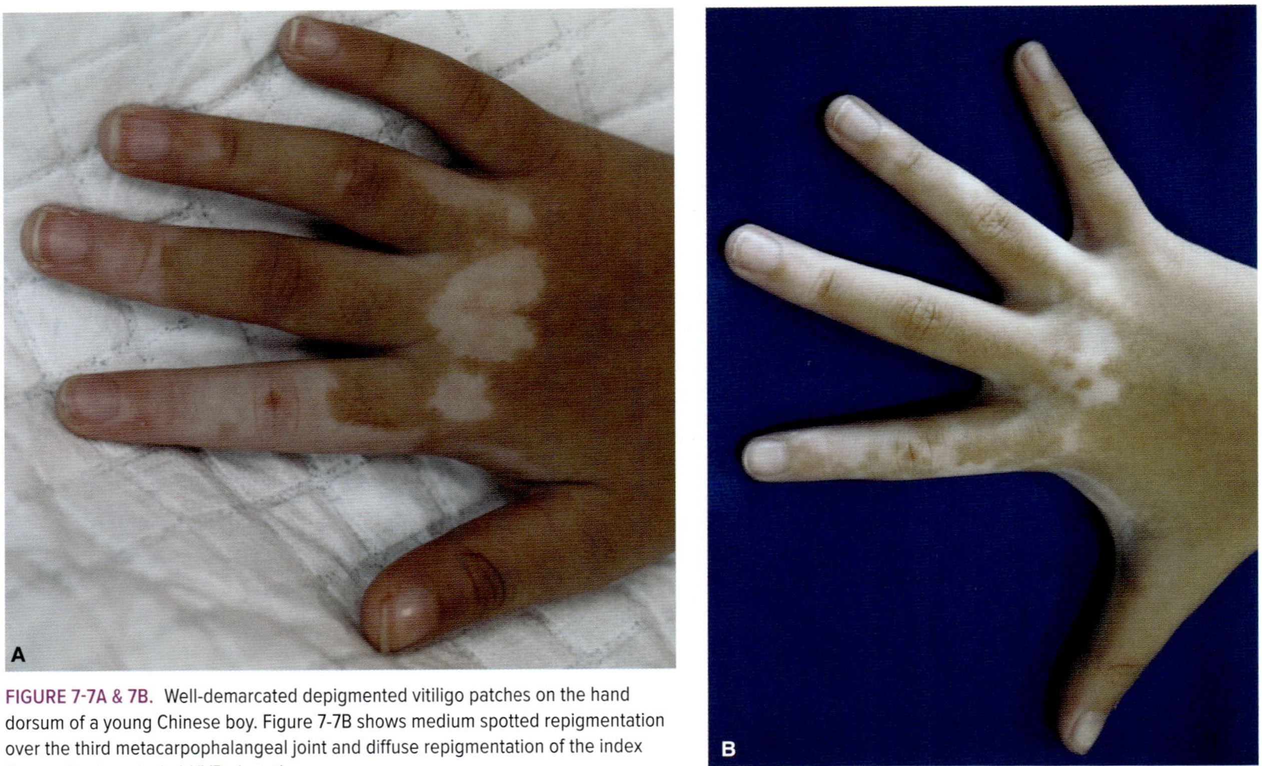

FIGURE 7-7A & 7B. Well-demarcated depigmented vitiligo patches on the hand dorsum of a young Chinese boy. Figure 7-7B shows medium spotted repigmentation over the third metacarpophalangeal joint and diffuse repigmentation of the index finger after targeted nbUVB phototherapy.

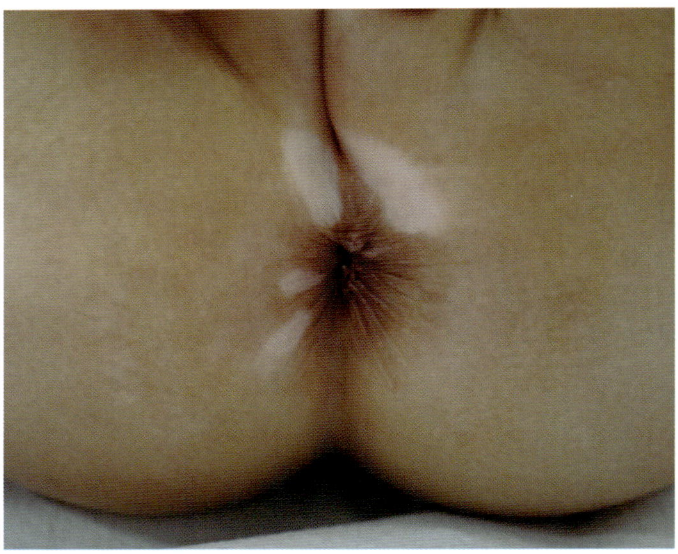

FIGURE 7-8. Perianal vitiligo in a 2-year-old Chinese girl.

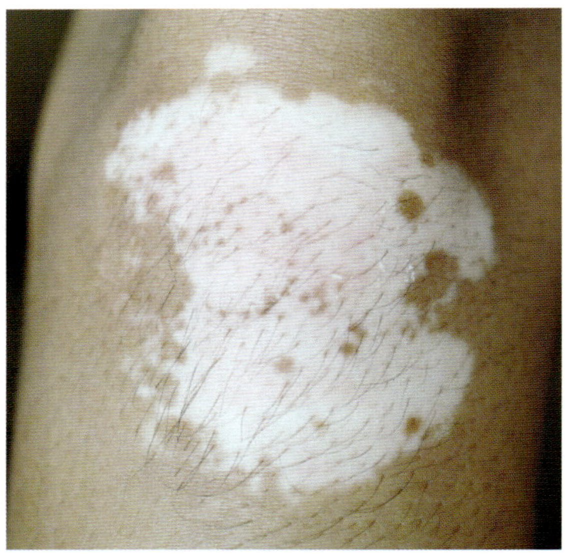

FIGURE 7-9. Mixed repigmentation (perifollicular and marginal) on the knee of a 7-year-old Sikh girl with non-segmental vitiligo.

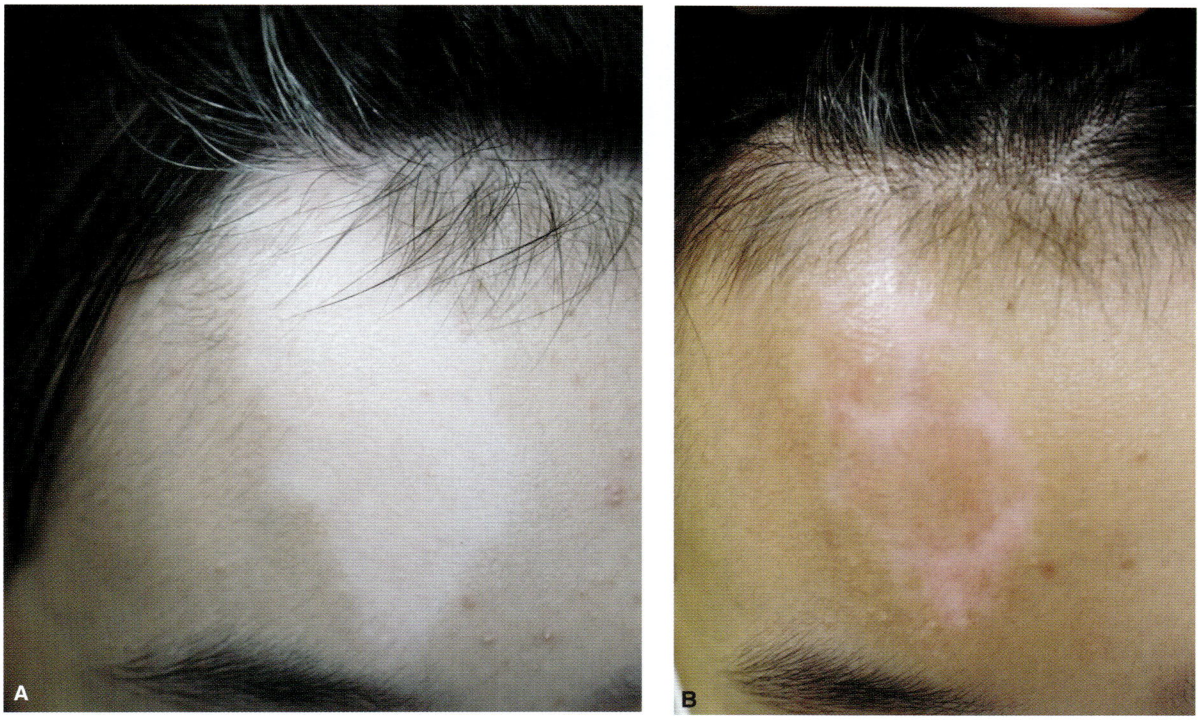

FIGURE 7-10A & 10B. Segmental vitiligo on the forehead with accompanying leukotrichia in a Chinese adolescent girl. Figure 7-10B shows excellent repigmentation after 6 months of targeted NBUVB phototherapy.

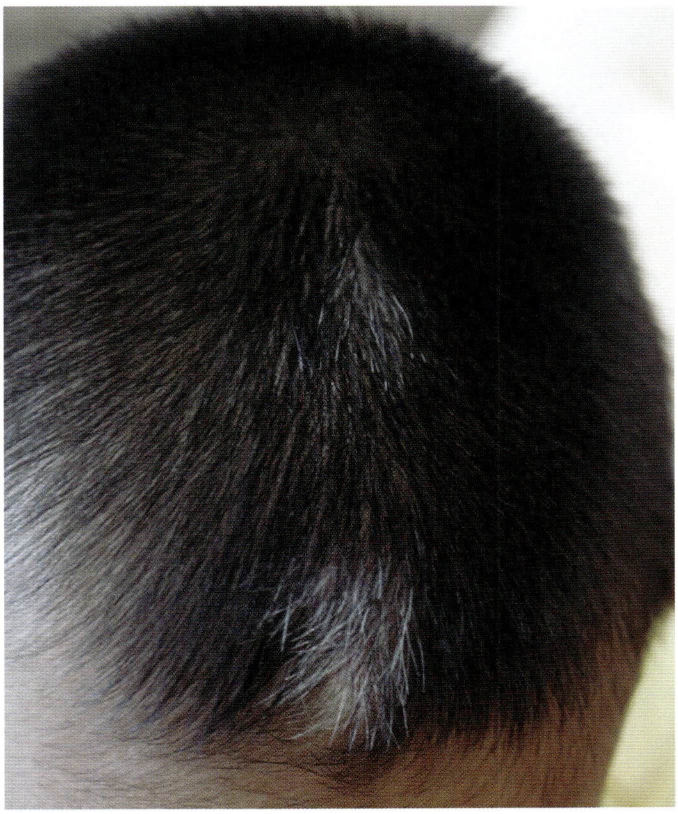

FIGURE 7-11. Patchy vitiligo on the scalp with accompanying leukotrichia in a young Chinese boy.

Differential Diagnoses

- Post-inflammatory hypopigmentation
  - Post-inflammatory pigmentation changes are transient. There is usually a history of preceding rash in the area of hypopigmentation. There is a lack of accentuation with Wood's lamp examination.
- Nevus depigmentosus
  - This occurs as a solitary lesion and appears more hypopigmented than depigmented. There is no change over time.
- Piebaldism
  - This is a rare, autosomal dominant condition, caused by mutations in the *KIT* or *SNAI2* genes. Patients typically present from birth or infancy with a white forelock and white patch on the forehead, with depigmented patches on other parts of the body, limbs, and face, usually following the midline.
  - Partial repigmentation may occur later in life with islands of normal or hyperpigmented skin appearing within the initial depigmented areas.
- Lichen sclerosus (LS)
  - This is an important differential diagnosis for vitiligo occurring in the genital area. LS presents with hypo- to depigmented patches typically on the genitalia and perineum, which may appear very similar to vitiligo.
  - Distinguishing features of LS include a shiny appearance, induration of active lesions, and symptoms of pain and itch.

Investigations & Treatment

- Management of vitiligo is threefold and involves halting the spread of depigmentation, inducing repigmentation, and maintaining the repigmentation.
- Topical corticosteroids and topical calcineurin inhibitors are used as first-line treatment. Topical vitamin D analogues may be considered for their steroid-sparing effects in chronic vitiligo.
- Phototherapy, surgical grafting, and cosmetic camouflage are other treatment options when first-line treatment has failed or is suboptimal.
- Pediatric patients with generalized vitiligo respond better to phototherapy than those with segmental vitiligo.
- A short course of systemic corticosteroids, or mini-pulse weekend therapy with systemic corticosteroids helps to stop the spread in rapidly progressive or worsening vitiligo.
- Oral antioxidants have been shown to be useful in limited studies. Topical or systemic Janus kinase (JAK) inhibitors have shown some promise in recent reports.

Pearls & Practical Tips

- Vitiligo patches in acral or bony areas exhibit lower rates of repigmentation compared to vitiligo of the face and trunk.
- Leukotrichia (whitening of the hair) can be seen in vitiligo. Depigmented areas with concomitant leukotrichia may be more resistant to treatment, as the reservoir of melanocytes and melanocyte precursors in the hair follicle has been affected.
- In a patient where the diagnosis of hypopigmented macules or patches is unclear, close follow-up is needed to observe for evolution into more typical depigmented patches of vitiligo.
- Vitiligo can be treated and should not be dismissed as a cosmetic condition in view of the significant psychological morbidity it is associated with.

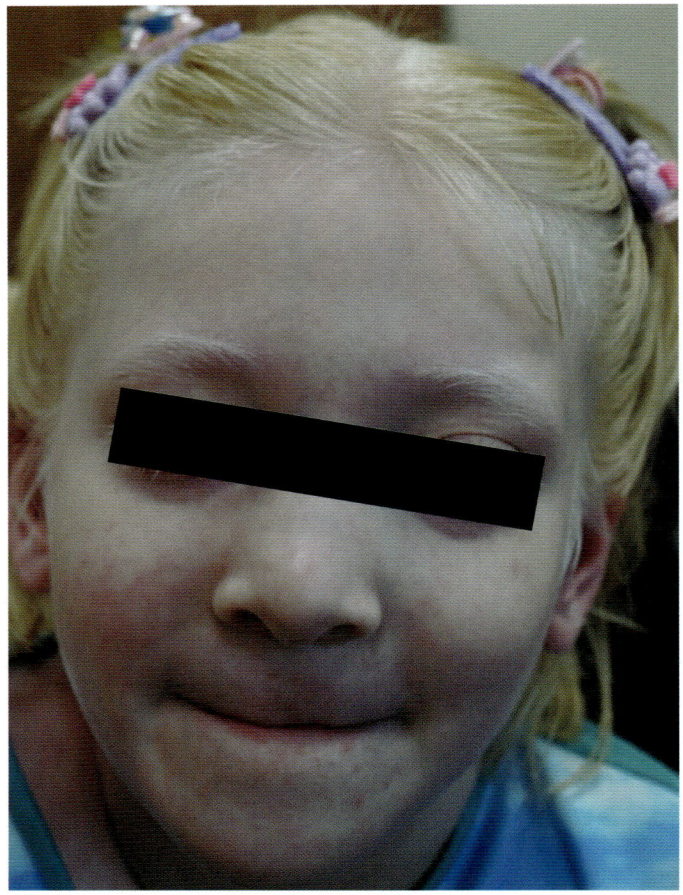

FIGURE 7-12. Light yellow hair, light brown irises, fair skin, and nystagmus in a 6-year-old Indian girl with oculocutaneous albinism.

OCULOCUTANEOUS ALBINISM

Oculocutaneous albinism (OCA) is the most common inherited disorder, resulting in diffuse hypopigmentation. It is characterized by the total or partial absence of melanin with a normal number of melanocytes in the skin, hair follicles, and eyes. The estimated global frequency is 1:20,000 and it is most frequently of an autosomal recessive inheritance pattern.

Clinical Features

- Eight subtypes of non-syndromic albinism have been described: OCA1-8 with multiple implicated genes (Figures 7-12 and 7-13A & 13B). OCA Type 1A is the most severe, with a total absence of melanin throughout life. In the other subtypes, the patients go on to acquire some pigmentation with age.
- The clinical phenotype depends on the degree of melanin absence. In complete absence of pigmentation, patients have a fair complexion with white hair and red eyes.
- People with OCA are highly susceptible to ultraviolet (UV) radiation— and are prone to sun damage, premalignant skin lesions (actinic keratoses), and early incidence of non-melanoma skin cancers (below the age of 30).
- Ophthalmologic abnormalities are common, and include photophobia, reduced visual acuity, refractive errors, nystagmus, fundus hypopigmentation, foveal hypoplasia, and abnormal decussation of optic fibers, resulting in strabismus and reduced stereoscopic vision.

Differential Diagnoses

- Rare, syndromic forms of OCA have other systemic manifestations, in addition to skin and hair hypopigmentation and ophthalmologic abnormalities.
  - Hermansky-Pudlak syndrome: platelet alterations, granulomatous colitis, interstitial pulmonary fibrosis.
  - Chediak-Higashi syndrome: frequent infections, bleeding diathesis, immunodeficiency, neurological abnormalities.
- Waardenburg syndrome type II
  - A rare condition due to an autosomal dominant mutation in the *MITF* gene.
  - Skin hypopigmentation, white forelock of hair, sensorineural hearing loss, and heterochromia of the iris.

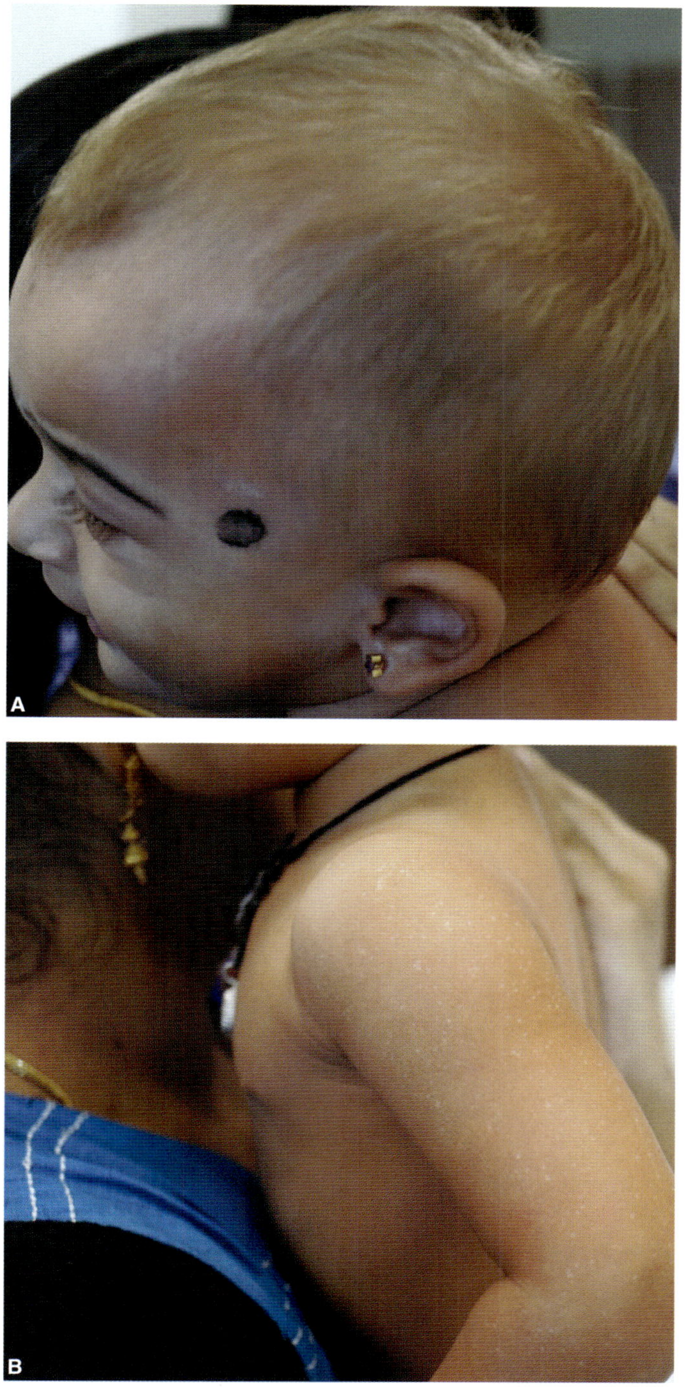

FIGURE 7-13A & 13B. This 1-year-old Indian girl has clinical features of OCA3, with light yellow-brown hair, tan-brown skin, brown irises, and widespread guttate hypopigmented macules on her skin. Her parents are consanguineous.

- Griscelli or Elejalde syndrome
  - Also known as the "silvery hair syndromes," these syndromes have autosomal recessive inheritance, and are extremely rare conditions of pigment dilution with systemic associations.
  - Griscelli syndrome is due to mutations in the *MYO5A*, *RAB27A*, and *MLPH* genes.

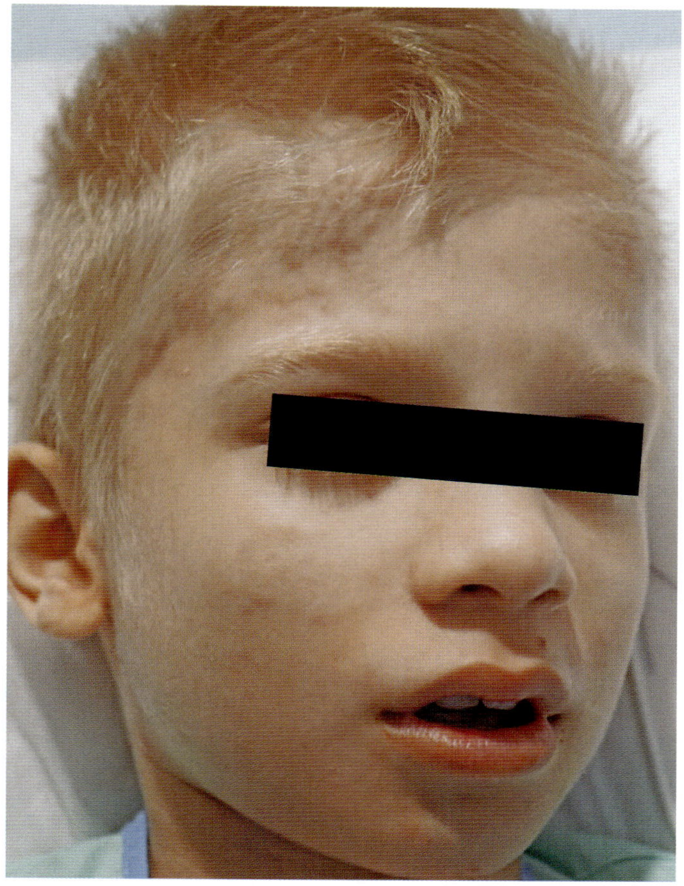

FIGURE 7-14. Oculocutaneous albinism in a Malay boy showing fair skin and fair hair. A congenital nevus on his left philtrum appears medium brown.

  - Elejalde syndrome is believed to correspond to Griscelli syndrome type 1, attributed to a mutation in *MYO5A*.
  - Both conditions present with skin hypopigmentation and silvery-grey hair. Other features include intellectual disability, neurological abnormalities, and immune dysfunction.

Investigations & Treatment

- Due to clinical overlap between the various OCA forms, molecular genetic testing is needed to identify the exact gene alteration and severity of mutation.
- Mutations in the *TYR*, *OCA2*, *TYRP1*, and *SLC45A2* genes are the most frequently implicated. *SLC24A5*, *C10orf11*, and *DCT* genes have been recently described.
- Education on photoprotection and sun avoidance are paramount. This includes—reducing UV exposure during peak sunlight hours (from 10:00 am to 4:00 pm), wearing UV-protective clothing (long-sleeved tops and long pants, wide-brimmed hats, sunglasses), applying broad-spectrum sunscreen with adequate SPF (at least 30+), and re-application of sunscreen every 2 hours when outdoors.

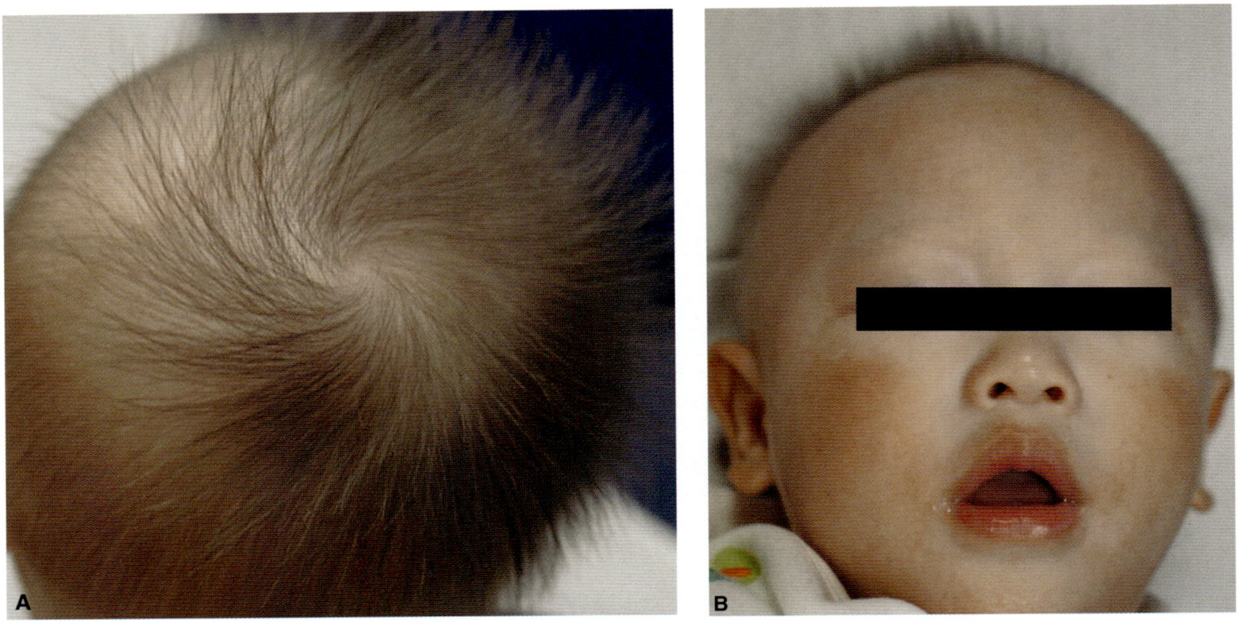

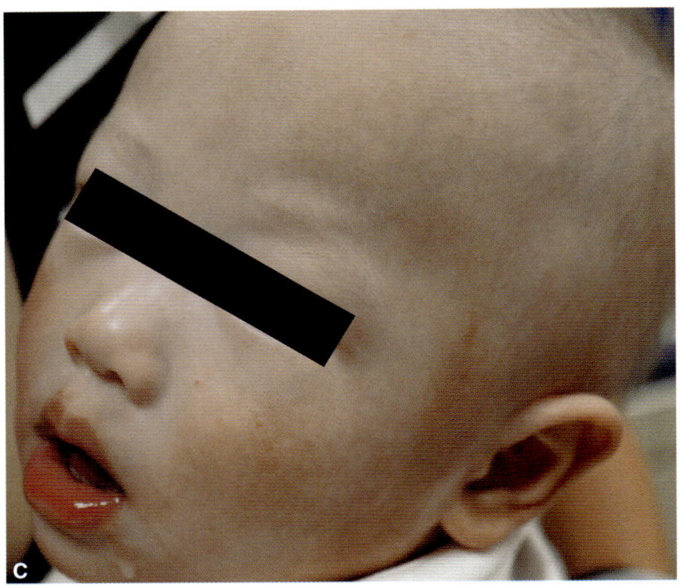

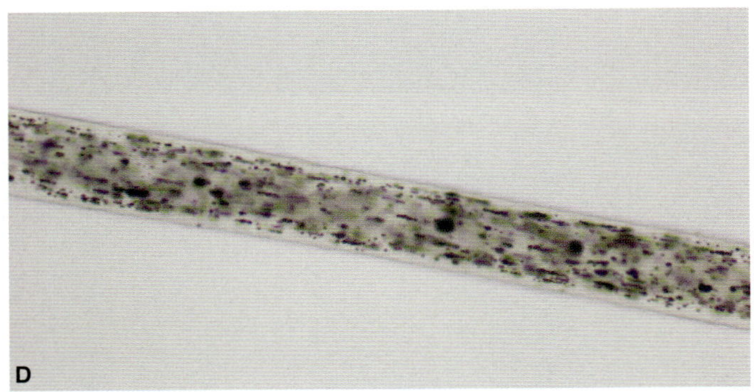

FIGURE 7-15A–15D. A young Chinese infant with Chediak-Higashi syndrome, presenting with grey-silvery hair and patchy hypopigmentation over his face, trunk, and limbs. A hair mount shows clumped melanin granules in the hair shaft (Figure 7-15D)

- Skin self-examination and regular skin examinations at least every 6 months for monitoring, and early intervention of premalignant and malignant skin lesions are recommended.
- Early ophthalmologic assessment and regular follow-up are also needed. Corrective lenses and surgical intervention may be necessary.

Pearls & Practical Tips

- Stress to the patient and parents the risk of premalignant and malignant skin lesions, especially in those with more severe phenotypes.
- Genetic testing and counseling should be offered to all patients and their parents so that they are aware of the risk of future offsprings having the same condition.
- Contacting and joining an albinism support group, such as The National Organization for Albinism and Hypopigmentation (NOAH) in the United States and Canada, can help patients better understand and cope with living with their condition.

NEVUS ANEMICUS

Nevus anemicus presents as a hypopigmented area of skin in children. This is due to increased sensitivity of the alpha-1-adrenergic receptors of dermal papillary blood vessels to catecholamines, resulting in sustained vasoconstriction.

Clinical Features

- Nevus anemicus presents at birth or in early childhood with hypopigmented, mottled, or coalescent macules with irregular, polycyclic borders.
- It most commonly occurs on the trunk, but may also occur on the limbs.
- Commonly seen with surrounding or adjacent erythema that becomes more prominent on rubbing or warming the skin.
- May be difficult to visualize without direct provocation.
- Diascopy causes the hypopigmented area to be less obvious due to vasoconstriction and blanching of the surrounding vasculature. This is performed by pressing a glass slide over the lesion.

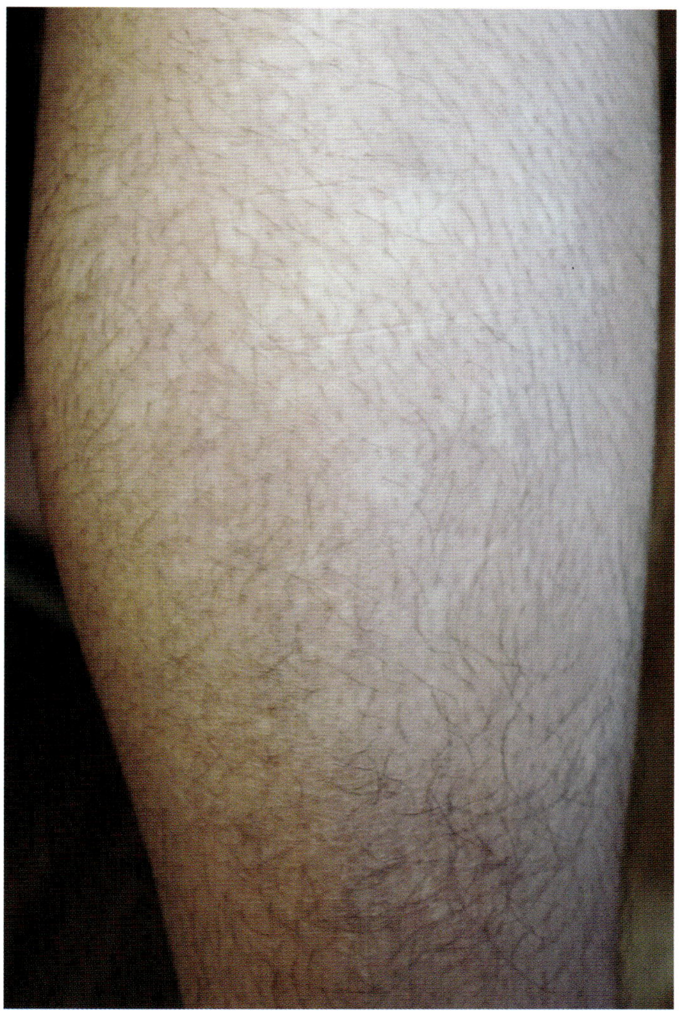

FIGURE 7-16. Nevus anemicus on the calf of a 12-year-old Chinese boy, presenting as patchy hypopigmented macules surrounded by mild erythema.

Differential Diagnoses

- Nevus depigmentosus
  - Nevus depigmentosus is not obscured or can become more apparent upon application of diascopy, with clear borders between the normal skin and hypopigmented lesion. It exhibits bluish-white fluorescence with Wood's lamp examination.

Investigations & Treatment

- Wood's lamp examination is unremarkable, as the hypopigmented area does not arise from a pigmentary disturbance.
- No treatment is effective or usually necessary.

Pearls & Practical Tips

- Nevus anemicus is more commonly seen in children with neurofibromatosis type 1[1] and has been described in 9% of such children, with 35% of those under 2 years of age.
- Nevus anemicus is more commonly found near or adjacent to other vascular anomalies, such as port wine stains.

Reference

1. Hernandez-Martin A, Garcia-Martinez FJ, Duat A, et al. Nevus anemicus: a distinctive cutaneous finding in neurofibromatosis type 1. Pediatr Dermatol 2015 May-Jun:32(3):342-7.

CONGENITAL MELANOCYTIC NEVUS

Congenital melanocytic nevi (CMN) refer to brown or black birthmarks due to proliferation of benign melanocytes in the skin. Many are visible at birth, although some may become apparent in the first year of life. Larger nevi have an increased risk of transformation to melanoma, and regular close surveillance is important for all patients with CMN.

Clinical Features

- The development of CMN has been associated with somatic mutations in the *NRAS* and *BRAF* genes.
- The appearance of CMN varies widely in morphology, texture, location, and size. They are usually round or oval in shape, brown, black, or variably pigmented macules, papules, patches, or plaques. CMN are traditionally classified based on their final size in adulthood (Table 7-1).
- Multiple satellite nevi,—smaller lesions found away from the principal lesion,—may accompany large and giant CMN.

TABLE 7-1. Traditional classification of congenital melanocytic nevi by size.

Size	Projected adult size (cm)
Small	<1.5
Medium	1.5–10
Large	11–20
Giant	
G1	21–30
G2	31–40
G3	>40

Ruiz-Maldonado, 2004.

- CMN may also become more pigmented, raised, or nodular, and acquire hair over time.
- Newer classifications include other features of CMN, including number of satellite nevi, anatomic location, color heterogeneity, skin rugosity, hypertrichosis, and presence of nodules (Table 7-2).
- Large and giant CMN are also associated with an increased risk of neurocutaneous melanosis and development of melanoma (see below).
- Large or giant CMN may lead to significant psychosocial morbidity.

Neurocutaneous Melanosis

- Large and giant CMN with multiple satellite nevi, especially those involving the head, neck, and back, may be associated with neurocutaneous melanosis (NCM), where there is a proliferation of melanocytes in the central nervous system (CNS).
- There is a predisposition to seizures, melanoma of the CNS, and complications relating to spinal cord compression and raised intracranial pressure.
- Other CNS abnormalities include Dandy-Walker malformation, corpus callosum agenesis, and lissencephaly.
- Patients often present with neurological symptoms within the first 2 to 3 years of life, such as headaches, seizures, irritability, vomiting, bulging anterior fontanelle, and photophobia.
- Prognosis for symptomatic NCM is poor, with a mortality rate of up to 90%.
- Patients with a suspicion for NCM should be referred to a pediatric neurologist for gadolinium-enhanced magnetic resonance imaging (MRI) and close follow-up.

TABLE 7-2. Newer proposed classification of congenital melanocytic nevi.

CMN Parameter	Terminology	Definition
CMN projected adult size	Small	<1.5 cm
	Medium	
	M1	1.5–10 cm
	M2	>10–20 cm
	Large	
	L1	>20–30 cm
	L2	>30–40 cm
	Giant	
	G1	>40–60 cm
	G2	>60 cm
	Multiple medium CMN	≥3 medium CMN without a single, predominant CMN
Localization		
CMN of the head	"Face," "scalp"	
CMN of the trunk	"Neck," "shoulder," "upper back," "middle back," "lower back," "breast/chest," "abdomen," "flank," "gluteal region," "genital region"	
CMN of the extremities	"Upper arm," "forearm," "hand," "thigh," "lower leg," "foot"	
Number of satellite nevi within first year of life	S0	No satellites
	S1	<20 satellites
	S2	20–50 satellites
	S3	>50 satellites
Additional morphological characteristics	C0, C1, C2	None, moderate, marked color heterogeneity
	R0, R1, R2	None, moderate, marked surface rugosity
	N0, N1, N2	None, scattered, extensive dermal/subcutaneous nodules
	H0, H1, H2	None, notable, marked hypertrichosis

Melanoma Risk

- All CMN should be considered as potential precursors of melanoma.
- The lifetime risk for malignant transformation of CMN is proportionate to their size.
  - Small and medium-sized CMN have a very low risk of <1%.
  - Lifetime risk of large and giant CMN is estimated to be higher, at 2% to 10%.
- Parents should be taught how to self-monitor for suspicious changes in their child's CMN with the "ABCDE rule" (Table 7-3).
- All patients with large and giant CMN should be regularly followed up by a dermatologist for long-term surveillance. Parents of patients with smaller CMN can be taught to self-monitor and to seek a dermatologist's opinion if suspicious changes occur.

Differential Diagnoses

Small/Medium CMN

- Acquired melanocytic nevus
  - Acquired melanocytic nevi are not present at birth.
  - They usually appear in early childhood and may increase in size and number until the third decade of life.

TABLE 7-3. The ABCDE rule of melanoma.

Clinical feature		Comment
A	Asymmetry	One half of the mole appears different from the other
B	Border irregularity	Edges of the mole are not well-defined—notched, blurred or irregular
C	Color variegation	Multiple colors, including blue, red, black, or white
D	Diameter >6 mm	May not always be applicable to CMN, which are often >6 mm or grow to be more than 6 mm
E	Evolution	Evolutionary change in shape, size, or color over time

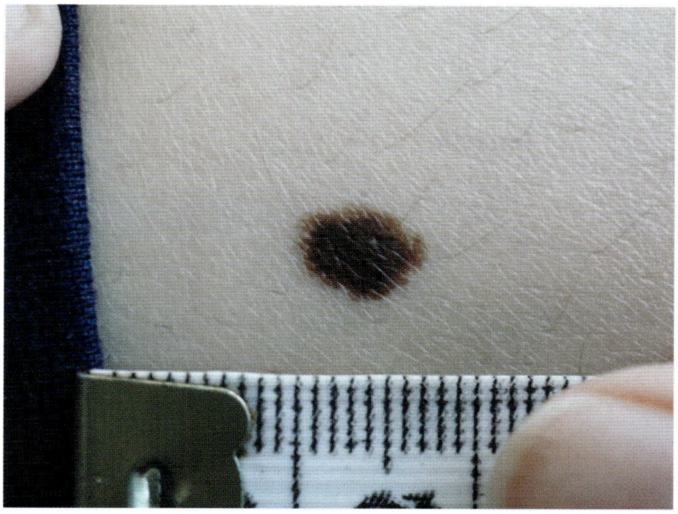

FIGURE 7-17. Small-sized congenital melanocytic nevus on the trunk presenting as a well-demarcated medium brown, slightly raised papule.

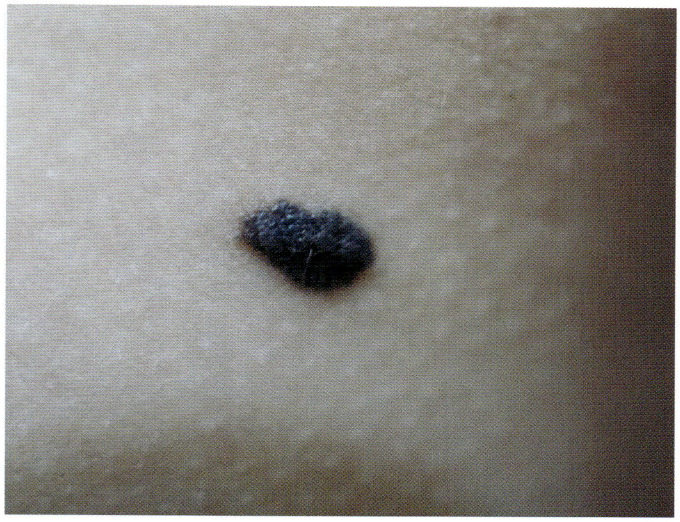

FIGURE 7-18. Small-sized intradermal melanocytic nevus on the trunk of a Chinese child. Note the well-demarcated borders and uniform color.

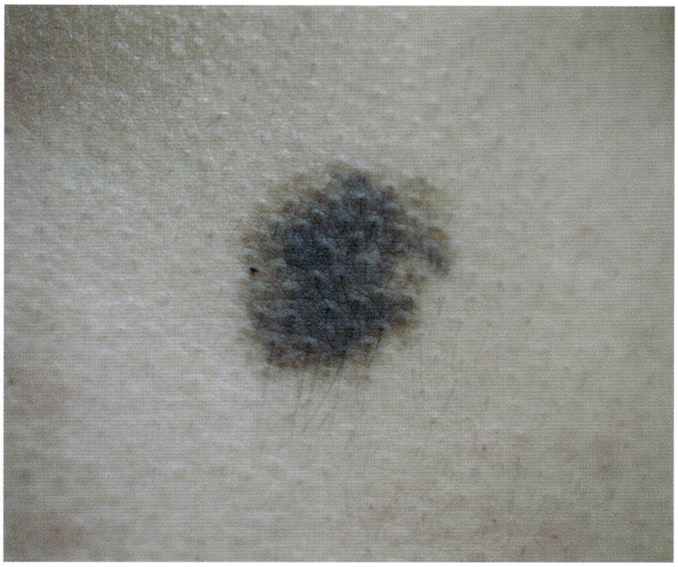

FIGURE 7-19. Congenital melanocytic nevus on the trunk of a teenage Filipino male with mild hypertrichosis.

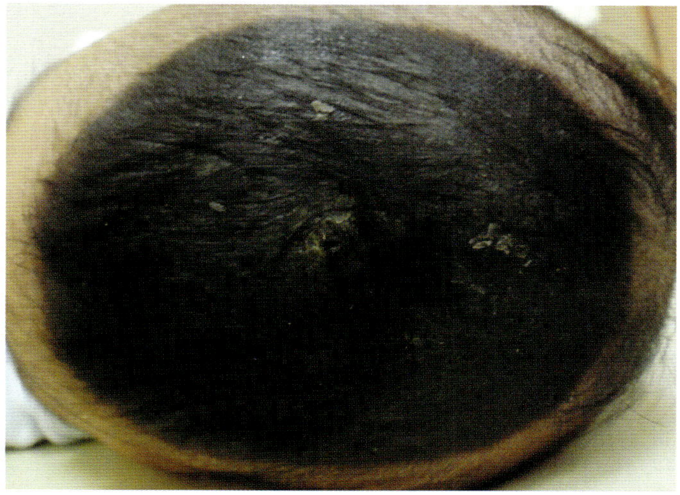

FIGURE 7-20. Large congenital melanocytic nevus on the scalp of a Chinese infant. There is concomitant seborrheic dermatitis of the scalp.

- Melanocytic nevus subtypes: blue nevus, Spitz nevus
  - The melanocytic nevus subtypes rarely present at birth, and tend to be present as solitary lesions.
  - Blue nevi appear more bluish grey compared to the typical brown-black pigmentation seen in CMN.
  - Spitz nevi present as rapidly growing raised papules or nodules, which are reddish-brown, tan, bluish, or black in color.

Large/Giant CMN

- Café-au-lait macules
  - A café-au-lait macule is a flat, light-brown uniformly hyperpigmented birthmark.
  - The brown hyperpigmentation seen in a café-au-lait macule is much lighter than that of a CMN.
- Becker's nevus
  - A Becker's nevus is a late-onset pigmented hamartoma, which occurs more commonly in males.
  - It develops during childhood or adolescence in contrast to CMN, which is present at birth. Patients present with a large unilateral brown patch or plaque, most commonly over the chest area, which may become darker and hairy over time.
- Dermal melanosis
  - Dermal melanosis appears as slate-brown or blue/gray macules or patches.
  - They may occur at birth in 50% of cases but may also appear during adolescence or in adulthood.
  - Nevus of Ota is classically located over the forehead and malar area, near the eye. Nevus of Ito is classically located on the shoulder and shoulder girdle. Mongolian spots usually occur on the back and buttocks.

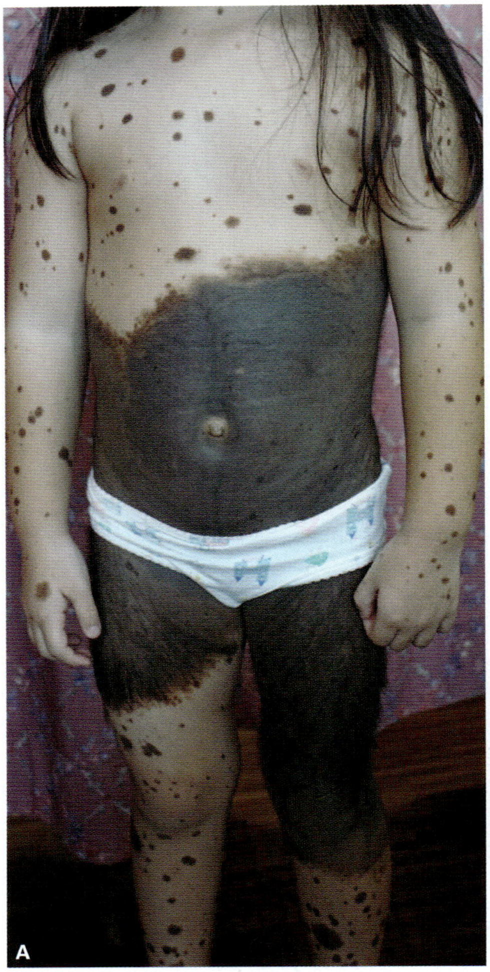

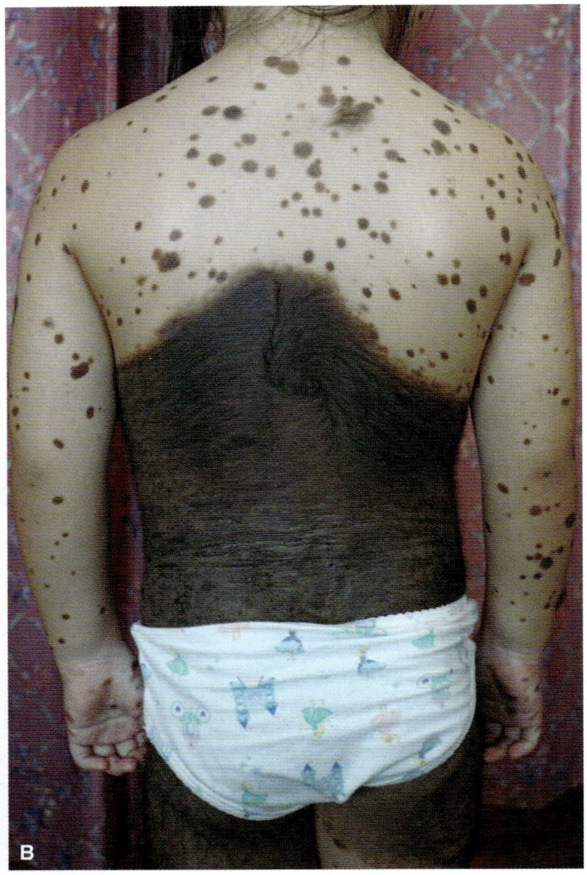

FIGURES 7-21A & 21B. Giant hairy congenital melanocytic nevus in a "bathing-suit distribution" of a 4-year-old Chinese girl, with multiple satellite nevi.

Investigations & Treatment

- CMNs are diagnosed by their clinical appearance.
- In cases of diagnostic doubt, examination with dermoscopy or biopsy for histopathology may be performed.
- Dermoscopy most commonly reveals a homogenous globular pigmentation pattern; other patterns include cobblestone, structureless, reticular, or mixed patterns.
- Features of disorganization are suggestive of atypia, and warrant histopathological examination. These include but are not limited to the appearance of irregular shape/structures, multiple colors, irregular vascularity, a blue-white veil, peripheral black dots/globules.
- Biopsy of benign CMN lesions demonstrates extension of melanocytes into the deep dermis and subcutis, between collagen bundles and surrounding appendages, nerves, and vessels. Single filing of melanocytes in between collagen bundles may be seen in the deep dermis.
- Biopsy for histopathology is also used to rule out melanoma in the event of rapid evolution, atypical features, or warning signs.
- MRI with contrast of the central nervous system, including the brain and spinal cord, is warranted for patients with suspicion of neurocutaneous melanosis. However, it neither rules out nor predicts those who will ultimately develop symptoms.
- Longitudinal observation with total body skin examination by a dermatologist is the mainstay of management in patients with CMN.
- Patients with NCM, or those at a high risk of NCM, should be regularly followed up by a pediatric neurologist.

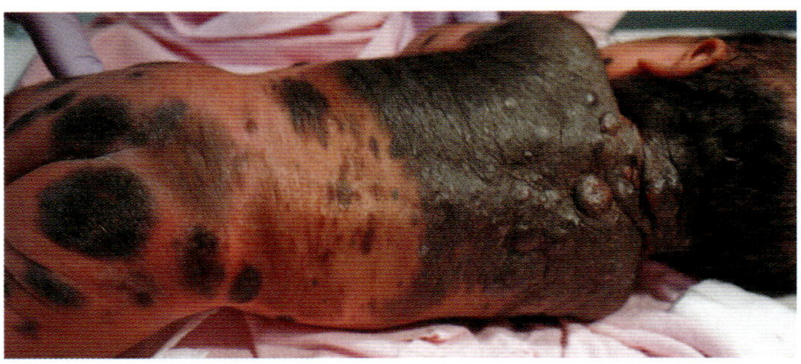

FIGURE 7-22. Giant congenital melanocytic nevus in an Indian newborn. Proliferating nodules are already seen at birth.

- Patient counseling regarding the following should be reinforced:
  - Sun protection
  - Regular skin self-examination
  - Detection of atypia/melanoma with the "ABCDE rule" (Table 7-3)
- Laser hair removal may be performed for overlying hypertrichosis.
- Laser excision/ablation of lesions
  - Limited efficacy with high risk of recurrence.
  - May result in lightening of the lesion but not complete removal. This can make the lesion more difficult to assess during long-term surveillance and in future biopsies.
- Surgical removal
  - Reasons to consider surgical removal include cosmesis with high psychosocial burden, suspicious evolution of the lesion, or features of atypia.
  - May be difficult, especially for large and giant CMN in which the extent of skin involvement is high. Staged excision with tissue expansion may be considered.
  - Parents should be counseled that removal of every nevus is often impossible.
  - A thorough discussion with consideration of the risks of surgery should be undertaken, including anesthetic risk and risk of worsening appearance due to scarring.
- Targeted molecular therapies focused on the MAPK pathway have shown some benefit in *BRAF* mutated giant CMNs, such as trametinib (MEK inhibitor).

Pearls & Practical Tips

- Patients with CMN may require multidisciplinary care management due to the various management challenges that they may face. Longitudinal follow-up with a pediatric dermatologist is encouraged for regular skin surveillance and for coordination of multidisciplinary care if required.
- The recurrence rate of melanocytic nevi after laser ablation is high, especially for compound or intradermal nevi. Laser ablation can result in surface scarring, leading to difficulty in differentiating from scarring seen in melanomas histologically.
- Melanomas that occur in large congenital melanocytic nevi usually occur as deep nodules, which can be confused clinically and histologically with proliferating nodules.

Bibliography

1. Levy R, Lara-Corrales I. Melanocytic nevi in children: a review. Pediatr Ann 2016;45(8):e293-8.
2. Moustafa D, Blundell AR, Hawryluk EB. Congenital melanocytic nevi. Curr Opin Pediatr 2020;32(4):491-7.
3. Krengel S, Scope A, Dusza SW, Vonthein R, Marghoob AA. New recommendations for the categorization of cutaneous features of congenital melanocytic nevi. J Amer Acad Dermatol 2013;68(3):441-51.
4. Nir A, Agim NG, Kane AA, et al. Giant congenital melanocytic nevus treated with trametinib. Pediatrics 2019;143(3):e20182469

ACQUIRED MELANOCYTIC NEVUS

Melanocytic nevi, frequently known as "moles," are extremely common benign skin neoplasms due to local proliferation of melanocytes in the skin. Acquired melanocytic nevi appear after birth, in contrast to congenital melanocytic nevi, which are mostly present at birth. Melanocytic nevi carry a small risk of transformation to melanoma, highlighting the importance of close monitoring and sun protection.

Clinical Features

- Acquired melanocytic nevi usually appear after infancy and may continue to increase in size and number throughout childhood and puberty.
- Predisposing factors to the development of melanocytic nevi include genetic predisposition, sun exposure, lighter skin phototypes, and immunosuppressive treatments.
- Melanocytic nevi are classified as junctional, compound, or intradermal, based on the microscopic location of nevus cells in the skin.
- Junctional nevi appear as small, flat, medium- to dark-brown macules. Compound nevi appear as flat or slightly raised medium- to dark-brown papules. Intradermal nevi present as skin-colored to medium- to dark-brown sessile or sometimes pedunculated papules or nodules.
- Acquired melanocytic nevi can occur anywhere on the skin or mucosal surfaces but are more common on the sun-exposed sites.

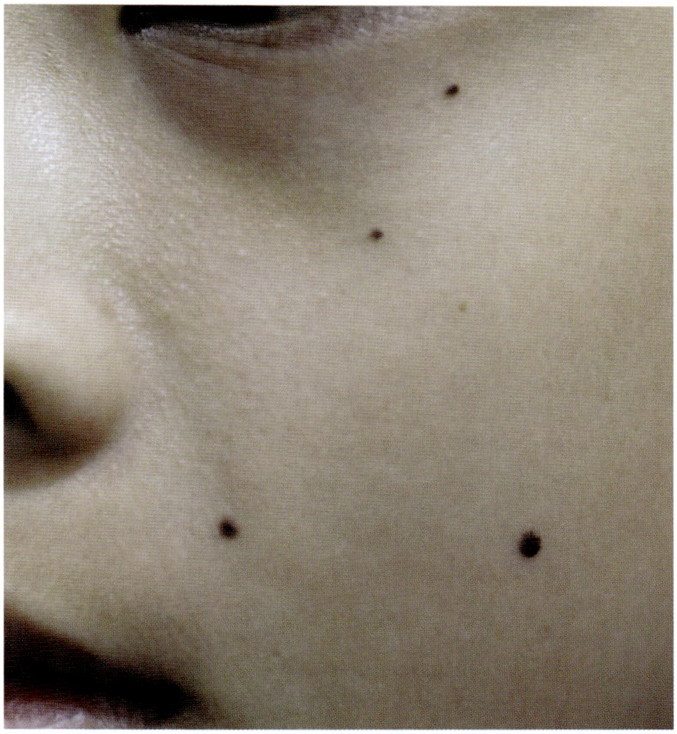

FIGURE 7-23. Multiple benign acquired melanocytic nevi on the face of a 12-year-old Chinese boy. He reported an increase in the number of facial melanocytic nevi in his adolescent years.

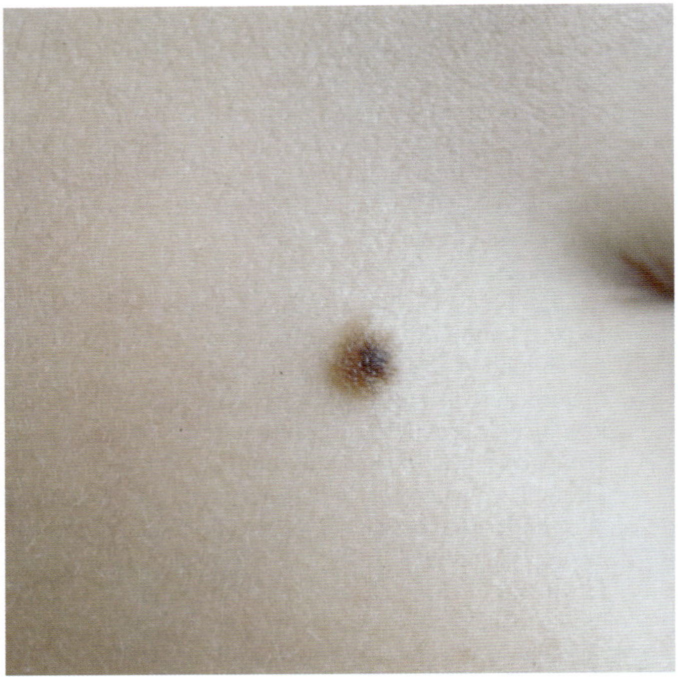

FIGURE 7-24. Junctional melanocytic nevus on the face of a child, presenting as a flat, demarcated, light brown macule.

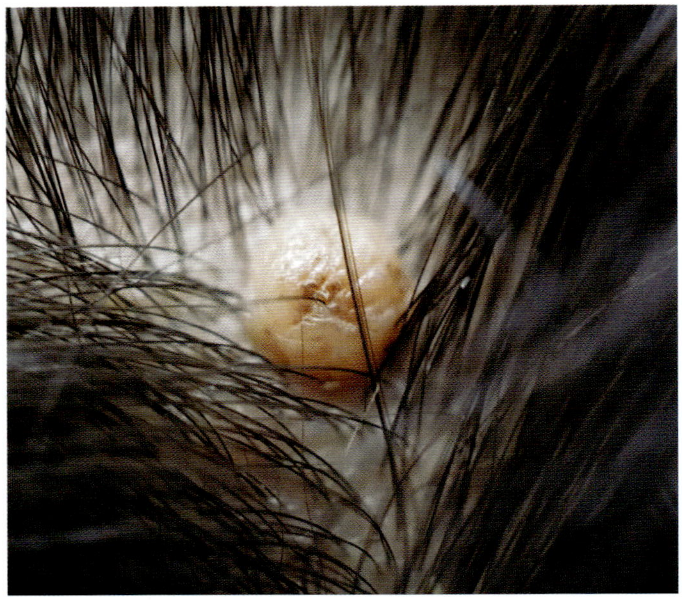

FIGURE 7-26. Intradermal melanocytic nevus of the scalp in an adolescent Chinese male, presenting as a pedunculated, soft, medium-brown nodule with demarcated borders.

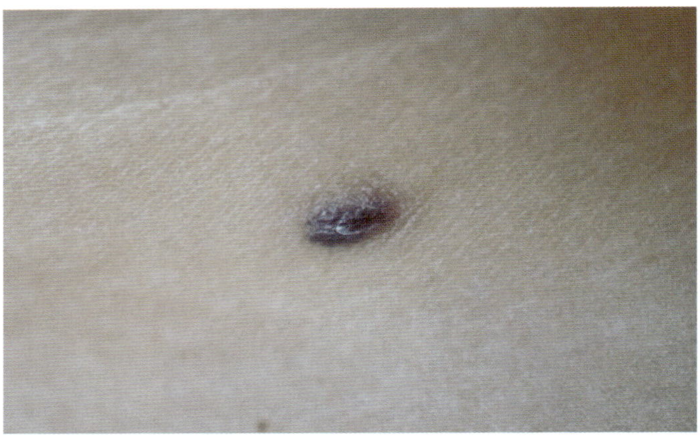

FIGURE 7-25. Compound melanocytic nevus on the neck of a Chinese child, presenting as a slightly raised, well-demarcated, dark brown papule.

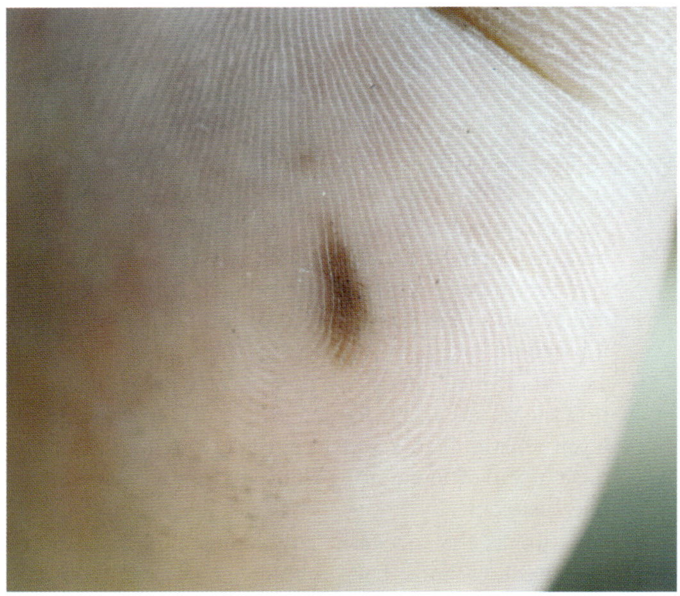

FIGURE 7-27. Acral junctional melanocytic nevus on the sole of a Chinese child.

- The risk of malignant transformation of melanocytic nevi is extremely rare in the pediatric population, especially in Asian skin types. Nevi that appear to have a stark difference in morphology from other nevi in an individual should be regarded as potentially abnormal ("ugly duckling" sign).

Differential Diagnoses

- Congenital melanocytic nevus
  - These are mostly present at birth or appear in the first few months of life. They vary in size and can affect large areas of skin.
- Atypical nevus
  - Atypical nevi are defined based on their clinical and histological appearances.
  - They tend to be larger in size than the common melanocytic nevus and demonstrate irregularities of color, texture, and borders.
- Café-au-lait macules
  - Café-au-lait macules appear as flat, light brown, hyperpigmented macules or patches that may be present at birth or occur in early infancy. They appear lighter than melanocytic nevi.

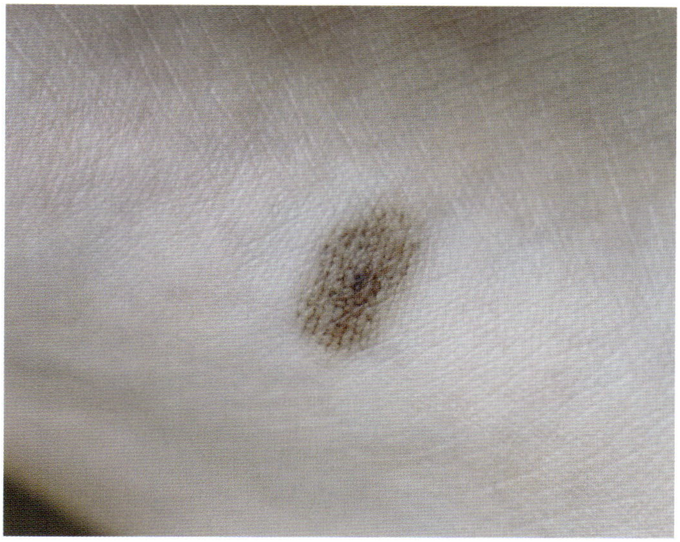

FIGURE 7-28. Acral junctional melanocytic nevus on the sole of a young Chinese child. It is often difficult to differentiate a congenital from an acquired acral melanocytic nevus.

- Lentigo simplex
  - Lentigo simplex presents as small round or oval shaped, flat macules which may have jagged or smooth edges. They may appear similar to junctional melanocytic nevi clinically and on dermoscopy. However, they are histologically different.
  - Histology of lentigo simplex shows proliferation of single melanocytes within the basal cell layer in the epidermis.
- Acrochordon (skin tag)
  - Skin tags are small, soft, sessile, or pedunculated skin growths and tend to be less pigmented or nonpigmented compared to melanocytic nevi. They commonly occur on the neck and axillae.
- Viral warts
  - Viral warts may appear as soft, skin-colored or hyperpigmented papules and often have overlying hyperkeratosis, pinpoint thrombosed capillaries, and disruption of skin lines.

Investigations & Treatment

- Acquired melanocytic nevi are diagnosed by their clinical appearance.
- Dermoscopic examination reveals a homogenous globular pigmentation pattern. Other patterns include cobblestone, structureless, reticular, or mixed patterns. Benign dermoscopic features include a well-organized structure, symmetry, and uniformity in structure and color. Features of disorganization are suggestive of atypia, including irregular shapes or structures, multiple colors, irregular vascularity, a blue-white veil, and peripheral black dots or globules.
- Biopsy of melanocytic nevi lesions demonstrates nests of proliferating melanocytes, which may extend from the epidermis into the dermis.
- Longitudinal observation with periodic total body skin examination by a dermatologist is the mainstay of management in patients with multiple acquired melanocytic nevi.
- Patient counseling should take place regarding sun protection, regular skin self-examination, and detection of atypia/melanoma with the "ABCDE rule."
- Acquired melanocytic nevi that require histological diagnosis or are causing cosmetic concern can be removed surgically by punch, excision, or shave biopsies.
- Laser ablation may be useful for junctional melanocytic nevi. However, there is a risk of recurrence.

Pearls & Practical Tips

- A common concern of parents is ongoing growth of existing nevi, and development of multiple new nevi in the child. Parents should be advised that this is common and nevi can even grow more rapidly during the child's growth spurts.
- Development of new nevi is known to continue up to the third decade of life.
- The recurrence rate of melanocytic nevi after laser ablation is high, especially for compound or intradermal nevi. Laser ablation can result in surface scarring, leading to difficulty in differentiating from scarring seen in melanomas histologically.

Bibliography

1. Levy R, Lara-Corrales I. Melanocytic nevi in children: a review. Pediatr Ann 2016;45(8), e293-8.

BLUE NEVUS

Blue nevi are melanocytic nevi that present with a characteristic dark blue or blue-black color. Blue nevi tend to remain static and persist throughout a person's life. Malignant transformation of a blue nevus is extremely rare.

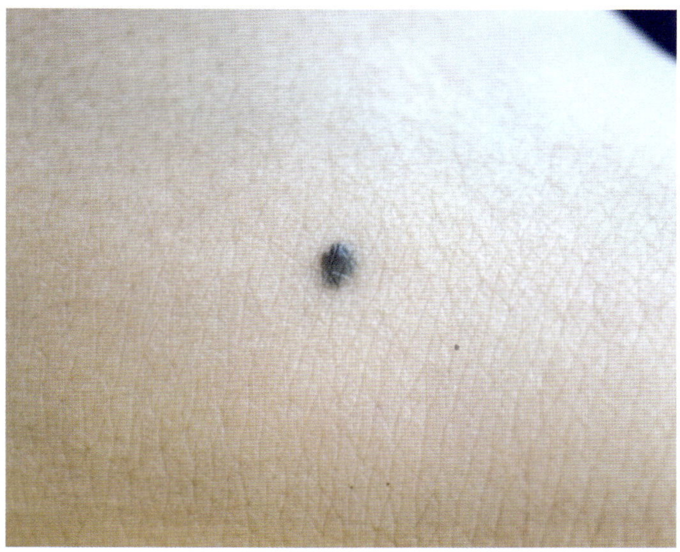

FIGURE 7-29. A small blue nevus on the wrist of a young Chinese child.

Clinical Features

- Blue nevi are caused by dermal proliferation of stellate or spindled melanocytes. They are postulated to be a result of incomplete migration of melanocytes from the neural crest.
- They may appear at any age, but more commonly in late childhood or adolescence.
- The two more common histological subtypes are the common blue nevus and the cellular blue nevus.
- Blue nevi usually present as acquired solitary, round, well-demarcated, blue-black, flat macules or dome-shaped papules. The blue color is attributed to the Tyndall effect, where shorter wavelengths of light are reflected by the dermal melanocytes.
- Blue nevi may appear anywhere on the body, including mucosal membranes. Areas of predilection include the buttocks, the dorsum of hands and feet, extensor aspect of the forearms, and the scalp.
- Congenital blue nevi are rare and may be associated with familial or other syndromes such as the epithelioid variant in Carney complex, a form of multiple endocrine neoplasia.
- Blue nevi tend to remain stable and persist throughout life.

Differential Diagnoses

- Dermatofibroma
  - Dermatofibromas are common and present as hyperpigmented, rubbery nodules that may clinically mimic the amelanotic variant of the blue nevus.
- Pencil lead tattoo
  - Pencil lead tattoo refers to graphite (usually from a pencil lead) that is traumatically implanted within the dermis, resulting in a blue-gray macule or papule.
  - A preceding history of traumatic implantation of a pencil lead tip will aid in differentiating.
- Vascular lesions (e.g., venous lake)
  - A venous lake is a common bluish soft macule or papule due to localized vascular dilatation.
  - Compression of a venous lake with a glass slide will cause its color to disappear due to clearance of blood from the dilated venule.

Investigations & Treatment

- Blue nevi can be diagnosed clinically by appearance.
- Dermoscopic features include homogeneity of color and smooth borders.
- In cases of diagnostic doubt, biopsy for histopathology may be performed. Histopathological examination will demonstrate elongated spindle-shaped melanocytes and dendritic melanocytes within the dermis, without the presence of atypia.
- Periodic monitoring of blue nevi is advised, given the potential for misdiagnosis and small risk of malignant transformation.
- Patients should be educated on performing regular skin self-examination and the "ABCDE rule" of melanoma (see section "Congenital Melanocytic Nevus").
- The definitive treatment of a blue nevus is surgical excision.

Bibliography

1. Austad SS, Athalye L. Blue Nevus. In: StatPearls [Internet]. Treasure Island, FL: StatPearls Publishing; 2021 Jan.e298.

HALO NEVUS

A halo nevus is a unique variant of melanocytic nevi in which there is a centrally placed melanocytic nevus surrounded by a 1- to 2-mm depigmented halo. The central pigmented brown nevus fades from dark brown to light brown to pink, and may eventually disappear.

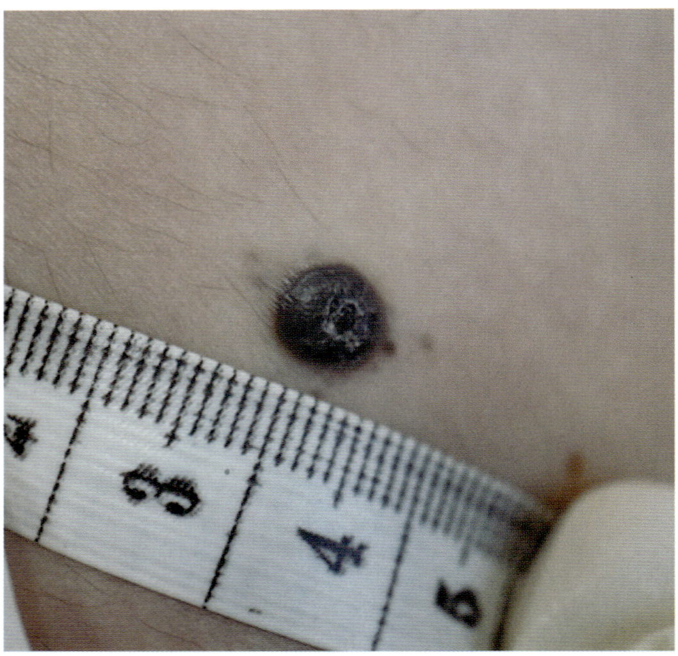

FIGURE 7-30. A blue nevus on a limb of an older Chinese child with a more papular morphology. Biopsy showed deeper dermal extension.

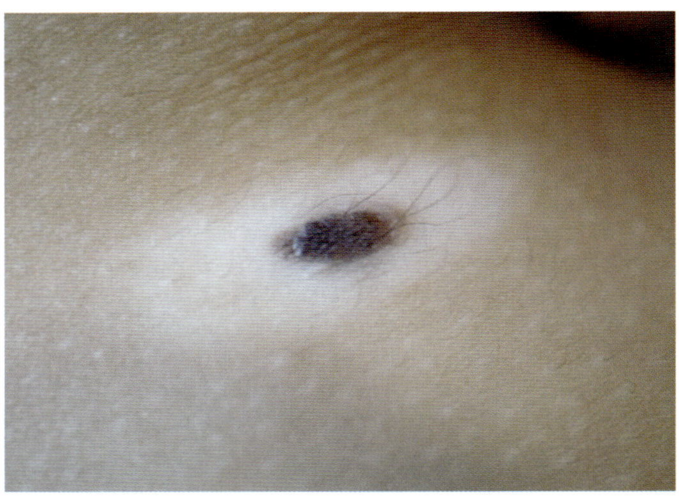

FIGURE 7-31. Halo nevus on the forearm of a 12-year-old Eurasian girl. There is a uniform, depigmented halo surrounding a centrally placed melanocytic nevus.

Clinical Features

- Halo nevus is a benign, mostly acquired variant of melanocytic nevi.
- It is common in children and adolescents, with a mean age of onset of 15 years.
- Halo nevi can appear anywhere on the body, but have a predilection for the trunk, particularly the back.
- Typical progression of a halo nevus is that of loss of pigmentation in the nevus, fading from dark brown (stage I) to light brown to pink (stage II), with eventual disappearance of the pigmented lesion (stage III).
- In most patients, eventual re-pigmentation of the remnant halo occurs over months to years (stage IV).
- Patients with a halo nevus, particularly those with multiple lesions, should undergo a total skin examination to assess for lesions with atypical features and to look for concomitant depigmented patches of vitiligo.
- The etiology of spontaneous depigmentation is unknown but is postulated to be autoimmune in nature, where there is immunologic destruction of melanocytes and nevus cells.

Differential Diagnoses

- Melanoma with halo phenomenon
  - This is extremely rare in Asian children.
  - Melanoma should be considered if the depigmentation is focal and not round/oval or uniformly surrounding the nevus or if the central nevus demonstrates suspicious features such as irregular structure and color.

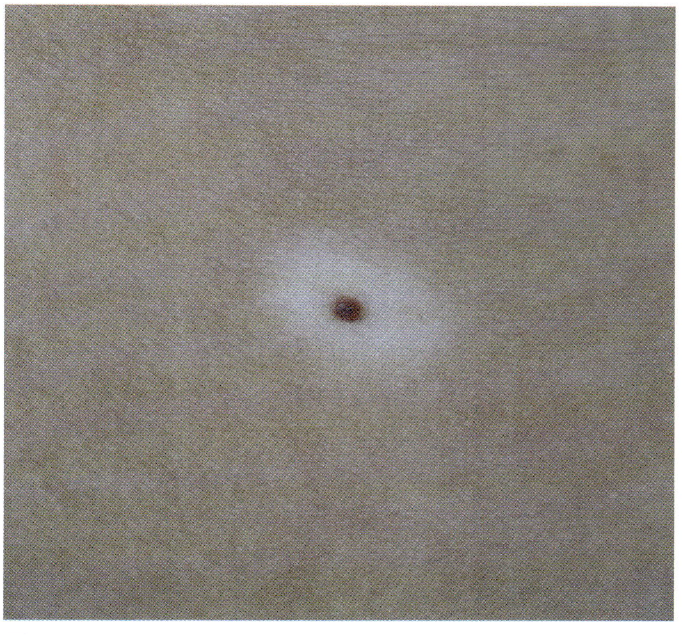

FIGURE 7-32. Halo phenomenon around a small melanocytic nevus on the back of a Chinese adolescent.

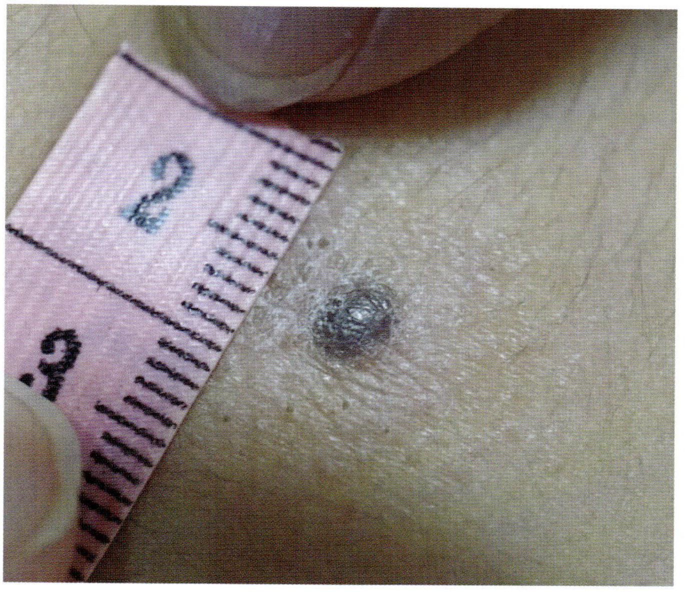

FIGURE 7-33. Meyerson phenomenon seen around a compound melanocytic nevus of an adolescent Chinese girl.

Investigations & Treatment

- Halo nevi are diagnosed by their clinical appearance.
- Benign dermoscopic features of the central melanocytic nevus should demonstrate a homogenous pigmentation pattern.
- In cases of diagnostic doubt or if melanoma is suspected, biopsy for histopathology should be performed, which will reveal a dense inflammatory infiltrate together with reduction or absence of melanin around a central nevus.
- Halo nevi with benign characteristics do not require excision and may be monitored at intervals until their resolution.
- The depigmented region of a halo nevus can develop a sunburn more easily than normal skin. Sun avoidance and/or protection should be advised.
- Complete excision is the definitive treatment for halo nevi with concerning or atypical features.

Pearls & Practical Tips

- Apart from the halo phenomenon, dermatitis can also be seen around melanocytic nevi (Meyerson phenomenon). This can be treated with moisturizers and topical corticosteroids or topical calcineurin inhibitors.
- Although more common in Caucasians, it is extremely rare for the halo phenomenon to be secondary to a melanoma in individuals with pigmented skin.

Bibliography

1. Patrizi A, Bentivogli M, Raone B, Dondi A, Tabanelli M, Neri I. Association of halo nevus/i and vitiligo in childhood: a retrospective observational study. J Eur Acad Dermatol Venereol 2012;27(2):e148–52.

SPITZ NEVUS

Spitz nevi are an uncommon and benign variant of melanocytic nevi. They occur primarily in childhood, adolescence, or early adulthood. They may resemble melanomas clinically and histologically, rendering diagnosis and management challenging.

Clinical Features

- There are three main morphological subtypes of Spitz nevi:
  - Classic Spitz nevus—dome-shaped, red or reddish-brown papule or nodule.
  - Pigmented Spitz nevus—tan or brown papule or nodule.
  - Pigmented spindle cell nevus of Reed—dark, bluish or black papule or nodule.
- It commonly occurs on the face or limbs as a solitary lesion. Multiple Spitz nevi in a segmental distribution is termed agminated Spitz nevi, which is extremely rare.
- Spitz nevi can grow rapidly for a few months, and subsequently may remain static for years.
- Up to 80% of Spitz nevi undergo spontaneous involution over a few years.

Differential Diagnoses

- Pyogenic granuloma
  - Pyogenic granulomas also present as brightly red friable papules or nodules, with surface bleeding from trauma.
- Juvenile xanthogranuloma
  - Juvenile xanthogranulomas can also present as reddish-brown papules, sometimes with surface ulceration after trauma. There is usually a yellowish-orange hue.

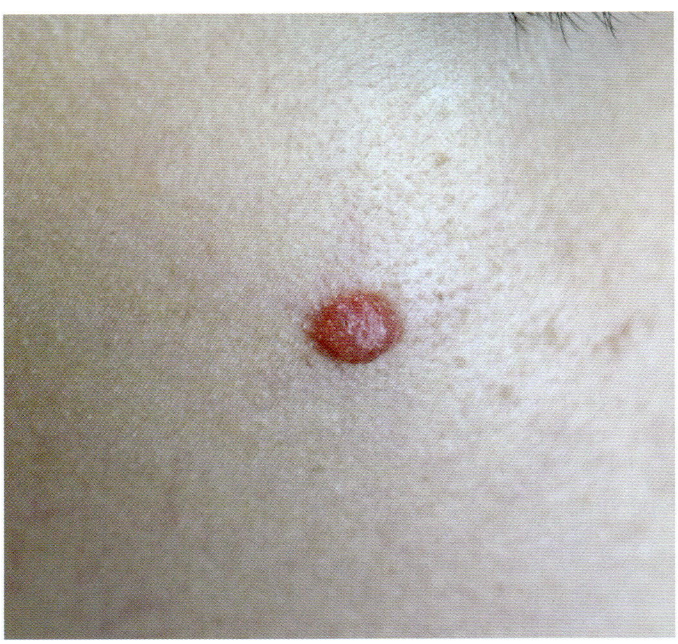

FIGURE 7-34. A reddish-brown, dome-shaped classic Spitz nevus on the cheek of an 11-year-old Chinese boy.

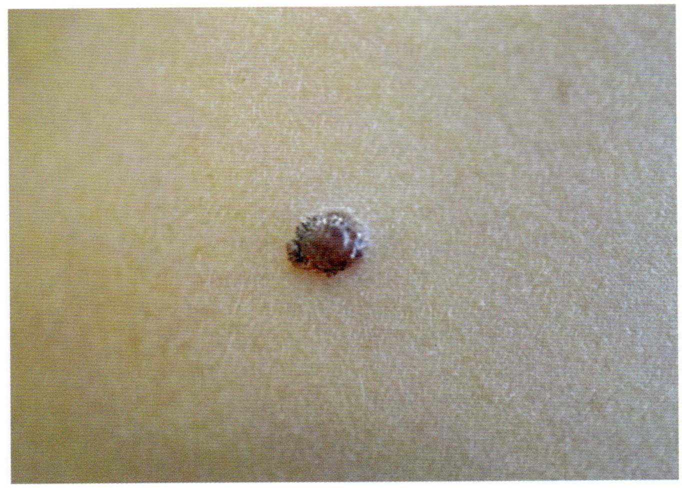

FIGURE 7-35. A darker red-brown pigmented Spitz nevus in a 9-year-old Chinese boy.

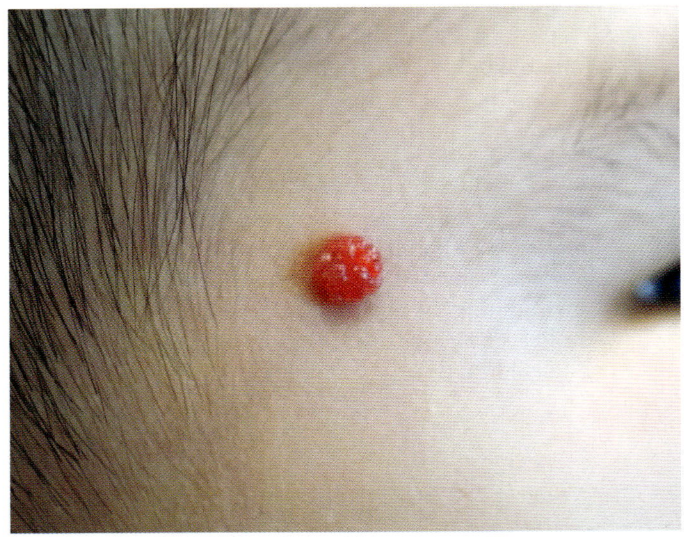

FIGURE 7-36. An intradermal Spitz nevus on the temporal area of a young Chinese boy. This lesion may be mistaken for a pyogenic granuloma.

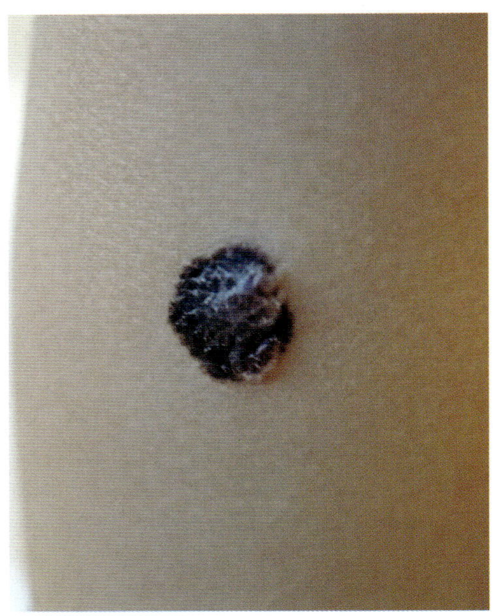

FIGURE 7-37. A pigmented spindle cell nevus of Reed, a variant of Spitz nevus that usually appears much darker than a classical Spitz nevus. This is on the arm of a Malay girl.

- Atypical Spitz tumor
  - Atypical Spitz tumors are usually larger (>10 mm), asymmetric with irregular borders, and may have surface ulceration.
  - Histologically, they resemble Spitz nevi but show some atypia that does not meet the criteria for melanoma.
- Spitzoid melanoma
  - Spitzoid melanomas are extremely rare but can present in childhood. They present as amelanotic or pigmented papules or nodules with color variegation and progressive growth larger than 1 cm, with surface ulceration.

Investigations & Treatment

- Making a clinical diagnosis of Spitz nevus can be difficult given its similarity with other skin tumors. Diagnosis can be confirmed with histopathological examination.
- Histologically, Spitz nevi are characterized by nests of epithelioid or spindle-shaped melanocytes with large, open nuclei. Other histological features of Spitz nevi include artefactual clefting, Kamino bodies, and maturation with depth. Rare mitoses may also be seen.
- Spitz nevi may be treated conservatively in children. However, if there are atypical features clinically, lesions should be excised.

Pearls & Practical Tips

- The most common differential diagnoses of Spitz nevi in children are pyogenic granuloma and juvenile xanthogranuloma.

Bibliography

1. Sainz-Gaspar L, Sánchez-Bernal J, Noguera-Morel L, Hernández-Martín A, Colmenero I, Torrelo A. Spitz nevus and other spitzoid tumors in children. Part 1: Clinical, histopathologic, and immunohistochemical features. Actas Dermosifiliogr (Engl Ed) 2020 Jan 2;111(1):7-19. English, Spanish.
2. Sainz-Gaspar L, Sánchez-Bernal J, Noguera-Morel L, Hernández-Martín A, Colmenero I, Torrelo A. Spitz nevus and other spitzoid tumors in children. Part 2: Cytogenetic and molecular features. Prognosis and treatment. Actas Dermosifiliogr (Engl Ed). 2020 Jan 2;111(1):20-5. English, Spanish.
3. A. Lallas, Z. Apalla, D. Ioannides, et al. Update on dermoscopy of Spitz/Reed naevi and management guidelines by the International Dermoscopy Society. Br J Dermatol 2017;177:645-55.

LENTIGO SIMPLEX AND LENTIGINOSIS

Lentigo simplex are common lesions and present with single or multiple flat, medium-brown macules which are not induced by sun exposure. The lesions may fade or disappear spontaneously over a few years. Multiple or extensive lentiginosis may be a component of an underlying syndrome and its presence warrants thorough evaluation and monitoring for the development of associated abnormalities.

Clinical Features

- Lentigines or lentigo simplex occur due to benign, linear proliferation of single melanocytes along the basement membrane of the epidermis. They are benign lesions and have no malignant potential.
- They typically develop in early childhood, or less commonly appear at birth, and may increase in number until adulthood.
- Lentigines can occur anywhere on the skin or mucous membranes and are generally asymptomatic.
- Multiple lentigines without associated abnormalities are termed *generalized lentigines*, or *lentigines profusa*. If the lentigines are clustered within a circumscribed area, the condition is termed *unilateral partial lentiginosis*.

Lentiginosis Syndromes

Peutz-Jeghers Syndrome

- Peutz-Jeghers syndrome is a rare lentiginosis syndrome with features of mucocutaneous lentiginosis and hamartomatous gastrointestinal polyps.
- It follows an autosomal dominant inheritance pattern, with the most commonly reported mutation in the serine-threonine kinase *STK11/LKB1* gene.
- The cutaneous hallmark of this syndrome is small lentigines commonly seen over the lips, oral mucosa, nasal and periorbital regions, elbows, hands/feet, periumbilical, and genital regions.

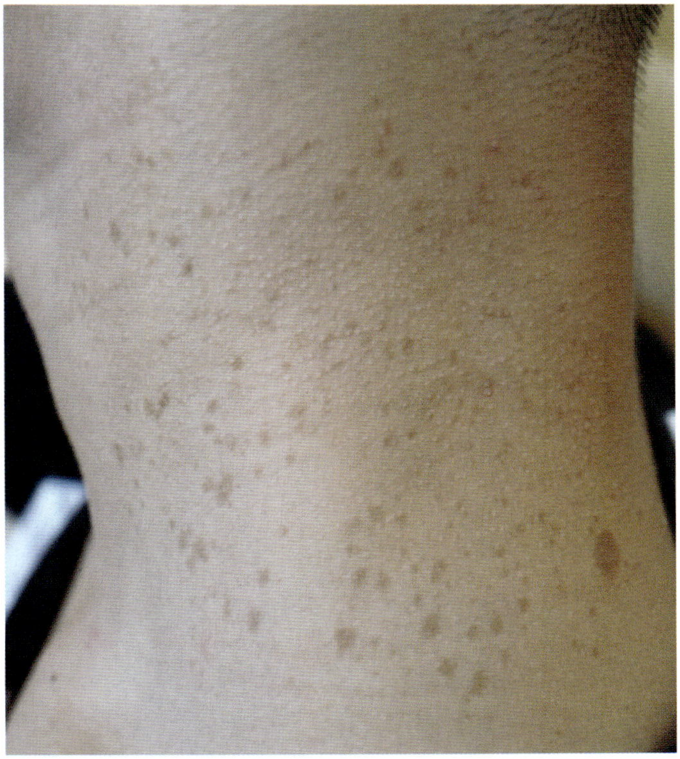

FIGURE 7-38. Multiple lentigines of varying sizes on the neck of a 13-year-old Chinese boy with unilateral partial lentiginosis.

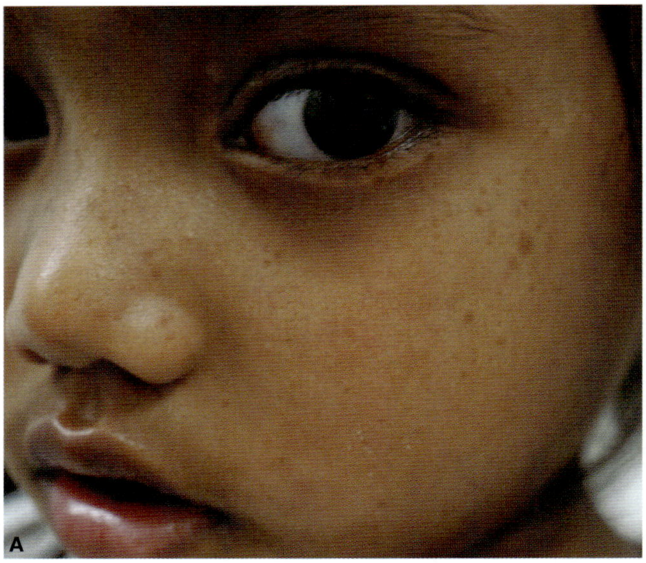

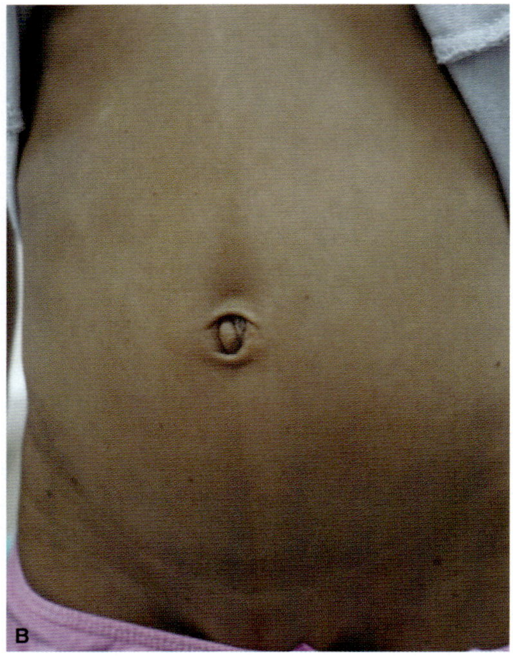

FIGURE 7-39A & 39B. A 7-year-old Malay girl with multiple lentigines over her face and trunk. She also has poor growth and learning difficulties, with suspicion for Noonan syndrome with multiple lentigines (LEOPARD syndrome).

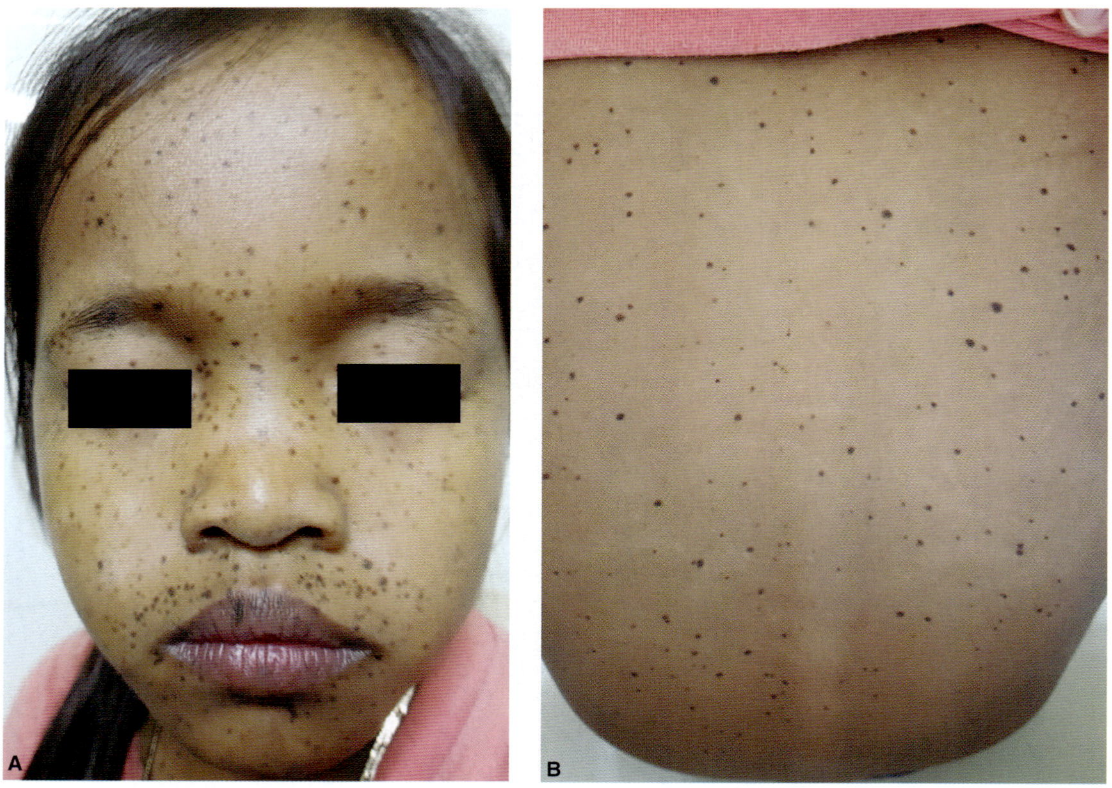

FIGURE 7-40A & 40B. Multiple lentigines in an adolescent Cambodian girl with Noonan syndrome with multiple lentigines (LEOPARD syndrome). She had concomitant heart disease.

- The lesions become apparent in infancy or early childhood and may fade in adulthood. Oral mucosa lesions, however, tend to be more persistent.
- Hamartomatous gastrointestinal polyps may be found anywhere from the stomach to the anal canal, with the small bowel being the most commonly involved portion. These polyps are generally benign and may occur in early childhood, presenting with symptoms of abdominal pain, melena, intestinal obstruction, or intussusception.
- The syndrome is associated with cancers of the gastrointestinal tract, breast, reproductive system, and respiratory system.

Noonan Syndrome with Multiple Lentigines

- Noonan syndrome with multiple lentigines is a RASopathy with an autosomal dominant pattern of inheritance. It is caused by pathogenic variants in one of four genes: *BRAF*, *MAP2K1*, *PTPN11*, or *RAF1*.
- The condition presents with multiple lentigines and features of Noonan syndrome.
- In addition, other findings (abbreviated by the acronym LEOPARD) include:
  - **L**entigines
  - **E**CG conduction defects
  - **O**cular hypertelorism
  - **P**ulmonary stenosis
  - **A**bnormal genitalia
  - **R**etardation of growth
  - **S**ensorineural deafness

Carney Complex

- Carney complex is a rare multiple endocrine neoplasia (MEN) syndrome characterized by pigmented lesions of the skin and mucosa, myxomas in the skin and heart, as well as endocrine abnormalities and tumors. The most commonly reported endocrine tumors include pituitary adenomas, ovarian tumors, testicular tumors, and adrenocortical disease.
- It follows an autosomal dominant pattern of inheritance, with mutations in the protein kinase A type I-α regulatory subunit (*PRKAR1A*) most frequently reported.
- Patients are usually diagnosed in late adolescence, but clinical manifestations may appear as early as infancy.
- Skin lesions are reported in up to 80% of patients, with lentigines the most commonly reported. Lentigines appear around the time of puberty and commonly involve the central face, perioral region, conjunctiva, and intraoral mucosa. Lesions typically fade in adulthood.
- Other cutaneous findings include multiple blue nevi, multiple cutaneous myxomas, and café-au-lait macules.

Differential Diagnoses

- Ephelides (freckles)
  - The pigmentation in ephelides is lighter than that seen in lentigo simplex.
  - The color of ephelides darkens with increased sun exposure. This is less so for lentigines.
- Café-au-lait macules
  - Café-au-lait macules also present as flat, light brown hyperpigmented macules or patches that may be present at birth or in early infancy. The pigmentation is usually darker, and the lesions are larger than lentigines.
- Junctional melanocytic nevi
  - Junctional melanocytic nevi present as smooth, flat, brown or black melanocytic lesions. They share very similar clinical and dermoscopic features with lentigo simplex.
  - Histologically, melanocyte nests are present at the dermal-epidermal junction of junctional nevi. In contrast, there is linear proliferation of melanocytes and no nesting in lentigo simplex.

Investigations & Treatment

- Lentigo simplex can be diagnosed clinically.
- Dermoscopy of lentigo simplex shows a dark uniform network across the entire lesion.
- If there is suspicion of associated syndromes in patients presenting with multiple lentigines, referral to a pediatric dermatologist and/or geneticist for further evaluation and investigation is warranted. Multidisciplinary management involving relevant pediatric specialties may be required, depending on the associated systemic complications.
- Lentigo simplex may be left alone. If treatment is required for cosmetic concern, lentigo simplex may be lightened or removed using the following modalities:
  - Topicals—retinoids, hydroquinone
  - Chemical peels
  - Cryotherapy
  - Laser ablation

Pearls & Practical Tips

- Lentigo simplex may spontaneously fade or disappear over a few years, especially those that appear early in life; those appearing later in life tend to persist.
- It is important to evaluate and monitor pediatric patients with multiple or extensive lentigines for the development of associated abnormalities. As some of the associated cutaneous or systemic features may not manifest until the child is older, genetic testing can be offered for early diagnosis.
- In patients with suspected Peutz-Jeghers syndrome but who test negative for *STK11/LKB1* gene variant, a diagnosis of Laugier-Hunziker syndrome is a differential. These patients present with diffuse oral hyperpigmentation associated with pigmentation of the nails. There are no systemic manifestations in Laugier-Hunziker syndrome.

CAFÉ-AU-LAIT MACULES AND ASSOCIATED SYNDROMES

Café-au-lait macules (CALMs) are common birthmarks which present with flat, medium brown, hyperpigmented skin lesions that may appear anywhere on the body. Most patients have solitary or few lesions. However, patients with an increased number of lesions may have associated genetic syndromes that warrant further evaluation.

Clinical Features

- CALMs arise from an increase in melanin production by melanocytes in the epidermis, with no increase in numbers of melanocytes.
- CALMs commonly present at birth or shortly after birth but may also increase in number or size over time.

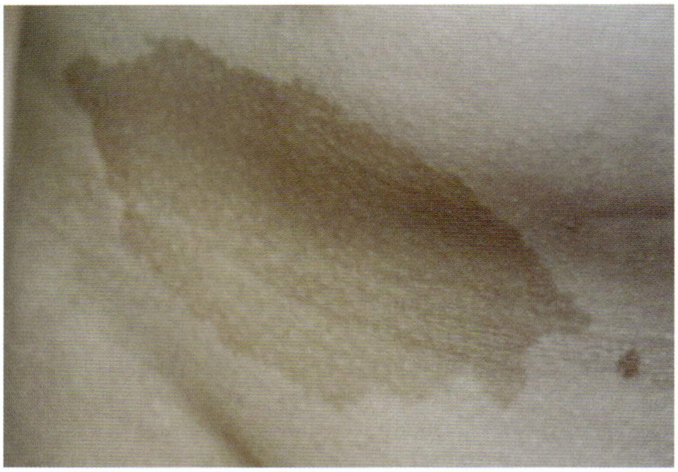

FIGURE 7-41. A large, solitary café-au-lait patch in a 4-year-old Chinese boy.

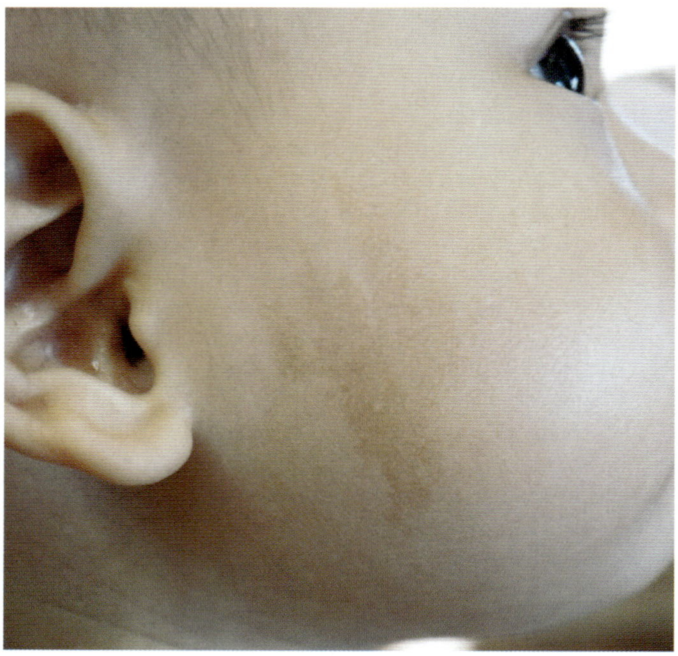

FIGURE 7-42. This café-au-lait patch in a young Chinese infant has a more irregular outline. A differential diagnosis is pigmentary mosaicism.

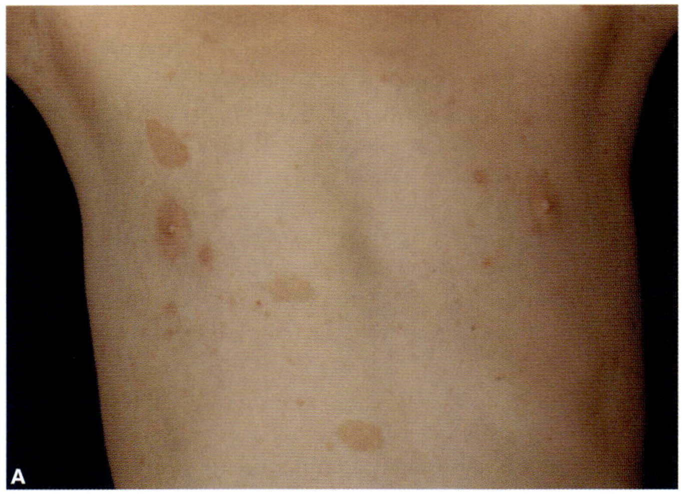

A

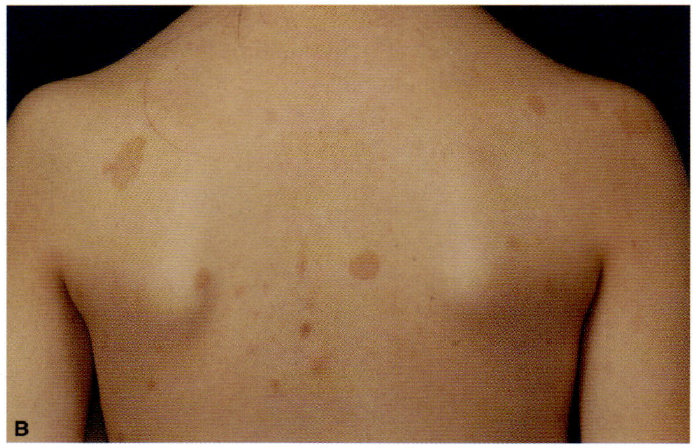

B

FIGURES 7-43A & 43B. A 3-year-old Chinese girl with neurofibromatosis type 1 and multiple café-au-lait macules over her trunk and limbs.

- They can occur anywhere on the skin but are more frequently found on the trunk and extremities, and less frequently on the face.
- Most solitary CALMs have no clinical significance, with their greatest concern being cosmesis.
- The presence of five or more CALMs is generally uncommon and should warrant evaluation for associated syndromes, including neurofibromatosis type-1 (see Chapter 12), neurofibromatosis type-2 (NF-2), Legius syndrome, and McCune-Albright syndrome.

Neurofibromatosis Type-2 (NF-2)

- NF-2 is a rare disorder distinct from NF-1, and arises due to a mutation in the *NF2* gene on chromosome 22, which produces merlin, a tumor suppressor protein. It follows an autosomal dominant pattern of inheritance.
- Apart from CALMs, other clinical features include bilateral acoustic schwannomas, cataracts, meningiomas, ependymomas, and gliomas.

Legius syndrome

- Legius syndrome (also known as NF-1-like syndrome) is characterized by multiple CALMs, axillary freckling, macrocephaly, learning disabilities, and Noonan-syndrome like facial features.
- It is a result of mutations in the *SPRED1* gene on chromosome 15q14. SPRED1 is a negative regulator of the RAS/MAPK signaling pathway, thereby affecting cell proliferation, differentiation and apoptosis.
- Patients with Legius syndrome do not have neurofibromas, central nervous system tumors, or skeletal and eye abnormalities as seen in NF-1.

McCune-Albright Syndrome

- McCune-Albright syndrome is a rare genetic condition secondary to a mosaic mutation in the *GNAS* gene occurring during early embryonic development.
- It classically presents with a triad of CALMs, bony fibrous dysplasia, and hyperfunctioning hormonal disorders (e.g., precocious puberty, hyperthyroidism, hypercortisolism).
- The CALMs in McCune-Albright syndrome are typically irregularly bordered ("coast of Maine" appearance), unilateral, and follow the lines of Blaschko.

Differential Diagnoses

- Lentigines
  - Lentigines present as small, pigmented, brown to black flat lesions on the skin with a clearly defined edge, which typically develop in early childhood. The pigmentation is generally darker than that seen in CALMs. CALMs are also larger than lentigines.
- Congenital melanocytic nevus
  - Congenital melanocytic nevi present with brown or black birthmarks that are mostly visible at birth. The pigmentation is generally darker than that seen in CALMs, and lesions can be papular.
- Nevus spilus
  - Nevus spilus are fairly common pigmented lesions that typically consist of a lighter brown background patch with scattered small, darker brown speckles within.
  - It may be differentiated from CALM by the presence of these darker brown speckles. However, at initial appearance, the darker brown speckles may not be obvious.
- Becker's nevus
  - This is a pigmented hamartoma, which occurs more commonly in males during childhood or adolescence. It presents with a large unilateral brown patch or plaque, most commonly over the upper chest or shoulder. It tends to darken during puberty, with increased hair growth.

Investigations & Treatment

- CALMs are diagnosed clinically. If performed, histology demonstrates an increase in melanin along the basal layer of the epidermis.
- Generally, if there are fewer than five lesions and there are no other clinical manifestations, no further investigations are required. If there are five or more lesions, further evaluation for an associated syndrome should be instituted, including referral to a pediatric dermatologist and/or geneticist.
- Treatment of CALMs is not clinically indicated.
- For cosmetic purposes, lasers such as the Nd:YAG, Alexandrite, or Ruby lasers may be used. Multiple treatment sessions are required, and results are highly variable.

Pearls & Practical Tips

- A thorough history and physical examination in the clinic plus a high index of suspicion for associated genetic syndromes is crucial when a patient presents with multiple CALMs.
- The risk of recurrence after laser therapy is high.

Bibliography

1. Anderson S. Café au lait macules and associated genetic syndromes. J Pediatr Health Care 2020;34(1):71-81.

DERMAL MELANOSIS

Dermal melanoses is a group of related conditions caused by spindled or stellate melanocytes found in the dermis. The distinctive bluish-gray color is attributed to the Tyndall effect, where shorter wavelengths of light are reflected by dermal melanocytes. They comprise Mongolian blue spots, nevus of Ota, and nevus of Ito. They are especially common in children of pigmented races, particularly Asians.

Clinical Features

- Common dermal melanoses include Mongolian blue spots, nevus of Ota, and nevus of Ito. In general, the dermal melanoses present with grayish-blue flat macules or patches.
- They are benign lesions with no malignant potential, and most are not associated with any syndromes.
- Mongolian blue spots
  - Also known as lumbosacral dermal melanocytosis.
  - Present with flat, grayish-blue, and often poorly circumscribed patches, typically located over the lumbosacral areas and buttocks, but may also present in extra-axial locations such as the ankles, wrists, legs, upper back, flanks, and shoulders of infants.
  - Mongolian blue spots are present at birth and tend to fade during the first years of life. However, they may persist in extra-axial locations, especially larger lesions (>10 cm) or if very extensive.
  - Rarely, large and extensive Mongolian spots may be associated with inborn errors of metabolism or appear in association with other vascular or pigmentary anomalies (e.g., phakomatosis pigmentovascularis).

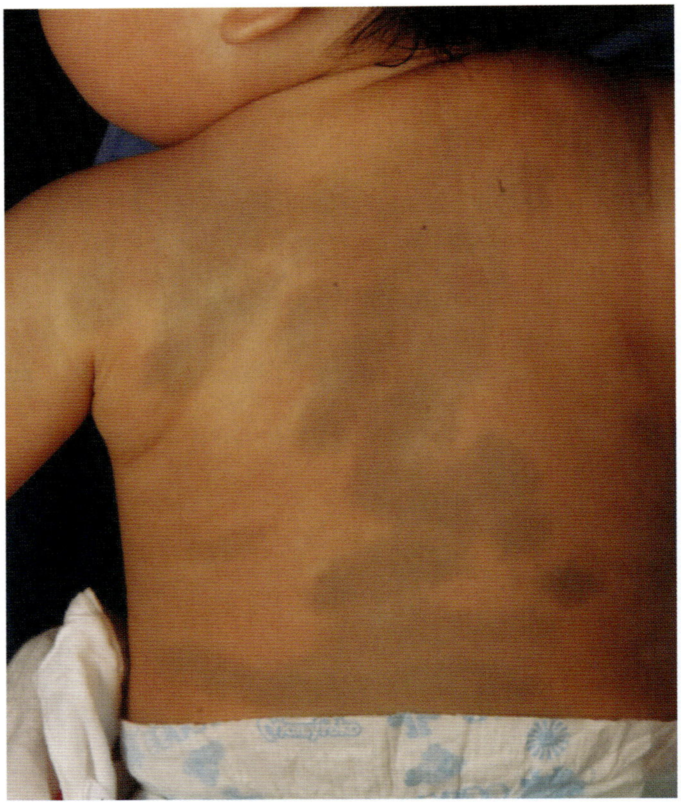

FIGURE 7-44. A 1-year-old baby girl with fairly extensive dermal melanosis/Mongolian spots over her back, presenting as flat, light gray patches.

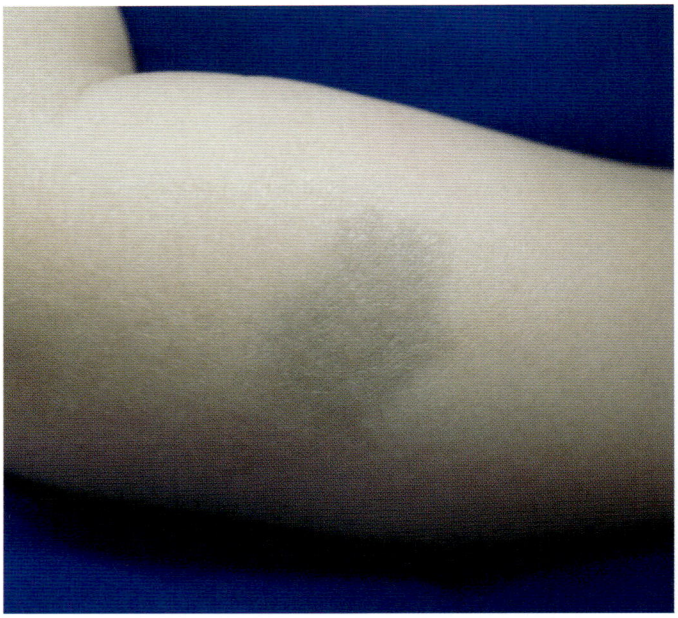

FIGURE 7-45. Dermal melanosis on the arm of a Chinese infant. This may not totally fade when the child is older.

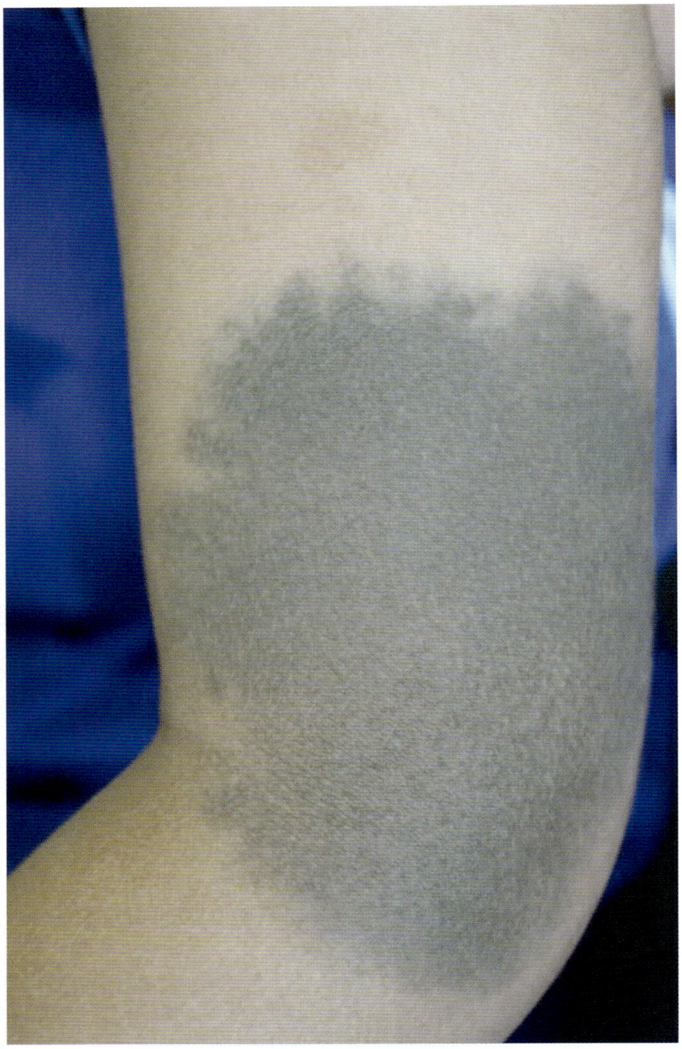

FIGURE 7-46. Dermal melanosis on the elbow and upper arm of an older child. As in the previous photograph, it is unlikely that this lesion will totally fade as the child grows older.

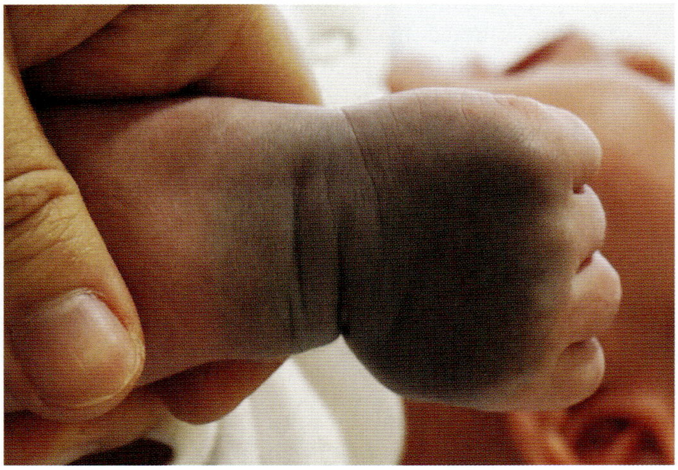

FIGURE 7-47. Dermal melanosis on the hand of a darker-skinned neonate at birth.

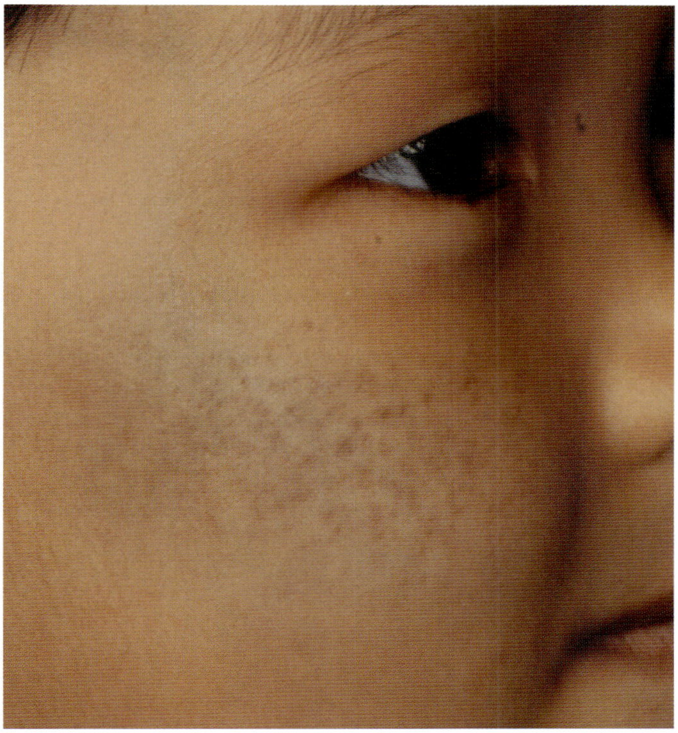

FIGURE 7-48. Nevus of Ota on the cheek of a 7-year-old Chinese girl. Note that apart from the bluish-gray pigmentation, there are also small macules that appear more light brown.

- Nevus of Ota and nevus of Ito
  - Nevus of Ota and nevus of Ito present with flat, grayish-blue and poorly circumscribed macular lesions which are often unilateral but may be bilateral. Some patients have lesions that are a combination of brown and grayish-blue hues.
  - They do not spontaneously fade, and can darken during puberty.
  - Nevus of Ota commonly involves the periorbital, temple, forehead, malar region, and nose.
  - About 60% of patients with Nevus of Ota have a patchy blue hyperpigmentation of the ipsilateral sclera. Melanocytosis may also occasionally affect the conjunctiva, cornea, and retina. There is an increased risk of uveal melanoma and glaucoma in these cases.
  - Nevus of Ito is less common and involves the shoulder girdle and upper arm area, following the territory of the lateral cutaneous brachial nerve and posterior supraclavicular nerves.

Differential Diagnoses

- Congenital melanocytic nevus
  - Large Mongolian spots may be confused with large congenital melanocytic nevi. The latter appear browner, have a rough surface, and are usually palpable.
- Bruises/ecchymoses
  - A thorough history of the skin lesions can help to differentiate bruises from dermal melanosis. Bruises are usually tender and their color evolves over time with resolution of the purpura.
- Venous or venolymphatic malformations
  - These may present as bluish patches on the skin. They are warmer than surrounding skin and are usually raised compared to lesions of dermal melanosis. In doubtful cases, imaging, such as ultrasound, may help to differentiate.
- Becker's nevus
  - Becker's nevus is a late-onset pigmented hamartoma, which occurs more commonly in males and generally develops during childhood or adolescence.
  - Patients present with a large unilateral brown patch or plaque over the shoulder girdle (similar in location to the nevus of Ito), which may become darker and hairy over time.

Investigations & Treatment

- No investigations are required for diagnosis, as the dermal melanoses are diagnosed clinically.

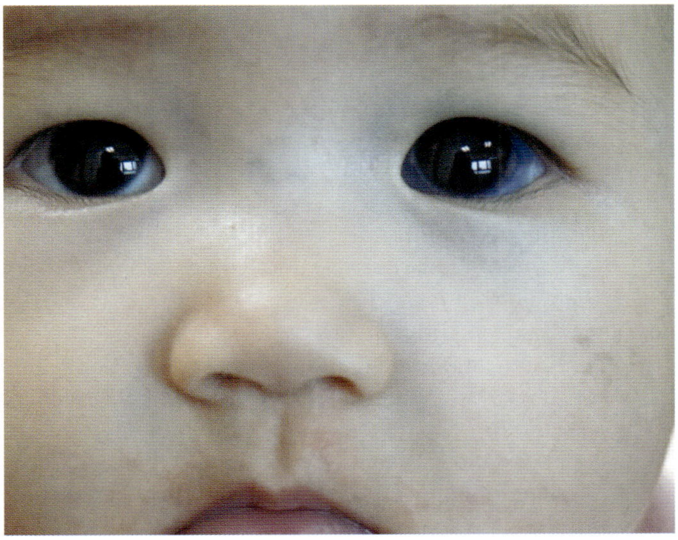

FIGURE 7-49. Nevus of Ota on the left cheek and temporal area in a 1-year-old Chinese girl. There is ipsilateral scleral pigmentation.

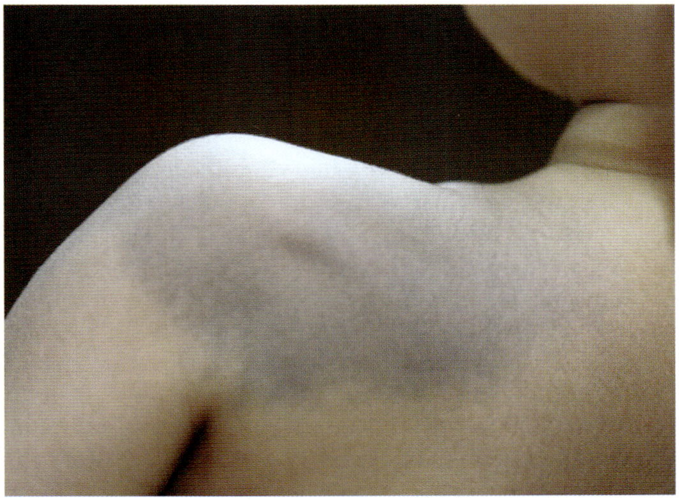

FIGURE 7-50. Nevus of Ito on the left shoulder in a 2-year-old Chinese boy.

- Skin biopsies are not required; however, if performed, demonstrate spindle-shaped melanocytes located deep in the dermis.
- Therapy is not necessary for Mongolian blue spots, as they are expected to fade with age. Pigment lasers may be considered in older children to treat any incompletely faded lesions, for better cosmesis.
- Laser therapy may improve the appearance of nevus of Ota and nevus of Ito. Common lasers used include the Nd:YAG nano- or picosecond laser and Q-switched alexandrite laser. Multiple sessions are often necessary, and there is a risk of recurrence after clearance.
- For patients with nevus of Ota, referral to a pediatric ophthalmologist for baseline eye examination and annual screening should be made.

Pearls & Practical Tips

- Addressing parental concerns regarding cosmesis, and reassurance regarding the benign nature and good prognosis of Mongolian spots is helpful.
- We generally start treating nevus of Ota early with lasers, even from a few months of life. Initially, this can be done without general anesthesia or sedation. However, this is required when the child becomes older.
- The use of metal internal ocular eye shields is important when lasering near the eyes, even if the child is under general anesthesia.

Bibliography

1. Alimi Y, Iwanaga J, Loukas M, Oskouian RJ, et al. A comprehensive review of Mongolian spots with an update on atypical presentations. Childs Nerv Syst 2018;34(12):2371-6.
2. Sinha S, Cohen PJ, Schwartz RA. Nevus of Ota in children. Cutis 2008;82:25-9.

PIGMENTARY DEMARCATION LINES

The skin of darker-skinned children differs physiologically from that of lighter-skinned children. The presence of pigmentary demarcation lines over the face and extremities is one example of this. Pigmentary demarcation lines, or Voigt-Futcher pigmentary demarcation lines, refer to physiologically normal, abrupt transitions between hyperpigmented and lighter skin.

Clinical Features

- Pigmentary demarcation lines are a physiological variant of normal skin and are found more commonly in darker-skinned individuals. They are classified based on their location (Table 7-4).
- They are usually persistent with the exception of those arising during pregnancy, which improve spontaneously after delivery.
- Patients may present with significant cosmetic concerns, especially when the lines involve the face.
- The pathogenesis is unclear, and there are several hypotheses, including hormonal causes, stimulation of peripheral cutaneous nerves, and pigmentary mosaicism.

TABLE 7-4. Classification of PDLs by anatomical location.[3]

PDL Type	Anatomical location
Type A	Lines along the upper limb with variable transpectoral extension
Type B	Lines along the lower limb
Type C	Paired lines in median or paramedian course on the chest with midline abdominal extension
Type D	Posteromedian demarcation
Type E	Bilaterally symmetrical, obliquely oriented hypopigmented macules on the chest
Type F (Facial)	Inverted cone-shaped patch extending from the lateral orbital rim and pointing inferiorly or inferolaterally
Type G (Facial)	Two inverted cones extending from the orbital rims and pointing inferiorly, with a rim of normal pigmentation in between, forming a W-shaped patch
Type H (Facial)	Linear and hyperpigmented, stretching from the lateral corners of the mouth

Differential Diagnoses

- Pigmentary mosaicism
  - Pigmentary mosaicism refers to varied patterns of pigmentation in the skin, which tend to follow the embryonic lines of Blaschko. Pigmentary demarcation lines do not follow any embryonic lines.
- Post-inflammatory hyperpigmentation
  - This is an acquired cause of pigmentary change.
  - The diagnosis of post-inflammatory hyperpigmentation may be established and differentiated from pigmentary demarcation lines with a supportive history of a previous inflammatory dermatosis in the affected areas, as well as the appearance of lesions corresponding to the location of the previous inflammatory dermatosis.
- Melasma
  - Melasma is a common acquired form of facial pigmentation that presents as bilateral, blotchy, brownish pigmentation over the malar region. This is a differential for pigmentary demarcation lines on the face.
- Nevus of Ota/Ito
  - Nevus of Ota and Ito are forms of dermal melanosis which have a slate-brown or blue/gray color and are commonly unilateral.
  - Nevus of Ota is classically located over the forehead and face, near the eye.
  - Nevus of Ito is classically located on the shoulder and shoulder girdle.

Investigations & Treatment

- No investigations are required for diagnosis, as pigmentary demarcation lines can be diagnosed by their clinical appearance.
- Skin biopsy is not required for diagnosis; however, biopsies done in some studies have demonstrated the following features:

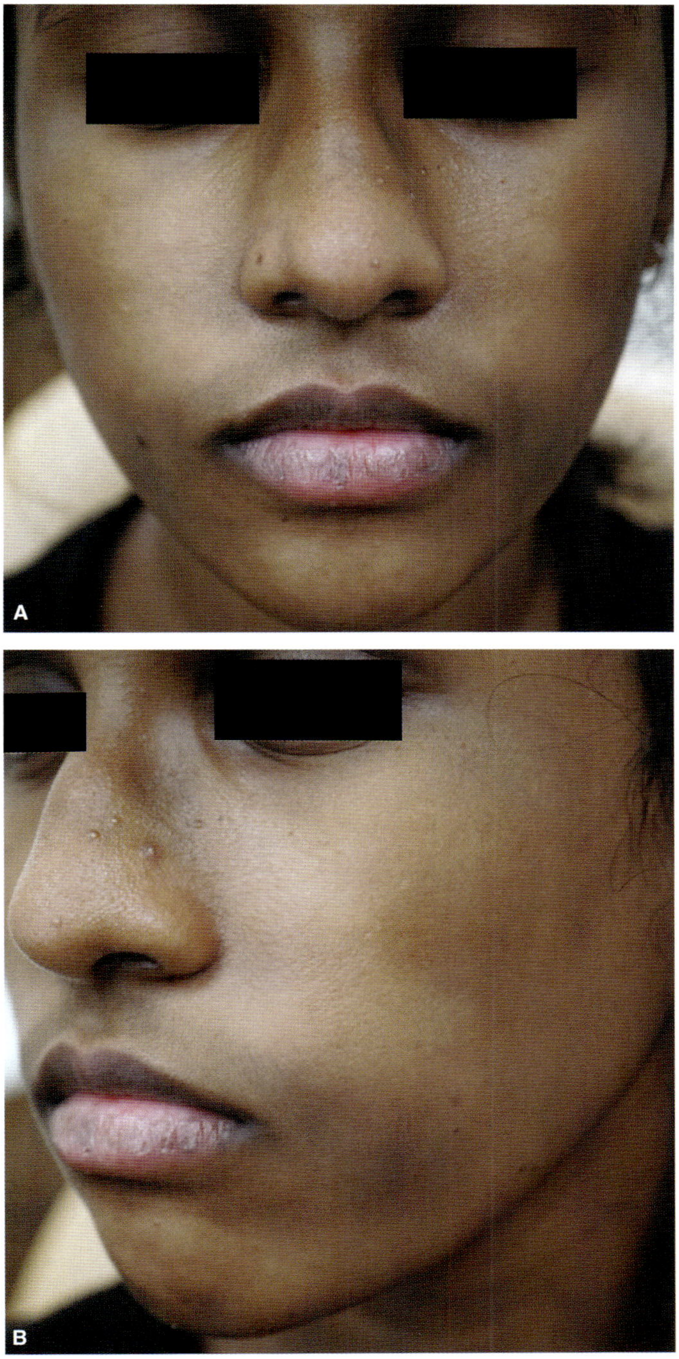

FIGURE 7-51A & 51B. Various pigmentary demarcation lines on the face of a 15-year-old Indian adolescent girl.

  - Lymphocyte infiltration around vessels in the upper dermis with mild basal layer hyperpigmentation. Basal and suprabasal pigmentation with mild pigment incontinence in the papillary dermis.
- Reassurance and addressing the patient's cosmetic concerns is important, as patients tend to be highly troubled by the condition.
- Camouflage makeup may be advised if there is cosmetic concern.
- Complete clearance of pigmentary demarcation lines may be challenging, and patient expectations should be managed.
- Suggested treatment modalities that may lighten the pigmentation include:
  - Kligman's regime—combination of topical hydroquinone, dexamethasone, and tretinoin
  - Chemical peels
  - Lasers, such as Q-switched alexandrite laser

Pearls & Practical Tips

- Pigmentary demarcation lines contribute to the presence of periorbital dark circles in some individuals. Recognize the pattern when there is extension beyond the orbit into the temple area.
- Sunscreen and sun avoidance are important to prevent further darkening.
- Recognizing this entity can help to manage patient's expectations with regard to treatment of facial hyperpigmentation.

References

1. Zieleniewski, L, Schwartz, RA, Goldberg, DJ, Handler, MZ. Voigt-Futcher pigmentary demarcation lines. J Cosmet Dermatol 2019;18:700-2.
2. Bukhari IA. Effective treatment of Futcher's lines with Q-switched alexandrite laser. J Cosmet Dermatol 2005;4:27-8.
3. Somani VK, Razvi F, Sita VN. Pigmentary demarcation lines over the face. Indian J Dermatol Venereol Leprol 2004;70:336-41.

PIGMENTARY MOSAICISM

Pigmentary mosaicism refers to a group of disorders characterized by various patterns of hyper- and/or hypopigmentation of the skin, distributed along the lines of Blaschko. This reflects somatic mosaicism of the affected skin cells and may arise from a wide range of genetic mutations. The majority of patients with pigmentary mosaicism do not have extracutaneous abnormalities and do not require long-term follow-up.

Clinical Features

- Pigmentary mosaicism is the term used to describe a group of conditions previously known as hypomelanosis of Ito, linear and whorled nevoid hypermelanosis, cutis tricolor, and segmental nevus depigmentosus.
- Pigmentary mosaicism is characterized as patterns of hypo- and/or hyperpigmentation, which follow the migration lines of embryonic keratinocytes and melanocytes, known as the lines of Blaschko.
- Solitary lesions are called nevus depigmentosus.
- The pattern of pigmentation may be noticed at birth or in early childhood, particularly after receiving sun exposure. The trunk is most affected, but it may also involve other areas such asthe limbs, and face.
- Various patterns of pigmentation have been described:
  - Narrow or broad bands in a Blaschkoid distribution
  - Phylloid (leaf-like) pattern

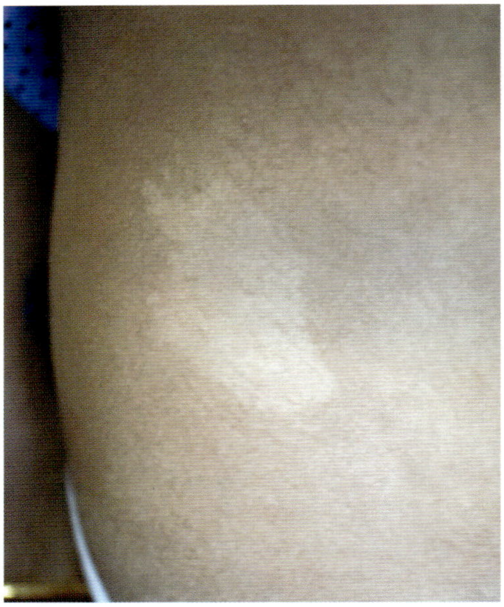

FIGURE 7-52. Nevus depigmentosus on the abdomen of a 4-year-old Indian girl, which was present at birth, and presenting as a well-demarcated hypopigmented patch with regular borders.

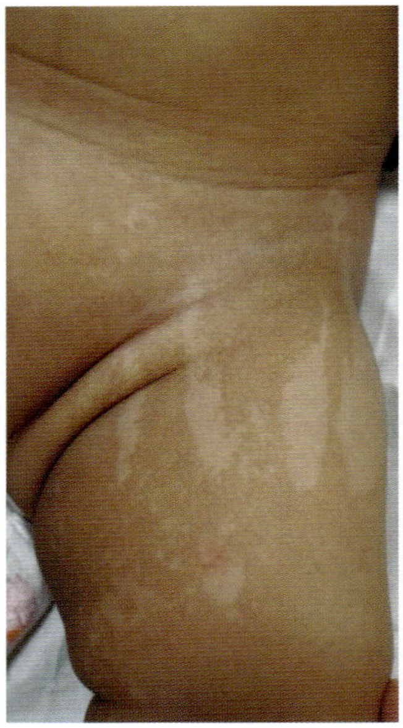

FIGURE 7-53. Pigmentary mosaicism presenting as broad hypopigmented streaks in a Blaschkoid distribution on the left thigh of a Chinese infant.

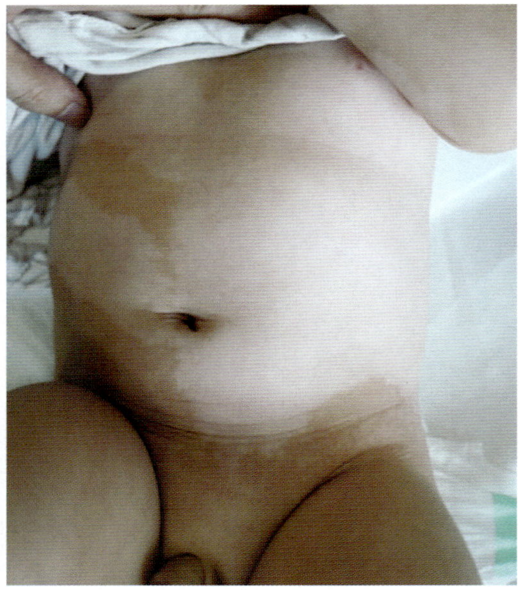

FIGURE 7-54. Hyperpigmented patches in a patchy pattern without midline separation in a Chinese infant with pigmentary mosaicism.

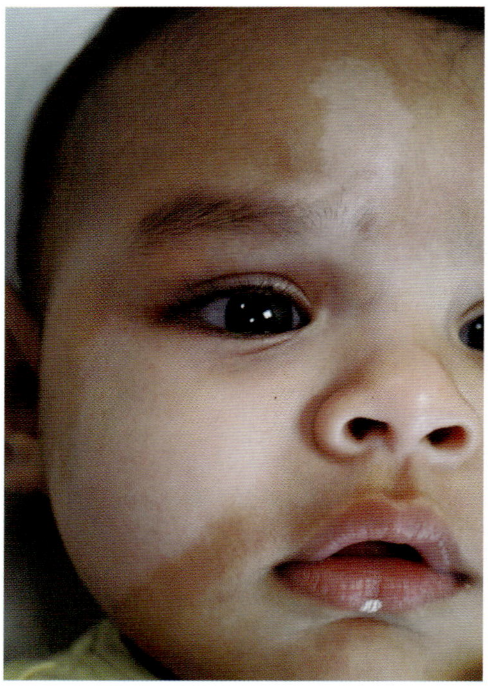

FIGURE 7-55. Hypopigmented patches on the face in an Indian infant with pigmentary mosaicism. Note the absence of leukotrichia.

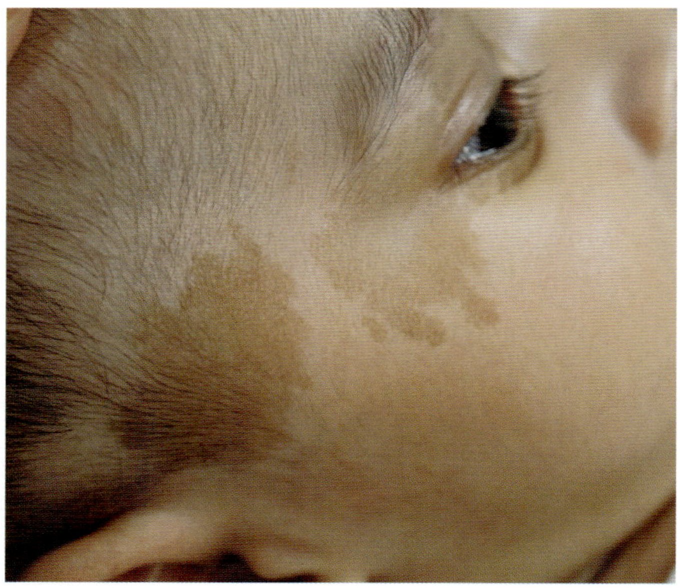

FIGURE 7-56. Irregular hyperpigmented patches on the upper eyelid and temporal region of an Indian infant with pigmentary mosaicism.

- Checkerboard/blocklike pattern
- Patchy pattern without midline separation
- Lateralization
- Sash-like pattern

- Pigmentary mosaicism has been associated with extracutaneous abnormalities, particularly in the musculoskeletal system, central nervous system, and eyes. However, the reported incidence of extracutaneous involvement varies widely and is generally considered to be uncommon.

Differential Diagnoses

- Vitiligo
  - Nevus depigmentosus is often confused with early hypopigmented lesions of vitiligo, as both fluoresce with Wood's lamp examination. However, congenital vitiligo is rare and controversial and should be a diagnosis of exclusion.
- Post-inflammatory dyspigmentation
  - More extensive post-inflammatory dyspigmentation in infants and young toddlers may be mistaken for pigmentary mosaicism. In younger children, the extensive post-inflammatory dyspigmentation is frequently secondary to atopic dermatitis, xerosis, or seborrheic dermatitis. A history of preceding rash or scaling would point to post-inflammatory pigmentary changes.
- Café-au-lait macules
  - These are coffee brown-colored macules or patches, which may be of different sizes. Larger or segmental lesions may resemble pigmentary mosaicism, as these are present from birth.
- Incontinentia pigmenti
  - An X-linked dominant condition due to a mutation in the *IKBKG* gene, predominantly affecting females. There are four stages of skin manifestations: verrucous, vesicular, hyperpigmentation, hypopigmentation. The hyper- or hypopigmented stages may be confused with pigmentary mosaicism. There is association with extracutaneous abnormalities including dental, hair, nail, skeletal, neurological, and ophthalmological manifestations.
- Tuberous sclerosis
  - An autosomal dominant, multisystem disorder associated with benign tumors in the kidneys, heart, lungs, and brain as well as neurodevelopmental issues. Hypopigmented macules present early in life and are usually oval-shaped with smooth regular borders (ash-leaf spots). They do not follow the lines of Blaschko. These ash-leaf spots can resemble nevus depigmentosus.

Investigations & Treatment

- Diagnosis is largely clinical, and investigations are usually not required for diagnosis. Careful skin examination helps to determine the extent and location of the cutaneous findings.
- Systematic history and clinical examination to identify extracutaneous signs and symptoms should pay attention to growth and development, neurological, musculoskeletal, and ophthalmological examinations.
- Routine follow-up for developmental milestones is important to detect early developmental and neurological issues.
- It is important to engage and reassure parents on the condition. The affected areas grow proportionately with the child and do not spontaneously resolve.
- Strategies to make pigmentary mosaicism less noticeable include sun protection and camouflage makeup. Lasers are typically not effective.

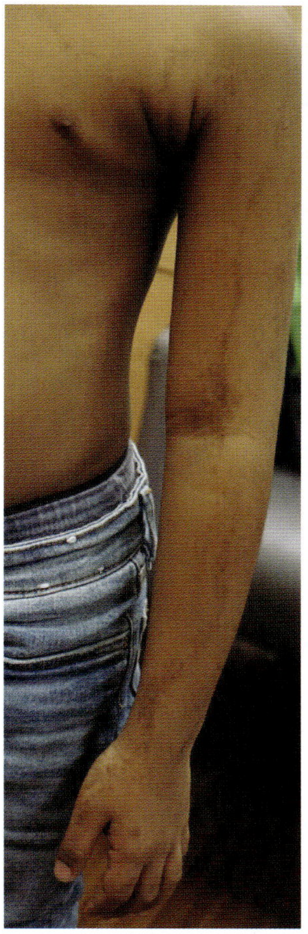

FIGURE 7-57. Hyperpigmented linear bands in a Blaschkoid pattern on the left arm and shoulder of an Indian boy with pigmentary mosaicism.

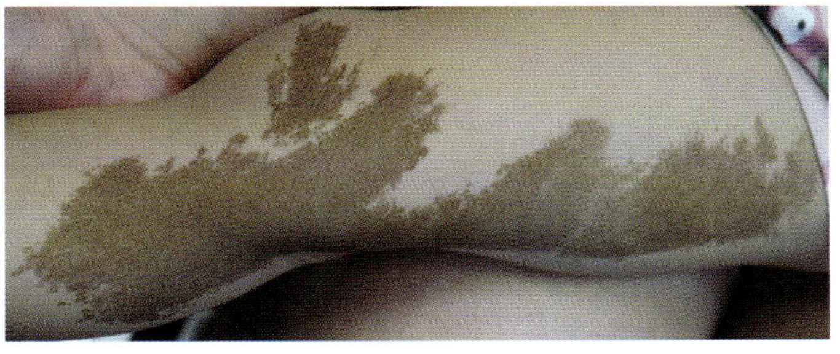

FIGURE 7-58. Pigmentary mosaicism on the leg of a young Chinese girl with hyperpigmented patches following a "phylloid" pattern.

Pearls & Practical Tips

- It may be difficult to distinguish between normal skin and hypopigmented lesions, particularly in lighter-skinned individuals. Similarly, in darker-skinned individuals it may be difficult to distinguish the normal from the affected areas. Examination with good, natural lighting and with the aid of a Wood's lamp is important.

POST-INFLAMMATORY DYSPIGMENTATION

Post-inflammatory dyspigmentation is one of the most common causes of hypo- and hyperpigmentation. The exact mechanism is unclear, but it is thought to be a reaction to cutaneous inflammation or trauma. Melanocytes may respond to this stimulus with either increased or decreased levels of melanin, and this tendency may be genetically and racially predetermined.

Clinical Features

- Post-inflammatory dyspigmentation can occur at any age and affects both males and females equally.
- It is more prevalent in darker-skinned phototypes (Fitzpatrick IV–VI).
- Cutaneous inflammation may be *endogenous* or *exogenous*. Endogenous causes include inflammatory dermatoses (e.g., atopic dermatitis, acne), drug-induced, or infections (e.g., impetigo, varicella). Exogenous causes occur due to external insults to the skin (e.g., trauma, chemical or thermal injuries).
- It presents as asymptomatic macules and/or patches with varying degrees of hypo- or hyperpigmentation (Figures 7-58 and 7-59).
- The distribution, size, and shape of the lesions corresponds to the areas affected by the previous insult. Often, the underlying dermatoses may still be present to aid diagnosis.

Differential Diagnoses

Post-inflammatory hyperpigmentation

- Idiopathic eruptive macular pigmentation
  - This condition is of unknown etiology and affects mainly younger individuals. It presents as an eruption of brown-black, discrete, non-confluent, asymptomatic macules that involve the neck, trunk, and proximal extremities. Unlike post-inflammatory dyspigmentation, there are usually no preceding inflammatory lesions or identifiable drug causes.
- Fixed drug eruption
  - An allergic reaction to a drug, in which well-defined, oval, or circular hyperpigmented macules characteristically recur in the same site(s) each time a particular drug is taken. Common sites include the hands and feet, lips, genitalia, and perianal regions. Positive history of drug intake preceding pigmentation is suggestive.
- Erythema dyschromicum perstans
  - Macules tend to be gray in color and are well-circumscribed, round to oval, or irregular patches on the face, neck, and trunk. Occurs more frequently in young adults than children. The exact cause is unknown.

Post-inflammatory hypopigmentation

- Early vitiligo
  - Early lesions of vitiligo exhibit hypopigmentation before progressing to complete depigmentation. A Wood's lamp examination may accentuate the early vitiligo lesions and distinguish from post-inflammatory hypopigmentation. Lack of preceding rash helps to distinguish from post-inflammatory hypopigmentation.
- Pityriasis alba
  - Some may consider pityriasis alba a form of post-inflammatory hypopigmentation occurring on the face secondary to a mild dermatosis that has resolved, such as atopic dermatitis. It most commonly occurs on the face of young children. There is often a history of worsening or appearance after a period of sun exposure.
- Tinea versicolor
  - The active lesions in tinea versicolor are typically scaly and may be accompanied by pruritus. They may range from hypopigmented to erythematous or hyperpigmented. Sites of predilection include the trunk, neck, and arms.
- Mycosis fungoides
  - This is the most common form of cutaneous T-cell lymphoma, and most commonly presents in Asian children as hypopigmented patches, mostly over the sun-covered sites of the trunk, especially the buttocks, but also over sun-exposed sites in more extensively affected individuals. There is often a slight scaling and mild erythema. In doubtful cases, punch biopsies may be performed to confirm the diagnosis.

Investigations & Treatment

- Post-inflammatory dyspigmentation is primarily a clinical diagnosis.
- A thorough history of any prior skin inflammation/rashes, drug use, or skin injury should be taken. Careful examination of the affected sites to exclude other causes is important.
- Early treatment and resolution of the initial insult can help to lessen the extent of dyspigmentation and aid in faster recovery.
- Adequate photoprotection is important to avoid aggravating the dyspigmentation.
- Gradual improvement over a period of months to years is expected and patients should be reassured and counselled appropriately.
- Active treatment for post-inflammatory hyperpigmentation (e.g., bleaching agents, chemical peels, lasers, and light therapy) is generally not recommended in children due to poor efficacy and a high risk of side effects.

Pearls & Practical Tips

- Emphasis should be placed on the prevention and/or early treatment of the underlying dermatosis or cutaneous insult, rather than the dyspigmentation itself.
- Sun avoidance and the use of sunscreens are important to reduce aggravation of the condition.

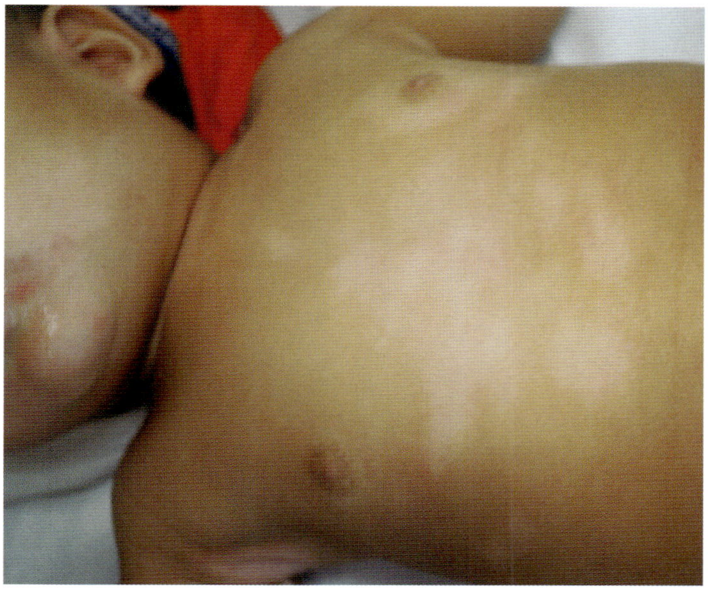

FIGURE 7-59. Post-inflammatory hypopigmentation on the trunk of a Chinese infant after atopic dermatitis. Residual mild erythema is still seen.

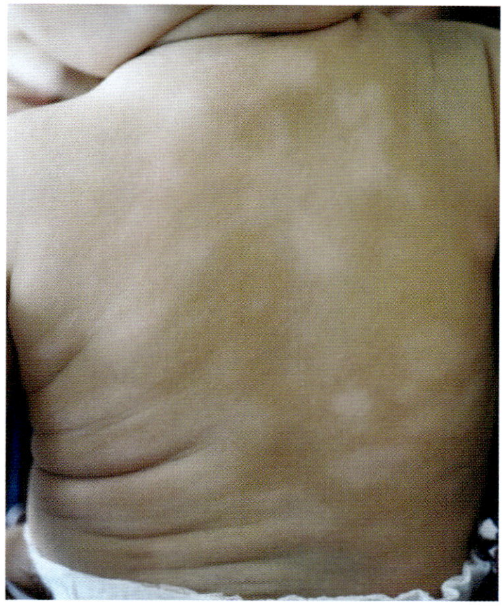

FIGURE 7-60. Extensive post-inflammatory hypopigmentation on the back of a Chinese infant with infantile atopic dermatitis.

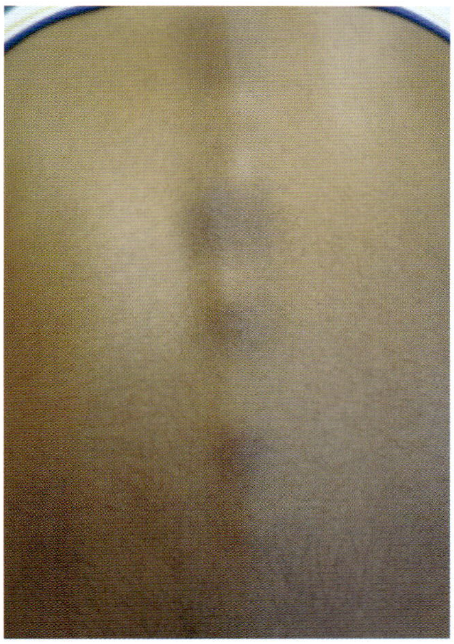

FIGURE 7-61. Post-inflammatory hyperpigmentation secondary to frictional dermatitis (Davener's dermatosis)

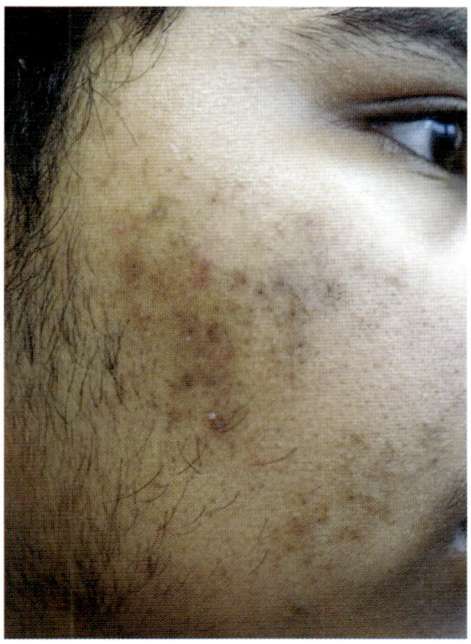

FIGURE 7-62. Indian adolescent male with post-inflammatory hyperpigmentation secondary to moderately severe acne vulgaris.

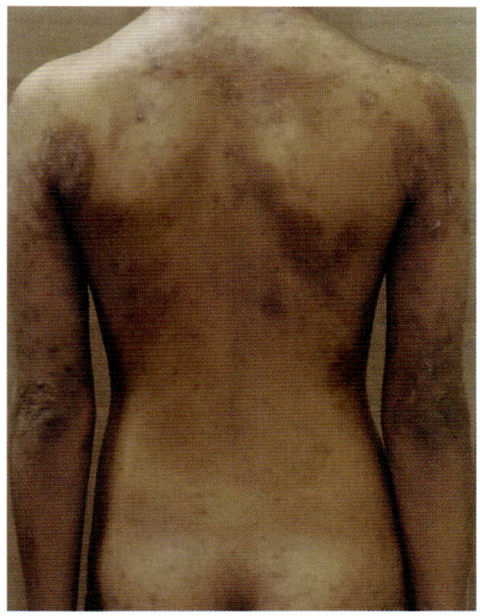

FIGURE 7-63. Extensive, patchy post-inflammatory hyperpigmentation in a Malay adolescent boy with chronic atopic dermatitis and prurigo nodules.

8

Vasculitis, Autoimmune and Photodermatology

LEUKOCYTOCLASTIC VASCULITIS & HENOCH-SCHONLEIN PURPURA

Leukocytoclastic vasculitis (LCV), also known as hypersensitivity vasculitis, is a fairly common disease process that involves vasculitic inflammation of small vessels in the skin. It can either be isolated to the skin or involve other organs such as the kidneys. In children, the most common variant is Henoch-Schonlein purpura (HSP). Other causes of LCV include infections, drugs, and connective tissue diseases. HSP is an acute, systemic IgA-mediated small vessel vasculitis that presents with palpable purpura variably associated with joint, abdominal, and renal involvement.

Clinical Features

- LCV, especially in children, usually occurs in response to an underlying infectious process (Streptococci, hepatitis, salmonella, and mycobacterial infection) or may be drug-induced (beta-lactam antibiotics, NSAIDs, antiepileptic drugs, and sulfur-containing drugs). Other causes include connective tissue disorders and rarely, malignancy.
- Palpable purpura is the hallmark manifestation of cutaneous LCV and HSP. Lesions usually appear over gravity-dependent areas such as the lower limbs, sacrum, or over areas of trauma. There may also be petechiae and ecchymoses, with associated pitting edema over these areas.
- Occasionally, urticated papules, vesicles, pustules, or necrotic lesions may be present. Smaller lesions may manifest as petechiae. In severe cases, hemorrhagic blisters may occur, resulting in erosion and ulceration of the skin.

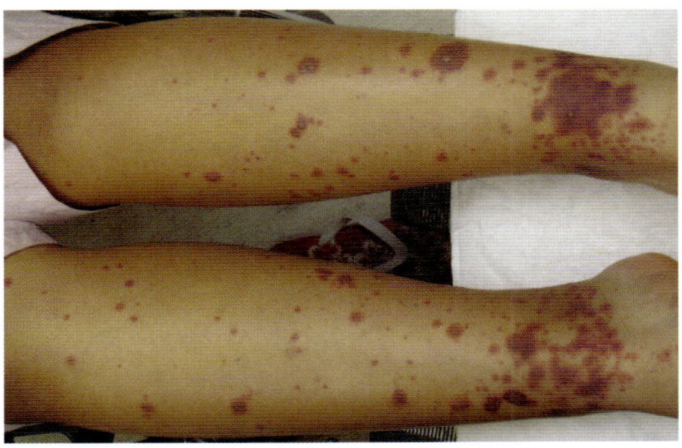

FIGURE 8-1. LCV in a Chinese adolescent girl, presenting with palpable purpura with small hemorrhagic bullae on her lower limbs.

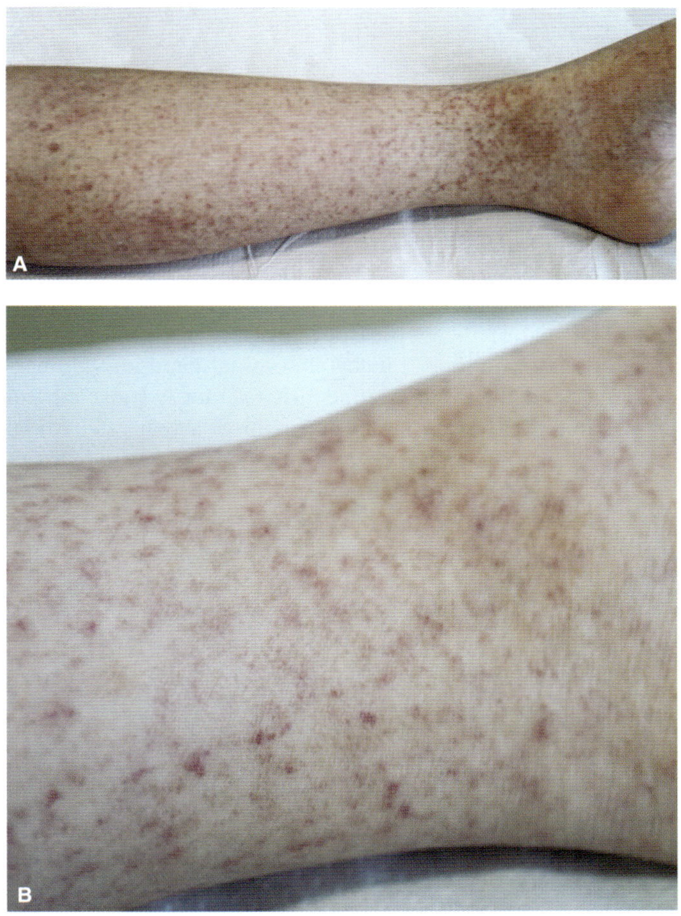

FIGURE 8-2A & 2B. LCV on the legs of a Chinese adolescent girl, presenting as small palpable purpura. She has underlying connective tissue disease.

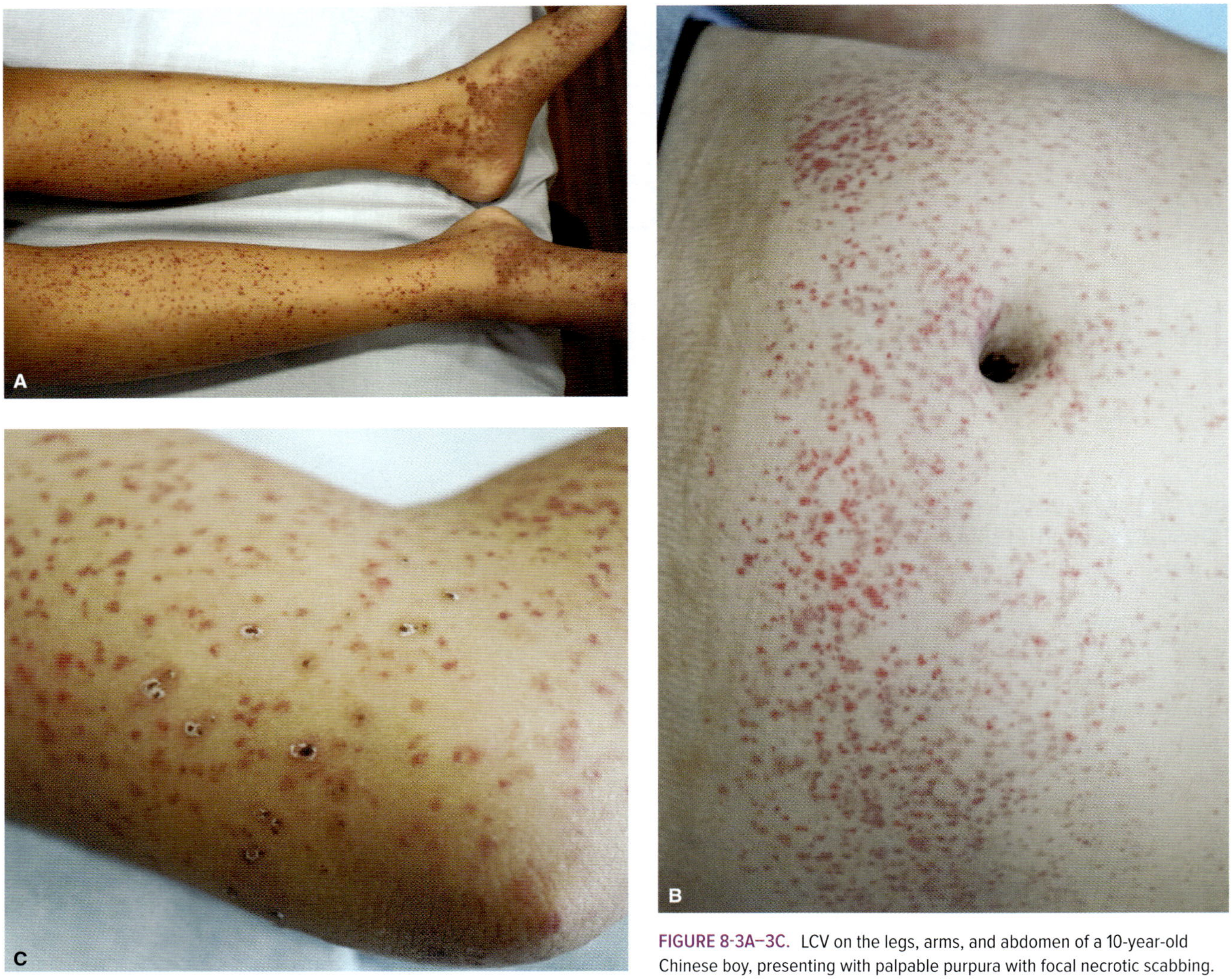

FIGURE 8-3A–3C. LCV on the legs, arms, and abdomen of a 10-year-old Chinese boy, presenting with palpable purpura with focal necrotic scabbing.

- Systemic involvement is variable, but is more common in HSP, with patients presenting with joint pain with periarticular swelling, colicky abdominal pain, and glomerulonephritis. Glomerulonephritis is mostly transient and benign. However, it can occur up to a year after initial presentation. Initial renal insufficiency is a predictor of prolonged HSP nephritis.
- It may be difficult to differentiate HSP from other forms of LCV solely on the cutaneous presentation, especially in the absence of other systemic features. Skin biopsy for immunofluorescence may help to differentiate, with IgA deposition seen within the vessel walls in HSP and IgG and C3 deposition in other forms of LCV.

Differential Diagnoses

- Pigmented purpuric dermatosis (PPD)
  - PPD is a form of capillaritis which often presents on bilateral lower limbs. It may be challenging to distinguish HSP from PPD, especially on initial presentation where lesions may first appear purpuric before turning into a characteristic reddish-brown hue. Histology and direct immunofluorescence may be required to differentiate between the two conditions.

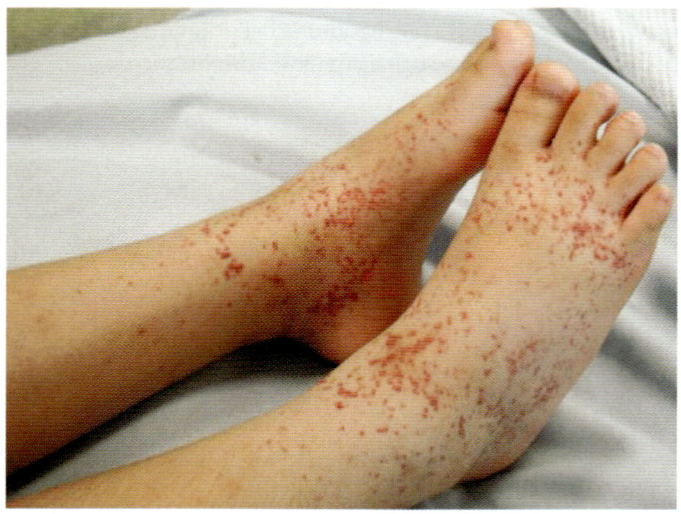

FIGURE 8-4. HSP in a young Chinese girl presenting as palpable purpura on the lower limbs. (Figure courtesy of Dr. Kumudhini Rajasegaran, Adolescent Medicine, KK Women's & Children's Hospital, Singapore.)

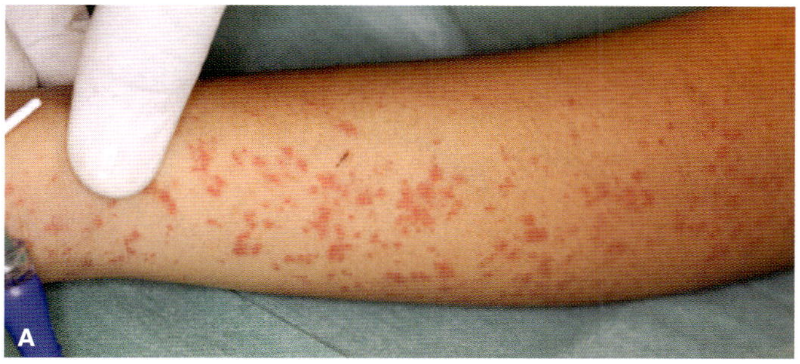

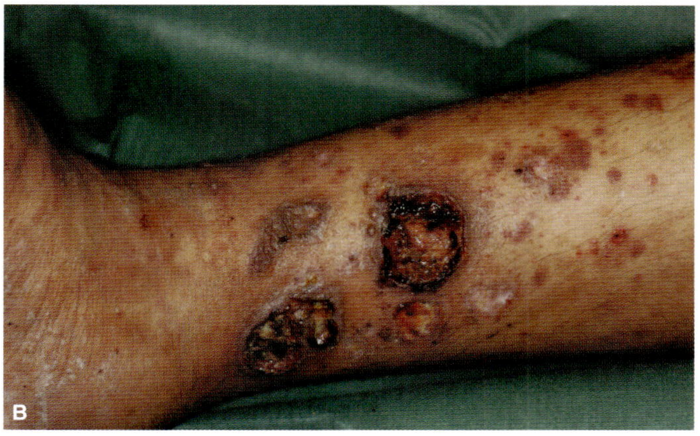

FIGURE 8-5A & 5B. LCV on the legs of a 12-year-old Malay boy with consequent blistering and ulceration (Figure 8-5B).

- Papular-purpuric gloves-and-socks syndrome
  - Acute swelling of hands and feet with erythema. Lesions are often purpuric with a sharp demarcation at both wrists and ankles, hence the term "gloves and socks." A generalized papular exanthem may be present on the body.
  - This condition is commonly associated with a parvovirus B19 infection, and it is usually self-limiting. Systemic features of fever, malaise, respiratory symptoms, and gastrointestinal upset may be present.

Investigations & Treatment

- Although LCV and HSP can be diagnosed clinically in children, a skin biopsy for histology and direct immunofluorescence will confirm the diagnosis. Skin biopsies should be performed on lesions that are less than 48 hours in appearance.

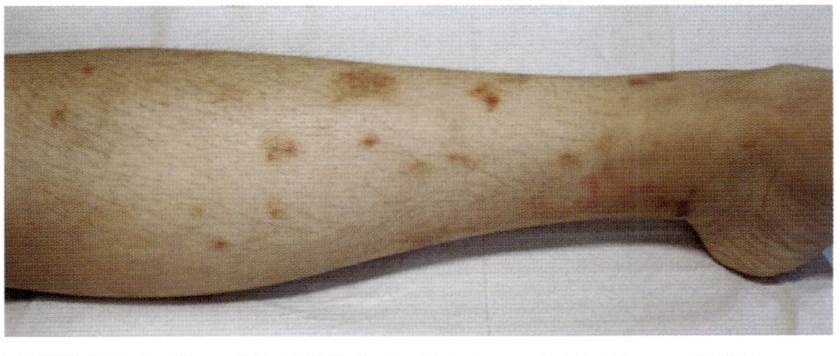

FIGURE 8-6. A differential of LCV is PPD which is seen in this 16-year-old Chinese girl presenting with areas of purpura associated with yellow-brown pigmentation, with a "cayenne pepper" appearance.

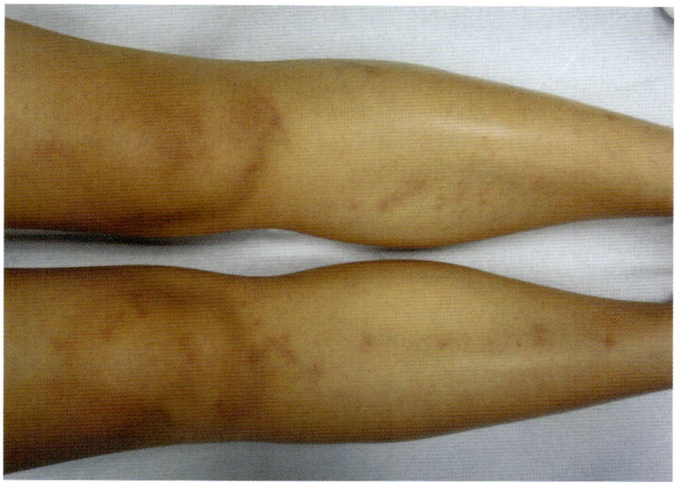

FIGURE 8-7. Another differential diagnosis of vasculitis is macular lymphocytic arteritis (MLA), also known as lymphocytic thrombophilic arteritis (LTA). This is a form of medium vessel vasculitis with mainly lymphocytic infiltrate in the walls of medium-sized cutaneous vessels. Clinically, it appears as reticulate, hyperpigmented patches, sometimes with more erythematous deep nodules.

- Histology will show neutrophilic inflammation around and within the walls of capillaries in the superficial and/or deep dermis. There is accompanying leukocytoclasis (neutrophil degeneration), nuclear dusting, red cell extravasation, and fibrinoid necrosis of small vessel walls.
- A thorough evaluation for culpable medications and occult infection should be performed. Other secondary causes, such as connective tissue disorders, should also be excluded if in the right clinical setting.
- Other laboratory and radiological investigations for joint, renal, and gastrointestinal involvement should be performed. Rarely, other organs may be affected, and serological and radiological tests may be required to investigate for other organ involvement.
- Treatment of cutaneous lesions is largely supportive, as symptoms usually resolve within a few weeks, often with residual hyperpigmentation. Topical corticosteroids may be used if lesions are extensive. If there is impeding necrosis, blisters, or ulceration, systemic corticosteroids may be required over a few weeks. Systemic medications, such as colchicine, dapsone, or immunosuppressants may be required if severe or recurrent.
- If there is significant systemic or renal involvement, systemic corticosteroids may also be used. The patient should be managed with a pediatric rheumatologist and/or pediatric nephrologist. Clinical recurrence may occur in a minority of patients.

Pearls & Practical Tips

- LCV and HSP in children are usually benign and self-limiting diseases with excellent prognosis. In younger children, the disease is milder, with less systemic involvement.
- Renal disease is the most important prognostic indicator in HSP, and patients are often followed for at least 1 year to screen for renal involvement.

URTICARIAL VASCULITIS

Urticarial vasculitis (UV) is a variant of cutaneous vasculitis that presents with urticaria-like features, with subtle differences in clinical presentation to common urticaria. It is often triggered by viral infections in children and has a favorable prognosis. However, it can rarely be associated with underlying systemic disease, such as other autoimmune conditions.

Clinical Features

- UV can be categorized into two forms – either normocomplementemic UV, which represents an idiopathic form, or hypocomplementemic UV, which may be associated with underlying systemic disease, such as systemic lupus erythematosus, Sjogren's syndrome, hepatitis C infection, cryoglobulinemia, or a drug-induced serum sickness-like disease.
- UV usually presents acutely with urticated wheals that evolve over a few days. More dusky and purpuric areas may also be present.
- Lesions often affect the trunk and limbs, and can be widespread.
- Compared to the presentation of urticaria, the lesions of UV often last beyond 24 to 48 hours and appear more dusky or purpuric. Lesions are also described as painful or "burning," in contrast to the pruritus seen in urticaria.
- The lesions of UV often resolve with post-inflammatory hyper- or hypopigmentation.

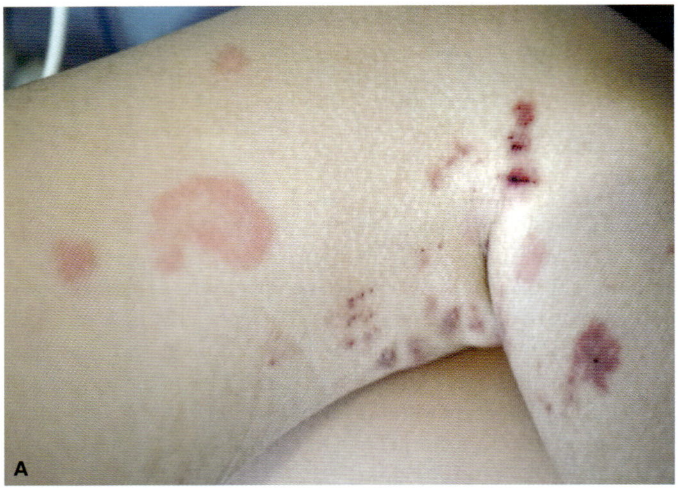

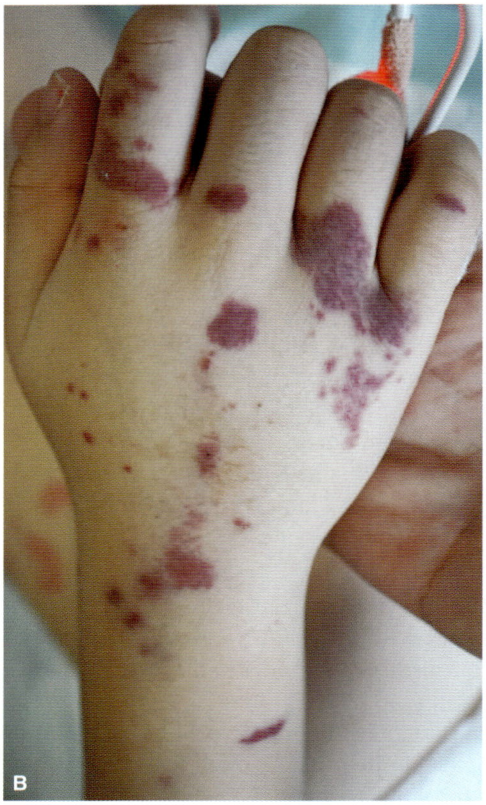

FIGURE 8-8A & 8B. Urticarial vasculitis in a 5-year-old Chinese girl, presenting with urticated plaques, as well as palpable purpura, scattered on her trunk and limbs.

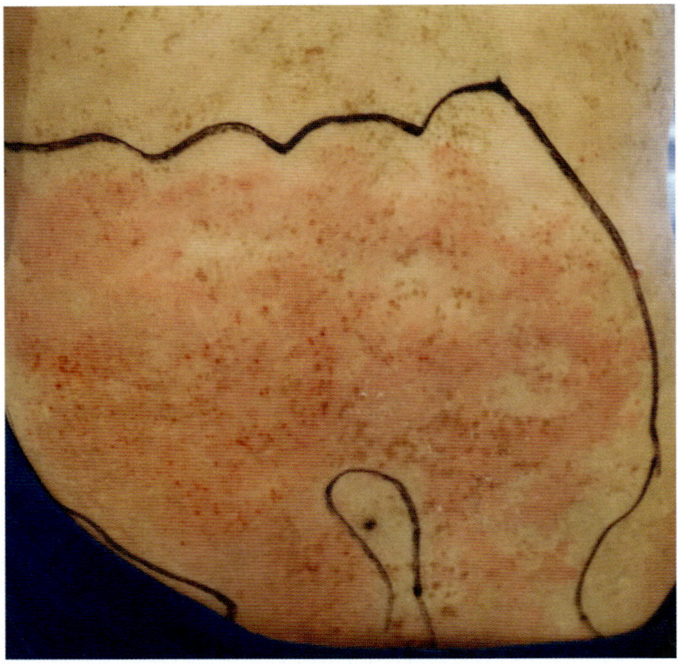

FIGURE 8-9. Urticarial vasculitis on the back of an 18-year-old Malay female who has a background of autoimmune hemolytic anemia, extensive vitiligo, and atopic dermatitis. There is a large, urticated plaque with concomitant purpura.

Differential Diagnoses

- Urticaria
  - Initially, the clinical features of UV may be similar to urticaria, especially during the acute presentation. Accurate and detailed history taking is essential to distinguish between the two conditions.
- Leukocytoclastic vasculitis (LCV)
  - LCV typically presents with palpable purpura. Occasionally, urticated papules, vesicles, pustules, or necrotic lesions may be present. Smaller lesions may be petechial in nature.
- Acute hemorrhagic edema of infancy
  - This condition presents with a clinical triad of fever, swelling, and purpura in infants. It is frequently preceded by an upper respiratory tract infection.

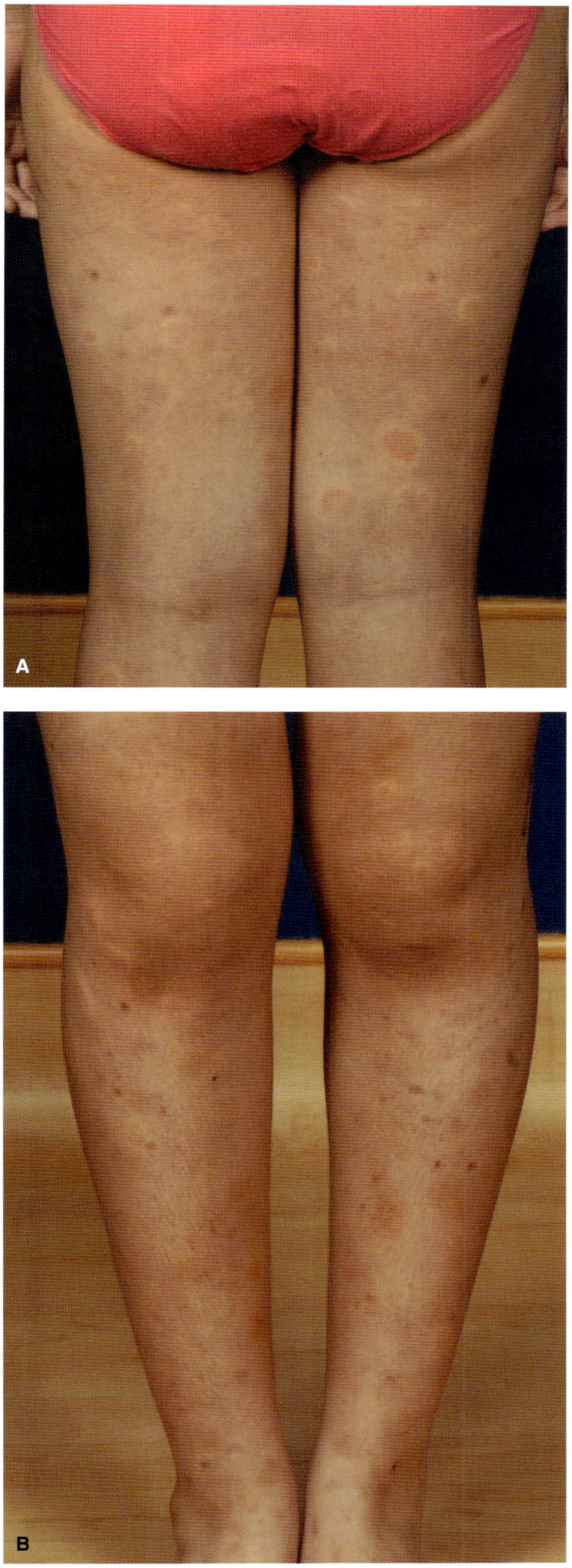

FIGURE 8-10A & 10B. Urticarial vasculitis on the legs of an 11-year-old Chinese girl, presenting as urticated plaques which resolve with post-inflammatory hyperpigmentation.

- In addition to urticated wheals, purpuric lesions are a characteristic feature. Atypical targetoid lesions and edema of the limbs may also be present.

- Viral exanthem
  - Viral exanthems usually appear more maculopapular, although more urticarial lesions may also be present. Viral exanthems usually last for a shorter duration compared to UV.

Investigations & Treatment

- UV in the pediatric population is usually benign and self-limiting, although in some patients lesions can be more chronic or recurrent over years. Histology and immunofluorescence studies are usually not required in children, especially if associated with acute infections.
- If performed, skin biopsies show subtle evidence of vessel wall damage, such as fibrinoid necrosis, red cell extravasation, neutrophils in the small vessel walls, and leukocytoclasis. Eosinophils are often conspicuous.
- Direct immunofluorescence may be positive with deposits of immunoglobulins, fibrin, and complement around blood vessels.
- If there is clinical suspicion, evaluation for connective tissue diseases such as systemic lupus erythematosus and Sjogren's syndrome should be performed. Serum C1q levels may be decreased.
- Treatment for UV includes oral antihistamines, topical anti-inflammatories, and oral colchicine in mild cases. In severe cases, oral corticosteroids or systemic immunosuppressants may be required. If associated with systemic disease, treatment is directed at the underlying condition.

Pearls & Practical Tips

- As the clinical differentiation between urticaria and UV can be subtle, and patients' and caregivers' history may not be reliable, the use of serial photography using mobile phones may be useful. Alternatively, urticated wheals can be demarcated with a surgical marker to monitor for resolution versus persistence.
- UV in the pediatric population is often triggered by viral infections and has a favorable prognosis compared to adults, resolving after a few weeks.

KAWASAKI DISEASE

Kawasaki disease (KD) is an acute childhood febrile disease primarily affecting children below the age of 5 years. It is postulated to be an immunological disorder triggered by an infectious or toxic agent. KD can mimic a viral exanthem and should be considered in a child with persistent fever, rash, and red eyes. KD can lead to potentially life-threatening cardiac complications.

Clinical Features

- The diagnostic criteria for KD includes fever for 5 or more days, in addition to four of five of the following features:
  1. Oral mucosal changes (strawberry tongue, lip fissures)
  2. Polymorphous skin exanthem

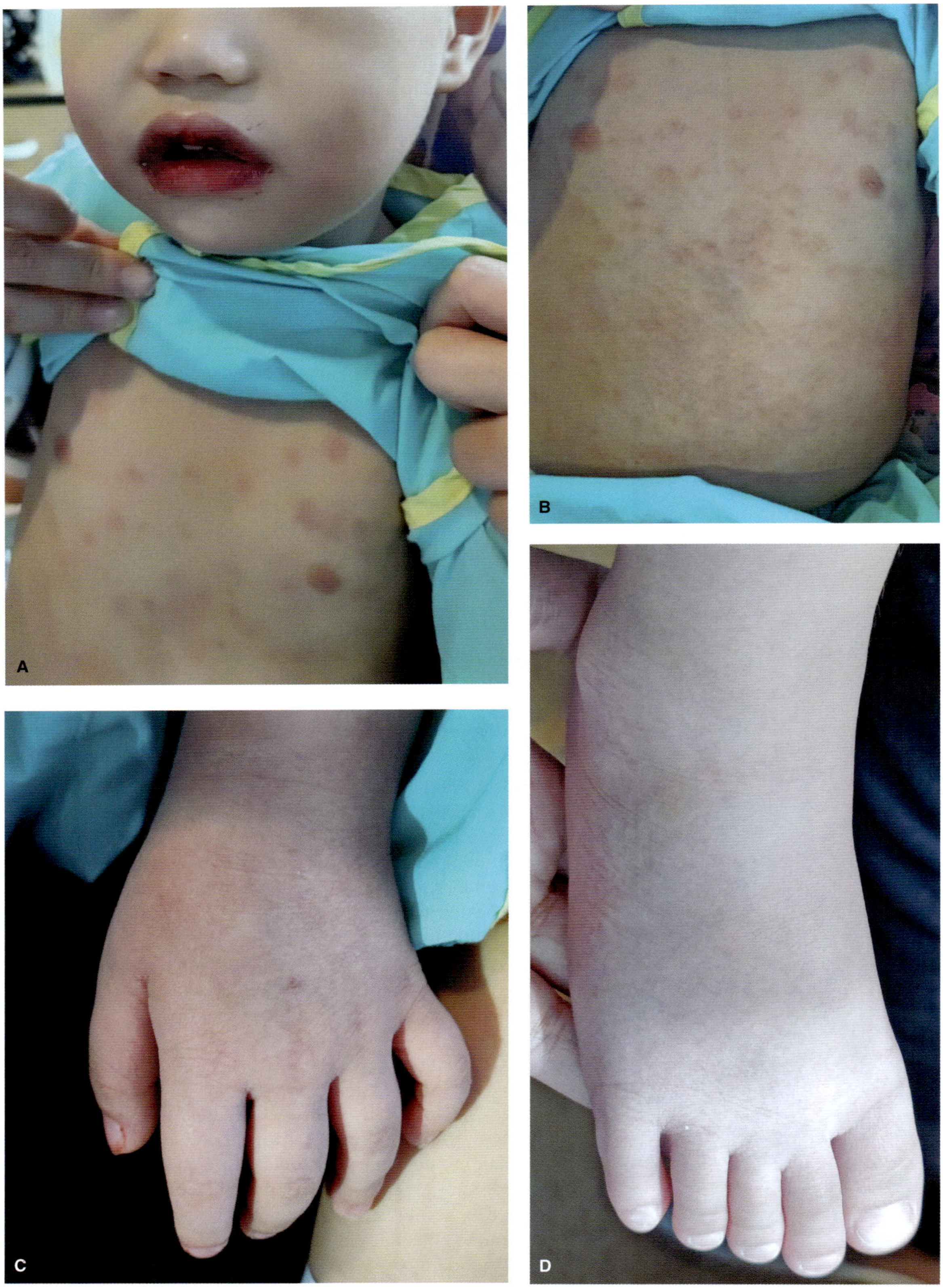

FIGURE 8-11A–11D. KD in a young Chinese boy presenting with red lips, polymorphous erythematous eruption on the trunk and swelling of the hands and feet.

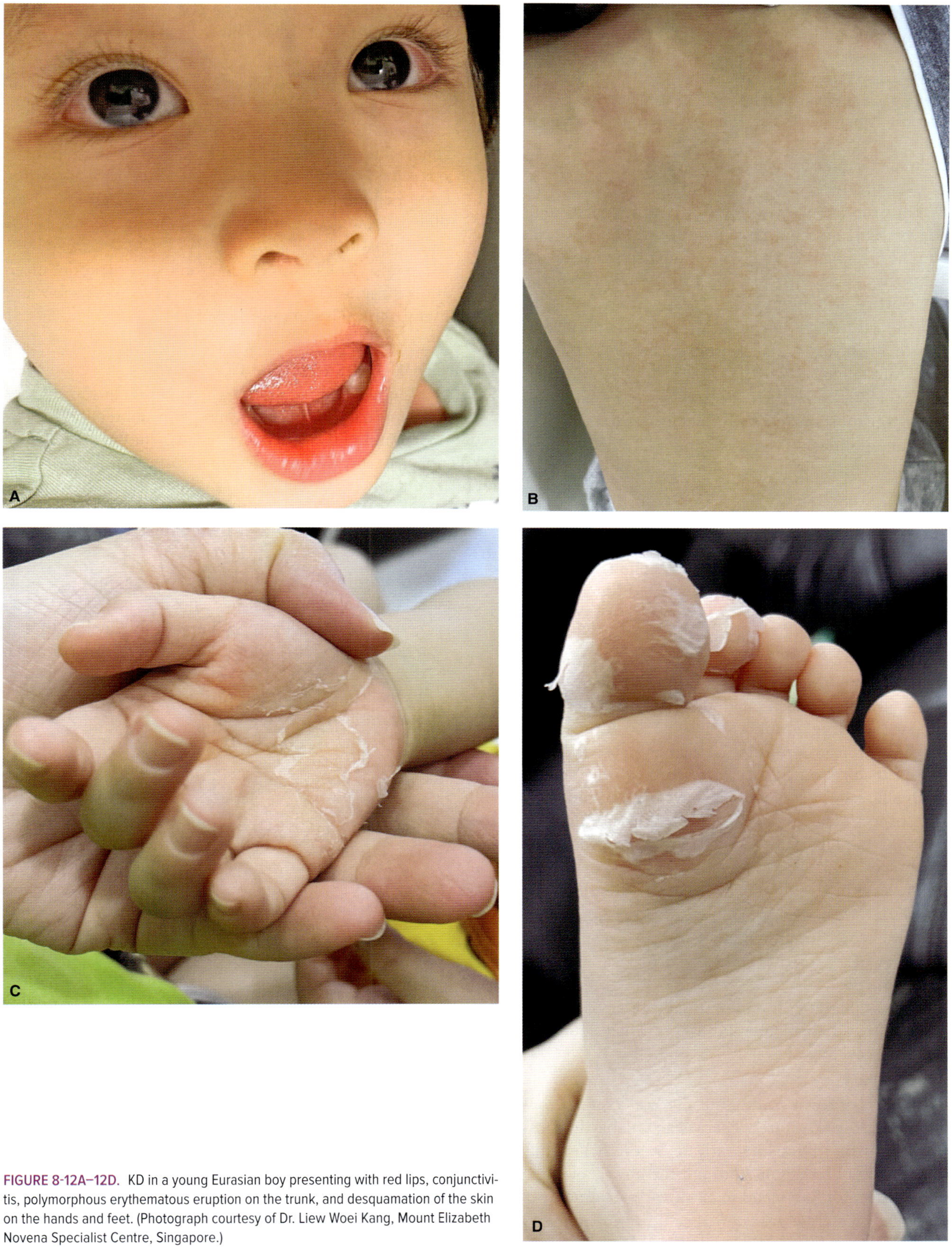

FIGURE 8-12A–12D. KD in a young Eurasian boy presenting with red lips, conjunctivitis, polymorphous erythematous eruption on the trunk, and desquamation of the skin on the hands and feet. (Photograph courtesy of Dr. Liew Woei Kang, Mount Elizabeth Novena Specialist Centre, Singapore.)

3. Skin changes over extremities
   - Erythema and edema of the hands and feet in the acute phase
   - Desquamation after the acute phase
4. Bilateral painless non-purulent conjunctival injection
5. Cervical lymphadenopathy (often unilateral, >1.5 cm in diameter)

- The clinical features can appear concurrently or sequentially, evolving over time.
- The skin eruption is polymorphous, although it commonly presents as a maculopapular morbilliform exanthem. The exanthem has a predilection for the perineum, and this may be an early finding in infants. Erythema of the BCG site is also often seen.
- Other clinical features include extreme irritability, lethargy, arthritis/myalgia, and neurological and gastrointestinal manifestations.
- Cardiac complications such as coronary artery aneurysm represent the most serious morbidity associated with KD.
- Recurrent episodes of skin peeling and nail changes (Beau's lines) may be present during the post-recovery period.

Differential Diagnoses

- Viral exanthems
  - Viral exanthems also appear polymorphous in nature, similar to KD. There may be associated mucosal and conjunctival changes. KD is often a diagnosis of exclusion of viral and other infections.
- Drug reactions
  - Various drug reactions may resemble KD clinically, especially in younger children. These include maculopapular drug eruptions, DRESS syndrome, and Stevens-Johnson syndrome. A comprehensive review of the medication history is essential to distinguish from KD, especially if patients have been commenced on suspect drugs, such as antiepileptics, antibiotics, sulfonamides, and NSAIDs, in the preceding few weeks.
- Scarlet fever
  - Scarlet fever can also present with fever, a sandpaper-like rash, sore throat, lymphadenopathy, swollen and red strawberry tongue, generalized malaise, myalgia, and anorexia.
  - Patients with scarlet fever are usually older than those with KD, and there may be a confirmed source of streptococcal infection.

Investigations & Treatment

- The diagnosis of KD is made clinically, based on the constellation of clinical features. There is no reliable diagnostic test to confirm KD, making early detection challenging. Any suspicion of KD should prompt the physician to get an early echocardiogram and institute early treatment.
- Histological features are non-specific. Inflammatory markers, such as ESR and CRP, are often raised.
- Management of KD includes systemic intravenous immunoglobulins (IVIG) and aspirin, with the aim to minimize inflammation and reduce the risk of cardiac complications. Long-term cardiac follow-up is required.

Pearls & Practical Tips

- "Incomplete" or "atypical" KD is more common in infants. This refers to fever and less than four of the clinical criteria. There is a higher risk of coronary artery abnormalities in this group of patients. A high index of suspicion is required for diagnosis, and early echocardiogram may be necessary to support the diagnosis. Other unusual features include seizures, stroke, nephritis, and acute hepatitis.
- "BCG-itis," which is inflammation with or without ulceration at the BCG vaccination site, has been described as a useful clinical feature in KD patients.

CUTANEOUS LUPUS ERYTHEMATOSUS

Cutaneous lupus erythematosus is generally uncommon in children. The various subtypes seen in this population include acute cutaneous lupus erythematosus, subacute cutaneous lupus erythematosus, discoid lupus erythematosus, tumid lupus, and lupus panniculitis. The cutaneous manifestations may present on its own or as part of systemic lupus erythematosus (SLE). Patients will need to be reviewed and evaluated for progression to SLE.

Clinical Features

- Acute cutaneous lupus erythematosus
  - Lesions of acute lupus erythematosus usually occur in the context of SLE, with the classical features of malar rash on the cheeks that spares the nasolabial folds. There is erythema and fine scaling. Sometimes purpuric lesions are also found.

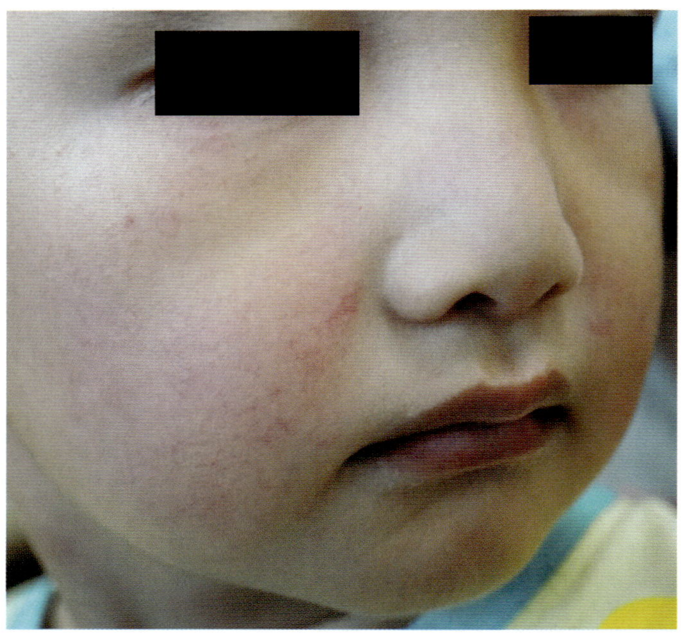

FIGURE 8-13. Chronic cutaneous lupus erythematosus affecting the cheeks of a 4-year-old Chinese boy, presenting as a chronic, erythematous, indurated plaque with minimal overlying scale.

- Other classical sites include the ears, nose, and other sun-exposed sites, such as the arms, hands, and fingers.

- Subacute cutaneous lupus erythematosus (SCLE)
  - The rash of SCLE appears as erythematous, annular, indurated plaques, with fine thin scale, or a psoriasiform pattern. Lesions may coalesce to form a polycyclic pattern.
  - Sites affected include photo-exposed areas of the upper trunk, arm extensors, and dorsum of hands. The face is usually unaffected.
  - SCLE can be drug-induced, and the common culprit drugs include terbinafine, calcium channel blockers, and thiazide diuretics.
- Discoid lupus erythematosus (DLE)
  - Lesions present as indurated raised erythematous plaques with overlying scale. Other features include telangiectasias, hyper- and hypopigmentation, and skin atrophy.

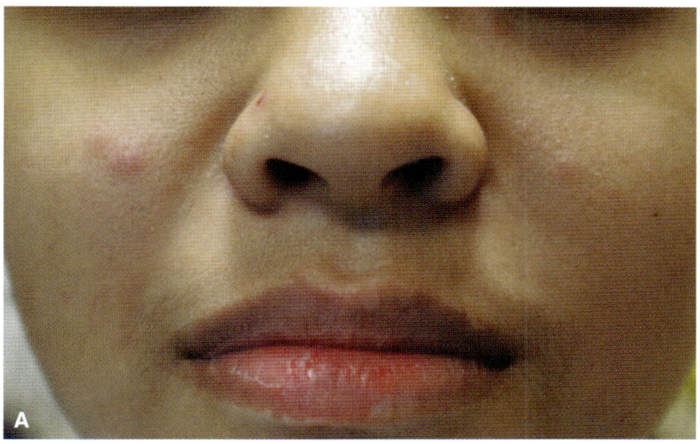

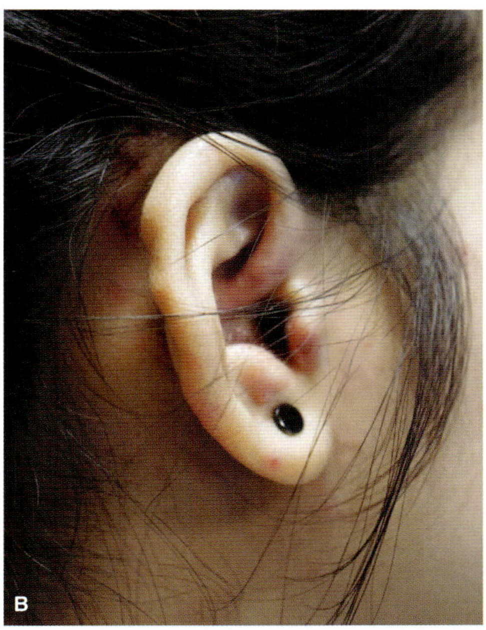

FIGURE 8-14A & 14B. Violaceous, mildly indurated papules on the cheeks and ear of a 16-year-old Malay girl with chronic cutaneous lupus erythematosus.

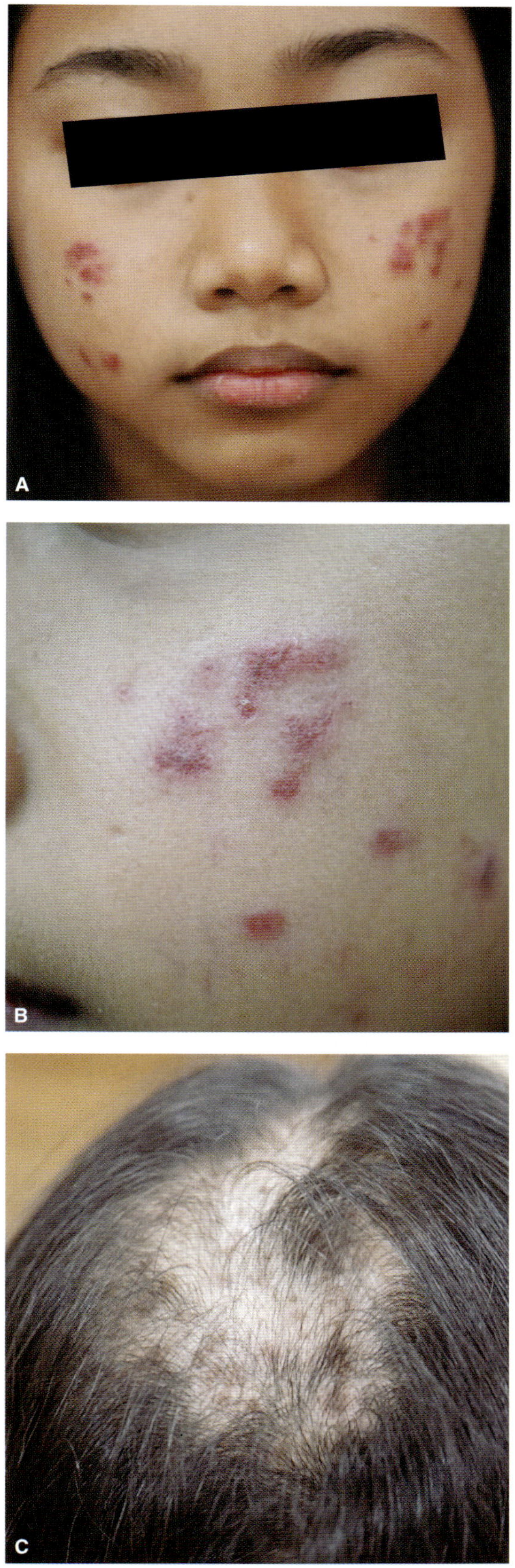

FIGURE 8-15A–15C. Chronic cutaneous lupus erythematosus on the cheeks of a 12-year-old Malay girl, presenting with violaceous, indurated papules and plaques with subtle scaling. She also has a patch of scarring alopecia on her scalp (Figure 8-15C).

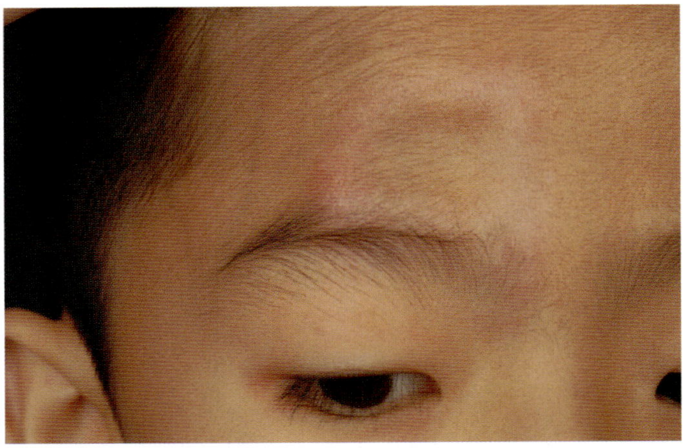

FIGURE 8-16. Lupus panniculitis on the forehead of a 7-year-old Chinese boy, presenting as a pink, deep, indurated annular plaque.

  - May exhibit the "carpet tack sign," where follicular plugging is visible once overlying scale is removed.
  - Photo-exposed areas such as the face, ears, scalp, neck, and exposed areas of the trunk and limbs are most commonly affected. Mucosal areas may also be involved. Lesions on the scalp may lead to scarring alopecia.

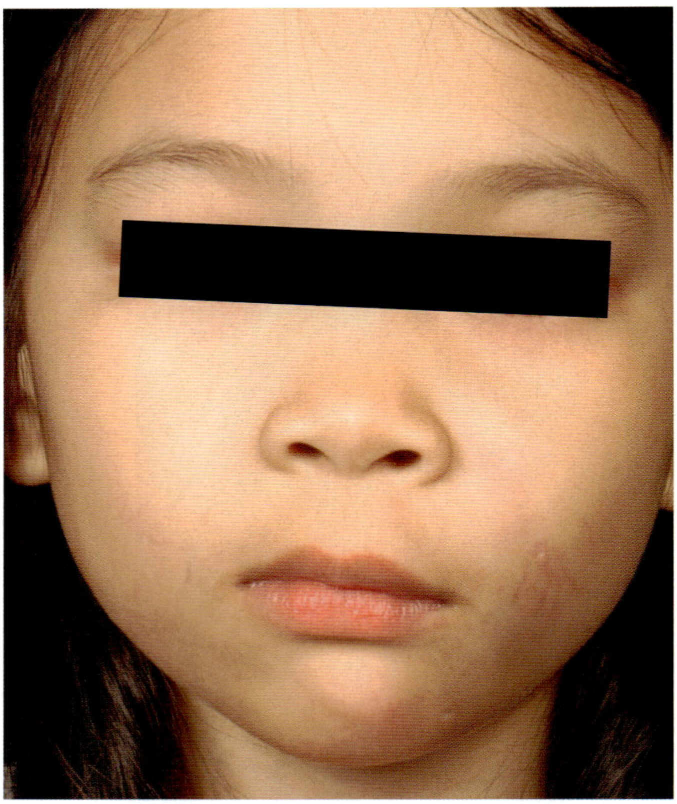

FIGURE 8-17. Lupus panniculitis on the left cheek of a 6-year-old Chinese girl, presenting with fullness of the left cheek with facial asymmetry and overlying telangiectasias.

- Tumid lupus (lupus tumidus)
  - This is a less common variant of chronic cutaneous lupus with lesions presenting as erythematous-to-violaceous, indurated, edematous, or urticated plaques. Unlike discoid lupus, there are minimal epidermal skin changes such as scaling or atrophy.
  - Lesions are usually found on photo-exposed areas of the face, neck, and trunk.
- Lupus panniculitis
  - This is a fairly common presentation in children and adolescents, with lesions presenting as deep, indurated plaques or nodules. The overlying skin may be normal or slightly erythematous.
  - It occurs most commonly on the face, upper arms/shoulders, breasts, thighs, and buttocks.
  - The lesions may persist for months or years, with eventual atrophy of the skin, leading to cosmetic disfigurement.

Differential Diagnoses

- Dermatomyositis and other connective tissue diseases
  - Lesions of dermatomyositis often have a more violaceous hue, compared to the intensely erythematous and scaly plaques of cutaneous lupus.
  - Even though both conditions occur over photo-exposed areas, dermatomyositis has a predilection for the periorbital area (heliotrope rash), shoulder (shawl sign), hip (holster sign), and hands (mechanic's hands, periungual telangiectasia).
- Lichen planus
  - Morphology of lichen planus may be described by "5Ps": polygonal, planar, purple, papular, and pruritic.
  - Features of Koebner's phenomenon are observed, where lesions appear in areas of trauma rather than being photo-aggravated.
- Photo-aggravated eczema
  - Features of telangiectasia, skin atrophy, and follicular plugging are not seen in photo-aggravated eczema.
  - Patient may have personal or family history of atopy, and xerosis may also be a prominent feature over the rest of the skin.

Investigations & Treatment

- Diagnosis of cutaneous lupus erythematosus is made clinically, supported by skin biopsies for histology and direct immunofluorescence.
- On histology, features of basal vacuolar alteration, lymphocytic exocytosis, necrotic keratinocytes and pigment incontinence are seen, associated with a superficial and deep perivascular and peri-adnexal lymphohistiocytic infiltrate. There is mucin deposition and occasionally a thickened basement membrane. Follicular plugging and epidermal atrophy may be more prominent in discoid lupus.

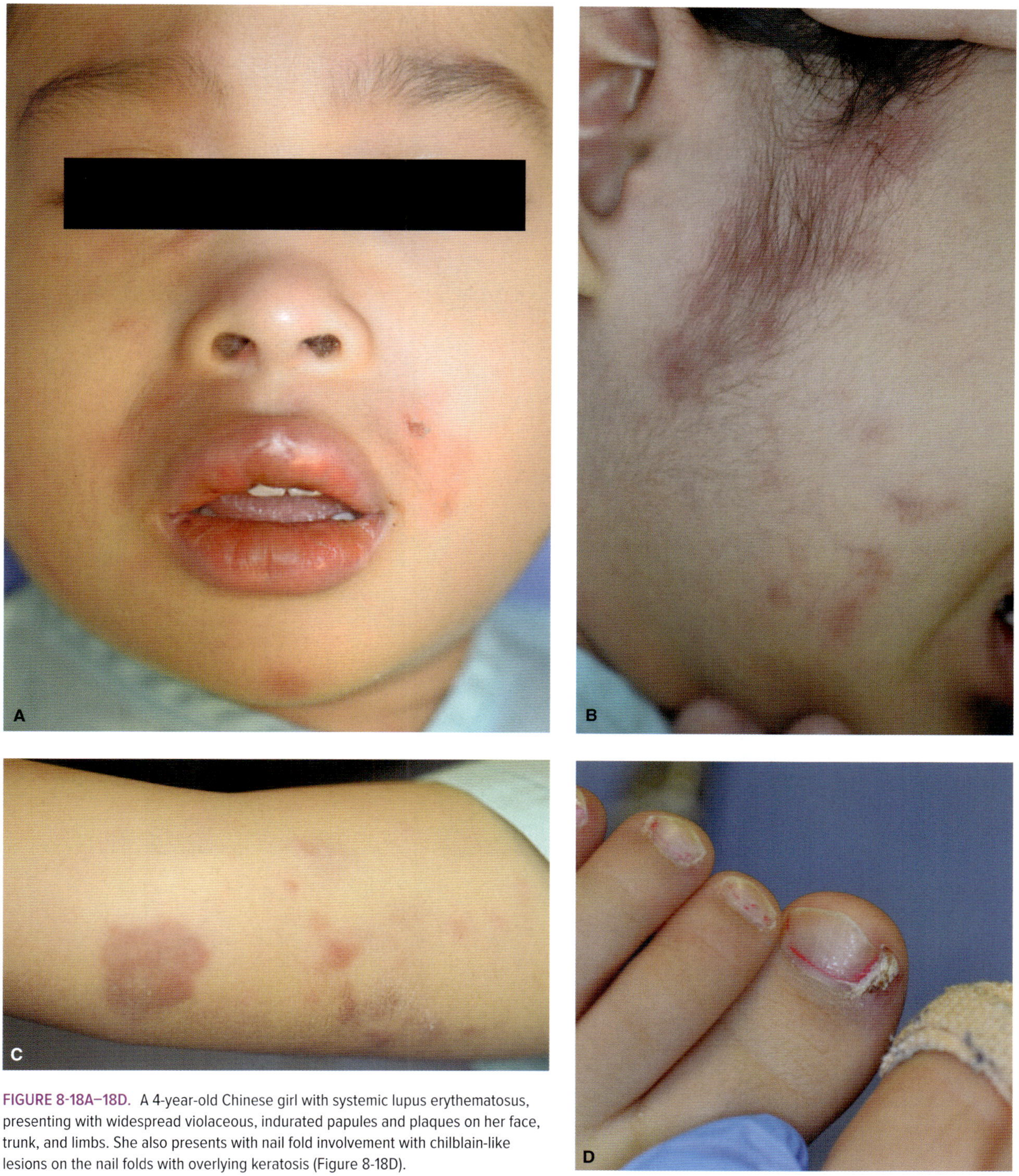

FIGURE 8-18A–18D. A 4-year-old Chinese girl with systemic lupus erythematosus, presenting with widespread violaceous, indurated papules and plaques on her face, trunk, and limbs. She also presents with nail fold involvement with chilblain-like lesions on the nail folds with overlying keratosis (Figure 8-18D).

- Direct immunofluorescence will show granular deposits of IgG, IgM, and C3 at the dermal–epidermal junction (lupus band).
- Serological testing and evaluation for SLE or systemic involvement is required, including antinuclear antigen (ANA), double-stranded DNA (dsDNA), and extractable nuclear antigen (ENA).
- Treatment includes non-pharmacological measures such as strict sun protection. Lesions may be treated with topical corticosteroids, topical calcineurin inhibitors, and intralesional corticosteroids. Systemic agents such as antimalarials (e.g., hydroxychloroquine, chloroquine), corticosteroids (e.g., prednisolone, methylprednisolone), and immunosuppressants (e.g., methotrexate, azathioprine) can be used for more severe or widespread disease.

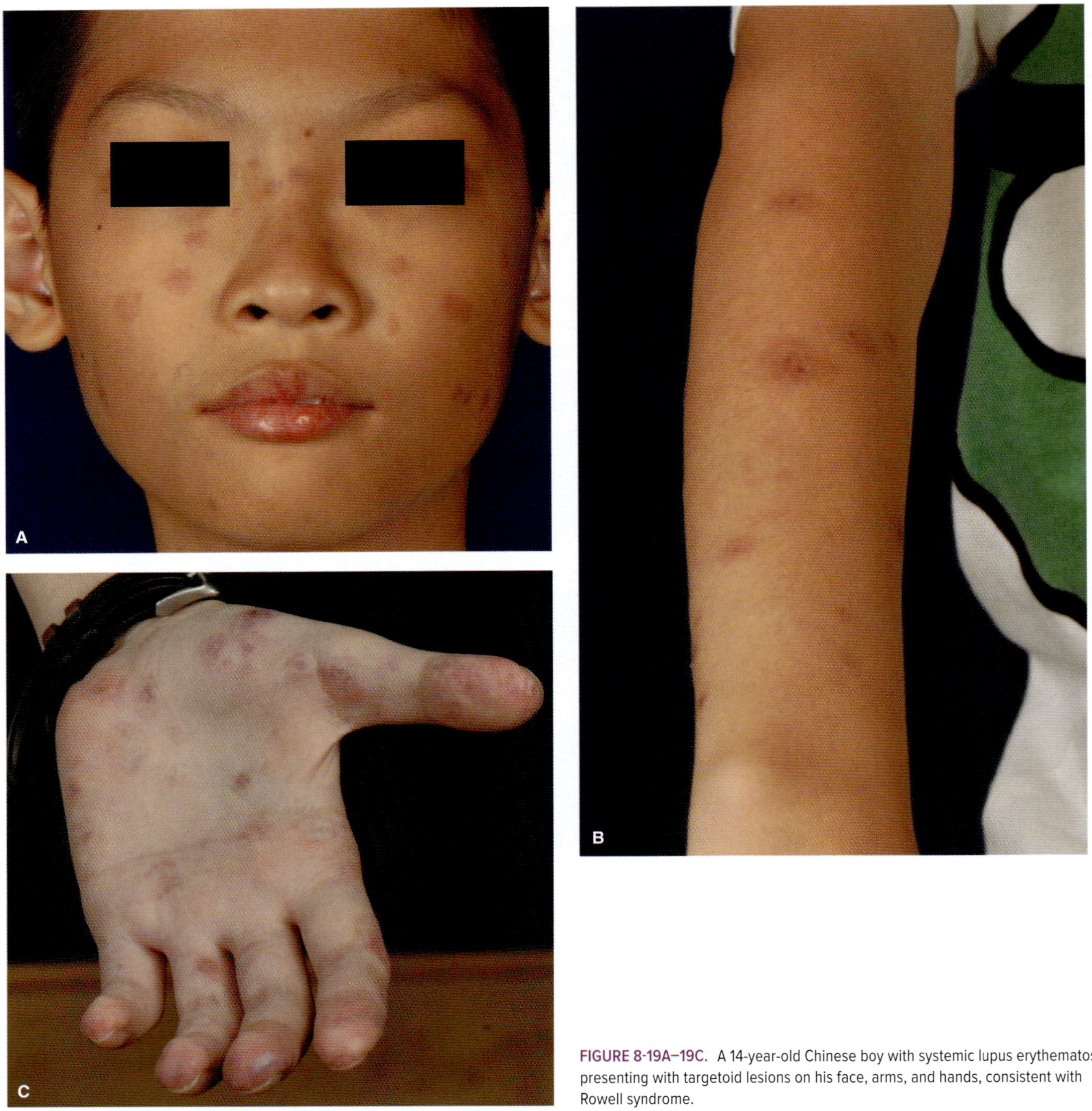

FIGURE 8-19A–19C. A 14-year-old Chinese boy with systemic lupus erythematosus presenting with targetoid lesions on his face, arms, and hands, consistent with Rowell syndrome.

Pearls & Practical Tips

- While cutaneous lupus is generally rare in children, a high index of suspicion is required due to possible systemic involvement. Untreated lesions may also lead to permanent cosmetic disfigurement and scarring alopecia.
- Localized lesions generally respond well to topical treatment and antimalarials. Sun protection includes the use of a broad-spectrum sunscreen, hats and protective clothing, and avoidance of direct sun exposure.
- Various subtypes of cutaneous lupus can occur in the same patient and at different time points during the course of disease.

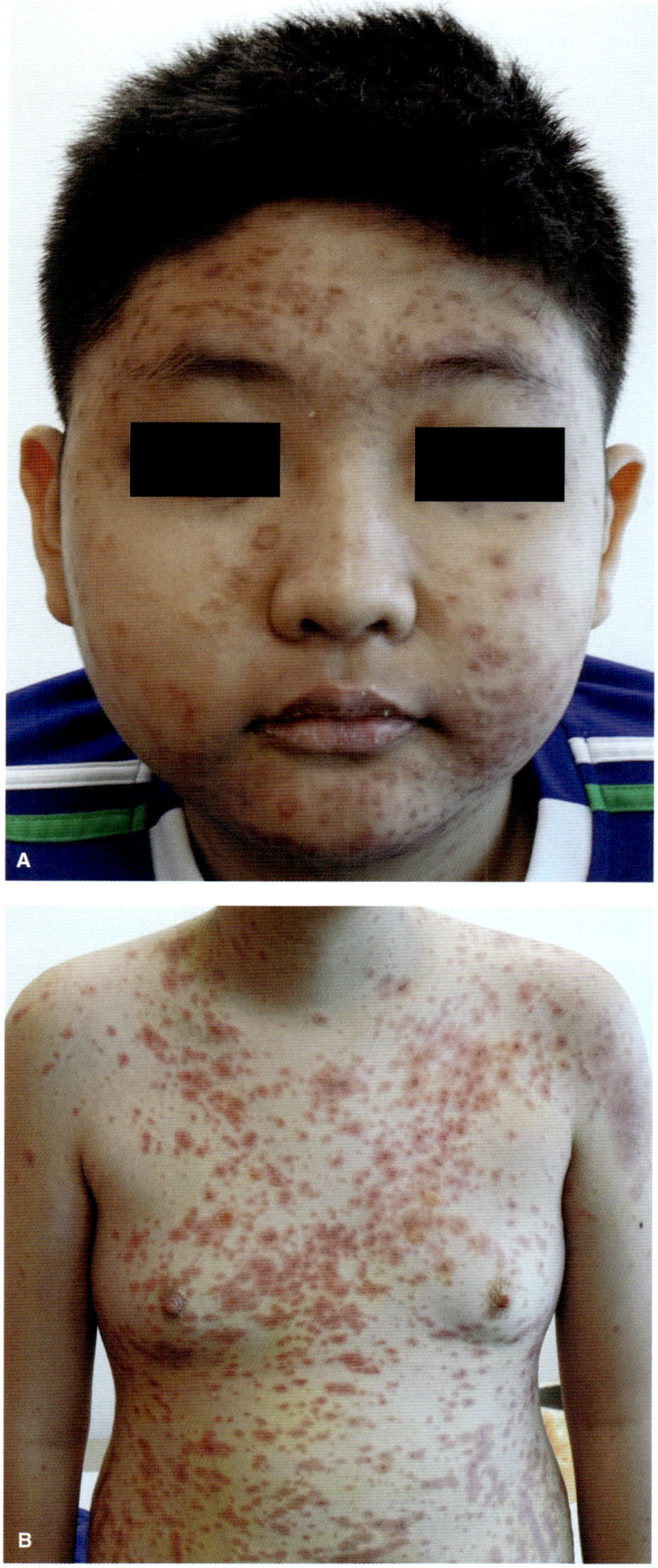

FIGURE 8-20A & 20B. A 14-year-old Chinese boy with systemic lupus erythematosus and lesions of chronic cutaneous lupus on his face. He presented with acute onset of violaceous, targetoid lesions with bullae formation on the trunk.

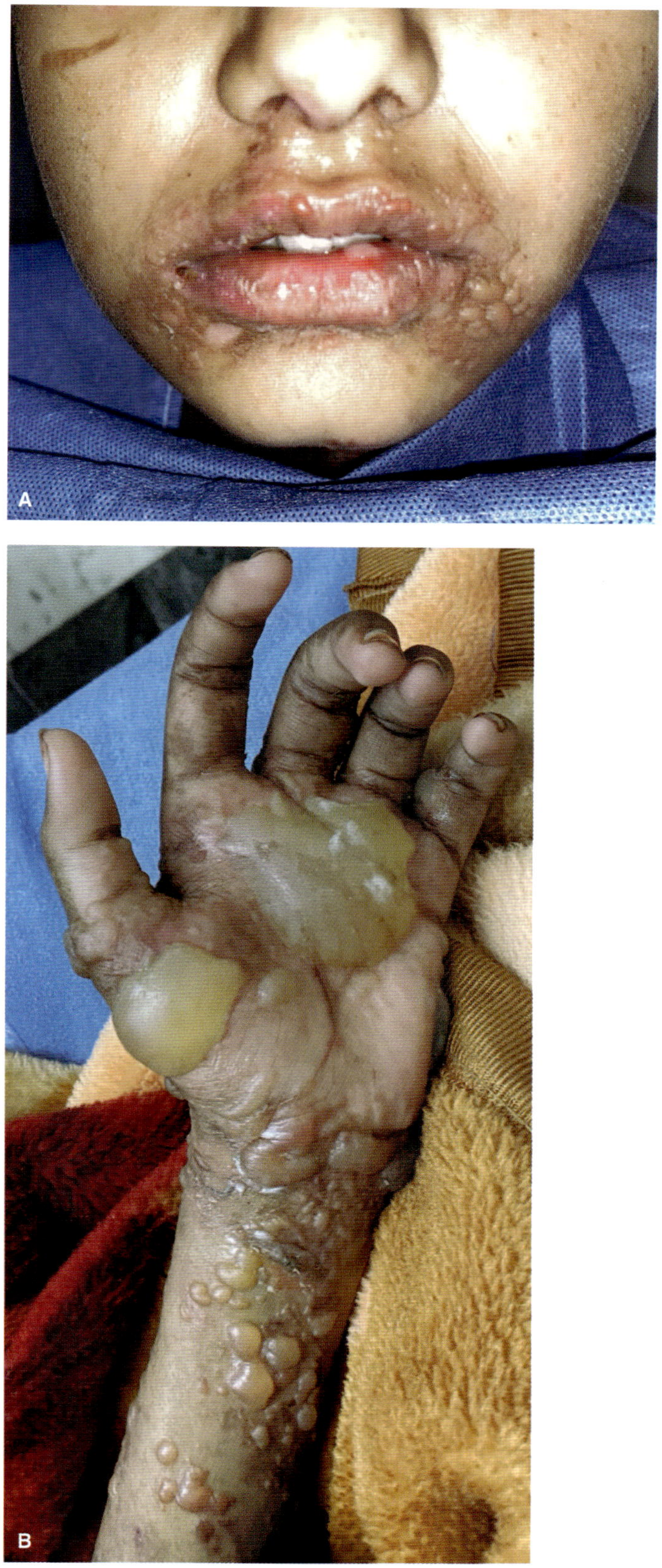

FIGURE 8-21A & 21B. An Indian teenager with bullous lupus, presenting with multiple bullae affecting his face and limbs. (Photo courtesy of Dr. Surabhi Sinha, Department of Dermatology, Dr. Ram Manohar Lohia Hospital & ABVIMS, New Delhi, India.)

NEONATAL LUPUS ERYTHEMATOSUS

Neonatal lupus erythematosus (NLE) is an uncommon condition caused by transplacental transfer of autoantibodies, in particular anti-Ro/SSA and anti-La/SSB. It is seen in infants whose mothers have a predilection for or have been diagnosed with systemic lupus erythematosus (SLE), Sjögren's syndrome, or mixed connective tissue disease. Approximately 50% of mothers are asymptomatic for autoimmune disease at the time of delivery.

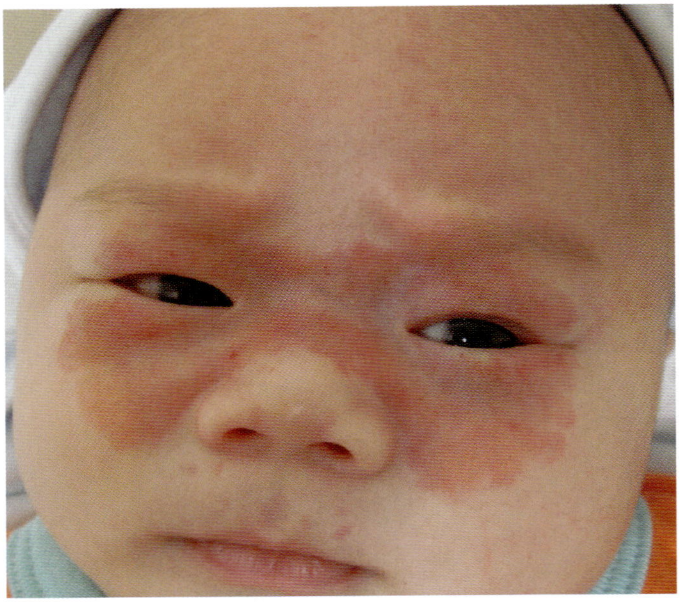

FIGURE 8-22. Neonatal lupus presenting with the classical "raccoon eyes" erythema, purpura, and telangiectasias on the periorbital region in a Chinese baby.

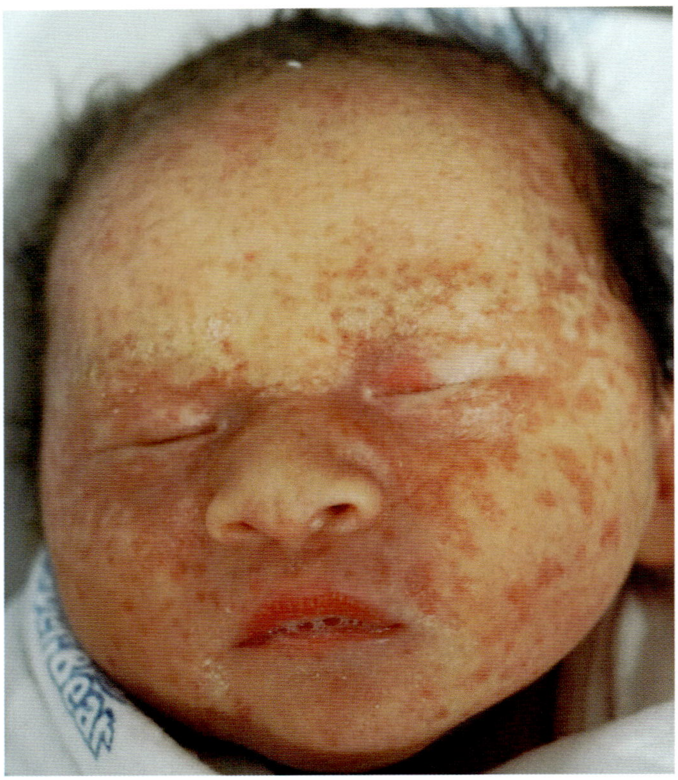

FIGURE 8-23. Neonatal lupus in a Chinese neonate, presenting with purpuric and erythematous macules and patches on the face, with telangiectasias and accentuation around the periorbital region.

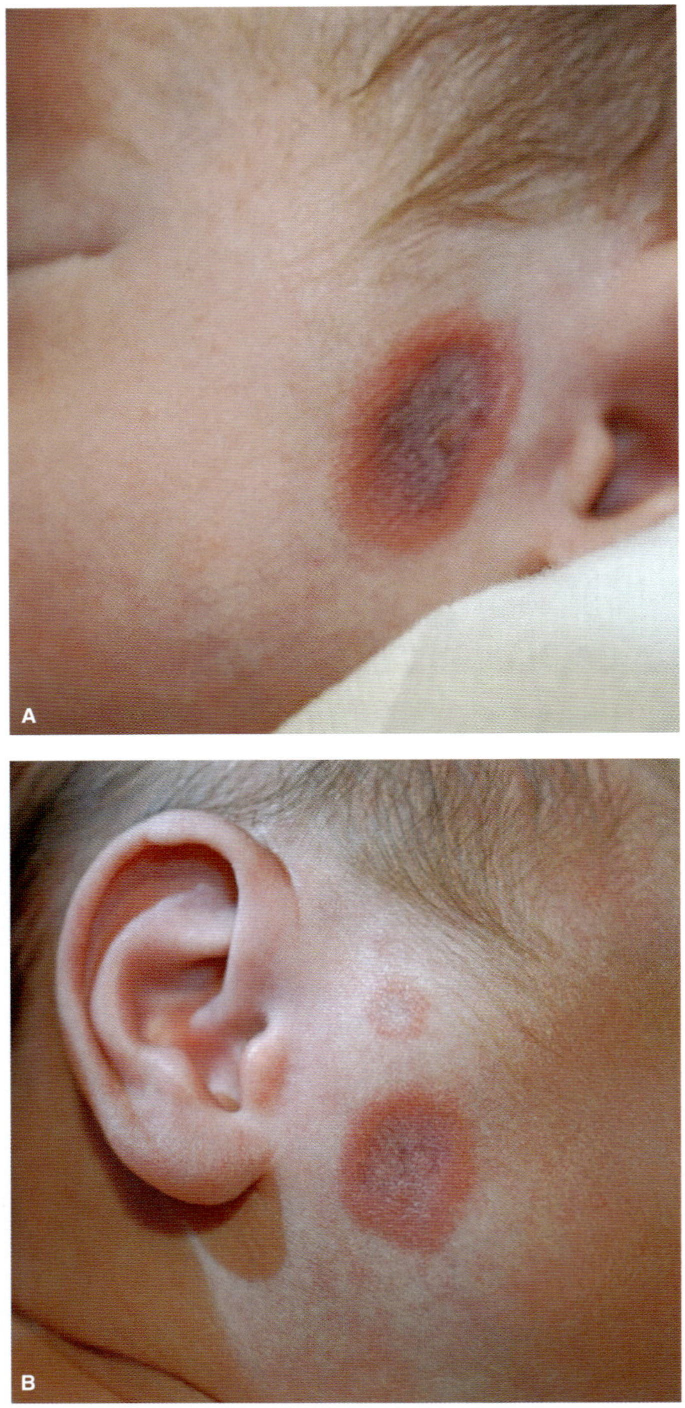

FIGURE 8-24A & 24B. Neonatal lupus presenting as annular, targetoid plaques on both lateral cheeks, in a Chinese-Malay neonate.

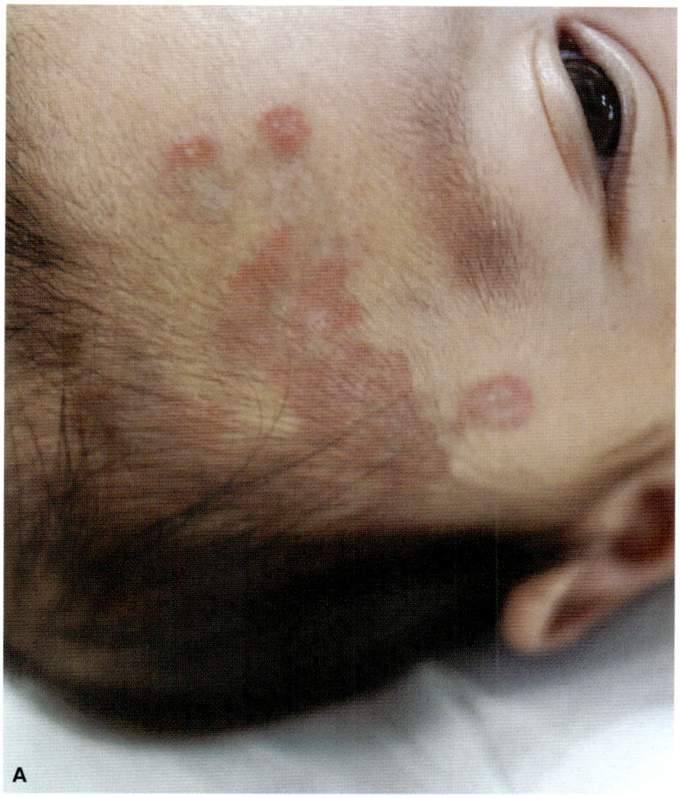

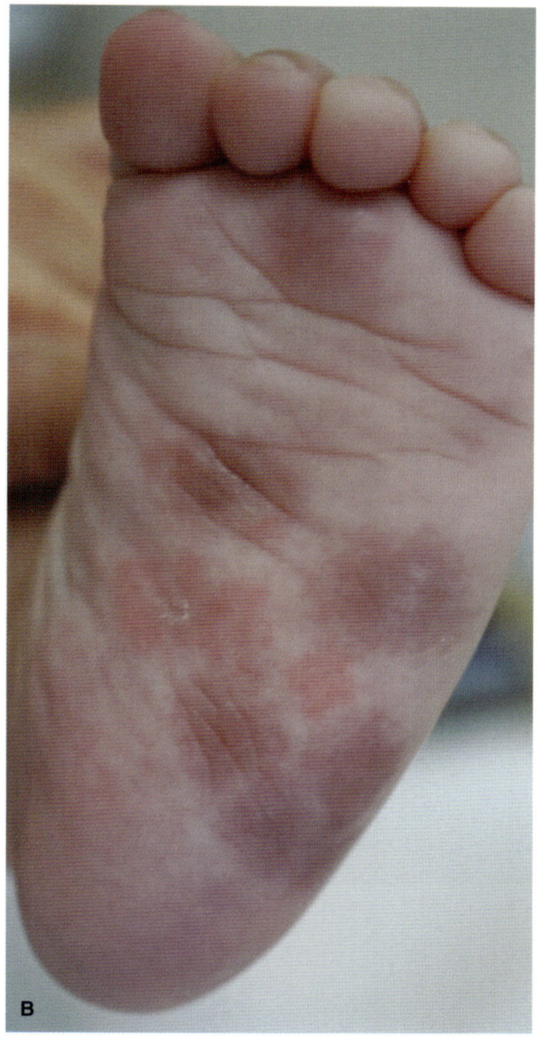

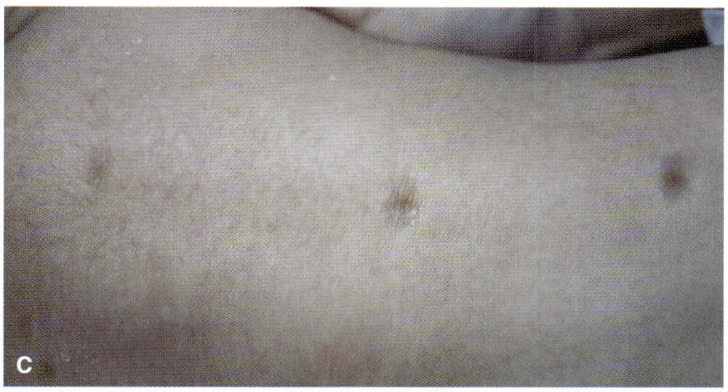

FIGURE 8-25A–25C. Congenital/neonatal lupus in an Indian neonate, with violaceous, annular plaques on the face, limbs, and trunk. Three atrophic, hyperpigmented papules were noted on his back at birth (Figure 8-25C).

Although the cutaneous findings are benign and self-limiting in NLE, a small proportion of babies can develop congenital heart block, and rarely, other systemic manifestations.

Clinical Features

- Most babies with NLE present after a few weeks of life. Less commonly, cutaneous manifestations may be present at birth, prompting the name "congenital lupus erythematosus."
- The classical features of NLE include bilateral periorbital annular erythematous patches ("racoon eyes"), annular erythematous-to-purpuric plaques with scaling, and telangiectasias.
- The eruption more often occurs over photo-exposed areas, such as the face, scalp, neck, and body. Follicular plugging or scarring is usually absent.
- Congenital heart block occurs in approximately 10% of patients, with inflammation of the AV node starting in utero. Congenital heart block is permanent.
- Other systemic complications of NLE include thrombocytopenia, anemia, hepatitis, and pneumonitis.
- Half of mothers who are undiagnosed or asymptomatic at time of delivery may develop SLE, Sjögren's syndrome, or mixed connective tissue disease within a median duration of 3 years. Hence, screening for autoimmune diseases and referral to a rheumatologist are essential.

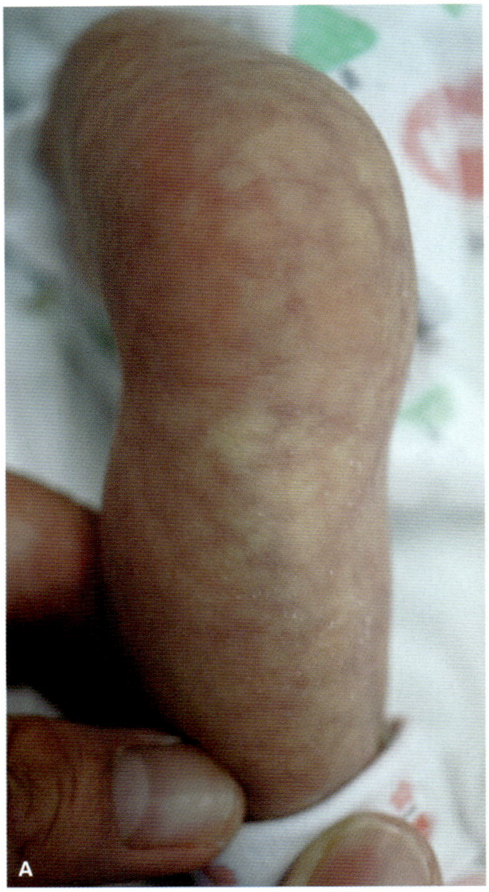

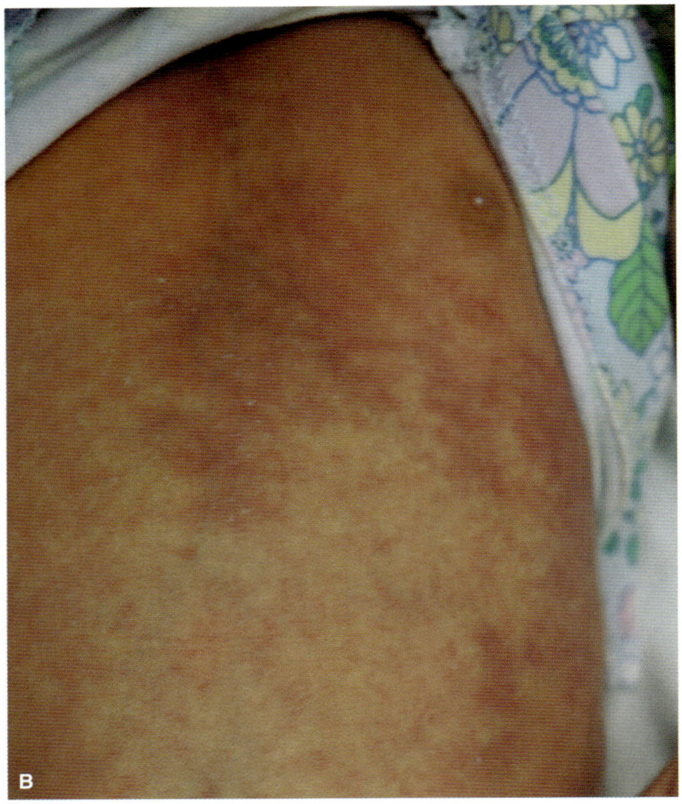

FIGURE 8-26A & 26B. Congenital lupus in a Chinese baby born to a mother with systemic lupus erythematosus, presenting with widespread patchy, reticulate, livedo racemosa-like patches on her trunk and limbs.

Differential Diagnoses

- Seborrheic dermatitis
  - Infantile seborrheic dermatitis has a similar distribution to and can present at approximately the same time as NLE.
  - Annular lesions and telangiectasias are not seen in seborrheic dermatitis, which presents with more greasy, thickened, yellowish scales. There may be a history of atopy.
- Infantile psoriasis
  - In infantile psoriasis, the scales tend to be large, thickened, and silvery. Non-exposed sites such as the groin are also commonly affected.
- Dermatophyte infection
  - Although rare, dermatophyte infection can occur in neonates and young infants, especially tinea faciei, corporis, and capitis. Scaly, annular plaques are often seen. There may be a contact history with an affected caregiver or pet.
  - Fungal scraping for microscopy and culture is useful to confirm dermatophyte infection.

Investigations & Treatment

- NLE is suspected usually on clinical grounds, with presentation of the classical annular rash or raccoon's eyes, especially if there is a history of autoimmune disease in the mother.
- In atypical cases, skin biopsies may help support the diagnosis. However, the histological features of NLE can be subtle and not as florid as biopsies from older patients with cutaneous lupus erythematosus.
- An electrocardiogram must be performed to evaluate for heart block, and if present, baby should be urgently referred to a pediatric cardiologist to evaluate for insertion of a pacemaker.
- Serology for autoimmune antibodies may be performed for baby and/or the mother. The antibody panel should include ANA, double-stranded DNA (dsDNA), and extractable nuclear antigen (ENA), which includes Anti-Ro, Anti-La, and Anti-U_1RNP antibodies.
- Other autoantibodies may also be screened for in the appropriate clinical setting.

- Other investigations include a complete blood count, liver function test, and renal panel.
- The cutaneous manifestations resolve spontaneously and gradually over 4 to 6 months, reflecting the waning levels of placentally transferred antibodies. Most lesions heal without scarring or dyspigmentation.
- Sun protection is important and should be emphasized.
- Mothers will require thorough evaluation and follow-up by a rheumatologist, as well as counseling on recurrence in subsequent pregnancies.

Pearls & Practical Tips

- The risk of having a child with NLE in mothers who test positive for autoantibodies is approximately 2% for first pregnancies or if previous babies were healthy. The risk increases by approximately tenfold in subsequent pregnancies. Weekly fetal echocardiograms are recommended between 16 and 26 weeks of gestational age.
- Although uncommon, prompt evaluation of congenital heart block is imperative to prevent infant mortality, especially if mothers are known to be positive for anti-Ro or anti-La antibodies.
- Maternal treatment with hydroxychloroquine has been shown to decrease cardiac complications in utero.
- Infants with neonatal lupus are at a higher risk of developing systemic autoimmune conditions later in life due to the familial risk.
- Although uncommon in neonatal lupus, scarring can be seen and can be extensive if lesions are present at birth (congenital lupus).
- Pleocytosis of cerebrospinal fluid may be found in babies presenting with NLE, especially if presenting with neonatal pyrexia.

JUVENILE DERMATOMYOSITIS

Dermatomyositis is an autoimmune inflammatory myositis affecting both children and adults, although it is much more common in adulthood. Juvenile dermatomyositis (JDM) is the most common type of juvenile idiopathic inflammatory myopathy, mainly affecting the skin and proximal muscles.

Clinical Features

- Characteristic skin lesions include purplish, telangiectatic patches over photo-exposed areas, especially the eyelids (heliotrope rash), scalp hairline, neck to anterior shoulders (shawl sign), and hip (holster sign).
- A classical sign of dermatomyositis is Gottron's papules, which refers to violaceous flat-topped lesions over the dorsal interphalangeal joints of the hands. The concurrent presence of ragged cuticles, hyperkeratosis, and fissuring of the hands gives rise to "mechanic's hands."
- Periungual telangiectasia is a characteristic feature of JDM and provides a good indication of cutaneous activity.
- Pitted ulcerations of the fingertips and pressure points such as the elbows are usually seen at presentation or with disease flares.
- Poikiloderma (areas of hyper- and hypopigmentation, skin atrophy, and telangiectasia) and calcinosis cutis occur in chronic JDM.
- Non-cutaneous findings include symmetrical proximal myopathy, large and small joint polyarthritis, exertional dyspnea, dysphagia, nasal speech, gastrointestinal bleeding, and pericarditis.
- Occasionally, overlap syndromes with other connective tissue disorders may be present and patients may have features of renal disease, neuropathy, and Raynaud's phenomenon.

Differential Diagnoses

- Cutaneous lupus erythematosus
  - Both conditions share features of photo-aggravation and the presence of telangiectasia, skin atrophy, and dyspigmentation. However, lesions of cutaneous lupus are usually more erythematous rather than violaceous. The typical sites of involvement for dermatomyositis will also be absent in cutaneous lupus.
  - The finger joints of the dorsal hand are usually spared in cutaneous lupus, while in dermatomyositis the finger joints will be involved.
  - Cutaneous lupus does not feature symmetrical proximal muscle weakness.
- Eczema
  - The heliotrope rash and photo-aggravated facial rash of JDM can be mistaken for an eczematous dermatitis. Similarly, initial minor hand findings may be attributed to hand eczema.
  - Physicians must have a high index of suspicion in patients with recalcitrant "eczematous" rash that does not respond to appropriate topicals or has atypical features.

Investigations & Treatment

- The diagnosis of JDM is made clinically, supported by various investigations, including histology and blood investigations.
- Skin biopsy will show evidence of interface dermatitis with increased mucin deposition, and a superficial and deep perivascular and peri-adnexal dermatitis. Direct immunofluorescence may be non-specific. It may be difficult to differentiate dermatomyositis from cutaneous lupus based on histology alone.
- Other investigations include muscle enzymes, myositis panel, magnetic resonance imaging and biopsy of the affected muscles, and relevant systemic workup. Unlike in adult dermatomyositis, presence of myositis-specific antibodies is not associated with malignancies.

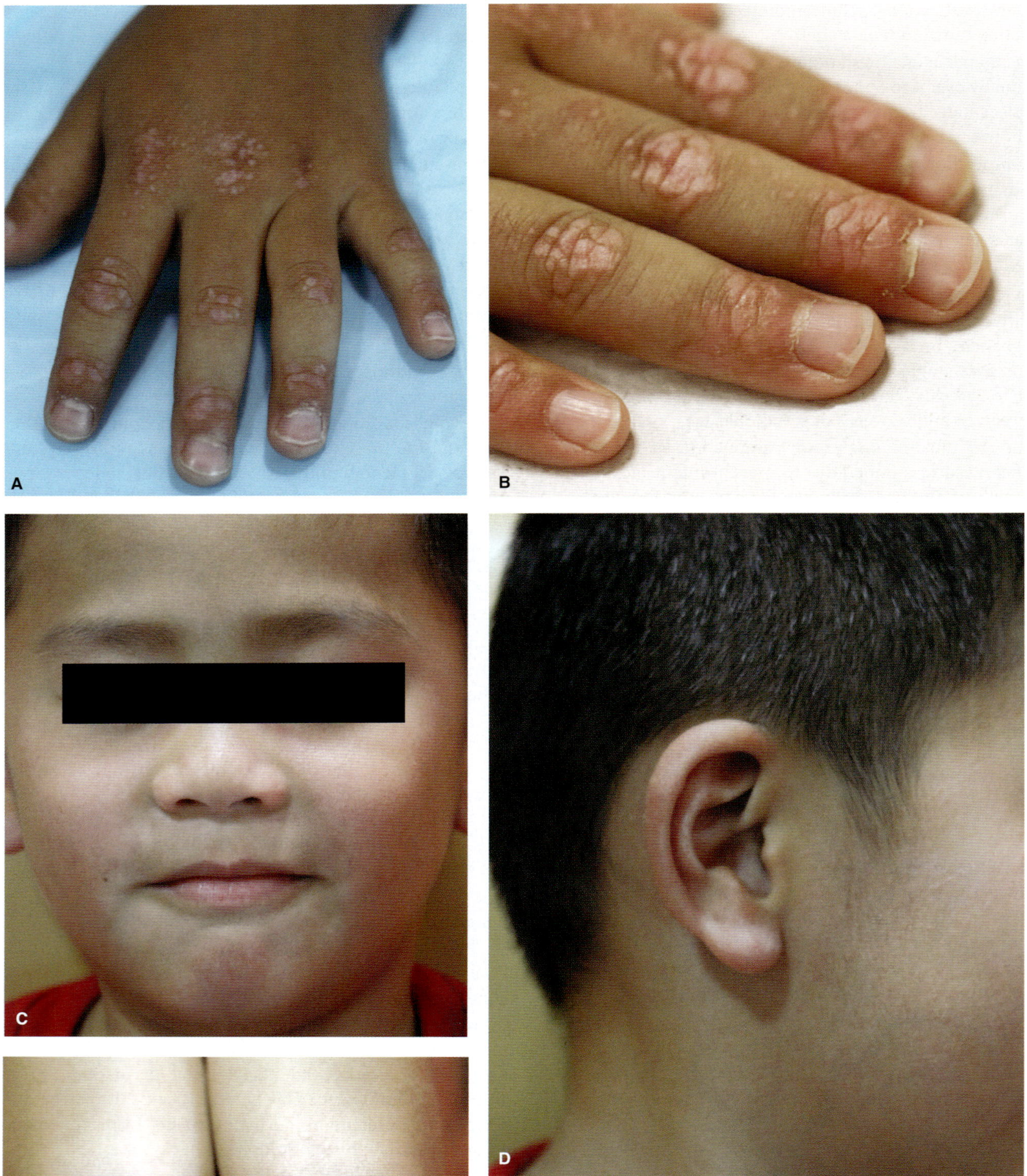

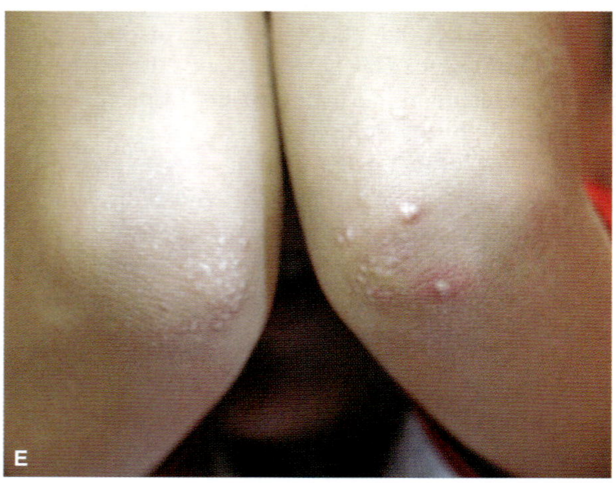

FIGURE 8-27A–27E. JDM in a 5-year-old Chinese boy, presenting with violaceous, flat-topped papules (Gottron's papules) over the dorsal interphalangeal and metacarpal-phalangeal joints of bilateral hands. In addition, he has ragged cuticles, faint heliotrope rash over his periorbital region, cheeks, and ears and calcinosis over the elbows.

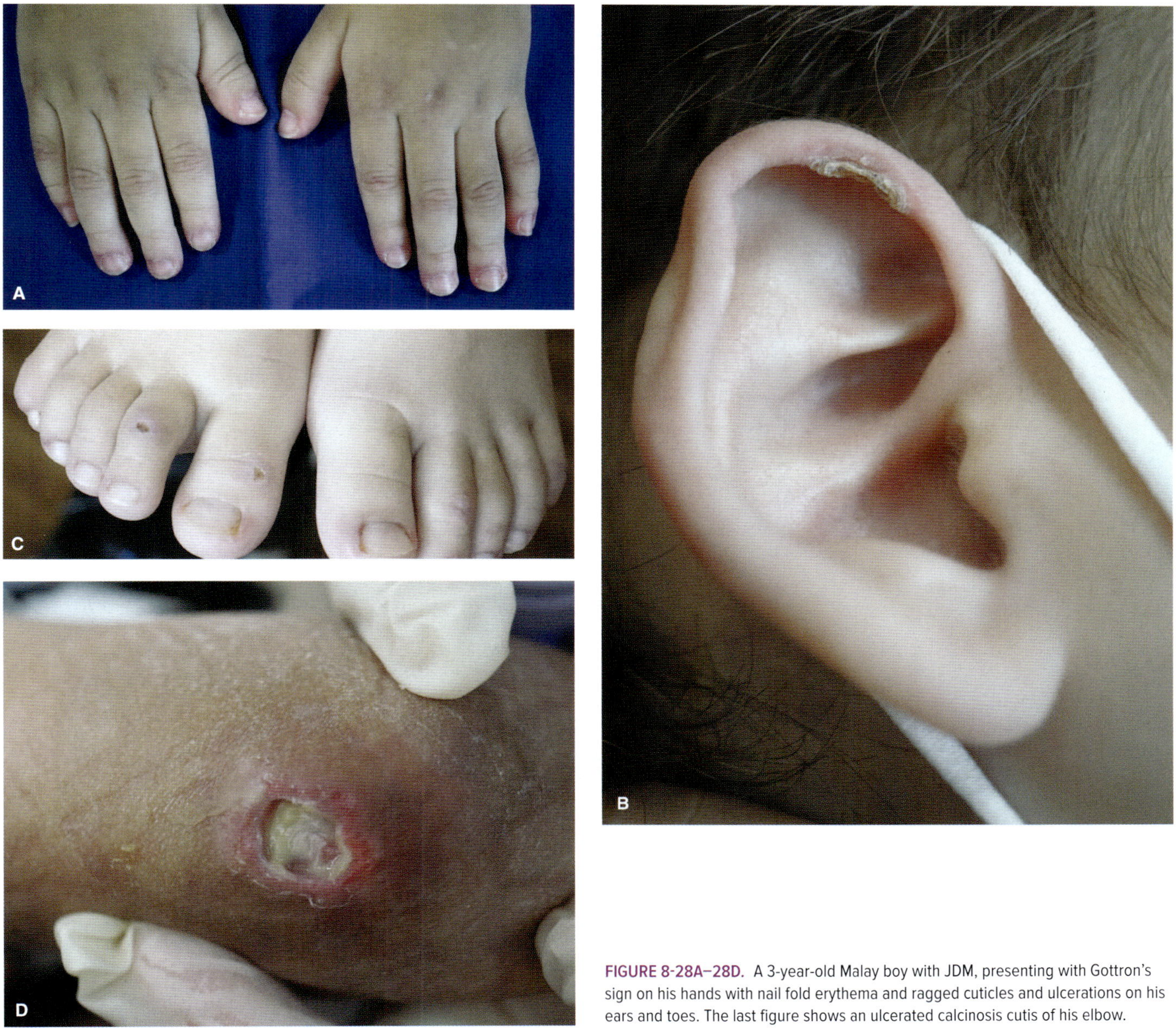

FIGURE 8-28A–28D. A 3-year-old Malay boy with JDM, presenting with Gottron's sign on his hands with nail fold erythema and ragged cuticles and ulcerations on his ears and toes. The last figure shows an ulcerated calcinosis cutis of his elbow.

- Management of JDM is complex and requires multidisciplinary care, preferably with a pediatric rheumatologist.
- Treatment of skin lesions includes sun protection, topical corticosteroids, topical calcineurin inhibitors, and oral antimalarials. High-dose systemic corticosteroids and disease-modifying antirheumatic drugs such as methotrexate are useful for muscle and internal organ involvement.

Pearls & Practical Tips

- In contrast to adults, children tend to have more inflammation and necrosis of muscle, more calcinosis, more small vessel vasculopathy, and a lower mortality.
- Unlike adult dermatomyositis, JDM is not associated with malignancy.
- Early and aggressive treatment may stabilize and prevent organ damage, hence a high index of suspicion and early referral is essential.

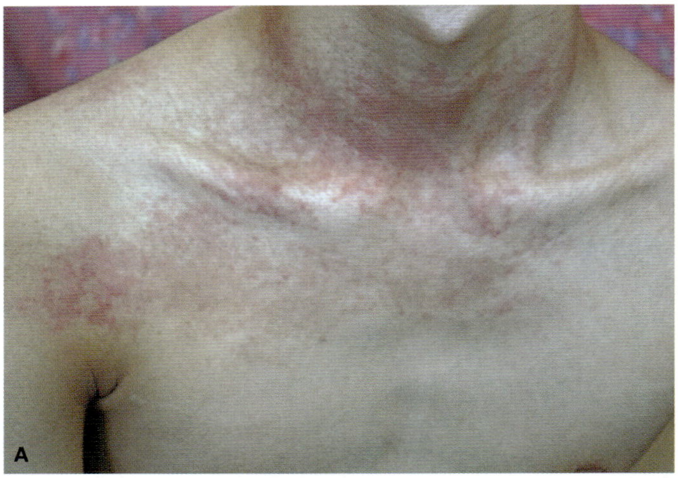

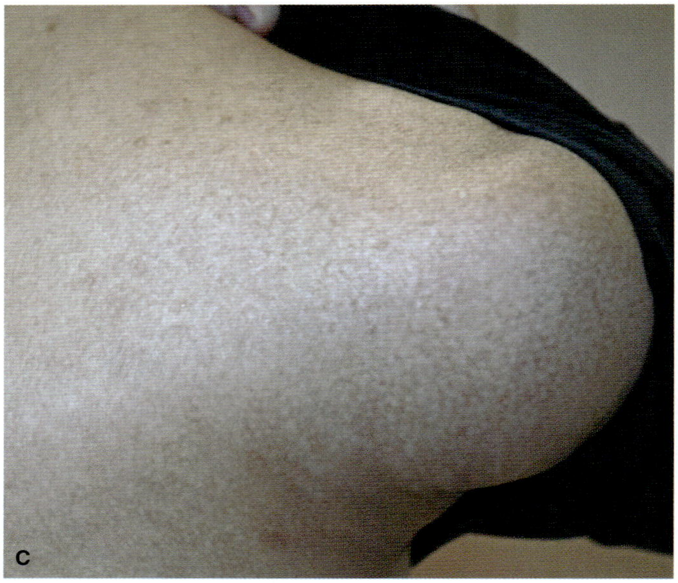

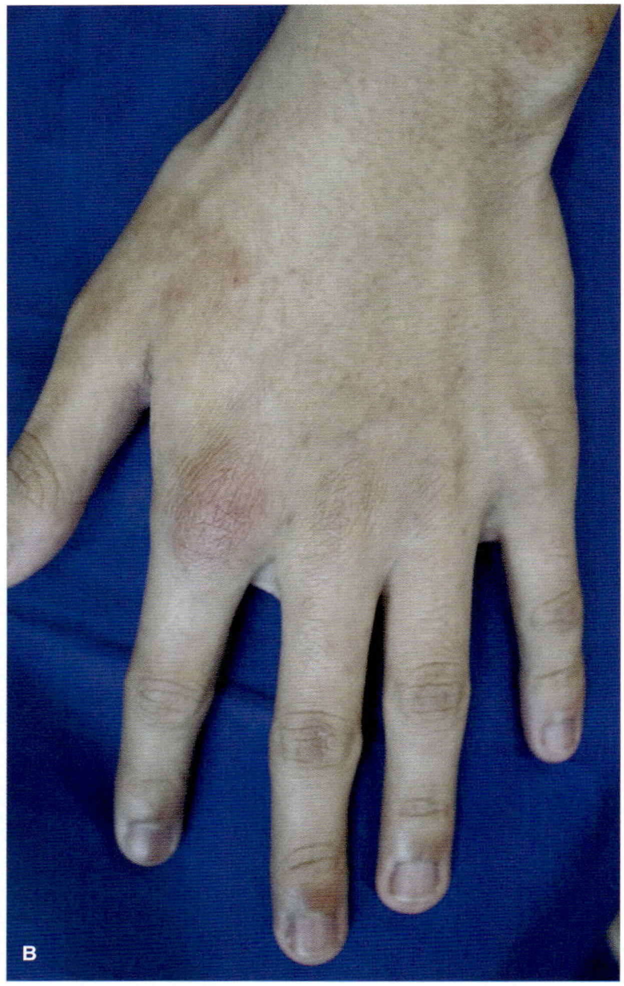

FIGURE 8-29A–29C. A 15-year-old Chinese male with JDM, with violaceous patches and plaques over the anterior chest (Shawl sign). He also exhibits Gottron's sign on the hands and poikiloderma over the shoulder.

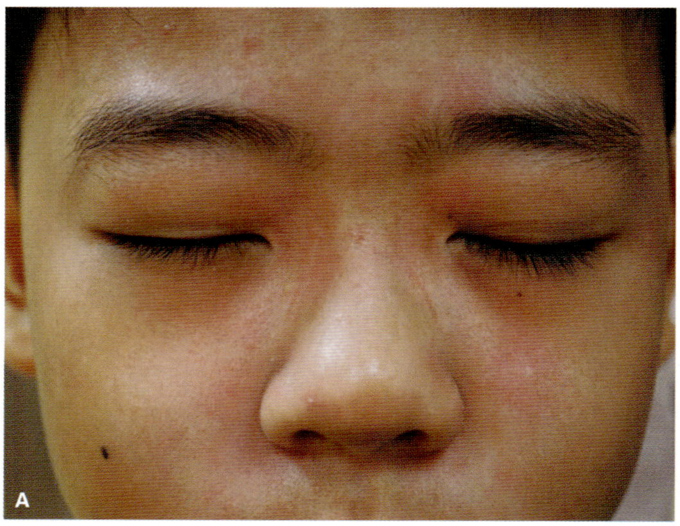

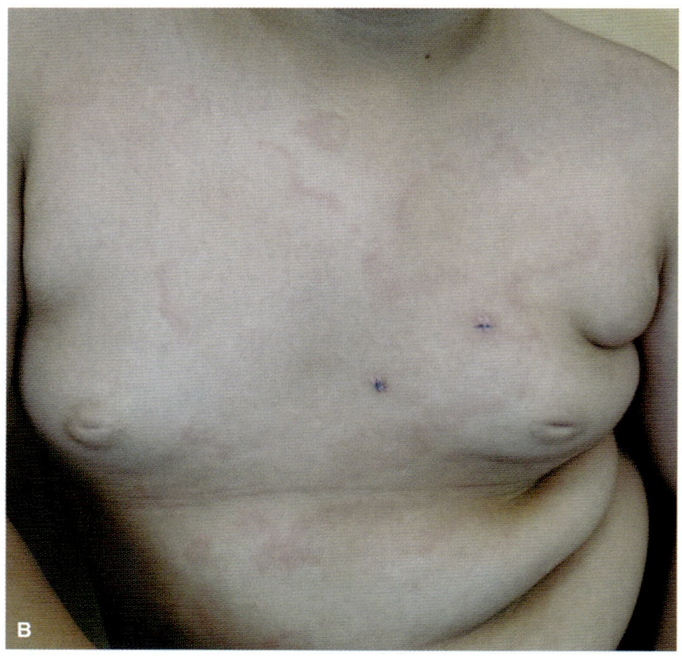

FIGURE 8-30A & 30B. A 12-year-old Chinese male with JDM, with classical heliotrope rash in the periorbital region and cheeks, associated with periorbital edema. He had initially presented with annular erythema on the trunk.

MORPHEA

Morphea is considered an autoimmune condition presenting with localized areas of hardening of the skin or sclerosis, leading subsequently to skin atrophy. It is uncommon in children. Linear morphea is the most common subtype in children, while plaque morphea is the commonest subtype in adults.

Clinical Features

- Morphea can be divided into five subtypes: plaque, linear, deep, generalized, and the rare bullous form.
- Affected areas present with indurated skin and overlying hypo- or hyperpigmentation. Peripheries of lesions often have a lilac-colored border. A shiny indurated appearance indicates active morphea.
- Linear morphea most commonly affects the limbs but can also affect the head and face (*en coup de sabre*, see below). Linear morphea with deep involvement can cause functional limitation, especially if it overlies a joint.
- In severe cases, the sclerosis can extend to underlying muscles, fascia, and bones to cause functional, mobility, and cosmetic issues.
- *En coupe de sabre* is a special variant of linear morphea, where the linear band is over the frontal or frontoparietal region of the scalp. There may be associated facial hemi-atrophy, known as Parry Romberg syndrome. *En coupe de sabre* may be associated with neurological manifestations such as seizures and migraines.

Differential Diagnoses

- Panniculitis
  - Various forms of panniculitis, especially autoimmune panniculitis, can also present with deep induration. Panniculitis lesions tend to be more painful, have an erythematous surface, and may ulcerate or discharge, depending on the cause. Biopsy will differentiate from morphea.

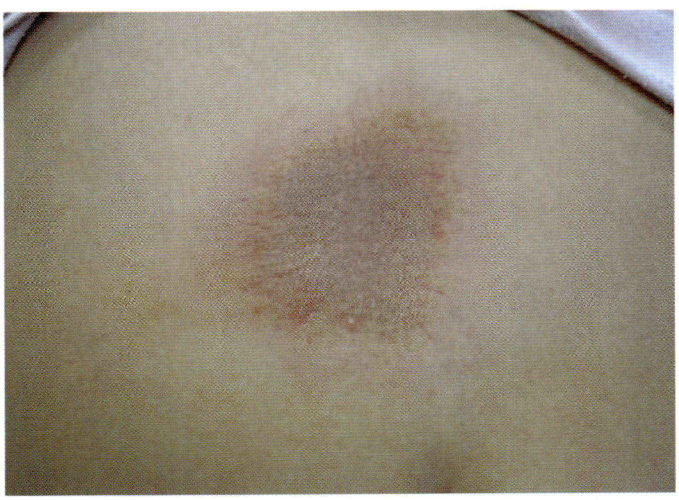

FIGURE 8-31. Early plaque morphea on the abdomen of an 8-year-old Chinese girl, presenting as a hyperpigmented, indurated plaque with a lilac ring along the periphery.

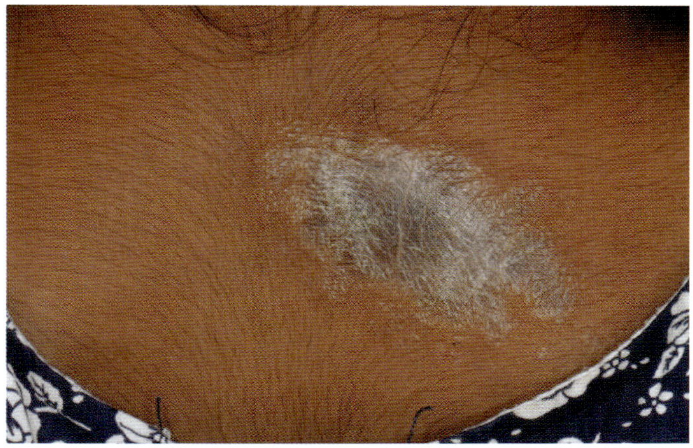

FIGURE 8-32. Plaque morphea on the upper back of an 11-year-old Indian girl, presenting as a hypo- and hyperpigmented, shiny, scaly, indurated plaque.

- Lichen sclerosus (extragenital)
  - Lichen sclerosus (LS) most commonly affects the genital areas in children but can also affect extragenital sites. The lesions of LS have a more shiny surface and are less indurated than morphea.
- Systemic sclerosis (scleroderma)
  - Systemic sclerosis can present with similar skin lesions as morphea. However, there are other facial features such as beaked nose and reduced mouth aperture, as well as systemic involvement, such as musculoskeletal, respiratory, or gastrointestinal tract.
- Atrophoderma (of Pasini and Pierini)
  - This is a rare form of skin atrophy characterized by slightly hyperpigmented depressed areas with a classical "cliff-drop" border. There is no preceding induration as seen in morphea.

Investigations & Treatment

- Diagnosis can be made clinically.
- If performed, histology will show a squared-off biopsy sample, epidermal flattening, thickened hyalinized

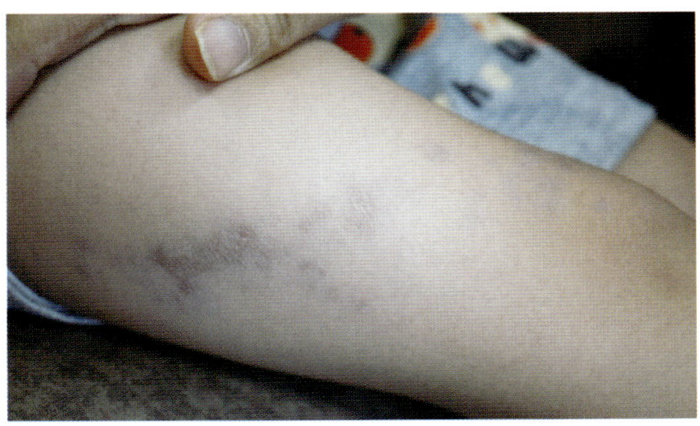

FIGURE 8-33. Linear morphea on the right thigh of a 3-year-old Chinese boy, extending to the right knee, presenting as a violaceous, indurated plaque with wrinkling of the surface.

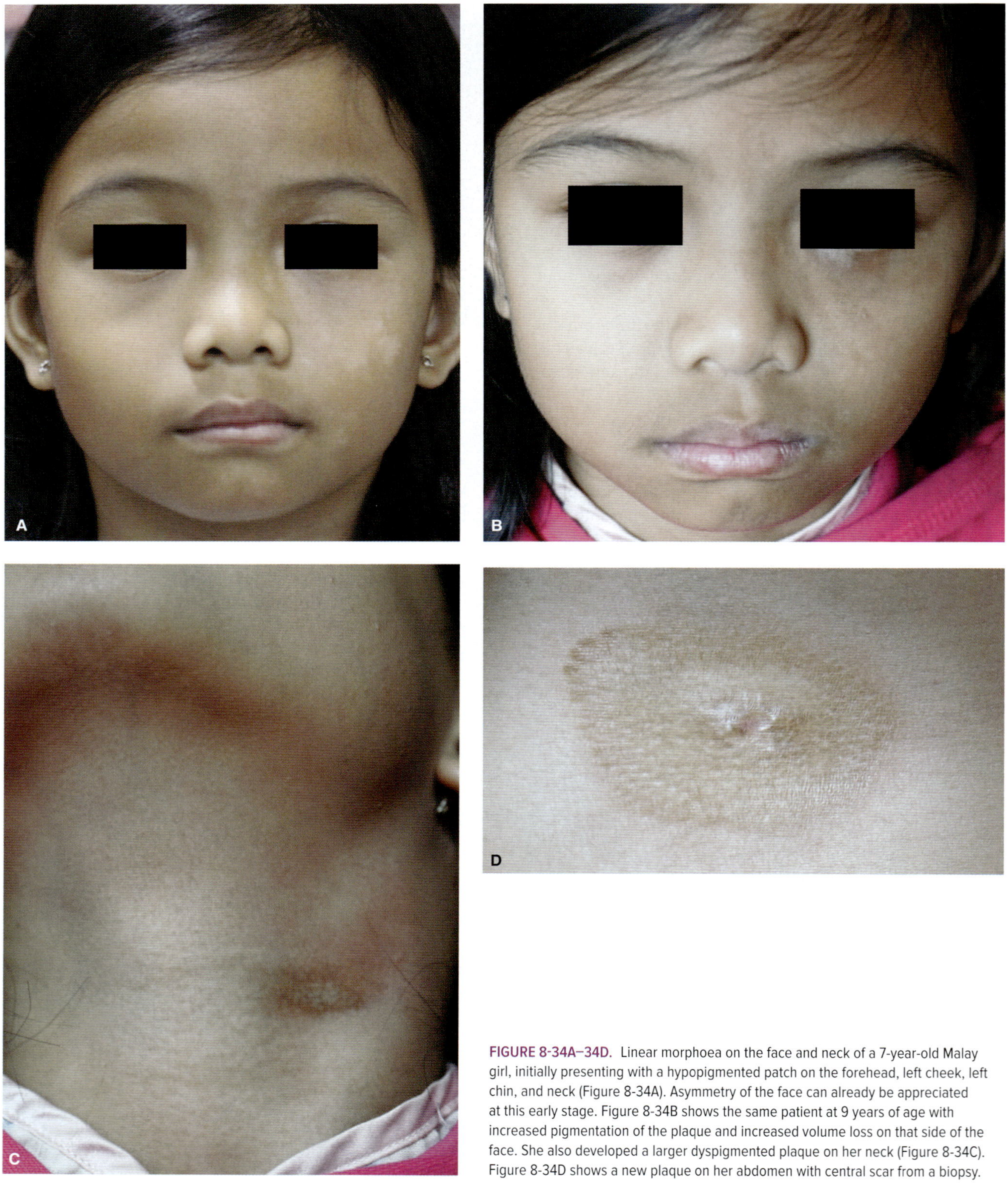

FIGURE 8-34A–34D. Linear morphoea on the face and neck of a 7-year-old Malay girl, initially presenting with a hypopigmented patch on the forehead, left cheek, left chin, and neck (Figure 8-34A). Asymmetry of the face can already be appreciated at this early stage. Figure 8-34B shows the same patient at 9 years of age with increased pigmentation of the plaque and increased volume loss on that side of the face. She also developed a larger dyspigmented plaque on her neck (Figure 8-34C). Figure 8-34D shows a new plaque on her abdomen with central scar from a biopsy.

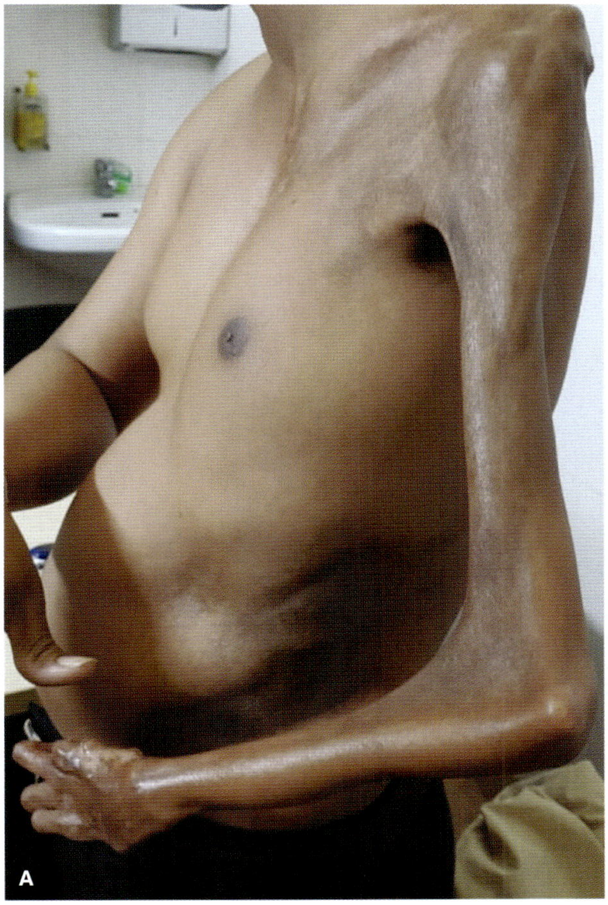

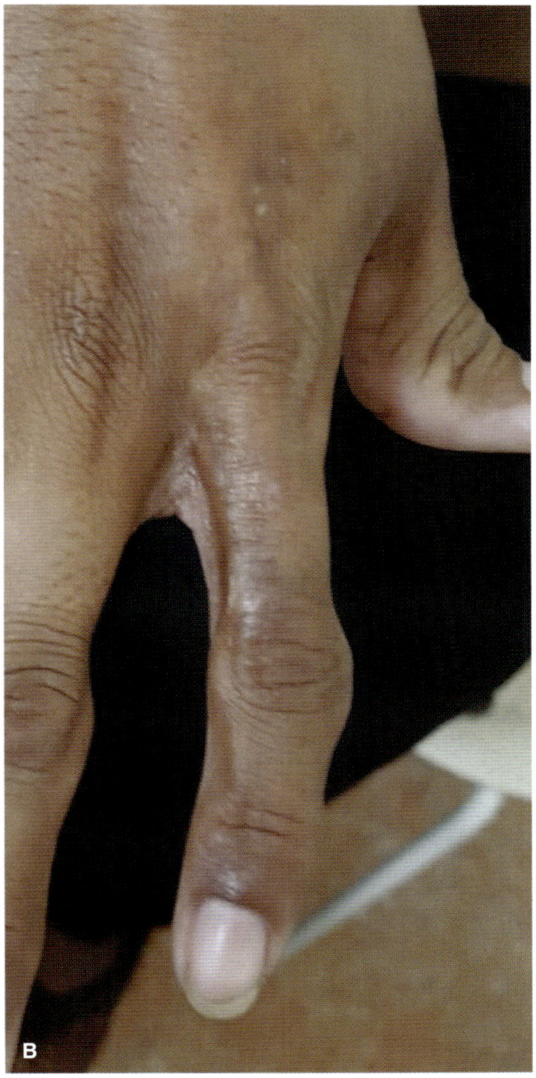

FIGURE 8-35A & 35B. Morphea affecting the entire upper limb of a young Cambodian adult male, leading to severe atrophy and contractures.

collagen in the dermis, and miniaturization of adnexal structures.

- Serological tests are not necessary for evaluation of morphea, although they may be useful in the workup of a mixed connective tissue disease.
- MRI scans may be required to evaluate the extent of involvement, particularly if lesions are over the limbs or head/face.
- Management is dependent on the site, type, severity, and activity. Treatment comprises topicals including topical corticosteroids, calcineurin inhibitors, and vitamin D analogues, such as calcipotriol. Phototherapy may also be considered, such as UVA1 phototherapy. Systemic treatment is advocated for more active lesions with potential for complications, such as joint contractures. Systemic corticosteroids and methotrexate are the most commonly used systemic therapies. Others include mycophenolate mofetil and ciclosporin.

Pearls & Practical Tips

- The initial onset of morphea may be insidious and easily missed. In active lesions, the lilac ring is a good morphological clue. Similarly, previously quiescent areas may show signs of reactivation with the appearance of the peripheral lilac ring.
- Linear morphea over the limbs or joints has to be treated aggressively to avoid limitation of range of movement.
- Parents should be counseled that the disease course may be prolonged over a few years, with a chance of relapse.
- Physiotherapy and occupational therapy may be required for lesions where there is functional impairment, such as linear morphea. Lesions may be also disfiguring, with subsequent psychosocial impairment. Multidisciplinary care is important for addressing the psychosocial aspects of the disease.

AUTOIMMUNE BULLOUS CONDITIONS IN CHILDHOOD

Autoimmune bullous conditions are generally very rare in childhood. They can occur do novo, or through transplacental transfer of antibodies from a mother with an underlying autoimmune bullous condition. In the latter, the blistering improves over a few months with waning maternal antibodies. Linear immunoglobulin A (IgA) bullous dermatosis (LABD) is rare but is by far the most common autoimmune bullous condition in children. Others, such as bullous pemphigoid, dermatitis herpetiformis, and the pemphigus group are extremely rare but should be suspected if a child or adolescent develops chronic, recurrent blisters. More common causes of blistering needs to be excluded, such as acute eczema (endogenous or exogenous), infections (e.g., impetigo, herpes, and varicella), trauma, and mechanobullous disorders, such as congenital epidermolysis bullosa.

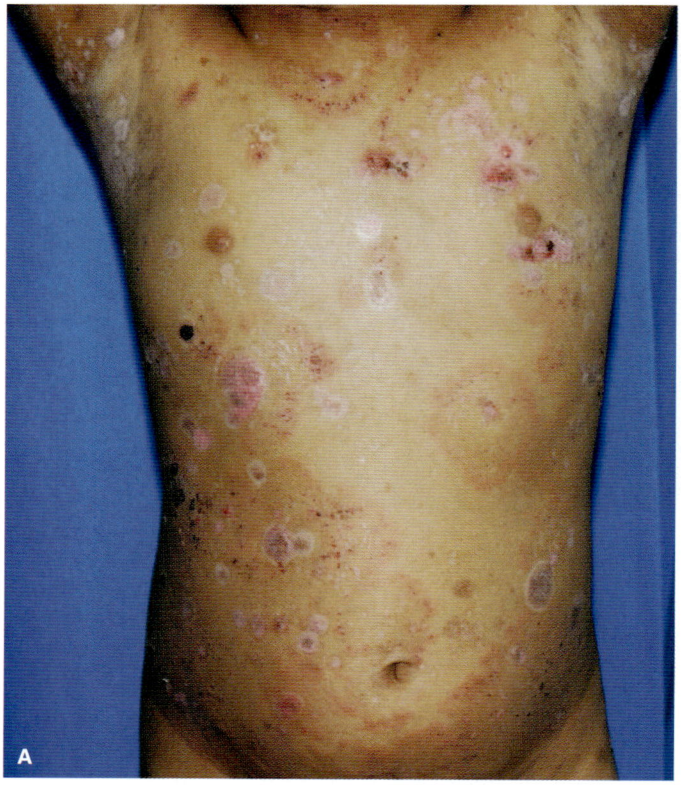

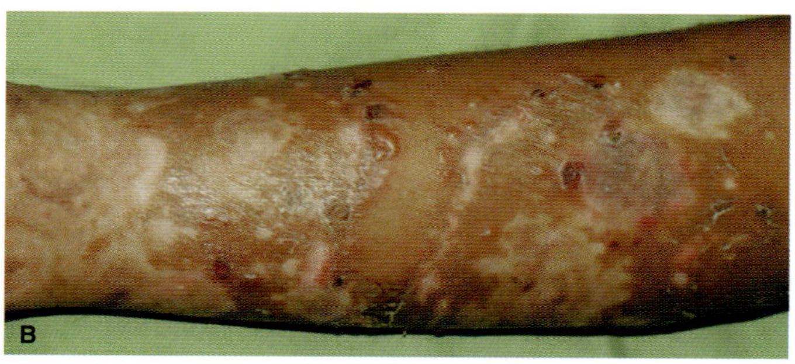

FIGURE 8-36A & 36B. Linear IgA bullous disease in a Malaysian child, presenting with tense blisters, erosions, and dyspigmentation (Photographs courtesy of Hospital Tunku Azizah Kuala Lumpur, Malaysia).

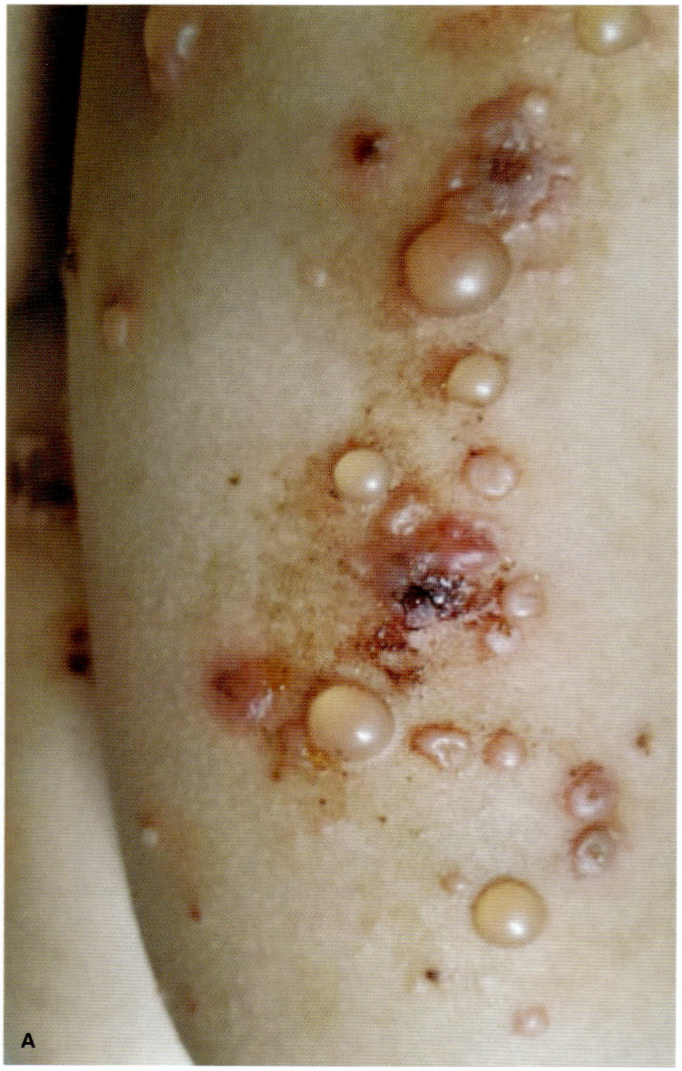

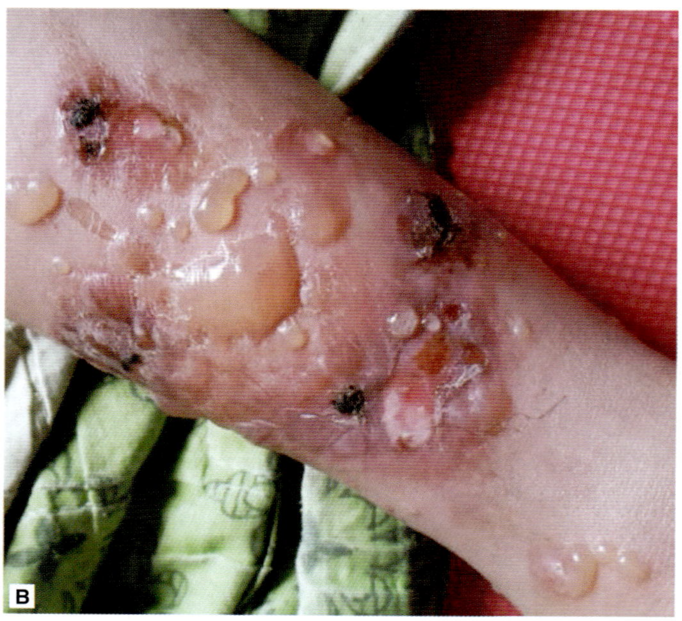

FIGURE 8-37A & 37B. Linear IgA bullous disease in a Vietnamese boy, presenting with widespread tense blisters in a “string-of-pearls” configuration, and crusted erosions.

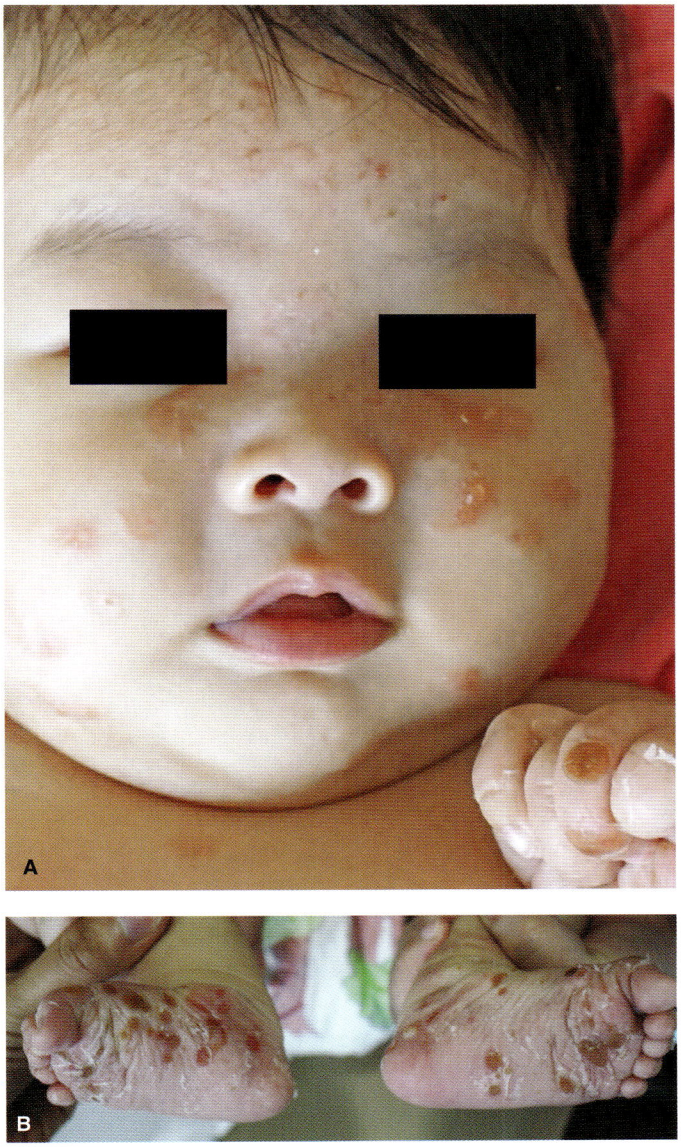

FIGURE 8-38A & 38B. Infantile bullous pemphigoid in a young Chinese infant girl who presented with urticarial plaques, tense blisters, and crusted erosions.

Clinical Features

- Apart from LABD, all other autoimmune bullous conditions are far more common in adults compared to children.
- The prognosis of all autoimmune bullous conditions in children is better than in adults, with most lasting for a few months to a few years before resolution.
- The pathogenesis, clinical features, and investigations results are summarized in Table 8-1.

Differential Diagnoses

- Cutaneous infections
  - These are a far more common cause of blistering in children and adolescents, and present more acutely than autoimmune blistering conditions.
  - Common skin infections that can cause blistering include bacterial infections (e.g., impetigo, cellulitis, and erysipelas), viral infections (e.g., herpes simplex, varicella-zoster, and hand-foot-mouth disease) and fungal infections (e.g., bullous tinea pedis).
- Acute eczemas
  - Various forms of acute eczemas can present with blistering. This can be both endogenous (e.g., pompholyx) or exogenous (e.g., allergic or irritant contact dermatitis).
  - There is usually a prior history of eczema or contact with a possible allergen.
- Bullous insect bite reactions
  - This is extremely common in children and presents very acutely, especially after an outdoor activity. Classical lesions of insect bites are usually also present.

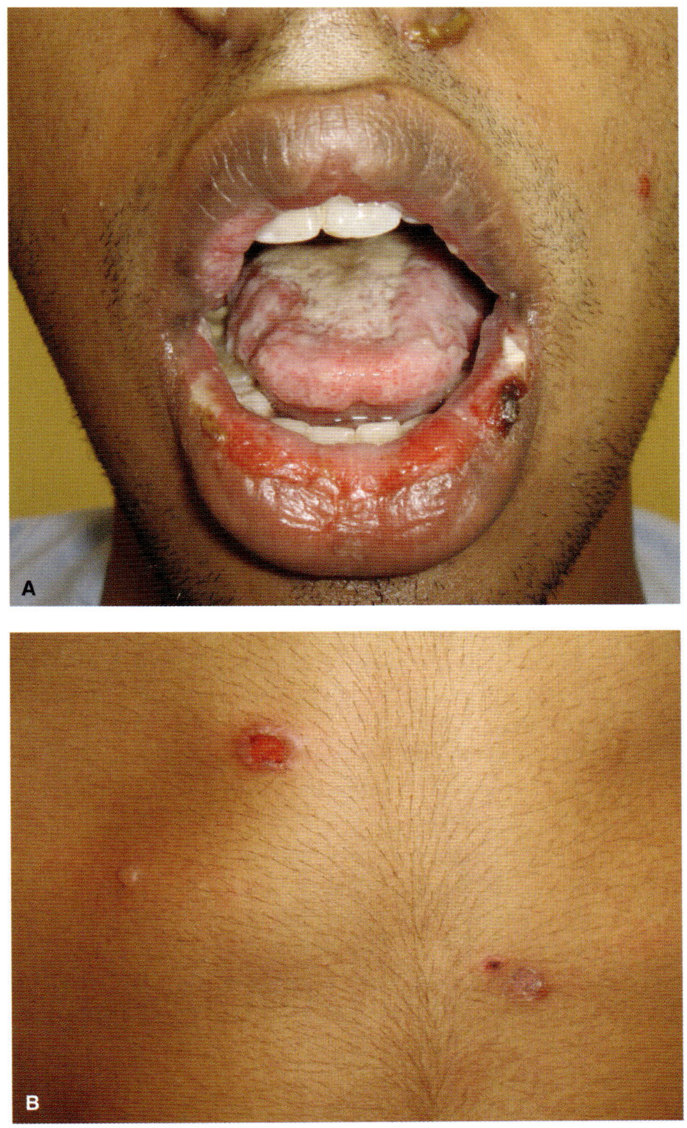

FIGURE 8-39A & 39B. Pemphigus vulgaris in an 18-year-old Malay male presenting with lip and oral erosions, and scattered blisters and erosions over the trunk.

TABLE 8-1. Pathogenesis & clinical presentation of autoimmune bullous conditions in childhood.

Condition	Auto-antibody	Target antigen	Presentation	Sites of predilection	Histology, DIF, IIF, and ELISA findings
Linear IgA bullous disorder (LABD)	IgA	BP180	Abrupt onset of tense vesicles and bullae arranged in an annular fashion with a tendency to form rings around older lesions ("string of pearls"); bullae can arise on normal or erythematous or urticated skin. Pruritus is variable.	Anogenital area, lower abdomen, lower limbs, head	H: Subepidermal blister, neutrophils D: Linear band of IgA at BMZ I: Roof pattern on salt split skin
Bullous pemphigoid	IgG	BP 180 or BP 230 (hemi-desmosomes)	Pre-bullous phase presents as edematous, erythematous plaques which resemble urticaria wheals, can occur months before the blistering occurs; bullous phase presents with crops of large, tense bullae appearing on erythematous/urticated skin.	Hands and feet in infants (infantile BP), can be generalized	H: Subepidermal blister, eosinophils D: Linear IgG, C3 at BMZ I: Roof pattern on salt split skin
Pemphigus foliaceus	IgG	Desmoglein-1	Small, flaccid blisters that rupture easily, leaving shallow, sometimes crusted plaques. There is no mucosal involvement.	Face, scalp, upper chest, abdomen	H: Intraepidermal blister with acantholysis D: Intercellular IgG, C3 in epidermis I: Same as DIF E: Anti-Desmoglein-1
Pemphigus vulgaris	IgG	Desmoglein-1 and 3	Vesicles or bullae on erythematous or normal skin. Blisters break easily, leaving erosions with crusting and scaling. Nikolsky sign is positive. Mucosal involvement is frequent.	Face, scalp, neck, axillae, groin (seborrheic areas), oral mucosa	H: Suprabasal blister with acantholysis D: Intercellular IgG, C3 in epidermis I: Same as DIF E: Anti-Desmoglein-1 and 3
Dermatitis herpetiformis	IgA	Tissue transglutaminase & endomysium	Symmetrical, grouped intensely pruritic, tense, small vesicles that rupture easily; small bowel abnormalities similar to celiac disease.	Extensor surfaces of elbows, knees, and buttocks	H: Small subepidermal blisters, neutrophils D: Granular IgA at BMZ E: Anti-endomysium, anti-epidermal transglutaminase, anti-gliadin antibodies

H, Histology; D, DIF; I, IIF; E, ELISA

- Inherited mechanobullous disorders
  - These include inherited epidermolysis bullosa (EB) and porphyria, although the latter is extremely rare in children.
  - EB presents with blisters at sites of trauma and there may be a family history of disease or consanguinity.

Investigations & Treatment

- Diagnosis of autoimmune bullous conditions in childhood can be difficult or delayed due to the rarity, and the clinical presentation can mimic many other childhood dermatoses.
- Investigations to exclude other more common causes of blistering should always be performed, especially bacterial cultures, viral PCR, fungal microscopy, or fungal culture.
- Investigations to confirm a diagnosis of autoimmune bullous conditions include skin biopsies for histology and direct immunofluorescence (DIF). Specimens for histology should be performed from the edge of a blister, while histology for DIF should be performed 0.5 to 1 cm away from an active blister.
- Autoantibodies may also be detected from blood by indirect immunofluorescence; ELISA or immunoblot can also be performed.
- Localized skin lesions may be treated with mid- to high-potency topical corticosteroid.
- Systemic medications may be required for more extensive disease. These include systemic corticosteroids and other immunomodulating agents, such as dapsone, mycophenolate mofetil, azathioprine, IVIG, and rituximab.

Pearls & Practical Tips

- Diagnosis of autoimmune bullous conditions in childhood can be difficult or delayed due to the rarity, and the clinical presentation can mimic many other childhood dermatoses.
- The prognosis of bullous disorders in childhood is variable, with some resolving after a few months or years and others continuing into adulthood.

Bibliography

1. Schwieger-Briel A, Moellmann C, Mattulat B, et al. Bullous pemphigoid in infants: characteristics, diagnosis and treatment. Orphanet J Rare Dis 2014;9:185.
2. Kong YL, Lim YL, Chandran NS. Retrospective study on autoimmune blistering disease in paediatric patients. Pediatr Dermatol 2015;32:845-52.

POLYMORPHOUS LIGHT ERUPTION

Polymorphous (or polymorphic) light eruption (PMLE) is the most common idiopathic immunologically mediated photodermatosis, especially in younger patients. The rash is postulated to be caused by a delayed-type hypersensitivity response to an unknown antigen and exposure to UV light in susceptible individuals.

Clinical Features

- The typical onset of PMLE is within the first three decades of life, with a female predominance.
- PMLE presents as pruritic, erythematous, 1- to 2-mm papules, macules, plaques, or vesicles on sun-exposed sites, such as the forehead, upper cheeks, ear helices, posterior and lateral neck, and the extensor surfaces of the forearms and legs.
- Characteristic areas of sparing are the shaded areas under the nose, lower lip, and chin, as well as the hairline, behind the earlobes, upper eyelids, and finger webs.
- Juvenile spring eruption is considered a localized form of PMLE, most commonly appears on the ears in boys, and presents as itchy, erythematous, small papules which may evolve into blisters with crusts. It resolves with minimal or no scarring after a few days to 2 weeks.
- Lesions classically appear within 30 minutes to a few hours following sun exposure. Resolution occurs within hours, or up to 2 weeks once light exposure is discontinued, without sequelae.

Differential Diagnoses

- Solar urticaria
  - Solar urticaria presents as urticarial wheals that develop within minutes after exposure to sunlight.
- Lupus erythematosus
  - Lesions are usually not itchy and persist for weeks to months.
  - Diagnosis may be made with skin biopsy and serology tests for lupus.
- Porphyria cutanea tarda
  - This is rare in children, and presents with vesicles and erosions that crust and heal with atrophic scarring and milia. Additional features include hypertrichosis, hyperpigmentation, and sclerodermoid changes.

Investigations & Treatment

- The diagnosis of PMLE is usually clinical with classical history and physical examination.

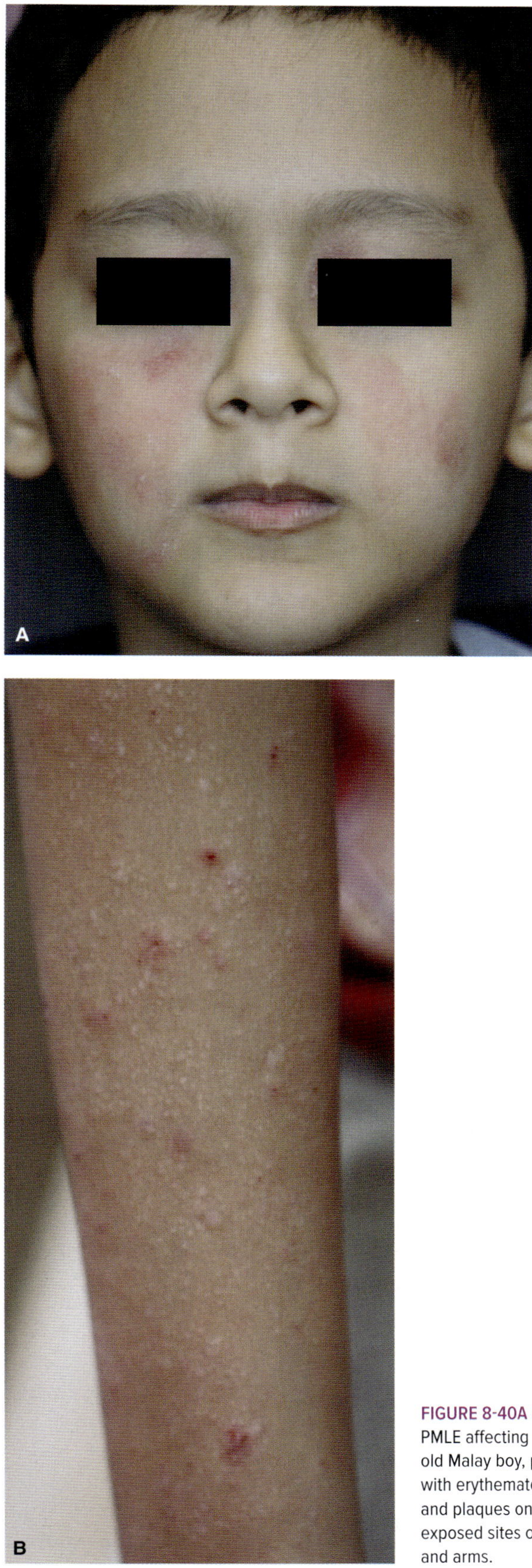

FIGURE 8-40A & 40B. PMLE affecting an 11-year-old Malay boy, presenting with erythematous papules and plaques on sun-exposed sites on his face and arms.

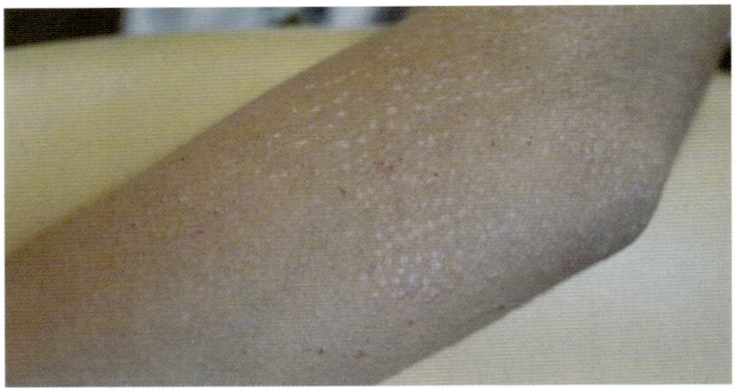

FIGURE 8-41. Lichen nitidus-like PMLE of the forearms and elbows of a 7-year-old Chinese boy, presenting as hypopigmented, flat-topped papules, with some excoriations.

- Phototesting, if performed, often provides equivocal results, although there may be reduced minimal erythema dose to UVA and less commonly UVB. Photoprovocation testing may reproduce the characteristic rash in the patient.
- Skin biopsy, if performed, shows spongiosis, vesicle formation, and mild interface changes.
- Screening for autoimmune antibodies, porphyrin levels, and complete blood counts may be performed in atypical presentations or if there is suspicion of other photosensitive disorders.
- Treatment is with photoprotection, including avoidance of excessive sun exposure, use of sun protective clothing, and sunscreens.
- Topical corticosteroids can offer symptomatic relief during acute episodes, while oral corticosteroids may be necessary for severe flares.
- In severe uncontrolled cases, phototherapy or systemic agents such as antimalarials, azathioprine, or cyclosporine may be helpful.

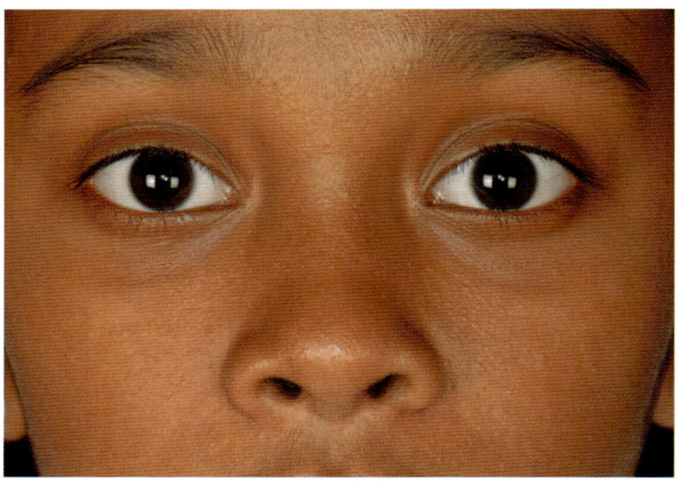

FIGURE 8-42. Lichen nitidus-like PMLE on the face of a 10-year-old Indian girl, presenting as skin-colored to hypopigmented 1- to 2-mm papules over the nose bridge and cheeks.

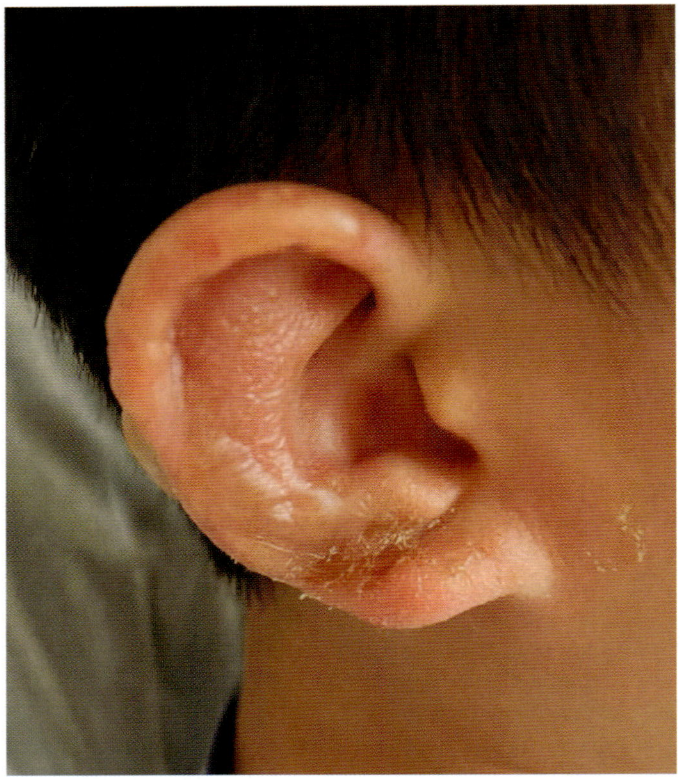

FIGURE 8-43. Juvenile spring eruption on the ear of a 7-year-old Chinese boy, presenting with erythematous papules, blisters, and crusting after sun exposure.

Pearls & Practical Tips

- The lichen nitidus–like PMLE variant is commonly seen in darker-skinned individuals, especially those of Asian descent. Unlike classical lichen nitidus, this variant of PMLE occurs secondary to UV exposure, occurs over sun-exposed sites, and resolves with sun avoidance.
- UVA, UVB, and visible light wavelengths have all been reported to trigger PMLE. Broad-spectrum sunscreens with both UVA and UVB filters and physical blockers containing titanium dioxide and zinc oxide are recommended.

OTHER PHOTODERMATOSES

Apart from polymorphous light eruption, the other photodermatoses are generally rare in children and adolescents. These include solar urticaria, hydroa vacciniforme, and juvenile spring eruption. Exogenous causes of photosensitivity also need to be excluded in patients presenting with a photo-distributed rash. These include photocontact dermatitis (phytophotodermatitis), phototoxic drug reactions, and photoallergic drug reactions.

Clinical Features

- The photodermatoses most commonly present with photo-distributed rashes, mostly affecting the face, neck, outer arms, and extensor surfaces of the legs. Secondary spread to sun-covered areas can also occur.

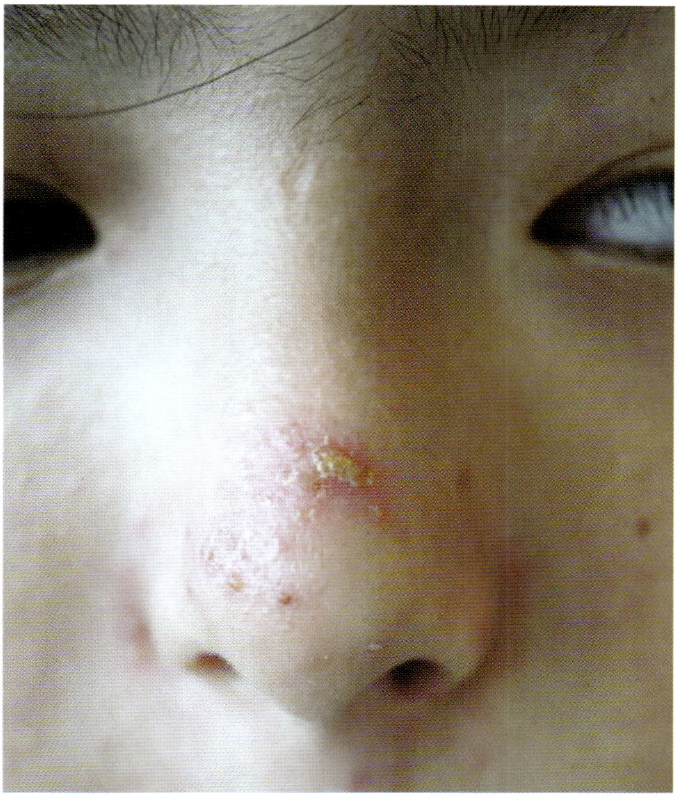

FIGURE 8-44. Hydroa vacciniforme on the sun-exposed sites of a 10-year-old Nepalese girl, presenting with recurrent small blisters after sun exposure. Some scarring is noted on the forehead.

- Occasionally, areas that are chronically exposed to the sun can develop "hardening" and do not develop the rash.
- Depending on the condition, the eruption can occur minutes, hours, to days after exposure to light. For example, in solar urticaria, the wheals appear minutes after light exposure, whereas in hydroa vacciniforme it can occur a few days after light exposure.
- Similarly, onset of photocontact dermatitis and photodrug eruption can occur days, months, or years after initial exposure, depending on the frequency and duration of application or drug ingestion.
- The causes, age at presentation, onset from exposure to light, clinical features, differential diagnoses, investigations, and treatment of the various idiopathic photodermatoses are summarized in Table 8-2.

Pearls & Practical Tips

- When faced with a photo-distributed rash, a thorough clinical history including a drug history and possible contactants is important. Investigations to exclude other more common causes of photosensitivity, such as connective tissue disorders, may be required, depending on the clinical picture. Certain dermatoses may also be photoaggravated, such as eczema.
- Often, lesions may occur on covered skin, as UVA and visible light can pass through thin clothing, or there may be secondary spread of the initial photosensitive rash.
- The initial inflammatory reaction in photocontact dermatitis may be mild and go unnoticed. These patients may only present weeks later with delayed "unexplained" hyperpigmentation. Patients frequently do not recall the inciting event.
- Photoactive drugs may continue to cause photosensitivity for up to 1 year after discontinuation of the drug.

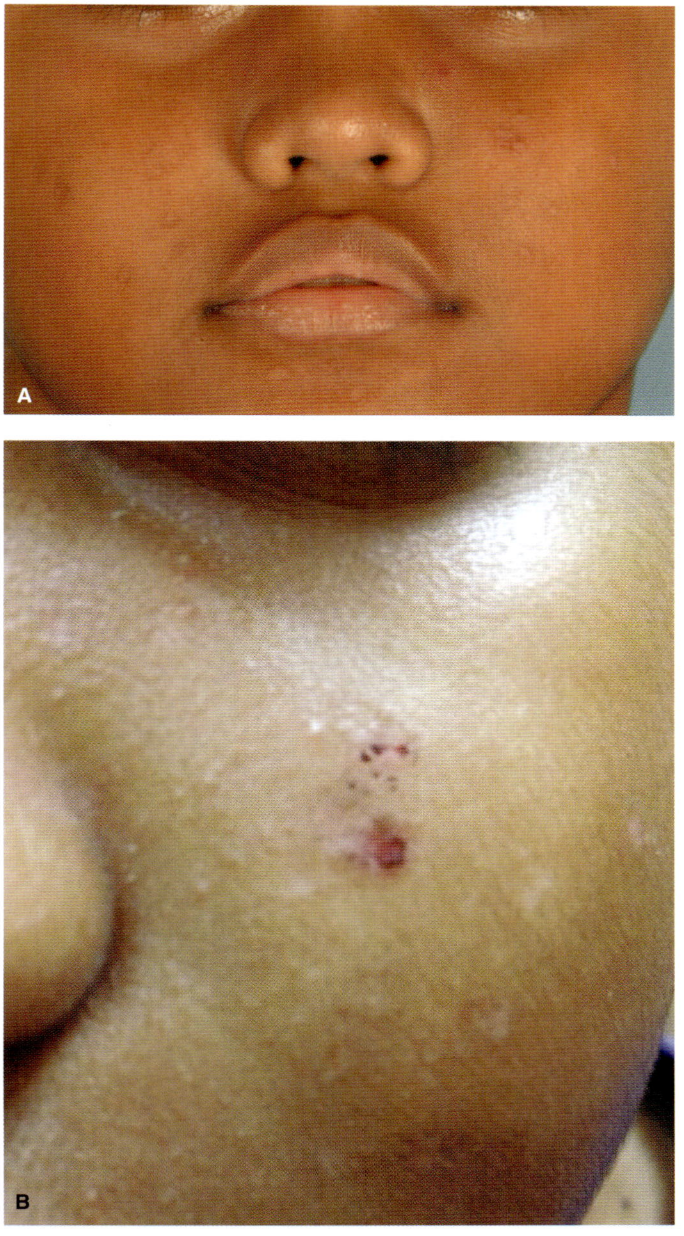

FIGURE 8-45A & 45B. Hydroa vacciniforme on the cheeks of a 14-year-old Malay boy with varioliform, depressed scars on both cheeks. Figure 8-45B shows an early crusted lesion on the right cheek.

TABLE 8-2. Pathogenesis & clinical presentation of autoimmune bullous conditions in childhood.

Condition	Causes	Age at presentation	Onset from light exposure	Presentation	Differential diagnoses	Investigations & Treatment
Solar urticaria	• None	• Any age • Peak 20–40 years	• Minutes	• Itchy or painful, erythematous wheals over sun-exposed sites • Eruption usually disappear within 30–60 minutes of sun avoidance, or within 24 hours • Intense light exposure to large areas of skin may lead to severe systemic anaphylactic-like reactions, such as giddiness, nausea, hypotension, bronchospasm, and syncope	• Polymorphous light eruption • Cholinergic urticaria • Heat urticaria	• Phototesting: wheals appear upon testing with visible light & UVA • Photoprotection • Antihistamines • Others: corticosteroids, anti-malarials, ciclosporin, omalizumab
Hydroa vacciniforme	• Ebstein-Barr virus	• Early childhood to adolescence	• 30 minutes to few hours	• Hemorrhagic papulovesicles with a burning and/or itching sensation • Symmetrically over the face, ears, and dorsum of the hands; there may be associated facial swelling • Crust and heal with pale, depressed scars, after 1–2 weeks • Associated mild fever and malaise • Most resolve by adolescence or early adulthood • Rarely, eye involvement, e.g., conjunctivitis, keratitis, corneal infiltration, uveitis, and photophobia can occur	• Polymorphous light eruption • Porphyria cutanea tarda • Cutaneous chronic lupus erythematosus • Hydroa vacciniforme–like lymphoma	• Histology: epidermal vesicles with epidermal necrosis, superficial & deep perivascular lymphocytic infiltrate • Photoprotection • Others: phototherapy for desensitization, anti-malarials, beta-carotene, azathioprine, cyclosporine, dietary fish oil supplementation
Photocontact dermatitis	• Sunscreens, e.g., oxybenzones • Plants and fruits, e.g., citrus • Fragrances, essential oils	• Any age • Uncommon in children	• 24–72 hours post-exposure	• Allergic reaction to chemicals that contact with skin, with subsequent exposure to light • Acute inflammatory phase presents as burning erythema, with vesicles and bullae on exposed skin • Post-inflammatory hyperpigmentation in linear or bizarre patterns, may persist for weeks to months • Most commonly affected areas are legs & hands	• Contact dermatitis • Nonaccidental injury • Jellyfish sting	• Photopatch testing, but can be difficult in children • Topical and/or systemic corticosteroids in acute phase • Photoprotection in hyperpigmentation phase • Avoidance of contactant
Phototoxic & photoallergic drug eruption	• Antibiotics, e.g., tetracyclines, fluoroquinolones • NSAIDs • Retinoids, e.g., isotretinoin, acitretin	• Any age • Uncommon in children	• Phototoxic: minutes to hours after exposure to drug & light • Photoallergic: 24–72 hours after exposure to drug & light	• Phototoxic reactions present as exaggerated sunburn reactions on sun-exposed surfaces; vesicles and bullae in severe reactions; limited to sun-exposed sites • Photoallergic reactions present as pruritic, eczematous reactions; post-inflammatory hyperpigmentation is common	• Sunburn • Airborne contact dermatitis • Lupus erythematosus	• Phototesting, but can be difficult in children, reduced minimal erythema dose to UVA • Identify & withdraw culprit drug • Moisturizers, topical corticosteroids, oral antihistamines • Severe reactions may require a course of systemic corticosteroids • Photoprotection with broad-spectrum sunscreens

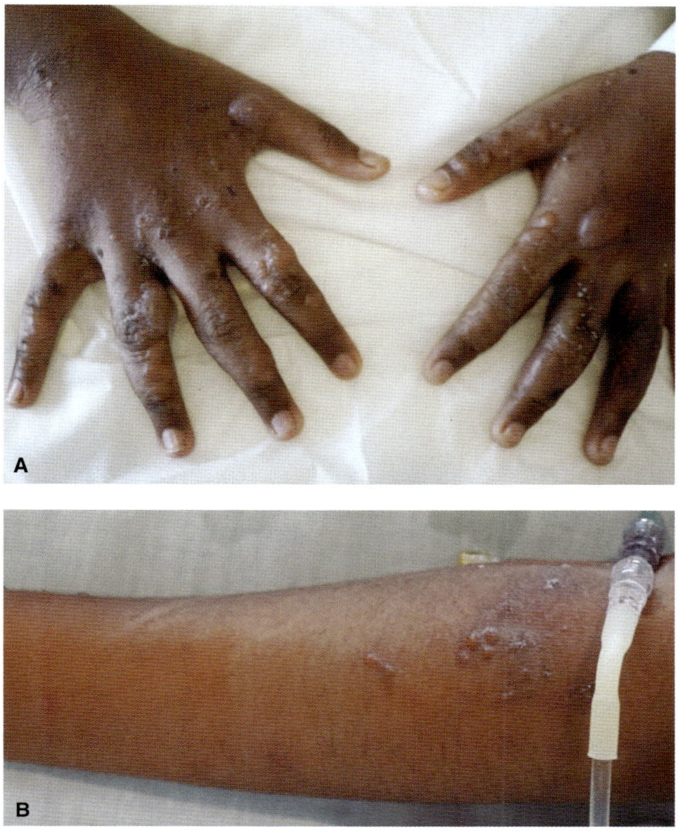

FIGURE 8-46A & 46B. Acute photocontact dermatitis in a 12-year-old boy, presenting with itchy blisters and papules on sun-exposed sites. He was in contact with plants 2 days before the eruption.

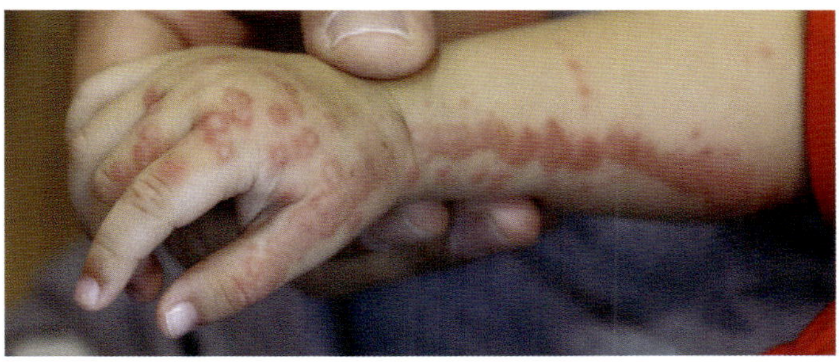

FIGURE 8-47. Photocontact dermatitis in a 15-month-old girl after playing with plants in the garden, presenting with pruritic, erythematous, linear plaques with vesicles on her right forearm and hand.

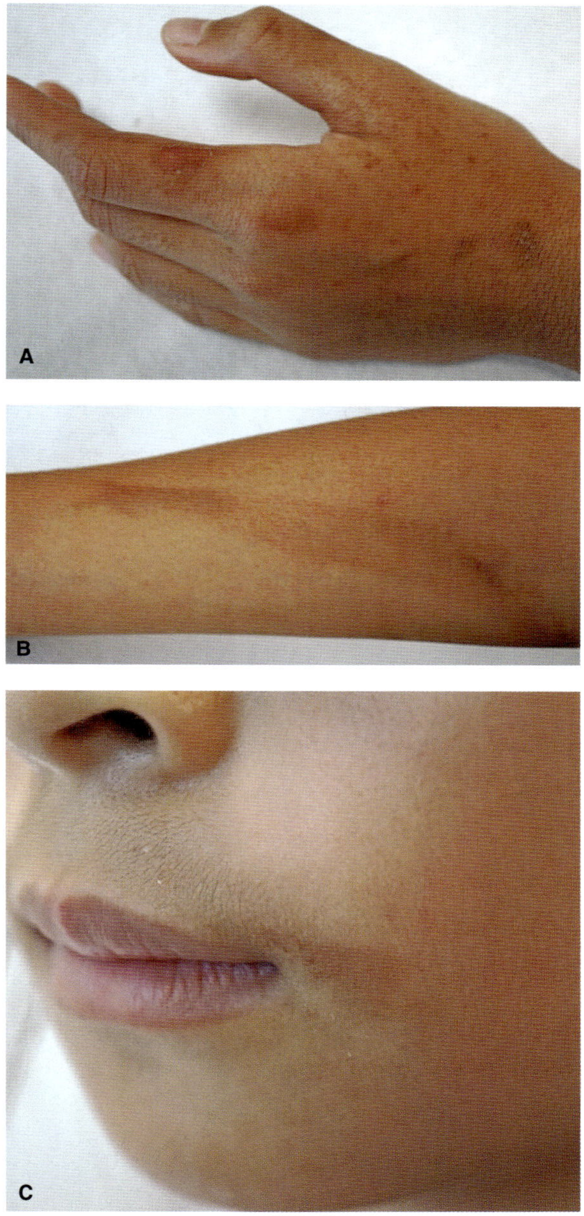

FIGURE 8-48A–48C. Photocontact dermatitis in an 11-year-old girl with linear hyperpigmented patch on her left arm, hyperpigmented macules over her thumb and index finger, and a patch on the left cheek, occurring after contact with citrus fruits at the beach. This form of photocontact dermatitis is also known as phytophotodermatitis.

9

Hair and Nail Disorders

APPROACH TO HAIR DISORDERS

The human body is comprised of approximately five million hair follicles. Lanugo hairs are found only in the fetal and neonatal life, which are then replaced by vellus hair after 3 to 4 months of age, followed by thicker, more pigmented terminal hairs.

HAIR GROWTH CYCLE

Hair growth occurs at an average rate of approximately 1 cm per month. There are three definitive stages in the terminal hair growth cycle:

1. Anagen phase—this is the growth phase of the hair cycle and lasts about 2 to 6 years (average 3 years). Approximately 85% to 90% of hairs are in this phase.
2. Catagen phase—this is the period of partial degeneration and lasts for about 3 weeks. Approximately 1% of hairs are in this phase.
3. Telogen phase—this is the resting phase and lasts between 3 and 4 months. Approximately 10% to 15% of hairs are in this phase.

Telogen hairs are pushed out of the hair follicles as new hairs are generated. The average number of hairs shed a day ranges from 50 to 100 in healthy individuals, higher on shampoo days.

Clinical History

Common complaints for patients presenting with hair problems include increased hair shedding or thinning of hair such that the scalp becomes more visible. These complaints usually point to a problem with the hair follicle. Some patients will complain of abnormal hair, such as twisted, curly, or irregularly shaped hair. These complaints usually point to a problem with the hair shaft. Some younger children may present with a history of not needing a haircut, or that their hair cannot "grow long." Differentials would include loose anagen or short anagen syndrome. Finally, some patients complain of scalp abnormalities, such as scaling or "dandruff." These patients most often have a scalp dermatosis that may be associated with hair loss such as psoriasis, eczema, or tinea capitis.

Other important points from the clinical history include:

- Presence of hair at birth
- Progression and rate of hair changes
- Diet and nutrition
- Environmental exposure, such as hair care products, toxins, and so forth
- Past medical history—especially atopic, autoimmune, and endocrine diseases
- Family history of hair and skin disorders

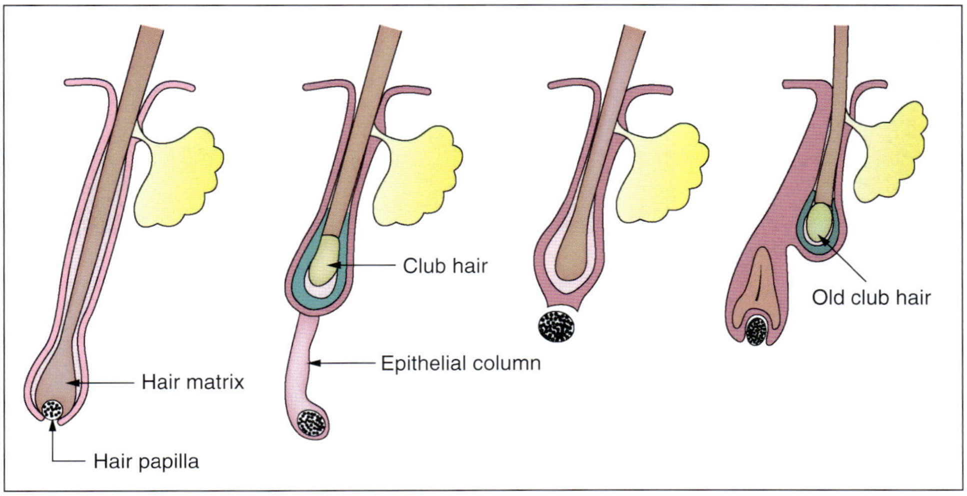

Normal hair cycle.

Clinical Examination

General hair examination should be performed, observing for color, texture, and length of hair. If there are concerns for alopecia, important aspects to examine for include the pattern of hair loss (diffuse, patchy, or focal), the extent of hair loss (e.g., scalp surface area), and the sites affected (e.g., vertex, occiput, temporal, eyebrows, eyelashes, beard area, axilla, groin, and other body hair sites). The scalp skin should be examined to observe for features of scarring, such as loss of hair follicles, smooth surface, and depression from surrounding skin. Features of inflammation should be examined for including erythema, scaling, crusting, and pustules. Pigmentary changes should also be noted.

The hair pull test should be performed in all cases of alopecia and involves gently pulling a bundle of 20 to 60 hairs between the thumb and forefinger from multiple locations. The test is positive if more than 10% of hairs are released. The hair tug test should be performed if a hair shaft abnormality is suspected, and involves grasping hair between the thumb and forefinger near its root and tugging the same strand at its distal end. Breakage of hair with this maneuver indicates hair shaft fragility. Trichoscopy using a dermatoscope should be employed to visualize the scalp and hair, if available.

Finally, a focused general examination should be performed and includes visualization of all skin sites, dentition, nails, growth parameters, dysmorphic features, and vision and hearing assessments.

ALOPECIA AREATA

Alopecia areata (AA) is a common cause of non-scarring, localized hair loss in the pediatric and adult population, with a prevalence of 0.1% to 0.2% of the population. Approximately 20% of patients present before 16 years of age, and 1% to 2% present before 2 years of age. It is usually limited and self-limiting, with spontaneous hair regrowth after several months. More severe cases can progress to alopecia totalis or alopecia universalis.

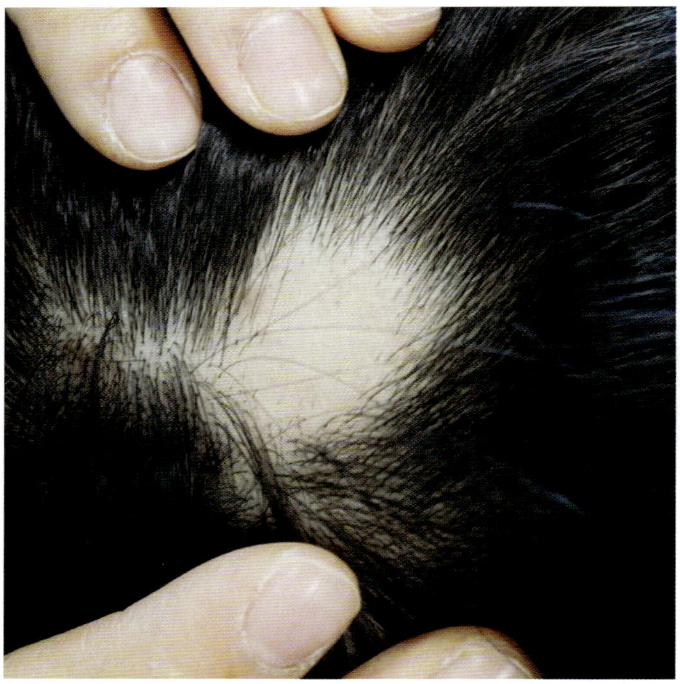

FIGURE 9-1. Alopecia areata on the scalp of a Chinese boy, presenting with a circular patch of non-scarring hair loss.

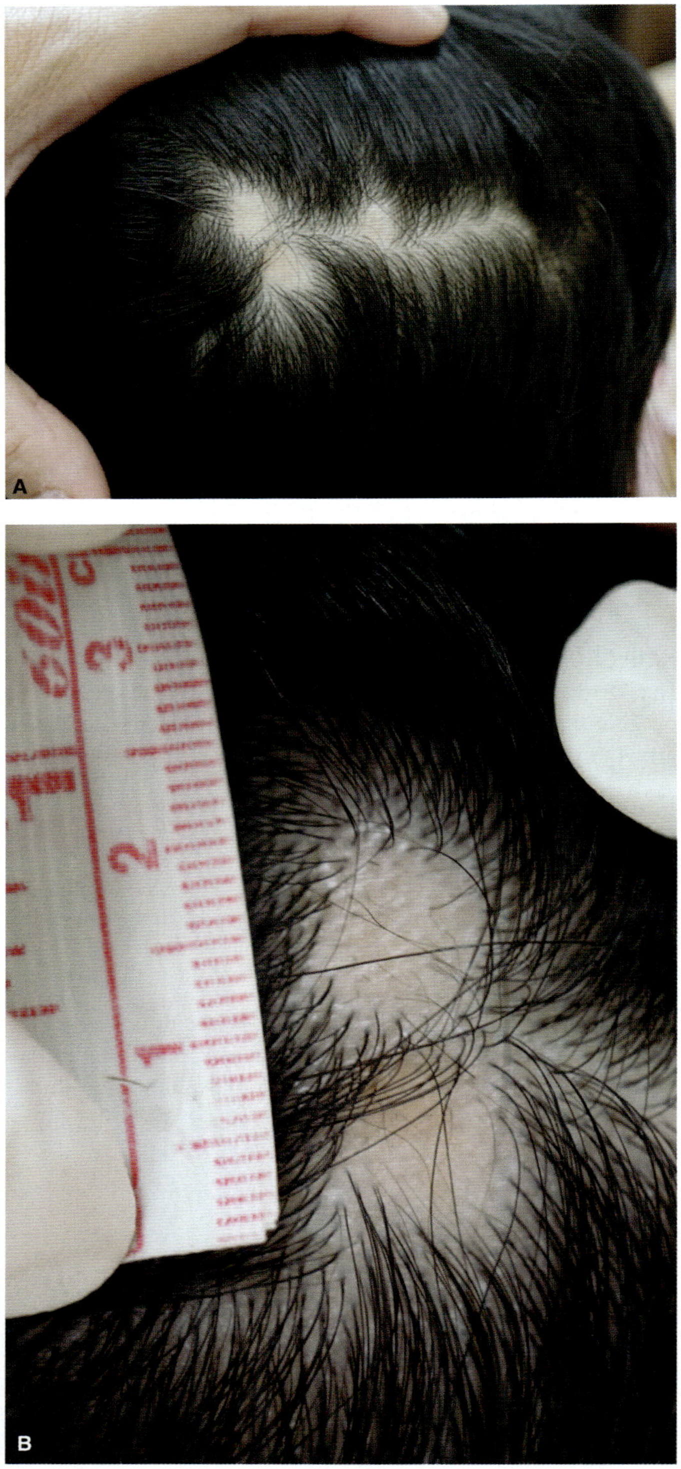

FIGURE 9-2A & 2B. Alopecia areata affecting the vertex scalp of a Chinese girl, presenting with circular, non-scarring patches of alopecia.

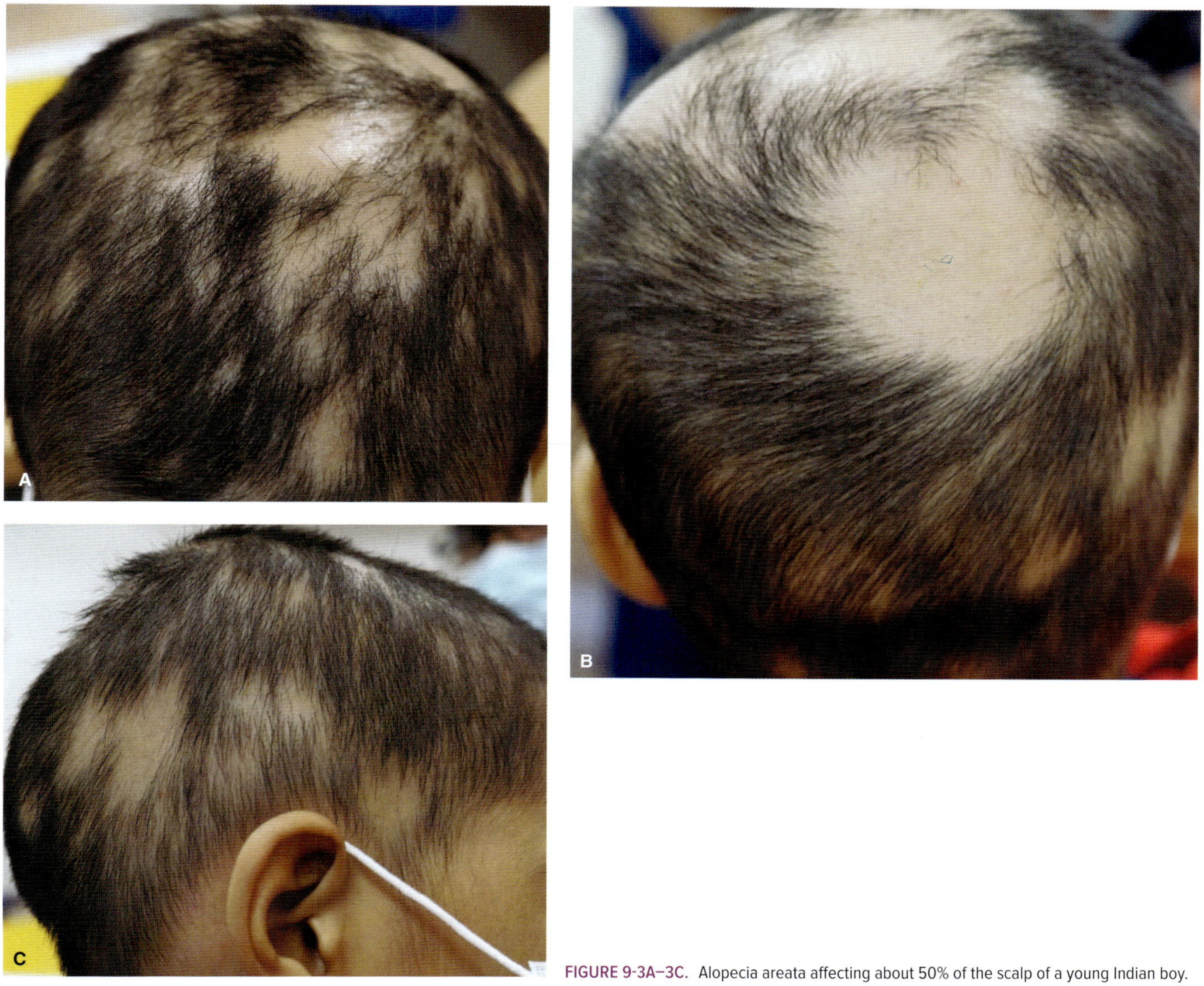

FIGURE 9-3A–3C. Alopecia areata affecting about 50% of the scalp of a young Indian boy.

Clinical Features

- The onset of hair loss is usually over days to several weeks, with single or multiple patches of non-scarring, well-demarcated areas of complete hair loss.
- AA most commonly affects the scalp, but can also affect the eyebrows, eyelashes, and beard area.
- The "ophiasis" pattern of alopecia presents with balding of the posterior occipital scalp in a band-like distribution.
- Alopecia totalis refers to total loss of scalp hair, and alopecia universalis refers to loss of all body hair.
- If the disease is still active, the hair pull test is positive, especially at the edges of the alopecic patches.
- Exclamation mark hairs may be observed at the periphery of lesions. This is better observed with a dermatoscope. Other features on dermoscopy include yellow dots, black dots, and short vellus hairs.
- Nail changes such as trachyonychia and fine pitting may be seen in some patients.

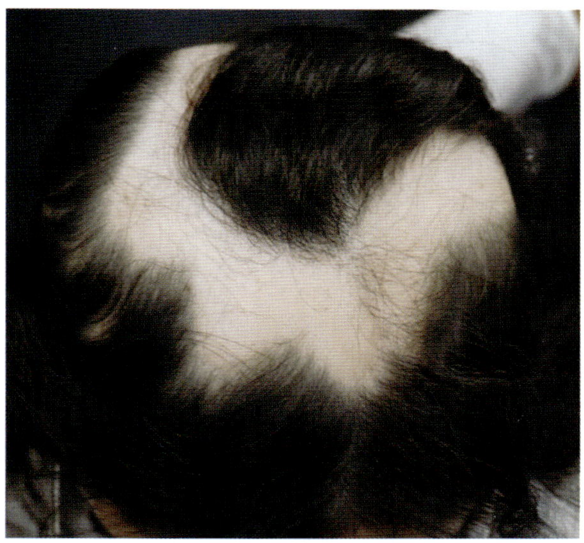

FIGURE 9-4. Extensive, progressive alopecia areata in a Malay teenage girl, despite treatment with topical immunotherapy.

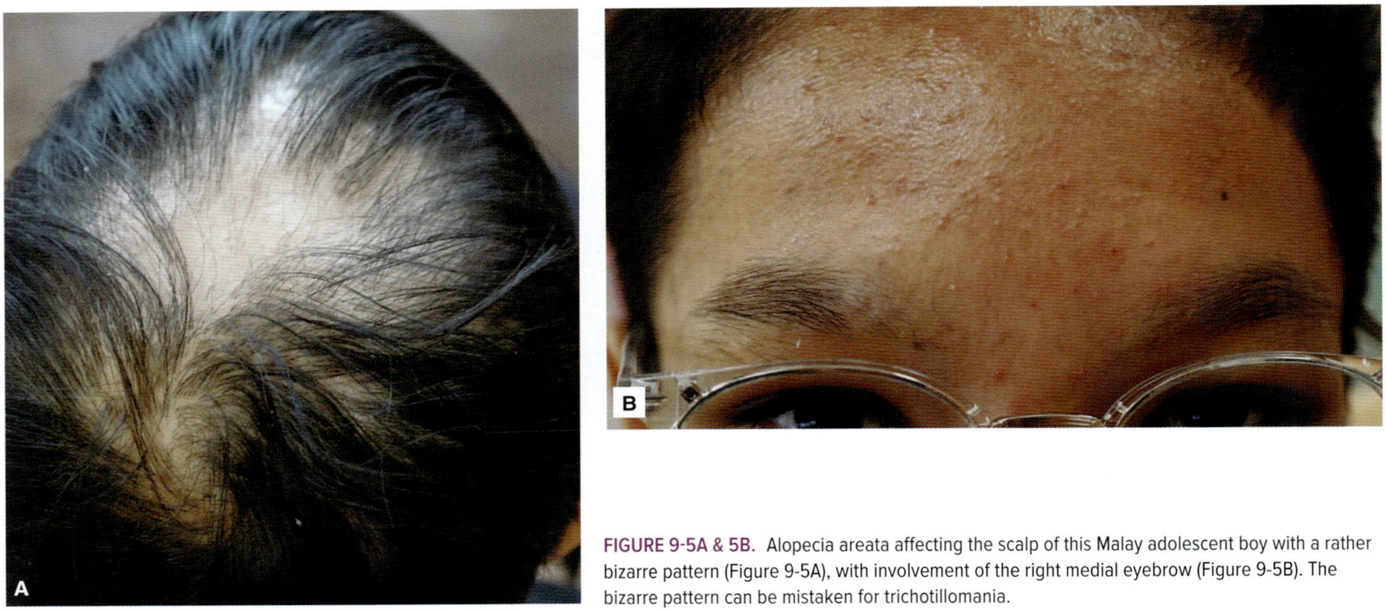

FIGURE 9-5A & 5B. Alopecia areata affecting the scalp of this Malay adolescent boy with a rather bizarre pattern (Figure 9-5A), with involvement of the right medial eyebrow (Figure 9-5B). The bizarre pattern can be mistaken for trichotillomania.

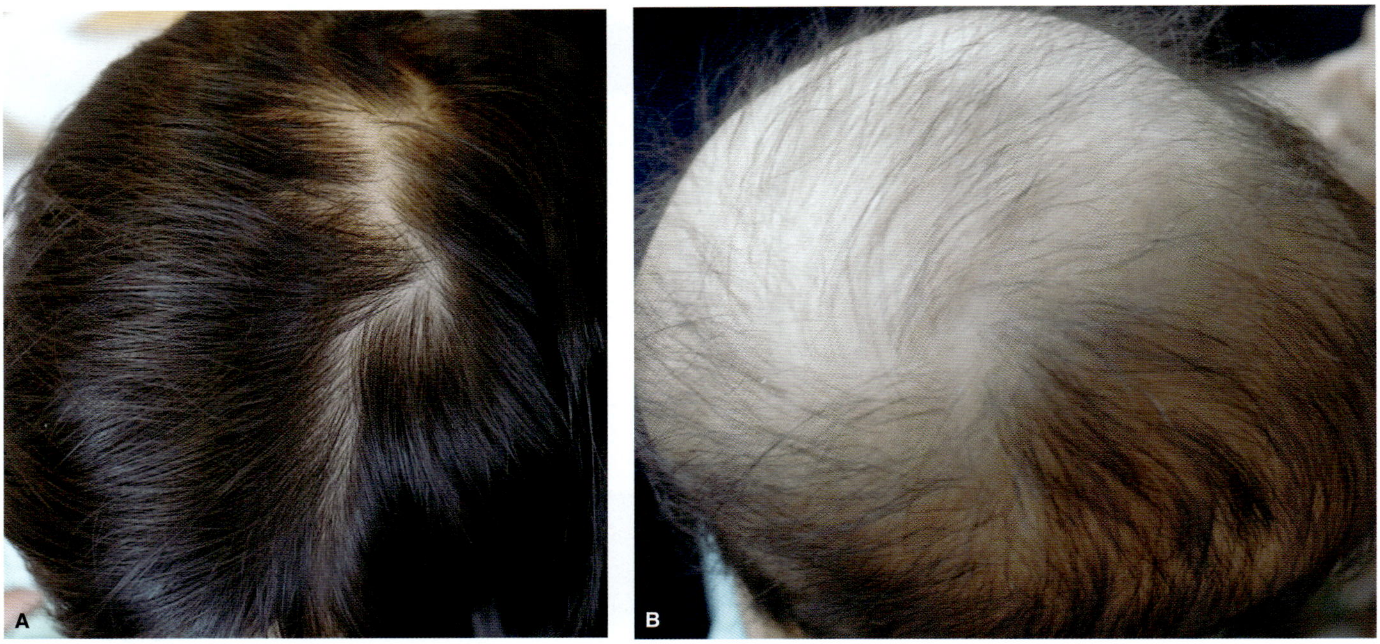

FIGURE 9-6A & 6B. Acute diffuse alopecia areata, initially presenting with diffuse hair loss with mild thinning of the vertex area (Figure 9-6A). Within a few weeks, there is rapid, diffuse hair loss affecting the entire scalp (Figure 9-6B).

Differential Diagnoses

- Trichotillomania
  - Trichotillomania is less common compared to AA in children and adolescents, and presents with irregular patches of scalp, eyebrow, or eyelash hair loss, usually in a bizarre fashion. Examination reveals hairs of different lengths, and the hair pull test is negative.
- Tinea capitis
  - Tinea capitis can also cause localized hair loss but is usually associated with signs of inflammation and scaling.
  - The condition can be confirmed by Wood's lamp examination, microscopic examination of hair shafts and skin scrapings after potassium hydroxide preparation, and fungal culture from hair and skin scrapings.

Investigations & Treatment

- AA is usually diagnosed by history and examination features. No further investigations are usually required for diagnosis.
- Hair mount examination of gently pulled hairs may show dystrophic, tapered proximal ends of hair shafts.

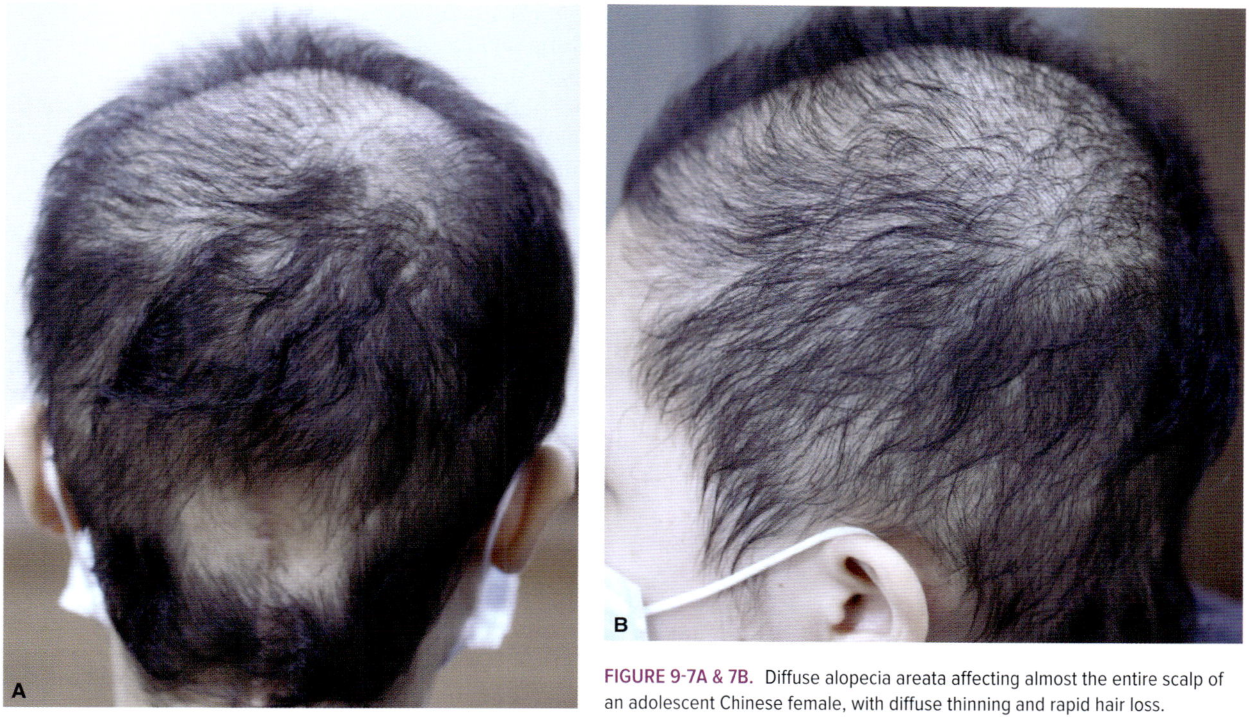

FIGURE 9-7A & 7B. Diffuse alopecia areata affecting almost the entire scalp of an adolescent Chinese female, with diffuse thinning and rapid hair loss.

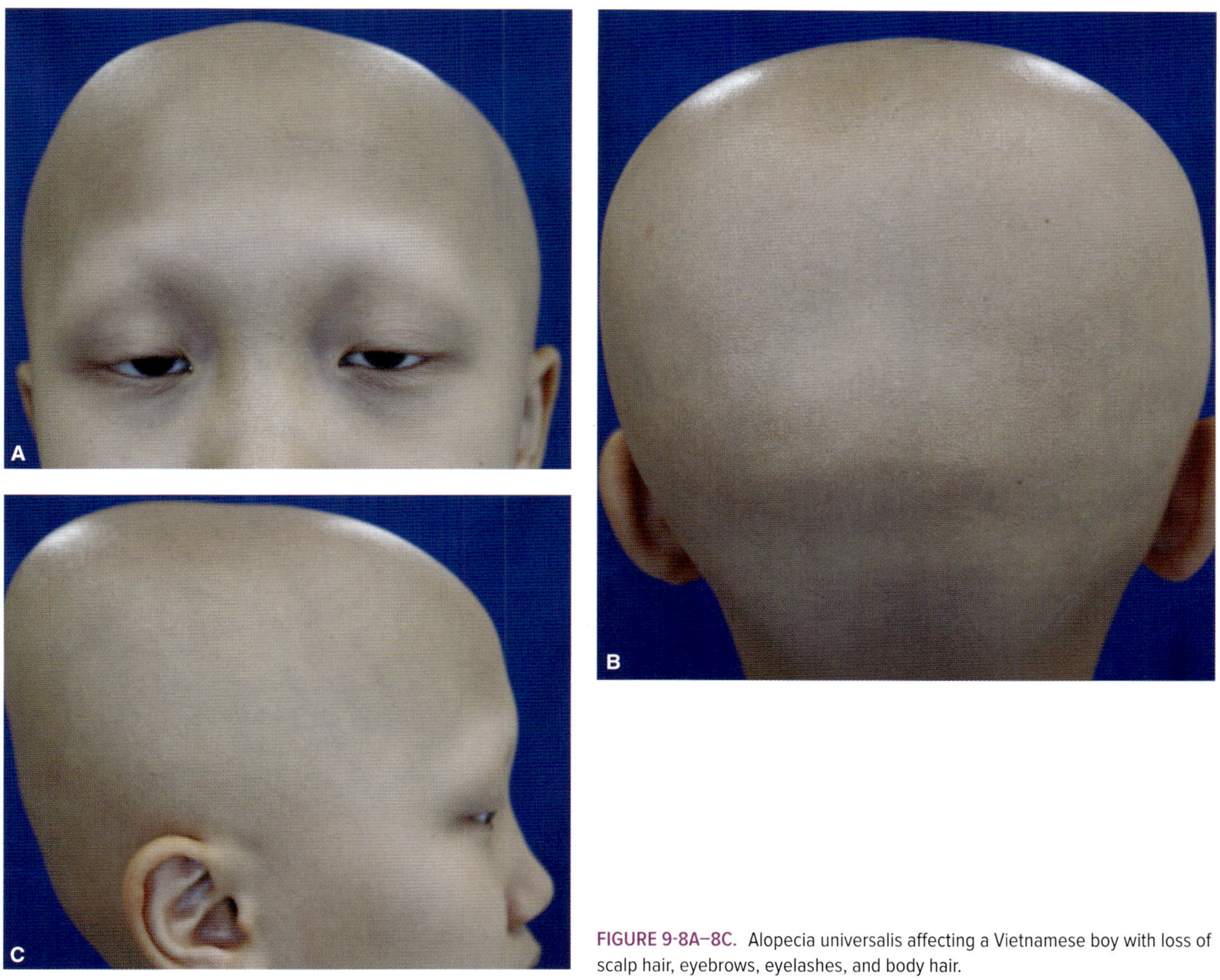

FIGURE 9-8A–8C. Alopecia universalis affecting a Vietnamese boy with loss of scalp hair, eyebrows, eyelashes, and body hair.

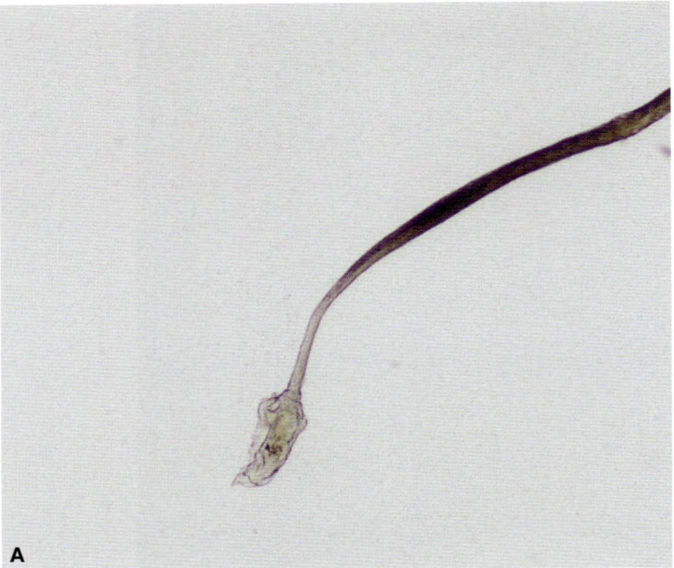

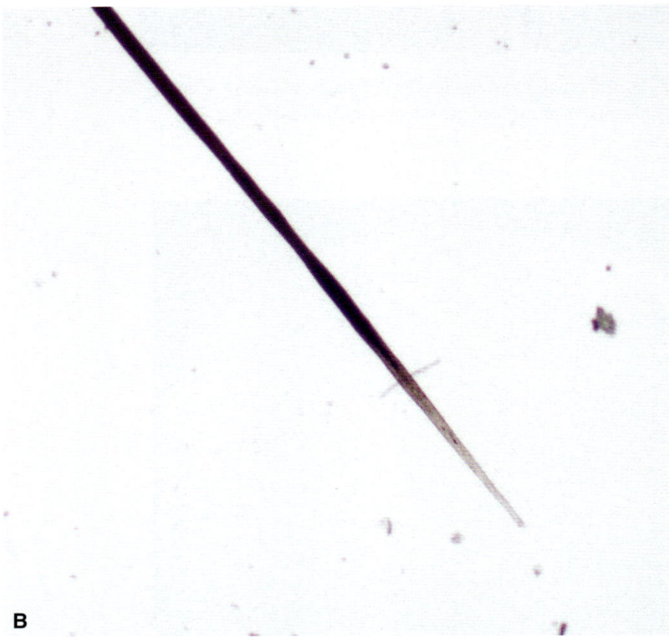

FIGURE 9-9A & 9B. Hair mount microscopy of gently pulled hair from a patient with alopecia areata. Figure 9-9A shows an "exclamation mark" hair, and Figure 9-9B shows a "pencil-point" hair.

- If performed, histological findings of scalp biopsy are a dense lymphocyte infiltration of anagen hair bulbs and dermal papillae.
- Watchful waiting is an option, as spontaneous regrowth can occur within 3 to 12 months.
- Topical corticosteroids, with or without occlusion, and/or topical minoxidil can be used for more limited AA.
- Topical immunotherapy can be used for more extensive disease, such as squaric acid dibutyl ester (SADBE) and diphenylcyclopropenone (DCP).
- Systemic corticosteroids may be used if the disease is progressing rapidly, but are not recommended for long-term use.
- Other forms of treatment that have been described to be useful to some extent in some patients include oral immunosuppressives, such as methotrexate, ciclosporin, and azathioprine, and JAK inhibitors.
- Psychological support and counseling are essential for patients and caregivers who exhibit psychosocial impairment. Hair wigs may also be helpful in this aspect.

Pearls & Practical Tips

- The course of AA is variable and difficult to predict, with limited disease an indicator of better prognosis, and earlier age of onset, more extensive involvement, personal history of atopy, nail abnormalities, and family history of autoimmune disease as indicators of worse prognosis.
- Diffuse AA is a rare condition and can be confused with other causes of diffuse alopecia, such as telogen effluvium. Progression can be rapid and can cause severe psychological distress in patients and caregivers. Underlying autoimmune disease needs to be excluded. Hair mounts may be useful to differentiate from other causes of diffuse hair loss.

Bibliography

1. Waśkiel-Burnat A, Kołodziejak M, Sikora M, et al. Therapeutic management in paediatric alopecia areata: a systematic review. J Eur Acad Dermatol Venereol 2021;35(6):1299-1308.

TRAUMATIC ALOPECIA

Traumatic or traction alopecia is due to the forceful extraction of hair, or breaking of hair shafts, by physical trauma such as friction, traction, and pressure. Common causes of traumatic alopecia in children and adolescents include trichotillomania, tight tying of ponytails, buns or braiding, and other cosmetic practices, such as hair straightening, frequent brushing with nylon bristles, and use of hot combs and oils.

Clinical Features

- Traction alopecia presents as oval or linear areas of hair loss, most commonly at the margins of the hairline or scattered throughout the scalp. Individuals who tie their hair tightly in ponytails or braids or use hair extensions may present with peripheral scalp hair loss, particularly the frontal, temporal, and preauricular area.
- Trichotillomania is a self-induced form of traction alopecia and involves various degrees of plucking, pulling, or cutting of hair. It is most common in prepubertal girls but can also occur in boys, and most commonly affects scalp hair but can also affect the eyebrows, eyelashes, and less commonly, hair from other areas of the body, in a bizarre pattern.
- Trichotillomania presents as irregular areas of partial hair loss that are never completely bald, in a bizarre configuration. Common areas affected are the frontal and frontoparietal areas, with the contralateral side of the dominant hand more commonly affected. The "tonsure" pattern or "Friar Tuck sign" may be seen. Hair pull test is negative.

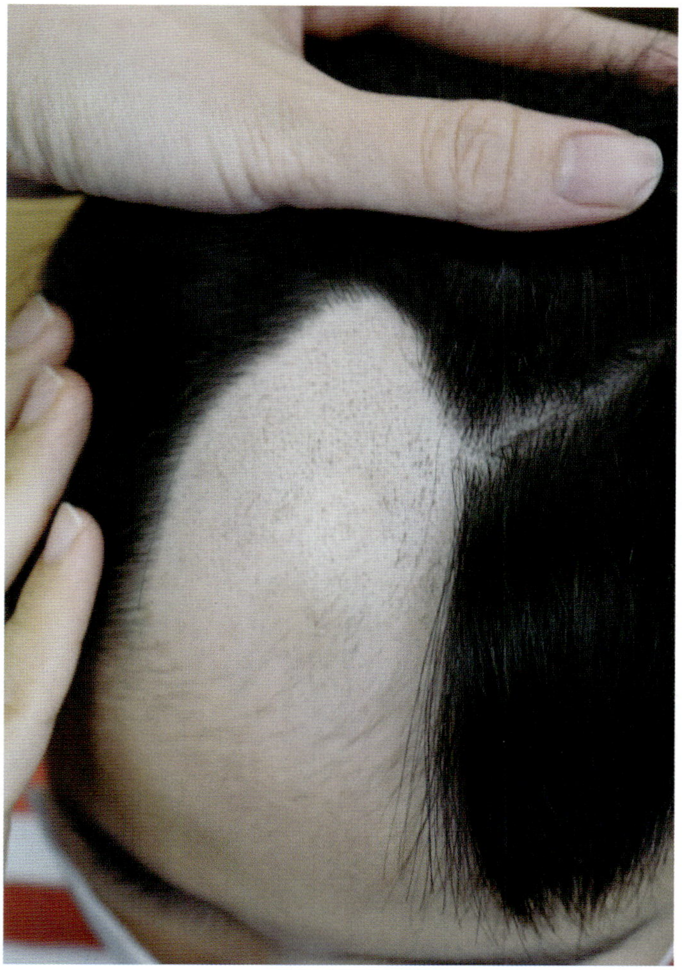

FIGURE 9-10. Trichotillomania in a Chinese boy presenting with a bizarre pattern of hair loss.

- Trichoscopy findings in traction alopecia include perifollicular erythema, pustules, scaling, and broken hairs. Trichoscopy findings in trichotillomania include irregularly broken hairs, coiled hairs, and flame hairs (wavy and cone-shaped hair residues).

Differential Diagnoses

- Alopecia areata
  - Alopecia areata is more common than trichotillomania and presents with non-scarring, well-demarcated, oval areas of complete hair loss. Hair pull test may be positive from the peripheries of the alopecic patches. Exclamation mark hairs are characteristic and can be better observed on dermoscopy.
- Tinea capitis
  - This is caused by dermatophyte infection of the hair and scalp skin. There may be scaling and erythema of the skin at the area of alopecia. Hair pull test may be positive.
  - Differentiation from trichotillomania may be aided by Wood's lamp examination, dermoscopy, microscopic examination with potassium hydroxide preparation, and fungal culture.

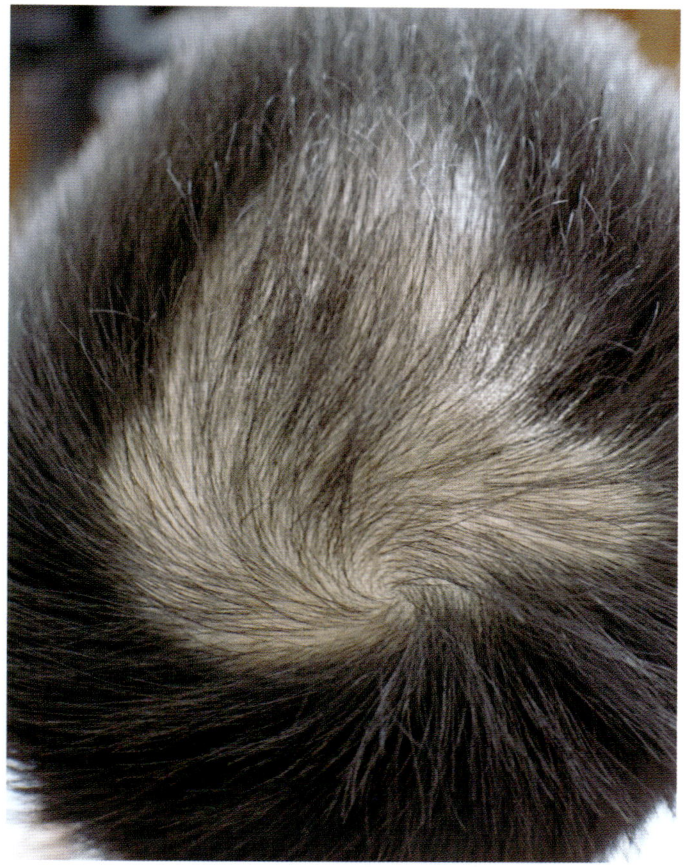

FIGURE 9-11. Trichotillomania in a Chinese boy affecting the vertex with a bizarre pattern of hair loss.

Investigations & Treatment

- Diagnosis of traumatic alopecia and trichotillomania in children is clinical, aided by adjuncts such as trichoscopy and hair mounts. Hair mount should be performed on hairs collected by patients or their caregivers, as the hair

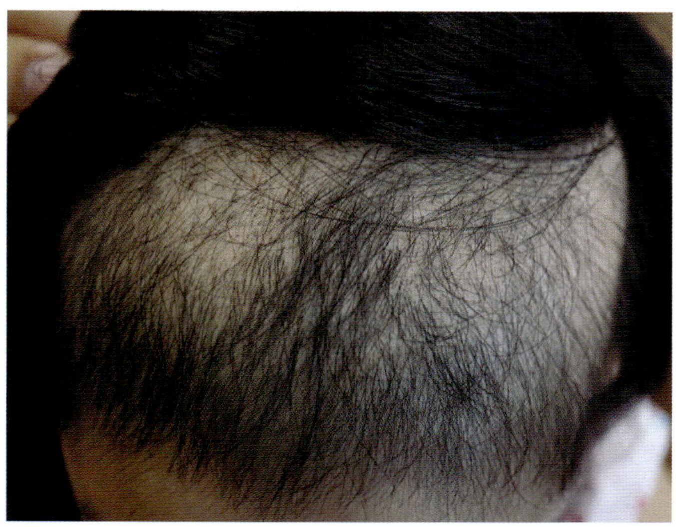

FIGURE 9-12. Trichotillomania in a young Chinese girl presenting with a bizarre pattern of hair loss. Close inspection of the bald area will reveal short hairs of deferring lengths.

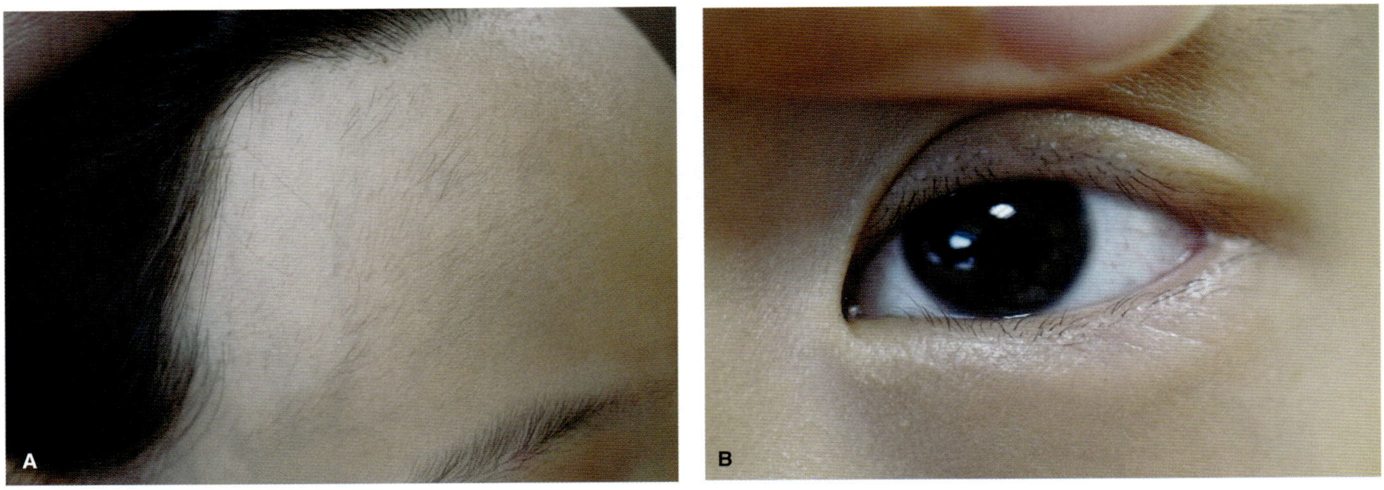

FIGURE 9-13A & 13B. This teenage Chinese girl has trichotillomania affecting the frontal hairline as well as her eyelashes. There are short broken hairs visible at the affected areas.

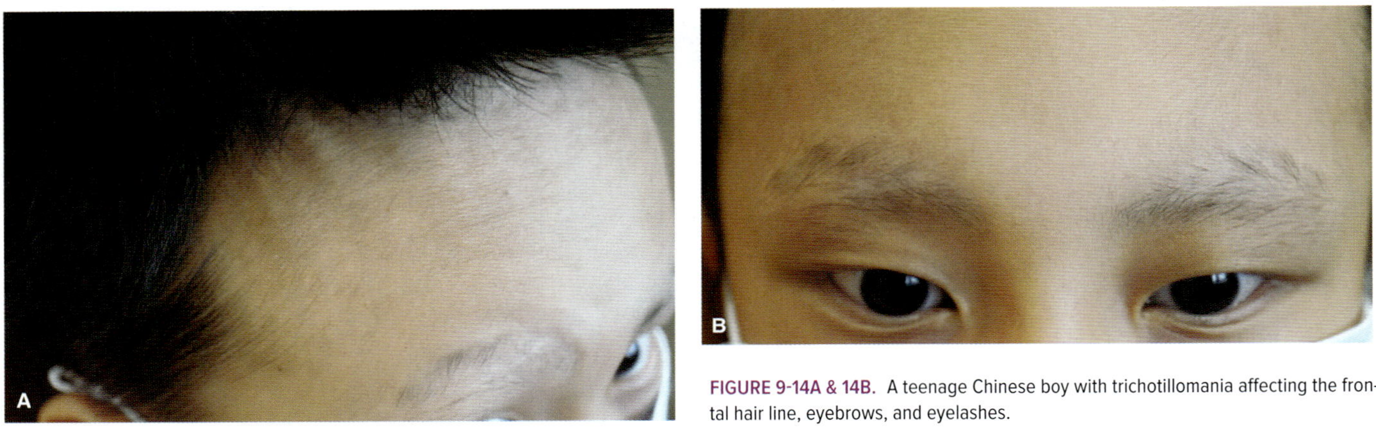

FIGURE 9-14A & 14B. A teenage Chinese boy with trichotillomania affecting the frontal hair line, eyebrows, and eyelashes.

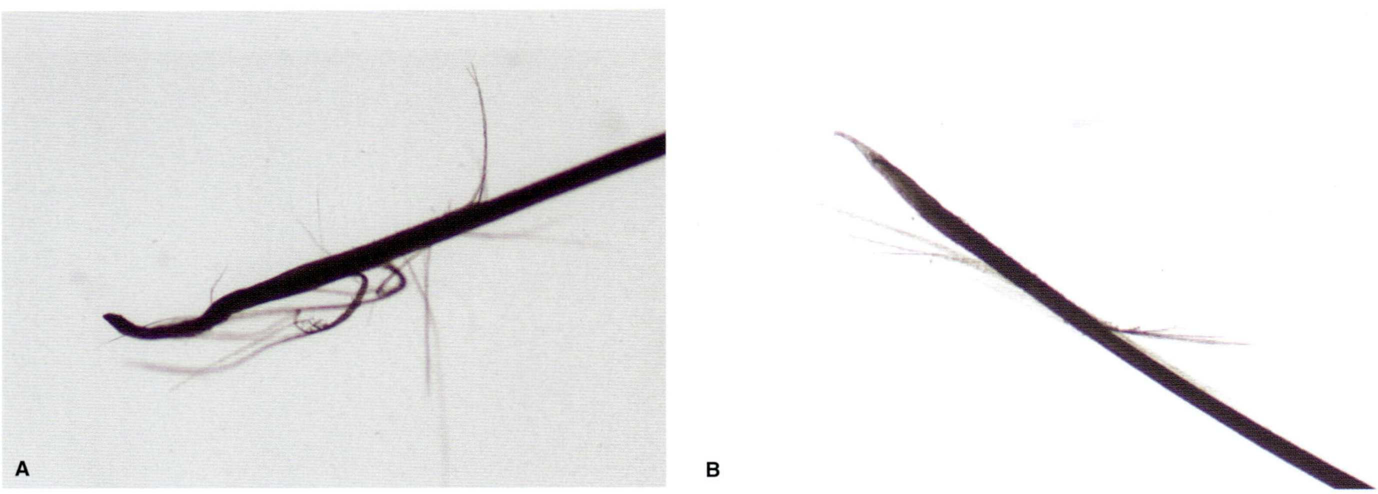

FIGURE 9-15A & 15B. Hair mount microscopy of hairs brought by patient with trichotillomania. The hair bulbs appear bizarrely dystrophic.

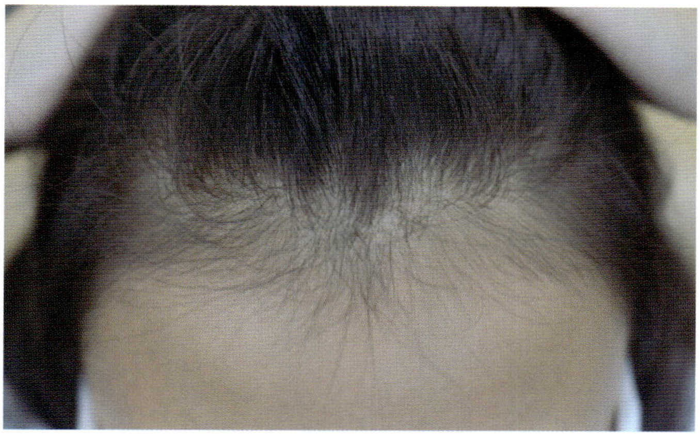

FIGURE 9-16. Traction alopecia affecting the frontal hair line of an adolescent girl caused by prolonged tight tying of hair.

pull is usually negative. Hair mount features include dysmorphic anagen bulbs as well as broken or traumatized proximal ends.

- Scalp biopsy may be required in atypical cases that are not easily diagnosed clinically. Histopathological features include empty follicles, incomplete disrupted follicular anatomy, trichomalacia, and pigment casts without significant inflammation.
- Management of trichotillomania requires a multifaceted approach, including behavioral modification techniques and psychiatric intervention such as cognitive behavioral therapy, and medications such as olanzapine and selective serotoninergic reuptake inhibitors in severe cases.
- Oral N-acetylcysteine has shown some effect in some patients.
- Psychological support and counseling are essential for patients and caregivers who exhibit psychosocial impairment. Hair wigs may also be helpful in this aspect.

Pearls & Practical Tips

- Patients with trichotillomania often do not admit to pulling or plucking their hair, and parents often do not witness these behaviors. There may be associated nail-biting (onychophagia), picking at acne (acne excoriee), and lip biting. We sometimes observe similar behaviors in other members of the family.
- Trichotillomania in younger children tends to have better outcomes than in older children and adolescents.
- Prolonged or forceful trauma may eventually lead to scarring alopecia.

Bibliography

1. Torales J, Ruiz Díaz N, Ventriglio A, et al. Hair-pulling disorder (trichotillomania): etiopathogenesis, diagnosis and treatment in a nutshell. Dermatol Ther 2021;34(1):e13466.
2. Henkel ED, Jaquez SD, Diaz LZ. Pediatric trichotillomania: review of management. Pediatr Dermatol 2019;36(6):803-7.

TELOGEN EFFLUVIUM

Telogen effluvium is one of the most common causes of diffuse alopecia in children and adolescents. It occurs as a result of a stressful event that stimulates anagen hairs to convert into telogen hairs, leading to the diffuse hair loss 1 to 3 months after the event. The condition is usually self-limiting in children and recovers fully after several months.

Clinical Features

- Telogen effluvium is usually preceded by a stressful event (such as acute illnesses, surgery, rapid weight loss, or other major physical or psychological trauma) or medications, such as isotretinoin, 1 to 3 months prior to the onset of alopecia.
- Patients present with diffuse hair loss without discrete alopecic patches.

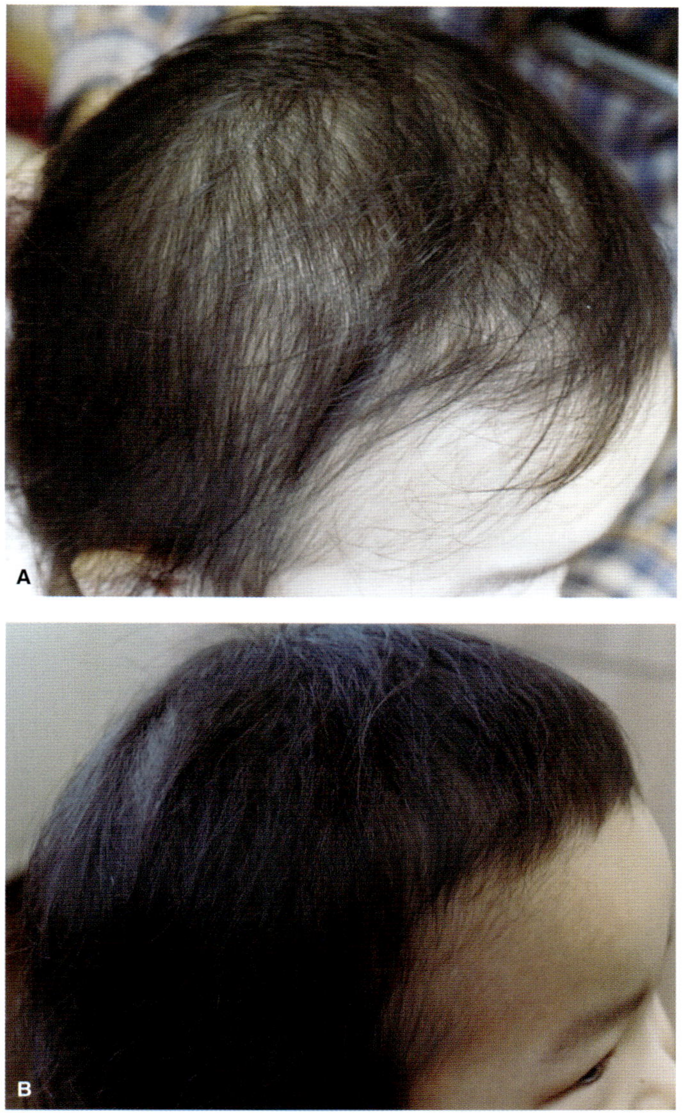

FIGURE 9-17A & 17B. Telogen effluvium in a toddler, occurring a few months after a viral illness. There is diffuse hair thinning (Figure 9-17A), with good regrowth of hair after 6 months (Figure 9-17B).

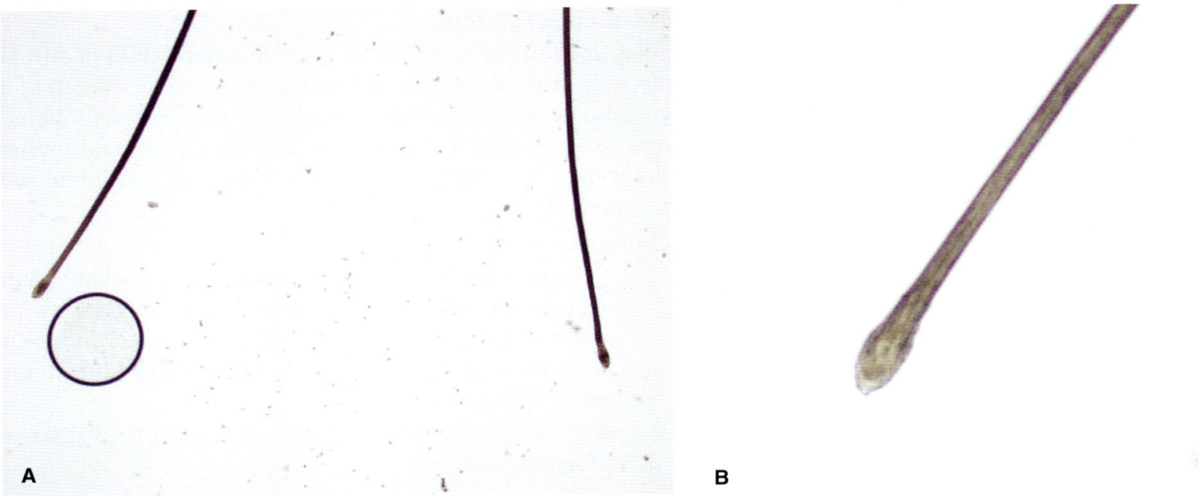

FIGURE 9-18A & 18B. Hair mount microscopy of gently pulled hairs in a patient with telogen effluvium. The majority of hair bulbs have telogen roots as shown in both figures.

- Hair pull test is positive when the disease is acute, but becomes negative after a few weeks to 1 to 2 months after the onset.
- Chronic telogen effluvium can be associated with chronic illness, thyroid disorders, nutritional disorders (e.g., iron deficiency anemia, zinc deficiency, hypervitaminosis A, malnutrition state in anorexia nervosa), malabsorption (e.g., celiac disease), and systemic connective tissue disorders.

Differential Diagnoses

- Diffuse alopecia areata
  - Diffuse alopecia areata is rare and can result in sudden or more gradual diffuse hair loss that can lead to alopecia totalis or alopecia universalis. The hair loss in this condition is usually more severe than in telogen effluvium. A hair mount will help to differentiate diffuse alopecia areata from telogen effluvium (see below).
- Androgenic alopecia
  - Androgenic alopecia can begin in post-pubertal adolescents, especially in males. There is usually a strong family history. Patients with androgenic alopecia usually complain of gradual hair thinning as compared to telogen effluvium, which presents with more easily visible hair loss. On dermoscopy, variation in hair shaft diameter may be seen in patients with androgenic alopecia.

Investigations & Treatment

- Telogen effluvium can be diagnosed if greater than 25% of gently pulled hairs are telogen hairs. This can be better visualized using a hair mount. Telogen hair roots appear as club-shaped, with decreased pigment and uniform shaft diameter.
- Trichoscopy may show empty follicles and short regrowing hairs of normal thickness.
- If chronic telogen effluvium is suspected, screening investigations should include full blood count, thyroid function tests, iron studies, and autoimmune screen.
- Complete regrowth occurs within months unless the stressful trigger recurs or is sustained.

Pearls & Practical Tips

- It is also important to obtain a medication history. Common drugs that can be associated with telogen effluvium include oral contraceptives, retinoids (e.g., isotreninoin), anticonvulsants, and angiotensin converting enzyme inhibitors (e.g., captopril, enalapril). The hair loss in patients undergoing chemotherapy is termed *anagen effluvium*.
- There is usually much anxiety on the part of caregivers of patients who present with telogen effluvium. Time should be spent reassuring them that telogen effluvium self-resolves and does not lead to total hair loss.
- A proportion of patients with telogen effluvium may not recall a preceding illness or traumatic event.

ANDROGENETIC ALOPECIA

Androgenetic alopecia (AGA) affects both males and females, although it is more common in males. Patients can present during adolescence or young adulthood and the condition is due to the effects of circulating androgens in genetically susceptible individuals.

Clinical Features

- Patients present with progressive, patterned hair loss from the scalp. The primary complaint is thinning of scalp hair, rather than shedding.
- There is usually a positive family history of AGA.
- In males, there is initially symmetrical bitemporal triangular recession of the hair line, followed by thinning at the vertex.

- In females, there is slow, diffuse thinning of the vertex and widening of the central hair parting. The frontal hairline is relatively unaffected.
- Hair pull test is negative.
- On dermoscopy, there is variability in hair shaft thickness, increased vellus hairs, and single hairs emerging from follicular ostia.

Differential Diagnoses

- Telogen effluvium
  - Telogen effluvium is common and presents with diffuse alopecia. There is usually an inciting cause 1 to 3 months prior to hair loss. Patients usually complain of increased hair shedding, rather than scalp thinning.
  - Chronic telogen effluvium can be difficult to differentiate from AGA, especially in women. Modalities to help differentiate include dermoscopy, hair mounts, and scalp biopsies.
- Diffuse alopecia areata
  - Diffuse alopecia areata is rare and can result in sudden or more gradual diffuse hair loss that can lead to alopecia totalis or alopecia universalis. Hair shedding is the main complaint and can be severe. Hair pull test is usually positive.

Investigations & Treatment

- AGA is usually diagnosed clinically, especially in men, where the pattern of hair loss is distinctive. Diagnosis can be more difficult in women, as clinical features may overlap with chronic telogen effluvium. Investigations including a full blood count, thyroid function tests, and iron studies, and autoimmune screens may be required to exclude a secondary cause of chronic telogen effluvium.
- Although not diagnostic, hair mounts may help to provide clues to differentiate AGA and chronic telogen effluvium. In AGA, there is variable hair shaft diameter. Increase in telogen bulbs is seen in both AGA and chronic telogen effluvium.
- Scalp biopsies may further differentiate between AGA and chronic telogen effluvium. In AGA, there are increased vellus hairs compared to terminal hairs (normal ratio 1:7; in AGA, this increases to 1:4) and miniaturization of hairs.
- The aim of treatment in AGA is to slow down further thinning of hair and promote hair growth.
- Topical minoxidil 2% or 5% twice daily can be trialed for a period of 6 to 12 months. Treatment has to be continued indefinitely if there is improvement. Halting treatment will result in progressive hair loss again.
- Oral antiandrogenic treatments can also be used. For males, finasteride 1 mg daily in combination with topical minoxidil has been shown to be useful. In females, oral spironolactone 50 to 200 mg daily has also been shown to be useful.

Pearls & Practical Tips

- In some patients, especially females, telogen effluvium may unmask an underlying androgenic alopecia.

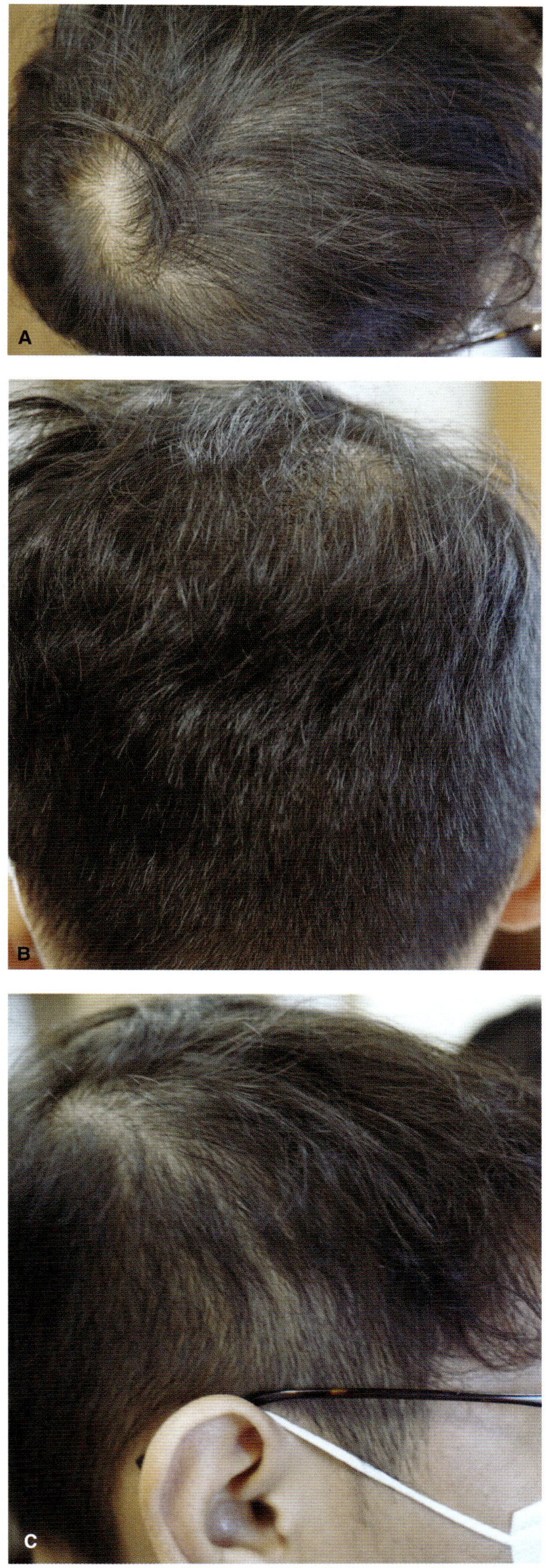

FIGURE 9-19A–19C. Early AGA in an adolescent Eurasian boy with slow, gradual thinning of the hair at the vertex.

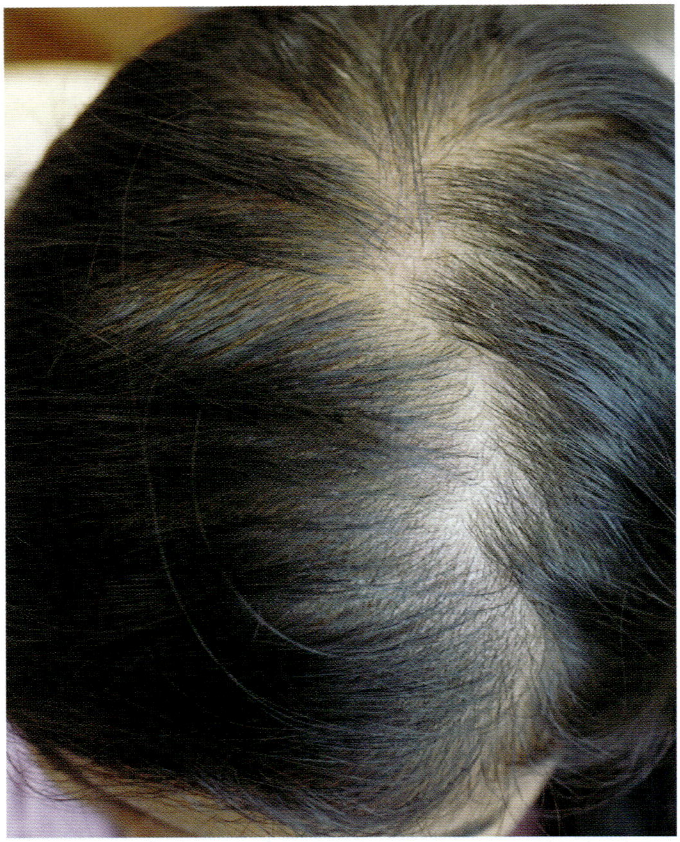

FIGURE 9-20. A Malay older teenage girl presenting with gradual thinning of the vertex. She has a strong family history of AGA.

- For treatment of AGA in women, we usually start with topical minoxidil 2%. In more severe cases, this may be increased to 5%. In men, we start with topical minoxidil 5%.
- In female patients, a hormonal evaluation may be required if there is severe acne with seborrhea, hirsutism, and menstrual irregularities.

APLASIA CUTIS CONGENITA

Aplasia cutis congenita (ACC) is a developmental defect hypothesized to be due to incomplete neural tube closure or an embryonic arrest of skin development. The occurrence is usually sporadic but can be associated with teratogens, maternal infections, and other developmental defects.

Clinical Features

- ACC presents at birth as an asymptomatic, well-demarcated, oval or circular alopecic erosion or ulceration of the scalp, sometimes covered by a thin membrane. ACC may also present as a scar or keloid at birth. Most ACC lesions measure between 1 and 3 cm in diameter.
- ACC is usually solitary but can be multiple or extensive in rare cases. It most commonly occurs on the vertex of the scalp, but other areas of the body may be affected in more extensive cases, such as the face, extremities, or trunk.
- The lesion heals with scarring, with no hair or appendages present in the scar.

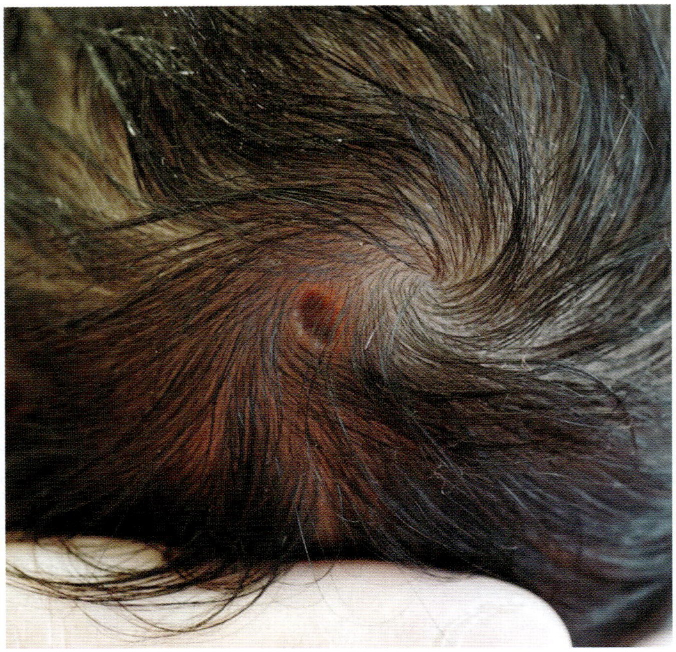

FIGURE 9-21. ACC presenting on the scalp of an Indian newborn, with central erosion and alopecia.

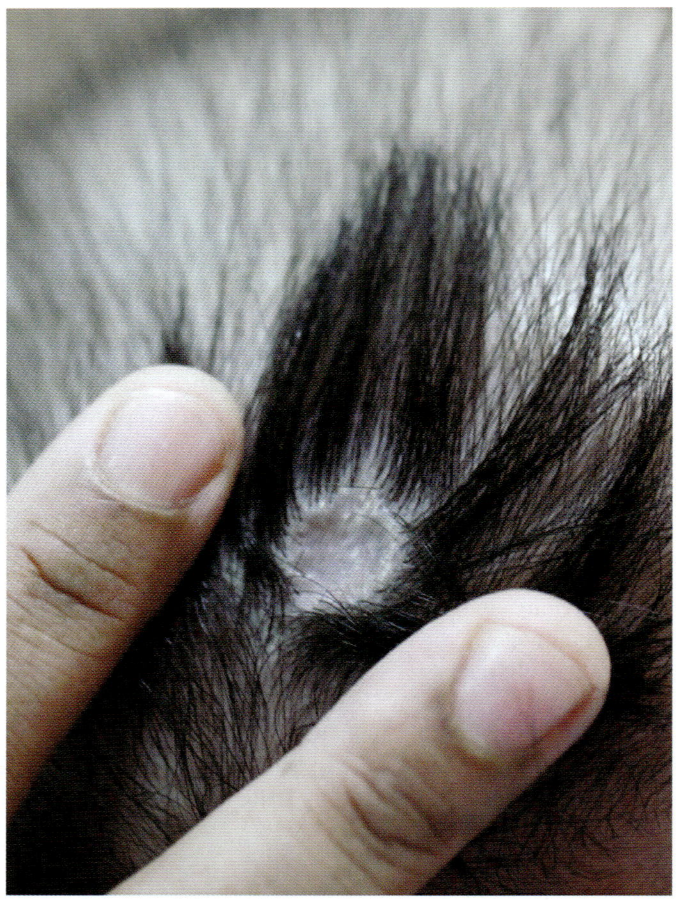

FIGURE 9-22. ACC on the scalp with central atrophy and surrounding hair collar sign.

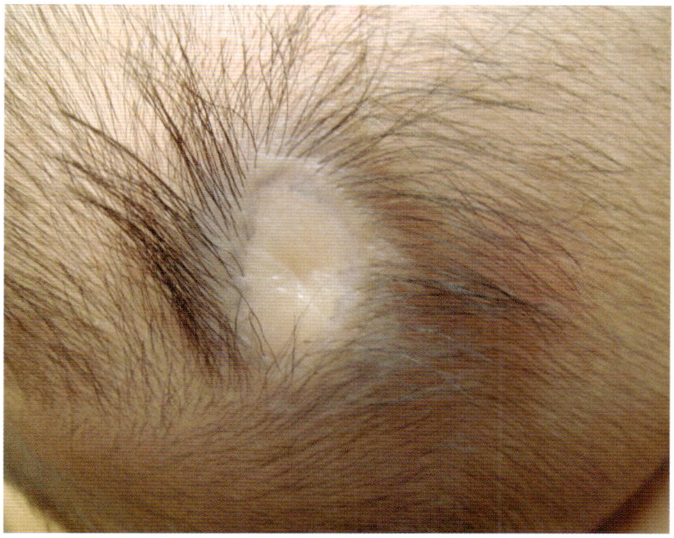

FIGURE 9-23. Relatively large ACC on the scalp of a Chinese infant with presence of the hair collar sign. There appears to be a membranous covering of the lesion of ACC.

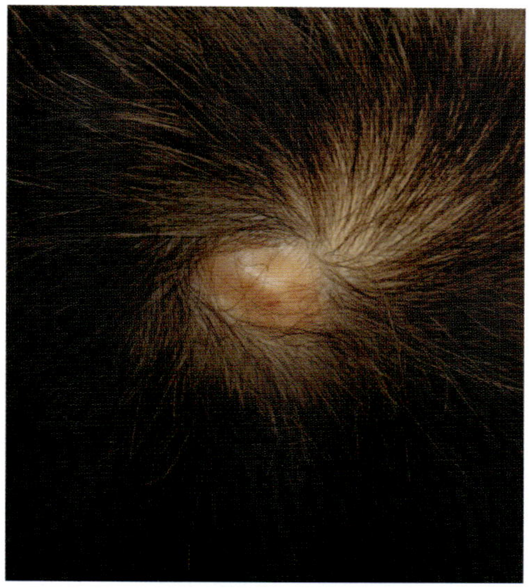

FIGURE 9-24. ACC on the scalp of a Chinese boy presenting with a hypertrophic scar.

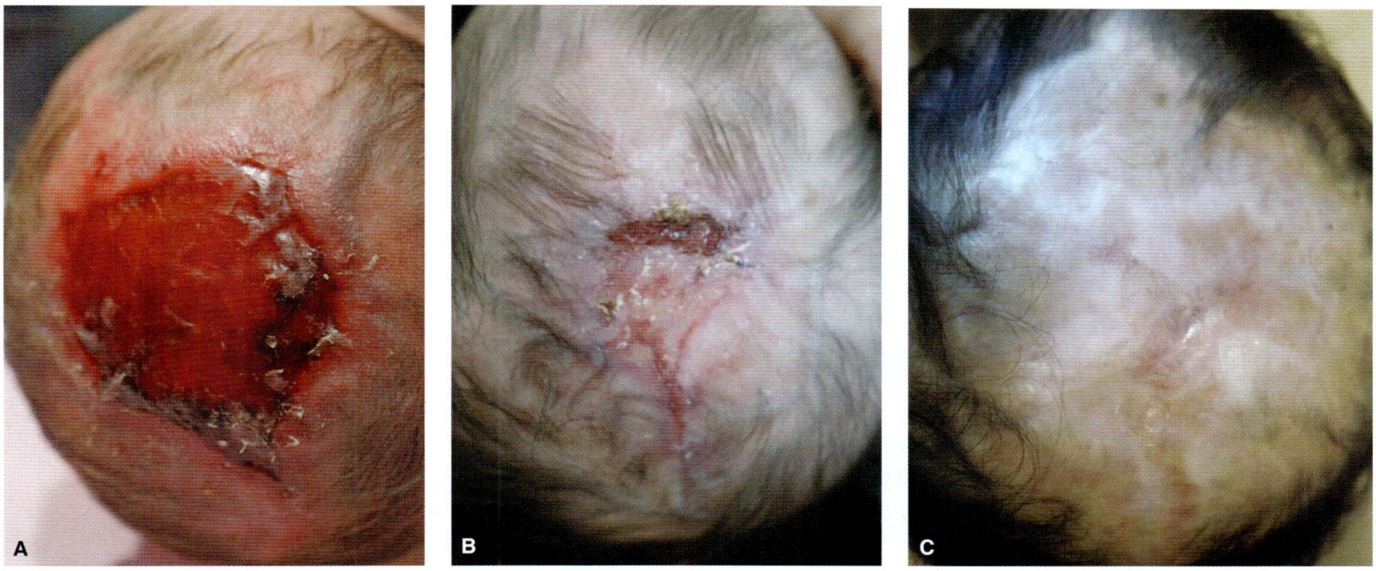

FIGURE 9-25A–25C. Large ACC with full thickness loss of skin on the vertex of a Chinese neonate. The lesion was allowed to heal by secondary closure, with re-epithelization seen after 3 months (Figure 9-25B) and full epithelization at 1.5 years with residual scarring, dyspigmentation, and alopecia (Figure 9-25C).

Differential Diagnoses

- Nevus sebaceous
  - These can also present at birth with an alopecic patch of skin on the scalp. However, the surface is usually more pebbly and has a yellow-orange hue. On dermoscopy, a pattern of yellow dots not associated with hair follicles may be seen.
- Iatrogenic peripartum birth injuries
  - These can occur secondary to electrode monitors or forceps.

Investigations & Treatment

- Diagnosis is clinical.
- Trichoscopy may show radially arranged elongated hair bulbs at the periphery of the lesion, with absence of follicular openings with prominent vasculature in the central parts of the lesion.
- If skin biopsy is done, histology shows an absence of epidermis and appendageal structures, decrease in the dermal elastic tissue, and in some cases, loss of all skin layers and subcutaneous tissues.

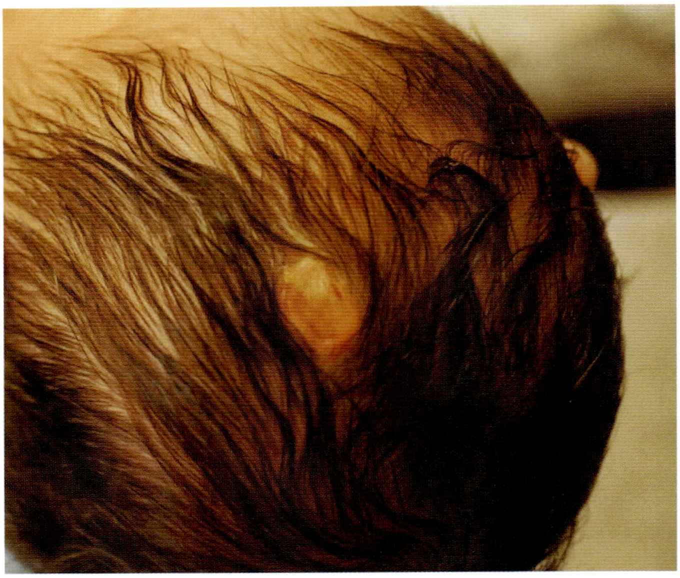

FIGURE 9-26. Rare presentation of bullous ACC on the scalp of a Chinese infant.

- Care of the ulcerated area at birth includes gentle cleansing, topical antibiotic ointments, and protective coverings to prevent further trauma to the area.
- The prognosis of aplasia cutis congenita as an isolated skin finding is good. The ulceration typically heals with scarring in a few weeks and becomes inconspicuous and covered with surrounding hair as the child grows.
- Large scalp lesions may require surgery with grafting, and hair transplant.

Pearls & Practical Tips

- ACC is often misdiagnosed as a traumatic defect or scar from peripartum instrumentation. Parents should be reassured that this is usually not the cause of ACC.

TABLE 9-1. Frieden classification of ACC.

Group	Features
1	Scalp aplasia cutis congenita without other anomalies
2	Scalp aplasia cutis congenita with limb anomalies, includes Adams-Oliver syndrome
3	Scalp aplasia cutis congenita with solitary epidermal or sebaceous nevus or an epidermal nevus syndrome
4	Aplasia cutis congenita overlying deep embryologic malformation
5	Stellate aplasia cutis congenita of trunk or limb associated with fetus papyraceus or placental infarct
6	Aplasia cutis congenita of lower limb associated with epidermolysis bullosa (Bart syndrome)
7	Aplasia cutis congenita of limb without epidermolysis bullosa
8	Aplasia cutis congenita due to teratogens such as intrauterine infection with herpes simplex or varicella, or drugs such as methimazole or carbimazole
9	Aplasia cutis congenita associated with malformation syndromes, e.g., Patau syndrome, Wolf-Hirschhorn syndrome, Setleis syndrome, Johanson-Blizzard syndrome, focal dermal hypoplasia (Goltz syndrome), and others

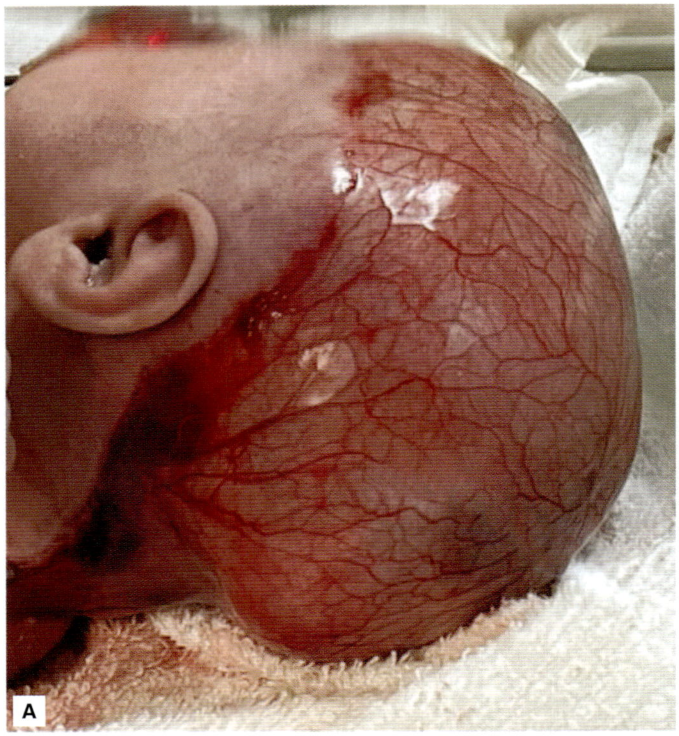

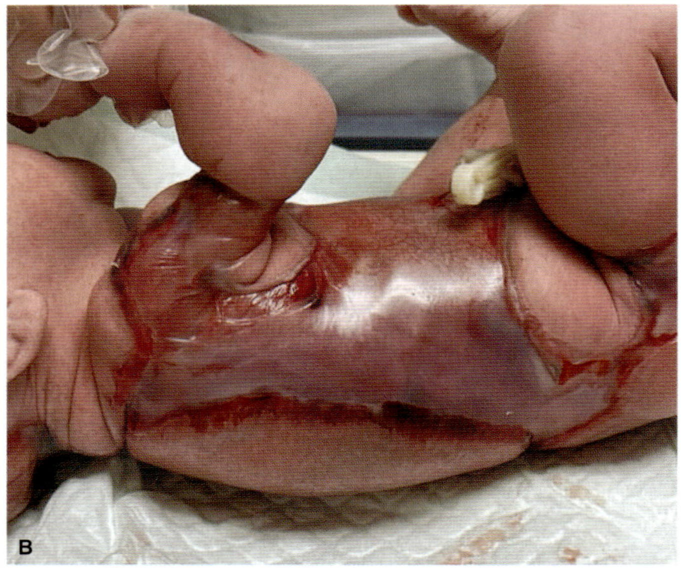

FIGURE 9-27A & 27B. Extensive ACC of the scalp, limbs, and trunk in this Malay neonate, most probably associated with fetus papyraceus or placental infarct (Group 5).

- The “hair collar sign” presents as a ring of dark, terminal hair surrounding an alopecic patch, and may be an indicator of an underlying neural tube defect. Brain imaging should be offered to evaluate for underlying central nervous system anomalies, such as encephaloceles, meningoceles, and soft tissue and bony defects.
- ACC is usually an isolated skin finding but in rare instances can be associated with developmental, neurologic, skeletal, and cardiac defects, and epidermolysis bullosa.

Bibliography

1. Swink SM, Castelo-Soccio L. Loose anagen syndrome: a retrospective chart review of 37 cases. Pediatr Dermatol 2016;33(5):507-10.
2. Oberlin KE, Maddy AJ, Martínez-Velasco MA, Vázquez-Herrera NE, Schachner LA, Tosti A. Short anagen syndrome: case series and literature review. Pediatr Dermatol 2018;35(3):388-91.

CONGENITAL TRIANGULAR ALOPECIA

Congenital triangular alopecia, also known as temporal triangular alopecia, is a benign non-scarring, non-progressive, localized pattern of hair loss. Although there is no gender predilection, it presents more often in boys than girls, probably related to the shorter hairstyles in boys making the condition more obvious than girls, who keep longer hair.

Clinical Features

- The condition may first be noticed at birth, in early infancy or early childhood. It most often affects the frontotemporal region but can also affect the temporoparietal or occipital scalp. It presents as a triangular, oval, or lancet-shaped patch of alopecia.
- It is usually unilateral, but about 20% of patients may present with bilateral, fairly symmetrical lesions.
- Although mostly devoid of any hair, close examination may reveal few normal terminal or vellus hairs within the affected patch. Sometimes, there may be a centrally localized hair tuft or small islands of hairs within the area of alopecia.

Differential Diagnoses

- Alopecia areata
  - This is an acquired condition and can be progressive or recurrent, whereas in congenital triangular alopecia, the area of hair loss is stable throughout life. Exclamation mark hairs can be seen in alopecia areata.
- Trichotillomania
  - Trichotillomania is also an acquired condition and presents with a bizarre pattern of hair loss. Examination reveals hairs of different lengths.

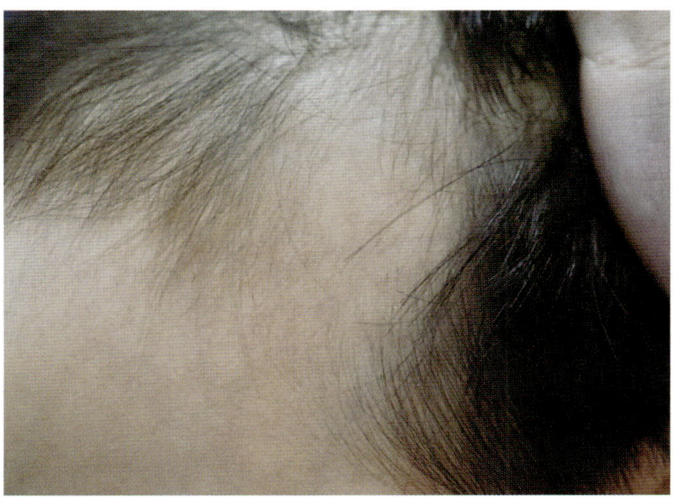

FIGURE 9-28. Large congenital triangular alopecia on the left frontotemporal region of an infant.

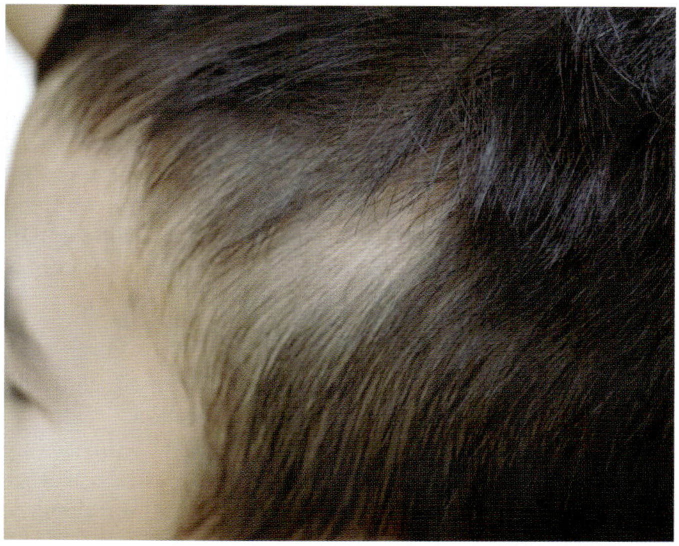

FIGURE 9-29. Classical presentation of congenital triangular alopecia affecting the left frontotemporal region.

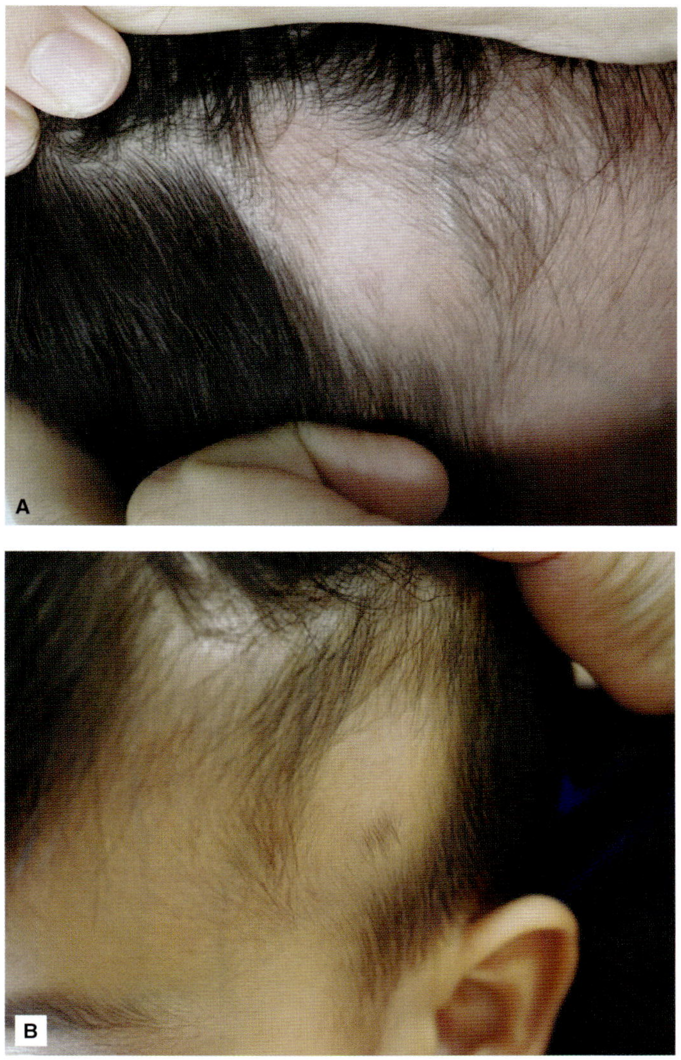

FIGURE 9-30A & 30B. Bilateral congenital aplasia cutis affecting both frontotemporal regions of this boy.

- Tinea capitis
  - Tinea capitis can also cause localized hair loss but is usually associated with signs of inflammation and scaling.
- Aplasia cutis congenita
  - Congenital triangular alopecia may be mistaken for aplasia cutis. The site of involvement and the condition of the overlying skin may provide clues to differentiate the two conditions. Scarring is not usually a feature of congenital triangular alopecia.

Investigations & Treatment

- Congenital triangular alopecia is diagnosed clinically, based on its distinct appearance and location.
- Trichoscopy may show short vellus hairs with varying hair length diversity, as well as white hairs, in the absence of diagnostic features for other types of localized alopecia.
- There is no specific treatment for congenital triangular alopecia, and most patients are asymptomatic. Hair follicular unit transplantation or surgical excision may provide patients with a satisfactory cosmetic result.

Pearls & Practical Tips

- As there is no definitive treatment for congenital triangular alopecia, parents and caregivers should be advised on the benign nature of the condition.

Bibliography

1. Yin Li VC, Yesudian PD. Congenital triangular alopecia. Int J Trichology 2015;7(2):48-53.

LOOSE ANAGEN SYNDROME & SHORT ANAGEN SYNDROME

Short anagen syndrome and loose anagen syndrome present in young children, usually girls, as short, fine hair that does not require haircuts. Loose anagen syndrome is probably more

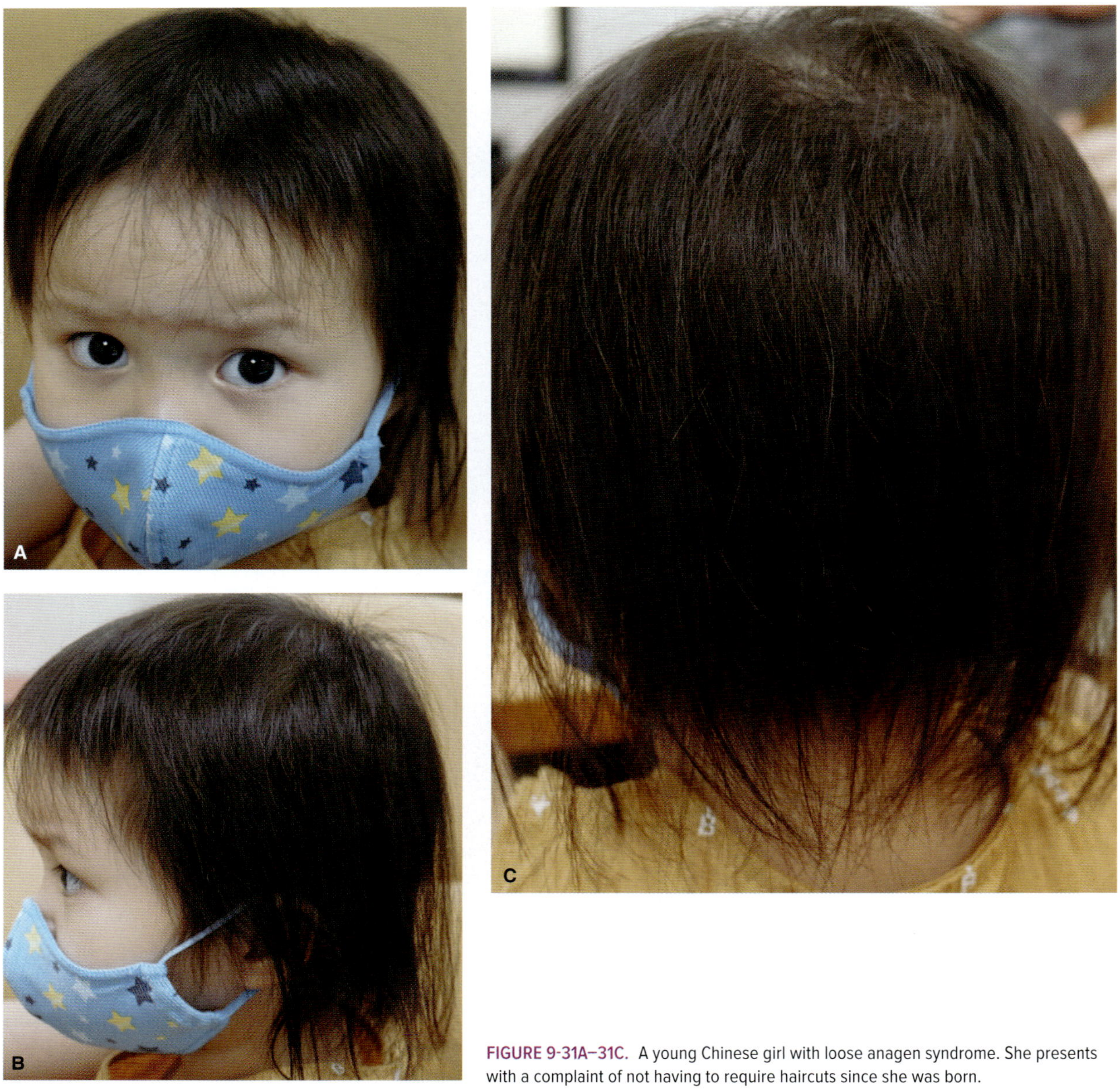

FIGURE 9-31A–31C. A young Chinese girl with loose anagen syndrome. She presents with a complaint of not having to require haircuts since she was born.

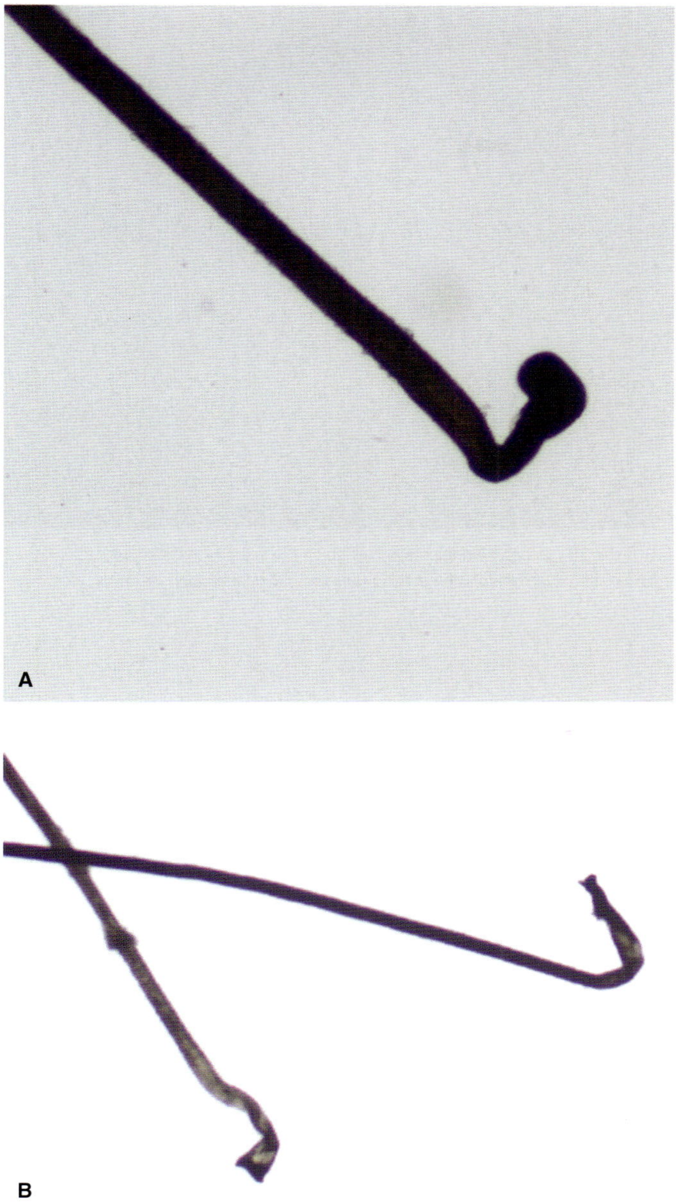

FIGURE 9-32A & 32B. Hair mount of gently pulled scalp hair of a patient with loose anagen syndrome with presence of dystrophic anagen roots that appear in the shape of a "hockey-stick with ruffled socks."

common than short anagen syndrome. In loose anagen syndrome, the actively growing anagen hairs are loosely anchored and can be easily and painlessly pulled from the scalp. In short anagen syndrome, the rate of growth is normal but there is shortening of the anagen phase, leading to a decrease in the maximal hair length and an increase in the number of hairs in telogen phase.

Clinical Features

- In loose anagen syndrome, the hair is sparse and short, and caregivers will provide a history of the child not or rarely requiring a haircut compared to other children of the same age. There is patchy or diffuse thinning with hair of uneven length, and the hair appears limp and matted. Hair pull test may be positive.
- In short anagen syndrome, similarly, scalp hairs remain short and are not able to grow long. There is increased shedding of hair with maximal hair length of about 6 cm. Hair density is normal and hair pull test may be positive.

Differential Diagnoses

- Loose anagen syndrome and short anagen syndrome are differential diagnoses. Hair mount examination will help to distinguish between the two diagnoses.
- Chronic telogen effluvium
  - Chronic telogen effluvium is a differential diagnosis of both conditions, especially short anagen syndrome, as both conditions can present with similar hair mount examination findings of increased telogen bulbs.
  - A thorough examination and specific investigations should be performed to exclude an underlying systemic cause of telogen effluvium.

Investigations & Treatment

- Trichoscopy of loose anagen syndrome will show rectangular granular structures (anagen follicles) and solitary yellow dots (follicular openings filled with sebum or keratin).
- Hair mount microscopy of loose anagen syndrome will show actively growing anagen hairs devoid of external root sheaths, with ruffled cuticles and pigmented misshapen bulbs ("hockey stick with rumpled sock" appearance).
- Hair mount microscopy of short anagen syndrome will show short hairs with telogen bulbs that have a club shape with decreased pigmentation.
- Topical minoxidil 2% or 5% may be useful in the treatment of both conditions. Both conditions are known to improve with age.

Pearls & Practical Tips

- We usually start with minoxidil 2% solution, with increase to 5% if no effect after a few months of treatment.

Bibliography

1. Swink SM, Castelo-Soccio L. Loose anagen syndrome: a retrospective chart review of 37 cases. Pediatr Dermatol 2016;33(5):507-10.
2. Oberlin KE, Maddy AJ, Martínez-Velasco MA, Vázquez-Herrera NE, Schachner LA, Tosti A. Short anagen syndrome: case series and literature review. Pediatr Dermatol 2018;35(3):388-91.

SCARRING ALOPECIA

Scarring or cicatricial alopecia results from inflammatory processes in and around the pilosebaceous units, causing irreversible destruction of tissue and permanent scarring alopecia. Scarring alopecia can be primary or secondary. Primary scarring alopecia has traditionally been classified as having a predominant lymphocytic, predominant neutrophilic, or mixed infiltrate. Secondary scarring alopecia is due to varied causes including trauma, malignancy, infection (e.g., kerion), connective tissue disease (e.g., morphea), and radiation.

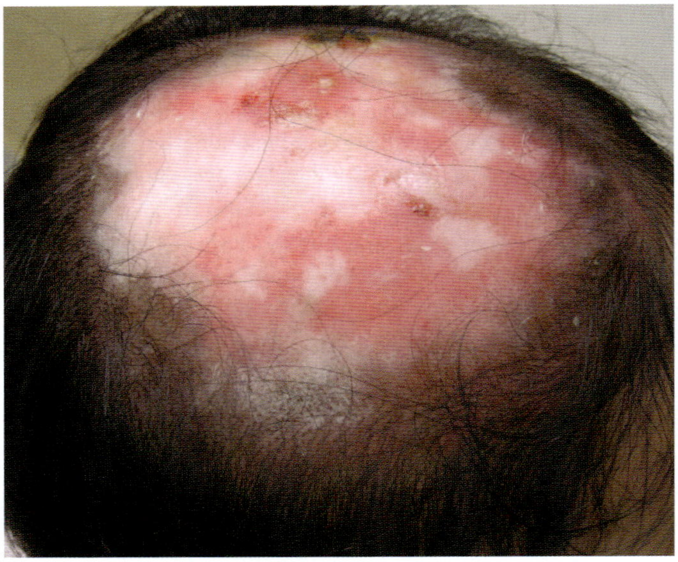

FIGURE 9-33. Severe scarring alopecia on the scalp of an older teenage girl with lupus erythematosus. There is loss of hair follicles, atrophy of the skin, dyspigmentation, and scaling present.

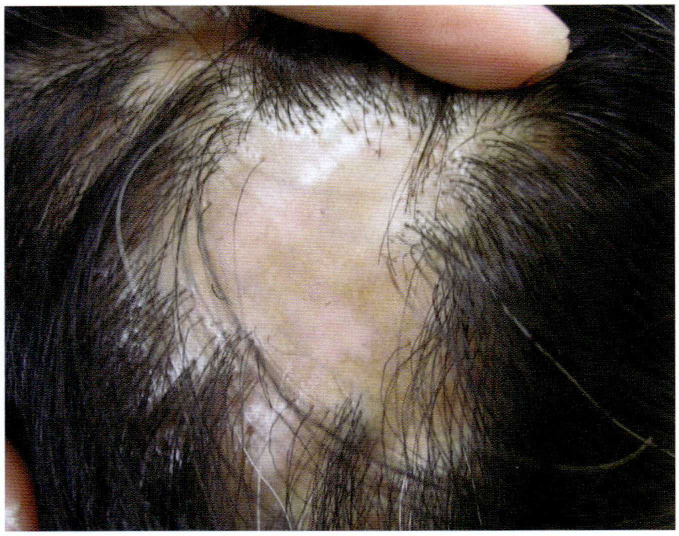

FIGURE 9-35. Lichen planopilaris occurring on the scalp with loss of hair follicles, scarring, and dyspigmentation in this teenager with lichen planus at other sites.

Clinical Features

- Conditions causing primary scarring alopecia with a predominant lymphocytic infiltrate include chronic cutaneous lupus erythematosus and lichen planopilaris. Both conditions are rare in children and adolescents. Both conditions can be isolated to the scalp, or more commonly, associated with similar disease elsewhere.
- Chronic cutaneous lupus erythematosus mostly affects females in late adolescence or early adulthood. Patients present with patchy or diffuse, alopecic, indurated, or atrophic papules and plaques with perifollicular scaling. Areas of scarring and dyspigmentation are also evident. Trichoscopy shows follicular plugging with perifollicular scale.
- Lichen planopilaris is a form of lichen planus that affects the scalp. The onset is insidious, with progression over months to years. The lesions may be asymptomatic, but itch, pain, or burning may often be present. Patchy keratotic follicular papules with erythema and scaling are seen, with active disease usually confined to the rim of the alopecic patches. Trichoscopy shows decreased follicular openings on a reddish background, perifollicular scaling, and tubular scaling.
- Conditions causing primary scarring alopecia with a predominant neutrophilic infiltrate include folliculitis

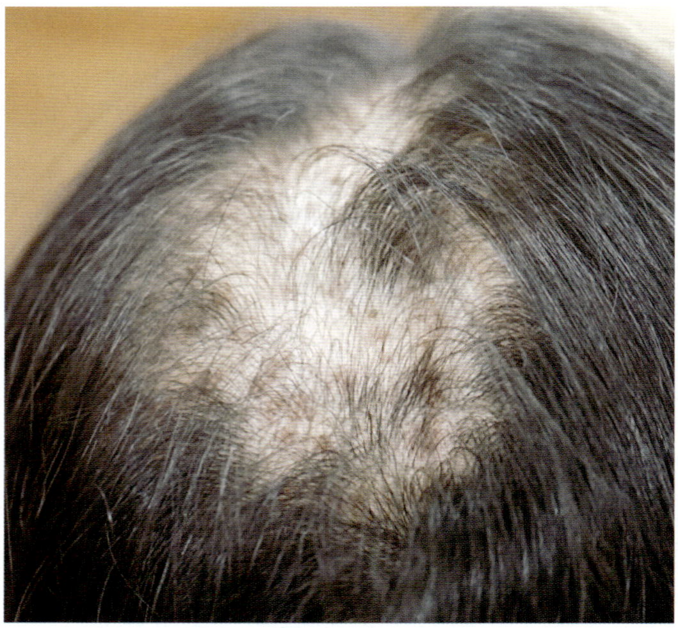

FIGURE 9-34. Cutaneous lupus erythematosus affecting the scalp of a Malay teenager presenting with scarring alopecia and scaling and atrophy of the scalp.

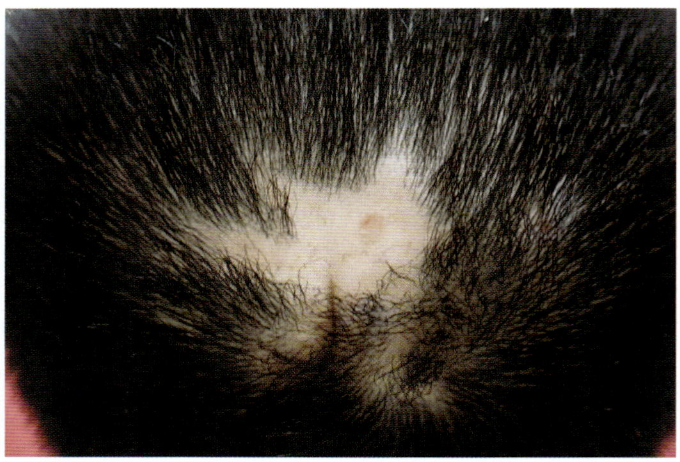

FIGURE 9-36. Secondary scarring alopecia on the scalp of a Chinese boy, secondary to previous folliculitis. Note the fallout of hair follicle openings.

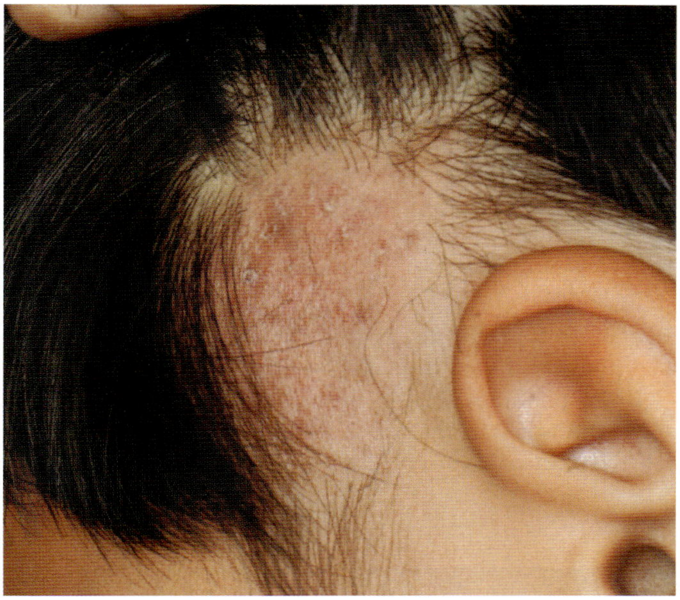

FIGURE 9-37. Secondary scarring alopecia on the temporal region of a Chinese boy, secondary to previous kerion.

decalvans and dissecting folliculitis. Both conditions are extremely rare in childhood but may occur in late adolescence.

- Folliculitis decalvans presents with successive crops of painful or itchy, patchy, follicular-based pustules and papules, with surrounding erythema, yellow scaling, and crusting. "Tufted hairs," whereby several follicles emerge from the same follicular ostium, are also seen. In later stages, irregular, atrophic, flesh-colored patches of scarring alopecia are seen. Lesions commonly affect the vertex and occipital area.

Differential Diagnoses

- Non-scarring alopecia
  - Scarring may not be evident if patients present early in the course of a scarring alopecia. Causes of non-scarring alopecia may then be considered, such as alopecia areata and trichotillomania. Observe for features of perifollicular scaling, erythema, dyspigmentation, pustules, and papules to provide clues to a diagnosis of scarring alopecia.
- Other scarring alopecias
  - Clinically, the various causes of scarring alopecia may be difficult to differentiate, especially in early disease, and there may be overlap of etiologies. Skin biopsy is essential if scarring alopecia is suspected.

Investigations & Treatment

- Scalp biopsies are essential in the diagnosis of scarring alopecia. At least two biopsies should be performed, with one processed vertically and the other horizontally. An additional biopsy for direct immunofluorescence should also be performed if chronic cutaneous lupus erythematosus is suspected. All biopsies should be performed at the edge of the alopecic patch, ideally an area with underlying erythema and scaling.
- Histopathological findings of chronic cutaneous lupus erythematosus include hyperkeratosis, follicular plugging, atrophy of the epidermis associated with basal vacuolar change, thickened basement membrane, superficial and deep perivascular lymphocytic infiltrate, and increased dermal mucin deposition. Direct immunofluorescence may be positive for a lupus band.
- Histopathological findings of lichen planopilaris include a band-like lymphohistiocytic infiltrate at the dermal–epidermal junction associated with basal vacuolar alteration and necrotic keratinocytes. No dermal mucin deposition is seen, and direct immunofluorescence is usually negative.
- Histopathological findings of folliculitis decalvans include a neutrophilic infiltrate principally affecting upper portions of hair follicles with destruction of sebaceous glands.
- Blood investigations to exclude systemic lupus erythematosus should be performed in patients diagnosed with chronic cutaneous lupus erythematosus.
- The mainstay of management is to control lesions and minimize scarring.
- Treatment of chronic cutaneous lupus erythematosus and lichen planopilaris includes topical treatments such as high-potency topical or intralesional corticosteroids, calcineurin inhibitors, and retinoids. Systemic therapies may be considered in more severe disease, and include antimalarials, methotrexate, mycophenolate, and azathioprine.
- Treatment of folliculitis decalvans includes antistaphylococcal topical antibiotics such as mupirocin and fusidic acid, with or without potent topical corticosteroids. Intralesional corticosteroids may be considered. Systemic treatments include oral antibiotics such as minocycline and doxycycline, rifampicin, clindamycin, or azithromycin, and oral retinoids such as isotretinoin.

Pearls & Practical Tips

- Primary scarring alopecia is very rare in children. Secondary scarring alopecia can occur, for instance secondary to bacterial or fungal infections.
- Early scalp biopsy and institution of early treatment is essential in the treatment of scarring alopecia to prevent or reduce inflammation and scarring.
- There is considerable overlap between chronic cutaneous lupus and lichen planopilaris both clinically and histologically.

Bibliography

1. Bolduc C, Sperling LC, Shapiro J. Primary cicatricial alopecia: Lymphocytic primary cicatricial alopecias, including chronic cutaneous lupus erythematosus, lichen planopilaris, frontal fibrosing alopecia, and Graham-Little syndrome. J Am Acad Dermatol 2016;75(6):1081-99.
2. Bolduc C, Sperling LC, Shapiro J. Primary cicatricial alopecia: Other lymphocytic primary cicatricial alopecias and neutrophilic and mixed primary cicatricial alopecias. J Am Acad Dermatol 2016;75(6):1101-17.

HAIR SHAFT DISORDERS

Hair shaft disorders can be categorized into conditions with increased hair fragility and conditions without increased hair fragility. Both can be congenital or acquired, with congenital hair shaft disorders presenting earlier than acquired disorders. Increased fragility can be demonstrated by a positive hair tug test.

Clinical Features

- The clinical features, associated disorders, investigation findings, and treatment are listed in Tables 9-2 and 9-3.

Investigations & Treatment

- Hair shaft disorders can be diagnosed using a combination of clinical features, including history and careful examination in conjunction with trichoscopy and microscopy of snipped hairs. Hairs should not be pulled for microscopy if hair shaft disorders are suspected, as the hairs will be broken at the abnormal area, leading to poor visualization of the abnormality.
- At present, there are no good treatments for most hair shaft disorders. Patients should be informed not to undergo excessive cosmetic hair treatments, such as perming or straightening, as this may lead to more damage to the already fragile hair.
- Treatment of monilethrix with oral retinoids or topical 2% minoxidil has been described, although results are variable.

Pearls & Practical Tips

- Most hair shaft abnormalities improve with age.
- In conditions with systemic associations, such as pili torti and wooly hair, a search for other organ involvement is important.

TABLE 9-2. Hair shaft disorders with increased fragility.

Condition	Clinical features	Associated disorders	Investigations
Trichorrhexis nodosa	• Dry, lusterless, short hair that is easily fractured • **Grey-white nodules** may be seen on hair; hair readily breaks off at the nodule sites	• Trauma, e.g., use of hot combs, hair dryers at high heat, hair straighteners, chemical treatments • Argininosuccinic aciduria • Citrullinemia • Trichothiodystrophy • Trichohepatoenteric syndrome	• Microscopy: appearance of two interlocking brushes (due to segmental longitudinal splitting of fibers without complete fracture)
Monilethrix	• Beaded hair with node-like deformities • Partial alopecia • Regrown hair after neonatal lanugo hair sheds is dry, lusterless, brittle, and fails to grow to any appreciable length • In severe cases, infant may be bald or have sparse scalp hair, easily fractured and stubble-like • Some have koilonychia	• Autosomal dominant disorder (most common): mutations in *KRT81* and *KRT86* • Autosomal recessive disorder: mutations in *DSG4* • Ectodermal dysplasia • Woolly hair with hypotrichosis	• Microscopy: variation in hair shaft thickness with small, node-like deformities
Trichorrhexis invaginata	• Due to abnormal keratinization of hair shaft • Dry, lusterless, easily fractured, sparse, and short hair	• Isolated • Characteristic of Netherton syndrome	• Microscopy: telescope-like invagination along the hair shaft (*resembles ball-and-cup joints of bamboo*)
Pili torti	• Dry and fragile hair, lighter in color • "Spangled" appearance (shimmers in reflected light due to hair twisting)	• Isolated with autosomal dominant or autosomal recessive inheritance • Mitochondrial disorders • Menkes syndrome • Crandall syndrome • Björnstad syndrome	• Trichoscopy: hair shafts that are irregularly bent at acute angles with 180-degree twists of flattened hair • Microscopy: 3–4 regularly spaced twists that occur at irregular intervals along the hair shaft, with flattening at the site of the twist

TABLE 9-3. Hair shaft disorders without increased fragility.

Condition	Clinical features	Associated disorders	Investigations
Pili annulati	• Hair appears colorful and shimmers, with alternating bright and dark bands	• Usually autosomal dominant • Has been seen in association with alopecia areata	• Trichoscopy: hair shafts with regular light bands
Woolly hair	• Tight, curly hair • Scalp hairs are dry and fine, light- colored, and corrugated at intervals • Usually present from birth	• Naxos disease • Carvajal syndrome • Cardiofaciocutaneous syndrome	• Trichoscopy: varying thickness of hair shafts, "crawling snake" appearance, kinking of hair shaft, and irregularity of shaft diameter

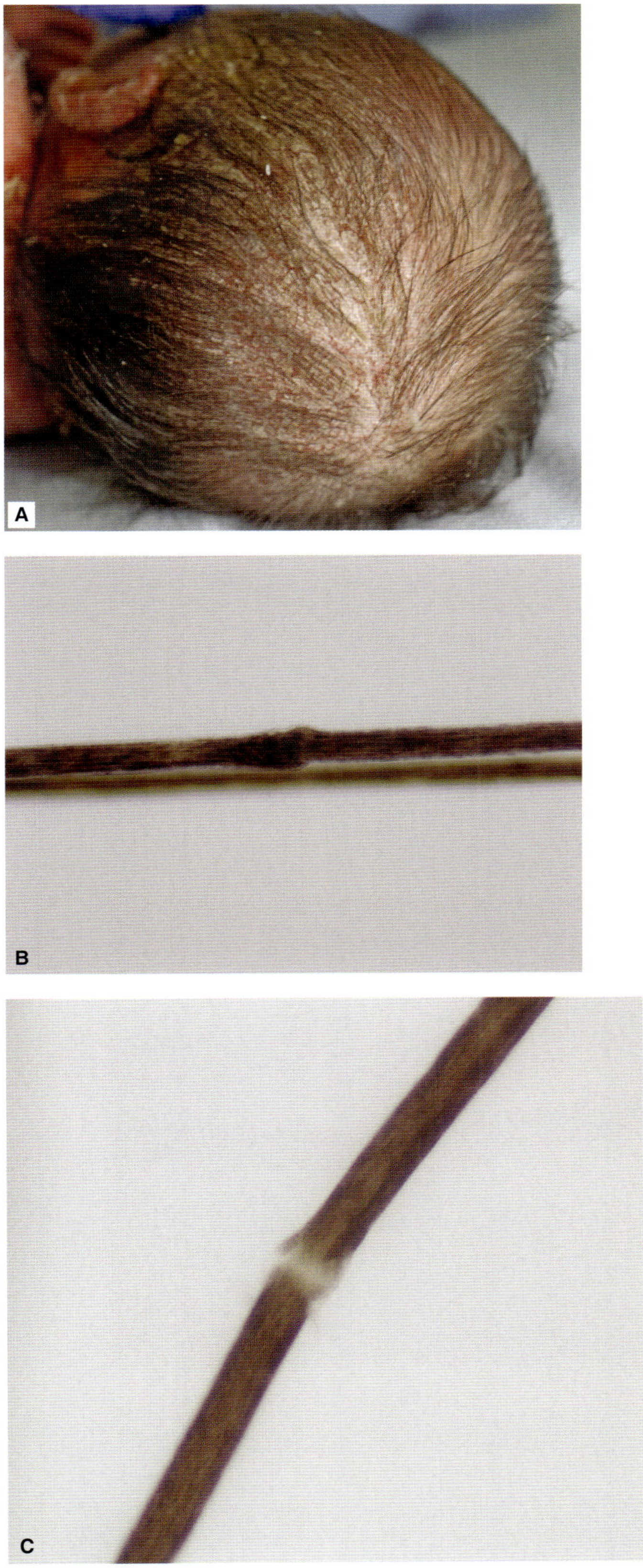

FIGURE 9-38A–38C. A neonate with Netherton syndrome with sparse scalp hair, generalized erythema, and scaling. Hair mount features include trichorrhexis invaginata (Figure 9-38B) and trichorrhexis nodosa (Figure 9-38C)

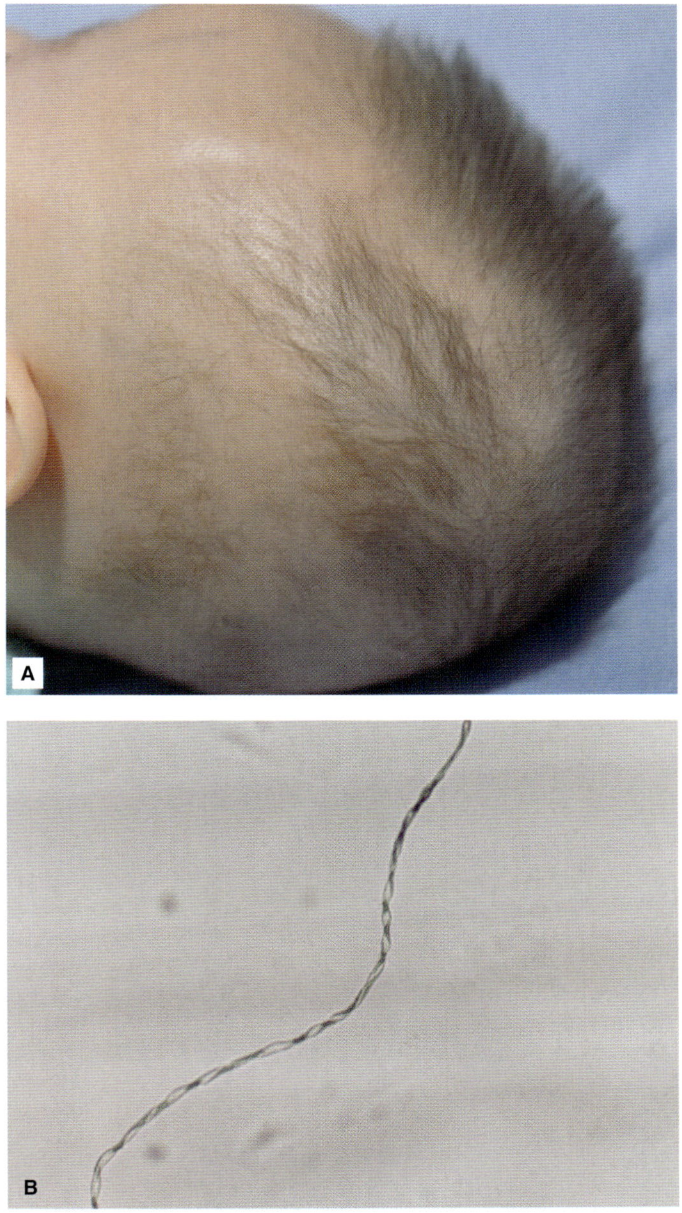

FIGURE 9-39A & 39B. A male infant with Menkes syndrome presenting with seizures, developmental delay, reduced skin pigmentation, and sparse and short hair. Hair mount showed features of pili torti (Figure 9-39B).

Bibliography

1. Rudnicka L, Olszewska M, Waśkiel A, Rakowska A. Trichoscopy in hair shaft disorders. Dermatol Clin 2018;36(4):421-30.
2. Singh G, Miteva M. Prognosis and management of congenital hair shaft disorders with fragility-Part I. Pediatr Dermatol 2016;33(5):473-80.
3. Singh G, Miteva M. Prognosis and management of congenital hair shaft disorders without fragility-Part II. Pediatr Dermatol 2016;33(5):481-7.

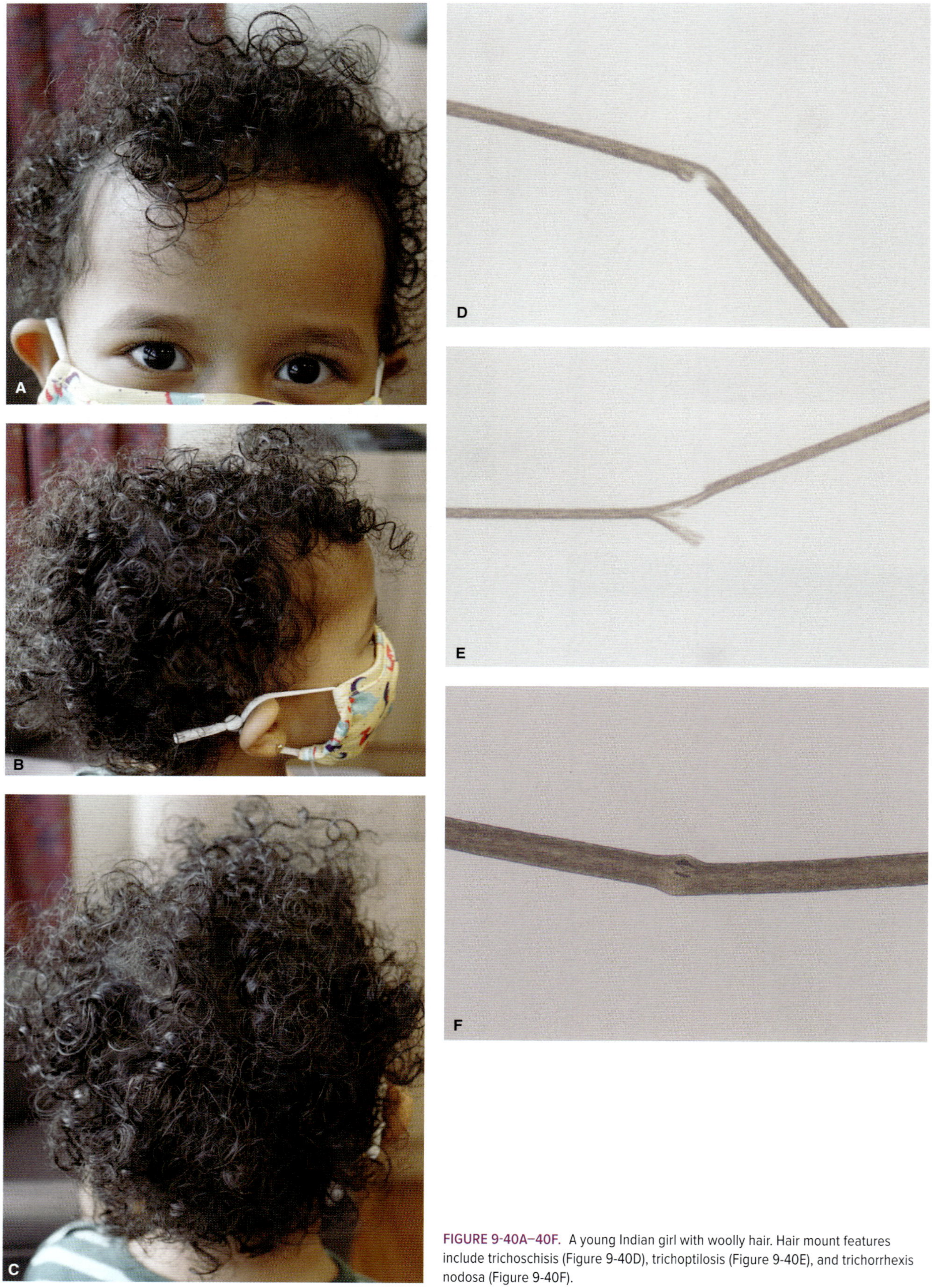

FIGURE 9-40A–40F. A young Indian girl with woolly hair. Hair mount features include trichoschisis (Figure 9-40D), trichoptilosis (Figure 9-40E), and trichorrhexis nodosa (Figure 9-40F).

APPROACH TO NAIL DISORDERS

NORMAL NAIL ANATOMY

The human nail consists of the nail plate and nail unit. The key components of the nail unit are the nail matrix, nail bed, hyponychium, cuticle, and nail folds.

- The nail plate is predominantly made of keratin and originates from the nail matrix. It is smooth in texture and translucent in appearance.
- The nail matrix consists of germinative epithelium and is responsible for keratinocyte differentiation to form the nail plate. The distal white part of the nail matrix is the lunula.
- The nail bed consists of cells located under the nail plate. It is pink in appearance because there is a rich vascular supply.
- The hyponychium is the layer of epithelium below the free edge of the nail plate and at the distal end of the nail bed.
- The nail folds enclose the nail plate and nail bed. The proximal and two lateral nail folds support and protect the nail.
- The cuticle is the distal horny layer, which is an extension of the proximal nail fold epidermis. It sticks to the nail plate and protects the nail from external irritants and infective organisms.

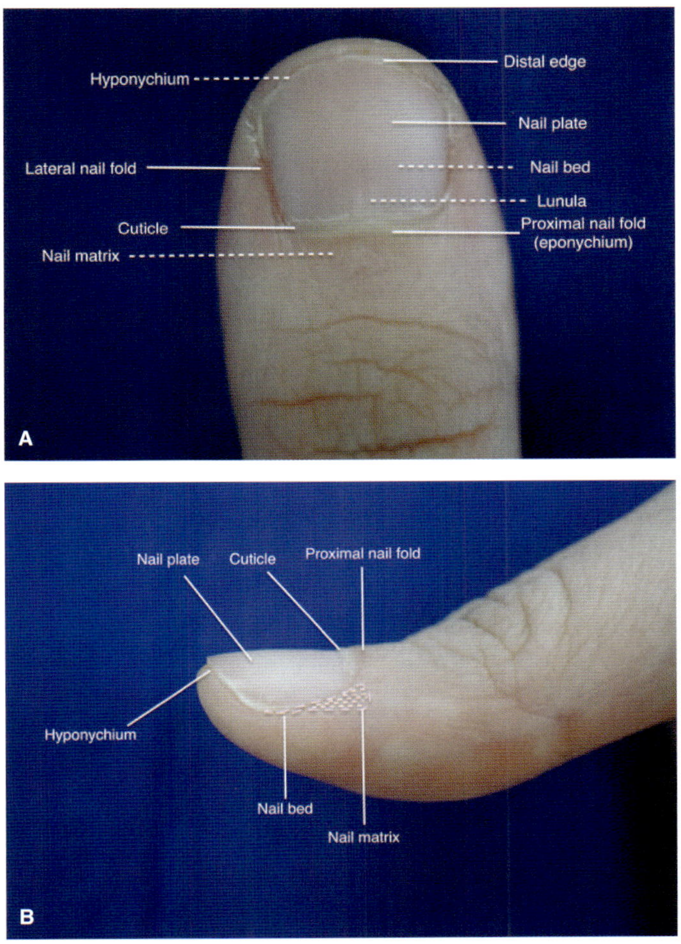

FIGURE 9-41A & 41B. Normal nail anatomy.

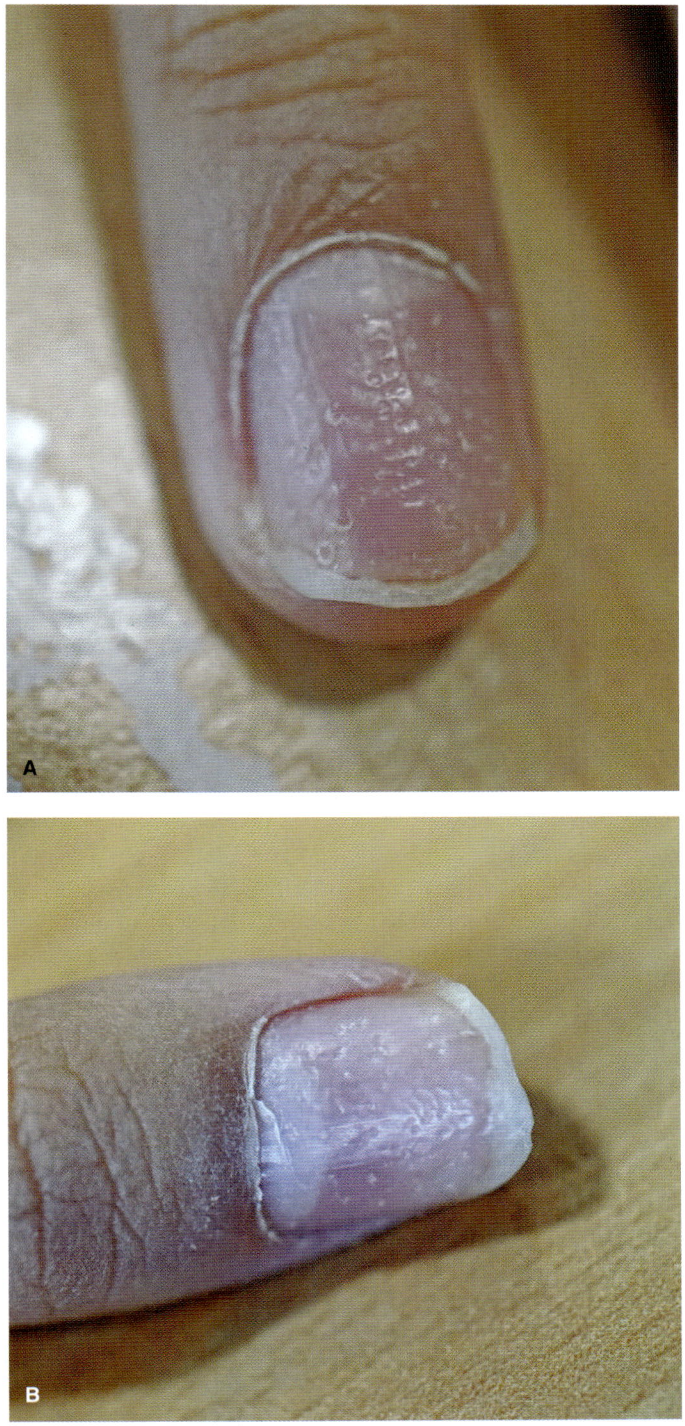

FIGURE 9-42A & 42B. Examples of nail pitting seen in two different patients.

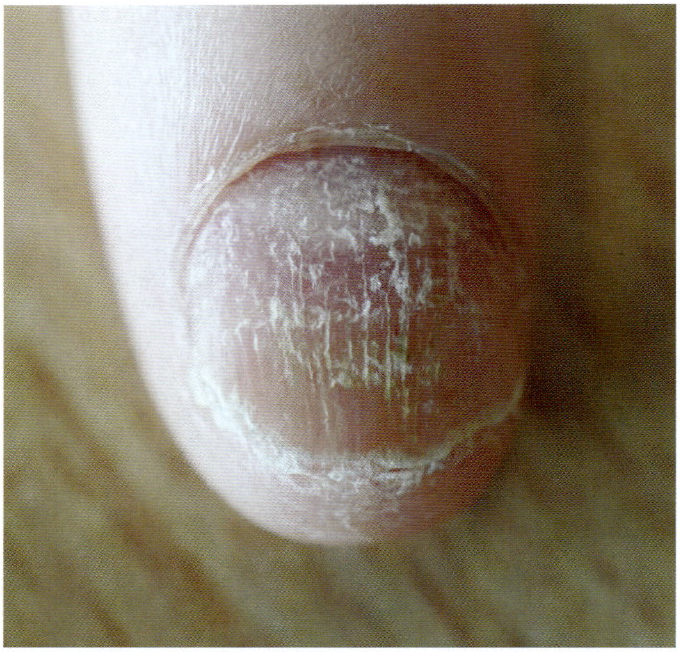

FIGURE 9-43. Longitudinal ridging of the nail plate, also known as trachyonychia.

NORMAL NAIL GROWTH

Fingernails grow at a faster rate than toenails, at an estimated rate of 0.5 to 1.2 mm per week (or approximately 2 to 4 mm per month), with complete nail plate growth occurring in approximately 6 months. Toenails grow at about one-third of the rate of fingernails. Factors that accelerate nail growth include young age, nail biting, and hyperproliferative skin diseases.

COMMON ABNORMAL NAIL PRESENTATIONS

Nail abnormalities can be broadly divided into three main categories.

Disfigured Nails

Nails may be "disfigured" due to changes in texture, shape, or structure. These changes may be physiological or pathological.

a. Changes in texture may be due to nail matrix abnormalities or nail plate abnormalities
   - Nail matrix abnormalities
     - Pitting: isolated pits, psoriasis, atopic dermatitis, alopecia areata
     - Ridging
       - » Transverse: Beau's lines/onychomadesis
       - » Longitudinal: lichen planus, lichen striatus, median nail dystrophy, twenty-nail dystrophy, Darier's disease
       - » Variable: onychotillomania
   - Nail plate abnormalities or abnormalities of the hyponychium
     - Nail plate: onychoschezia
     - Hyponychium: onycholysis

b. Changes in shape or structure
   - Abnormal nail curvature/shape: Clubbing, koilonychia, wedge-shaped nails, pincer nails
   - Other structural nail abnormalities: Congenital malalignment of great toenails, brachyonychia

c. Loss of nail
   - Temporary loss without scarring: Trauma
   - Permanent loss with scarring: Pterygium (lichen planus), congenital anonychia, nail-patella syndrome

Nail Pigmentation

Nail pigmentation refers to the presence of melanin in the nail plate. This usually presents as a pigmented longitudinal band along the entire length of the nail (melanonychia). It is important to differentiate between benign and malignant nail pigmentation. Benign causes of melanonychia include melanocyte activation, nail matrix lentigo, and nail matrix melanocytic nevus. Nail matrix melanoma is rare in children but is a malignant cause of melanonychia.

Discolored Nails

Nails may be discolored due to abnormalities in the nail bed or nail plate. For the latter, there may be associated nail thickening as well. Nail bed abnormalities leading to discolored nails include leukonychia, glomus tumor, splinter hemorrhage, and subungual hematoma. Nail plate abnormalities include yellow nail syndrome and onychomycosis.

ASSESSMENT OF PATIENTS WITH NAIL CONCERNS

History

A comprehensive history is important for accurate diagnosis. The key components of the history include a good characterization of the presenting complaint and thorough evaluation of potential causes.

a. Characterization of presenting complaint
   - Onset and duration
   - Progression (rapidly evolving, stable, or improving)
   - Associated symptoms (pain, cutaneous involvement, and systemic manifestations)

b. Evaluation of underly etiology
   - Congenital or acquired
   - Presence of comorbidities, including other dermatological conditions such as psoriasis, atopic dermatitis, alopecia areata, and lichen planus
   - Presence of trauma
   - Family history of similar symptoms or diseases
   - Lifestyle, nail care routines, and environmental exposures
   - Medication history

Physical Examination

Thorough inspection of all nails, including fingernails and toenails. This should be done under optimal lighting, ideally natural sunlight. The nails should be examined from three different angles: from above, from the side, and from the end. This will facilitate identification of the type of nail abnormality and the number of nails affected.

a. Nail examination from above
   - Surface texture: pitting, transverse and longitudinal ridges
   - Discoloration and pigmentation: discoloration of the nail bed and nail plate, presence of warning signs (e.g., Hutchinson's sign) in nail pigmentation
   - Nail fold and cuticle changes

b. Nail examination from the side
- Shape of nails: presence of koilonychia or wedge-shaped nails, abnormal nail curvature, ingrowing of nails
- Nail dystrophy, loss of nails and associated scarring
- Abnormalities around the nail, such as paronychia

c. Nail examination from the end
- Nail plate thickening or splitting
- Presence of subungual hyperkeratosis
- Nail bed detachment (onycholysis)

Examination of the rest of the skin, hair, and genitalia should be performed, as nail conditions may be manifestations of underlying dermatological diseases. A focused systemic examination should also be performed, as nail conditions may occur in underlying systemic diseases (e.g., chronic disease with digital clubbing, psoriatic arthropathy, tuberous sclerosis).

Bibliography
1. Smith RJ, Rubin AI. Pediatric nail disorders: a review. Curr Opin Pediatr 2020;32(4):506-15.
2. Starace M, Alessandrini A, Piraccini BM. Nail disorders in children. Skin Appendage Disord 2018;4(4):217-29.

BEAU'S LINES & ONYCHOMADESIS
Beau's lines are linear transverse grooves on the nail plate and are due to temporary disruption of nail matrix growth. As the fingernail grows, Beau's lines gradually progress more distally on the nail. Onychomadesis occurs when there is complete disruption of nail growth and is considered a more severe variant of Beau's lines.

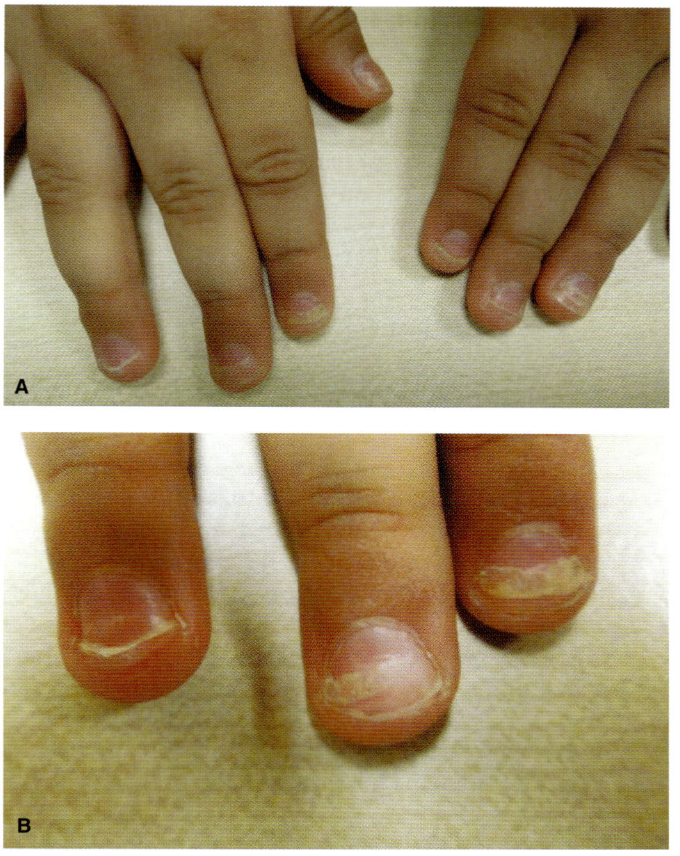

FIGURE 9-45A & 45B. Beau's lines and onychomadesis affecting several nails in a Chinese girl.

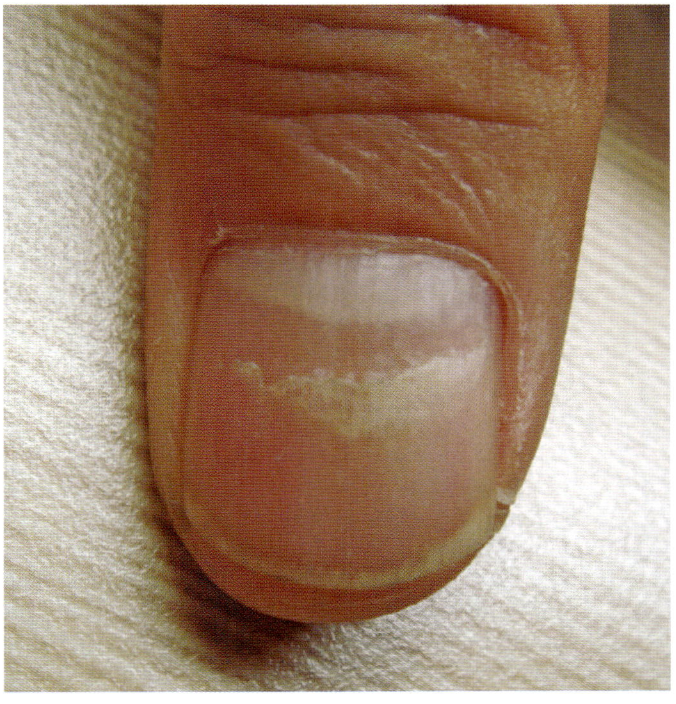

FIGURE 9-44. Beau's lines affecting the nail in an adolescent patient after illness.

Clinical Features
- Beau's lines can be a normal physiological variant but may also indicate underlying pathology. In newborns, causes of Beau's lines include intrauterine or perinatal distress. In older children, causes include trauma, acute illness, poor nutrition, drugs, and post-surgery stress.

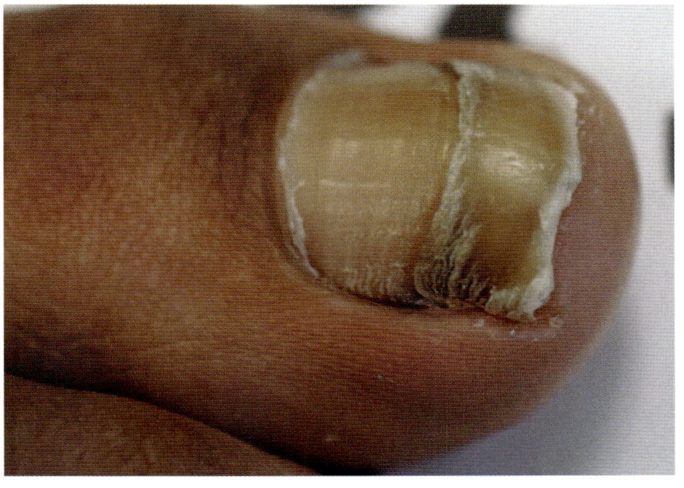

FIGURE 9-46. Onychomadesis affecting the big toe of an Indian adolescent.

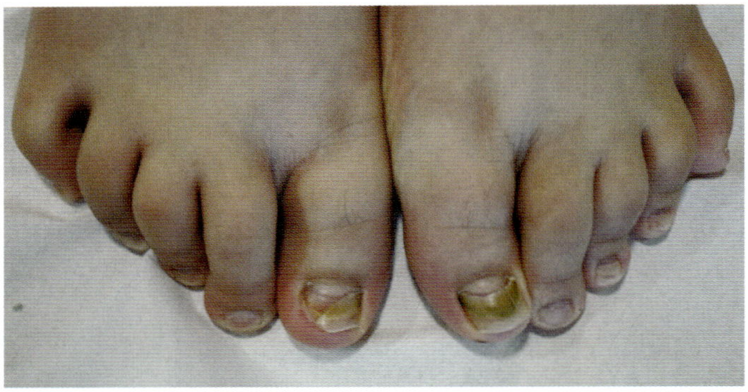

FIGURE 9-47. Onychomadesis affecting the bilateral big toes of a Chinese boy.

- Clinically, there is a single transverse depression extending from one lateral nail fold to the other. They occur more commonly on fingernails than toenails. In cases due to underlying systemic illness, they are found on multiple digits. If found on a single digit, trauma needs to be considered.
- Onychomadesis occurs when there is complete disruption of nail growth. Due to detachment of the nail plate from the proximal nail fold, there is full-thickness disruption of the nail plate and subsequent shedding of the nail.
- Causes of onychomadesis include systemic infections and drug reactions.
- In onychomadesis, nail regrowth usually occurs spontaneously within 12 weeks.

Differential Diagnoses

- Mees' lines
  - These are non-blanchable white-colored transverse bands on the nail bed parallel to the lunula. Unlike Beau's lines, there are no palpable grooves.
  - They may be caused by chemotherapy, systemic illnesses, or poisoning with arsenic and heavy metals.

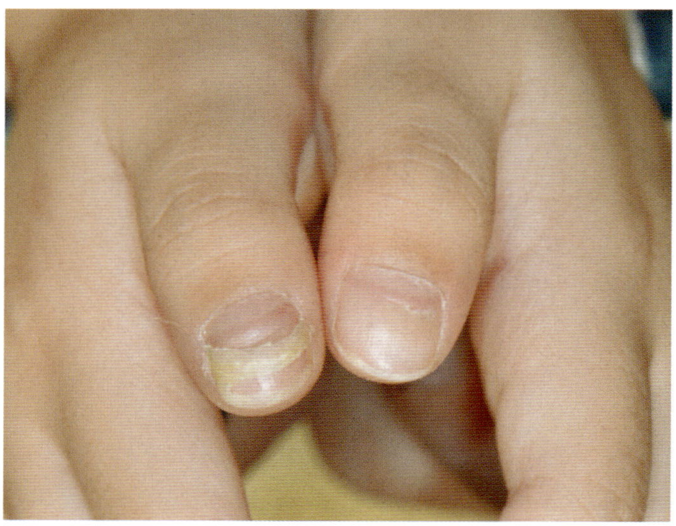

FIGURE 9-48. Onychomadesis affecting the right thumbnail and Beau's line affecting the left thumbnail of a young Chinese boy.

- Muehrcke lines
  - These are paired, transverse white lines. They are blanchable and smooth, with no palpable grooves.
  - Muehrcke lines are specific for chronic hypoalbuminemia.
- Onychoschizia
  - There is horizontal peeling of the lamellar and splitting within the nail plate at the free edges of the nail.
  - In young children with lamellar dystrophy present in one thumb, it is likely due to thumb sucking.

Investigations & Treatment

- Consider evaluation for underlying systemic illness if clinically indicated. Otherwise generally self-limiting and does not require investigations.
- The condition is managed conservatively. No specific treatment is required apart from reassurance.

Pearls & Practical Tips

- Beau's lines are common in neonates and progress distally over 3 to 4 months before resolving.
- Beau's lines and onychomadesis are both commonly seen after hand-foot-mouth disease and sometimes after dengue fever.
- Predicting when the episode of illness causing the Beau's line or onychomadesis occurred may be possible by measuring the distance of the line from the proximal nail fold. Fingernails grow about 1 mm per week, while toenails grow about 0.5 mm per week.

Bibliography

1. Smith RJ, Rubin AI. Pediatric nail disorders: a review. Curr Opin Pediatr 2020;32(4):506-15.

TWENTY-NAIL DYSTROPHY

Twenty-nail dystrophy, also known as trachyonychia, is a fairly common acquired inflammatory condition involving the nail matrix that can involve some or all nails. There is excessive longitudinal ridging of the nails, resulting in a rough sandpaper texture. It can occasionally be associated with other dermatoses.

Clinical Features

- Twenty-nail dystrophy usually occurs in children between 2 and 12 years of age. It has a slow, insidious course and can involve a few or all fingernails and toenails.
- The clinical features can be divided into two main categories:
  - The first presents as excessive longitudinal nail ridging, resulting in a diffusely rough texture. There is nail thinning, and the cuticles may be hyperkeratotic. The nails are opaque and lose their natural luster.
  - In the second type of presentation, the nails retain their luster and the nail plate is shiny, with superficial ridging and multiple small nail pits.
- The condition usually occurs in isolation but may be associated with other dermatological conditions like alopecia areata, atopic dermatitis, psoriasis, and lichen planus.

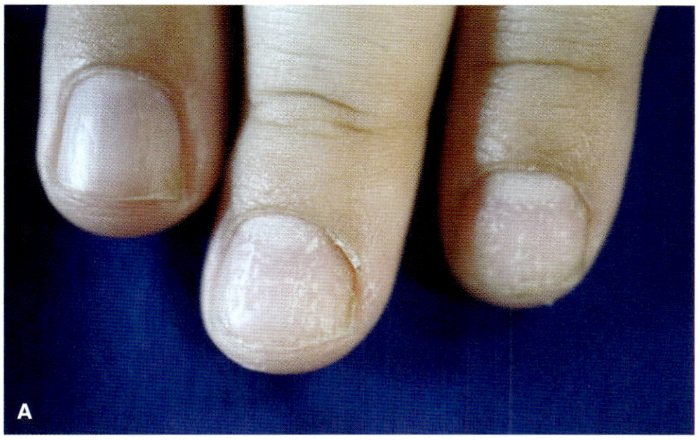

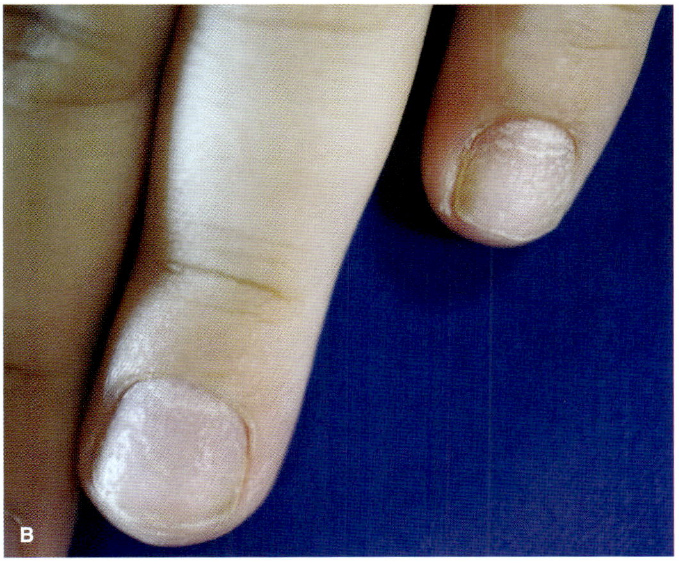

FIGURE 9-49A & 49B. Classical features of twenty-nail dystrophy in this Chinese girl with features of pitting and trachyonychia.

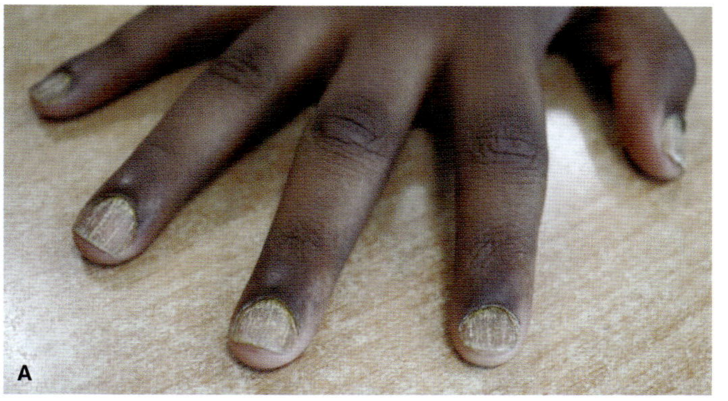

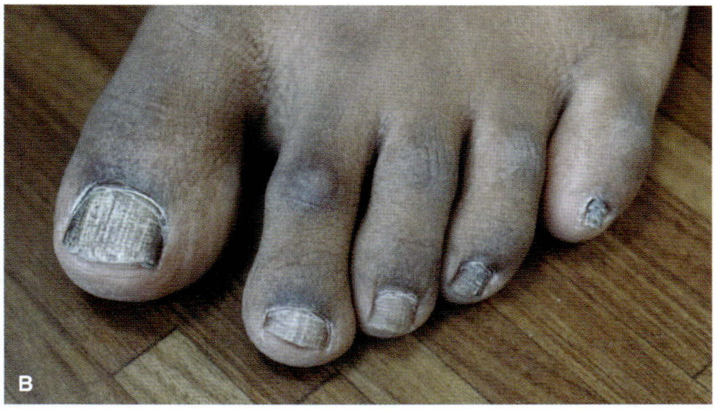

FIGURE 9-50A & 50B. Twenty-nail dystrophy affecting an Indian adolescent with concomitant alopecia areata. There is marked longitudinal ridging seen affected all the nails.

Differential Diagnoses

- Onychomycosis
  - Onychomycosis represents fungal infection of the nails. This is very rare in children and usually involves only single nails.
- Psoriasis nails
  - Nail involvement in psoriasis may present rather similarly to twenty-nail dystrophy. However, the classic features of nail psoriasis are nail pitting, onycholysis, subungual hyperkeratosis, and oil-drop pigmentation. Other cutaneous features of psoriasis should be examined for in the patient.
- Eczema nails
  - Nail involvement is commonly seen in children with eczema affecting the fingers and toes. These changes include irregular transverse ridging, pitting, thickening, and discoloration. Eczematous papules and plaques will be seen on the affected fingers and toes.
- Pachyonychia congenita
  - This is a rare autosomal dominant condition affecting keratin genes, resulting in hypertrophic nail dystrophy and palmoplantar keratoderma. Other associated features include paronychia, palmoplantar keratoderma, and white patches on mucous membranes.

Investigations & Treatment

- Nail biopsies are not routinely required for diagnosis. However, if performed, either spongiotic or psoriasiform features may be seen on histological examination.
- Treatment involves reassurance and supportive management with emollients and nail polish. The condition usually spontaneously improves over years.
- Although efficacy is unclear, other treatments that may be prescribed include:
  - Topical corticosteroids, tazarotene gel, 5-fluorouracil
  - Intralesional triamcinolone acetonide to the proximal nail folds or intra-matrix
  - Phototherapy with psoralen UVA (PUVA)
  - Systemic medications: biotin, cyclosporin, retinoids, systemic steroids

Pearls & Practical Tips

- Although cosmetically concerning, twenty-nail dystrophy is asymptomatic and does not lead to nail scarring. Spontaneous improvement is anticipated in most cases.

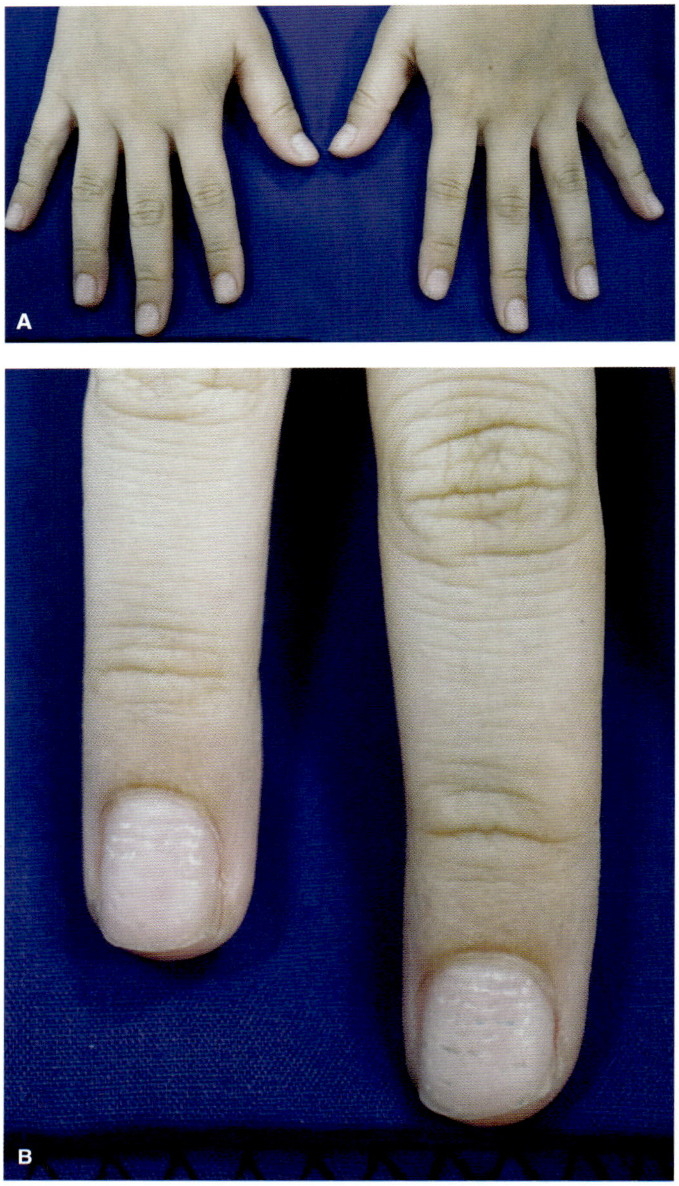

FIGURE 9-51A & 51B. Twenty-nail dystrophy affecting the fingernails of a Chinese girl. There are rough pits in a transverse distribution throughout the affected nails.

- For biopsies, a punch biopsy of the nail matrix or longitudinal nail biopsy should be performed to ensure appropriate tissue sampling.
- If there is evidence of an associated disease (e.g., psoriasis), treatment should be directed at treating the associated condition.

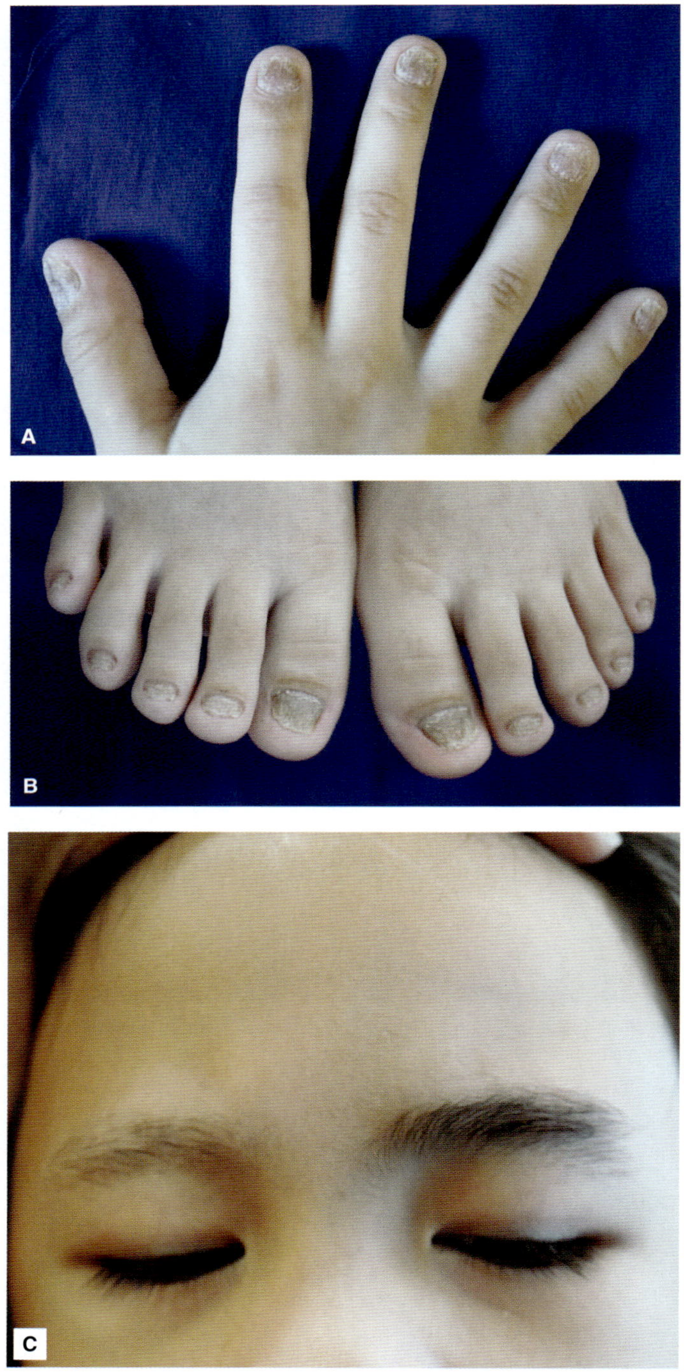

FIGURE 9-52A–52C. Twenty-nail dystrophy affecting a Filipino girl with concomitant alopecia areata affecting her right eyebrow (Figure 9-52C).

Bibliography

1. Smith RJ, Rubin AI. Pediatric nail disorders: a review. Curr Opin Pediatr 2020;32(4):506-15.

MEDIAN NAIL DYSTROPHY

Median nail dystrophy is an uncommon, acquired nail condition presenting as longitudinal midline splitting in the nail plate. Although the pathogenesis is not fully understood, it is believed to be due to microtrauma leading to a transient defect in the nail matrix. A similar appearance can be seen in association with habitual picking of the nail fold.

Clinical Features

- Although mostly idiopathic, other associated etiologies include habitual trauma, subungual tumors (e.g., glomus and myxoid tumors), and oral retinoid use. Familial cases have also been described.
- The condition presents as a median longitudinal groove and small ridges extending laterally from the central split, resembling a fir tree.
- The thumbnails are most commonly involved, although other fingernails or toenails may be affected as well.
- The condition spontaneously resolves after months to years, although recurrence is possible.

Differential Diagnoses

- Habit tic deformity
  - This refers to nail dystrophy due to habitual trauma to the nail matrix. The thumbnails are usually affected, although it can affect any nail.
  - Typical features include a centralized longitudinal depression and irregularly spaced transverse ridges. There may also be lunula hypertrophy and absent cuticles. In contrast, the cuticles are usually unaffected in median nail dystrophy.
  - Treatment involves habit reversal and use of physical barriers (e.g., tape) to prevent manipulation of the nail. In some cases, it may be associated with anxiety or obsessive-compulsive disorder (OCD), which should be addressed.

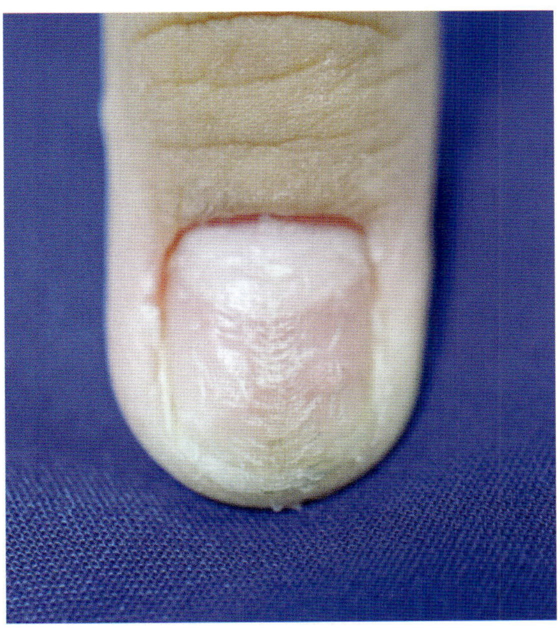

FIGURE 9-53. Median nail dystrophy presenting as a central groove on this thumb nail of a child.

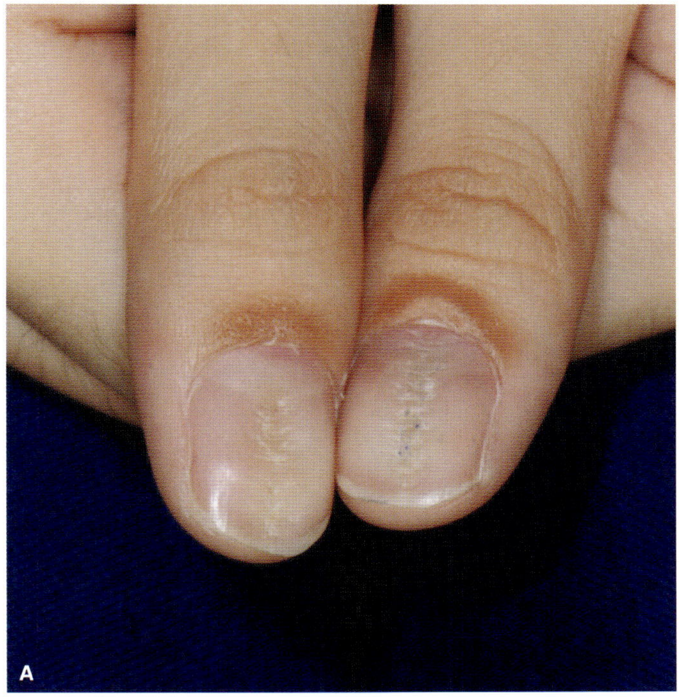

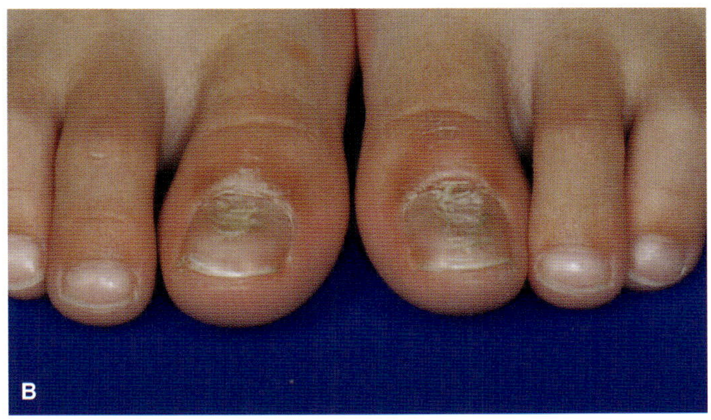

FIGURE 9-54A & 54B. Median nail dystrophy affecting bilateral thumbs and big toes of this Chinese girl.

- Nail lichen striatus
  - Clinical signs include involvement of a single nail with longitudinal ridging over a medial or lateral aspect of the nail. These nail changes may be isolated, or more commonly occurs with cutaneous lesions.
- Pterygium unguis/nail lichen planus
  - Also known as dorsal pterygium, this is a manifestation of nail lichen planus. Unlike median nail dystrophy, this condition can lead to permanent scarring of the nail unit.

Investigations & Treatment

- Nail biopsies are not required for diagnosis. If performed, histopathological features include parakeratosis and melanin accumulation within and between the nail bed keratinocytes.
- Possible therapeutic options include topical corticosteroids, topical tacrolimus, and topical retinoids. Treatment results are usually disappointing.

- If there are concerns of an underlying habitual tic disorder or other psychiatric disorder, management with a psychologist or psychiatrist may be considered.

Pearls & Practical Tips

- In patients with median nail dystrophy, it is important to consider repetitive nail trauma and associated psychiatric conditions such as depression and OCD. In these cases, management with behavioral counseling or antidepressants may be necessary.
- Nail care methods, such as keeping short nails, buffing the nail surface, and covering the nail plate may help protect the nail from further damage by preventing its edges from catching on other objects.

ECZEMA NAILS

Nail changes may occur in patients with eczema from atopy or chronic irritation that affects the nail unit. Nail matrix inflammation results in various changes, such as transverse ridging and nail pitting.

Clinical Features

- Patients may have underlying chronic atopic dermatitis, pompholyx, or contact dermatitis involving the fingertips and nail folds.
- Perionychium involvement results in nail matrix inflammation and associated nail changes, such as irregular transverse ridging, pitting, onycholysis, discoloration, and subungual hyperkeratosis.
- Other features include absent or ragged cuticles and swollen proximal or lateral nail folds, with associated chronic paronychia due to bacteria or fungal superinfection.
- Chronic eczematous lesions are usually evident over the hands and/or feet, in addition to other more classical sites, such as the flexures.

Differential Diagnoses

- Twenty-nail dystrophy
  - Twenty-nail dystrophy can present with similar nail features as eczema nails, such as longitudinal nail ridging and rough nail texture. Eczematous changes are usually not apparent.

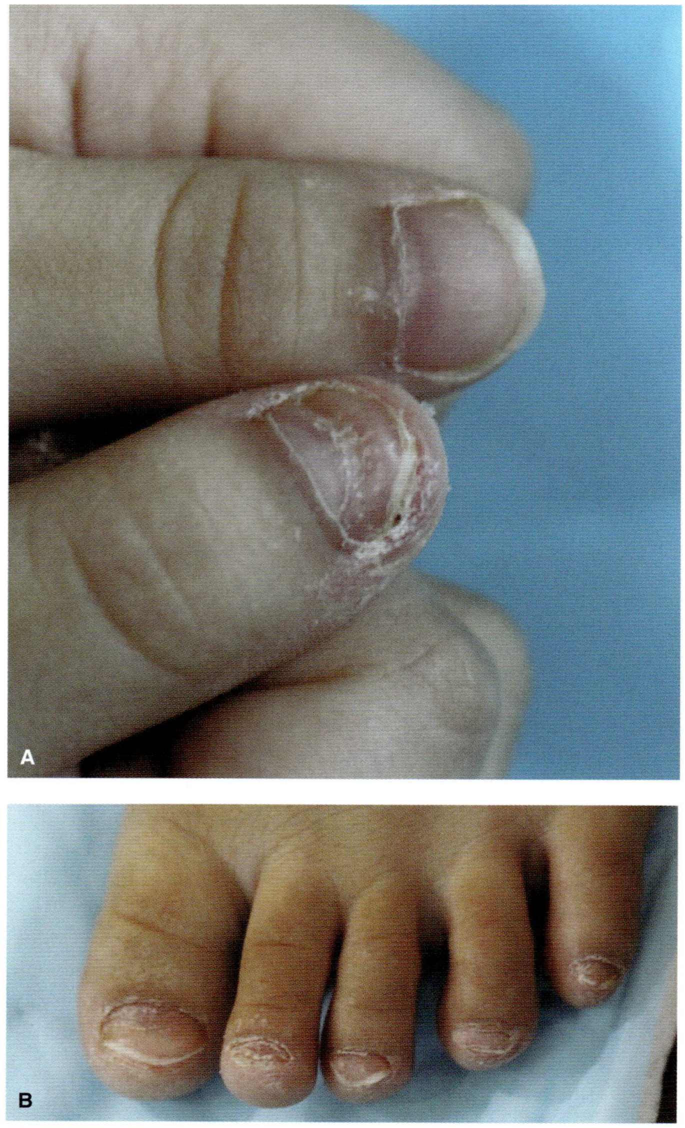

FIGURE 9-56A & 56B. Dystrophic nail changes seen in a young Chinese boy with eczema affecting his nail folds with concomitant chronic paronychia.

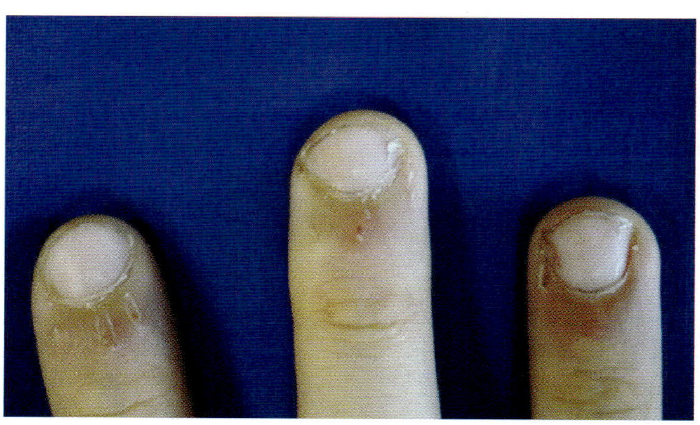

FIGURE 9-55. Early nail fold eczema presenting as mild erythema and scaling, with minimal nail changes.

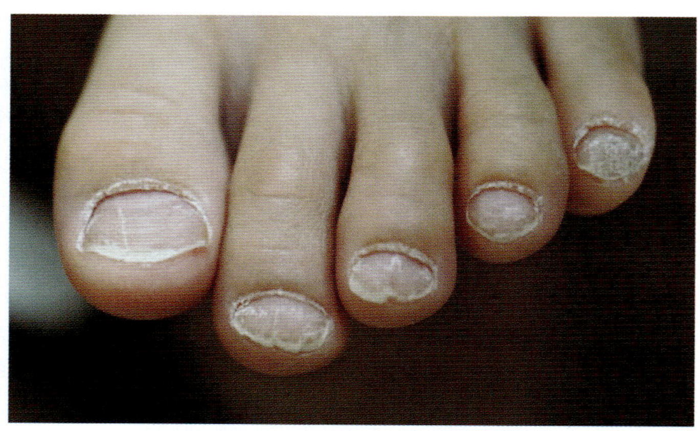

FIGURE 9-57. Nail dystrophy secondary to nail fold eczema in a Chinese boy.

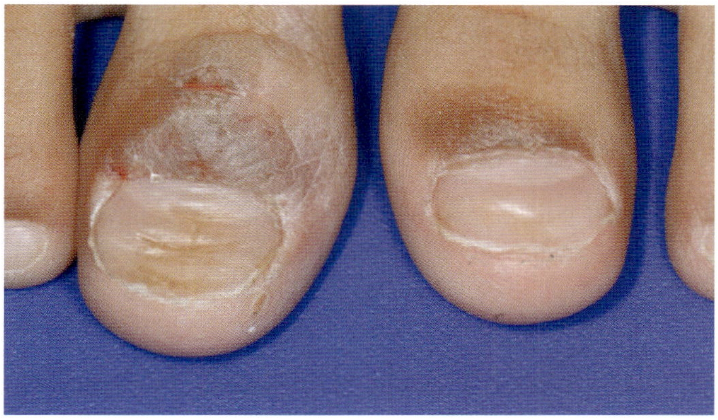

FIGURE 9-58. Nail fold eczema causing a central groove on both big toenails of a child with atopic dermatitis.

- Psoriasis
  - Psoriatic nail changes include pitting, onycholysis, subungual hyperkeratosis, and oil drop pigmentation. Nail pitting is usually deep and irregular. Chronic paronychia may also occur. Features of psoriasis are seen at other cutaneous sites.
- Alopecia areata nail changes
  - These include nail pitting and trachyonychia, which may be confused with eczema nails. The nail pitting in alopecia areata is more regular, shallower, and smaller than in eczema. Cutaneous features of eczema are not seen.

Investigations & Treatment

- Management involves optimizing treatment of the underlying skin and nail eczema. This includes patient education, avoidance of potential triggers, regular emollients, and potent topical corticosteroids or tacrolimus ointment.
- For more severe cases that do not respond to topical treatments, phototherapy (e.g., soak PUVA), systemic steroid-sparing immunosuppressants (e.g., azathioprine, methotrexate, ciclosporin), or newer biologics may be indicated.
- Antimicrobial therapy may be required if there is secondary infection.

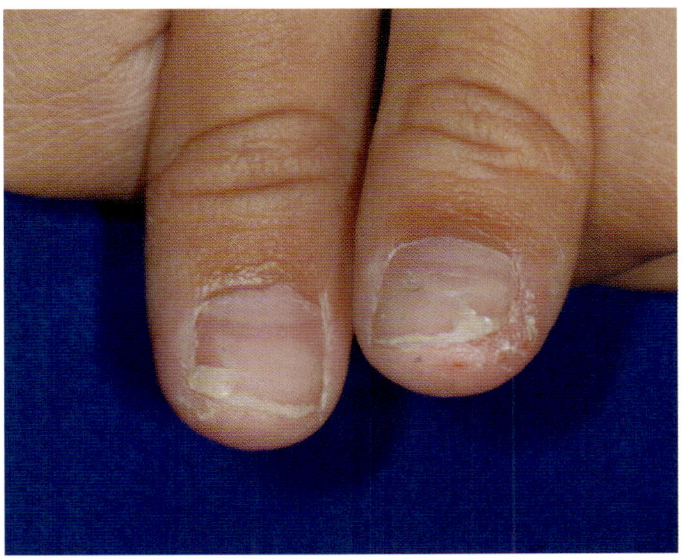

FIGURE 9-59. Nail dystrophy affecting the left thumb associated with eczema on the pulp and hyponychium.

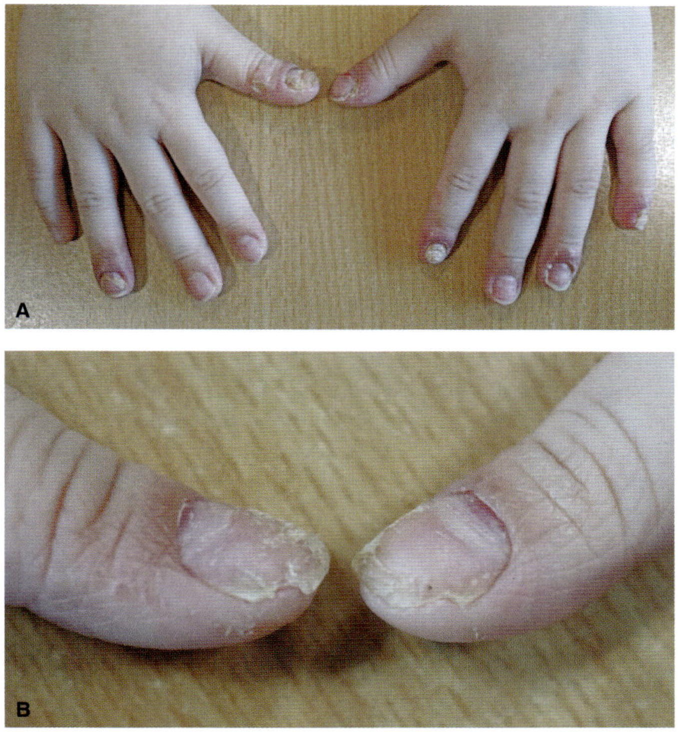

FIGURE 9-60A & 60B. Nail dystrophy associated with chronic eczema and paronychia in a young child with discoid eczema.

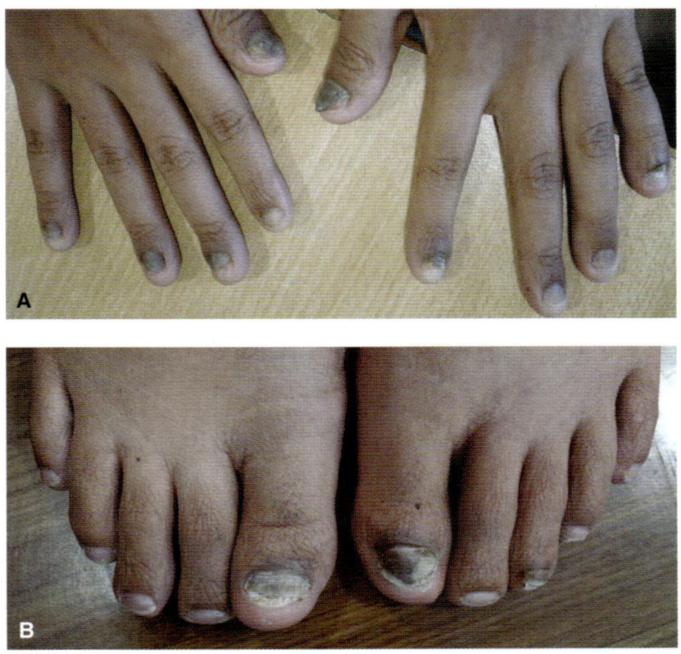

FIGURE 9-61A & 61B. Chronic nail changes, including discoloration, in a Malay teenager with chronic hands and feet eczema.

Pearls & Practical Tips

- Nail changes associated with eczema usually resolve when the underlying eczema is well controlled.
- Habitual picking of the nail unit can worsen the nail changes associated with eczema and should be adequately addressed.
- In cases of irritant contact dermatitis, patients may need to wear gloves if unable to avoid exposure to the underlying cause.

NAIL PSORIASIS

Nail involvement is common in psoriasis, although it is more common in adults compared to children with psoriasis. In some cases, nail changes may occur without cutaneous lesions for months or years, often leading to misdiagnosis. Nail involvement is strongly associated with psoriatic arthritis.

Clinical Features

- Typical clinical features of nail psoriasis include large and deep irregular pits, onycholysis with a distinct erythematous border, yellow-brown discoloration of the nail bed (known as "oil-drop" or salmon patch), and an erythematous border.
- Other less common and less specific nail changes include subungual hyperkeratosis, onychorrhexis (brittle nails), splinter hemorrhages, and chronic paronychia.
- Acrodermatitis continua of Hallopeau is a form of localized pustular psoriasis and is rare in children. It may occur as part of generalized pustular psoriasis (of von Zumbusch) or occur in isolation. Patients present with recurrent painful inflammation and sterile pustular eruptions around and under the nail plate, associated with marked paronychia.

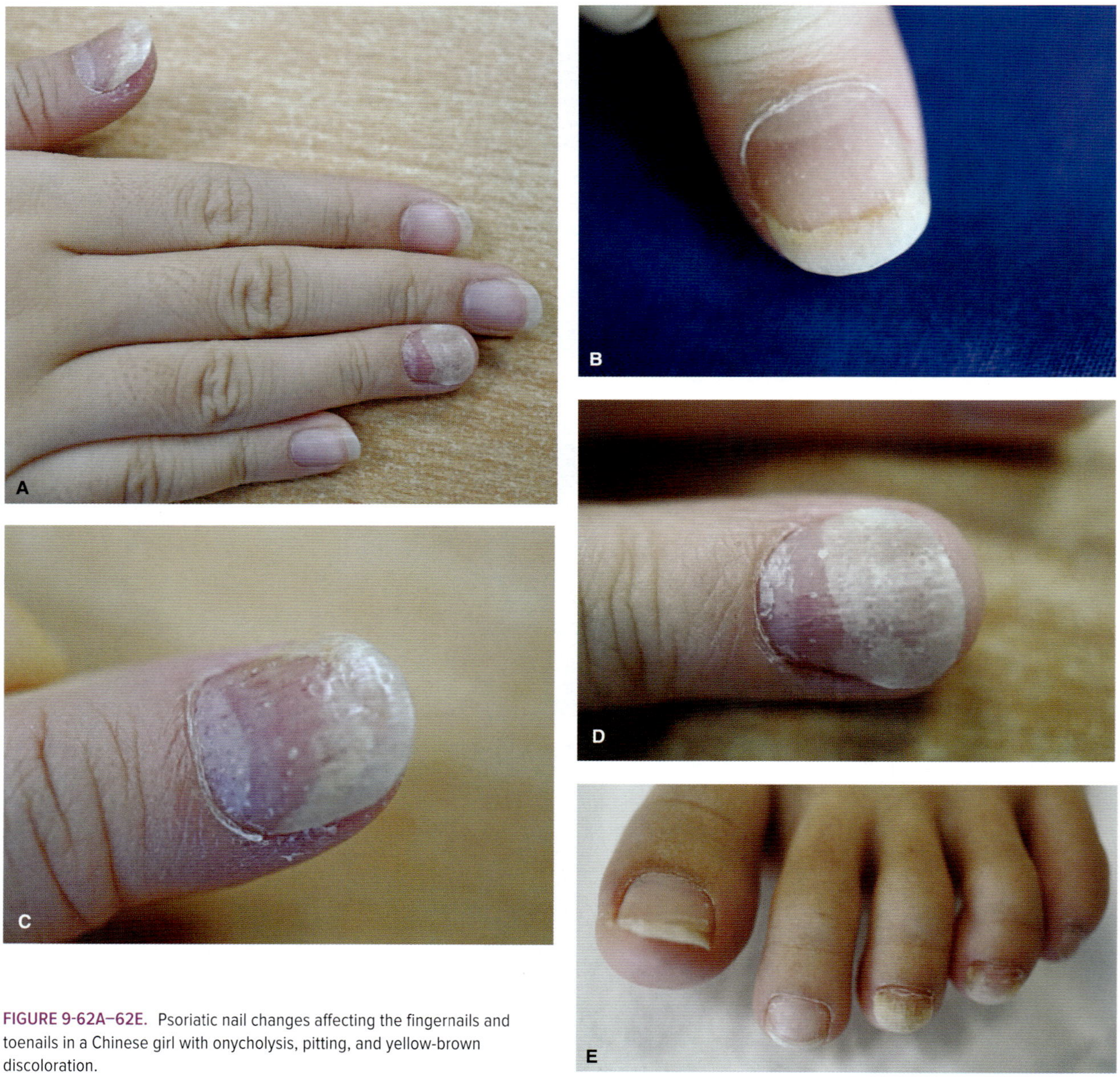

FIGURE 9-62A–62E. Psoriatic nail changes affecting the fingernails and toenails in a Chinese girl with onycholysis, pitting, and yellow-brown discoloration.

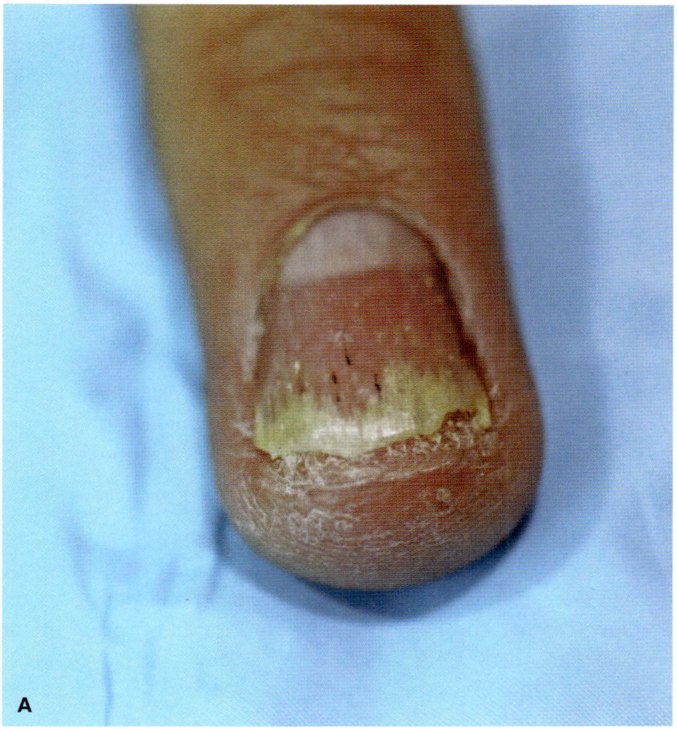

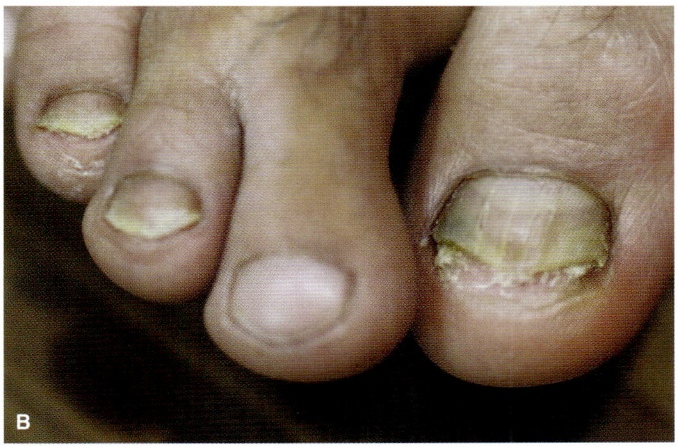

FIGURE 9-63A & 63B. Psoriatic nail changes affecting several fingernails and toenails of this Malay adolescent, presenting with features of onycholysis, pitting, splinter hemorrhages, brown discoloration, and subungual debris.

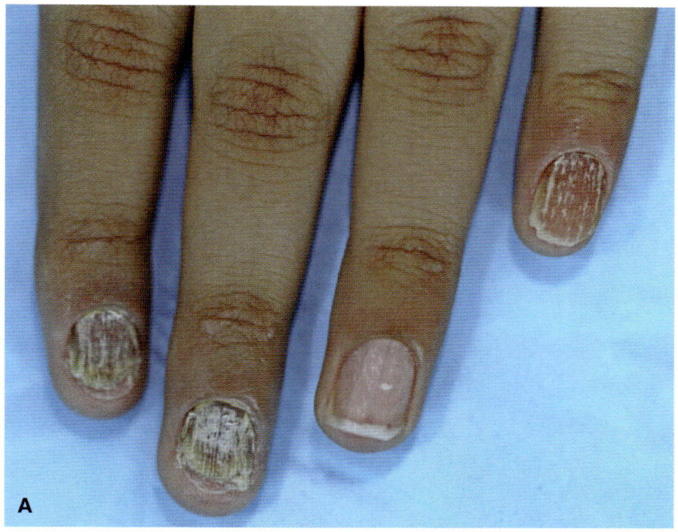

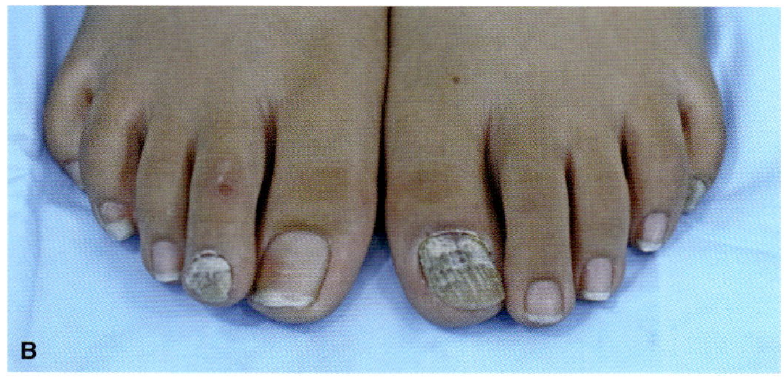

FIGURE 9-64A & 64B. Psoriatic nail changes affecting multiple fingernails and toenails of a Malay adolescent. There are features of onycholysis, pitting, trachyonychia, and crumbling. These cases can have a similar presentation to twenty-nail dystrophy in the early stages.

Differential Diagnoses

- Nail changes secondary to eczema or atopic dermatitis
  - Atopic dermatitis or eczema affecting the fingertips or nail folds may also lead to nail changes such as pitting and onycholysis.
- Onychomycosis
  - Fungal nail infections in children are rare and usually affect only one or two nails, unlike psoriasis, which affects multiple nails.
- Infective paronychia
  - Acute paronychia presents with swelling, induration, and pus in a nail fold. The history is usually short, and there may be a history of trauma. If chronic or recurrent, underlying dermatoses affecting the nail folds (e.g., eczema or psoriasis) needs to be excluded.

Investigations & Treatment

- Nail biopsies are not routinely performed but may aid in diagnosis if there are no associated cutaneous lesions. Histopathological findings include hyperkeratosis with parakeratosis, and neutrophilic infiltrates of the nail bed epithelium.
- Management of nail psoriasis is challenging. Topical or intralesional corticosteroids and topical vitamin D3 analogues can be used as first-line treatment, but response is usually suboptimal due to limited penetration into the nail matrix.
- Systemic treatment may be offered for psoriasis patients with both skin and nail disease, although it may not be recommended in patients with isolated nail involvement. Methotrexate is usually prescribed in patients with moderate to severe disease. Other medications include acitretin and cyclosporin. In recalcitrant cases, biologics (e.g., tumor necrosis factor alpha inhibitors or IL-17 inhibitors) may be indicated.

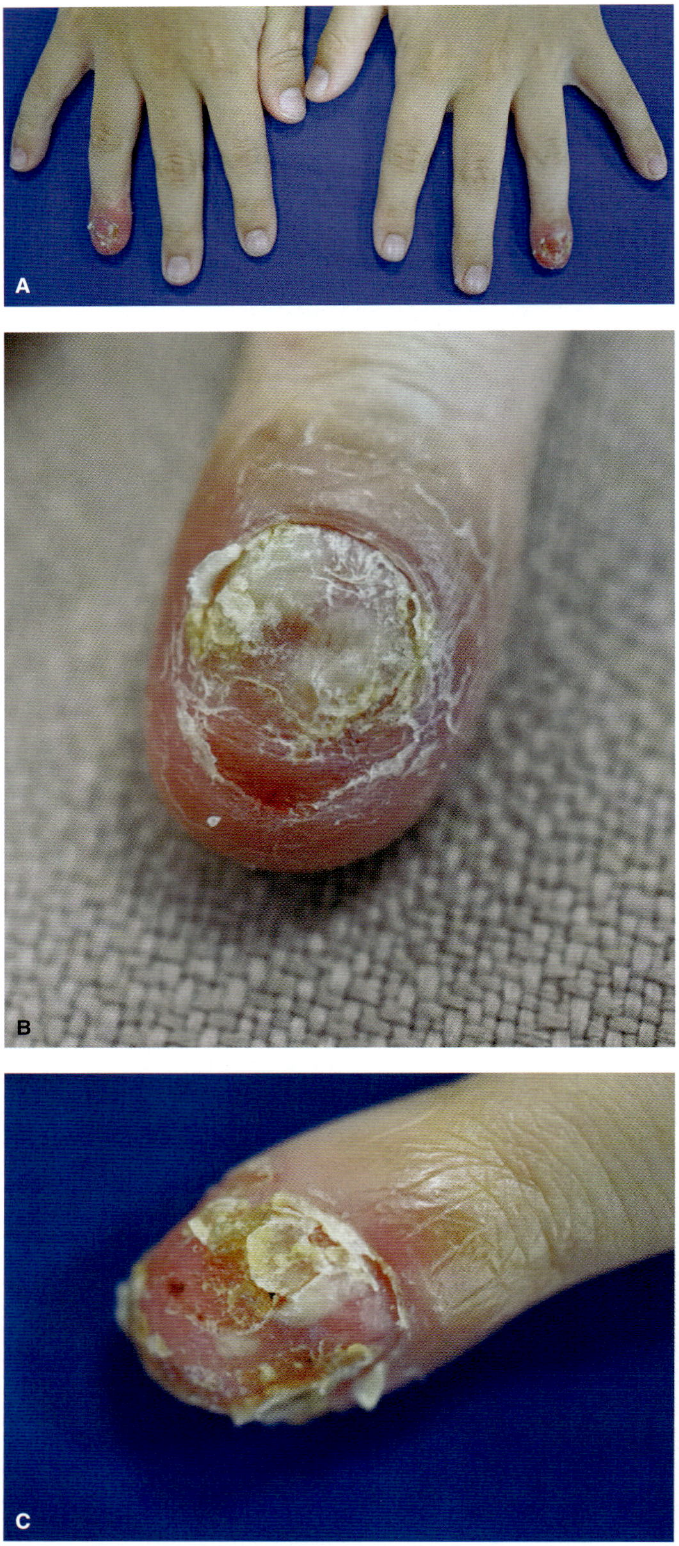

FIGURE 9-65A–65C. Pustular nail psoriasis at various stages with features of paronychia, lakes of pus, and thick crusts with total loss of nail, occurring in a Chinese boy.

Pearls & Practical Tips

- A dermatoscope may be helpful to facilitate identification of specific nail abnormalities. For example, it may help with visualization of an erythematous border in patients with psoriasis.
- Onycholysis may be concealed with nail varnish. Keeping nails short also prevents worsening of onycholysis.
- Nail manipulation should be avoided, as this may result in koebnerization and worsening of the nail abnormalities.

Bibliography

1. Smith RJ, Rubin AI. Pediatric nail disorders: a review. Curr Opin Pediatr 2020;32(4):506-15.
2. Pourchot D, Bodemer C, Phan A, Bursztejn AC, Hadj-Rabia S, Boralevi F, et al. Nail psoriasis: a systematic evaluation in 313 children with psoriasis. Pediatr Dermatol 2017;34(1):58-63.

NAIL LICHEN PLANUS

Lichen planus is a chronic inflammatory condition that can affect the skin, nails, scalp, and mucosa. Nail lichen planus can occur in isolation without other cutaneous manifestations. Permanent scarring and loss of nails can occur, and prompt intervention is important.

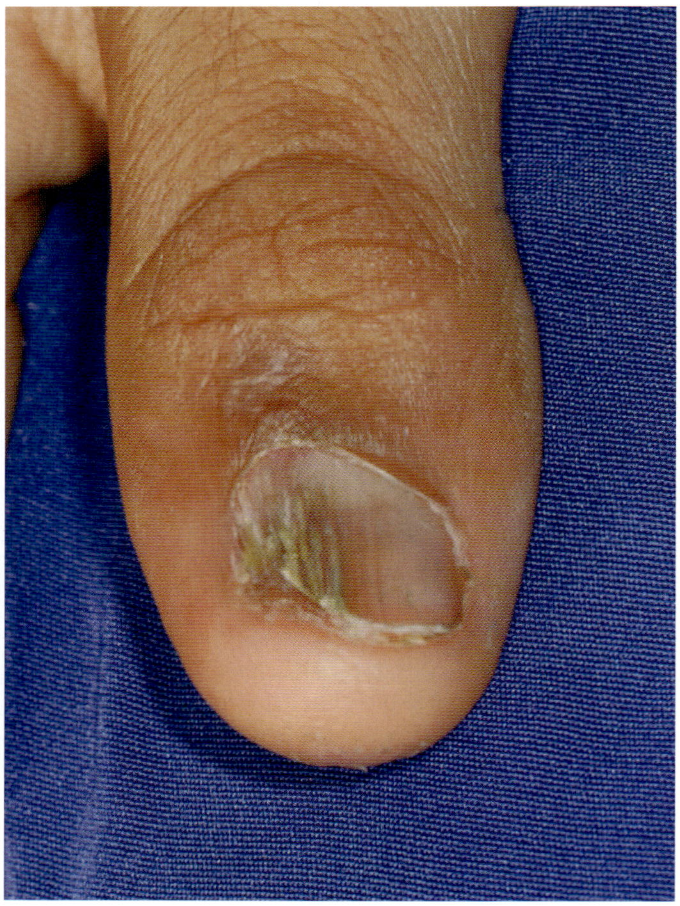

FIGURE 9-66. Lichen planus affecting just the thumb in this Indian male with lichen planus. There is longitudinal ridging and early pterygium formation at the proximal nail fold.

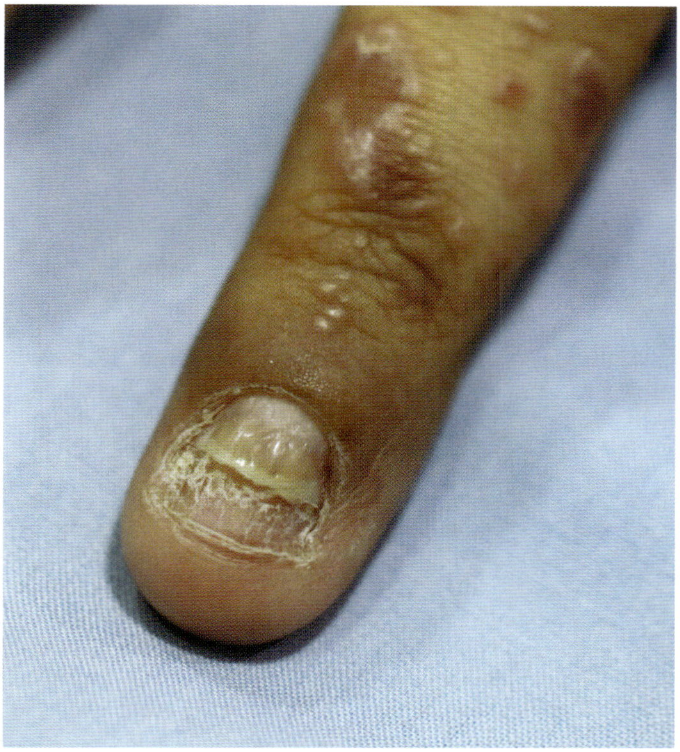

FIGURE 9-67. Lichen planus affecting the finger and nail of this Malay child.

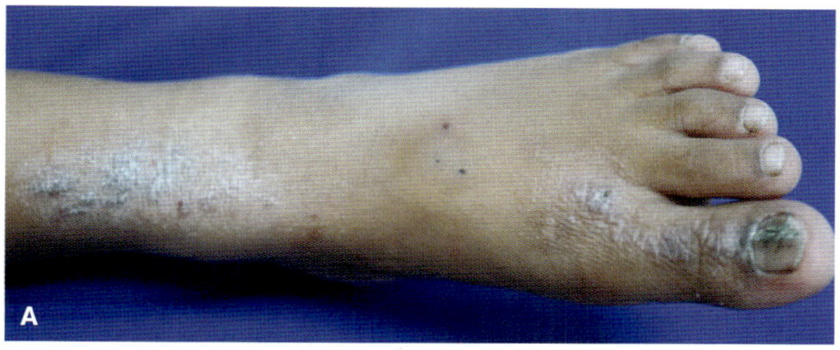

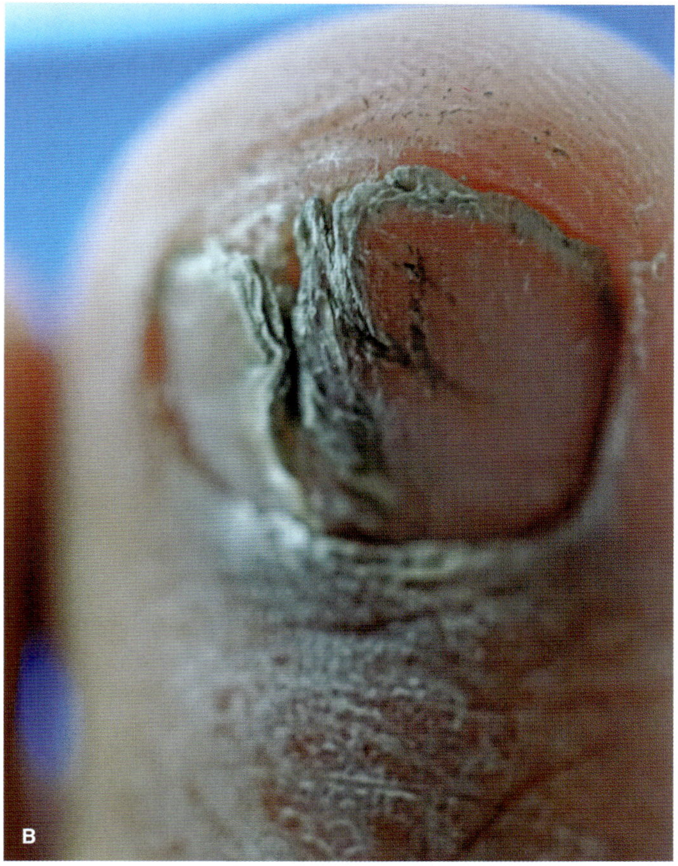

FIGURE 9-68A & 68B. Linear lichen planus on the leg of this Indian girl associated with nail ridging.

Clinical Features

- Although usually affecting isolated nails, all nails may potentially be affected.
- Typical features include nail thinning, longitudinal ridging and fissuring, and dorsal pterygium formation. Other nonspecific signs include onycholysis, nail thickening, and discoloration.
- In addition to typical nail lichen planus, other presentations of nail lichen planus in children include twenty-nail dystrophy and idiopathic nail atrophy. The latter occurs fairly acutely, resulting in painless nail destruction and scarring. The nail eventually stops growing and disappears, resulting in anonychia.

Differential Diagnoses

- Lichen striatus
  - Lichen striatus can also involve nails, in addition to the cutaneous findings. Clinical signs include longitudinal ridging over the medial or lateral aspect of a single nail. Unlike lichen planus, it is usually self-limiting, and scarring is uncommon.
- Twenty-nail dystrophy
  - Rare cases of twenty-nail dystrophy may be associated with lichen planus. Examination for cutaneous and mucosal lichen planus may help to differentiate from isolated twenty-nail dystrophy.
- Nail psoriasis
  - Nail psoriasis presents with pitting, onycholysis, and oil-drop discoloration, which differentiates it from nail lichen planus.

Investigations & Treatment

- A biopsy may be performed to confirm the diagnosis. Typical histopathological features include a band-like lymphocytic infiltrate at the dermal–epidermal junction of the nail matrix and nail bed. Other findings include hyperkeratosis, hypergranulosis, and acanthosis of the nail matrix epithelium.
- Treatment depends on the extent of disease. If only a few nails are affected, topical or intralesional steroids may be administered. Systemic corticosteroids may be indicated if there are multiple nails involved, or to prevent pterygium formation and permanent nail scarring. In more severe cases, other systemic treatments such as retinoids, antimalarials, and methotrexate may be required.
- In cases with significant nail atrophy, systemic steroids are ineffective, as scarring has already occurred.

Pearls & Practical Tips

- A thorough examination of the skin surfaces, scalp, and mucosa (oral, genitalia) should be performed if nail lichen planus is suspected. Sometimes isolated nail lichen planus may be the only manifestation for years before the appearance of other skin or mucosal signs.
- Lichen striatus should be considered as a differential diagnosis if only one or two digits are involved.
- Twenty-nail dystrophy usually spontaneously resolves over time and without treatment.

Bibliography

1. Smith RJ, Rubin AI. Pediatric nail disorders: a review. Curr Opin Pediatr 2020;32(4):506-15.

PARONYCHIA

Paronychia refers to soft tissue inflammation around a nail, affecting the proximal and/or lateral nail folds. It can be acute, lasting for less than 6 weeks, or chronic if persistent for more than 6 weeks.

Clinical Features

- Acute paronychia
  - This usually occurs when there is trauma to the cuticle or proximal nail fold, resulting in inoculation of infective pathogens.
  - The most common infective agents are bacteria such as *Staphylococcus aureus* and *Streptococcus pyogenes*, and viruses like herpes simplex virus, causing herpetic whitlow.
  - It usually affects one nail fold, which becomes tender, erythematous, and indurated, with pus under the cuticle and occasional blistering. In herpetic whitlow, there may be multiple tender vesicles.
  - In severe cases, the infection may progress and result in abscess formation, cellulitis, and tendonitis.
- Chronic paronychia
  - This occurs gradually and often involves multiple digits. It usually starts in the proximal nail fold and progresses laterally.

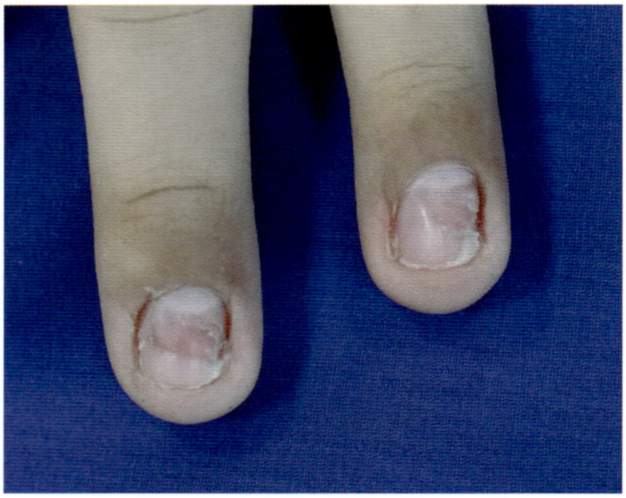

FIGURE 9-69. Chronic paronychia affecting the lateral and proximal nail folds of both fingers shown here. There is associated nail dystrophy.

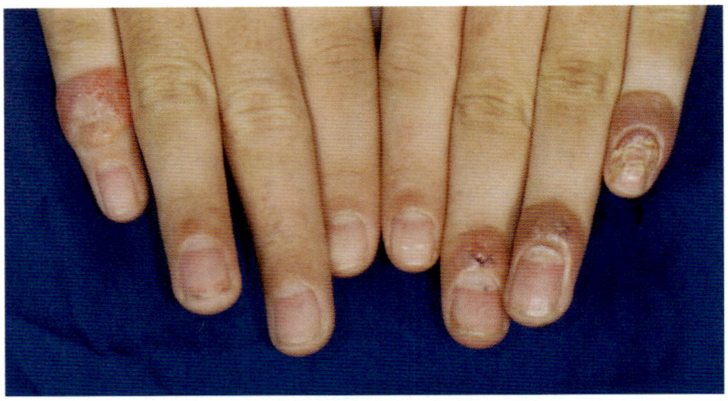

FIGURE 9-70. Paronychia affecting several fingers on the left hand of this Chinese adolescent male with discoid eczema. A classical discoid lesion is seen on the little finger of his right hand. There are secondary nail changes from the paronychia, especially affecting the little finger of the left hand.

  - Patients usually have hand dermatitis, which may be endogenous, exogenous, or both. It is associated with chronic infection with *Pseudomonas aeruginosa* or *Candida*.
  - Clinically, the affected skin is erythematous and tender, and there may be small collections of pus under the cuticle. The nail plate is often thickened and distorted, with transverse ridges.

Differential Diagnoses

- Periungual warts
  - Caused by human papillomavirus, these that appear as periungual keratotic, verrucous papules that often extend onto the contiguous nail folds.

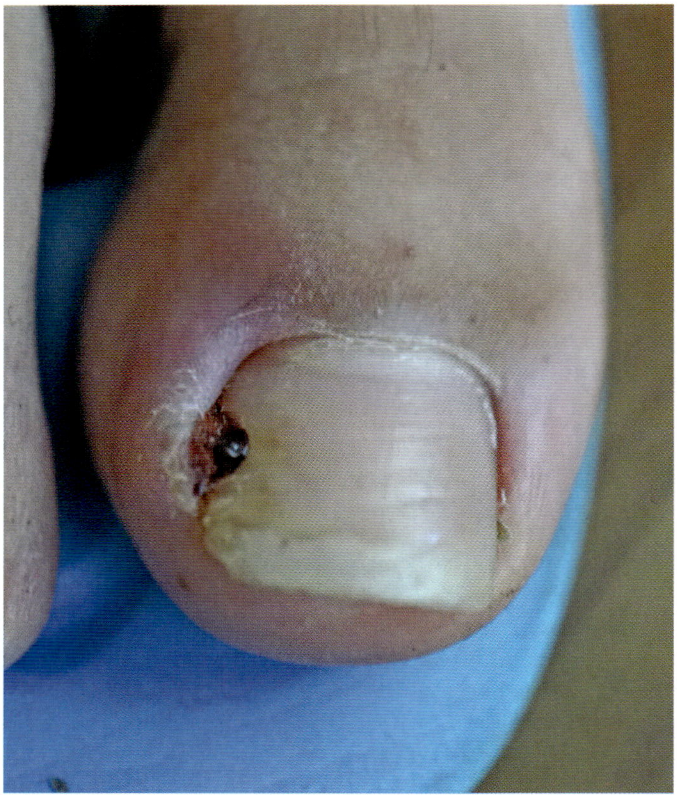

FIGURE 9-71. Paronychia associated with an ingrown toenail.

- Contact dermatitis (allergic/irritant)
  - Contact dermatitis of the nail folds may occur following exposure to chemicals, such as detergents and nail polish. It presents as nail fold erythema and inflammation.
- Felon
  - This represents a compartmentalized infection of the fingertip, resulting in erythema, swelling, and severe tenderness. Unlike paronychia, this involves the pulp of the fingertip and not the nail folds.

Investigations & Treatment

- The diagnosis of paronychia is made clinically. Supportive microbiological investigations may be performed to identify any underlying infective pathogen.
- Management of acute paronychia involves warm water soaks, topical antiseptics, and in more severe cases, oral antibiotics. Surgical incision and drainage may be required if there is abscess formation. Herpetic whitlow can be treated with oral acyclovir.
- Chronic paronychia requires management of underlying triggers. This includes good hand hygiene, keeping hands dry and warm, and management of hand dermatitis with emollients and topical corticosteroids. Antiseptic solutions and topical or oral antifungal medication may be required if secondarily infected.

Pearls & Practical Tips

- Acute paronychia usually resolves completely over a few days and seldom recurs in healthy patients.
- Predisposing factors such as onychophagia, thumb sucking, habitual nail fold picking, and ingrown toenails may result in recurrent paronychia. Thumb sucking often results in candidal paronychia.
- Paronychia may be seen with other dermatological conditions such as psoriasis and eczema affecting the nail folds. Paronychia affecting the big toe may be associated with ingrown toenails, which should be addressed.

STRUCTURAL NAIL DISORDERS

Structural nail deformities are uncommon in children but may lead to pain and functional difficulties. Pincer nail deformity predominantly affects the hallux toenails. Other nail deformities are koilonychia, brachyonychia, congenital malalignment of great toenails, and ingrown toenails.

Clinical Features

- Pincer nail deformity
  - This presents as nail thickening with increased transverse curvature along the longitudinal nail axis with narrowing of the distal end of the nail bed. This deformity may result in pain, recurrent infections, and chronic inflammation.
  - The condition may be hereditary or acquired. Acquired cases are associated with poorly fitting shoes, systemic diseases (e.g., Kawasaki disease, systemic lupus erythematosus, renal failure), onychomycosis, nail tumors, and recurrent trauma.

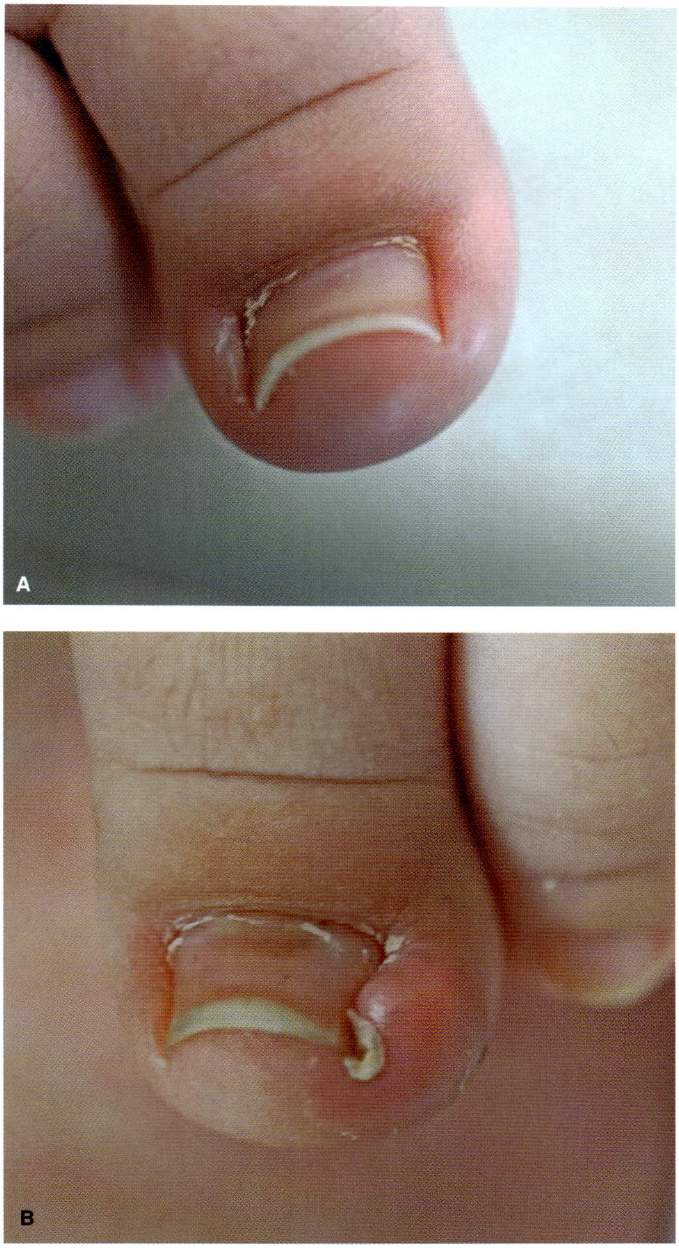

FIGURE 9-72A & 72B. Pincer nail deformity affecting bilateral big toes of this toddler, with secondary paronychia affecting the left big toe.

  - Hereditary pincer nails are usually symmetrical, whereas acquired cases tend to be asymmetrical.
- Koilonychia
  - Nails are "spoon-shaped" in appearance, as the free edges of the nails are everted.
  - The condition may be physiological in young children, as nails are soft and thin, and will spontaneously resolve with time when the nail plate thickens.
  - Koilonychia can be associated with iron deficiency anemia, connective tissue disease, and thyroid disorders. In these cases, further investigations and management of the underlying cause is required.

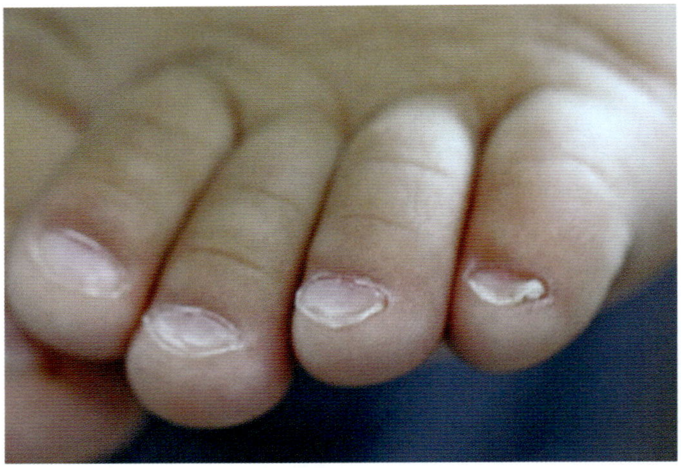

FIGURE 9-73. Koilonychia of the toenails in a Chinese toddler.

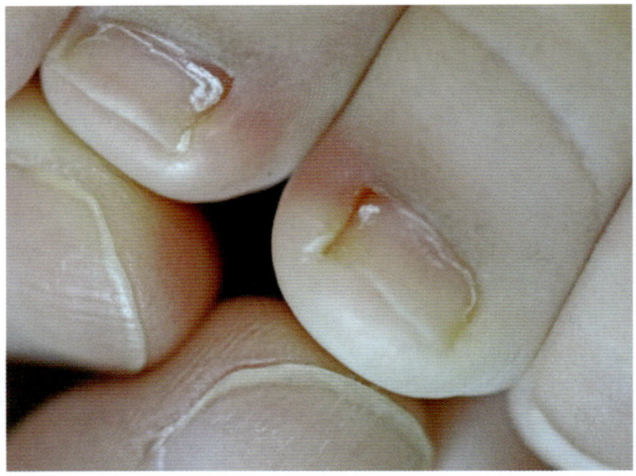

FIGURE 9-75. Ingrown toenails affecting both big toes of this toddler with associated mild paronychia.

- Brachyonychia
  - Also known as racquet thumb, brachyonychia is a fairly common malformation. The distal phalanx and thumbnails are abnormally short and wide.
  - It is an autosomal dominant condition, and patients are otherwise well. No further intervention is required. Rarely, it may be associated with genetic syndromes such as Rubinstein-Taybi syndrome.
- Congenital malalignment of great toenails
  - This condition is due to abnormalities in the ligament connecting the nail matrix to the periosteum, resulting in lateral deviation of the nail plates.
  - In cases with marked deviation, toenails may be deformed, with nail thickening, ridging, and brown discoloration. There is also an increased risk of developing ingrown toenails.
  - While spontaneous improvement may occur, surgical correction may be indicated in persistent, severe, or complicated cases.
- Ingrown toenails
  - Ingrown toenails are common in adolescents but can also be seen in children. The condition occurs due to the nail plate growing into the lateral nail folds and acting as a foreign body to induce inflammation. The great toenail is most commonly affected.
  - Predisposing factors include tight-fitting footwear, persistent trauma, and incorrect nail trimming techniques.

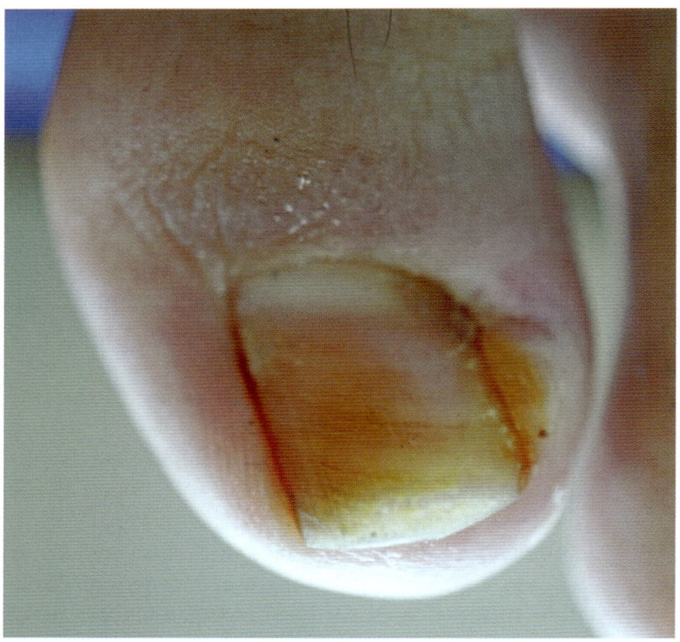

FIGURE 9-74. Congenital malalignment of great toenail associated with paronychia in an adolescent.

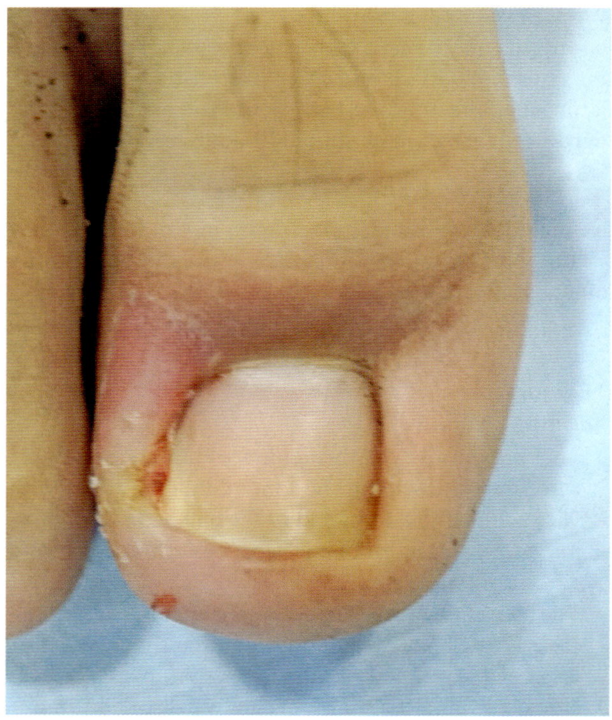

FIGURE 9-76. Ingrown toenail affecting the big toe of this Chinese boy with accompanying paronychia.

Investigations & Treatment

These nail deformities are mostly diagnosed clinically. Sometimes radiographic images may be required to exclude abnormalities of the underlying phalangeal bone.

- Pincer nails
  - Management can be conservative or surgical.
  - Conservative methods include nail grinding to increase the nail width and decrease its height, and use of various devices to correct the nail curvature.
  - Surgical intervention involves either laser surgery or surgical excision with reconstruction. The nail matrix may be preserved in some of these surgical techniques.
- Ingrown toenails
  - Management can be conservative or surgical.
  - Conservative treatment includes soaks with an antiseptic solution (e.g., potassium permanganate) and application of topical antibiotic ointments with or without topical corticosteroids. Avoidance of tight-fitting footwear is advised, and nails should be clipped so that the distal corners are visible beyond the nail folds.
  - Surgical treatments include nail avulsion with or without destruction of the nail matrix (e.g., phenol application or wedge resection) or surgical excision of the affected nail matrix.

Bibliography

1. Smith RJ, Rubin AI. Pediatric nail disorders: a review. Curr Opin Pediatr 2020;32(4):506-15.

MELANONYCHIA

Melanonychia refers to brown-black pigmentation of the nail plate due to melanin. Longitudinal melanonychia, also known as melanonychia striata, is the most common morphological type, and is very common in patients of Asian descent, especially those with darker skin types.

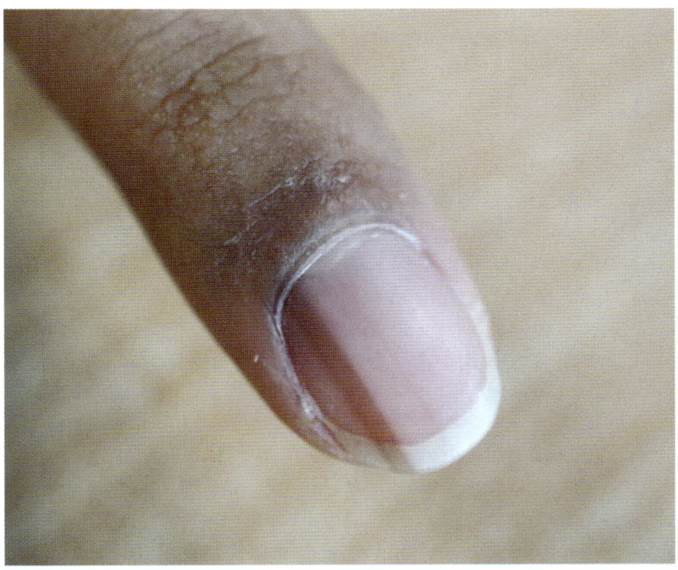

FIGURE 9-77. Longitudinal melanonychia in a Nepalese boy presenting as a uniform, light-brown band with parallel edges and uniform color.

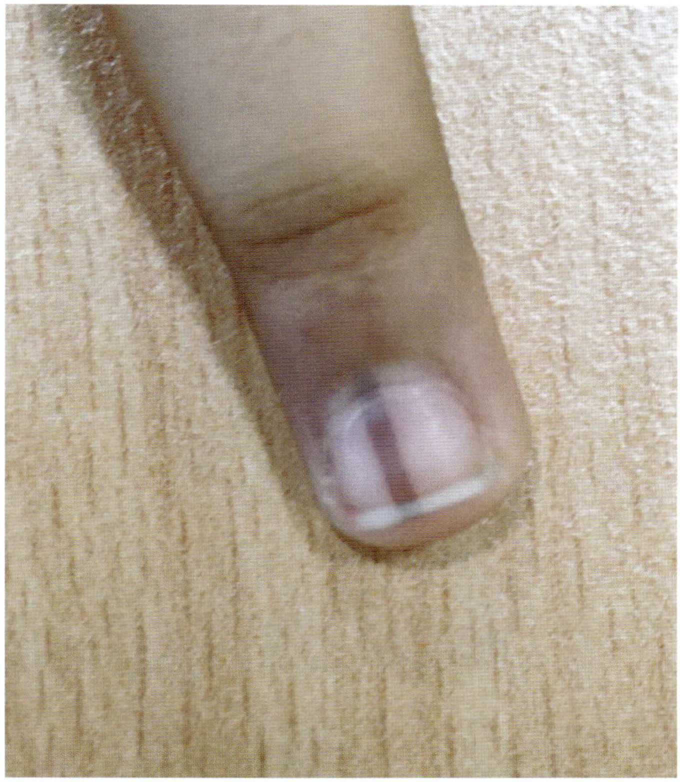

FIGURE 9-78. Longitudinal melanonychia in a Nepalese girl presenting as a uniform, medium-brown longitudinal band, with pseudo-Hutchinson sign.

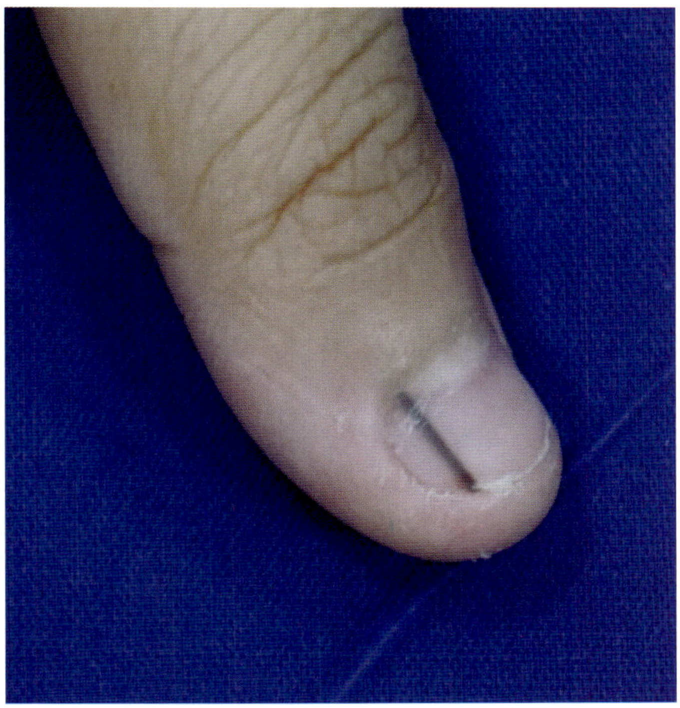

FIGURE 9-79. Longitudinal melanonychia on the thumb of a Chinese girl due to a nail matrix nevus. Note the dark brown color of the band and the presence of pseudo-Hutchinson sign under the thin cuticle at the proximal nail fold.

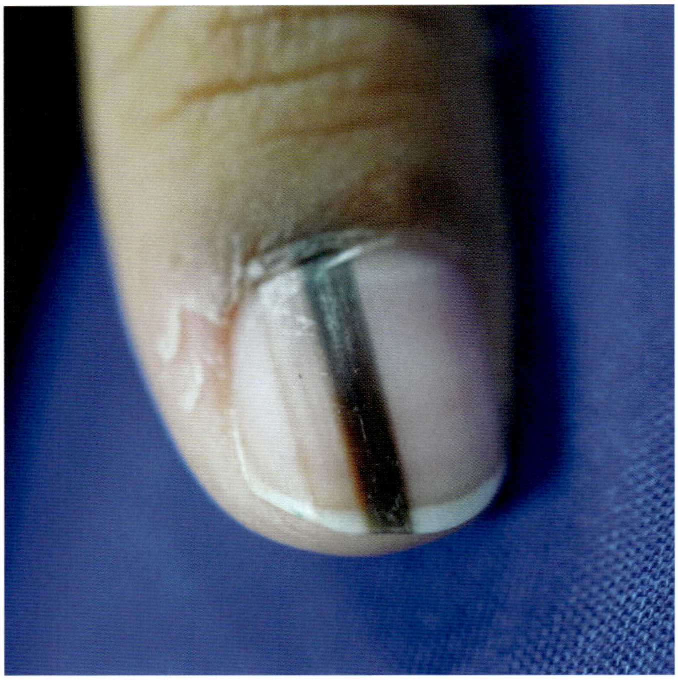

FIGURE 9-80. Longitudinal melanonychia in an Indian boy due to a nail matrix nevus. Note the dark color with some irregularity of pigmentation.

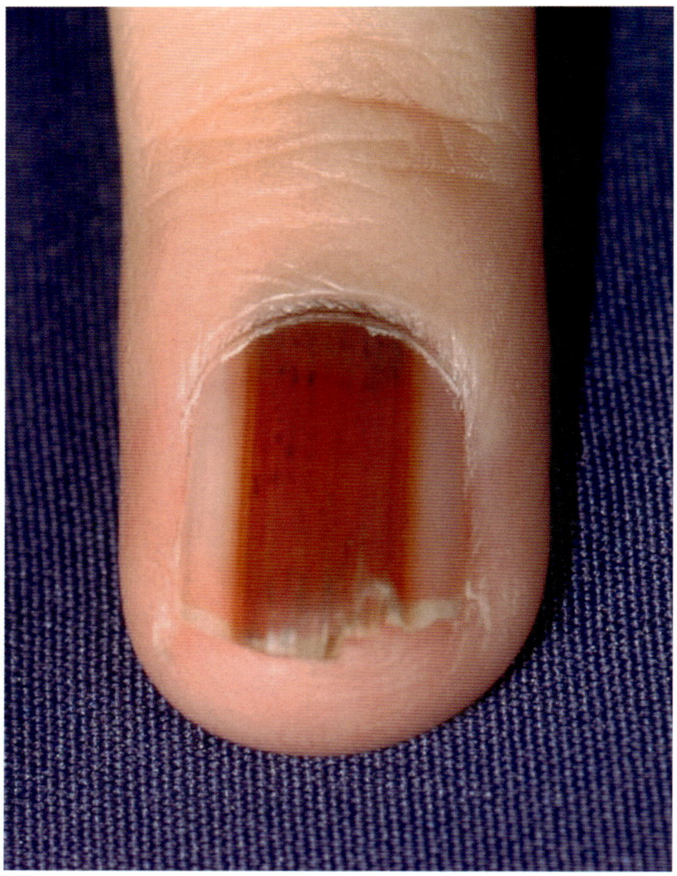

FIGURE 9-81. Longitudinal melanonychia secondary to a compound melanocytic nevus with atypical features affecting the nail matrix in this young Chinese girl. Note the irregular pigmentation and pseudo-Hutchinson sign. The lesion was removed but recurred.

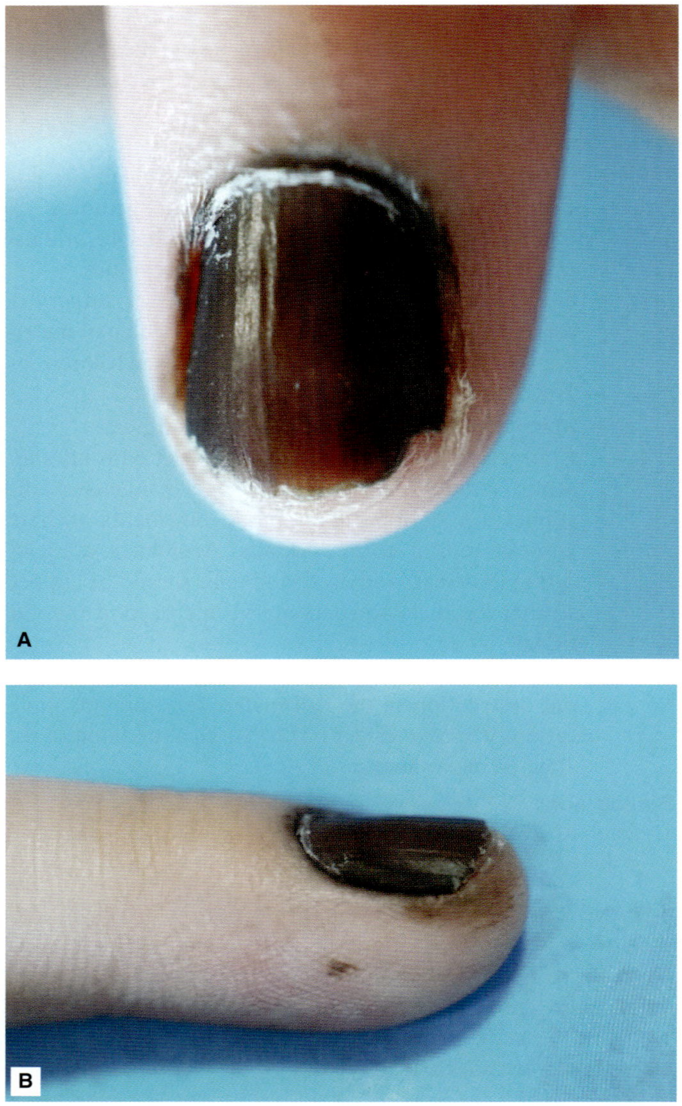

FIGURE 9-82A & 82B. An extremely rare case of melanoma-in-situ occurring in a young Chinese boy that presented with total melanonychia. Hutchinson sign is positive with extension of pigmentation onto the nail folds as well as the finger pulp.

Clinical Features

- Melanonychia occurs as a result of either melanocyte activation or melanocyte hyperplasia, which can be benign or malignant.
- Causes of melanocyte activation include physiological (e.g., racial), trauma, infections (e.g., HIV), inflammatory or systemic disorders, endocrinopathies (e.g., Addison disease), nutritional deficiencies (e.g., B12, folate) and drugs (e.g., chemotherapy, antimalarial medications).
- Melanonychia can be divided into three morphological subtypes: longitudinal melanonychia, diffuse melanonychia, and transverse melanonychia.
- Melanonychia striata presents as a linear pigmented band over the nail. Causes include melanocyte activation, lentigo, melanocytic nevus, and melanoma of the nail matrix.

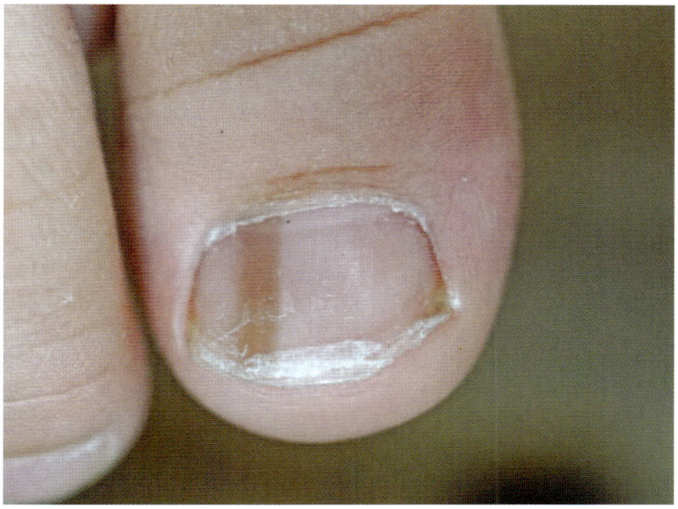

FIGURE 9-83. Longitudinal melanonychia affecting the big toe of a young Chinese boy presenting with a light-brown band.

In children, the majority of cases of melanonychia striata are benign. Nail matrix melanoma is extremely rare in children, especially in Asian races.

- Clinically, melanonychia caused by benign melanocytic lesions have a uniform brown or dark brown pigmentation and are usually less than 3 mm in width. The edges of the band are usually uniform, with the width at the base similar to the width at the free edge.

Differential Diagnoses

- Subungual hematoma
  - This develops following traumatic bleeding under the nail plate, and most commonly affects the toenails.

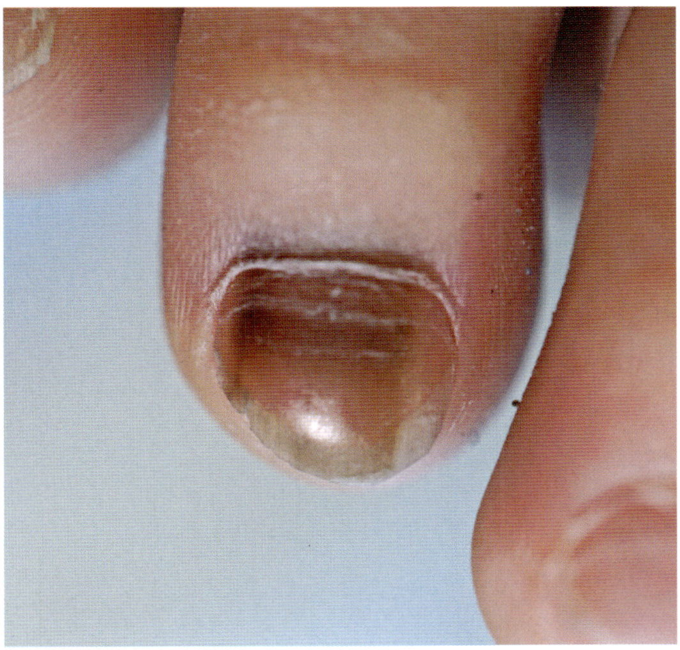

FIGURE 9-84. Near-total melanonychia affecting the fourth toe of a young Chinese boy caused by a nail bed melanocytic nevus. Pseudo-Hutchinson sign may be appreciated.

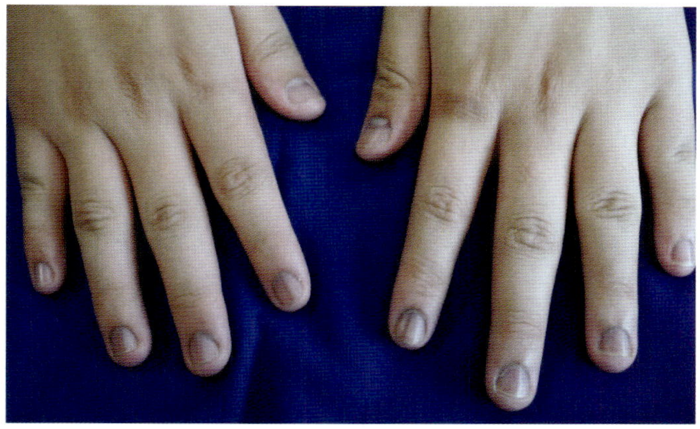

FIGURE 9-85. Frequent nail biting can lead to multiple grayish-brown "melanonychia," as seen in this Chinese adolescent.

It is usually dark red or purple in color initially and becomes brown or black with time. There may be nail plate dystrophy if the hematoma compresses on the nail matrix.

  - Unlike melanonychia, subungual hematomas grow out at the same rate as the nail growth.
- Splinter hemorrhages
  - Damage to the nail bed capillaries results in thin longitudinal red-brown streaks, which are mainly located at the distal part of the nail.
  - Causes of splinter hemorrhages include trauma, psoriasis, infective endocarditis, autoimmune disease, and vasculitis.
- Pseudomonas nail infection
  - *Pseudomonas aeruginosa* infection of the nail plate causes excretion of pyocyanin pigment, resulting in green-black nail discoloration.
  - Causes include constant exposure to water and mechanical trauma. This is rare in children but may occur in immunosuppressed individuals.

Investigations & Treatment

- When examining a patient with nail pigmentation, a dermatoscope is helpful to differentiate between melanin and non-melanin pigmentation, and to distinguish between benign and malignant melanocytic lesions. Typical features suggestive of melanin pigmentation include brown-black pigmentation within the nail plate and a longitudinal appearance.
- A full-thickness nail matrix biopsy should be performed if there is suspicion of malignancy. Although punch biopsies are easier to perform, they frequently do not provide enough tissue for diagnosis. An incisional biopsy after nail avulsion and reflection of the proximal nail fold is recommended for better tissue sampling.
- If malignant melanoma is confirmed, the Breslow thickness should be assessed, and the primary tumor needs to be completely excised with adequate margins.
- In benign causes of melanonychia, no active treatment is required. The patient may be followed up to monitor for changes in clinical appearance.

Pearls & Practical Tips

- When viewed under a dermatoscope, the presence of globules of different sizes and colors is suggestive of a subungual hematoma. However, presence of subungual hemorrhage does not exclude a melanoma.
- Hutchinson sign is an important feature of nail melanoma. It refers to extension of pigmentation to involve the periungual skin. Other features of nail melanoma include widening of the proximal end of the pigmented band, irregular pigmentation, nail dystrophy, nodule formation, and ulceration.
- Pseudo-Hutchinson sign refers to pigmentation present under the cuticle, and is commonly seen in children presenting with melanonychia due to the thinness of the cuticle. This sign is indicative of a benign cause of the melanonychia.
- A nail matrix biopsy can cause nail scarring and deformity. It should be performed only if indicated, and patients and families should be counseled on the potential complications.

Bibliography

1. Smith RJ, Rubin AI. Pediatric nail disorders: a review. Curr Opin Pediatr 2020;32(4):506-15.
2. Colin Tan W, Wang DY, Seghers AC, Koh MJA, Nicholas Goh SG, Joyce Lee SS. Should we biopsy melanonychia striata in Asian children? A retrospective observational study. Pediatr Dermatol 2019;36(6):864-8.

10

Histiocytoses and Other Cutaneous Immune Cell Proliferations

HISTIOCYTOSES

The histiocytoses represent a group of disorders characterized by the abnormal proliferation of histiocytes, such as macrophages, dendritic cells, or monocyte-derived cells, in various tissues and organs. The clinical presentation and histological features of histiocytoses vary widely. Based on clinical, radiographic, pathological, phenotypic, genetic, and molecular features, the histiocytoses are now classified under five broad groups: (1) Langerhans-related (L-group), (2) cutaneous and mucocutaneous (C group), (3) malignant histiocytoses (M group), (4) Rosai-Dorfman disease (R group), and (5) hemophagocytic lymphohistiocytosis and macrophage activation syndrome (H group). They have different prognosis and treatment strategies. Only conditions in the L-group and C-group will be discussed in this textbook, as they commonly present with cutaneous lesions in the pediatric age group.

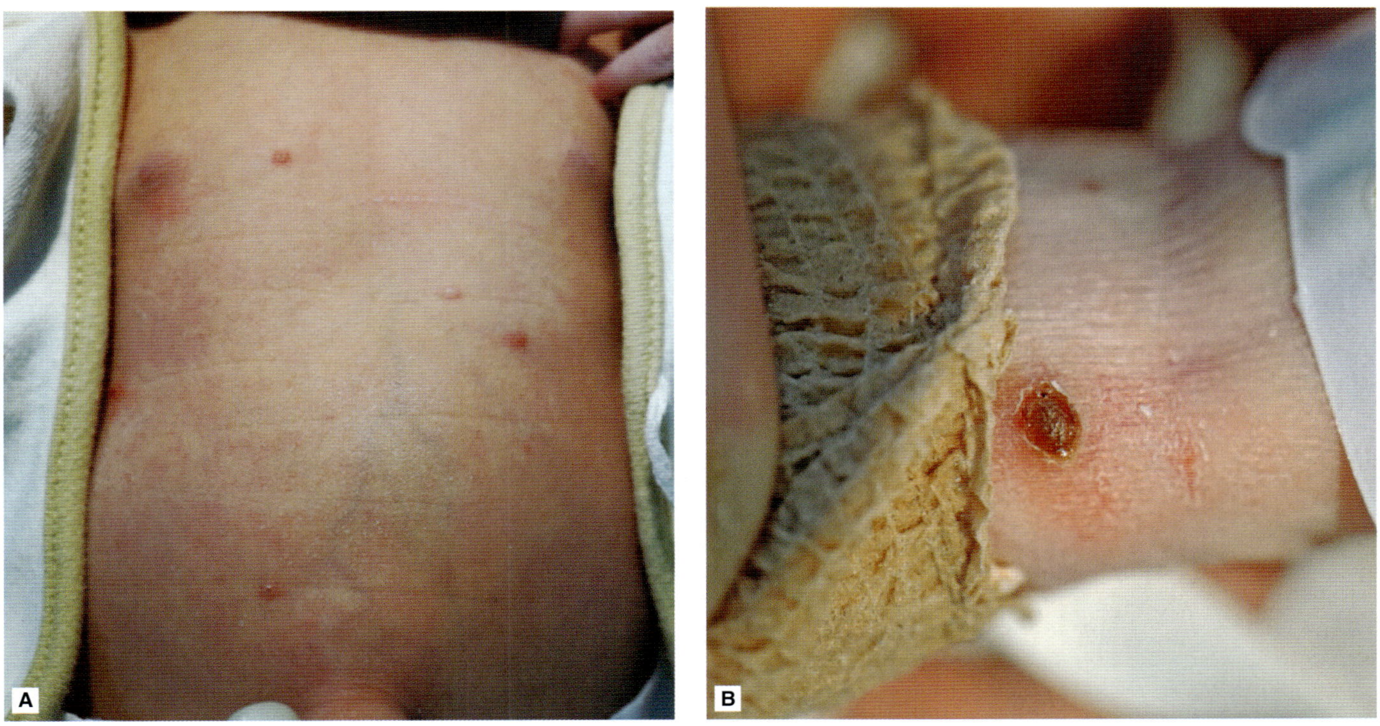

FIGURE 10-1A & 1B. Self-healing reticulohistiocytosis or neonatal LCH presenting in a newborn with scattered discrete, crusted, hemorrhagic papules on the face, trunk, and limbs. The lesions resolved after a few months.

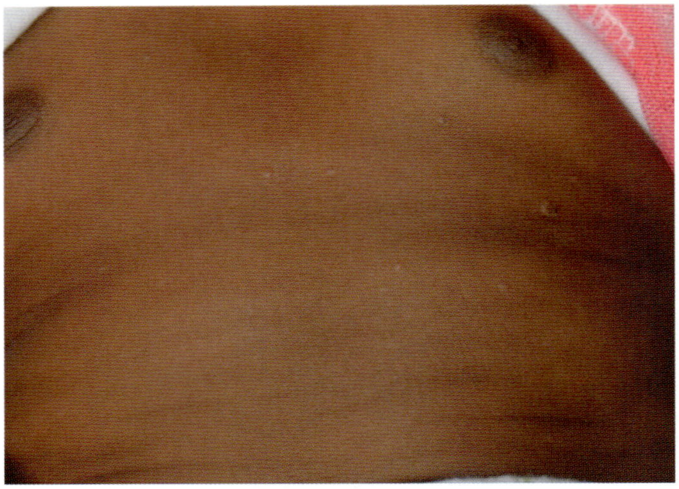

FIGURE 10-2. Self-healing reticulohistiocytosis in an Indian neonate presenting with scattered, discrete, skin-colored, and hypopigmented macules and papules on the trunk.

LANGERHANS CELL HISTIOCYTOSIS

Langerhans cell histiocytosis (LCH) is a rare disorder. It is more common in children compared to adults, presenting usually in the first few years of life. The exact pathophysiology of LCH is not well understood, but mutations in the proto-oncogene *BRAF*, especially the common V600E mutation, have shown to result in hyperactivation of the RAS-RAF-MEK kinase pathway. Mutations in *MAP2K1* have also been found.

Clinical Features

- LCH most commonly presents in infancy or early childhood.
- Clinical manifestations vary widely, from self-healing single-system involvement to life-threatening disseminated disease involving multiple organ systems. The skin and bones are the most commonly affected sites.
- Cutaneous LCH lesions usually occur on intertriginous and "seborrheic" sites, such as the scalp, face, neck, upper trunk and back, axillae, and groin. Other common sites include the palms and soles, nails, and oral mucosa.

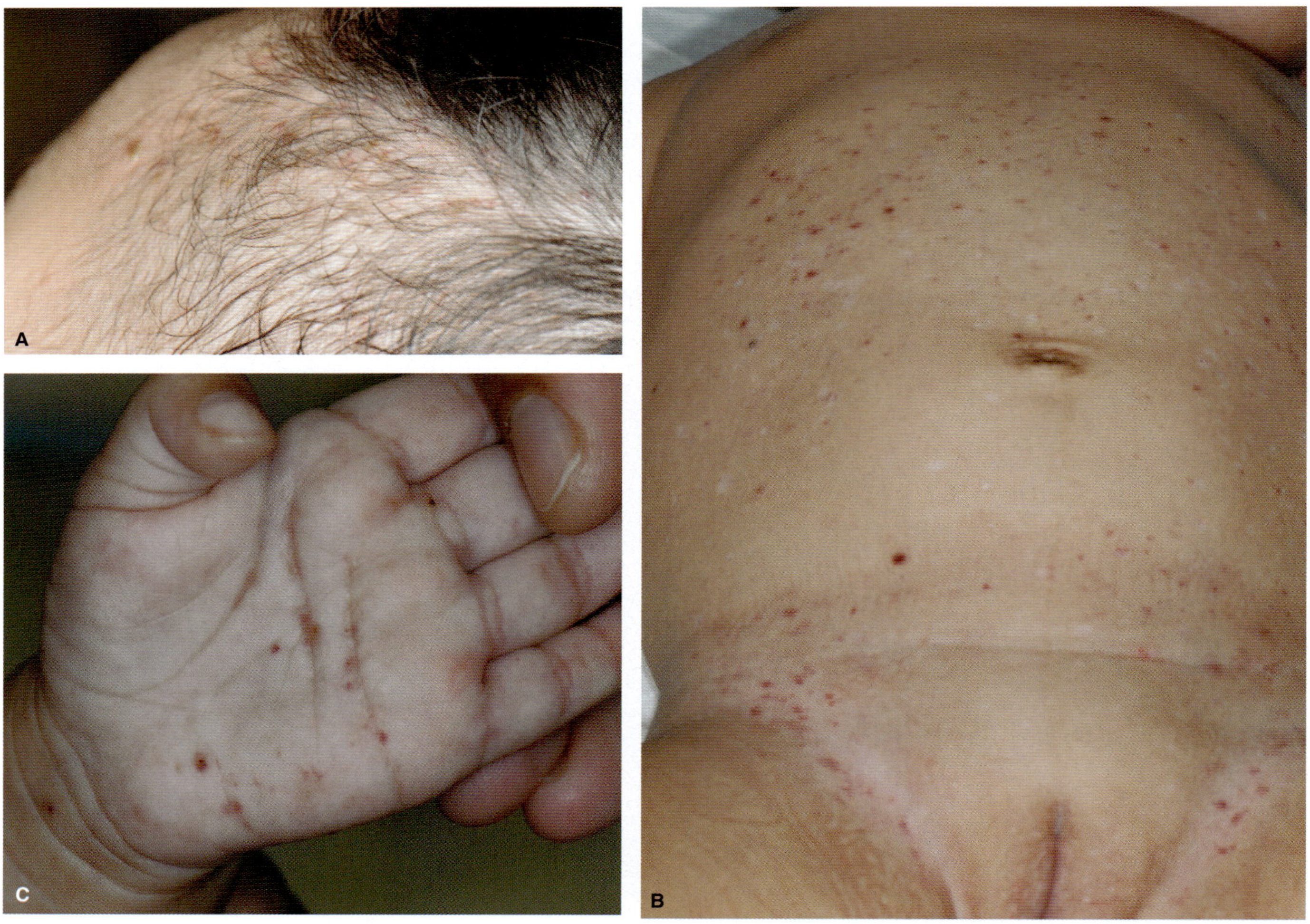

FIGURE 10-3A–3C. LCH in a Vietnamese infant girl presenting with multiple crusted, hemorrhagic, red-to-brown papules with erosions over the scalp, intertriginous sites, trunk, and acral sites.

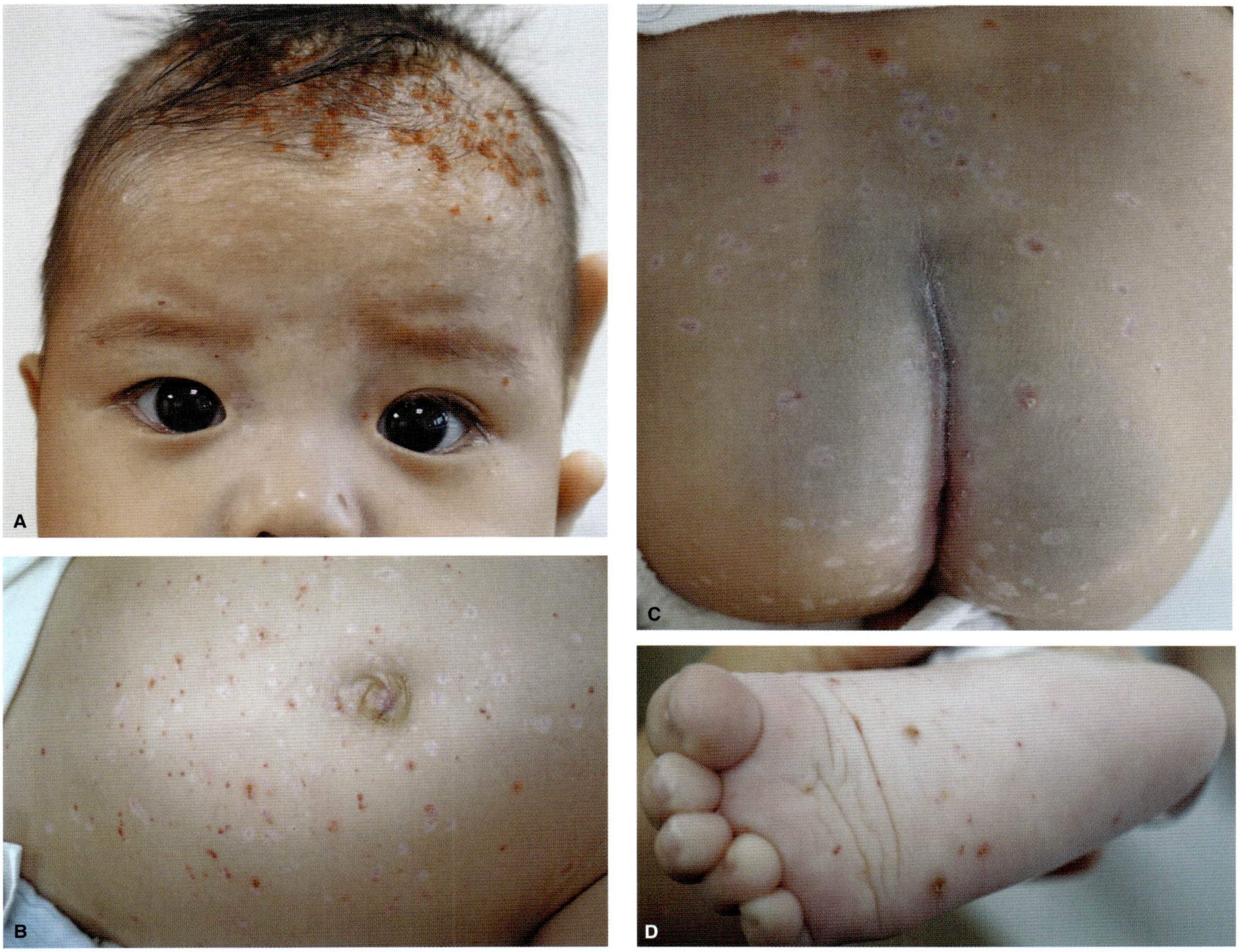

FIGURE 10-4A–4D. LCH in a 1-year-old Chinese boy presenting with multiple crusted, yellow-orange-brown papules on the scalp, face, trunk, and limbs. The patient had systemic involvement.

- The morphology of cutaneous lesions can vary from eczematous, crusted papules and nodules to petechiae and hemorrhagic papules. Erosions and small ulcers, especially in the intertriginous areas and perineum, can sometimes be seen. Bullous lesions have rarely been reported.
- Neonatal LCH, or congenital self-healing reticulohistiocytosis, is a type of LCH presenting in newborns or in the neonatal period, with a solitary or multiple small red-brown papules, nodules, or vesicles, often with surface crusting. The lesions tend to involute spontaneously within several months. Progression to systemic involvement is rare, but long-term follow-up is recommended.
- Nail involvement includes paronychial erythema, subungual hyperkeratosis, subungual pustules and/or purpura, onycholysis and nail plate loss, longitudinal grooving, and nail plate thickening.
- Oral involvement includes gingival hyperplasia and chronic ulcers, especially of the buccal mucosa, palate, or tongue.
- Bone involvement can present with swelling, pain, or pathological fractures. They may, however, be asymptomatic, and only detected radiologically. The skull is the most commonly affected site, although the long bones and axial skeleton may also be involved.
- Hormonal complications include diabetes insipidus and growth hormone and thyroid hormone deficiencies.
- Other systemic involvements include hepatosplenomegaly, elevated liver enzymes, sclerosing cholangitis, lymphadenopathy, pulmonary and central nervous system abnormalities.

Differential Diagnoses

- Diaper dermatitis
  - LCH can present similarly to other causes of diaper dermatitis, including irritant contact dermatitis, frictional dermatitis, diaper candidiasis, zinc deficiency, and psoriasis.
  - Persistent diaper dermatitis, especially if not responding to treatment, should prompt investigations for LCH.

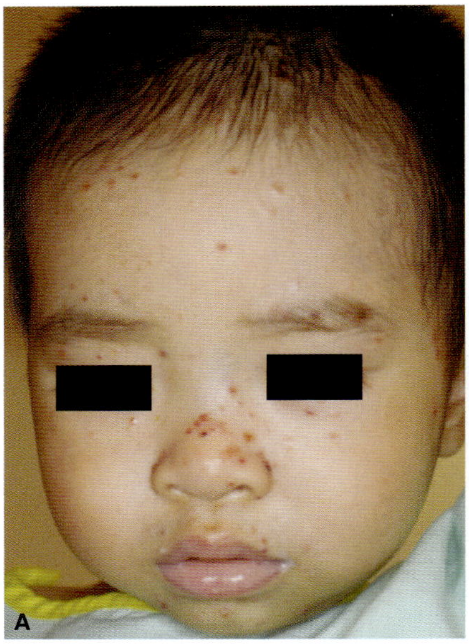
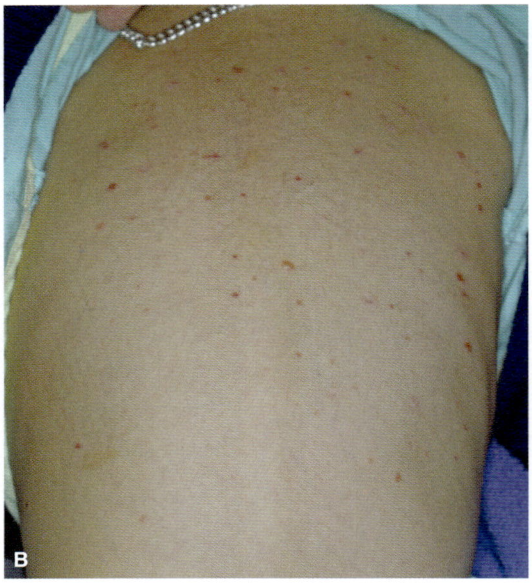
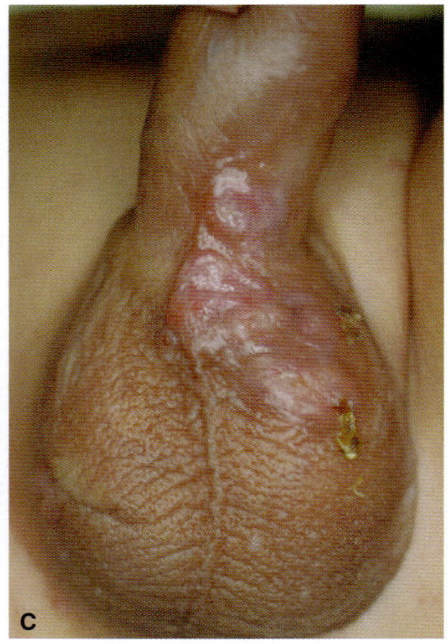
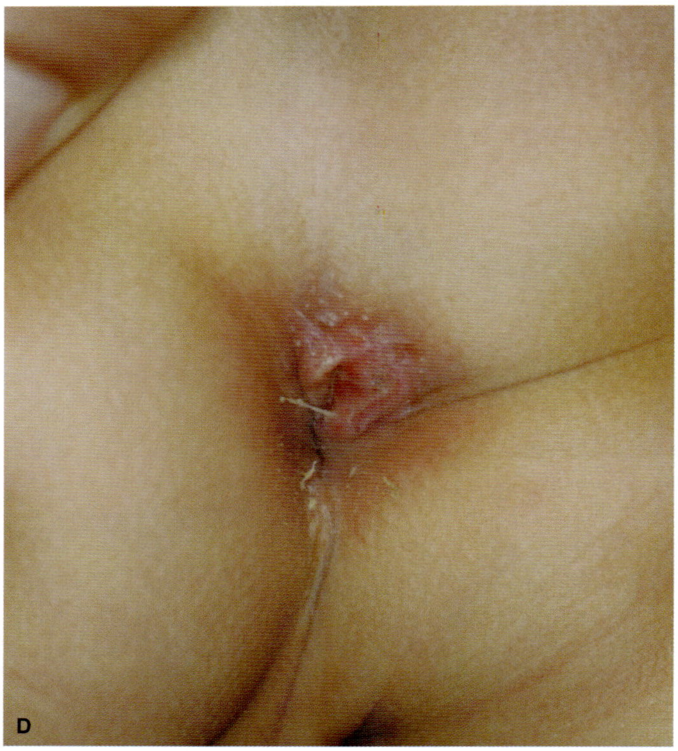
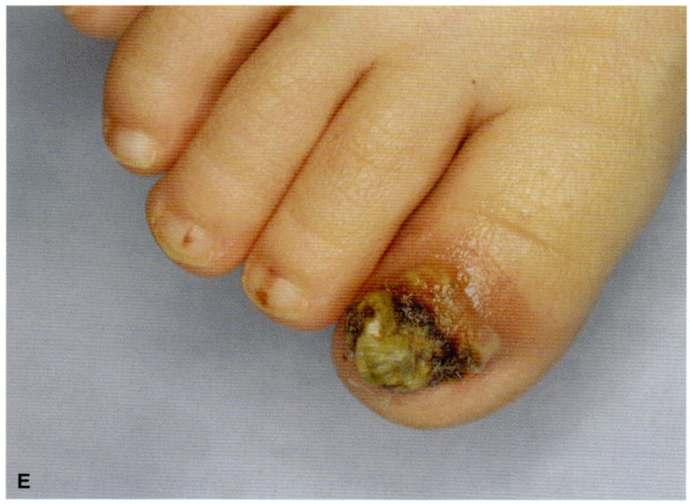

FIGURE 10-5A–5E. LCH in a Vietnamese toddler presenting with crusted, hemorrhagic papules on his face, trunk, and limbs. There are infiltrated plaques on the genitalia and perianal region (Figures 10-5C & 5D), and nail fold involvement with dystrophic nails (Figure 10-5E).

- Seborrheic dermatitis
  - LCH can affect similar sites as infantile seborrheic dermatitis. Persistence or poor response to treatment should prompt investigations for LCH. LCH eruptions are also more petechial or hemorrhagic, with erosions and ulcers.
- Atopic dermatitis (AD)
  - Infantile AD can also affect the scalp, face, and intertriginous sites. There is usually a family history of atopy. Similar to seborrheic dermatitis, petechial or hemorrhagic lesions should not be seen in AD.
- Other forms of histiocytosis, most commonly juvenile xanthogranuloma (JXG).
  - JXG lesions range from a solitary nodule to multiple papules that are yellow-orange-brown in color, as compared to the hemorrhagic crusted papules in LCH. Histology and immunohistochemical stains can differentiate JXG from LCH lesions.

Investigations & Treatment

- Skin biopsy is required to confirm the diagnosis of LCH. Histological features include epidermal ulceration and spongiosis with epidermal and dermal infiltrate of histiocytes

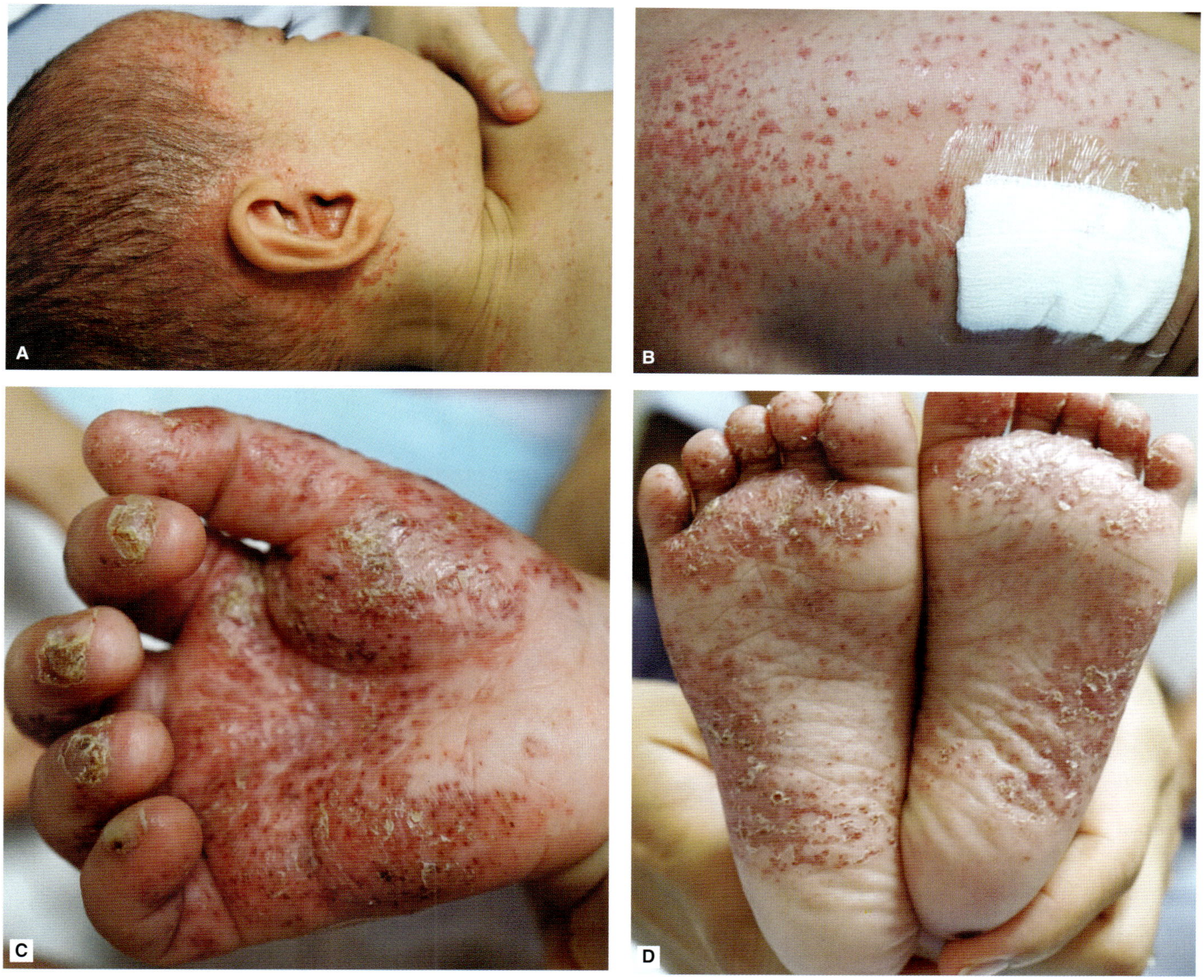

FIGURE 10-6A–6D. LCH in an Indonesian toddler presenting with widespread, crusted, hemorrhagic papules and plaques, affecting the scalp, face, intertriginous areas, trunk, and acral sites. Note the paronychia with nail involvement. The patient also had mucosal involvement.

with large, open nuclei, some with reniform or coffee bean-shaped nuclei. These cells stain positively for langerin (CD207), S100, and CD1a immunohistochemical stains.

- Staging investigations include ultrasound of the hepatobiliary system, liver function test, full blood count and coagulation studies, paired urine and serum osmolality and sodium, and a skeletal survey. Further investigations depend on the clinical features and results of the initial evaluation.
- Treatment depends on the organ systems involved and disease stratification.
- Cutaneous lesions can be treated with topical corticosteroids and topical calcineurin inhibitors. Phototherapy has also been used for more widespread disease.
- Systemic therapy will be required if there is extensive cutaneous disease, especially if unresponsive to topical therapies or if there is systemic organ involvement. This usually involves chemotherapy with the current LCH-IV protocol, or stem cell transplant for refractory disease. Recently, BRAF-inhibitors, such as vemurafenib, have been used to treat refractory or recurrent LCH.

Pearls & Practical Tips

- LCH should be considered in young children with extensive "eczematous" or "seborrheic dermatitis" eruptions, especially if there is involvement of atypical sites such as the palms, soles, and genitalia, or is refractory to regular treatment for eczema.
- Infants with LCH are also often clinically irritable with poor growth, at lower weight centiles.
- Patients with the *BRAF* V600E mutations have been associated with more severe multi-organ disease.

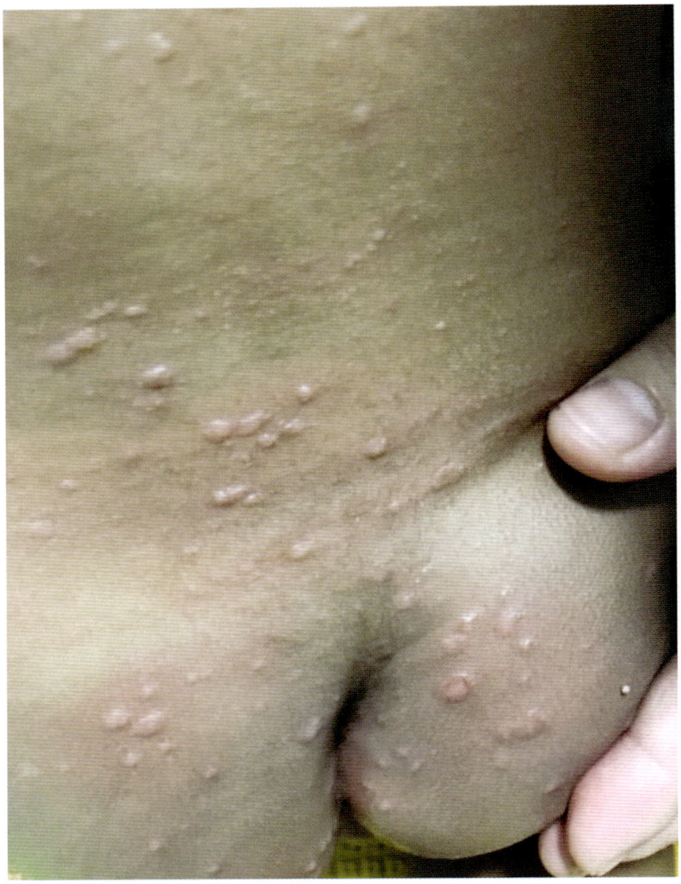

FIGURE 10-7. A rare case of bullous LCH in a 3-month-old child who developed multiple small bullae on his trunk. Skin biopsy confirmed the diagnosis. The lesions self-resolved after 6 months.

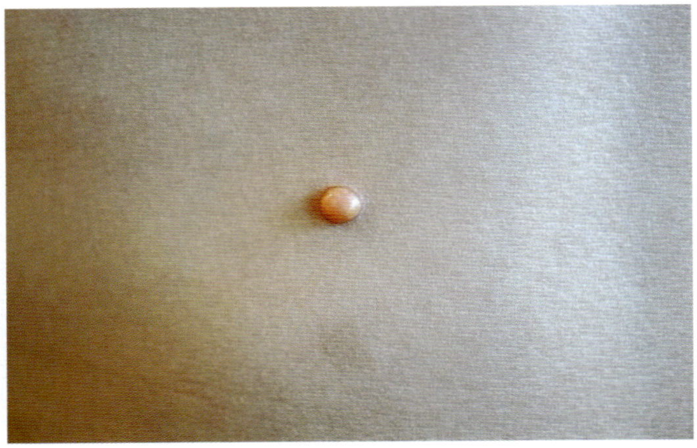

FIGURE 10-8. JXG on the abdomen of a Chinese child, appearing as a sessile yellow-brown papule.

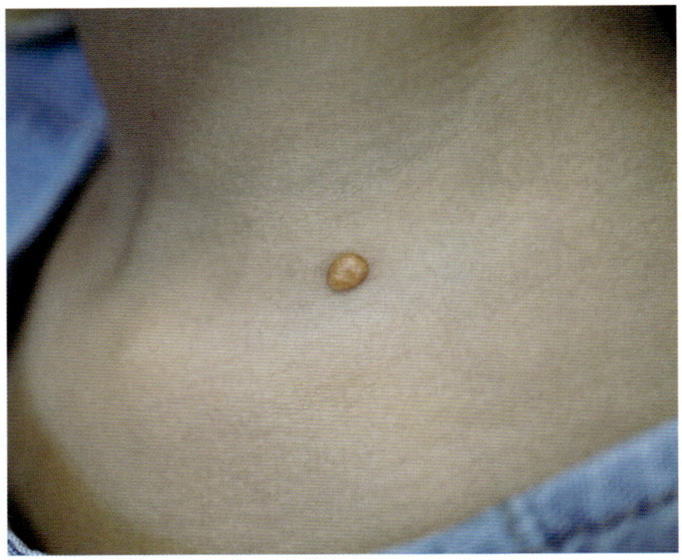

FIGURE 10-9. JXG in an older Chinese girl presenting as a sessile, soft, yellow-brown papule on the upper chest.

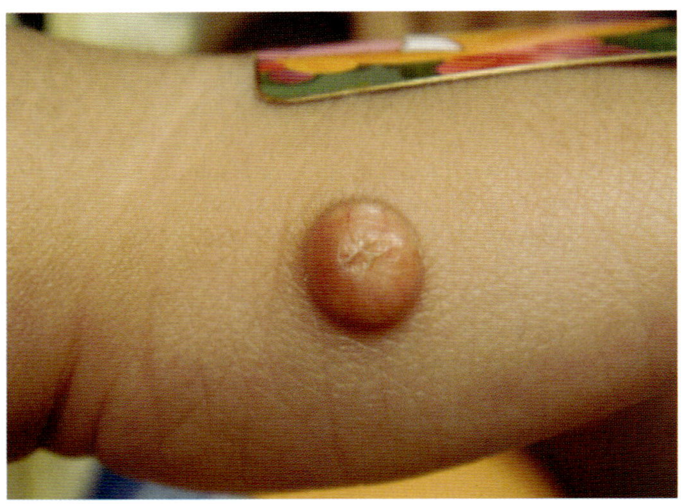

FIGURE 10-10. A larger JXG on the side of the palm of a Chinese child, presenting as a firm, yellow-brown papule with a central depression and scales. Telangiectasias are visible on the surface.

Bibliography

1. Aricò M. Langerhans cell histiocytosis in children: from the bench to bedside for an updated therapy. Br J Haematol 2016 Jun;173(5):663-70.
2. Héritier et al. BRAF mutation correlates with high-risk Langerhans cell histiocytosis and increased resistance to first-line therapy. J Clin Oncol 2016 Sep 1;34(25):3023-30. doi: 10.1200/JCO.2015.65.9508.

NON-LANGERHANS CELL HISTIOCYTOSIS

The xanthogranuloma group of conditions is the most common form of non-Langerhans cell histiocytosis. Juvenile xanthogranulomas (JXG) are by far the most common clinical presentation of this group of conditions, especially in children. The pathogenesis of JXG is not fully elucidated but has been postulated to be a result of disordered macrophage response to non-specific tissue injury, resulting in a granulomatous reaction. Other less common presentations of the xanthogranuloma group include benign cephalic histiocytosis (BCH), generalized eruptive histiocytosis (GEH), xanthoma disseminatum (XD), and progressive nodular histiocytosis (PNH). Although generally considered to be variants of JXG, these other rare forms are differentiated by their age of presentation, clinical involvement, and prognosis.

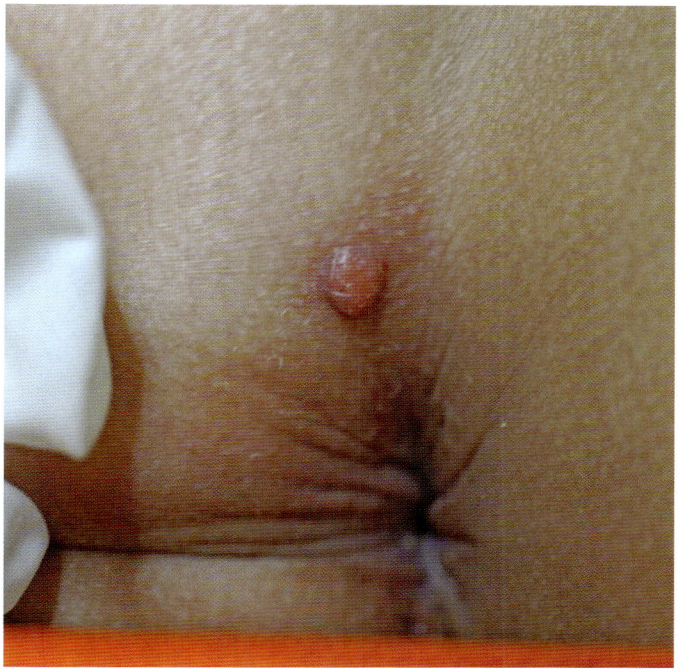

FIGURE 10-11. Perianal JXG in a Chinese infant presenting as a red-brown nodule.

Clinical Features

Juvenile Xanthogranuloma (JXG)

- JXG commonly presents in infancy or early childhood. Congenital lesions may also occur, but rarely.
- JXG presents as one to multiple small, yellowish-brown, dome-shaped, sessile papulonodules. The surface is usually smooth but may have overlying scale. And may occasionally erode after trauma.
- The skin is the most commonly affected organ, and lesions can occur anywhere but most frequently occurring on the head and neck region.

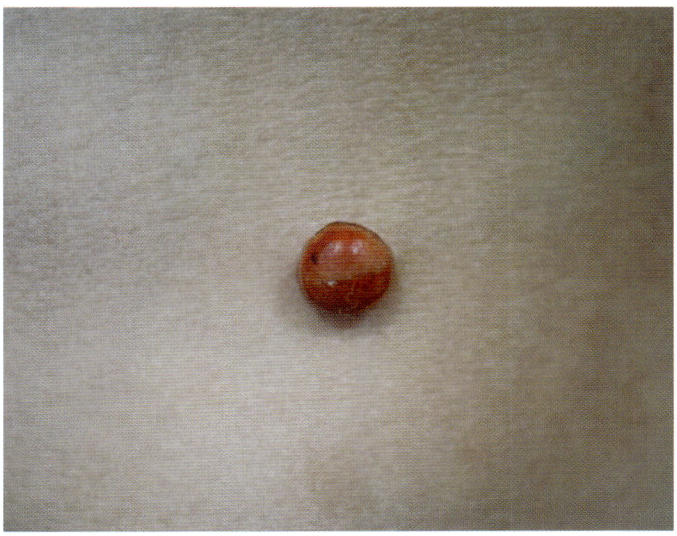

FIGURE 10-12. JXG on the trunk of a Chinese child presenting as a firm, red-brown nodule with some overlying scaling.

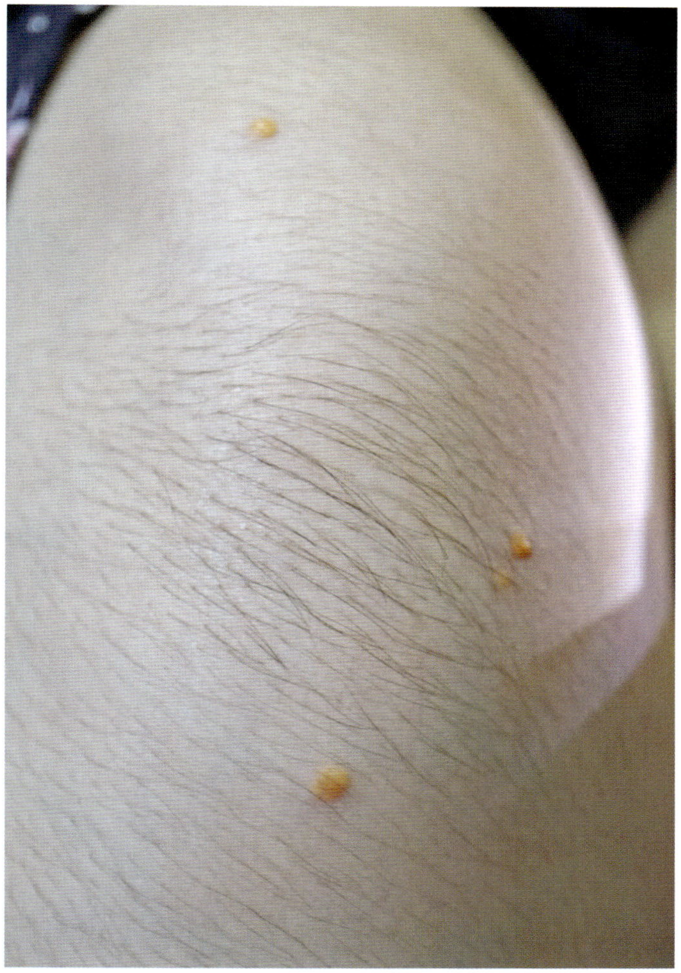

FIGURE 10-13. Multiple discrete JXG on the knee of a Chinese child presenting as several yellow papules.

- The eye is the most common extracutaneous site of involvement. The involvement of bones, liver, lung, and brain has also been rarely reported.
- An uncommon but important association of multiple JXG is juvenile myelomonocytic leukemia (JMML), a rare leukemia predominantly affecting young children under the age of 5 years, characterized by the uncontrolled proliferation of monocytes that accumulate in the bone marrow, resulting in marrow suppression. The risk is higher in neurofibromatosis type 1 patients with concomitant JXG.
- Benign cephalic histiocytosis (BCG) is a variant of JXG that presents with multiple small, yellowish-brown papules affecting the head and neck region. Lesions can occasionally coalesce to give a reticulate pattern. It usually affects young infants and toddlers.

Differential Diagnoses

- Langerhans cell histiocytosis (LCH)
  - There is some overlap between the LCH and JXG groups of disorders. Some patients may present with concomitant lesions. Systemic involvement is far more common in LCH compared to JXG.

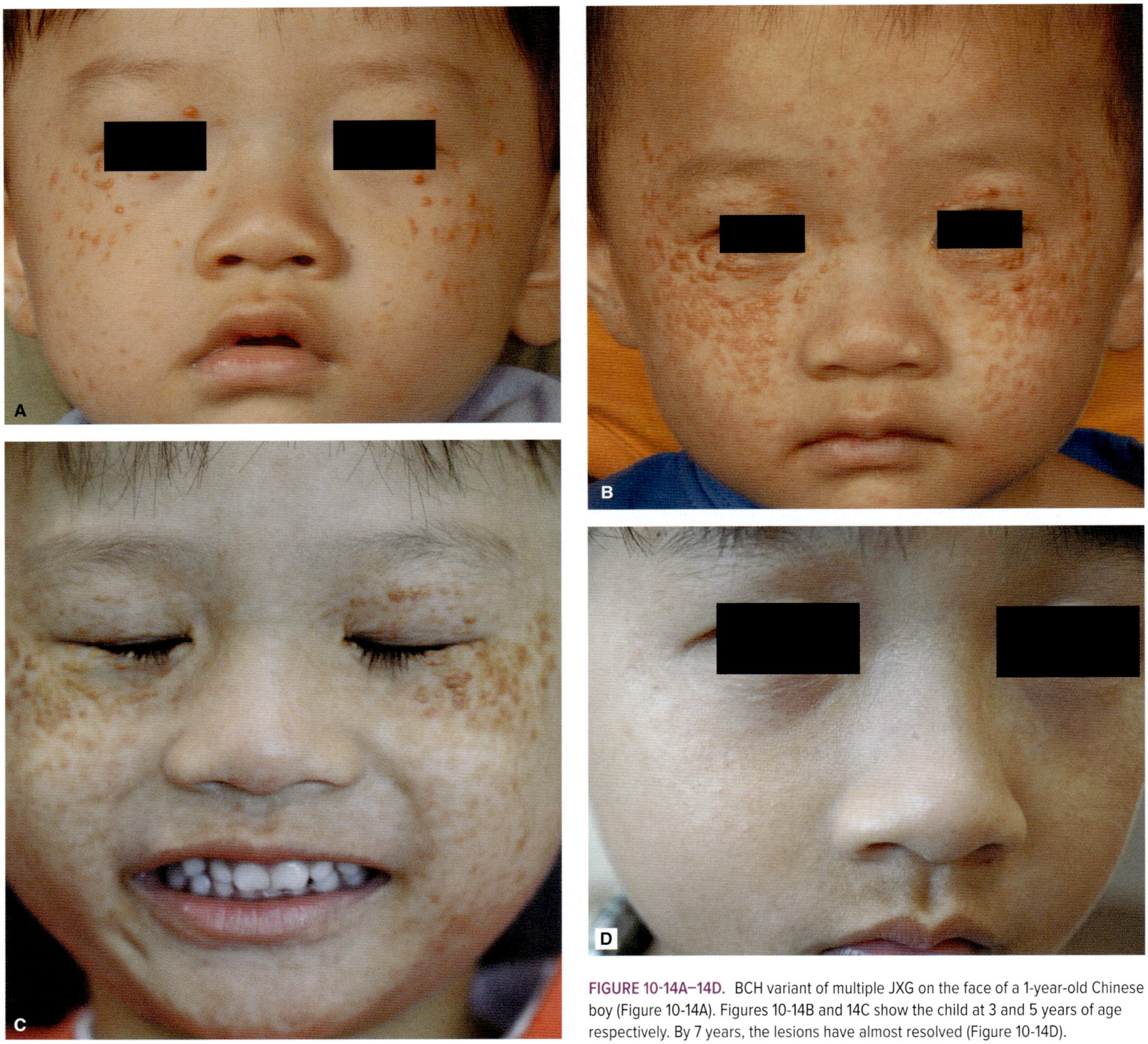

FIGURE 10-14A–14D. BCH variant of multiple JXG on the face of a 1-year-old Chinese boy (Figure 10-14A). Figures 10-14B and 14C show the child at 3 and 5 years of age respectively. By 7 years, the lesions have almost resolved (Figure 10-14D).

- Clinically, LCH presents with more scaly, eroded, and hemorrhagic macules and papules that coalesce to form patches and plaques. They can, however, present with discrete papules, especially in younger infants.
- Skin biopsy for histology and immunohistochemical stains may be required to differentiate between LCH and JXG. The histiocytes in JXG lesions stain positively for factor XIIIa, CD68, CD163, and CD14 and negatively for S100, CD1a, and Langerin, while LCH stains positively for S100, CD1a, and Langerin immunohistochemical stains.

- Mastocytosis
  - Mastocytosis also presents in infancy and early childhood. Lesions present as solitary or multiple red-brown, hyperpigmented macules, papules, or plaques with a more irregular surface. Darier sign may be positive.
- Spitz nevus
  - Spitz nevi usually occur in childhood and are common on the head and neck region. They present as solitary dome-shaped, red-brown papules. They usually appear redder compared to JXG.

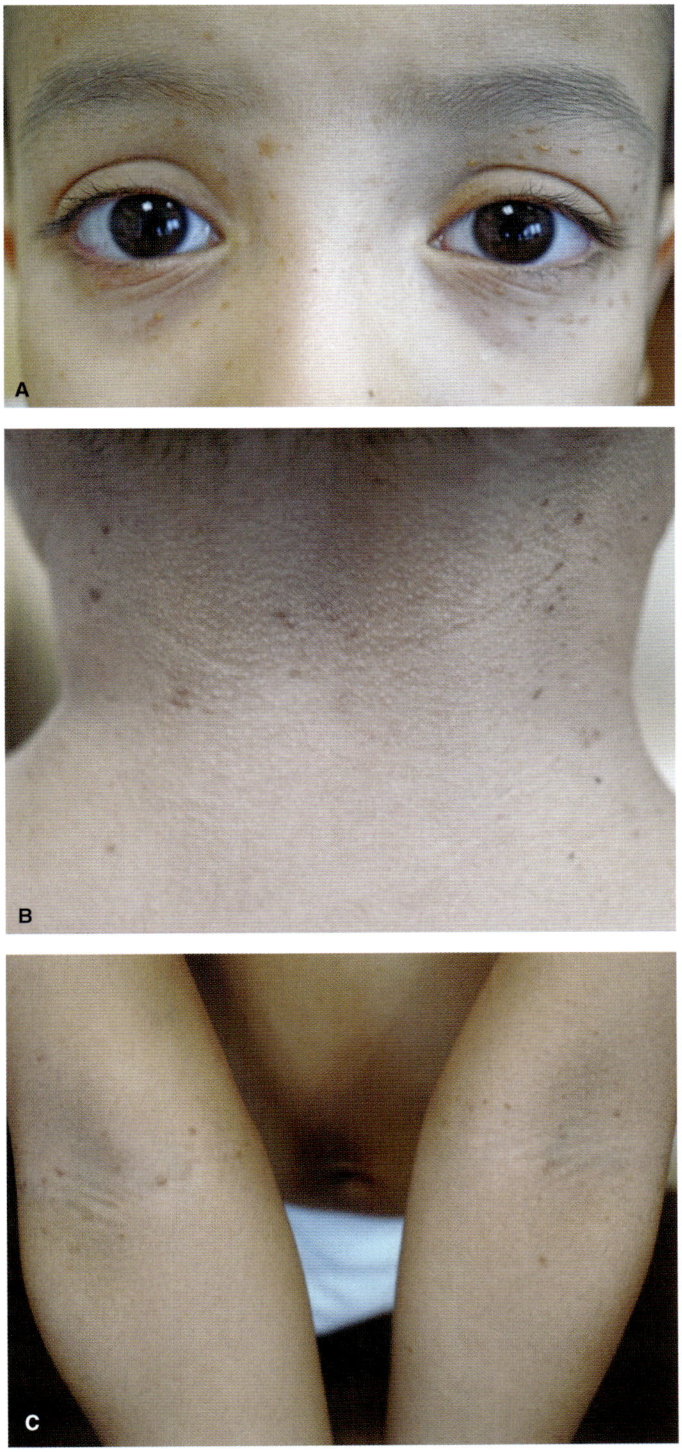

FIGURE 10-15A–15C. Multiple JXG affecting an Indian boy, presenting with multiple yellow-brown papules on his face, with multiple discrete, hyperpigmented macules and papules over his trunk and limbs.

- Dermatofibroma
  - Dermatofibroma usually occurs in older children and is more common on the trunk or limbs. It is characterized by a hyperpigmented grayish-brown nodule with a lighter, depressed center.
- Flat warts
  - Flat warts are a differential for BCH. However, they occur in older children and have a flatter surface as compared to the dome shape of BCH lesions.

Investigations & Treatment

- JXG can be diagnosed clinically. For less typical cases, a skin biopsy can be diagnostic.
- The histologies of JXG, BCH, and other conditions in the xanthogranuloma group are very similar. They consist of a nodular proliferation of histiocytes, often with foamy cytoplasm. Variable numbers of Touton giant cells are seen, although they could be absent.
- JXG and BCH are generally limited to the skin and are rarely associated with systemic involvement, with most lesions resolving spontaneously after a few years, sometimes leaving atrophic scars with dyspigmentation. They do not require treatment, but clinical follow-up for progress is recommended given the clinical variation and overlap with other histiocytic conditions.
- Routine laboratory screening for JMML and systemic manifestations is generally not recommended unless there is clinical suggestion of extracutaneous involvement.

Pearls & Practical Tips

- Routine ophthalmological screening is now less frequently recommended for patients with multiple JXG, even on the head and neck region, unless there are signs and symptoms of eye involvement, including painful, red eyes or visual disturbances.
- Although most cases regress spontaneously, surgical excision can be performed for larger lesions, which are frequently traumatized.

Bibliography

1. Wee LWY, Ling HY, Ho VPY, Foong AYW, Koh MJA. Juvenile xanthogranulomas in Asian children. Dermatol Ther 2021 Nov 24;e15224.
2. Samuelov L, Kinori M, Chamlin SL, et al. Risk of intraocular and other extracutaneous involvement in patients with cutaneous juvenile xanthogranuloma. Pediatr Dermatol 2018;35:329-35.

MASTOCYTOSIS

Mastocytosis occurs when there is excessive accumulation of mast cells in one or more organs, with the skin being the most common site of involvement (cutaneous mastocytosis), especially in pediatric patients. Systemic mastocytosis is rare in childhood but can lead to systemic involvement, such as the bone marrow, spleen, and liver. Most forms are caused by somatic *c-KIT* gene mutations. Mastocytosis usually present in early infancy but can also occur in older children and rarely, adults.

Clinical Features

- Cutaneous macrocytosis in children can present as solitary mastocytomas, maculopapular cutaneous mastocytosis (urticaria pigmentosa), and diffuse cutaneous mastocytosis. Mastocytoma and maculopapular cutaneous mastocytosis are the more common forms. Bullous lesions may be seen in all forms of mastocytosis.

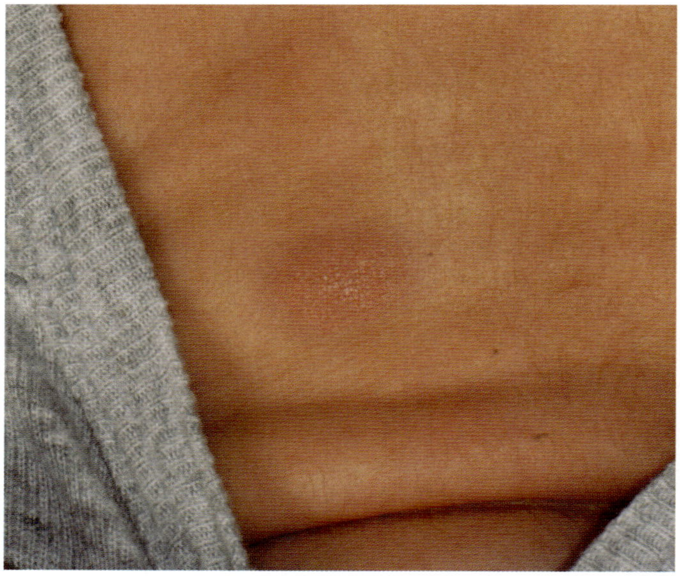

FIGURE 10-16. Solitary mastocytoma on the back of a Chinese infant, presenting as a yellow-brown plaque with peau d'orange surface.

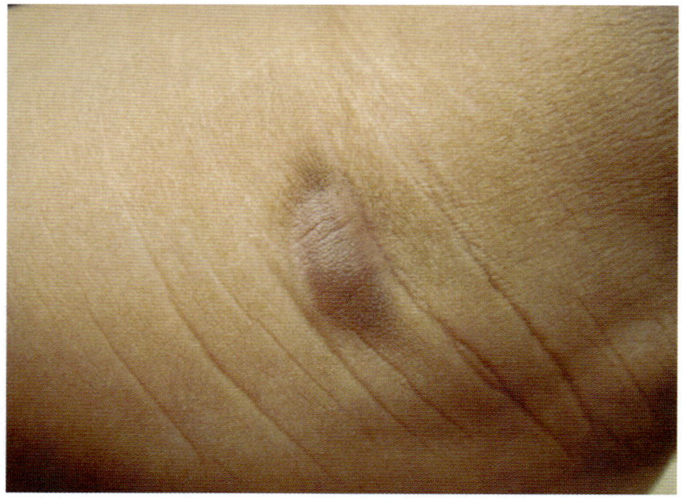

FIGURE 10-18. Solitary mastocytoma on the ankle of a Chinese infant.

- A positive Darier sign is the hallmark of cutaneous mastocytosis, in which mechanical irritation of skin lesions results in redness and/or swelling due to release of mast cell mediators. More generalized urticarial lesions can also occur in patients with more widespread involvement.
- Solitary mastocytomas present as localized, itchy, erythematous-to-brown, thickened plaque, with an irregular, pebbly surface, likened to a "peau d'orange" appearance.

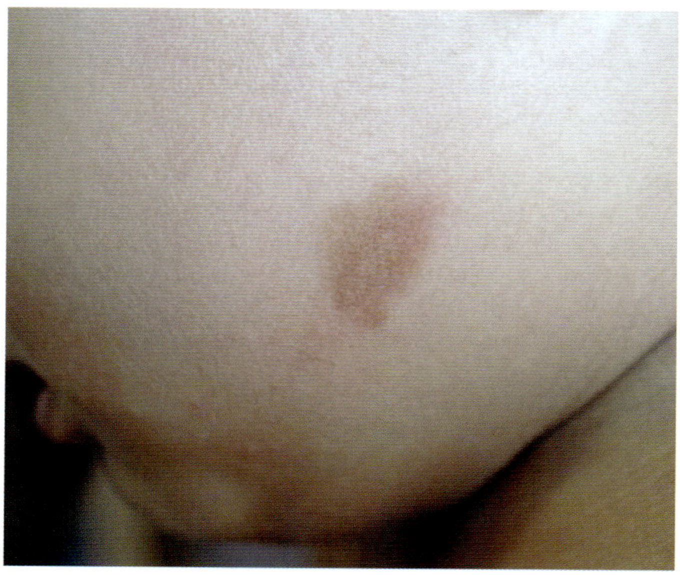

FIGURE 10-17. Solitary mastocytoma on the jawline of a Chinese infant with surrounding erythema after rubbing (Darier sign).

- Maculopapular cutaneous mastocytosis, formerly known as urticaria pigmentosa, presents as multiple red-to-brown macules, papules, and plaques, which can affect the trunk, limbs, and head.
- Diffuse cutaneous mastocytosis (DCM) is the rarest variant of cutaneous mastocytosis and can present with extensive blisters in a neonate or young infant. The skin subsequently develops a thickened, leathery appearance with yellowish discoloration, accentuation of hair follicles, and increase folding ("peau d'orange"). Blistering, flushing, erythema, edema, pruritus, and dermographism can also be seen. Due to the widespread mast cell infiltration in the skin with subsequent mast cell degranulation, systemic symptoms such as diarrhea, flushing, shock, and other anaphylactic symptoms can occur.

Differential Diagnoses

- Café-au-lait macules
  - These can also present in infancy with hyperpigmented lesions. However, the surface is usually smooth, and Darier sign is negative.
- Congenital melanocytic nevus
  - Melanocytic nevi can also present as a hyperpigmented plaque during infancy, but the color is usually darker and Darier sign is negative.
- Juvenile xanthogranulomas (JXG)
  - JXG can also present as solitary or multiple small, brown papules during infancy. However, there is usually a yellowish-orange hue and the surface is smooth unless traumatized.
- Post-inflammatory hyperpigmentation
  - This can occur secondary to common dermatoses, such as atopic dermatitis, seborrheic dermatitis, or psoriasis, and is more common in darker-skinned infants. A thorough history and physical examination will help to differentiate from mastocytosis.

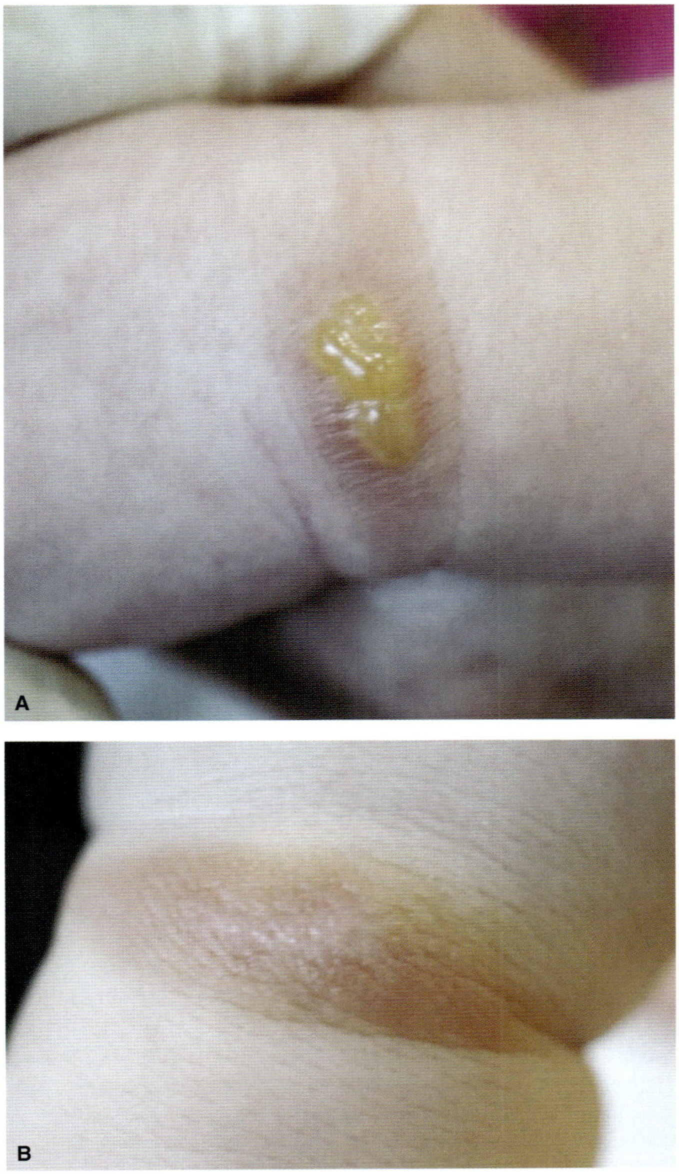

FIGURE 10-19A & 19B. Bullous mastocytoma on the wrist of a Chinese infant, presenting with tense blisters with surrounding erythema and pigmentation. Figure 10- 19B shows the same lesion after the blister resolved.

- Insect bite reactions/papular urticaria
  - Insect bite reactions, or papular urticaria, is common in infants and children and can present with blisters which heal with residual hyperpigmentation.

Investigations & Treatment

- Diagnosis of mastocytosis can often be made based on clinical features. A thorough examination to exclude systemic involvement (lymph nodes, liver, spleen) should be performed.
- In the absence of characteristic skin findings, a skin biopsy can be performed for histological confirmation, which shows characteristic mast cell accumulation within

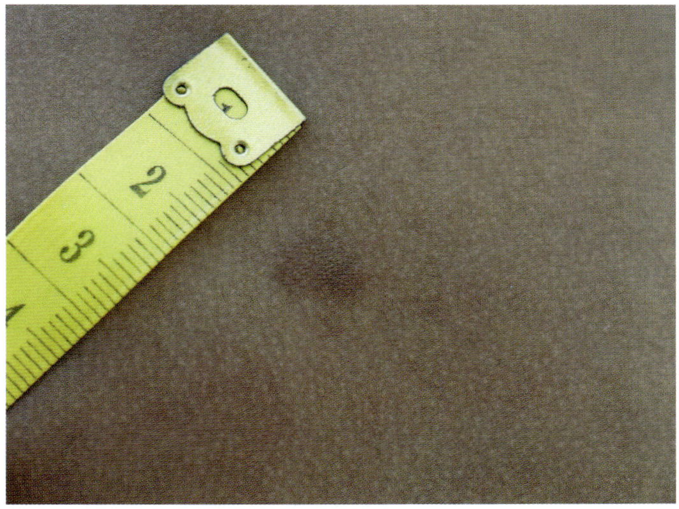

FIGURE 10-20. Peau d'orange surface can be appreciated in this case of scattered mastocytomas on the trunk of an Indian child.

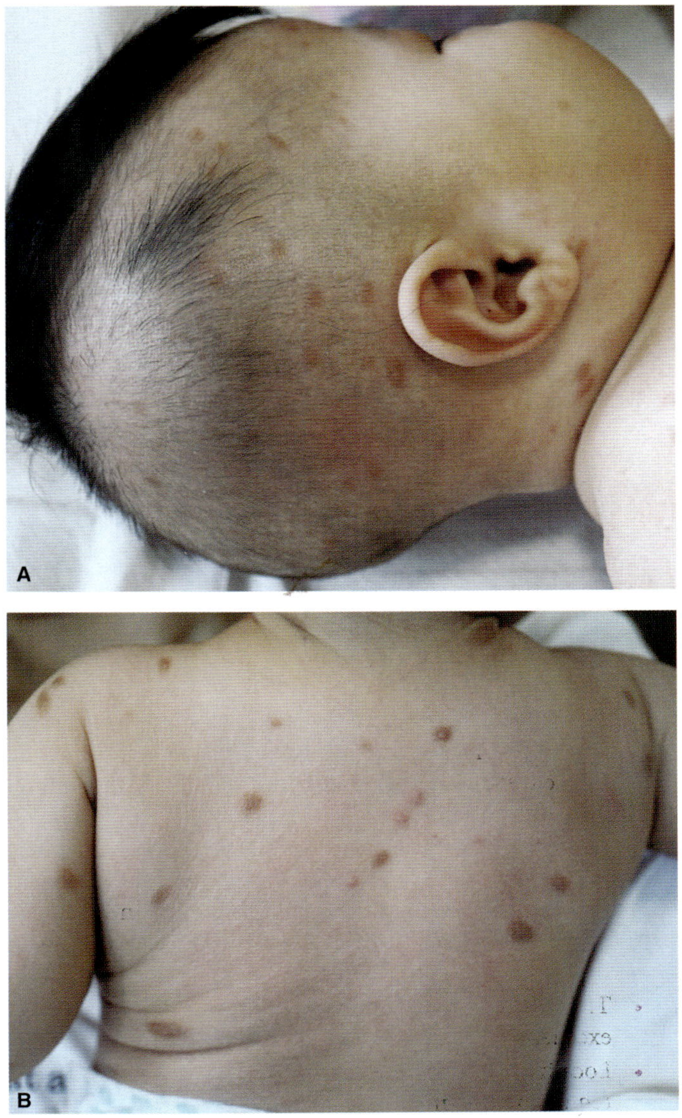

FIGURE 10-21A & 21B. Maculopapular cutaneous mastocytosis presenting as multiple discrete, red-brown papules on the trunk and face of this Chinese infant.

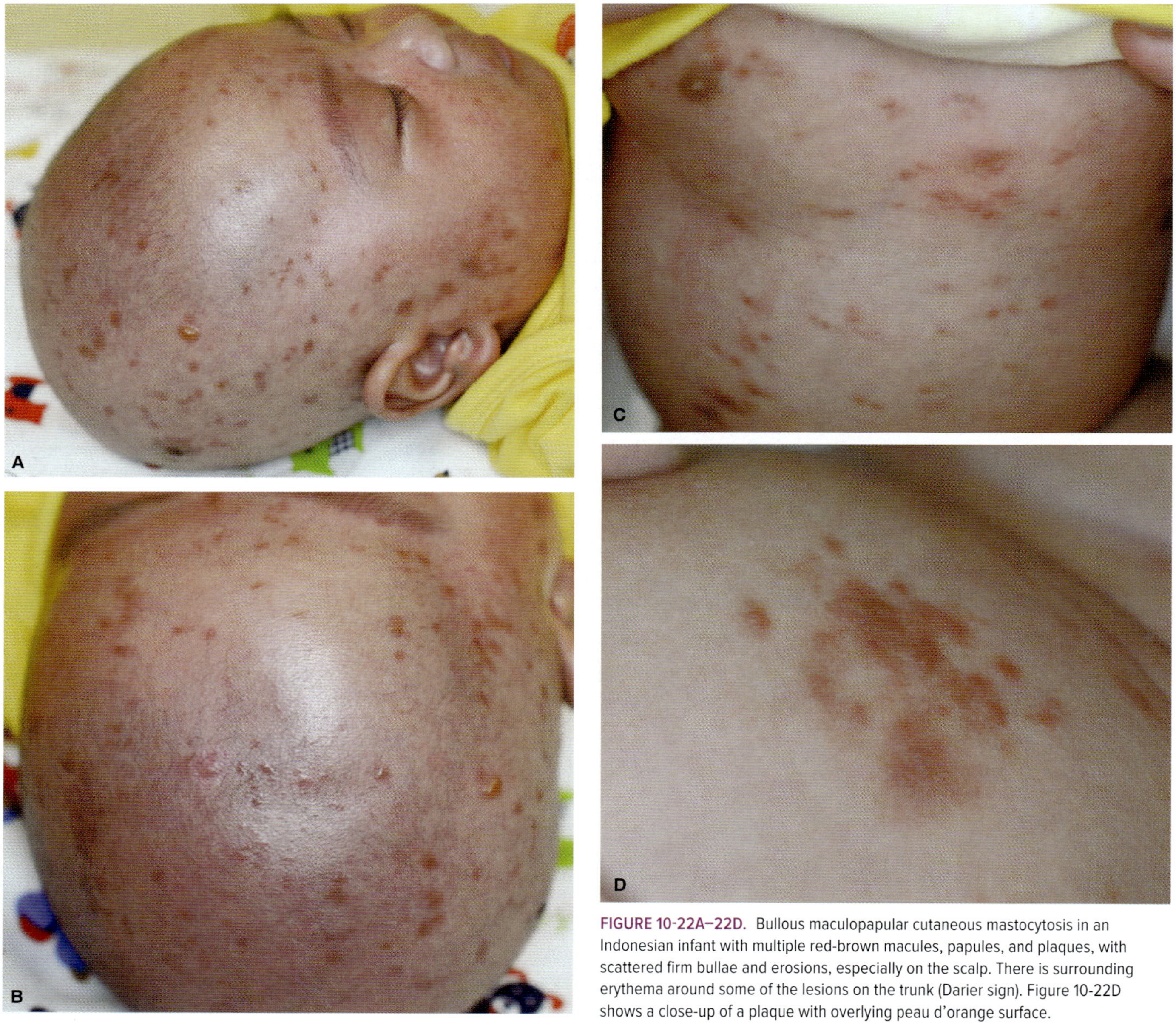

FIGURE 10-22A–22D. Bullous maculopapular cutaneous mastocytosis in an Indonesian infant with multiple red-brown macules, papules, and plaques, with scattered firm bullae and erosions, especially on the scalp. There is surrounding erythema around some of the lesions on the trunk (Darier sign). Figure 10-22D shows a close-up of a plaque with overlying peau d'orange surface.

the dermis. These mast cells have a "fried egg" appearance and may be highlighted using Giemsa, toluidine blue, and chloroacetate-esterase stains, and CD117 (c-kit) immunochemical stain.

- In patients with extensive disease, investigations including full blood count, liver function tests, and serum tryptase can be performed to exclude systemic involvement. Tryptase levels can correlate with mast cell numbers in the skin.
- The prognosis of childhood mastocytosis is generally excellent, with most cases undergoing self-resolution.
- Localized forms of cutaneous mastocytosis usually require no treatment.
- Oral antihistamines may be prescribed if symptoms are present.
- Other pharmacological treatments that have been described include mast cell stabilizers (e.g., sodium cromoglycate), leukotriene antagonists, and omalizumab. The use of phototherapy has also been described.
- Multidisciplinary management with pediatricians, allergists, and hematologists is required in the event of systemic mastocytosis, where other forms of systemic therapy may be required.
- Patients with extensive lesions or known anaphylactic reaction may benefit from carrying an adrenaline autoinjector (e.g., EpiPen).

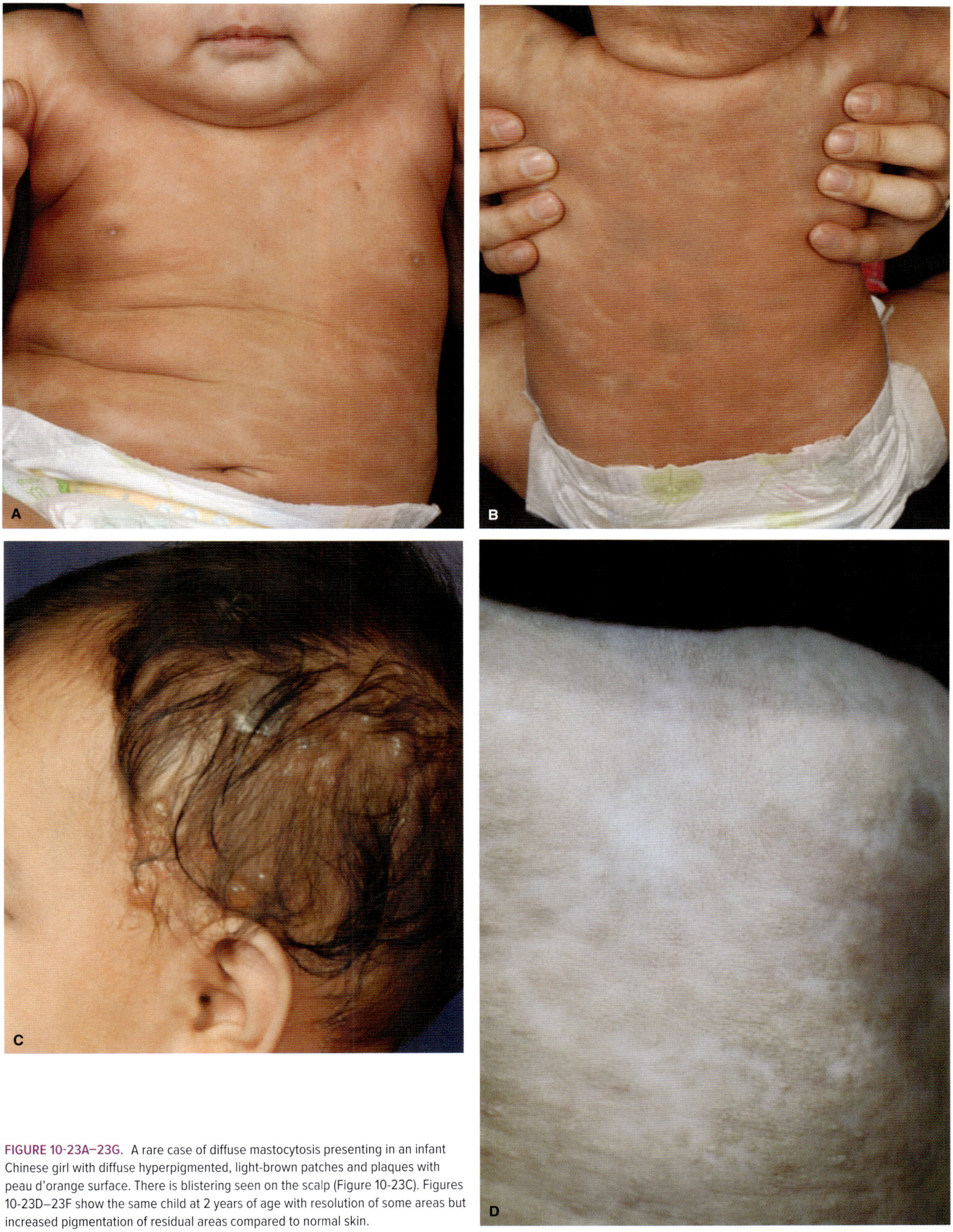

FIGURE 10-23A–23G. A rare case of diffuse mastocytosis presenting in an infant Chinese girl with diffuse hyperpigmented, light-brown patches and plaques with peau d'orange surface. There is blistering seen on the scalp (Figure 10-23C). Figures 10-23D–23F show the same child at 2 years of age with resolution of some areas but increased pigmentation of residual areas compared to normal skin.

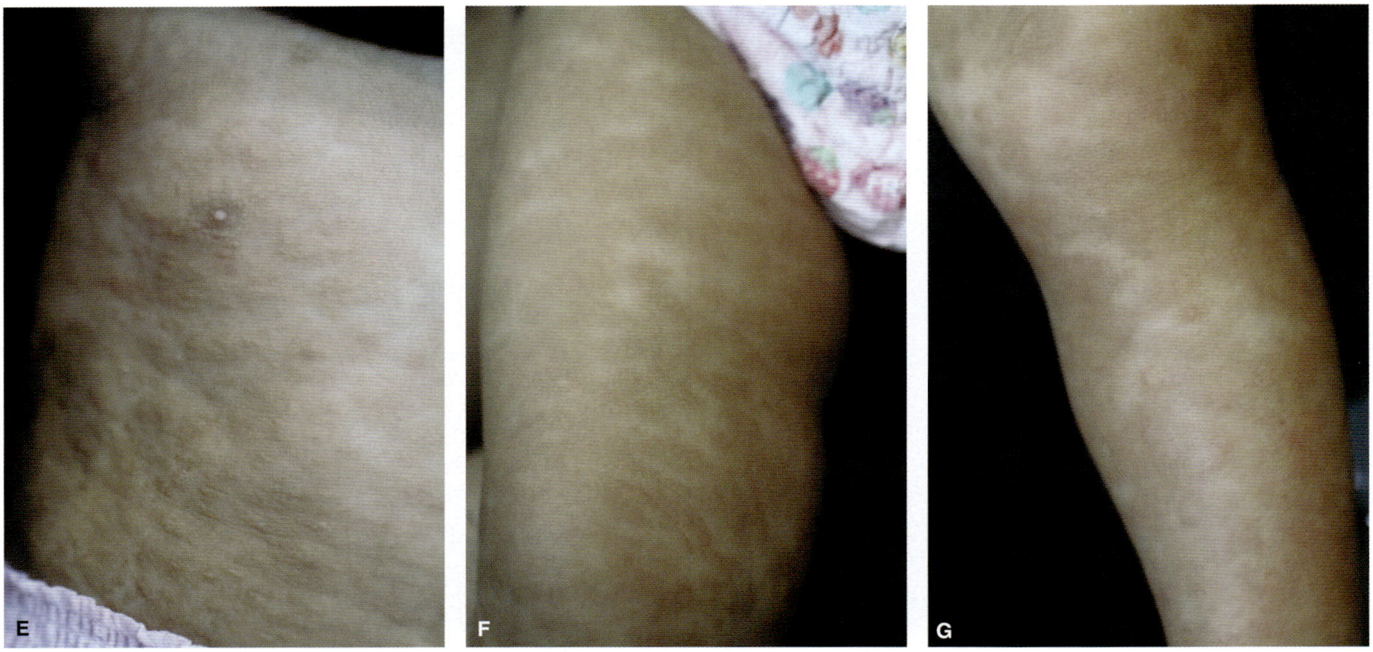

FIGURE 10-23A–23G. (Continued)

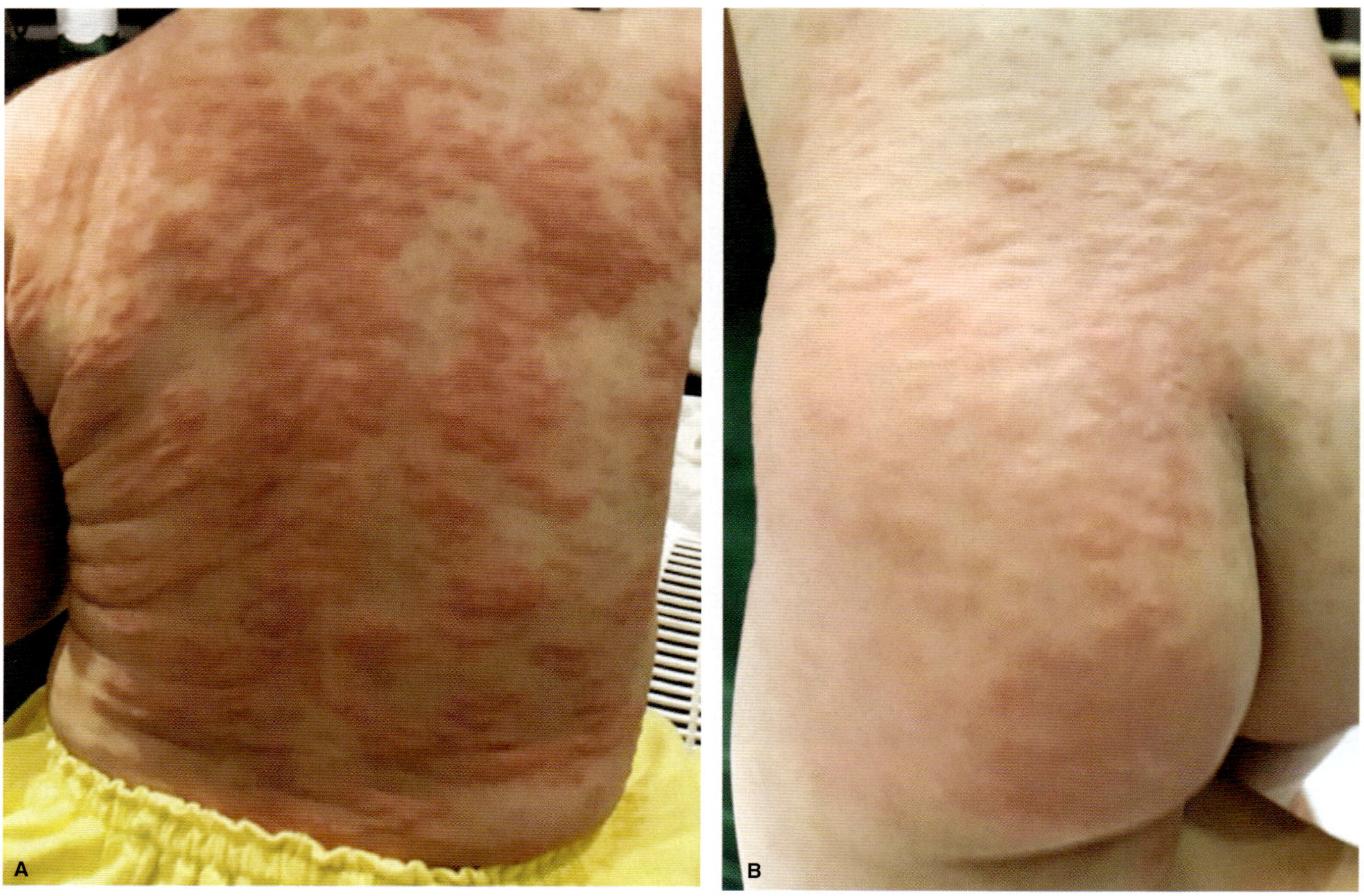

FIGURE 10-24A & 24B. A young child with mastocytosis presenting with widespread urticarial reaction. (Photos courtesy of child's parents.)

TABLE 10-1. Possible triggers of mast cell degranulation.

Drugs	• Non-steroidal anti-inflammatory drugs (NSAIDs), including aspirin and ibuprofen • Local anesthetics: esters e.g., tetracaine, procaine; (*amides can be used safely e.g. lidocaine, bupivacaine, prilocaine) • Neuromuscular blocking agents: D-tubocurarine, decamethonium, gallamine, metocurine, pancuronium • Narcotics: codeine, morphine, pethidine, and all derivatives • Iodine-containing radiographic dyes • Other medications: amphotericin B, thiamine, polymyxin B
Physical	• Excessive exercise, heat, hot baths, hot beverages • Excessive cold • Excessive stress
Venom	• Insects such as bees, wasps, and fire ants • Snakes • Jelly fish
Foods	• Alcohol • Seafoods: crayfish and lobster • Less common: egg white, chocolates, strawberries, tomatoes, citrus

Pearls & Practical Tips

- It is important to advise parents/patients to avoid potential triggers that can cause histamine release from mast cells, especially certain medications. A list of triggers is provided in the Table 10-1.
- All physicians, particularly anesthetists, should be informed of the patient's condition prior to any surgical procedure to avoid the risk of mast cell degranulation secondary to the use of certain anesthetic agents.
- Although almost all cases of childhood mastocytosis self-resolve, the amount of time for resolution can vary among patients. Solitary mastocytosis usually resolves after a few years, while maculopapular cutaneous mastocytosis and diffuse mastocytosis may resolve only in late childhood, adolescence, or early adulthood.

Bibliography

1. Matito A, Azaña JM, Torrelo A, Alvarez-Twose I. Cutaneous mastocytosis in adults and children: new classification and prognostic factors. Immunol Allergy Clin North Am 2018;38(3):351-63.
2. Hussain SH. Pediatric mastocytosis. Curr Opin Pediatr 2020;32(4):531-8.

MYCOSIS FUNGOIDES

Mycosis fungoides (MF) is the most common primary cutaneous T-cell lymphoma, although it is rare in children. It is an indolent disease with slow progression. Most children and adolescents present with early-stage disease with good prognosis and excellent response to skin-directed therapies. Diagnosis is often delayed, as it can mimic other inflammatory dermatoses.

Clinical Features

- More commonly diagnosed in older children and adolescents, MF has been described in young children below the age of 4 years.

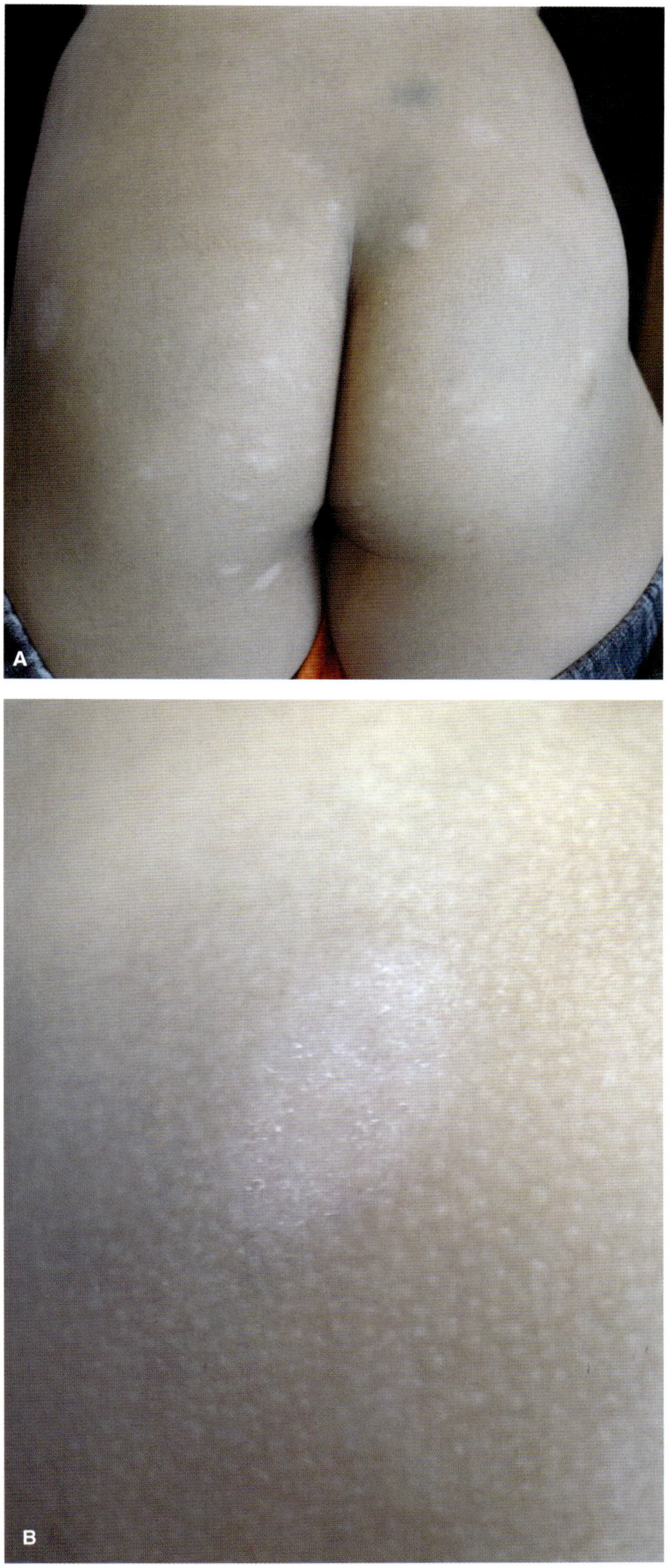

FIGURE 10-25A & 25B. Hypopigmented MF in a 4-year-old Chinese boy with scattered hypopigmented patches on mostly sun-covered sites. Close inspection reveals fine scaling on these patches (Figure 10-25B).

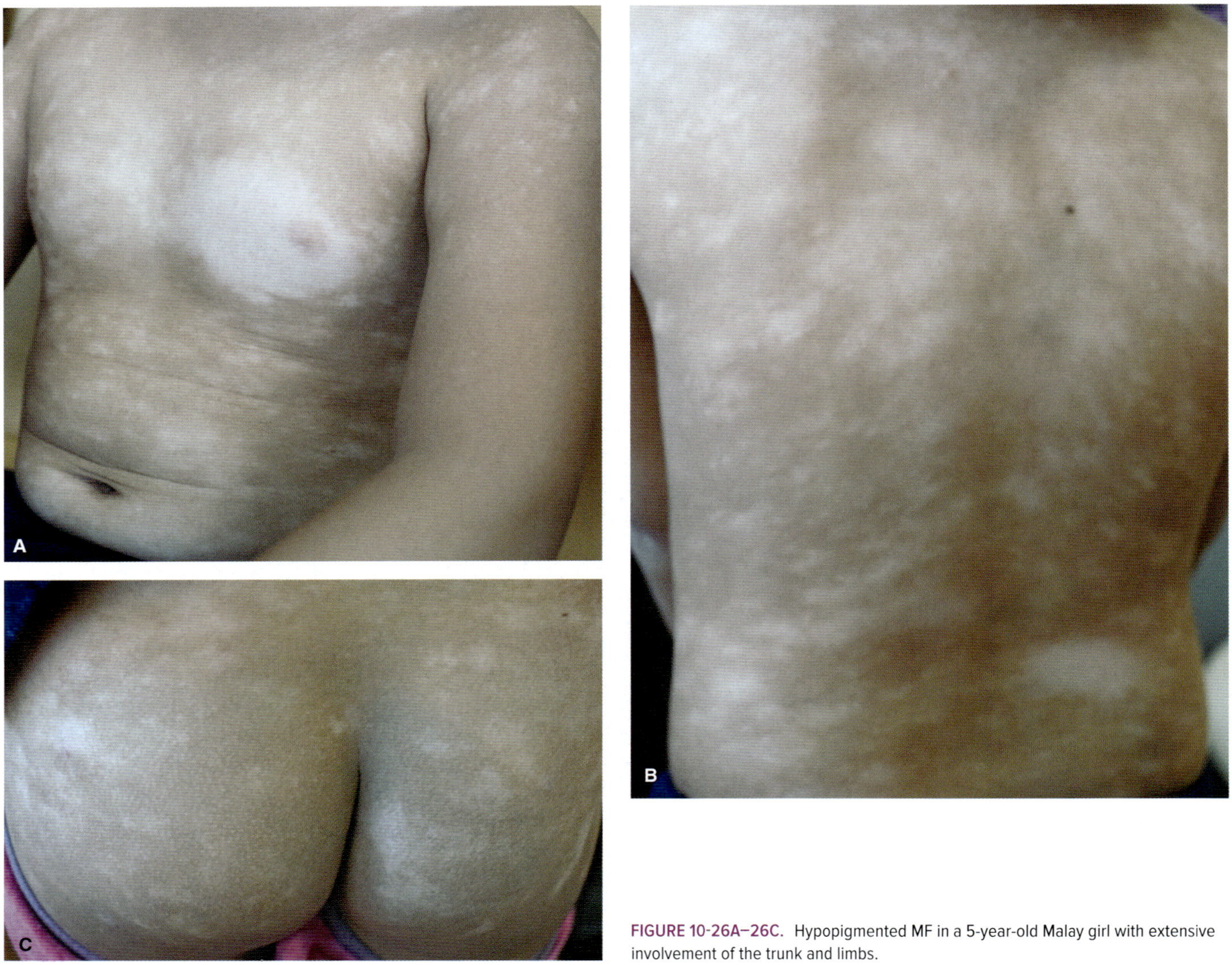

FIGURE 10-26A–26C. Hypopigmented MF in a 5-year-old Malay girl with extensive involvement of the trunk and limbs.

- The clinical presentation of MF in children is variable, although the most common presentation in Asian children is the hypopigmented variant.[1] Patients present with multiple variably sized hypopigmented macules and patches, most commonly affecting the sun-covered sites, such as the buttocks, trunk, and abdomen. However, involvement of sun-exposed sites may also be seen, such as the face, arms, and legs. Fine scales or subtle atrophy may sometimes be appreciated within these lesions.
- Some patients may present with lesions more classically seen in adolescents and adults, with erythematous, scaly macules, papules, patches, and plaques. Lesions may or may not be pruritic. Atrophy may sometimes be seen, and annular lesions can occur with central clearing.
- Tumor-stage MF is rare in children and adolescents but has been reported. Other rare variants that have been reported in children include unilesional MF, granulomatous MF, granulomatous slack skin, and follicular mucinosis.
- The presence of systemic symptoms, lymphadenopathy, and other systemic involvement in pediatric MF is extremely rare. However, if these are present, adequate staging investigations are necessary.

Differential Diagnoses

- Eczemas and other papulosquamous conditions
  - MF in children is often misdiagnosed as other papulosquamous disorders, including atopic dermatitis, psoriasis, parapsoriasis, pityriasis rosea, and pityriasis lichenoides.
  - If there are atypical features, skin biopsies should be performed to exclude MF, especially before commencing systemic treatments for these conditions.
- Post-inflammatory hypopigmentation
  - Post-inflammatory hypopigmentation is common in children, especially if there is a history of an underlying dermatosis, such as atopic dermatitis or psoriasis, and if there is significant sun exposure.
  - It is important to examine for other features of these underlying benign dermatoses. If in doubt, and if sun-covered areas are predominantly affected, skin biopsies should be offered to exclude MF.

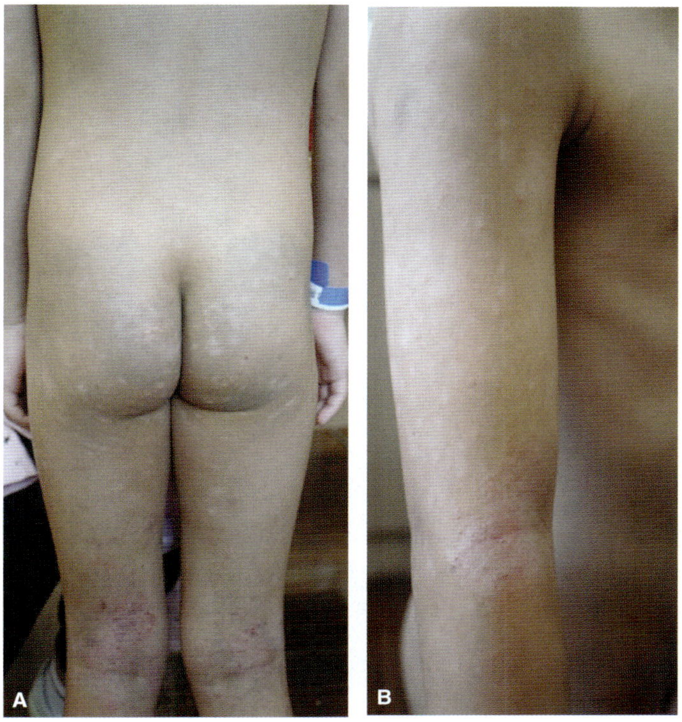

FIGURE 10-27A & 27B. Hypopigmented MF in a 7-year-old Chinese girl with a background of atopic dermatitis with predominantly flexural involvement. She presents with new hypopigmented macules and patches on areas without prior eczematous involvement, especially over the buttocks and limb extensor areas.

- Pityriasis alba
  - Pityriasis alba is most commonly seen on the face and usually does not affect sun-covered areas, and there may be other signs of atopic dermatitis.
- Tinea versicolor
  - Tinea versicolor usually occurs in adolescents and commonly affects the upper trunk, shoulders, and upper arms. It can be scaly and is more well demarcated. Fungal scrapings may show the characteristic "spaghetti and meatballs" appearance of the fungus.
- Vitiligo
  - Vitiligo also presents with decreased pigmentation. However, the lesions of vitiligo are more starkly depigmented and well defined, compared to lesions of hypopigmented MF. The lesions in vitiligo are also not pruritic.

Investigations & Treatment

- Diagnosis of MF requires histological confirmation, with close clinical-pathological correlation. Often, serial biopsies from different sites may be required for diagnosis. We usually offer biopsies 6 to 12 months apart if there is continued suspicion for MF despite prior negative biopsies. It is also important to stop treatments (e.g., topical corticosteroids, phototherapy) a few weeks before biopsy for optimal results.
- The classical histological findings of small or medium-sized T lymphocytes tagging the basal epidermis and

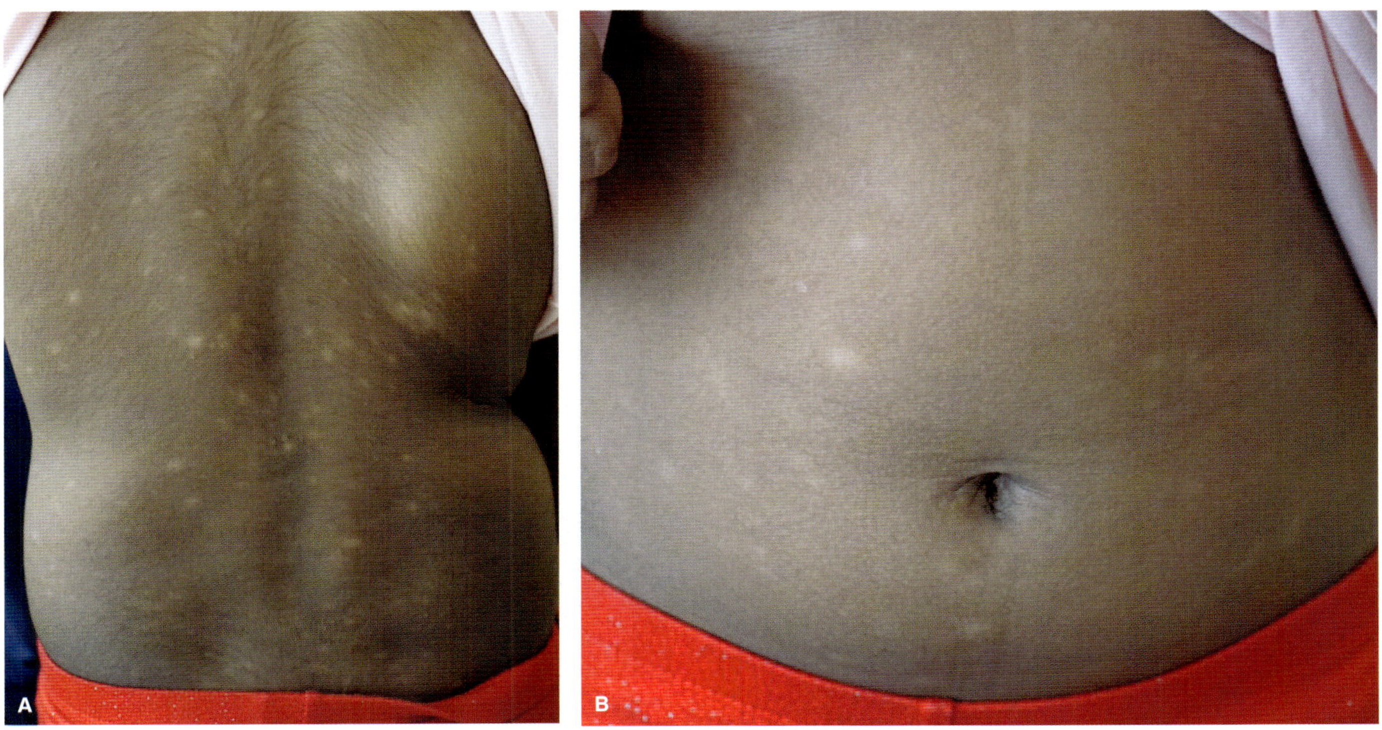

FIGURE 10-28A & 28B. Hypopigmented MF in a 7-year-old Indian girl with multiple hypopigmented macules and patches.

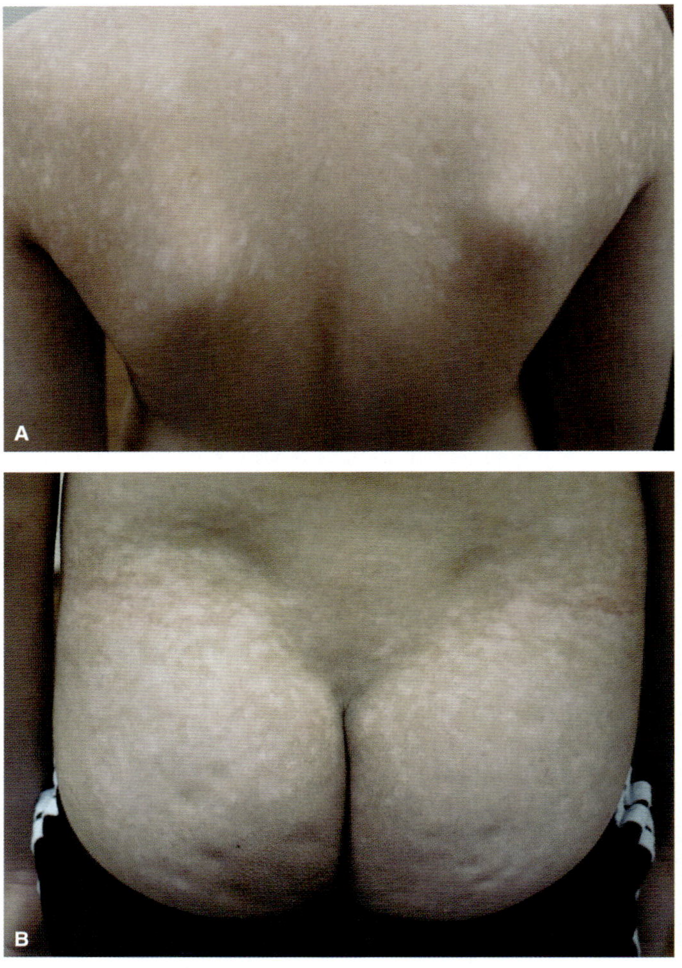

FIGURE 10-29A & 29B. Hypopigmented MF in a 9-year-old Indian boy, with multiple hypopigmented macules, papules and patches over the trunk, buttocks, and limbs.

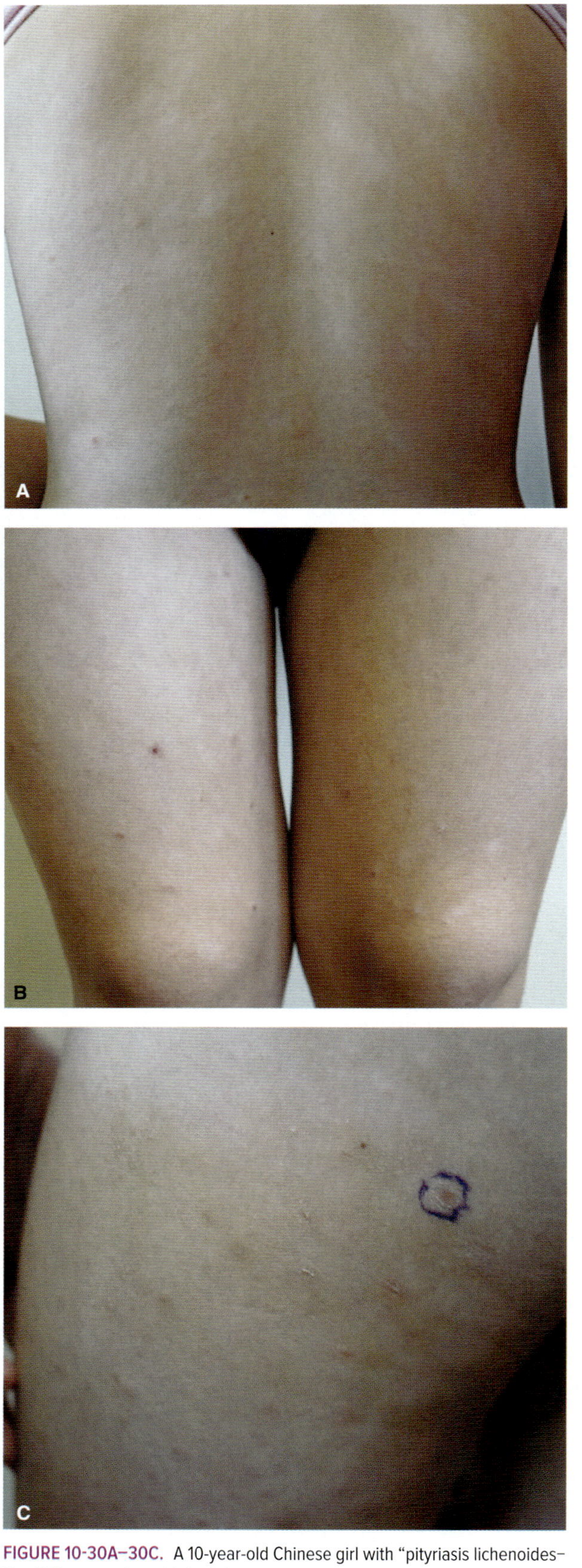

FIGURE 10-30A–30C. A 10-year-old Chinese girl with "pityriasis lichenoides-like MF" presenting with both hypopigmented patches and pityriasis lichenoides chronica–like small papules with peripheral scale.

moving up the epidermis with minimal surrounding spongiosis are classical for MF. Some of these lymphocytes are seen lying in a clear vacuole, sometimes with a few lymphocytes within the vacuole (Pautrier's microabscesses).

- Patients presenting with early-stage MF do not require extensive staging. Staging investigations are indicated for stage IIB and above, and include imaging, such as PET-CT (position emission tomography and computed tomography), bone marrow biopsy, and lymph node biopsies.
- Treatment of early-stage MF is with skin-directed treatment. Limited disease may be treated with topical therapies such as topical corticosteroids and calcineurin inhibitors, topical retinoids, and topical nitrogen mustard.
- MF responds very well to treatment with phototherapy. Thinner lesions may be treated with narrow-band ultraviolet B (nbUVB) phototherapy. Thicker lesions, such as plaque-stage MF, may require treatment with oral or topical psoralen with ultraviolet A (PUVA) phototherapy. Rarely, tumor-stage MF in children may require

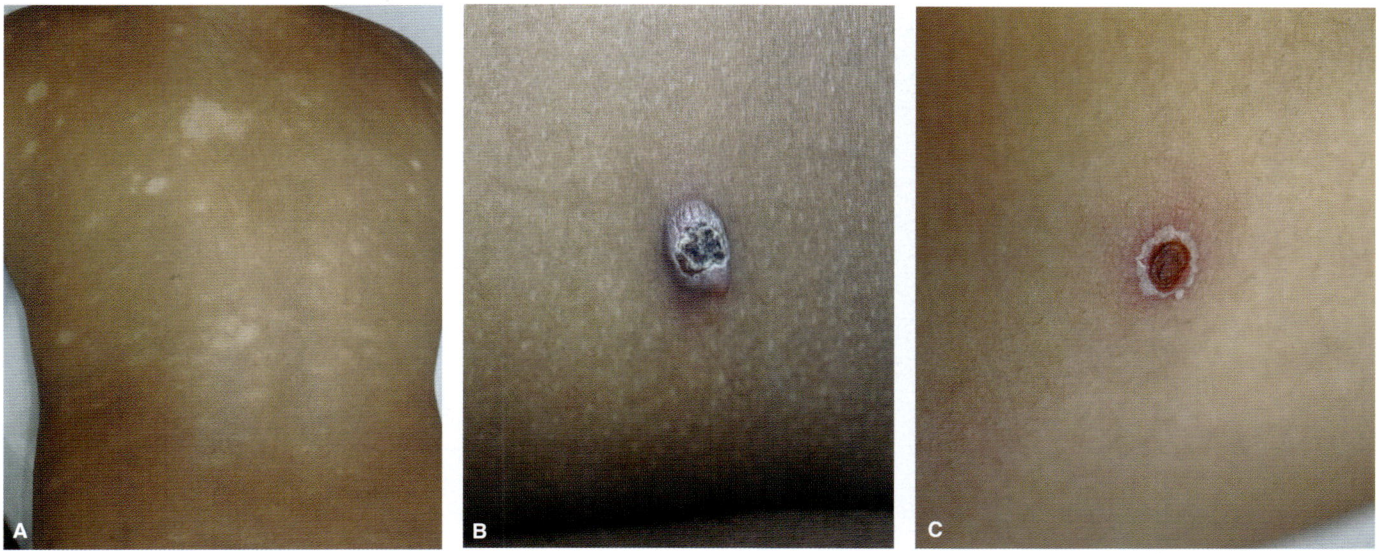

FIGURE 10-31A–31C. A 12-year-old Indian boy presenting with both hypopigmented MF and lymphomatoid papulosis. The latter presents with crusted nodules and hemorrhagic papules (Figures 10-31B & 31C).

treatment with radiotherapy or total skin electron beam therapy (TSEBT).

- Systemic treatments may be considered if there is suboptimal response to topical therapies or phototherapy, or for extensive and late-stage disease. These include systemic retinoids, such as acitretin or bexarotene, methotrexate, interferon, denileukin diftitox, photopheresis, chemotherapy, and bone marrow transplant.

Pearls & Practical Tips

- MF is often misdiagnosed as other papulosquamous or conditions associated with hypo- or depigmentation. A consideration for MF has to be entertained if there are unusual features such as presence of atrophy, poor response to classical treatments, or presence in only sun-covered areas.
- Pityriasis lichenoides-like lesions have been described in patients with MF. In patients presenting with pityriasis lichenoides, it is important to examine for larger patches which may raise the suspicion for MF.
- As MF is not curable, and MF patients have higher risk of developing other lymphomas or other malignancies, these patients should be followed up for life.
- Other cutaneous T-cell lymphomas are extremely rare in children and adolescents, with the two more common ones being lymphomatoid papulosis and subcutaneous panniculitis-like T-cell lymphoma (SPTCL).

Bibliography

1. Heng YK, Koh MJA, Giam YC, Tang MBY, Chong WS, Tan SH. Paediatric mycosis fungoides in Singapore: a series of 46 children. Pediatr Dermatol 2014;31(4):477-82.
2. Wu JH, Cohen BA, Sweren RJ. Mycosis fungoides in pediatric patients: clinical features, diagnostic challenges, and advances in therapeutic management. Pediatr Dermatol 2020;37(1):18-28.

GRANULOMA ANNULARE

Granuloma annulare (GA) is a benign, self-limiting inflammatory skin condition characterized by the accumulation of histiocytes or skin macrophages within the dermis or subcutaneous fat, forming characteristic granulomas. The etiology is unknown, although a delayed-type hypersensitivity reaction to a trigger has been postulated. Although conditions such as diabetes mellitus, dyslipidemia, hematological malignancies, systemic infections (e.g., hepatitis, HIV), and thyroid disorders are known associations in adults, this is not a known association in pediatric patients. Rare cases of drug-induced GA have been reported, including to allopurinol, topiramate, vaccinations, and TNF-alpha inhibitors.

Clinical Features

- GA can occur at any age and is fairly common in children and young adults.
- Patients present with raised, skin-colored to erythematous papules or plaques, with an annular configuration with a central depression, and no epidermal or surface change.
- The lesions most commonly occur on the hands and feet, although they may occur at almost any skin site.
- The lesions are generally asymptomatic, but can be mildly pruritic.
- There are four main variants:
  - **Localized GA** is the most common and often occurs on the lateral or dorsal aspects of the hands and feet. Lesions spontaneously resolve over a few years.
  - **Disseminated or generalized GA** presents with 10 or more lesions, typically affecting the extremities and trunk. Lesions may be more persistent.
  - **Subcutaneous GA** most often occurs in children and presents as rapidly enlarging, deep nodules on the extremities, scalp, buttocks, pretibial, or periorbital region.

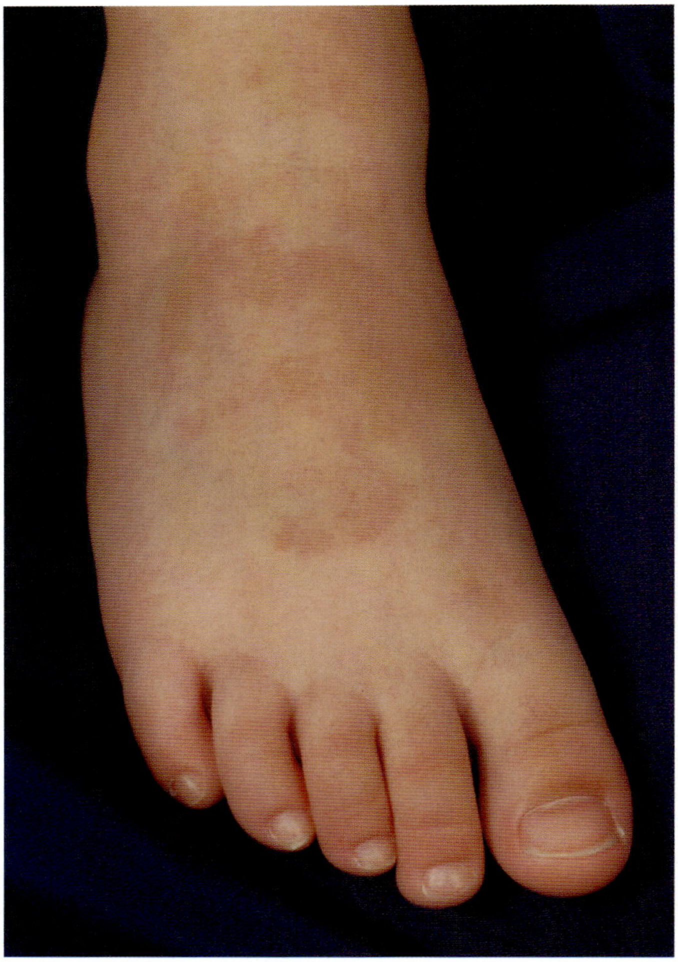

FIGURE 10-32. Localized GA on the dorsum of the right foot of a 3-year-old Chinese boy, presenting as an annular, slightly erythematous plaque.

Lesions may be solitary or in clusters and resolve over years.

- **Perforating GA** is rare. Lesions can be localized or generalized, and present as 1- to 4-mm umbilicated papules with a central keratotic core. Lesions may be painful or pruritic.

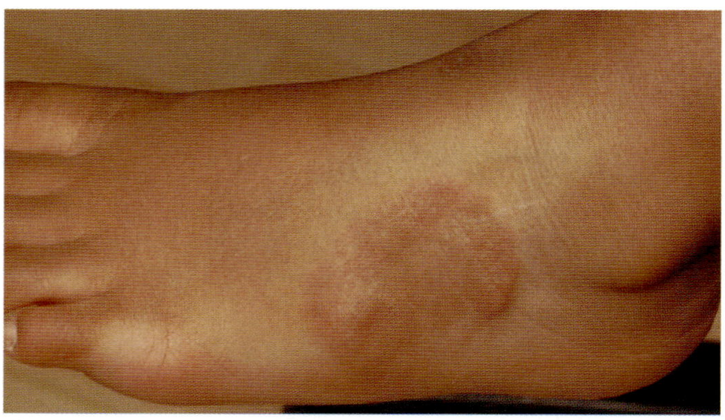

FIGURE 10-33. Localized GA on the lateral aspect of the foot of an Indian child, presenting as a soft, raised, skin-colored, annular plaque.

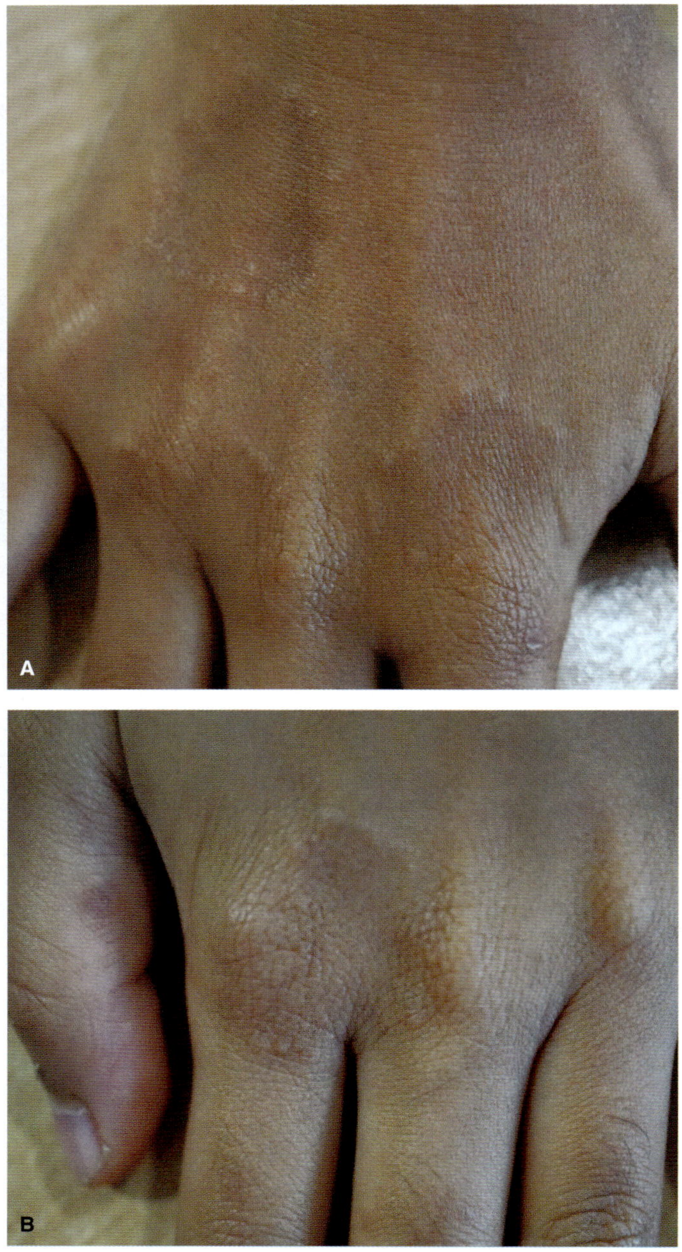

FIGURE 10-34A & 34B. Several lesions of GA on the dorsum of both hands of a Malay boy, presenting as skin-colored, annular plaques with no overlying epidermal changes.

Differential Diagnoses

- Tinea
  - Tinea also presents with annular plaques. However, the lesions are usually more pruritic, with peripheral scaling and central hyperpigmentation.
- Other annular eruptions
  - Other conditions that can present with annular lesions include eczema, psoriasis, pityriasis rosea, subacute lupus erythematosus, and erythema annulare centrifugum, usually with associated epidermal changes such as erythema and scaling.

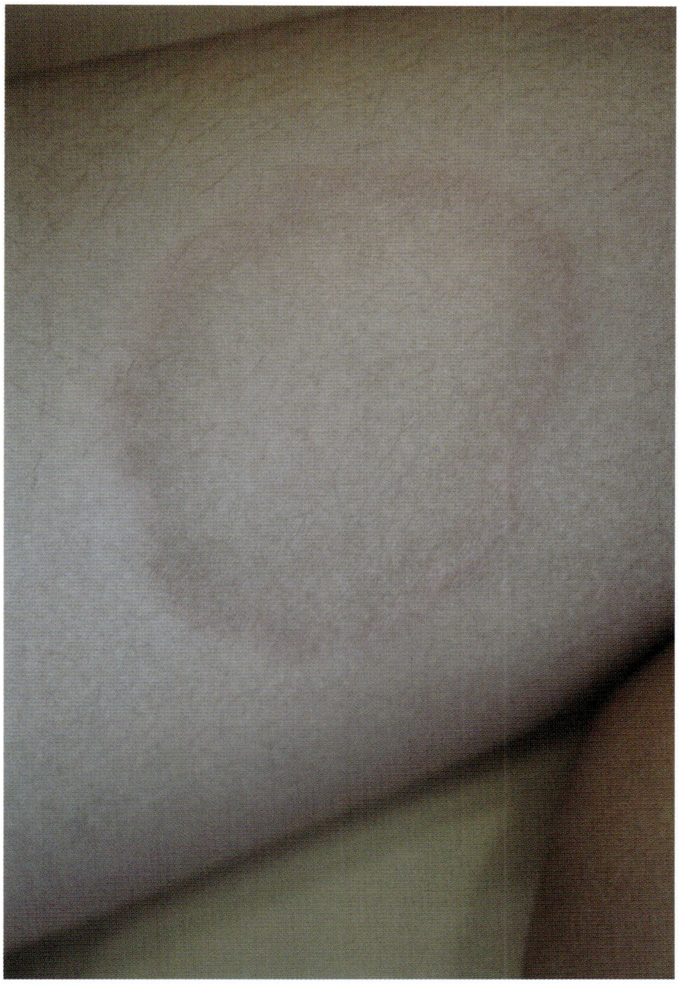

FIGURE 10-35. GA on the thigh of a 6-year-old Indian girl, presenting with a mildly erythematous, non-scaly plaque with central clearing.

- Other granulomatous conditions
  - Other granulomatous conditions can also present with lesions that resemble GA. These include sarcoidosis, necrobiosis lipoidica, foreign body granulomas, and atypical infections, such as deep fungal and mycobacterial infections.
  - The annular configuration is usually absent in these lesions and there may be more surface change, such as scaling and erythema.
  - Biopsy for histology and microbiological investigations may be required to differentiate these lesions.

Investigations & Treatment

- Diagnosis can be made based on clinical features, especially in solitary or localized GA presenting with classical features.
- Skin biopsies may be required in atypical cases, especially of the subcutaneous or perforating type.
- Histological features include palisading or diffuse granulomatous reaction, with surrounding or adjacent to areas of necrobiotic collagen and mucin accumulation. The infiltrate consists mostly of histiocytes with varying numbers of lymphocytes. There is an accompanying perivascular lymphohistiocytic infiltrate. Epidermal changes are usually absent, except in cases of perforating GA.
- Most cases of GA are self-limiting and do not require treatment. Localized GA has been reported to spontaneously remit within 2 years, although recurrences may occur.

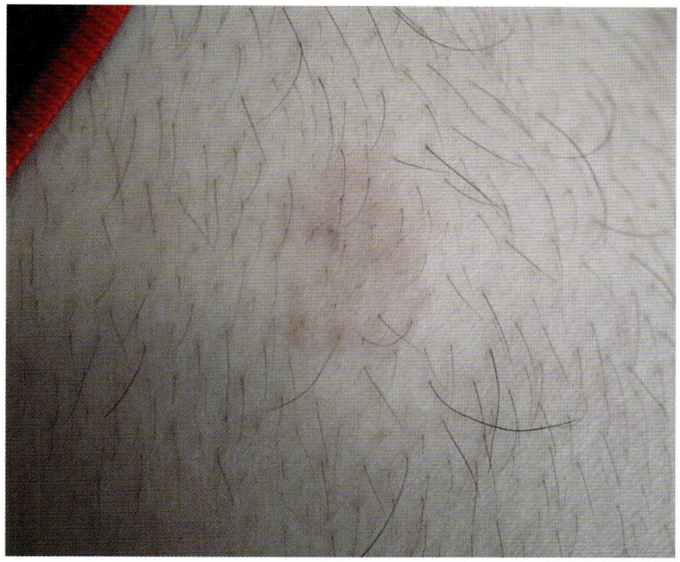

FIGURE 10-36. GA on the thigh of a 16-year-old Chinese boy, presenting with a mildly indurated erythematous plaque with central clearing. Histology showed a interstitial type of granulomatous infiltrate.

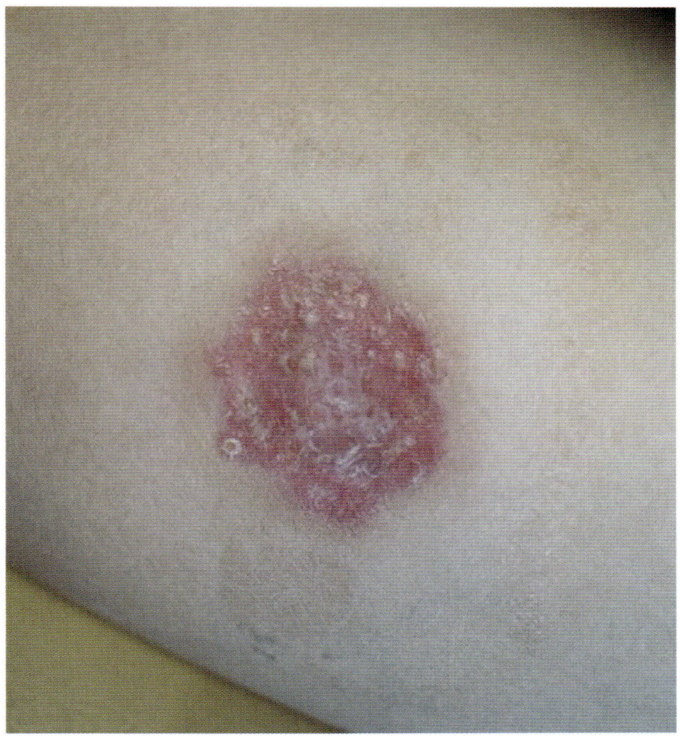

FIGURE 10-37. Perforating GA on the thigh of a 5-year-old Chinese boy, presenting with an erythematous plaque with overlying scale and crusting. There is a vague annular configuration. Diagnosis was confirmed on a skin biopsy.

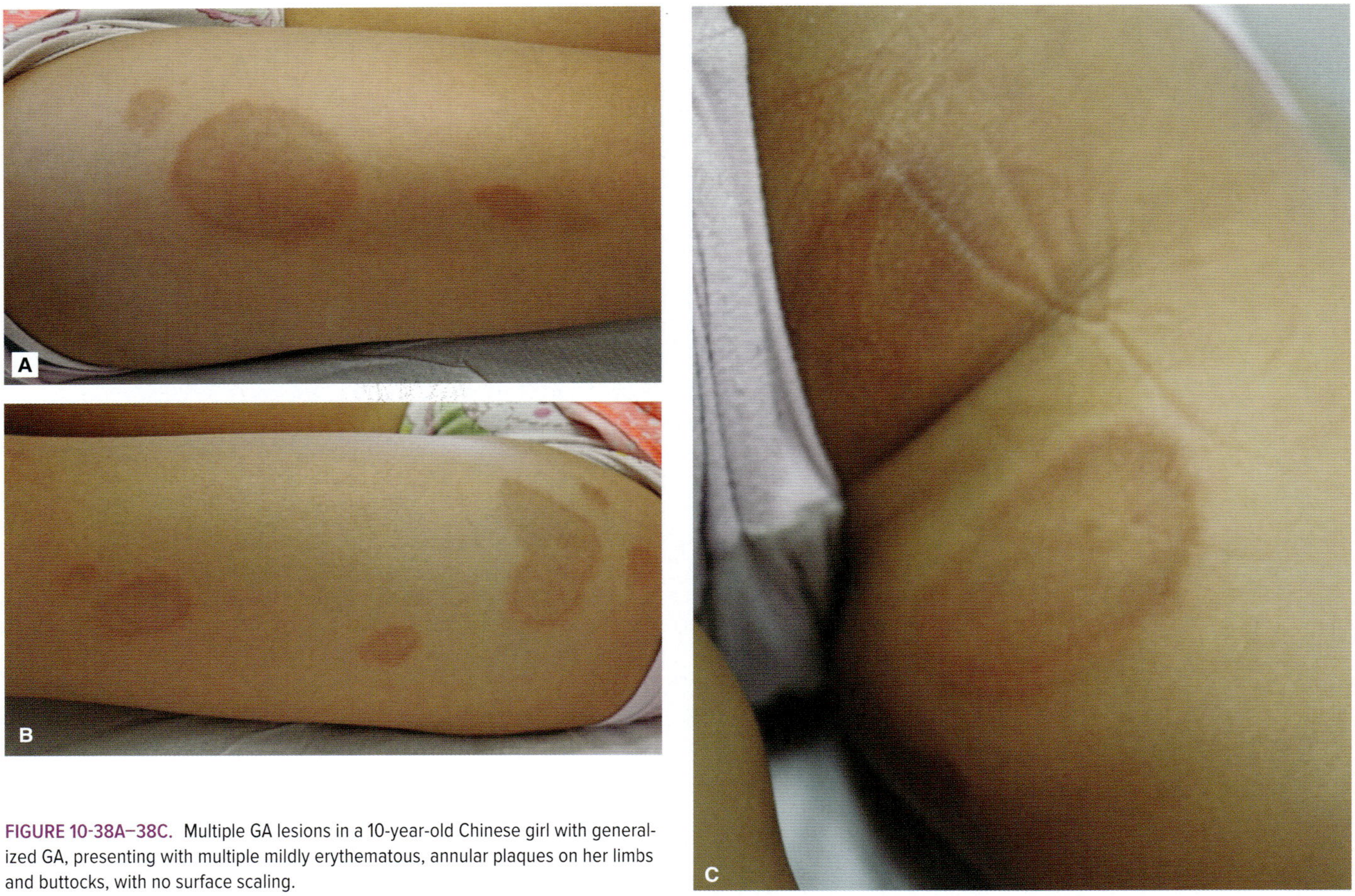

FIGURE 10-38A–38C. Multiple GA lesions in a 10-year-old Chinese girl with generalized GA, presenting with multiple mildly erythematous, annular plaques on her limbs and buttocks, with no surface scaling.

- Topical corticosteroids or calcineurin inhibitors may be used to treat symptomatic lesions.
- Other forms of local treatment include intralesional corticosteroids and cryotherapy.
- Treatments for disseminated GA include phototherapy and systemics such as dapsone, retinoids, antimalarials, ciclosporin, and biologics. However, the evidence is limited, and the lack of symptoms may not justify the potential side effects of these systemic agents.

Pearls & Tips

- The prognosis of GA in children, especially the more common localized variant, is good, with most cases undergoing spontaneous resolution within a few years. It is important to educate and reassure parents.
- Cases of disseminated or generalized GA may be more persistent and challenging to treat. A screen for systemic associations may be considered, especially in recalcitrant, atypical, or evolving cases.

Bibliography

1. Thornsberry LA, English JC 3rd. Etiology, diagnosis, and therapeutic management of granuloma annulare: an update. Am J Clin Dermatol 2013 Aug;14(4):279-90.
2. Piette EW, Rosenbach M. Granuloma annulare: clinical and histologic variants, epidemiology, and genetics. J Am Acad Dermatol 2016 Sep;75(3):457-65.
3. Piette EW, Rosenbach M. Granuloma annulare: pathogenesis, disease associations and triggers, and therapeutic options. J Am Acad Dermatol 2016 Sep;75(3):467-79.

11

Drug Eruptions and Other Hypersensitivity Disorders

MACULOPAPULAR DRUG ERUPTION

Maculopapular or morbilliform drug eruptions are the most common cutaneous adverse drug reaction in children, characterized by generalized erythematous macules and/or papules. It is a form of delayed T-cell hypersensitivity reaction (Type IV).

Clinical Features

- Commonly implicated drugs include antibiotics (penicillins, sulfonamides, cephalosporins), anti-epileptics, and nonsteroidal anti-inflammatory drugs (NSAIDs).
- Maculopapular drug eruptions usually begin 4 to 14 days after initiation of the culprit drug but may also occur a few days after cessation of the drug.
- The exanthem starts as erythematous macules and papules on the trunk in a symmetric distribution, progressing to the face and extremities within 1 to 2 days. There is variable itch and patients may have low-grade fever.
- The palms and soles may be affected, but mucous membranes are classically spared.

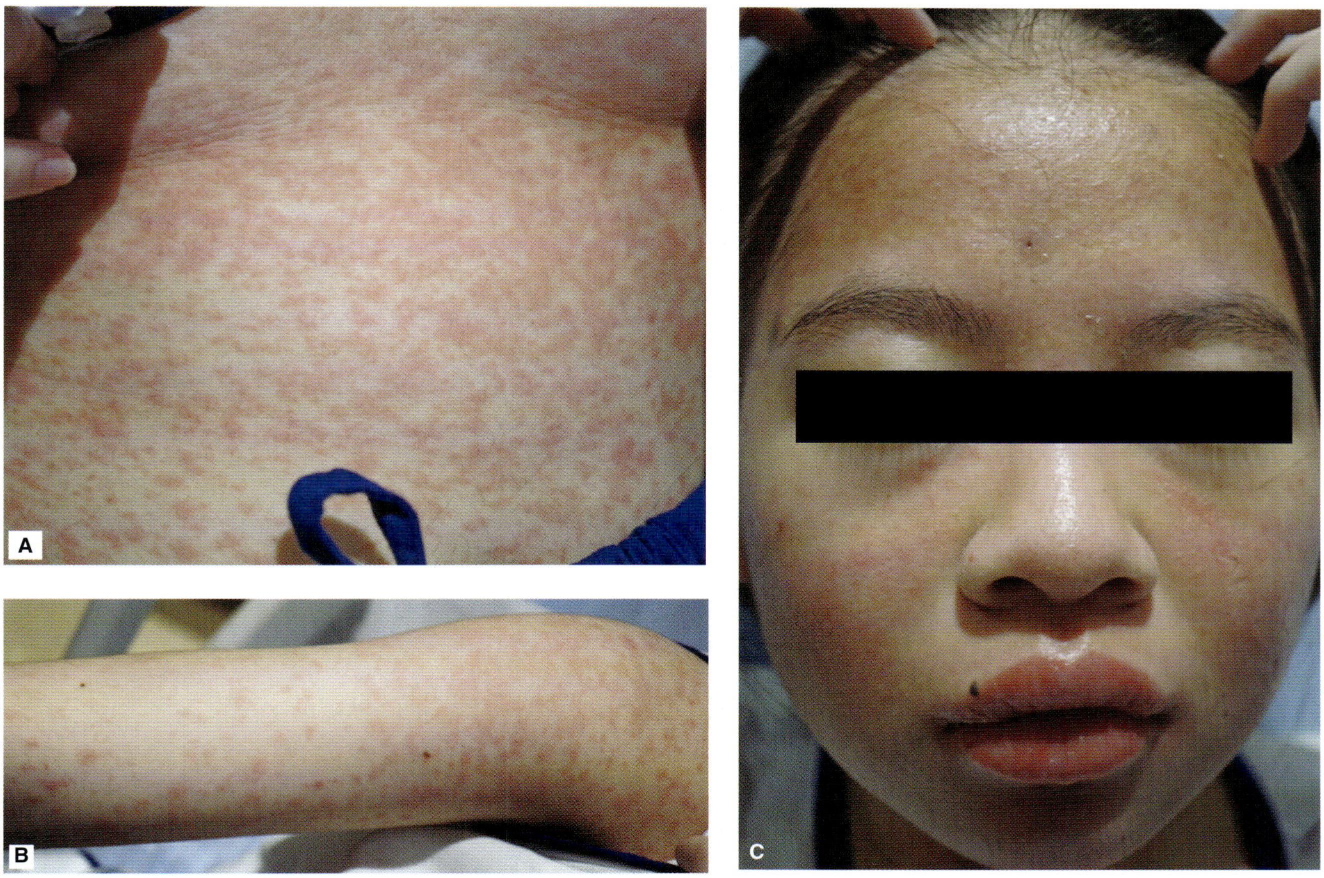

FIGURE 11-1A–1C. Maculopapular drug exanthem presenting in a Thai adolescent girl with erythematous macules and papules affecting the trunk, proximal limbs, and face.

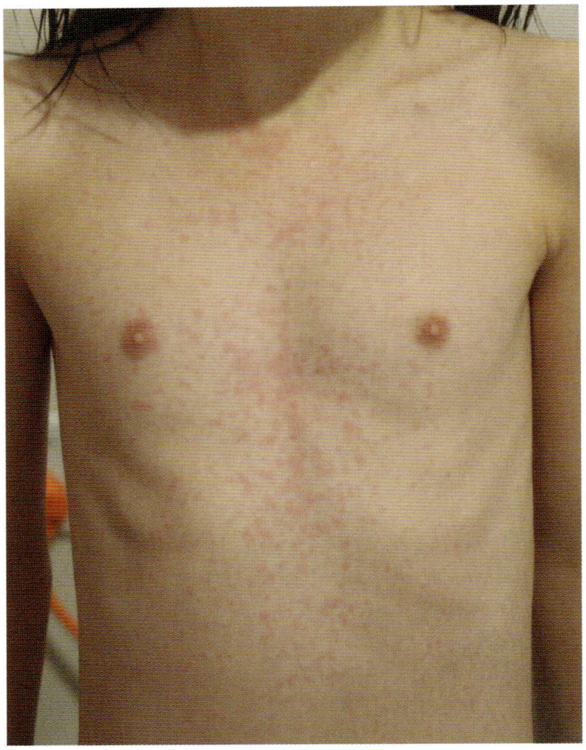

FIGURE 11-2. Mild maculopapular drug exanthem presenting with rather localized erythematous macules and papules on the trunk of this Chinese girl.

- The eruption fades spontaneously in 1 to 2 weeks with post-inflammatory hyperpigmentation, especially in darker-skinned patients. Desquamation is variable.

Differential Diagnoses

- Viral exanthems
  - Viral exanthems are common in children. The rash commonly begins on the face and progresses in a cephalocaudal manner. A history of prodromal symptoms such as fever, rhinorrhea, sore throat, and cough points more to a viral exanthem. Viral exanthems are usually also more monomorphic, while drug eruptions tend to be more polymorphic, with atypical skin lesions like urticaria or targetoid lesions.
  - Complete blood counts may show lymphopenia or lymphocytosis in viral exanthems, while eosinophilia generally favors drug exanthem. Skin biopsies are not helpful to differentiate between drug and viral exanthems.
- DRESS syndrome (drug reaction with eosinophilia and systemic signs and symptoms)
  - DRESS is a more dangerous drug eruption. The cutaneous eruption in DRESS may look similar to a maculopapular exanthem; however, there is usually more facial edema and more severe and extensive rash in DRESS. There are often also systemic manifestations, such as fever, lethargy, and lymphadenopathy in DRESS syndrome.

Investigations & Treatment

- Diagnosis is mainly clinical, with a definite time course between initiation of drug and onset of eruption. Skin biopsy is not routinely done but if performed usually shows non-specific features of mild basal vacuolar alteration and superficial perivascular mononuclear infiltrates, with occasional eosinophils.
- Complete blood count, liver function test, and renal panel may help to differentiate from DRESS syndrome.
- Discontinuation or substitution of the culprit drug helps in the resolution of the exanthem. Topical corticosteroids, moisturizers, and antihistamines can be prescribed for symptomatic relief.

Pearls & Practical Tips

- The two most important differentials to consider when a child presents with fever and rash are viral exanthem and drug eruption. It is also common that children with viral infections may develop an exanthem on exposure to antibiotics, especially the beta-lactams. These children should not be labeled as allergic to the antibiotics.
- It is important to examine for ocular, oral, or genital erosions, lymphadenopathy, and organomegaly in all cases of fever with rash, to exclude more dangerous drug eruptions such as Stevens-Johnson syndrome and DRESS syndrome.

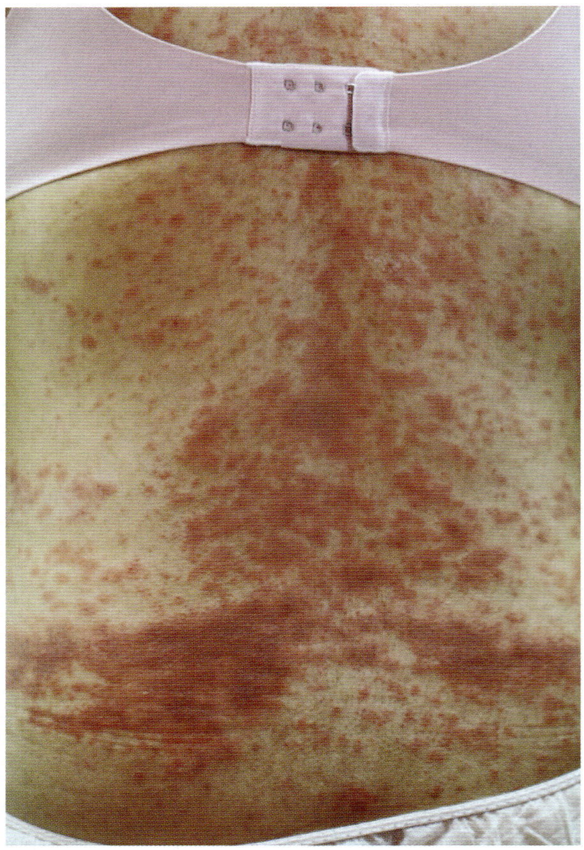

FIGURE 11-3. This adolescent Chinese girl presents with rather extensive maculopapular eruption, with some areas appearing more purpuric.

FIXED DRUG ERUPTION

Fixed drug eruption (FDE) is a common cutaneous adverse drug reaction in children. It is postulated to be due to antigen from the drug activating CD8 + cytotoxic T cells in the epidermis which release cytokines such as interferon-γ, granzyme B, and perforin, leading to keratinocytes apoptosis. These cells then remain in the epidermis as memory T cells and release more cytokines when re-exposed to the causative drug.

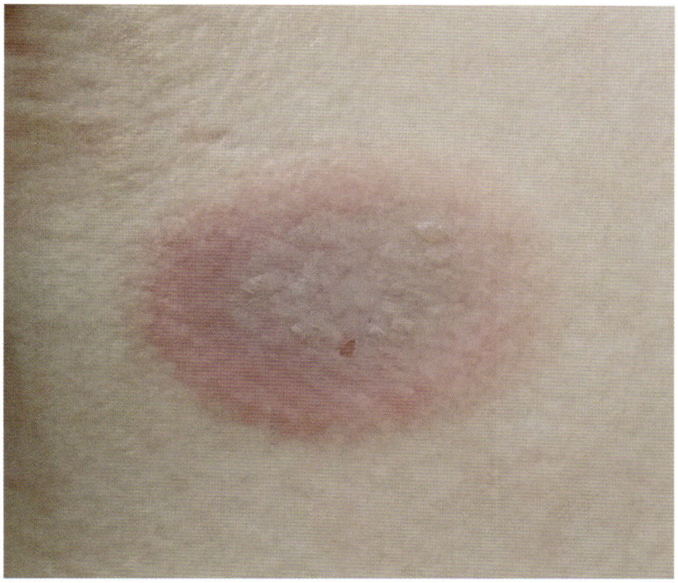

FIGURE 11-4. FDE on the back of a young Chinese boy presenting with a targetoid lesion with a central dusky area surrounded by an annular ring of erythema.

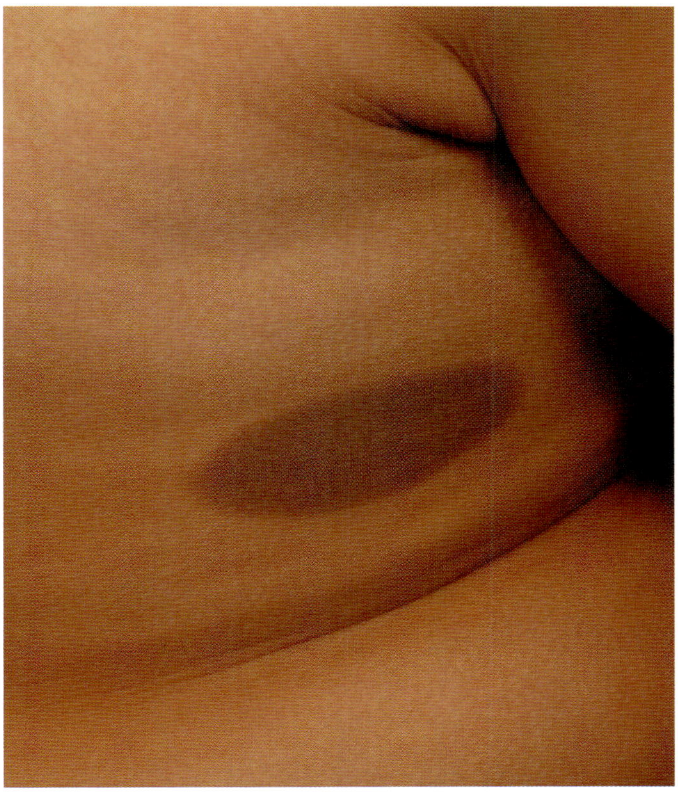

FIGURE 11-6. Pigmented FDE presenting as a well-demarcated, ovoid, brown patch on the flank of this Malay boy.

Clinical Features

- Many drugs have been implicated to cause FDE, but the common ones include antibiotics (sulfonamide, penicillins, tetracyclines), analgesics (paracetamol, ibuprofen, naproxen), pseudoephedrine, and antihistamines (diphenhydramine, hydroxyzine, loratadine).
- FDE usually develops a few weeks after the initial exposure to the culprit drug but recurs within 24 hours with subsequent exposure.

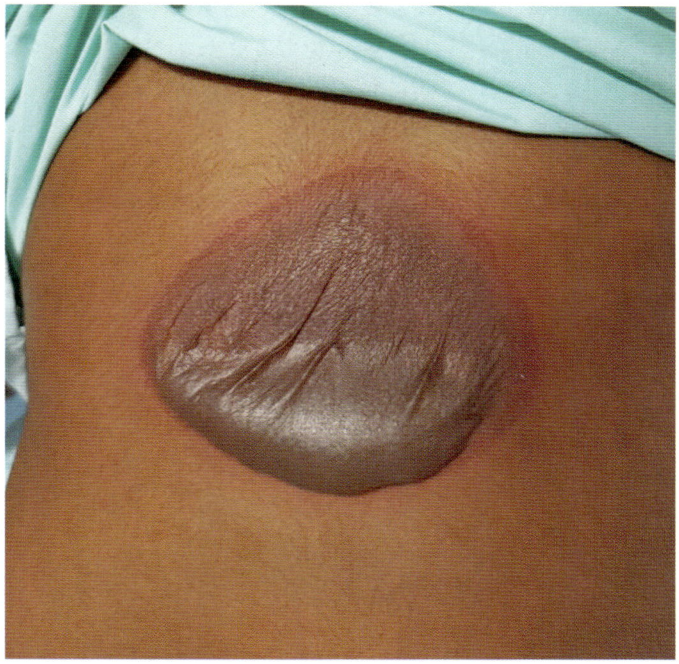

FIGURE 11-5. Bullous FDE on the back of a young Malay boy presenting with a central dusky blister with surrounding erythematous ring.

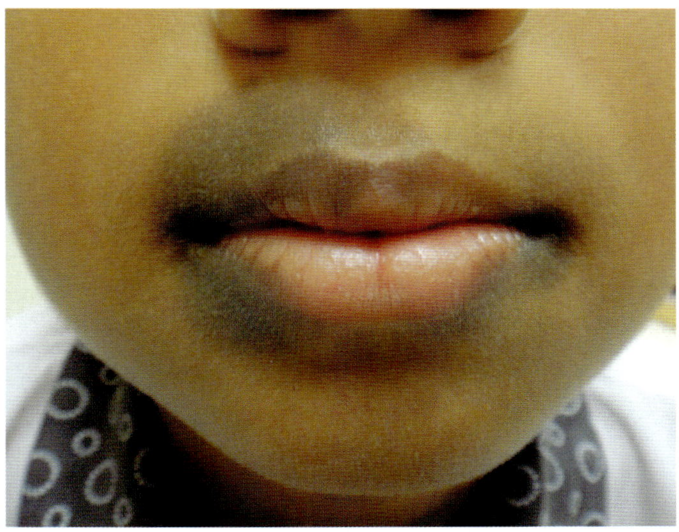

FIGURE 11-7. Pigmented FDE presenting as ovoid hyperpigmented patches in a perioral distribution in this Malay child.

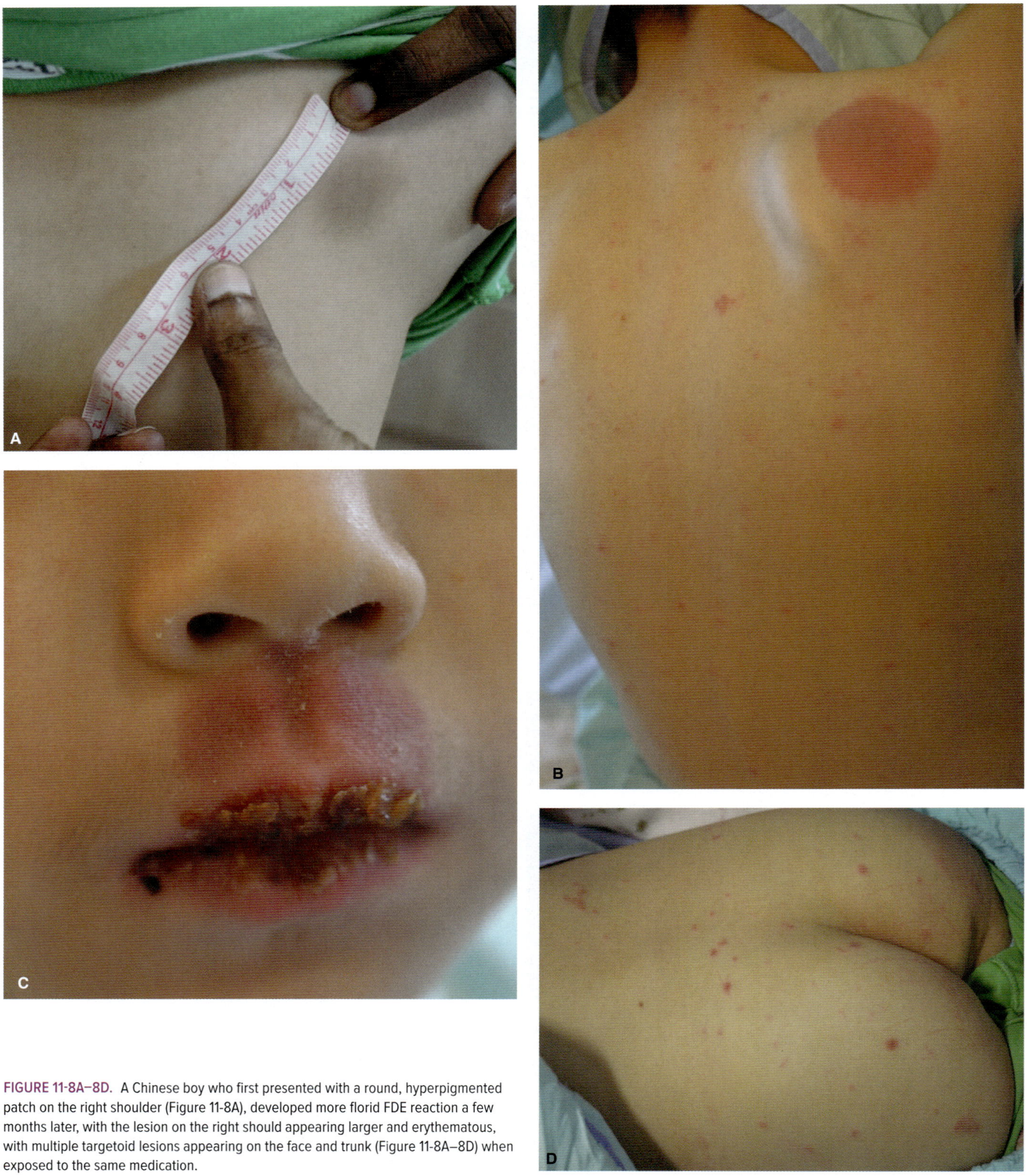

FIGURE 11-8A–8D. A Chinese boy who first presented with a round, hyperpigmented patch on the right shoulder (Figure 11-8A), developed more florid FDE reaction a few months later, with the lesion on the right should appearing larger and erythematous, with multiple targetoid lesions appearing on the face and trunk (Figure 11-8A–8D) when exposed to the same medication.

- Clinically, it presents as single or a few round to oval-shaped well-demarcated erythematous edematous plaques with central duskiness or vesicle formation. Upon re-exposure, it appears at the same sites but can develop at new sites with repeated exposures.
- The sites of predilection include the lips, perioral region, hands, feet, and genitalia.
- The rash resolves in 7 to 14 days with residual gray-brown pigmentation, which may persist for months.
- Generalized bullous FDE is rare in children.

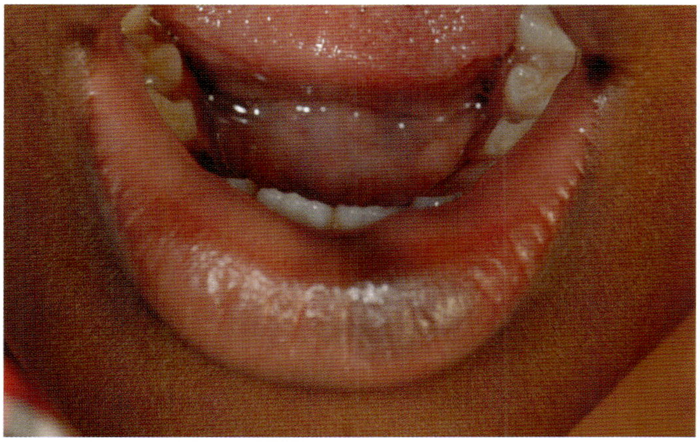

FIGURE 11-9. FDE presenting in an Indian adolescent with hyperpigmented, round patch on the lip.

Differential Diagnoses

- Arthropod bites
  - Arthropod bites are common in children and generally occur on exposed sites such as distal extremities. They are usually associated with severe itch and do not recur at the same site.
- Stevens-Johnson syndrome/toxic epidermal necrolysis (SJS/TEN)
  - If the involvement of FDE is more extensive and generalized, it can mimic SJS and TEN. However, patients with generalized FDE are generally well, without severe mucosal involvement.
- Genital herpes
  - If it occurs on the genitalia, FDE can be confused with genital herpes, especially if the bullae and erosions are painful. Tests for herpes simplex virus (e.g., PCR) can aid in the diagnosis.

Investigations & Treatment

- The diagnosis of FDE is usually clinical, based on history and clinical findings.
- A skin biopsy may aid in the diagnosis, especially when taken in the early stages. It will show necrotic keratinocytes with vacuolar alteration of the basal layer.
- Drug challenge may be offered to confirm the offending drug, especially if there is a list of suspected medications.
- Avoidance of the offending drug is the key to management. Patients and caregivers should be counseled on avoiding the offending drug and any cross-reacting drugs.
- Symptomatic treatment can be instituted with topical corticosteroids and oral antihistamines.

Pearls & Practical Tips

- The diagnosis of FDE is often delayed due to inadequate history or suspicion by patients, caregivers, or healthcare providers.
- We have seen a few patients who had a negative drug challenge when they were well but reacted when the drug was taken when the child was unwell with a viral infection.
- Patch testing has been used to diagnose FDE. However, we do not find this method of testing very useful.

ACUTE GENERALIZED EXANTHEMATOUS PUSTULOSIS

Acute generalized exanthematous pustulosis (AGEP) is a delayed-type hypersensitivity reaction that presents with generalized pustules. It is less common in children compared to adults. In children, AGEP is triggered more commonly by infections rather than drugs.

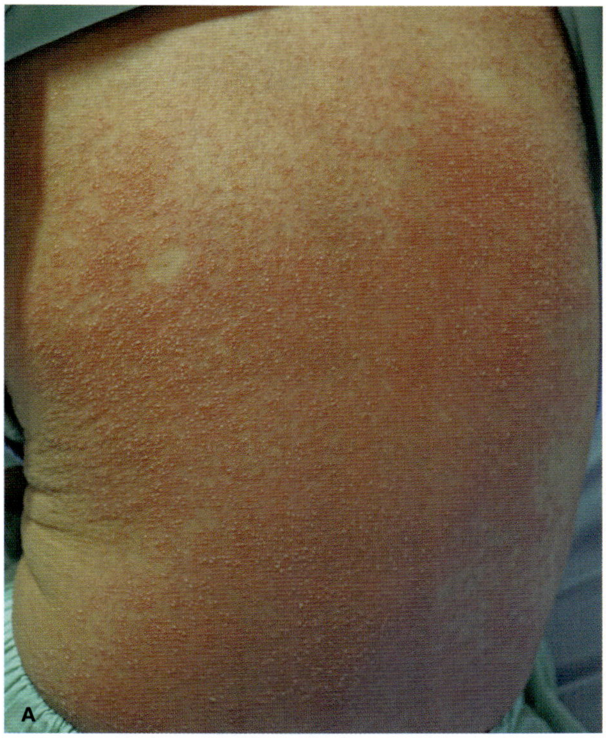

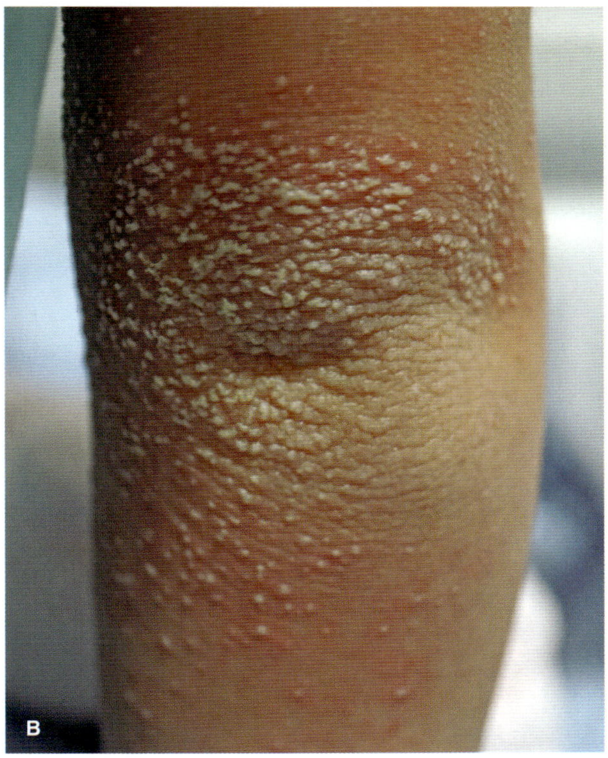

FIGURE 11-10A & 10B. AGEP in a 6-year-old Chinese boy with widespread erythema with multiple pinpoint pustules that coalesce into lakes of pus and superficial desquamation.

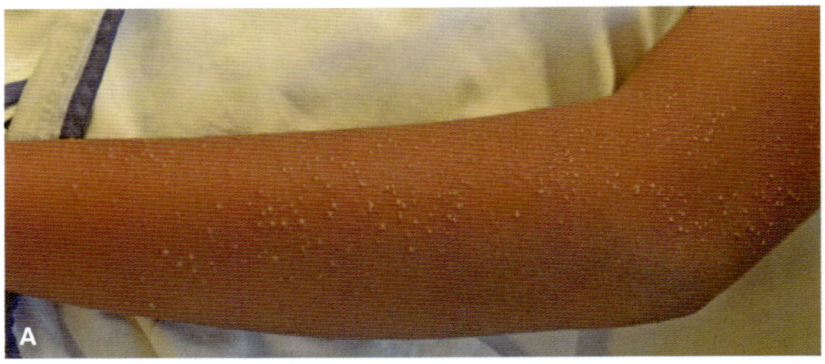
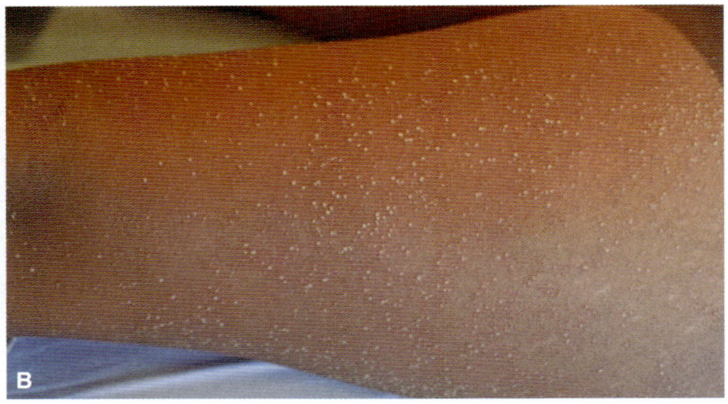

FIGURE 11-11A & 11B. AGEP in an older 15-year-old Malay female with extensive small pustules.

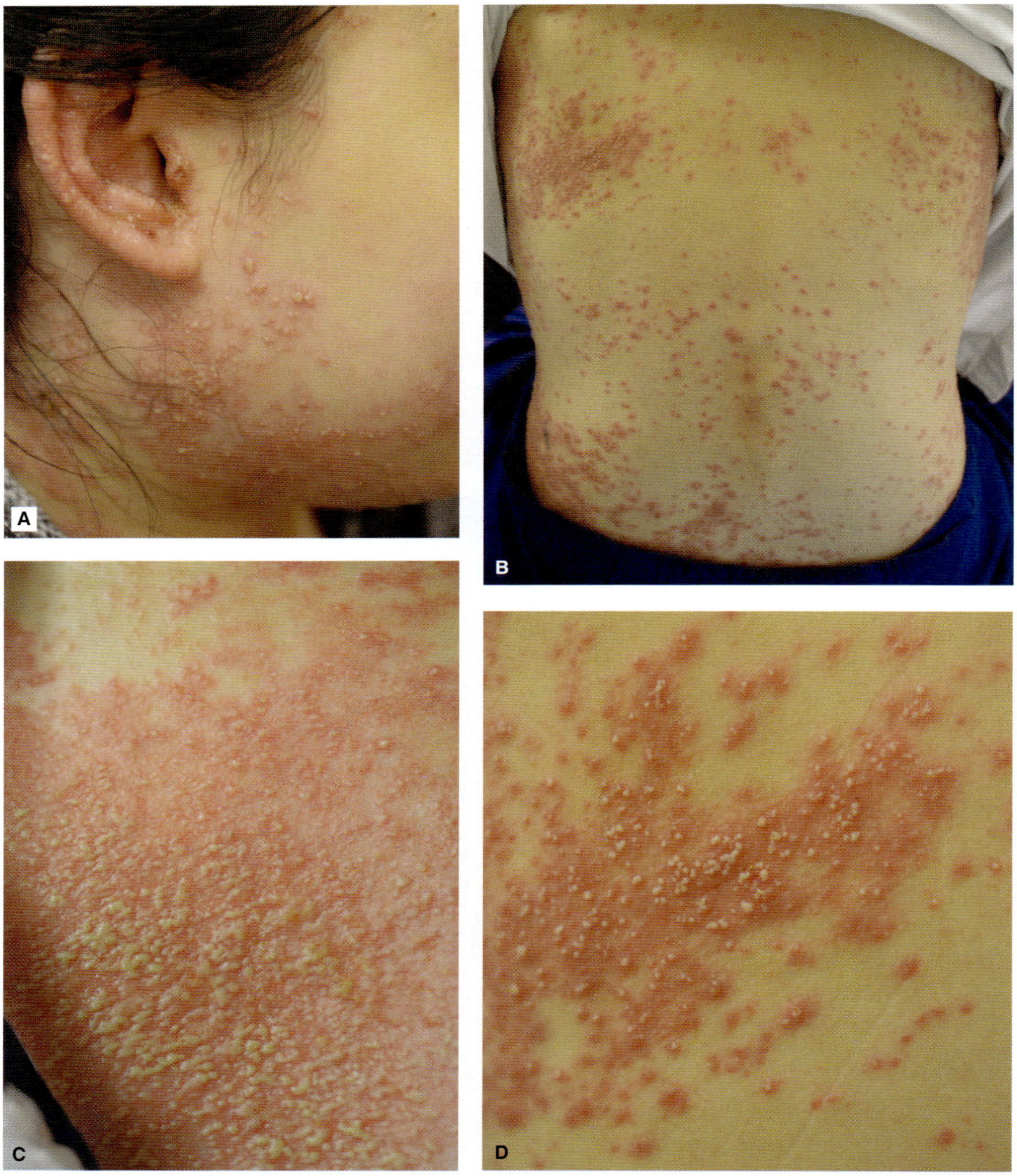

FIGURE 11-12A–12D. AGEP in a 15-year-old Chinese adolescent female with underlying immunodeficiency secondary to interferon-γ antibodies (ISIGA syndrome) with extensive erythema and pustulation.

Clinical Features

- Common inciting drugs for AGEP include antibiotics (beta-lactam antibiotics, macrolides, clindamycin), antifungals (terbinafine, fluconazole), and contrast agents.
- AGEP has a rapid onset, with an average of 48 hours after drug exposure.
- It presents with a mildly pruritic erythematous rash studded with multiple tiny sterile non-follicular-based pustules with accentuation at the intertriginous areas like the axilla and groin. The mucous membranes are usually spared.
- Patients may have an associated high-grade fever and neutrophilic leucocytosis.
- Systemic involvement in the form of hepatic, pulmonary, and renal dysfunction is rare, especially in children.
- The eruption resolves with classical fine desquamation within 1 to 2 weeks.

Differential Diagnoses

- Pustular psoriasis
  - AGEP and pustular psoriasis may be difficult to differentiate. In fact, AGEP has been considered a drug- or infection-induced form of pustular psoriasis. Clinically, pustular psoriasis has a chronic protracted course compared to the acute eruption of AGEP. Patients with pustular psoriasis may have clinical signs of plaque psoriasis before the appearance of pustules, sometimes with nail changes and joint involvement. Both conditions also show similar histological features.
- DRESS syndrome (drug reaction with eosinophilia and systemic signs and symptoms) and Stevens-Johnson syndrome/toxic epidermal necrolysis (SJS/TEN)
  - Pustular lesions have been reported with DRESS syndrome and SJS/TEN. Other features differentiating these two diagnoses need to be examined for to exclude these more serious drug eruptions.

Investigations & Treatment

- The diagnosis of AGEP is made clinically. Skin biopsy, if performed from a pustule, will show subcorneal neutrophilic collections, edema of the papillary dermis and perivascular mixed inflammatory infiltrate (neutrophils, eosinophils, and lymphocytes).
- Baseline complete blood count, liver function tests, and renal panel should be sent in patients with extensive AGEP and high-grade fever.
- In most cases of AGEP, discontinuing or substituting the inciting medication is all that is required.
- Moderate-potency topical steroids along with oral antihistamines can be prescribed for symptomatic relief.
- If systemic manifestations are marked, a short course of oral steroids in the dose of 0.5 to 1 mg/kg/day may be warranted.

Pearls & Practical Tips

- In rare cases, children with AGEP may present with overlapping features of DRESS and SJS/TEN. These cases have a higher risk of systemic involvement and should be referred earliest to a specialist for inpatient care.
- A variant of AGEP is acute localized exanthematous pustulosis, in which patients present with only localized areas of pustulation. Management is similar to AGEP.
- If the pustular rash does not resolve in a few weeks, consider a diagnosis of pustular psoriasis instead.

Bibliography

1. Lee EY, Koh MJA. Acute generalized exanthematous pustulosis in children and adolescents in Singapore: a ten-year retrospective review. Pediatr Dermatol 2021 Mar;38(2):424-30.

ERYTHEMA MULTIFORME

Erythema multiforme (EM) is a self-limiting immune-mediated skin reaction pattern distinguished by the presence of hallmark "target" and "targetoid" lesions. It occurs in all age groups. The majority of cases presenting in the pediatric age group are precipitated by infections like herpes simplex virus and mycoplasma. Some cases may be precipitated by medications.

Clinical Features

- Common inciting drugs include antibiotics such as penicillins, cephalosporins and sulfonamides, and nonsteroidal anti-inflammatory drugs (NSAIDs).
- EM is characterized by acute onset of target and targetoid (or atypical target) lesions. Target lesions consist of round, palpable lesions with three well-defined concentric zones: a central dusky or violaceous zone, a pale edematous zone, and an outer red zone. Targetoid lesions consist of two zones: a central dusky zone surrounded by a paler zone.
- The lesions are symmetrically distributed, mostly on acral sites such as the palms and soles, but can also be found on the face and limbs, and less commonly on the trunk.
- There may be mucosal involvement, generally limited to a single mucosa. Oral mucosal involvement is the most common, affecting the lips, tongue, and buccal mucosa. The conjunctiva or genitalia are less often affected by EM.
- Systemic manifestations are generally mild. Patients may experience low-grade fever, myalgia, and malaise, but are otherwise well.

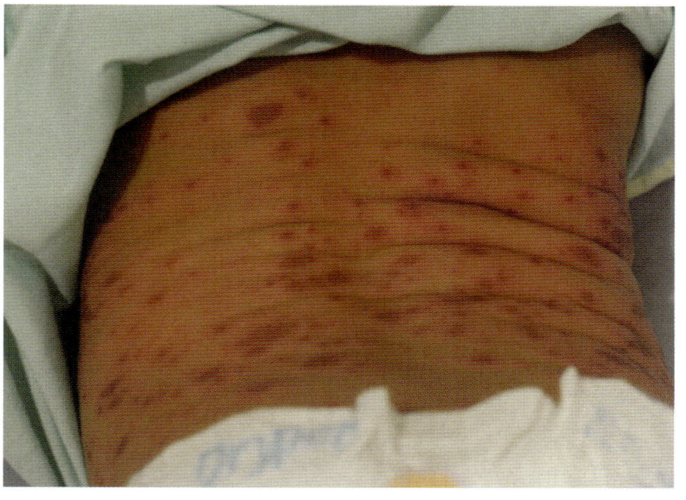

FIGURE 11-13. An uncommon case of EM in a young infant Malay girl after vaccination, presenting with extensive target and targetoid lesions on the face, trunk, and limbs with central duskiness.

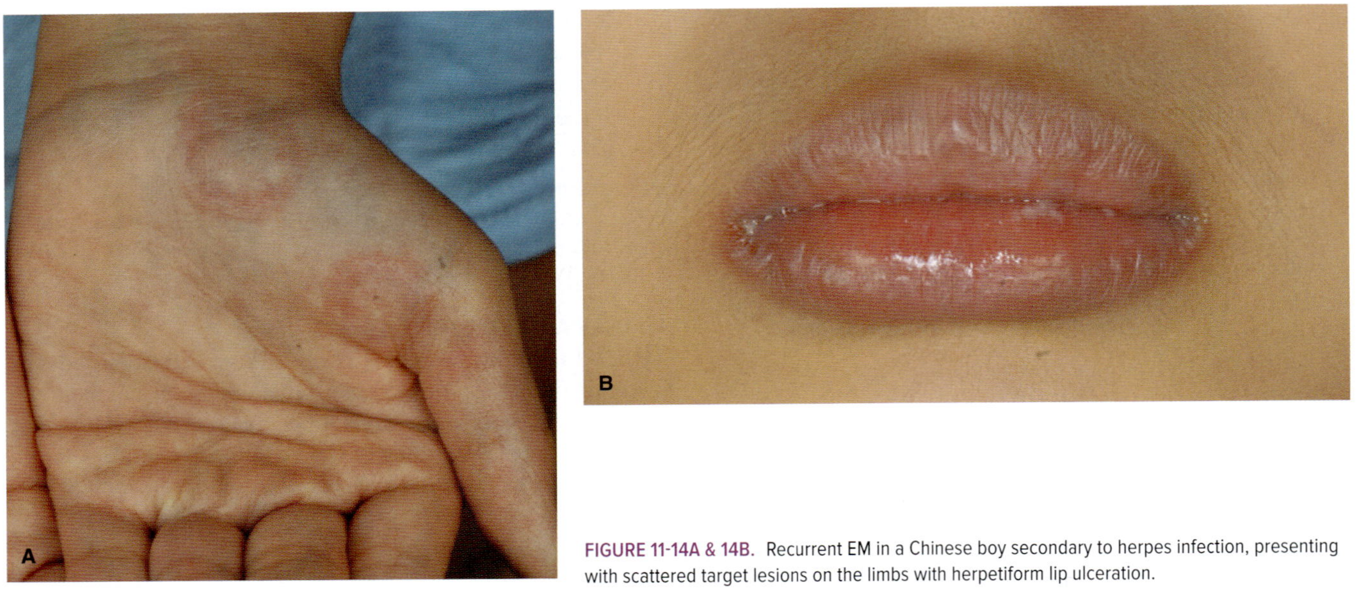

FIGURE 11-14A & 14B. Recurrent EM in a Chinese boy secondary to herpes infection, presenting with scattered target lesions on the limbs with herpetiform lip ulceration.

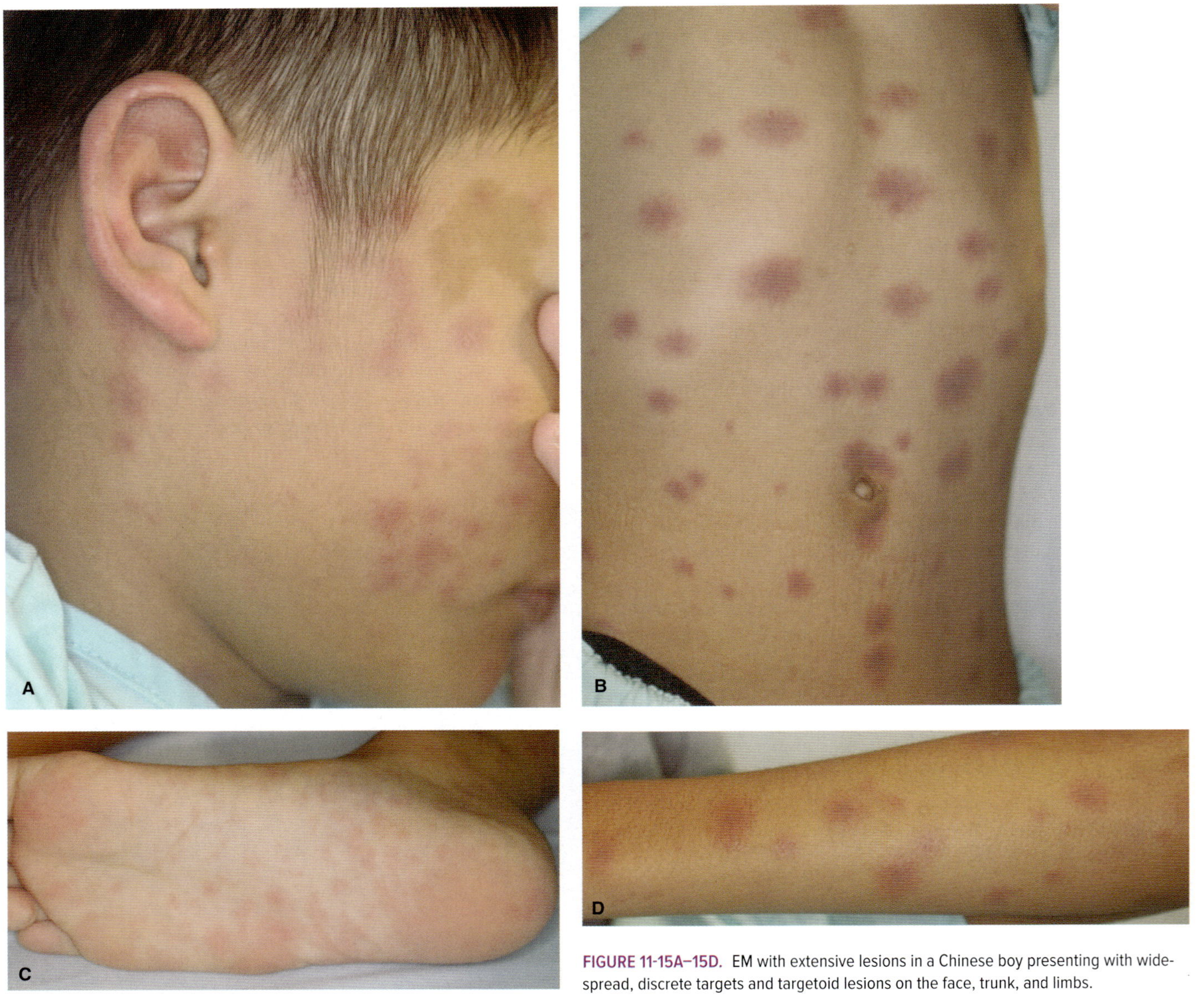

FIGURE 11-15A–15D. EM with extensive lesions in a Chinese boy presenting with widespread, discrete targets and targetoid lesions on the face, trunk, and limbs.

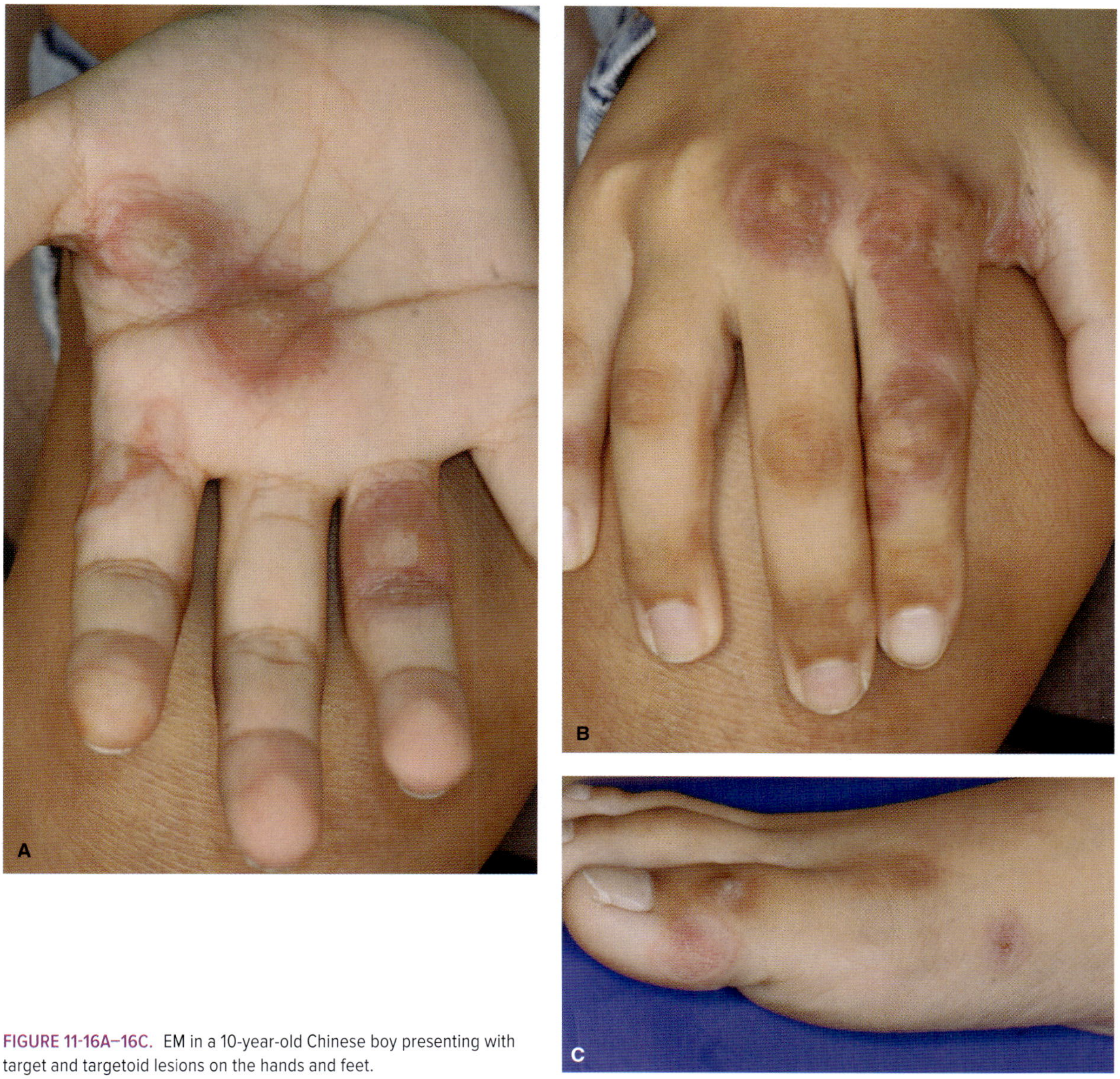

FIGURE 11-16A–16C. EM in a 10-year-old Chinese boy presenting with target and targetoid lesions on the hands and feet.

- Most episodes resolve within 2 to 3 weeks, with post-inflammatory hyperpigmentation.
- Some patients may experience recurrent episodes, which are generally linked to herpes virus infection known as herpes-associated EM.

Differential Diagnoses

- Steven-Johnson syndrome (SJS)
  - Although previously thought to be on a similar continuum of EM, SJS is increasingly being considered a separate disease process.
  - The rash in SJS is more widespread with more than one mucosal involvement.
- Leukocytoclastic vasculitis
  - EM can be confused with small-vessel vasculitis, as EM lesions tend to also be purpuric and fixed. Mucosal involvement is not seen in vasculitis, but may be associated with other systemic manifestations, such as arthritis, and renal and gastrointestinal involvement.
  - A skin biopsy can be useful to differentiate EM from vasculitis.
- Urticaria multiforme
  - Urticaria multiforme is considered a variant of urticaria with targetoid lesions. The central area of the targetoid lesions in urticaria multiforme is lighter than the periphery. The duration of each lesion usually lasts for less than 24 hours in urticaria multiforme and there is no mucosal involvement.

Investigations & Treatment

- The diagnosis of EM is clinical. If required, skin biopsies will show interface dermatitis with keratinocyte necrosis and exocytosis of lymphocytes.
- In the right clinical context, investigations to exclude infections, such as herpes simplex virus PCR, mycoplasma serologies, and chest radiographs, should be performed.
- The first-line therapy is to treat any underlying infection and stop any inciting drugs.

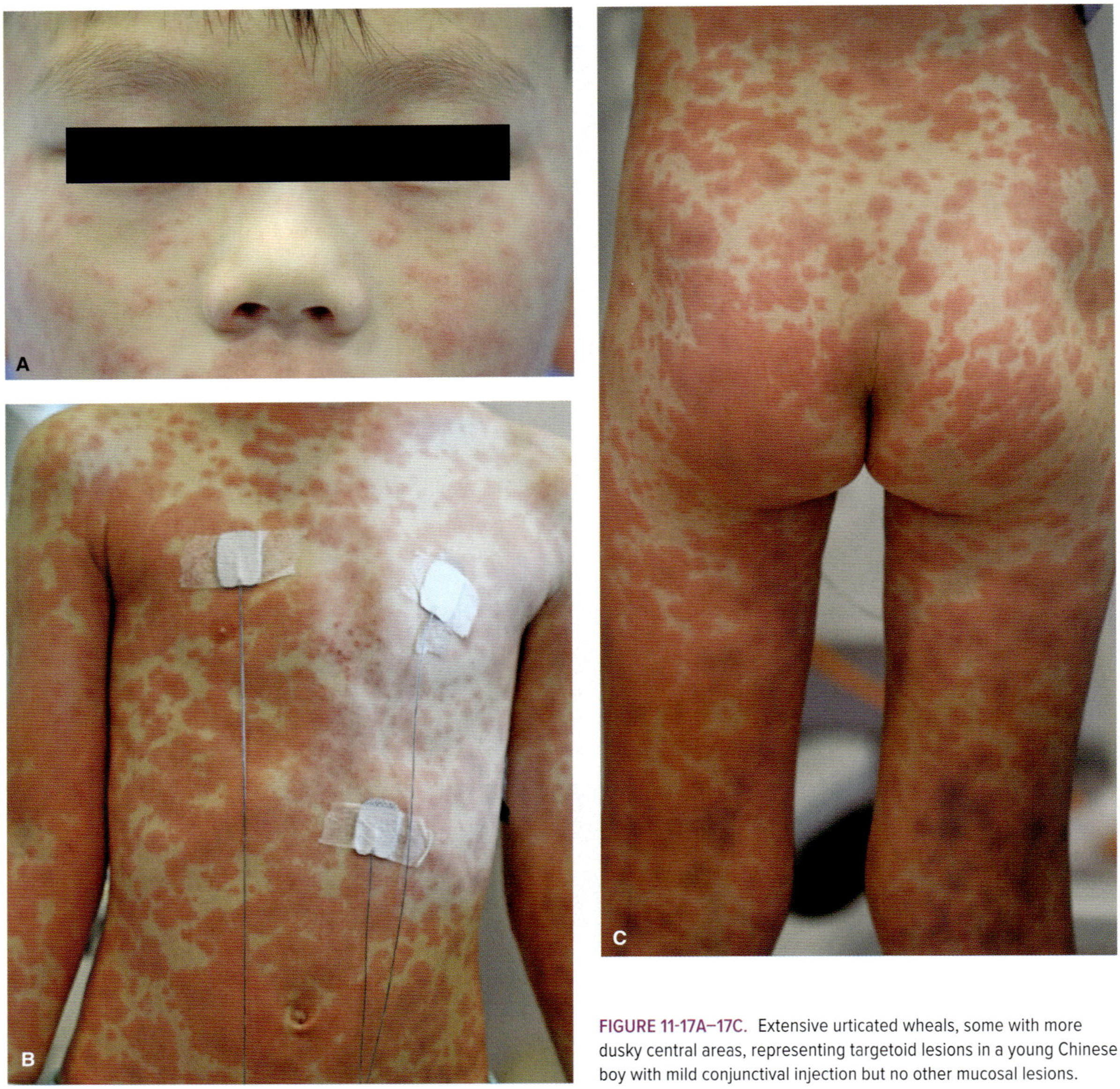

FIGURE 11-17A–17C. Extensive urticated wheals, some with more dusky central areas, representing targetoid lesions in a young Chinese boy with mild conjunctival injection but no other mucosal lesions.

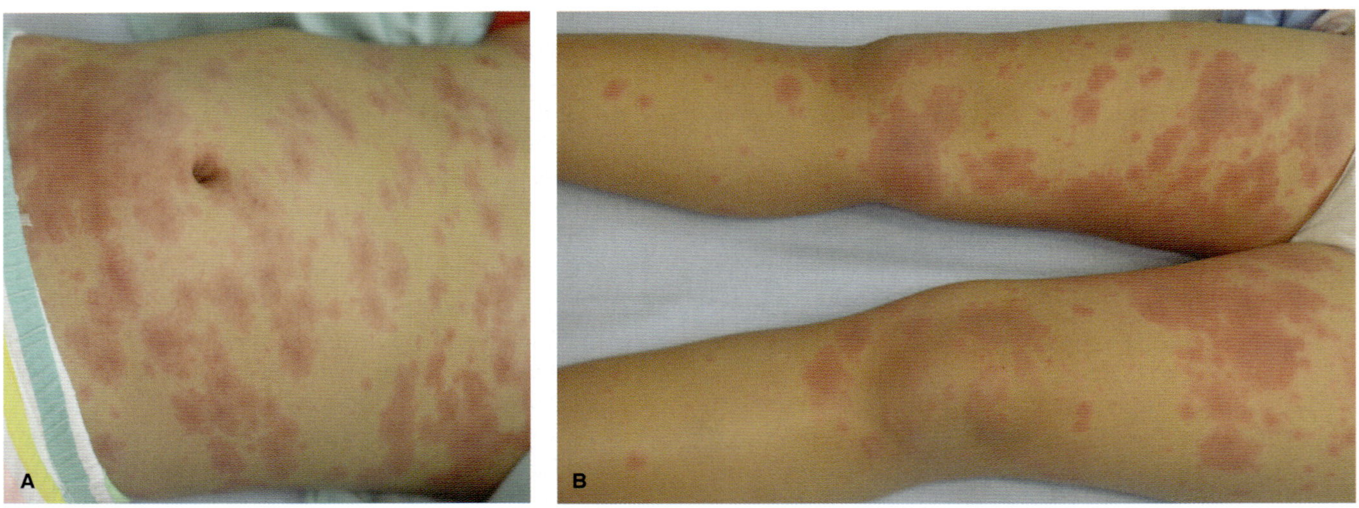

FIGURE 11-18A & 18B. This 3-year-old Chinese girl, also with urticaria multiforme, presents with urticarial wheals and targetoid lesions affecting the face, trunk, and limbs. There is no mucosal involvement.

- Topical corticosteroids and oral antihistamines may be given for symptomatic relief.
- Oral corticosteroids should be avoided, as they may prolong the duration of illness.
- Acyclovir prophylaxis (5 to 10 mg/kg/day) for 6 to 12 months can be considered in patients with recurrent herpes-associated EM (HAEM).

Pearls & Practical Tips

- EM used to be classified into EM major and EM minor, with EM minor having one mucosal involvement and EM major having two or more. The latter is now considered to be SJS.
- In children, EM may also be incited by arthropod bites and vaccinations.

DRUG REACTION WITH EOSINOPHILIA AND SYSTEMIC SYMPTOMS/DRUG HYPERSENSITIVITY REACTION

Drug reaction with eosinophilia and systemic symptoms (DRESS), also known as drug hypersensitivity syndrome, is considered a severe cutaneous adverse drug reaction (SCAR). It is characterized by a maculopapular rash, fever, and systemic signs or symptoms. DRESS is considered a delayed drug hypersensitivity reaction caused by an interplay between drug metabolites and certain viruses like HHV 6 in a genetically predisposed individual.

Clinical Features

- Common inciting drugs for DRESS include anticonvulsants (phenytoin, phenobarbital, carbamazepine), antibiotics (trimethoprim-sulfamethoxazole, beta-lactams), nonsteroidal anti-inflammatory drugs (NSAIDs), allopurinol, and antituberculous drugs (rifampicin, ethambutol).
- The onset of symptoms is typically 2 to 6 weeks after drug initiation.
- The symptoms usually begin with high-grade fever and malaise followed by the development of widespread maculopapular exanthem, which typically starts on the face and progresses in a cephalocaudal manner. Facial edema is characteristic. Mucus membranes are usually spared.
- Systemic manifestations that can occur in pediatric patients include lymphadenopathy, hematological abnormalities (eosinophilia, thrombocytopenia, or atypical lymphocytes), and transaminitis.
- Complications like nephritis, pneumonitis, heart failure secondary to myocarditis, thyroiditis, or meningitis/encephalitis have been described, but these are rare in children.
- The recovery in patients with DRESS is slow, and the illness may persist for weeks to months after medication withdrawal.
- The prognosis of DRESS in the pediatric population is better compared to adults, and mortality is rare.

Differential Diagnoses

- Viral exanthems with hepatitis
  - Viral exanthems that are associated with liver transaminitis can also present with a similar rash with abnormal liver enzymes. These include Epstein-Barr virus (EBV) and cytomegalovirus (CMV) infections.
  - Acute viral hepatitis may present with an exanthem with transaminitis. Viral serologies can help differentiate.
- Kawasaki disease
  - Kawasaki disease can also present with fever, maculopapular rash, and lymphadenopathy, especially in younger children. Other features of Kawasaki disease include strawberry tongue and non-exudative conjunctivitis.
- Connective tissue disorders
  - Autoimmune conditions, such as systemic lupus erythematosus, can also present with generalized exanthematous rash with fever and lymphadenopathy. An autoimmune screen may have to be performed if suspected.

Investigations & Treatment

- The diagnosis of DRESS is made with a combination of clinical history, examination findings, and investigation results.
- Laboratory tests, including complete blood count, liver enzymes, renal function, urine microscopy, and thyroid function test, should be performed in patients with DRESS.
- A skin biopsy is usually not required for diagnosis, but if performed will show variable interface dermatitis with perivascular lymphocytic infiltrate in the papillary dermis, with eosinophils.
- Use of the Regi-SCAR score can aid in the diagnosis of DRESS (Table 11-1).
- Prompt withdrawal of the offending drug is of paramount importance.
- Topical corticosteroids and oral antihistamines are sufficient in the majority of mild cases without internal involvement.
- Systemic corticosteroids in the dose of 1 to 2 mg/kg/day can be initiated if there are signs of visceral involvement (hepatitis, myocarditis, interstitial pneumonitis) and are gradually tapered over a few months to avoid relapse.

TABLE 11-1. RegiSCAR criteria for diagnosis of DRESS.

1. Acute rash
2. The rash is suspected to be drug related
3. Hospitalization
4. Fever (>38°C)
5. Enlarged lymph nodes greater than two sites
6. Involvement of at least one internal organ
7. Blood cell abnormality (at least one of four: lymphopenia, eosinophilia, thrombocytopenia, atypical lymphocytes)

The presence of the first three criteria is essential for diagnosis and the presence of any three of the last four.

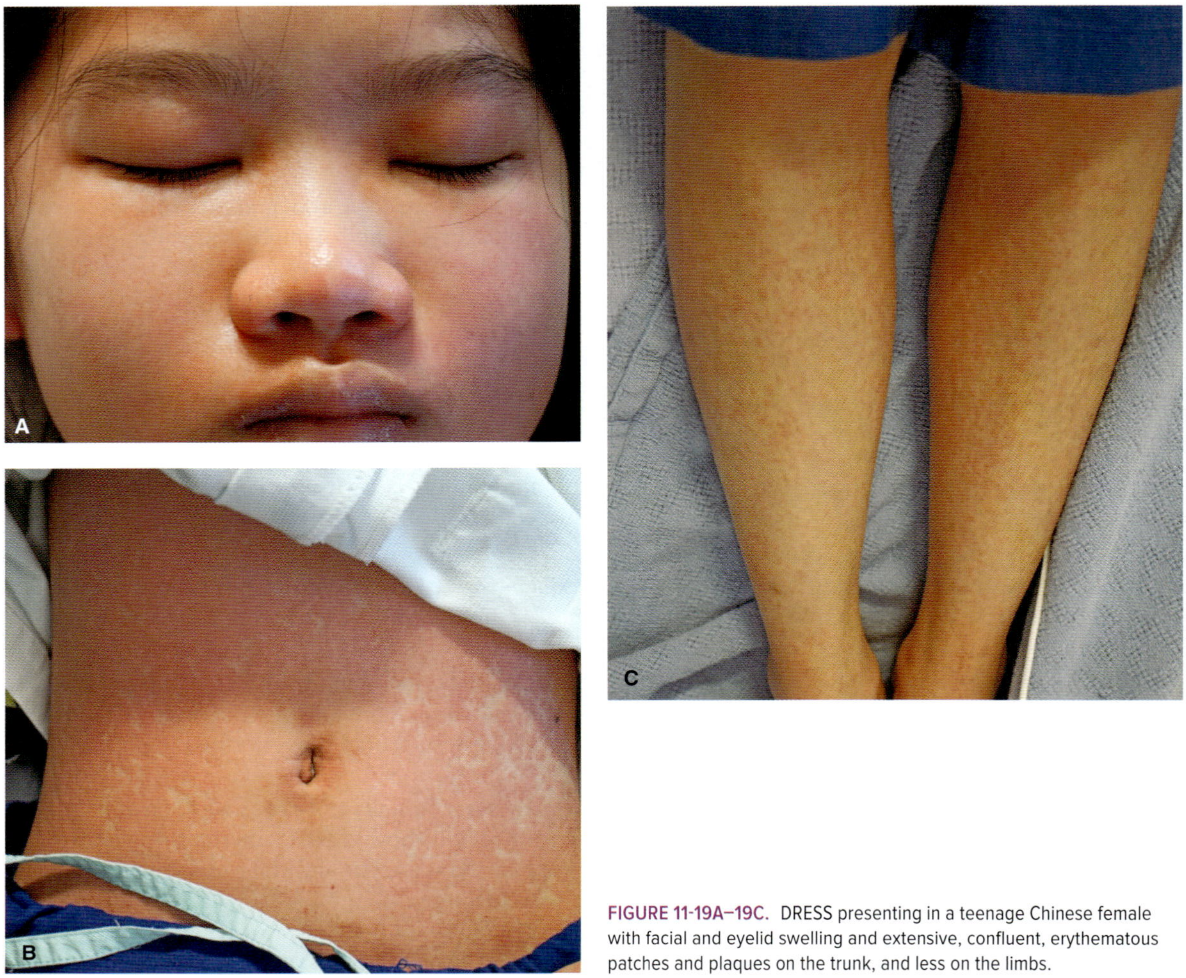

FIGURE 11-19A–19C. DRESS presenting in a teenage Chinese female with facial and eyelid swelling and extensive, confluent, erythematous patches and plaques on the trunk, and less on the limbs.

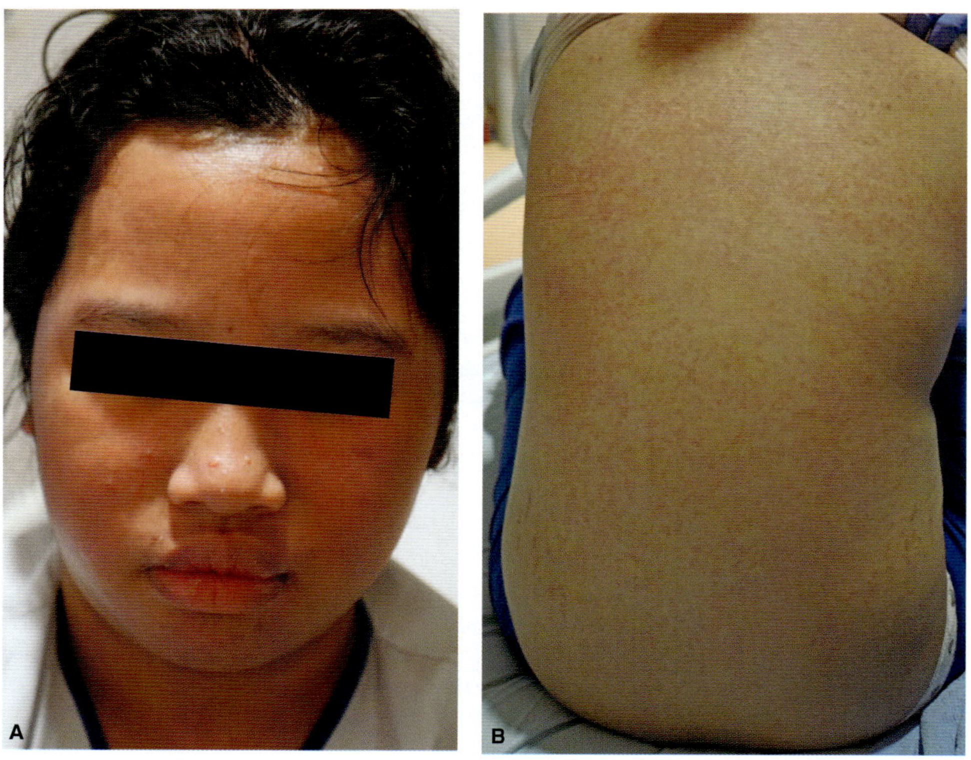

FIGURE 11-20A & 20B. DRESS in a Chinese adolescent presenting with mild facial swelling and patchy, erythematous macules and papules over the trunk and limbs.

Pearls & Practical Tips

- The aromatic anti-epileptics can cross-react, so affected patients should avoid all aromatic anti-epileptics, including phenobarbital, phenytoin, carbamazepine, lamotrigine, and oxcarbazepine. Alternative anti-epileptics include valproate, levetiracetam, gabapentin, and topiramate.
- Trimethoprim-sulfamethoxazole is one of the most common offending drugs causing DRESS in the pediatric population. It should be avoided as a first-line oral antibiotic in teenagers with acne.
- First-degree relatives of patients with DRESS are at higher risk of developing similar drug reactions.

Bibliography

1. Han XD, Koh MJA, Wong SMY. Drug reaction with eosinophilia and systemic symptoms in a cohort of Asian children. Pediatr Dermatol 2019 May;36(3):324-9.

STEVENS-JOHNSON SYNDROME/TOXIC EPIDERMAL NECROLYSIS

Stevens-Johnson syndrome (SJS) and toxic epidermal necrolysis (TEN) are on a spectrum of the most severe cutaneous adverse reactions (SCAR). They are characterized by keratinocyte apoptosis and widespread epidermal detachment. The incidence of SJS/TEN increases with age and is uncommon in children. In the pediatric age group, SJS occurs more often than TEN and may be triggered by infections or drugs. TEN is predominantly precipitated by drugs.

Clinical Features

- Common inciting drugs for SJS and TEN include antibiotics, such as sulfonamides and penicillins, antiepileptics, such as phenobarbital, carbamazepine, and lamotrigine, nonsteroidal anti-inflammatory drugs (NSAIDs), and allopurinol. SJS can also be associated with mycoplasma and herpes simplex virus infections.
- The illness typically begins with prodromal symptoms, such as fever, malaise, headache, cough, sore throat, diarrhea, arthralgia, and myalgia that begin 1 to 3 weeks after initiation of the inciting drug. However, the latent period can be up to 2 months.
- The patient then develops painful, irregularly shaped, symmetrically distributed purpuric macules initially over the face and upper trunk. These coalesce to form large targetoid lesions with flaccid bullae that rupture to leave superficial painful erosions.
- Epidermal detachment is an important clinical hallmark of SJS/TEN. Based on the degree of epidermal detachment, the condition is classified as SJS if detached epidermis affects <10% of body surface area, SJS/TEN overlap if detached epidermis affects between 10% and 30% of body surface area, and TEN if detached epidermis affects >30% of body surface area.
- Nikolsky sign is invariably positive, demonstrated by exerting mechanical pressure with a finger on the border of an intact blister, resulting in the dislodgment of the normal epidermis and extension of the blister.
- Extensive mucous membrane involvement occurs in almost all cases of SJS and TEN, with at least two mucosal surfaces involved, which may include the oral mucosa (lips, tongue, buccal mucosa), eyes, and genitalia. These areas show painful superficial erosions and ulcerations with varying degrees of hemorrhagic crusting.
- Oral mucosa is almost always involved, leading to difficulty in eating and drinking.
- Eye involvement may range from mild conjunctivitis to severe erosive keratitis that can lead to blindness.
- Genital erosions lead to difficulty in micturition.
- Systemic involvement may occur in the form of lymphadenopathy, pneumonitis, acute kidney injury, myocarditis, or transaminitis.
- The compromised skin barrier and extensive epidermal denudation may lead to excessive fluid loss, electrolyte imbalance, impairment of temperature regulation, bacterial superinfection or sepsis, and excessive energy expenditure.
- The course of SJS/TEN is generally protracted, lasting over a month. However, milder cases may heal in 10 to 15 days. Mortality and morbidity in children is much lower compared to adults.
- Long-term sequelae may occur in the form of cutaneous hyperpigmentation or scars, dry eyes, trichiasis, symblepharon, dystrophic nails, or synechia formation in the genitalia.

Differential Diagnoses

- Erythema multiforme (EM) and multiple fixed drug eruptions (FDE)
  - EM is more common in children than SJS or TEN. It is usually caused by infections but can also be caused by drugs. Children with EM tend to be generally well.
  - Similarly, multiple FDE can also present with targetoid lesions with central blistering and erosion. Mucosal involvement can also occur. However, as with EM, patients are generally well.
- Staphylococcal scalded skin syndrome (SSSS)
  - SSSS is a superficial blistering disorder caused by exfoliative toxin produced by *Staphylococcus aureus*. It is more common below the age of 5 years, and can occur in the neonatal period, which is extremely rare for SJS/TEN.
  - The blisters in SSSS are also very superficial and break easily, leading to superficial erosions. Nikolsky sign is also positive, and patients with SSSS can also appear ill. The rash in SSSS is usually more pronounced in the intertriginous areas, such as the neck, axilla, and inguinal folds.
  - In SSSS there is also no mucosal involvement.
- Autoimmune bullous disorders
  - Autoimmune bullous disorders such as pemphigus vulgaris can also present with flaccid blisters and mucosal erosions. However, the onset is usually more gradual over weeks to months, and patients are generally not unwell.

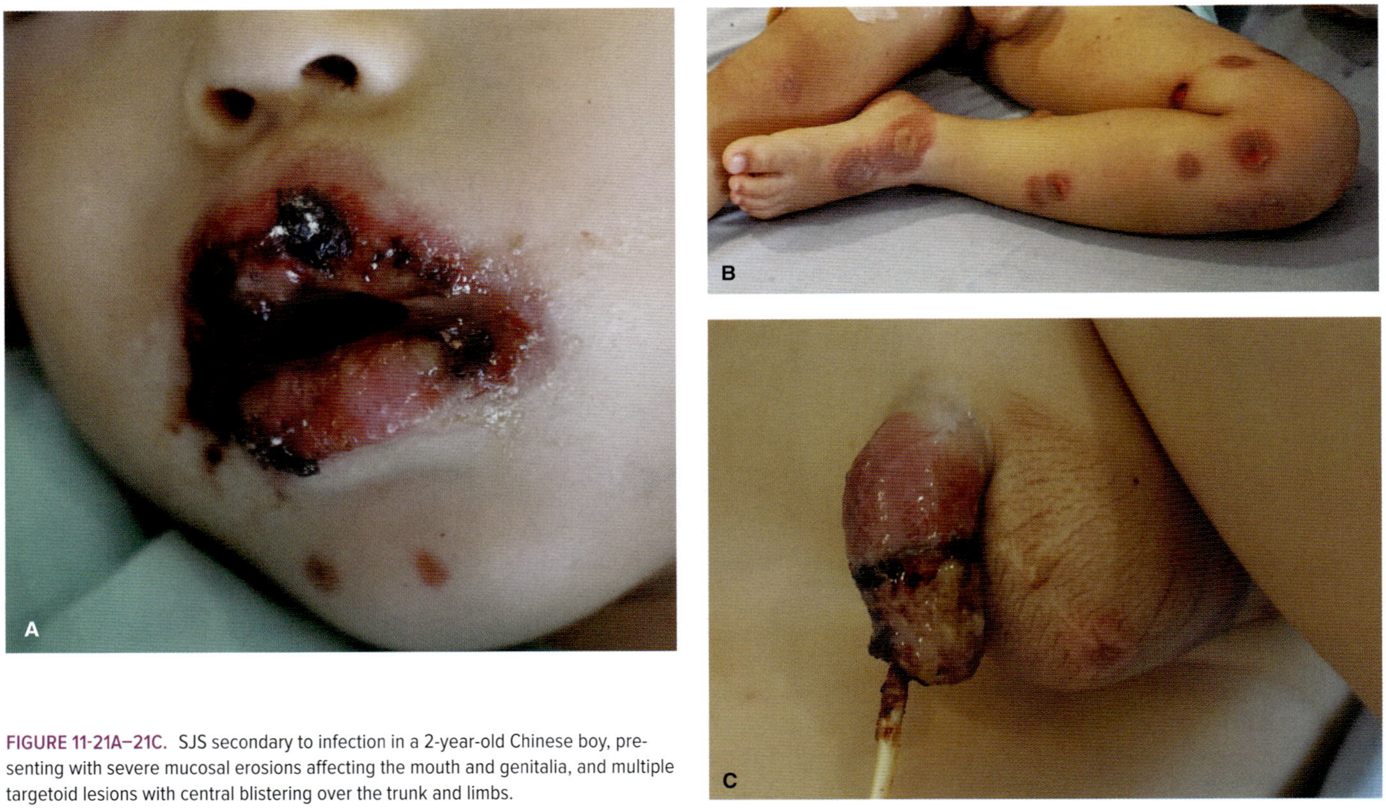

FIGURE 11-21A–21C. SJS secondary to infection in a 2-year-old Chinese boy, presenting with severe mucosal erosions affecting the mouth and genitalia, and multiple targetoid lesions with central blistering over the trunk and limbs.

- Bullous lupus erythematosus can also present with blisters and erosions, with mucosal ulceration. Other features of lupus erythematosus may be present.
- Skin biopsies, immunofluorescence studies, and autoimmune serologies can help to differentiate from SJS/TEN.

Investigations & Treatment

- The diagnosis of SJS/TEN is usually clinical. Skin biopsies will show full-thickness epidermal necrosis, subepidermal cleft, interface change, and a sparse inflammatory infiltrate in the superficial dermis, sometimes with eosinophils.
- SCORTEN score (Tables 11-2 and 11-3) is a prognostic score that helps to predict the mortality rate but has only been validated in adults. It is to be calculated within 24 hours of admission and at day.
- Laboratory investigations, including complete blood counts, renal and liver function tests, and serum glucose, should be monitored regularly.
- Prompt cessation of the culprit drug is of paramount importance.
- The patient should be nursed in an intensive care or burns unit.
- Supportive care to maintain fluid and electrolyte balance, nutritional support, wound dressings, analgesia, and avoidance of skin infection is crucial in the management.
- Eye care by an ophthalmologist is critical to prevent long-term sequalae.
- Specific treatment in the form of intravenous Ig (IVIG), oral cyclosporine, oral corticosteroids, and TNF-α inhibitors has been used with varying degree of success in more severe cases.

TABLE 11-2

SCORTEN score
1. Age > 40 years
2. Heart rate >120 bpm
3. Cancer or hematologic malignancy
4. BSA involved on day 1 above 10%
5. Serum urea level (>10 mmol/L)
6. Serum bicarbonate level (<20 mmol/L)
7. Serum glucose level (>14 mmol/L)

TABLE 11-3

SCORTEN	Mortality rate
0–1	3.2%
2	12.1%
3	35.8%
4	58.3%
≥5	90%

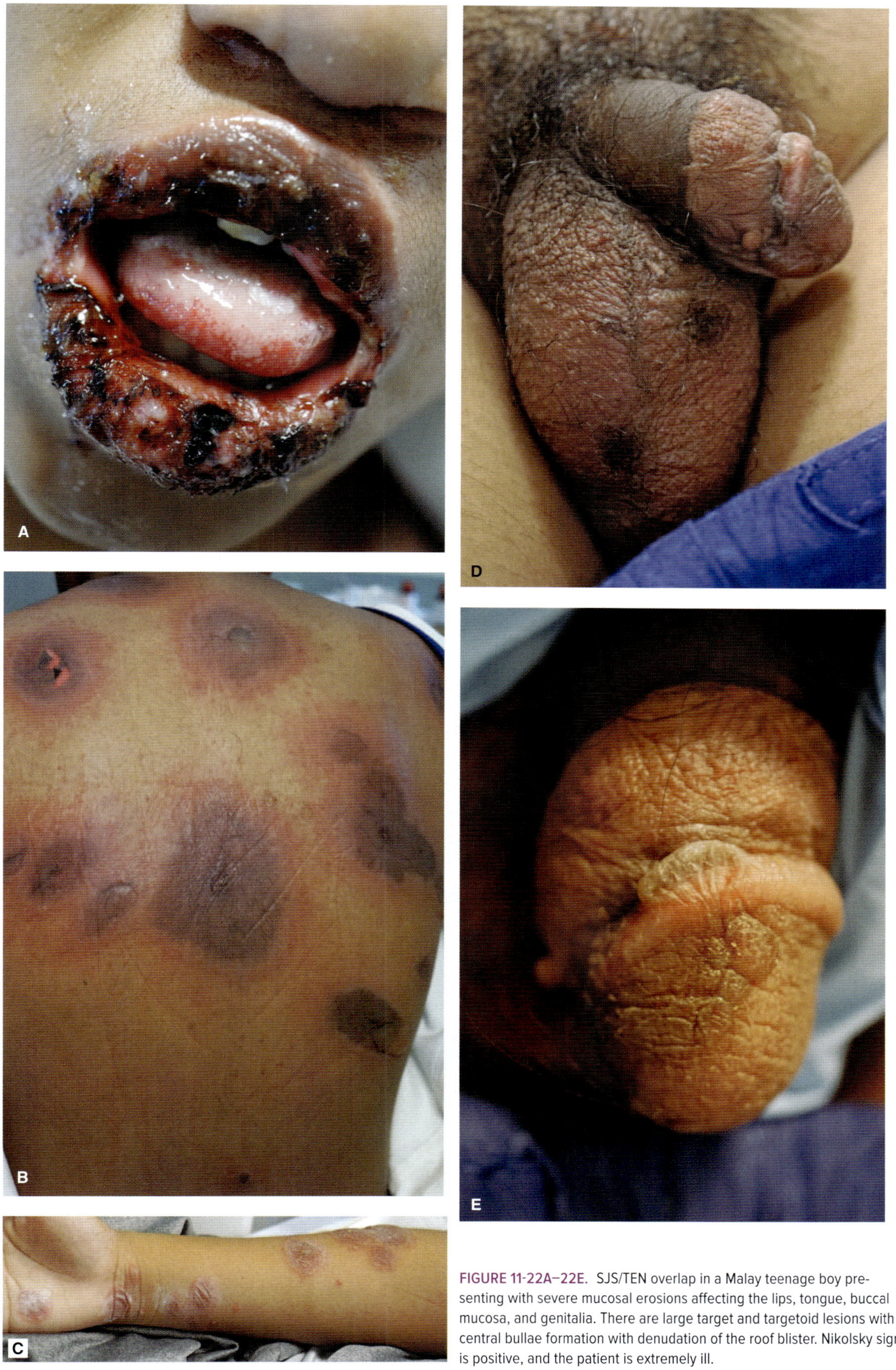

FIGURE 11-22A–22E. SJS/TEN overlap in a Malay teenage boy presenting with severe mucosal erosions affecting the lips, tongue, buccal mucosa, and genitalia. There are large target and targetoid lesions with central bullae formation with denudation of the roof blister. Nikolsky sign is positive, and the patient is extremely ill.

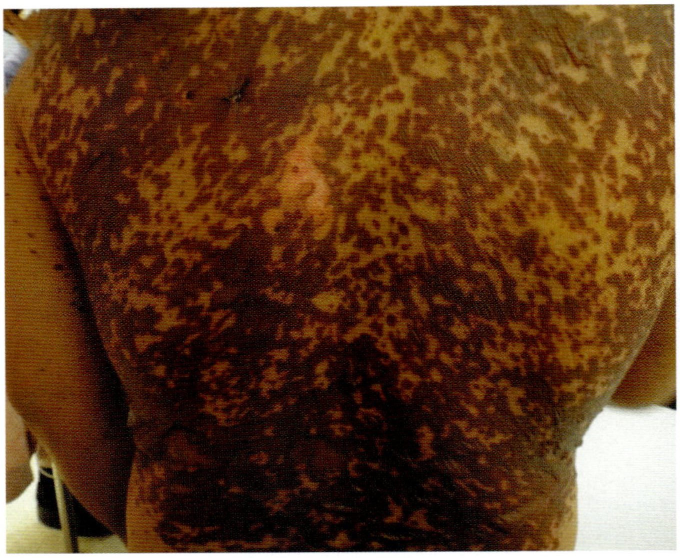

FIGURE 11-23. TEN in an 20-year-old Malay male presenting with extensive dusky patches and plaques with blistering and extensive epidermal detachment. Nikolsky sign is positive.

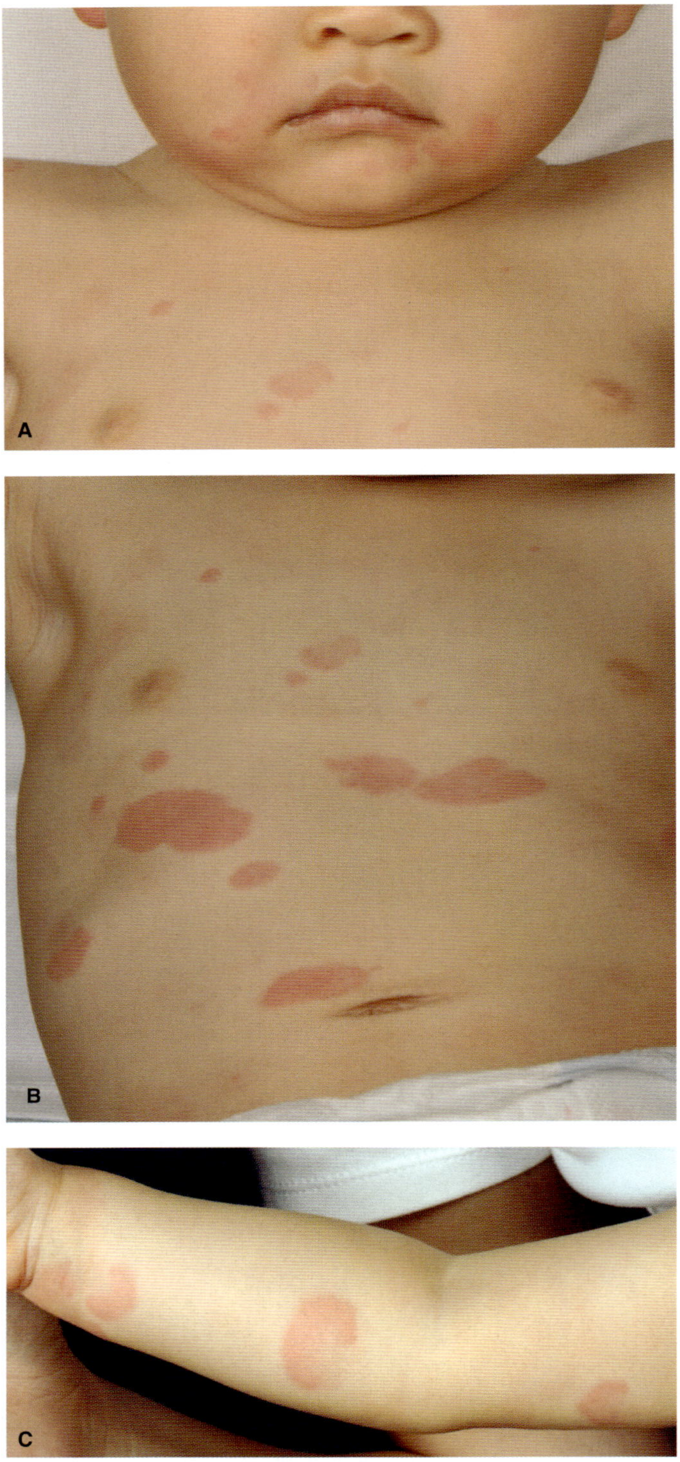

FIGURE 11-24A–24C. Acute urticaria in a Chinese infant presenting with scattered, itchy, erythematous wheals on the face, trunk, and limbs.

Pearls & Practical Tips

- Patients with SJS and TEN are generally unwell. This is in contrast with EM, where patients are generally otherwise well. The skin is also more painful in SJS and TEN as compared to other dermatoses, which tend to be itchy.
- Our center has found systemic ciclosporin to be useful in the treatment of more severe cases of SJS/TEN.
- Mycoplasma pneumonia-induced rash and mucositis (MIRM), also known as reactive infectious mucocutaneous eruption (RIME), is a recently described entity that occurs mostly in children, presenting with severe mucosal involvement but minimal cutaneous rash.
- The incidence of SJS and TEN associated with carbamazepine has seen a dramatic decrease with HLA-B*1502 testing in many countries.

Bibliography

1. Koh MJA, Tay YK. An update on Stevens-Johnson syndrome and toxic epidermal necrolysis in children. Curr Opin Pediatr 2009;21(4):505-10.
2. Koh MJ, Tay YK. Stevens-Johnson syndrome and toxic epidermal necrolysis in Asian children. J Am Acad Dermatol 2010;62(1):54-60.
3. Canavan TN, Mathes EF, Frieden I, Shinkai K. Mycoplasma pneumoniae-induced rash and mucositis as a syndrome distinct from Stevens-Johnson syndrome and erythema multiforme: a systematic review. J Am Acad Dermatol 2015;72(2):239-45.

URTICARIA

Urticaria is a common skin condition that can affect children and adults. The majority are acute, lasting for less than 6 weeks, while only a small number will have a more chronic course lasting more than 6 weeks. Acute urticaria in children is most often related to infections, especially viral infections. Other causes include drugs, food, and insect bites. Chronic urticaria in children is mostly idiopathic. Rarely, urticaria can be associated with systemic disease such as connective tissue disorders.

Clinical Features

- Urticaria is characterized by wheals, which are transient superficial skin-colored or erythematous swellings that are itchy and evanescent, with each wheal lasting for less than 24 hours.

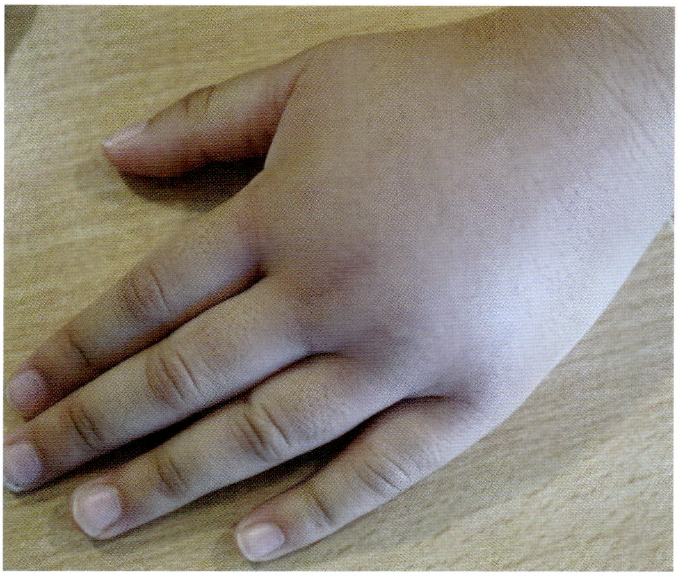

FIGURE 11-25. Urticaria affecting the dorsum of the hand presenting with angioedema.

- Angioedema may also be present and represent deeper involvement of the lower dermis. It may lead to a burning sensation and resolves more slowly than urticaria.
- If food or drug allergies are suspected, there should be a constant temporal relationship between ingestion or contact and appearance of symptoms, usually within minutes to an hour after exposure.
- Chronic urticaria is almost never due to allergies. About 20% of patients may report physical triggers such as dermographism (appearance of wheals when the skin is stroked or scratched), pressure (e.g., clothing, chairs, toweling, cold weather/objects) or sweating (cholinergic urticaria). Rare physical urticarias include solar and cold urticaria.
- Some patients with chronic urticaria may produce autoantibodies against IgE receptors on mast cells, or against IgE. This is more common in adults than children. These patients may have an associated risk of other autoimmune conditions, such as thyroiditis.
- Although acute urticaria may resolve in a few weeks, patients with chronic urticaria may experience remission only after months or even years.

Differential Diagnoses

- Urticarial vasculitis
  - Urticarial vasculitis is rare in childhood and presents with painful, urticarial-like plaques which persist for more than 24 hours and resolve with bruising or post-inflammatory hyperpigmentation. Skin biopsy will reveal the presence of vasculitis.
- Papular urticaria
  - This is common in children and represents a hypersensitivity reaction to insect bites, which tend to occur more on the exposed parts of the body, and persists for days to weeks.

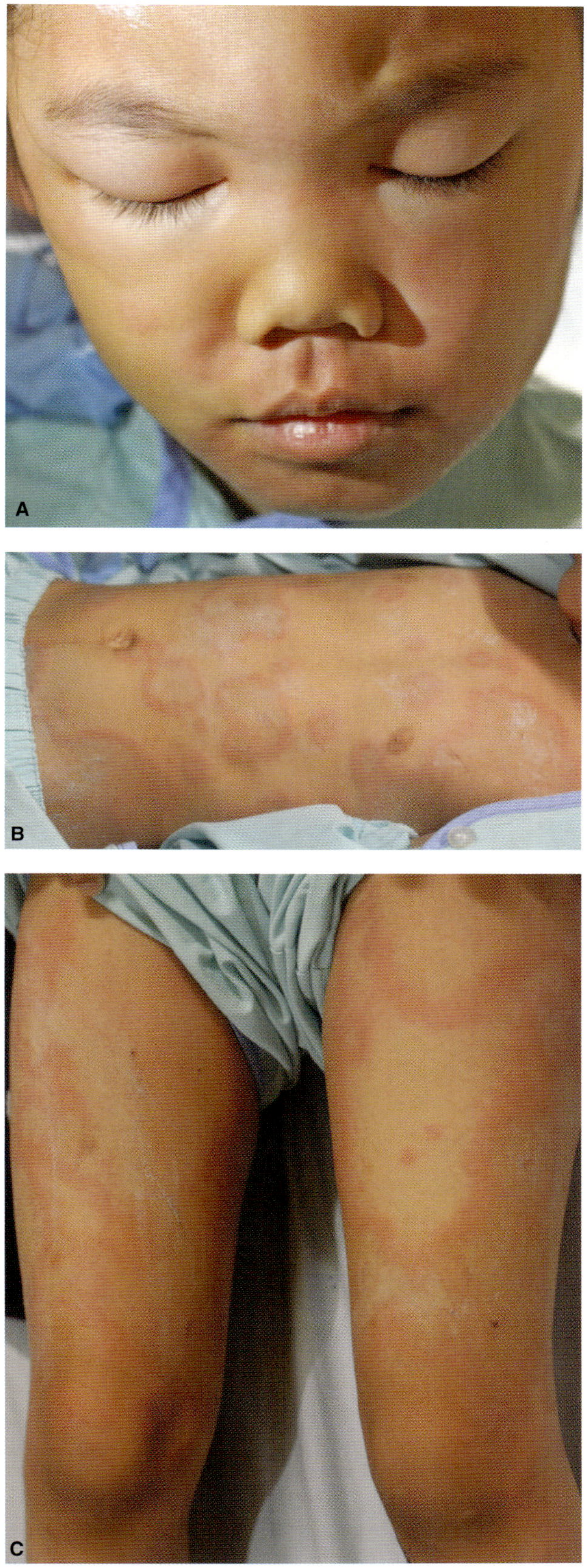

FIGURE 11-26A–26C. Acute urticaria in a young Malay child presenting with large erythematous wheals on the face, trunk, and limbs. There is accompanying mild angioedema of the eyelids.

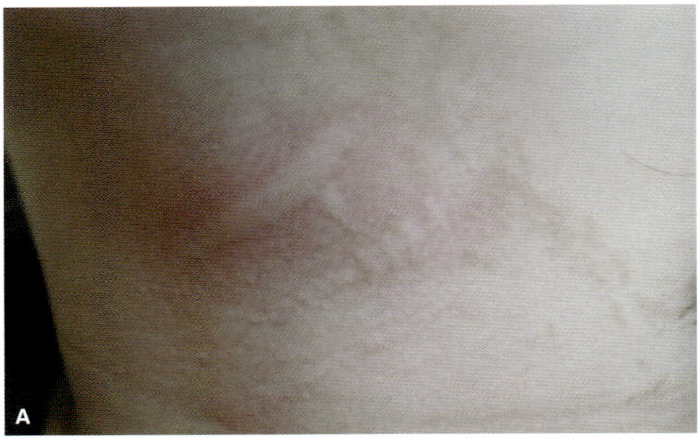

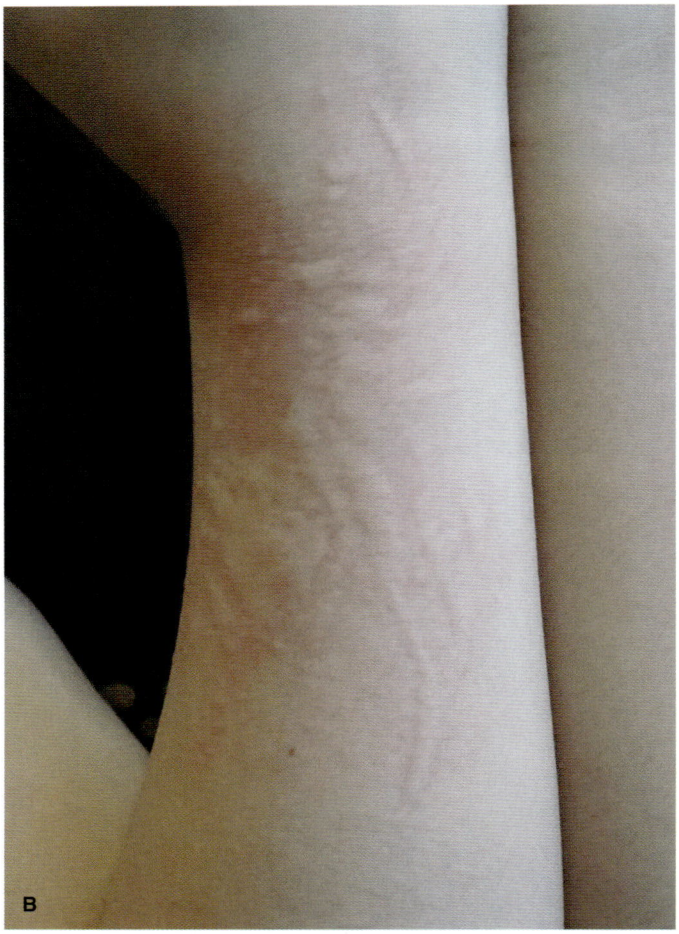

FIGURE 11-27A & 27B. Urticaria with dermographism on a 10-year-old girl, presenting with linear wheals.

- Mastocytosis
  - Mastocytosis is uncommon and usually occurs in younger children. It presents with persistent, itchy, brown-red patches or plaques which can urticate, especially when rubbed (Darier sign). Urticaria can become generalized in more severely affected patients (e.g., urticaria pigmentosa).

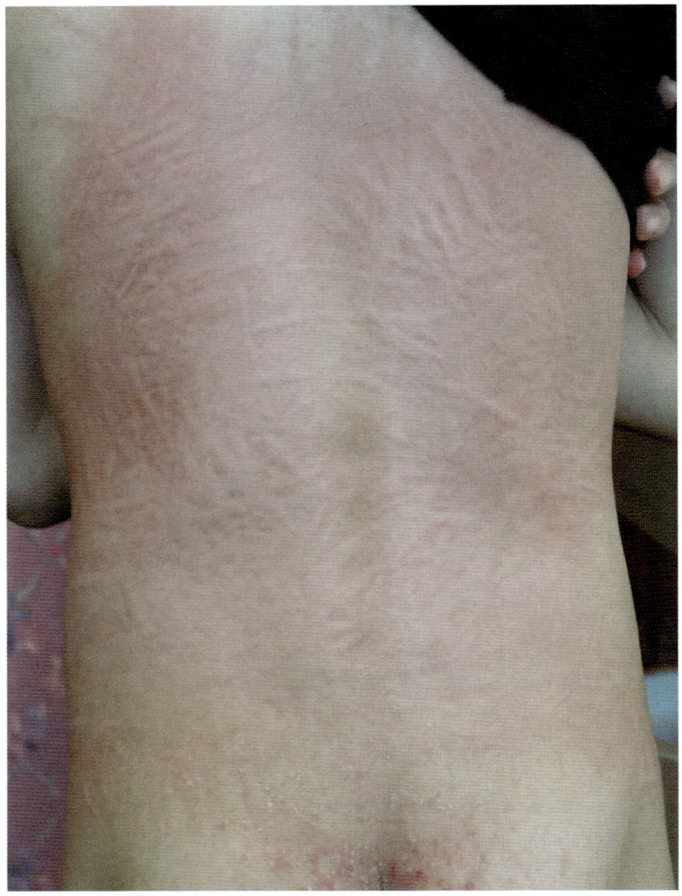

FIGURE 11-28. Dermographism demonstrated on the back of a teenage Chinese boy with chronic physical urticaria.

- Hereditary angioedema
  - This is an extremely rare inherited condition caused by deficiency of C1 esterase inhibitor. It presents with recurrent angioedema rather than urticaria.

Investigations & Treatment

- Urticaria is diagnosed clinically, and investigations are usually not necessary.
- Allergy tests for type 1 hypersensitivity to foods or drugs are only required if the history is suggestive.
- Thyroid autoantibody testing may be considered in patients with chronic urticaria.
- Most pediatric patients respond to oral antihistamines. Second-generation non-sedating antihistamines are recommended. Doses of up to four times the regular dose may be required for control of urticaria in some children. First-generation antihistamines should be avoided due to their risk of central nervous system and anticholinergic side effects.
- Treatment should be aimed at complete symptom relief, bearing in mind the patient's age and safety profile of medications. Antihistamines should be avoided in children less than 6 months of age.

- For severe urticaria not responding to antihistamines, omalizumab (anti-IgE monoclonal antibody) or cyclosporine may be considered.

Pearls & Practical Tips

- The use of oral antihistamines should be regular and continuous for at least 1 to 2 weeks during episodes of acute urticaria, until the child is asymptomatic.
- A short course of oral corticosteroids may be required if symptoms are severe.
- Evaluation for underlying systemic illness, such as connective tissue disorders, should be considered in patients who present with systemic symptoms, such as fever and joint pain, during the episodes of urticaria.

Bibliography

1. Kudryavtseva AV, Neskorodova KA, Staubach P. Urticaria in children and adolescents: an updated review of the pathogenesis and management. Pediatr Allergy Immunol 2019 Feb;30(1):17-24.
2. Wang EA, Chan SK. Chronic urticaria in children: an update on diagnosis and treatment. Curr Allergy Asthma Rep 2020 Jun 6;20(8):31.

ERYTHEMA ANNULARE CENTRIFUGUM

Erythema annulare centrifugum (EAC) is an idiopathic chronic or recurrent dermatosis postulated to represent a delayed-type hypersensitivity reaction, most commonly idiopathic, although a wide variety of triggers have been implicated, such as drugs (e.g., hydroxychloroquine, finasteride, amitriptyline), infections (fungal, bacterial, viral, parasitic), foods (e.g., tomatoes, blue cheese), and autoimmune disorders. Other rare associations are with malignancy and endocrine disorders.

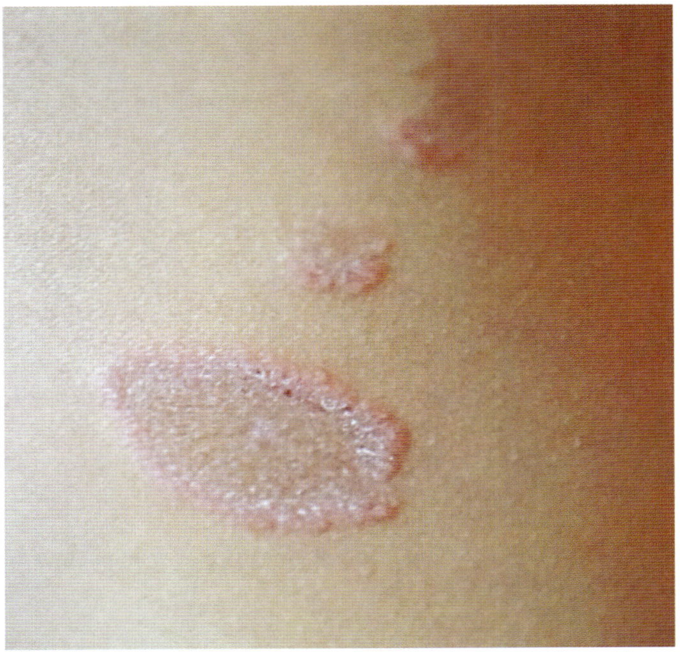

FIGURE 11-29. EAC in a young Chinese girl presenting with annular plaques with peripheral erythema and scaling with central clearing and hyperpigmentation.

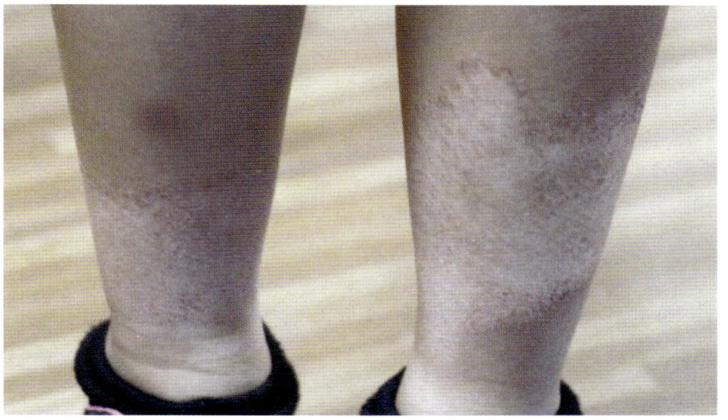

FIGURE 11-30. EAC in a young Chinese male with a more epidermal component, presenting with annular plaque with peripheral erythema and scaling with central clearing.

Clinical Features

- EAC is more common in adults but may occur in children and adolescents.
- Patients typically present with small urticaria-like or erythematous papules that enlarge over several weeks into annular plaques with central clearing. Itch is variable.

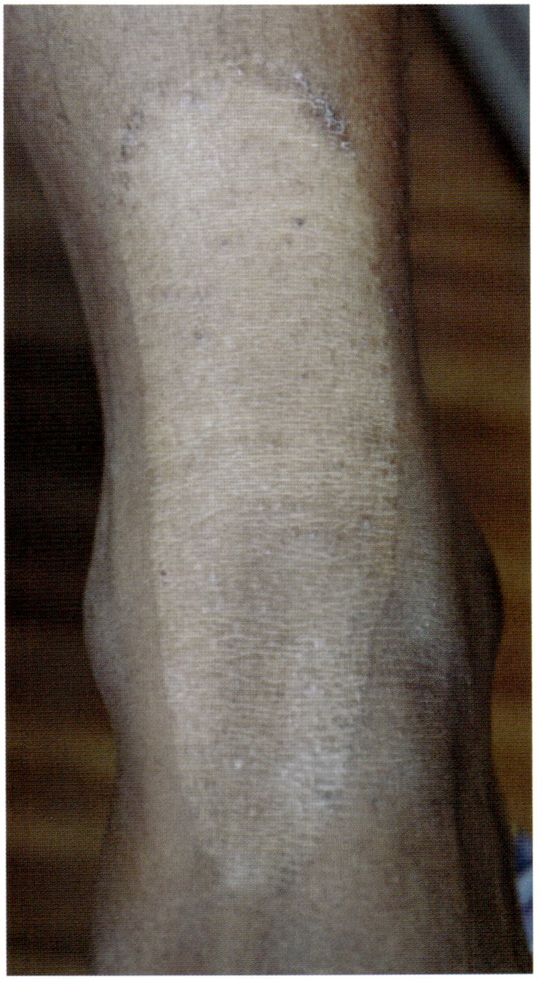

FIGURE 11-31. EAC on the leg of an Indian girl presenting with a hypopigmented patch with annular erythema and scaling.

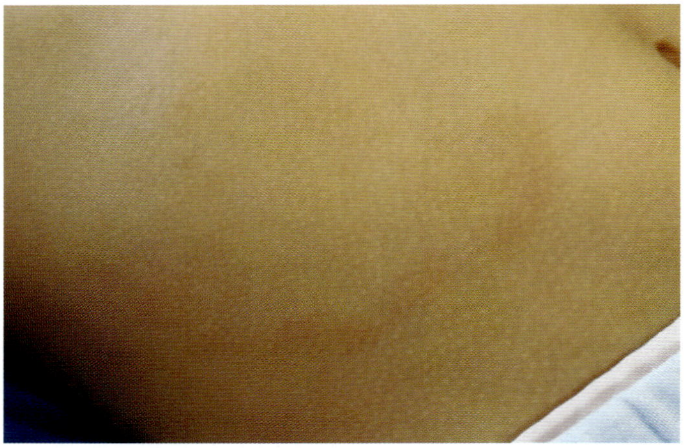

FIGURE 11-32. EAC in a young Chinese girl with a more dermal component. Clinically there is an annular erythematous-to-hyperpigmented plaque, with minimal surface scaling.

- Lesions may range from a few millimeters to several centimeters in size. They may be partial (arcuate) or may coalesce to form various polycyclic or serpiginous patterns.
- Classically, the advancing outer edge is slightly raised and erythematous, while the trailing (inner) edge may be scaly.
- Lesions commonly occur on the trunk, thighs, and buttocks, but any part of the body may be involved.
- EAC usually has a waxing and waning course over months to years, with each lesion typically lasting for several months. However, most cases eventually resolve spontaneously.

Differential Diagnoses

- Tinea (dermatophyte infection)
  - Tinea tends to be scalier and itchier than EAC. Tinea scales are on the leading edge of the annular plaques, compared to the trailing scales in EAC.
  - Skin scrapings for fungal microscopy and culture can be performed from the scaly edge to exclude tinea infection.
- Erythema multiforme (EM)
  - Early lesions of EAC may resemble EM lesions, which classically present with target or targetoid lesions, with central dusky areas surrounded by a lighter erythematous rim. Blisters and mucosal involvement may be seen in EM but not in EAC.
- Granuloma annulare (GA)
  - GA also presents with a chronic, expanding, annular plaque. However, it is usually less erythematous or scaly, and feels more "rubbery" than EAC. Doubtful cases can be differentiated on biopsy.
- Subacute cutaneous lupus erythematous (SCLE)
  - SCLE can also present with scaly, annular plaques that are more pronounced in sun-exposed sites. Serum autoantibodies (e.g., ANA, anti-Ro, and anti-La) and skin biopsies for histology and immunofluorescence can be performed to exclude SCLE.
- Erythema migrans
  - Erythema migrans is due to *Borrelia burgdorferi* infection, acquired through tick bites. There may be associated fatigue and lymphadenopathy. If there is travel or contact in endemic areas, serological tests can be performed.
- Secondary syphilis
  - Secondary syphilis can also present with annular nonpruritic scaly plaques, although this is rare in children. Serological tests for syphilis can be performed to exclude this diagnosis.

Investigations & Treatment

- EAC may be diagnosed clinically with the typical waxing and waning course and characteristic trailing scales are present, and other causes of annular rashes are excluded.
- Skin scraping for fungal microscopy and culture may be performed to exclude tinea.
- Skin biopsies may be useful if the clinical assessment is unclear, and may show one of two possible histologic subtypes: (1) deep subtype, in which there is a dense lymphocytic perivascular infiltrate in a coat-sleeve pattern in the superficial and deep dermis, without epidermal changes; and (2) superficial subtype, in which there is a perivascular lymphocytic infiltrate limited to the superficial dermis, and epidermal parakeratosis and spongiosis.
- Investigations for other associated conditions such as infections and autoimmune conditions should be carried out if the clinical history and physical examination are suggestive.
- Treatment of the underlying trigger can lead to resolution of EAC.
- In most patients, even if a trigger is not identified, spontaneous resolution may occur after several months to years, with an average duration 1 year.
- Topical steroids or calcineurin inhibitors may be applied to pruritic lesions. However, they do not prevent new lesions from appearing.
- Systemic therapies that have been described for refractory cases include azithromycin, erythromycin, fluconazole, metronidazole, and etanercept. The efficacy of these treatments remains unclear.

Pearls & Practical Tips

- EAC is generally a diagnosis of exclusion. Differential diagnoses as listed above need to be excluded before arriving at a diagnosis of EAC.
- Even though the identification and treatment of an underlying trigger is important, an underlying cause is not found in most cases.
- Treatments for EAC do not appear to alter the course of the condition.

ERYTHEMA NODOSUM

Erythema nodosum (EN) is the most common form of panniculitis in children. It is considered to be a delayed hypersensitivity response to various inciting agents. In children, Group A β-hemolytic streptococcal infection accounts for most of the cases. The peak incidence is in the adolescent age group.

Clinical Features

- Common implicated triggers of EN include infections (streptococcus, yersinia, tuberculosis), drugs (antimicrobials, oral contraceptive pills), inflammatory conditions (inflammatory bowel disease, sarcoidosis, celiac disease) or rarely, malignant diseases (haematological malignancy).
- EN is characterized by an acute onset of tender, 1- to 3-cm, erythematous, warm subcutaneous nodules, occurring symmetrically on the pretibial region and lateral shins. Less commonly, it can also occur on the thighs, arms, and trunk.
- Associated systemic symptoms include low-grade fever, sore throat, malaise, arthralgia, and ankle swelling.
- Over a few days or weeks, the lesions slowly flatten, leaving behind a purple or blue-green discoloration.

Differential Diagnoses

- Erythema induratum
  - Erythema induratum is a rare panniculitis in children and adolescents and is commonly associated with tuberculosis in endemic regions. It usually presents with lesions on the calves rather than on the shins in EN. Unlike EN, lesions of erythema induratum can ulcerate.
- Infective panniculitis
  - Especially in immunocompromised patients, opportunistic infections can present with panniculitis. These include opportunistic fungal and mycobacterial infections. In these patients, microbiological cultures are mandatory when performing skin biopsies.
- Arthropod bite reactions
  - Arthropod bite reactions are common in children and can often present with indurated nodules, especially on the exposed limbs. Unlike EN, lesions are usually itchy and there may be a central punctum. Lesions also resolve faster than EN, within a few days.

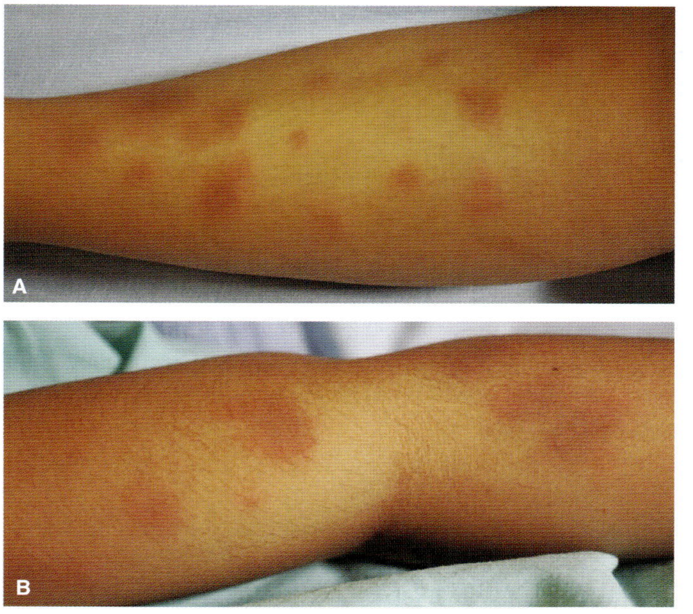

FIGURE 11-34A & 34B. EN occurring in a Malay adolescent girl, presenting with erythematous, tender nodules over the extensor aspects of the lower legs and upper legs.

- Other rare forms of panniculitis
  - These include lupus panniculitis and subcutaneous panniculitis–like T-cell lymphoma. Biopsies will be required to exclude these diagnoses.

Investigations & Treatment

- The diagnosis of EN is usually made clinically. Skin biopsies are not necessary unless the presentation is atypical.
- When performed, skin biopsy shows septal panniculitis, characterized by inflammatory infiltrate affecting the septa of the subcutaneous fat. In the acute stage, neutrophils predominate, while in later stages, mononuclear cells and histiocytes are predominant.
- Tissue for microbiological investigations, including bacterial, fungal, and mycobacterial cultures, may be required if chronic infections are suspected.
- The management of EN is mainly to identify and treat any underlying triggers.

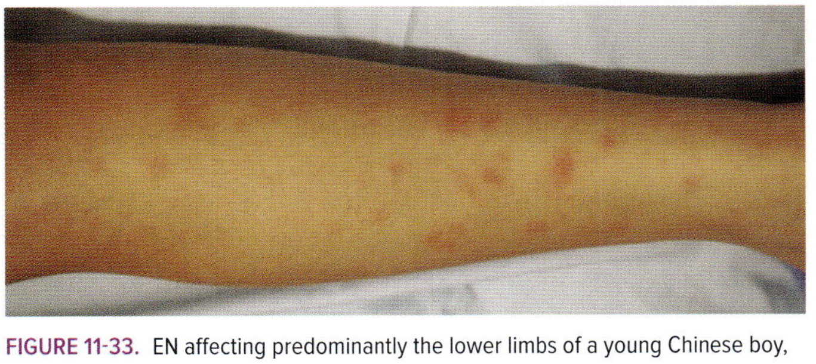

FIGURE 11-33. EN affecting predominantly the lower limbs of a young Chinese boy, presenting with multiple erythematous, deep papules and nodules.

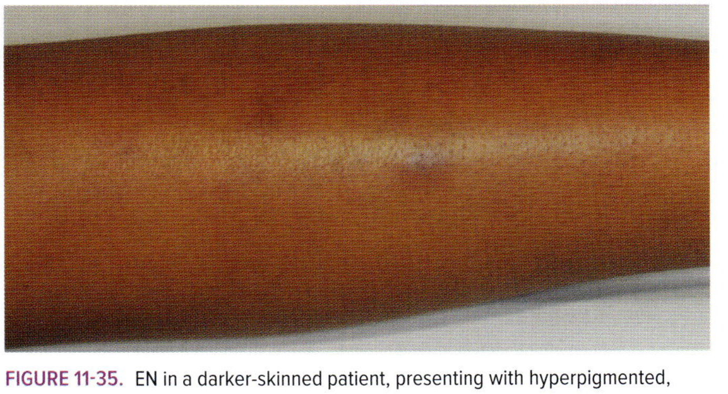

FIGURE 11-35. EN in a darker-skinned patient, presenting with hyperpigmented, indurated nodules on the shin.

- Complete blood count (CBC), c-reactive protein (CRP), erythrocyte sedimentation rate (ESR), anti-streptolysin O antibodies (ASOT), throat swab, tests for tuberculosis, and chest radiographs may be required depending on the clinical context.
- Bed rest and nonsteroidal anti-inflammatory drugs (NSAIDs) like ibuprofen or naproxen can be prescribed for pain and arthralgia and are sufficient in the majority of the cases.
- Persistent painful lesions may require systemic corticosteroids in the dose of 0.5 to 1 mg/kg/day for 4 to 6 weeks.
- Potassium iodide, which has been used historically in the treatment of EN, is not recommended in children.

Pearls & Practical Tips

- Pregnancy tests may can required in adolescent females, as pregnancy is a possible trigger.
- EN is the most common tuberculid in many tuberculosis-endemic areas. Investigation to exclude tuberculosis is mandatory in these endemic areas.

ERYTHEMA INDURATUM

Erythema induratum is a type of lobular panniculitis characterized by the presence of plaques or nodules on the calves, which may ulcerate and drain. It is most often associated with mycobacterial infections, especially tuberculosis (TB). Whether it is due to direct infection with mycobacteria or a hypersensitivity response is debatable. The term "nodular vasculitis" is used in cases that have the same clinical and histopathological presentation but are of non-tuberculous origin. These cases may be idiopathic or secondary to drugs or non-tuberculous infections like pseudomonas or nocardia.

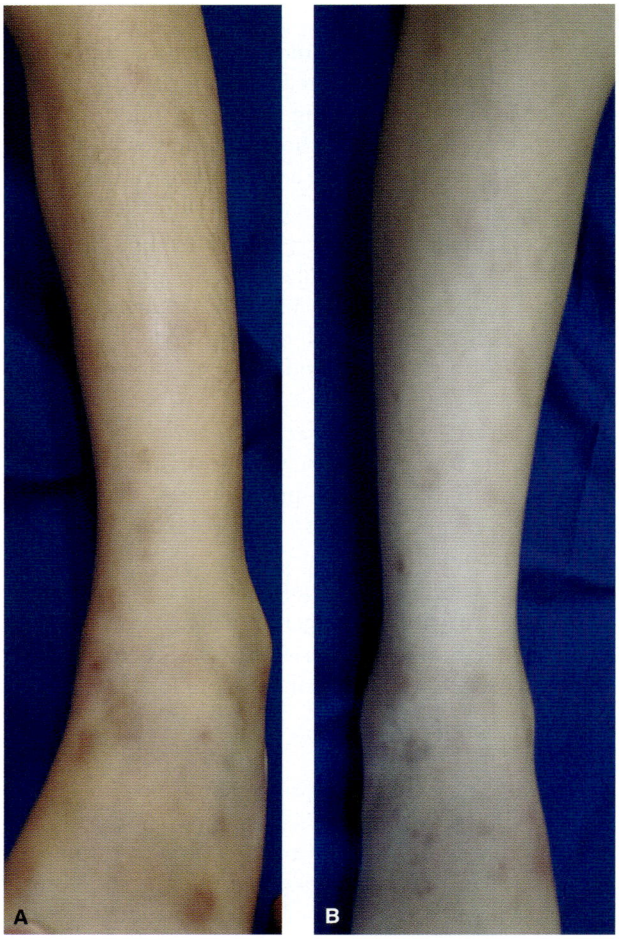

FIGURE 11-36A & 36B. Erythema induratum in a Chinese boy presenting with irregular, erythematous-to-dusky, deep nodules, affecting mostly the lower limbs.

Clinical Features

- Erythema induratum most commonly occurs in middle-aged to elderly females, but children and adolescents can also be affected.
- It is characterized by chronic or recurrent eruptions of erythematous to violaceous, deep nodules or plaques, which can be asymptomatic or painful and occur predominantly on the bilateral lower legs, especially the calves. The trunk and upper limbs may also be less commonly affected.
- The nodules can ulcerate and drain an oily material.
- Lesions can persist for months and heal with scarring. Recurrence is common unless the underlying infection is treated.

Differential Diagnoses

- Erythema nodosum
  - Erythema nodosum is more common than erythema induratum, and occurs predominantly on the shins rather than the calves. Ulceration does not occur. In doubtful cases, skin biopsies will show a septal panniculitis.
- Infective panniculitis
  - Especially in immunocompromised patients, opportunistic infections can present with panniculitis. These include opportunistic fungal and mycobacterial infections. In these patients, microbiological cultures are mandatory when performing skin biopsies.
- Arthropod bite reactions
  - Arthropod bite reactions are common in children and can often present with indurated nodules, especially on the exposed limbs. Lesions are usually itchy and there may be a central punctum.
- Other rare forms of panniculitis
  - These include lupus panniculitis and subcutaneous panniculitis-like T-cell lymphoma. Biopsies will be required to exclude these diagnoses.

Investigations & Treatment

- Skin biopsy is usually required to confirm the diagnosis of erythema induratum, especially in children and adolescents. Histology shows a septal-lobular panniculitis with medium-vessel vasculitis in the subcutaneous fat. The inflammatory infiltrate is often mixed with neutrophils, lymphocytes, histiocytes, and multinucleated giant cells. Coagulative necrosis may occur, which clinically appears as suppuration.

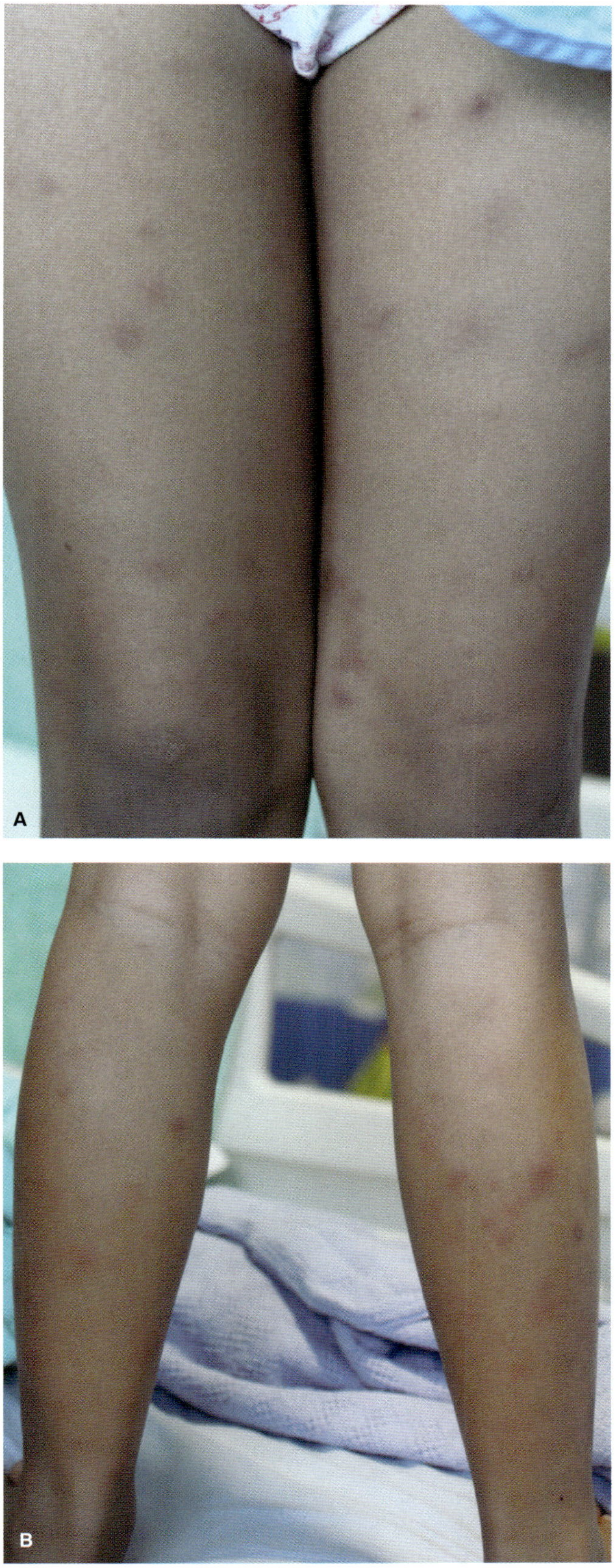

FIGURE 11-37A & 37B. Erythema induratum affecting mostly the legs of a Malay girl, with erythematous hyperpigmented deep nodules.

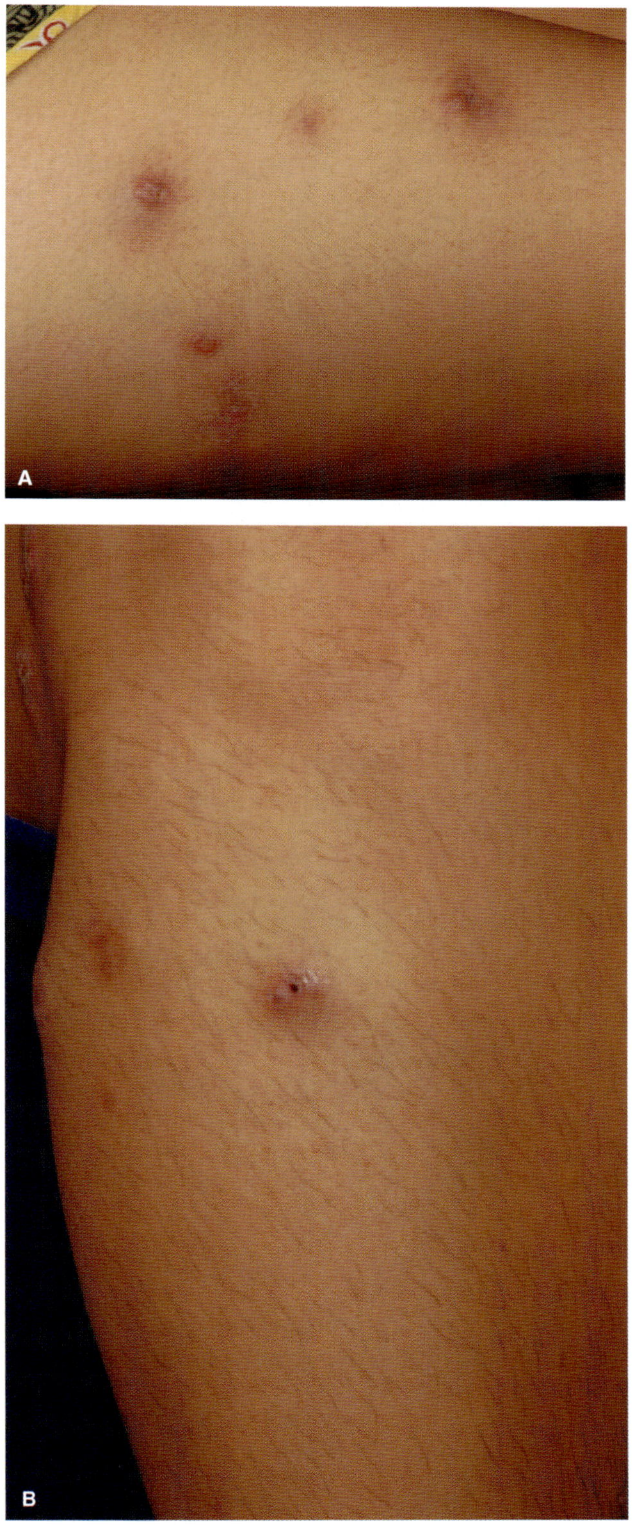

FIGURE 11-38A & 38B. Erythema induratum in an Indian adolescent female presenting with multiple ulcerated, erythematous, indurated nodules on her legs.

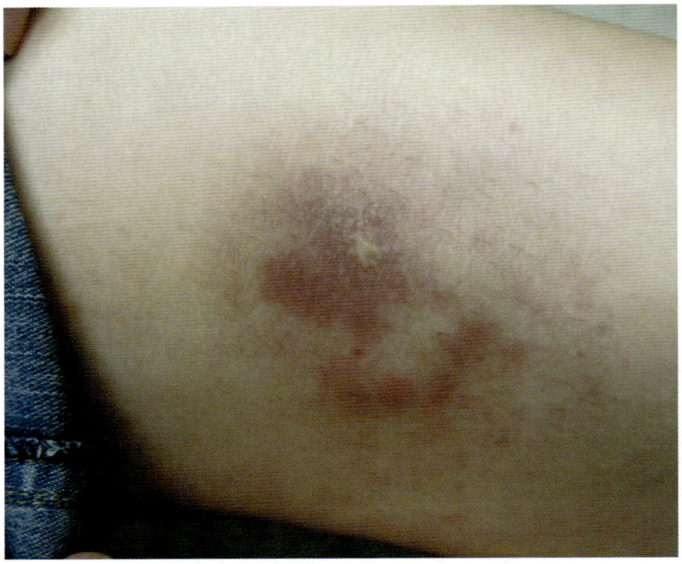

FIGURE 11-39. Erythema induratum on the thigh of a Chinese adolescent female, presenting with indurated, hyperpigmented, deep nodules and plaques. A biopsy scar is seen in the center of the lesion.

- Investigation to exclude infection with TB is mandatory, especially in endemic areas. These include chest radiograph, Mantoux test, and interferon-γ release assays (IGRA), such as the Quantiferon-TB Gold test and TB-T-spot tests.
- Treatment should be directed at the underlying cause. Cases with evidence of active TB will need multidrug antituberculous therapy.
- Supportive care includes nonsteroidal anti-inflammatory drugs, bed rest, and wound care.

Pearls & Practical Tips

- Even if results of investigations for TB return negative, if lesions are chronic or recurrent and the patient resides in a TB-endemic area, we have patients who improve with anti-TB treatment.

NEUTROPHILIC DERMATOSES

Neutrophilic dermatoses are a heterogenous group of skin conditions characterized by dense neutrophilic infiltrate on histologic examination, in the absence of infection. They are rare in the pediatric age group, and are often associated with underlying systemic disease. Neutrophilic dermatoses include Sweet syndrome (acute febrile neutrophilic dermatosis), pyoderma gangrenosum, Behçet disease, and neutrophilic eccrine hidradenitis.

Clinical Features

- Neutrophilic dermatosis can present with various skin findings, including papules, pustules, nodules, or ulcerated lesions.
- A commonly seen feature is pathergy, in which lesions occur at sites of minor injury such as scratches, insect bites, needle pricks, or biopsies.

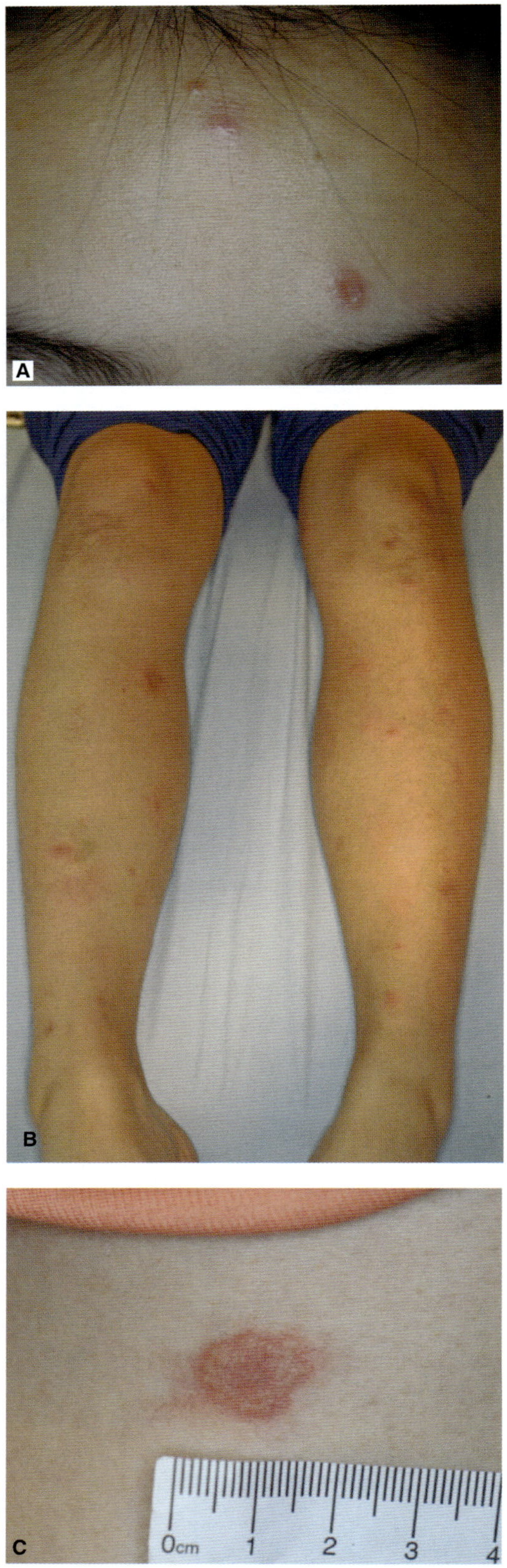

FIGURE 11-40A–40C. A Chinese adolescent female with underlying immunodeficiency secondary to anti-interferon-γ antibodies (ISIGA syndrome) presenting with lesions of Sweet syndrome, with juicy, erythematous papules (Figure 11-40A & 40C) on the face, trunk, and limbs and lesions of erythema nodosum (Figure 11-40B) on her shins.

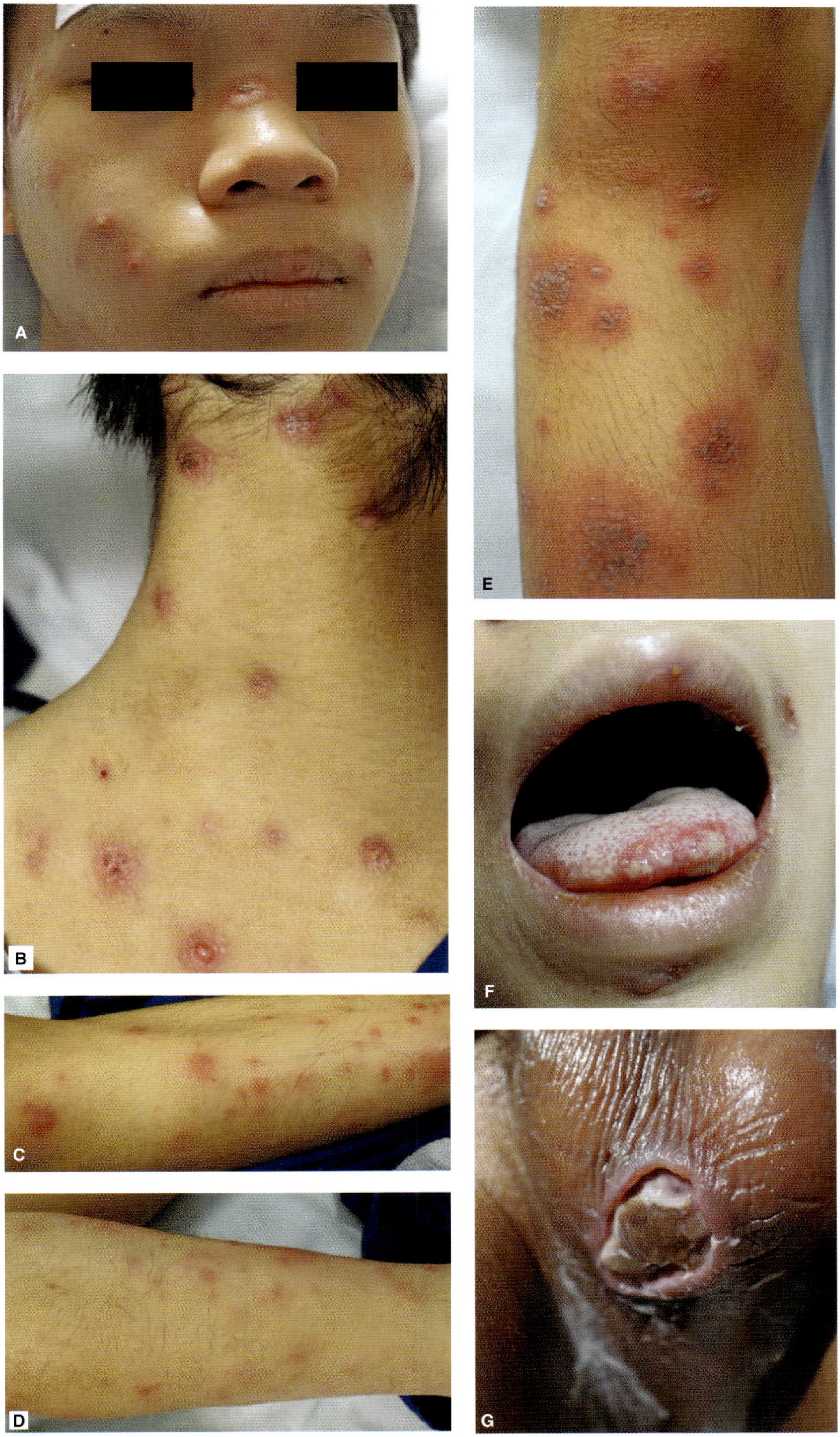

FIGURE 11-41A–41G. Sweet syndrome in a Chinese teenage male presenting with bright red, juicy papules over his face, trunk, and limbs (Figure 11-41A–41C), with central blistering and necrosis. There are also erythema nodosum–like lesions on the legs (Figure 11-41D). The lesions on the legs developed overlying pustules over a few days (Figure 11-41E). He also developed recurrent mouth (Figure 11-41F) and genital ulcers (Figure 11-41G).

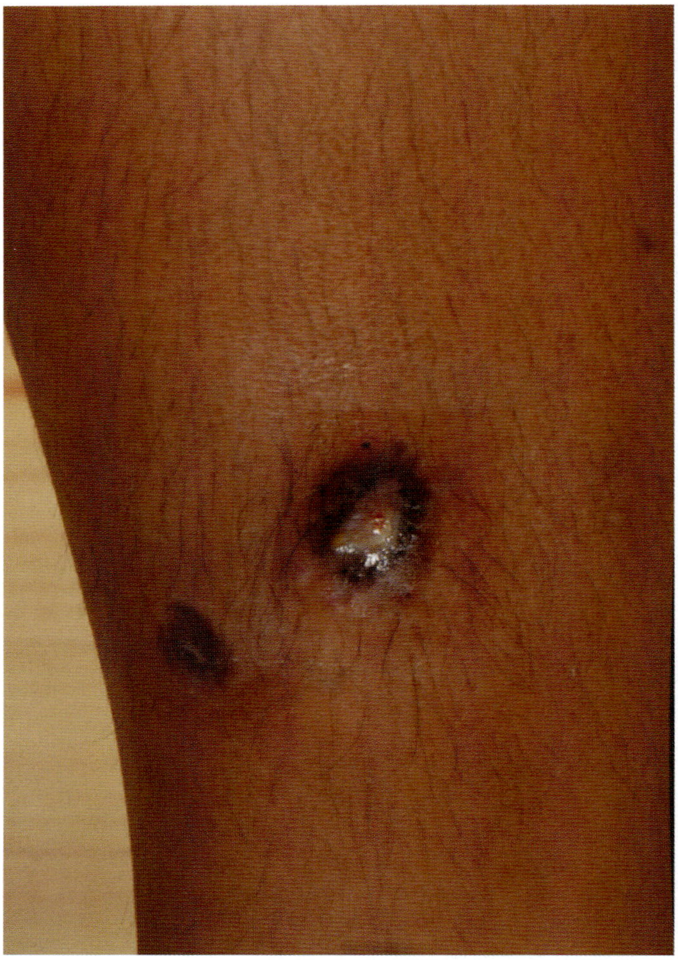

FIGURE 11-42. Pyoderma gangrenosum on the leg of a Malay boy presenting with deep ulcer with dusky borders.

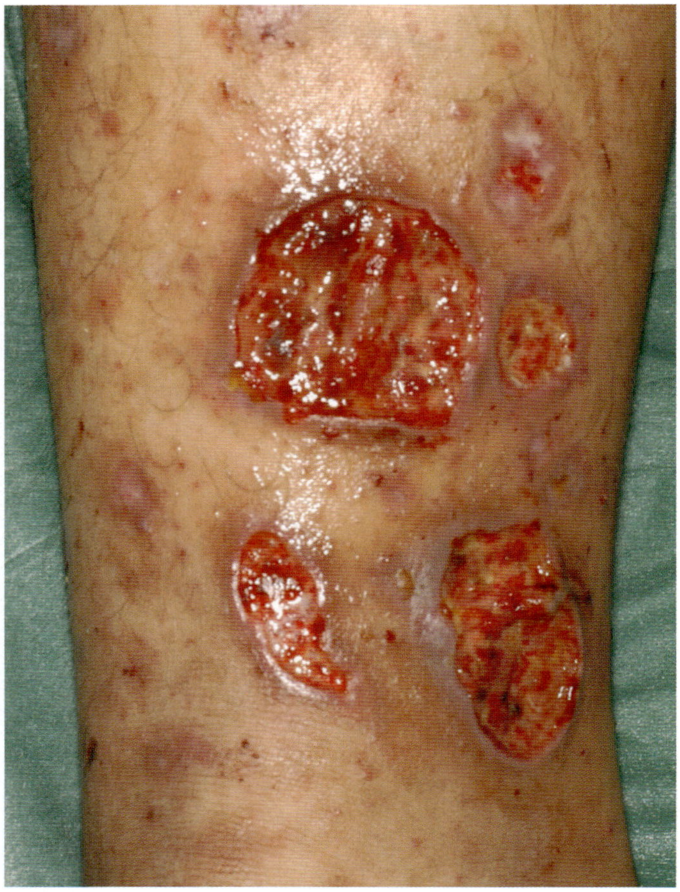

FIGURE 11-43. Pyoderma gangrenosum on the legs of a Malay boy.

- **Sweet syndrome**
  - Characterized by tender, erythematous to violaceous papules, which may coalesce to form plaques. Pseudovesicles, pustules, bullae, and ulcers may also be seen.
  - Common sites include the face, neck, and upper limbs, especially the hands, although any part of the body may be involved.
  - Fever is a common associated symptom.
  - Associated conditions in pediatric patients include infections (upper respiratory tract infection, gastrointestinal infection), malignancies (hematologic or solid organ), autoimmune conditions (rheumatoid arthritis, inflammatory bowel disease), and drugs.[1]
- **Pyoderma gangrenosum**
  - Characterized by an inflammatory papule or pustule that develops into a painful, rapidly enlarging ulcer with violaceous "gunmetal" borders. Ulcers may be solitary or multiple.
  - The most common sites affected are the lower limbs, perineum, and head. Mucosal lesions have also been reported.
  - Associated conditions in pediatric patients include inflammatory bowel disease, hematologic disorders, vasculitis, and immunodeficiencies. However, most cases are idiopathic.[2]
- **Behçet disease**
  - This is a chronic, relapsing condition that presents with recurrent oral and genital ulcers, uveitis, and skin lesions that resemble acne, folliculitis, pustules, plaques, and erythema nodosum.[3,4]
  - There is association with HLA-B51, 52, A26, and B27.
- Other organs may also be involved in the neutrophilic dermatoses, such as the eyes, heart, central nervous system, lungs, kidneys, liver, spleen, and joints.

Differential Diagnoses

- Other neutrophilic dermatoses
  - There is considerable overlap between the various neutrophilic dermatoses, both clinically and histologically. They are also associated with similar systemic conditions, such as infections, autoimmune disease, inflammatory bowel disease, malignancy, and drugs.
- Leukocytoclastic vasculitis (LCV)
  - LCV may also present with purpuric papules, which can also blister and ulcerate. It can also be associated with systemic manifestations. LCV predominantly affects the legs and tends to be more symmetrical.

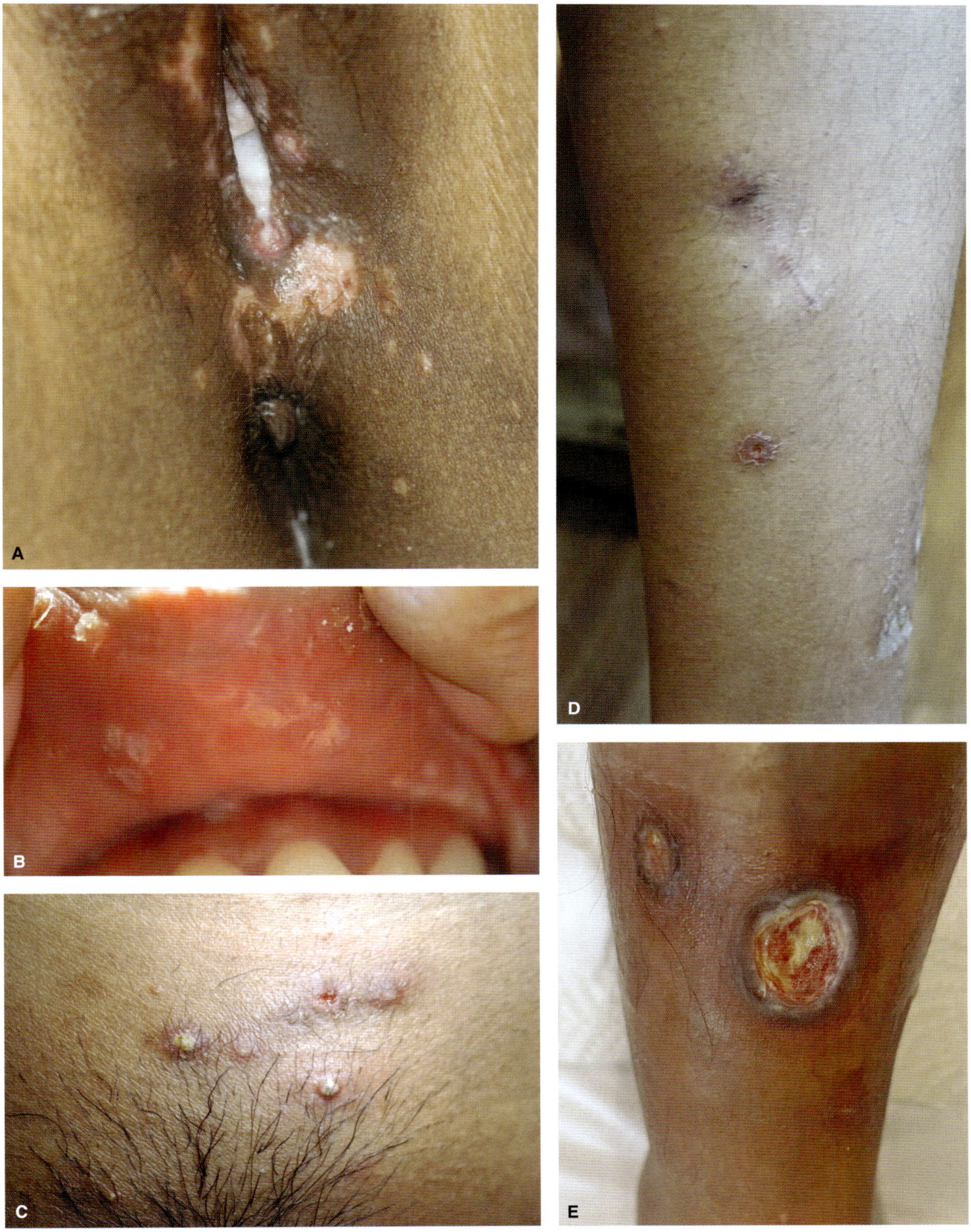

FIGURE 11-44A–44E. Behçet disease in a young Indian adult patient presenting with recurrent genital and oral ulcers (Figure 11-44A & 44B), papulopustular lesions (Figure 11-44C & 44D), as well as pyoderma gangrenosum lesions (Figure 11-44E) which developed after incisional biopsies were performed on erythema nodosum lesions, a sign of pathergy.

- On biopsy, there is also a dense neutrophilic infiltrate. However, there is evidence of vessel damage including fibrinoid necrosis of blood vessels and red cell extravasation in LCV, which should not be seen on biopsies of neutrophilic dermatoses.

- Leukemia cutis
  - This is extremely rare and represents infiltrate of leukemic cells into the skin. The underlying leukemia may sometimes be undiagnosed at the time of diagnosis of leukemia cutis.
  - Lesions of leukemia cutis can also appear as violaceous and purpuric papules, nodules, and plaques, and are usually multifocal.
  - Close correlation with biopsies from the skin and bone marrow can help to differentiate from neutrophilic dermatoses.

Investigations & Treatment

- Leukocytosis is seen in many patients with neutrophilic dermatosis.
- A positive pathergy test can help in the diagnosis of Behçet disease, but is also seen in patients with the other neutrophilic dermatoses.
- Skin biopsies in all neutrophilic dermatoses show predominant neutrophilic infiltrate in the dermis, which can extend into the epidermis and subcutaneous fat. Features of vasculitis should not be seen. Infective causes should be excluded by performing the appropriate special stains, such as periodic acid–Schiff (PAS), Gomori methenamine silver (GMS), and Ziehl-Neelsen (ZN) stains. If required, tissue for microbiological cultures should also be performed.
- Treatment often requires the use of systemic, intralesional, and topical corticosteroids as well as other immunomodulatory agents, such as colchicine, dapsone, nonsteroidal anti-inflammatory drugs (NSAIDs), ciclosporin, mycophenolate, and thalidomide. Newer biologics including TNF-α inhibitors and anakinra (IL-1 inhibitor) have also been recently described.
- Investigating and treating the associated systemic illness is essential.

Pearls & Practical Tips

- Although neutrophilic dermatosis in children may be idiopathic, associations with other systemic disease may be seen in more than 50% of patients. These should be excluded by clinical history, examination, and investigations.
- There is considerable overlap between the neutrophilic dermatoses, and sometimes the disease can evolve over time. Close clinical correlation is important to arrive at a final diagnosis.
- Immunodeficiency secondary to anti-interferon-γ autoantibodies (ISIGA syndrome) is a recently described condition that has been reported mostly in Asians, especially from East and Southeast Asia. The condition presents with lesions resembling Sweet syndrome, but patients are also susceptible to various opportunistic infections, such as mycobacterial infections.[5]

References

1. Uihlein LC, Brandling-Bennett HA, Lio PA, Liang MG. Sweet syndrome in children. Pediatr Dermatol 2012 Jan-Feb;29(1):38-44.
2. Kechichian E, Haber R, Mourad N, et al. Pediatric pyoderma gangrenosum: a systematic review and update. Int J Dermatol 2017;56(5):486-95.
3. Yıldız M, Köker O, Adrovic A, et al. Pediatric Behcet's disease—clinical aspects and current concepts. Eur J Rheumatol 2019;7(Suppl 1):1-10.
4. Batu ED. Diagnostic/classification criteria in pediatric Behcet's disease. Rheumatol Int 2019;39(1):37-46.
5. Liew WK, Thoon KC, Chong CY, et al. Juvenile-onset immunodeficiency secondary to anti-interferon-gamma autoantibodies. J Clin Immunol 2019;39(5):512-18.

Genodermatoses

EPIDERMOLYSIS BULLOSA

Epidermolysis bullosa (EB) is a rare genetic disorder of skin fragility characterized by blisters and erosions that develop spontaneously or with minimal mechanical stress. Based on the level of defect within the skin and clinical manifestations, they have been divided into four major types: EB simplex, junctional EB, dystrophic EB, and Kindler syndrome.

Clinical Features

- Epidermolysis bullosa simplex (EBS)
  - EBS is the most common subtype of EB and is most often inherited in autosomal dominant fashion, although autosomal recessive inheritance has also been rarely reported. The most commonly associated genes are *KRT5* and *KRT14*, encoding keratin 5 and keratin 14 proteins, found in the basal epidermis.
  - Patients with EBS present with variable severities of blistering. Most patients have localized lesions, although less commonly, intermediate or severe blistering disease is encountered.
  - Onset of blistering can be seen at birth but most commonly occurs from early childhood. Rarely, patients can present later in life.
  - The hands and feet are the most common sites involved, especially at sites of constant trauma. In more severe patients, other sites such as the arms and legs are also involved. Mucosal surfaces are either not affected or minimally involved. Nail involvement is limited.
- Junctional epidermolysis bullosa (JEB)
  - JEB is extremely rare, with autosomal recessive inheritance pattern and mutations found in proteins of the basement membrane zone, namely laminin 332, collagen XVII (BP180), and integrins α6 or β4.
  - The clinical subtypes are localized, intermediate, and severe JEB, with features ranging from mild cutaneous involvement to extensive blistering. Blisters and erosions are usually seen at birth. In severe cases, granulation tissue in the peri-oral region, tips of fingers, and ears is classical.

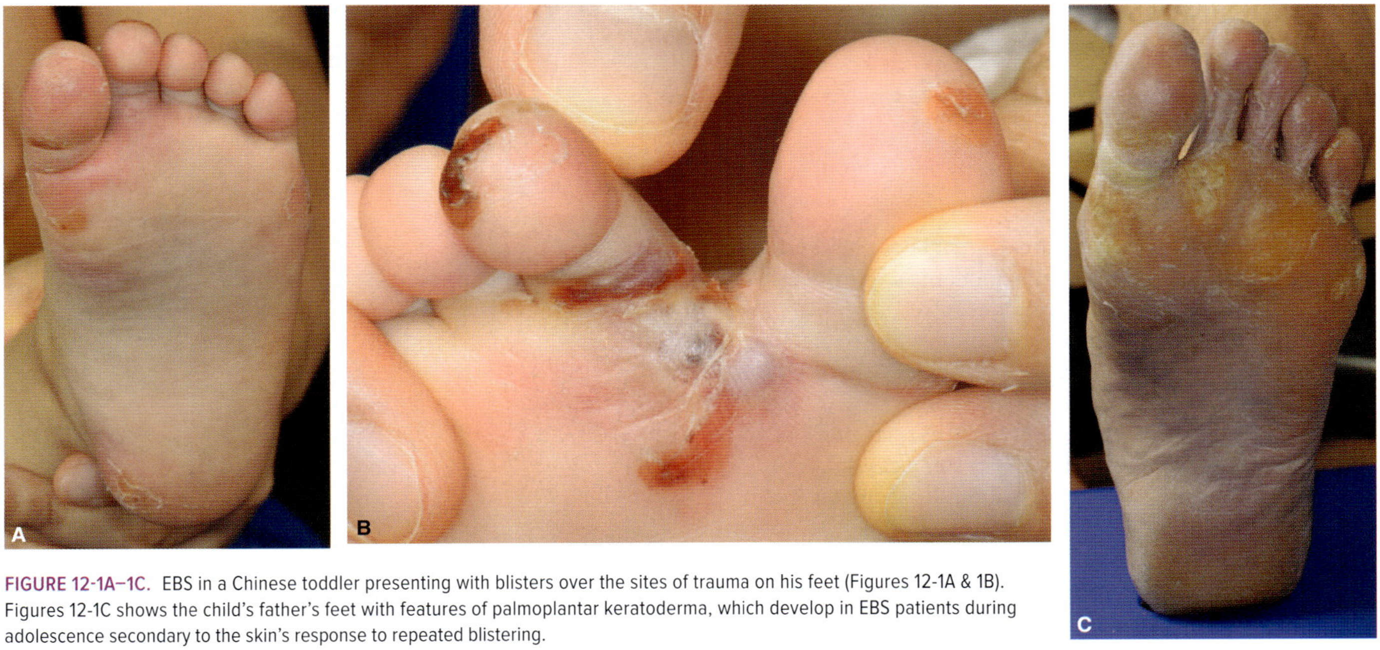

FIGURE 12-1A–1C. EBS in a Chinese toddler presenting with blisters over the sites of trauma on his feet (Figures 12-1A & 1B). Figures 12-1C shows the child's father's feet with features of palmoplantar keratoderma, which develop in EBS patients during adolescence secondary to the skin's response to repeated blistering.

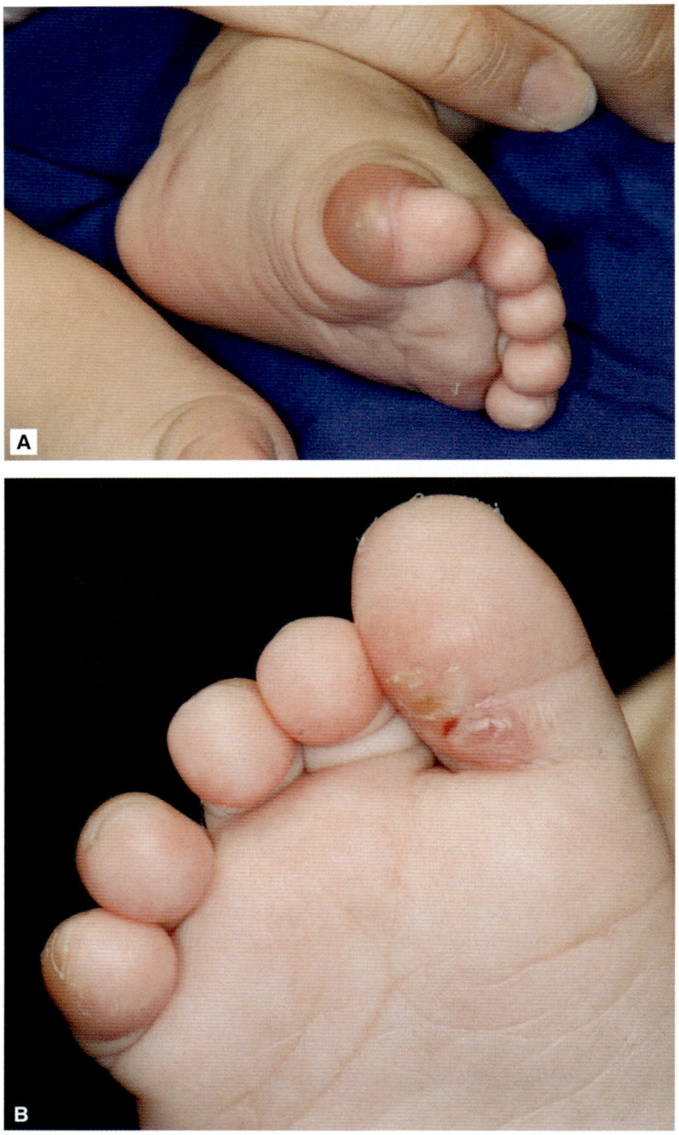

FIGURE 12-2A & 2B. Tense and flaccid blisters on the soles of the feet and toes in an infant with EBS.

- Involved skin may heal with atrophy and post-inflammatory pigmentary changes. However, milia formation is not a common feature.
- Mucosal involvement is common, with the oral mucosa being the most typical site affected. Eye involvement is also seen frequently.
- Laryngeal involvement presents as hoarseness of voice, and can be life-threatening in some cases.
- Genitourinary and gastrointestinal involvement is seen in severe cases. Cases associated with integrin mutations often present with pyloric atresia.
- Dental enamel dysplasia with pitted teeth is also a common finding.
- Prognosis is poor, especially in severe cases, with high mortality in the first few years of life. Intermediate and

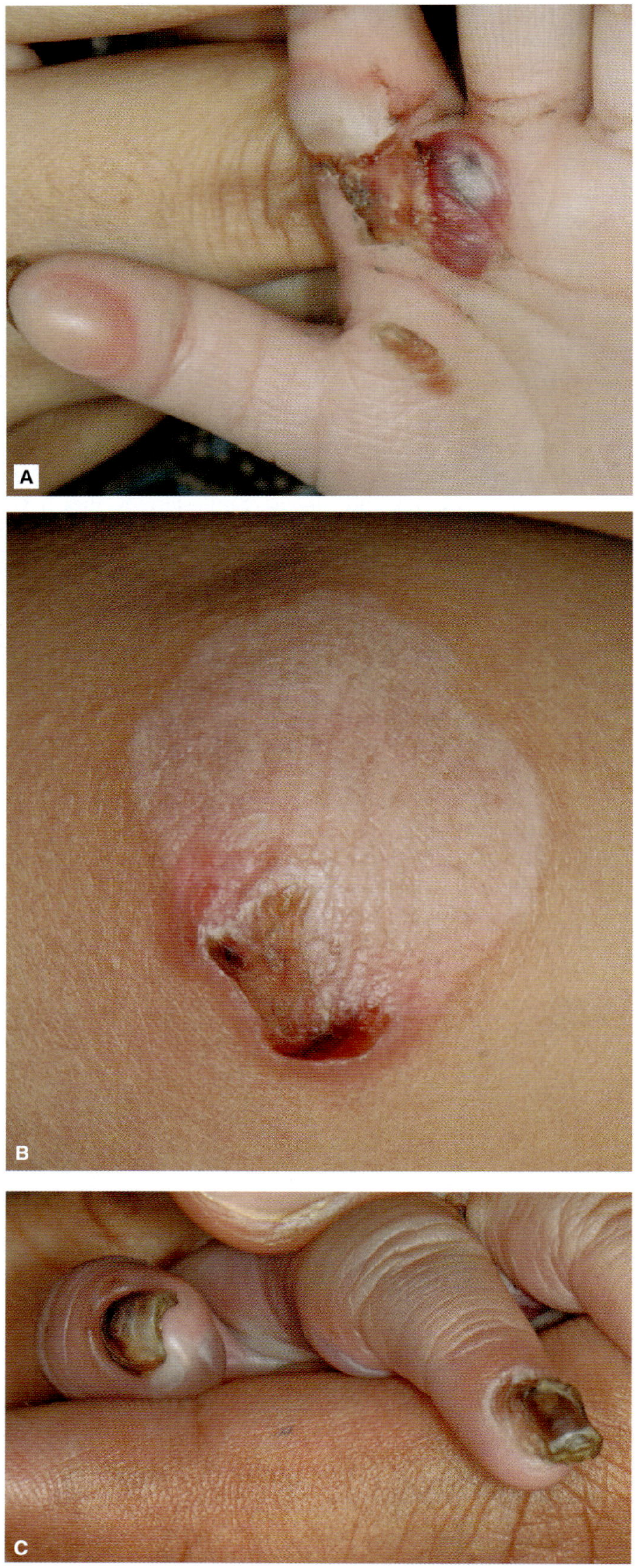

FIGURE 12-3A–3C. EBS in an Indian infant associated with *KRT14* mutation, presenting with flaccid and tense blisters and erosions, mainly over the acral sites. There is accompanying dyspigmentation (Figure 12-3B) and abnormal nails (Figure 12-3C).

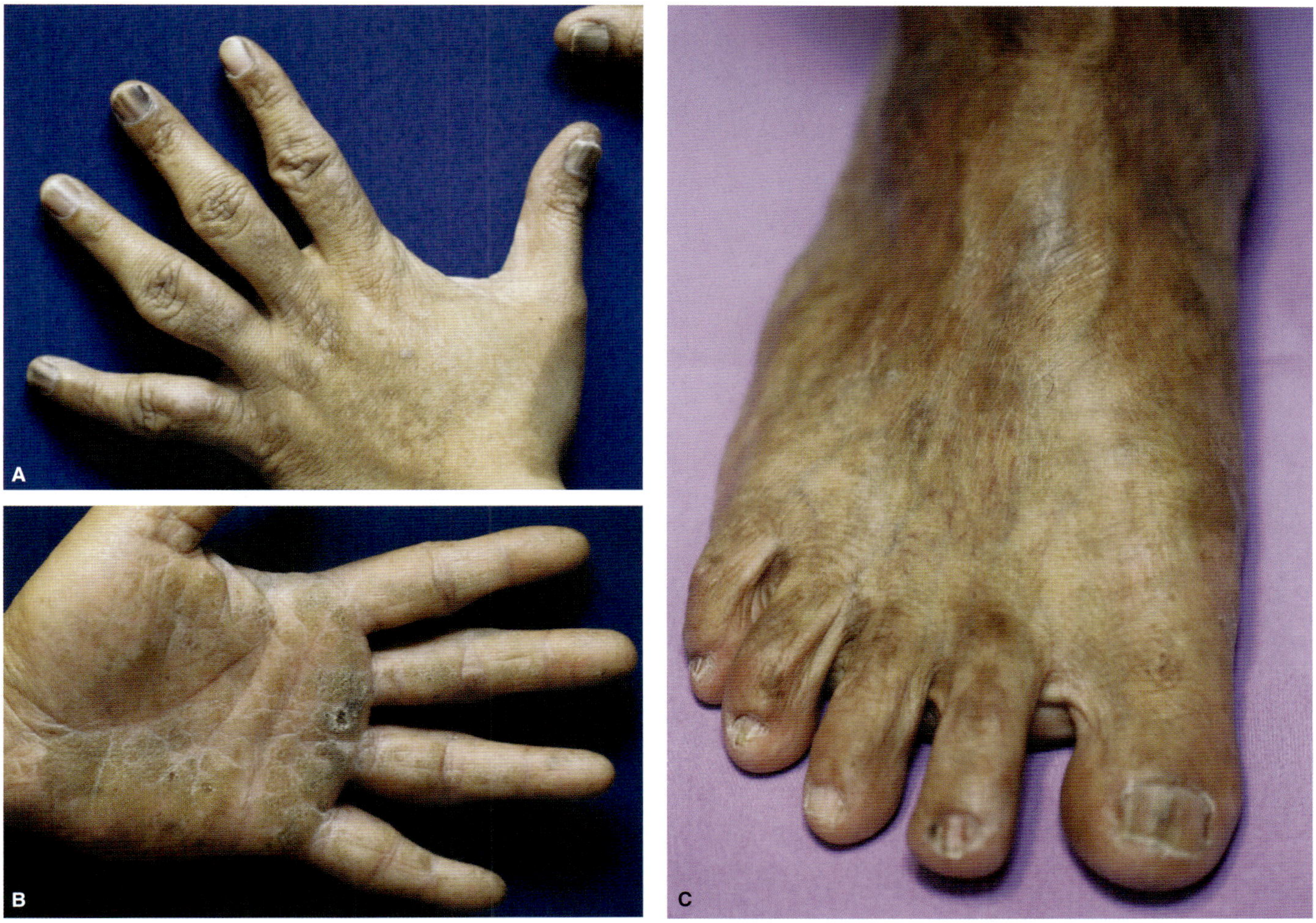

FIGURE 12-4A–4C. EBS with mottled pigmentation associated with *KRT14* mutation in a Malay adolescent male. There is minimal blistering at this age, but hyperkeratosis of the palms is evident. There is widespread mottled hyperpigmentation and there are abnormal nails (Figure 12-4C).

mild subtype have better prognosis, but patients have blistering throughout life.

- Dystrophic epidermolysis bullosa (DEB)
  - All forms of DEB are associated with mutations in type VII collagen, which is an important component of the anchoring fibrils in the superficial dermis.
  - DEB can be inherited as autosomal dominant or recessive traits, with the recessive forms presenting with more severe disease.
  - Blisters and erosions are commonly seen on areas prone to trauma and friction such as the hands and feet, elbows, and knees. Involvement can be more widespread in the recessive type of DEB.
  - Scarring and milia formation at the site of healed blisters and erosions are classical.
  - Nail dystrophy may be seen in about 80% of cases.
  - Other features in severe recessive DEB include extensive mucosal involvement, fusion of digits, joint contractures, and growth retardation.
  - Development of squamous cell carcinoma is a common complication in adolescents and early adulthood, and can lead to early mortality.
- Kindler syndrome
  - Kindler syndrome is an extremely rare subtype of EB caused by mutation in *FERMT1* gene, and has autosomal recessive inheritance.
  - Clinical features include early acral blisters that improve with age, photosensitivity, diffuse skin atrophy, and poikiloderma.
  - Mucosal involvement is common and presents as mucositis, gingivitis, periodontal disease, and premature loss of teeth.

Differential Diagnosis

- Friction blisters
  - Friction blisters are common in newborns and can often be mistaken for early EB. These occur at sites that are accessible to the fetus' mouth in-utero, such as over the fingers, hands, and even the feet. They may also

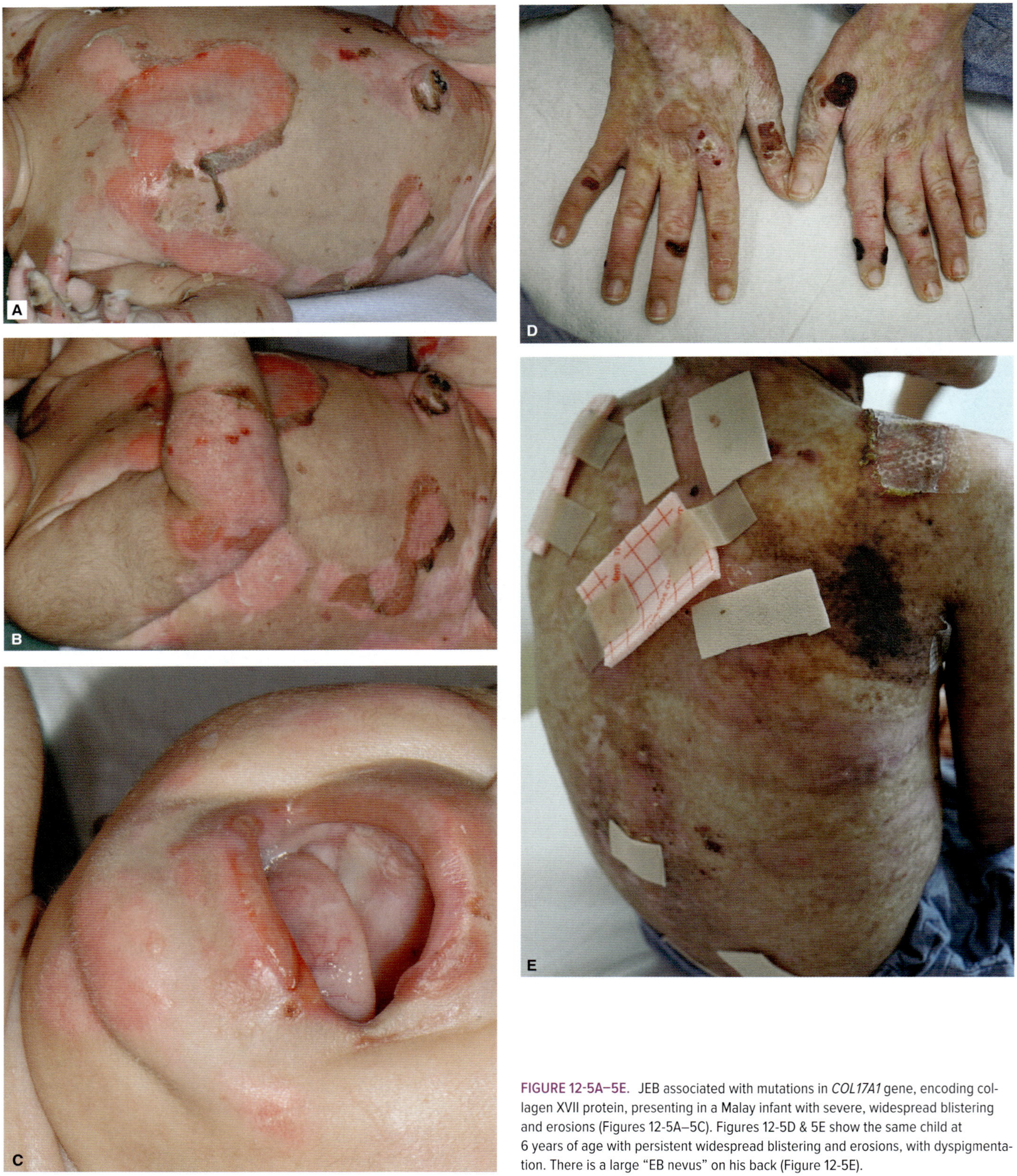

FIGURE 12-5A–5E. JEB associated with mutations in *COL17A1* gene, encoding collagen XVII protein, presenting in a Malay infant with severe, widespread blistering and erosions (Figures 12-5A–5C). Figures 12-5D & 5E show the same child at 6 years of age with persistent widespread blistering and erosions, with dyspigmentation. There is a large "EB nevus" on his back (Figure 12-5E).

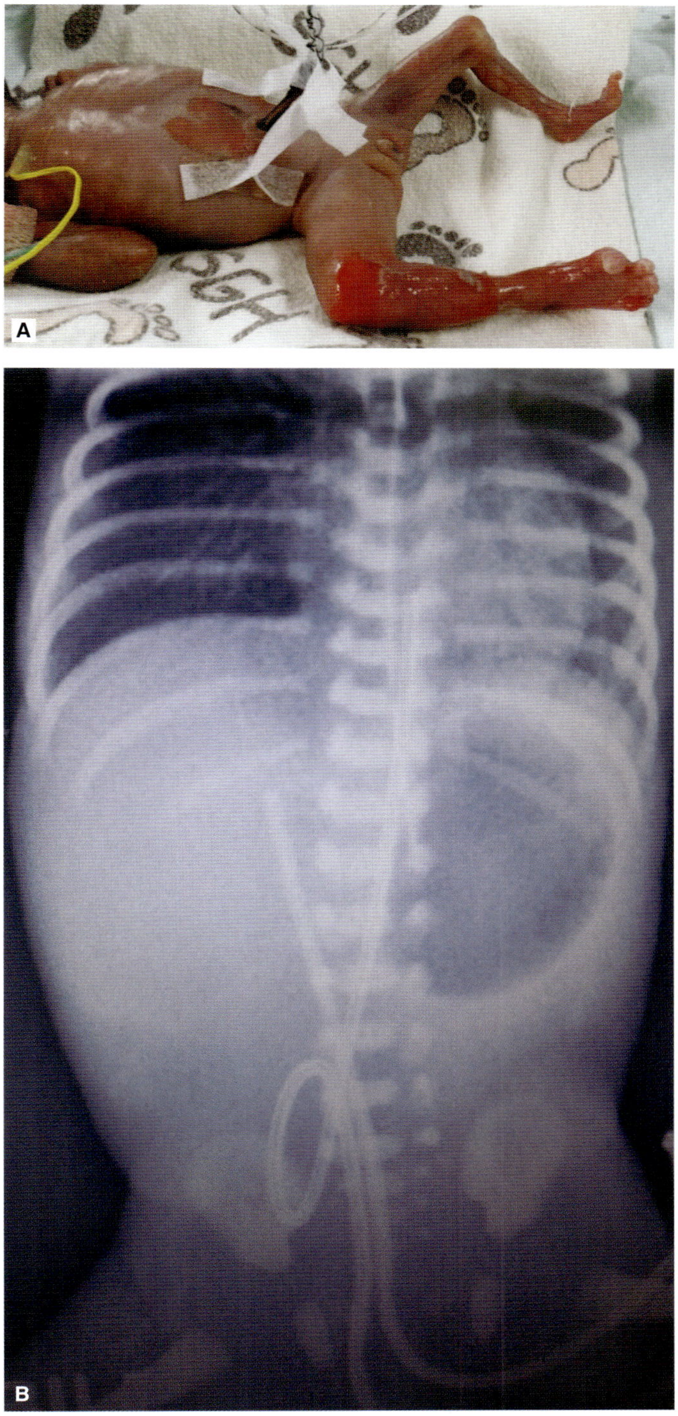

FIGURE 12-6A & 6B. JEB with pyloric atresia, associated with mutation in *ITGB4* gene, encoding integrin β4 protein, presenting in a premature neonate with widespread erosions on the limbs, face, and trunk. Abdominal radiograph reveals the "gas-bubble" sign (Figure 12-6B).

sometimes occur on the lips. Observation for more blisters will differentiate it from EB.

- Infections
  - Common infections that present with blisters in the neonatal period include bullous impetigo or staphylococcal scalded skin syndrome and herpes infections (herpes simplex virus or varicella-zoster virus).
  - These can be excluded by appropriate microbiological investigations. Empirical systemic antimicrobials should be initiated before results return if there is suspicion for infections.
- Immune mediated blistering disorders
  - Very rarely, immune-mediated blistering disorders occurring in the mother, such as bullous pemphigoid and epidermolysis bullosa acquisita, can also occur transiently in the newborn due to transplacental transfer of autoantibodies.
  - De novo occurrence of immune-mediated blistering disorders is very rare in infants and early childhood. These can be excluded by appropriate investigations, such as direct immunofluorescence and indirect immunofluorescence.
- Keratinopathic ichthyosis (KI)
  - Patients with KI, an autosomal condition caused by mutations in KRT1 or KRT10 genes, may also present with superficial blisters and may be confused with EB. With time, the skin of these patients thickens and becomes more ichthyotic.
  - A skin biopsy will show the characteristic finding of epidermolytic hyperkeratosis, with the superficial stratum granulosum appearing vacuolated with coarse keratohyalin granules.
- Mastocytosis
  - Patients with mastocytosis can present with bullae. However, the underlying skin is usually hyperpigmented with a slightly irregular "peau-de-orange" surface.
  - A skin biopsy will help to confirm the diagnosis of mastocytosis.

Investigations & Treatment

- Regular skin biopsies are not useful to delineate the level of cleavage to determine the EB subtype. Instead, performing skin biopsies for immunofluorescence mapping (IFM) will help to ascertain the level of cleavage. Skin biopsy for IFM should be taken from a freshly induced blister.
- Mutation analysis for molecular confirmation is useful for accurate diagnosis, prognostication, and for prenatal or perinatal diagnosis for future pregnancies.
- Treatment of EB is multidisciplinary and mostly palliative. Treatment should focus on avoidance of trauma and chronic wound management. Ideally, the use of nonadherent dressings should be advised (e.g., silicone dressings).
- Management of extracutaneous complications includes monitoring and treatment of pain, eye and dental

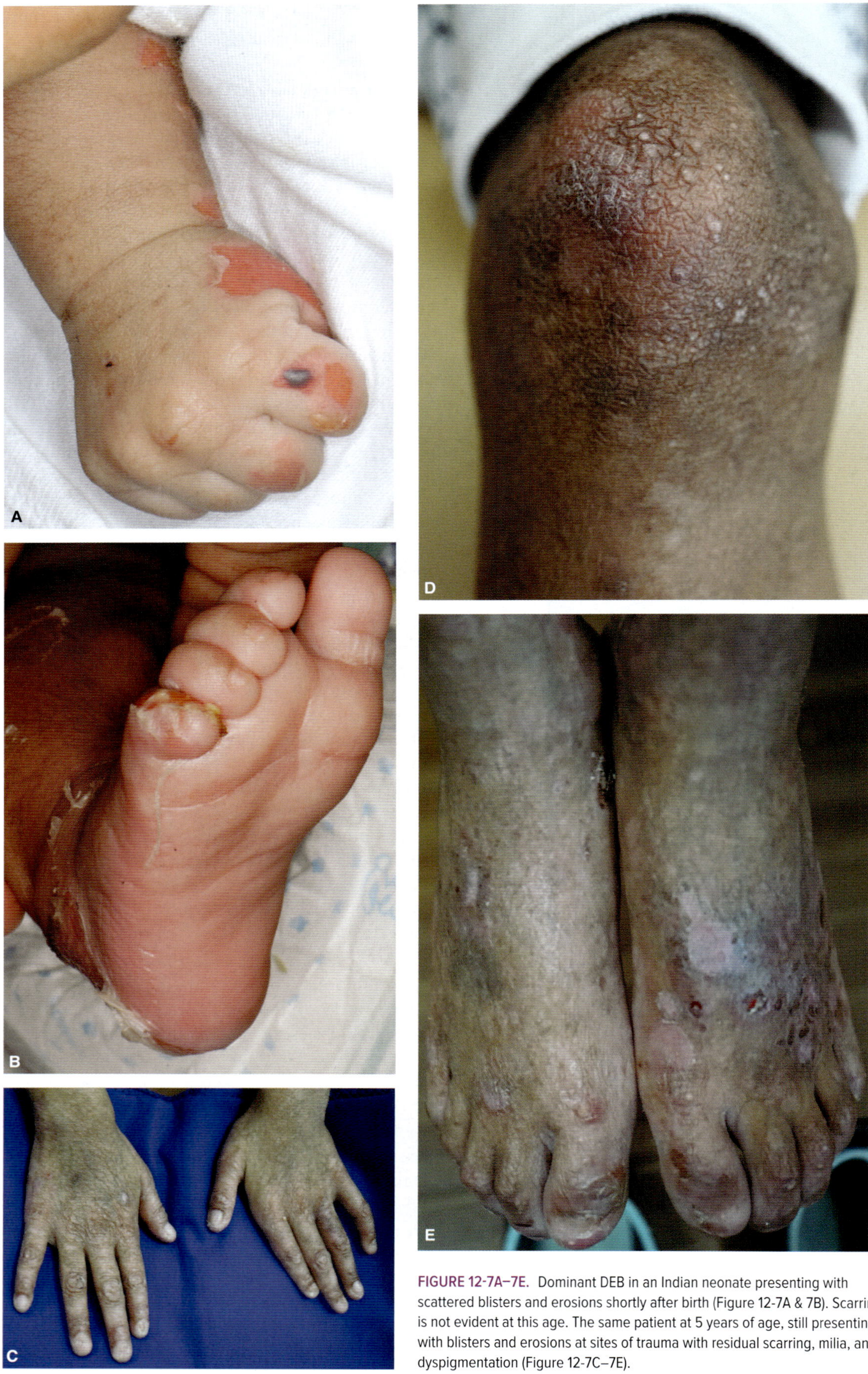

FIGURE 12-7A–7E. Dominant DEB in an Indian neonate presenting with scattered blisters and erosions shortly after birth (Figure 12-7A & 7B). Scarring is not evident at this age. The same patient at 5 years of age, still presenting with blisters and erosions at sites of trauma with residual scarring, milia, and dyspigmentation (Figure 12-7C–7E).

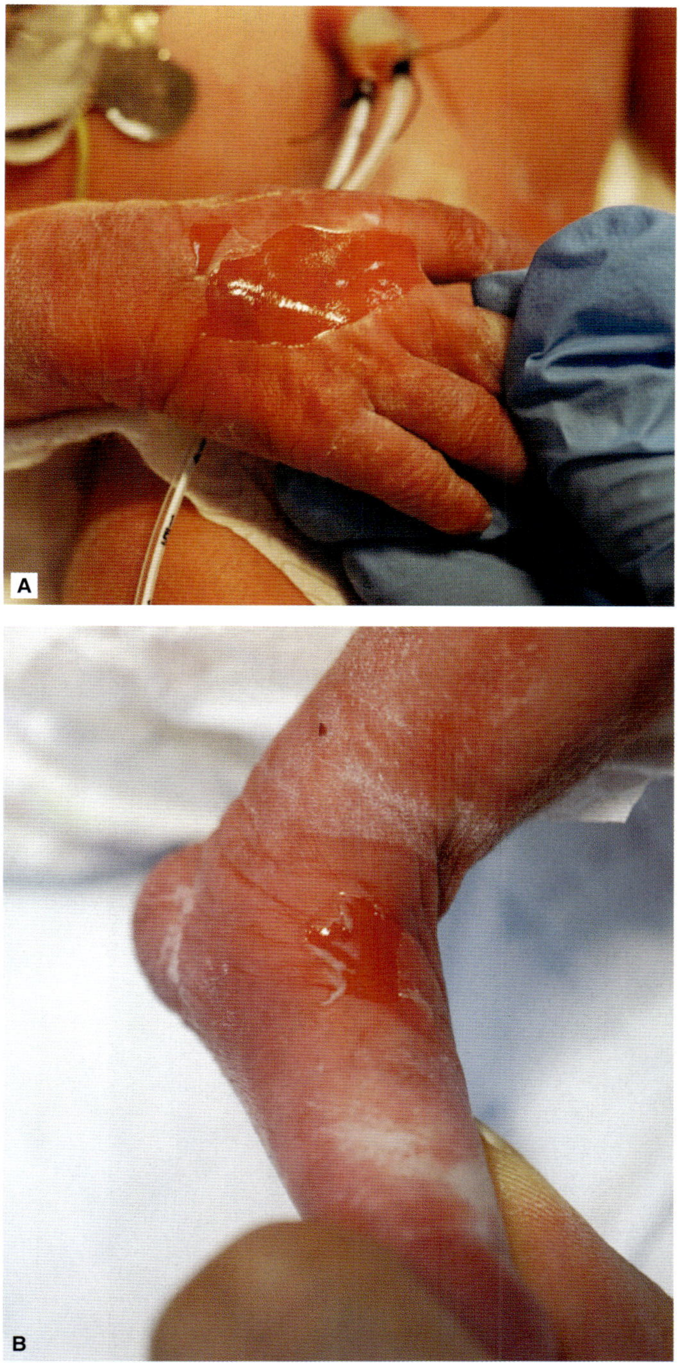

FIGURE 12-8A & 8B. An uncommon case of self-healing DEB presenting in a Malay neonate with scattered blisters and erosions within a few days of life. Blistering improved within the first 2 years of life.

complications, nutritional issues, and orthopedic and growth problems.

Pearls & Practical Tips

- Differentiating the various subtypes of EB in the neonatal and infantile period can be extremely difficult. Apart from clinical features, early IFM and genetic testing can be useful in early diagnosis and prognostication.

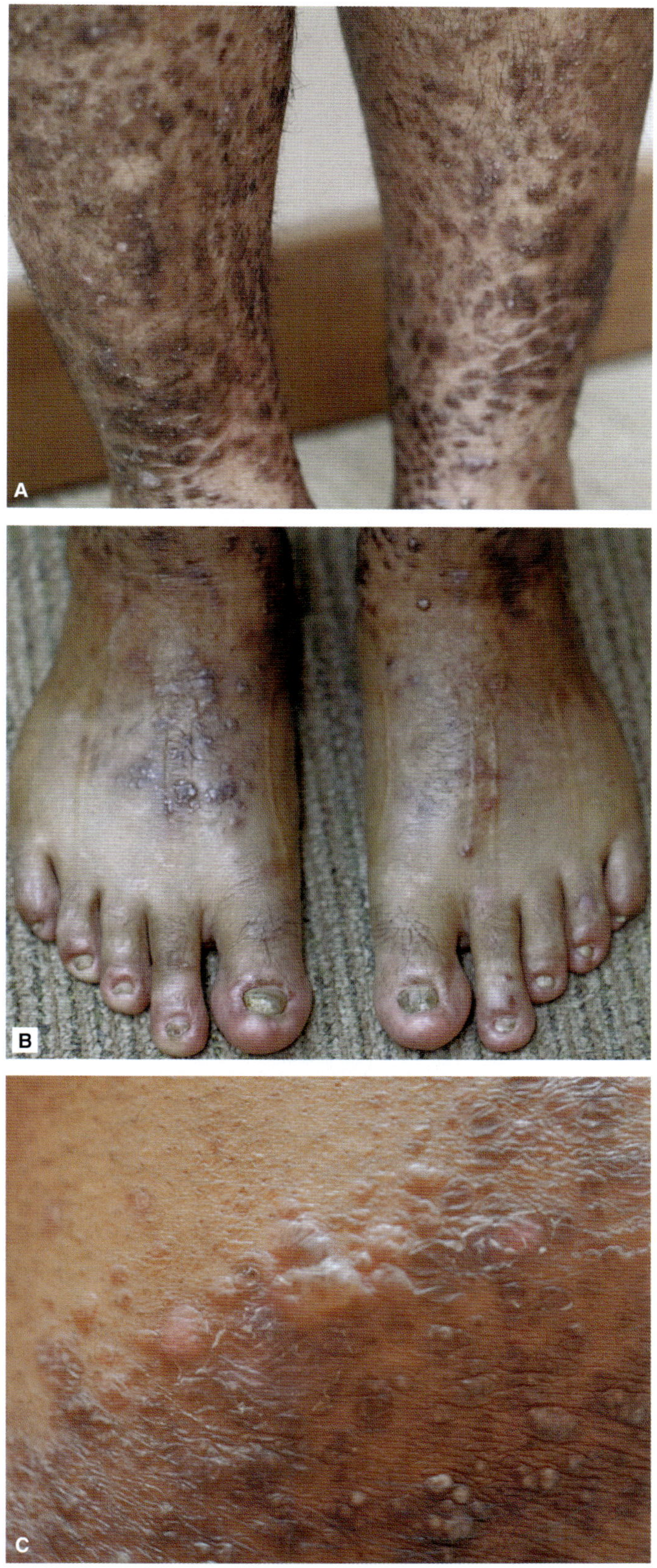

FIGURE 12-9A–9C. DEB pruriginosa is a distinct form of DEB that presents with blisters that heal to form hyperpigmented, extremely pruritic papules, mimicking prurigo nodularis, affecting mainly the extensor surfaces. This is seen in this Indian adult female with *COL7A1* mutation.

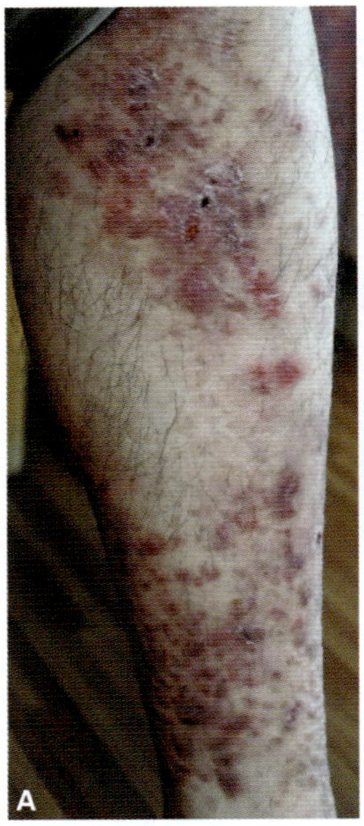

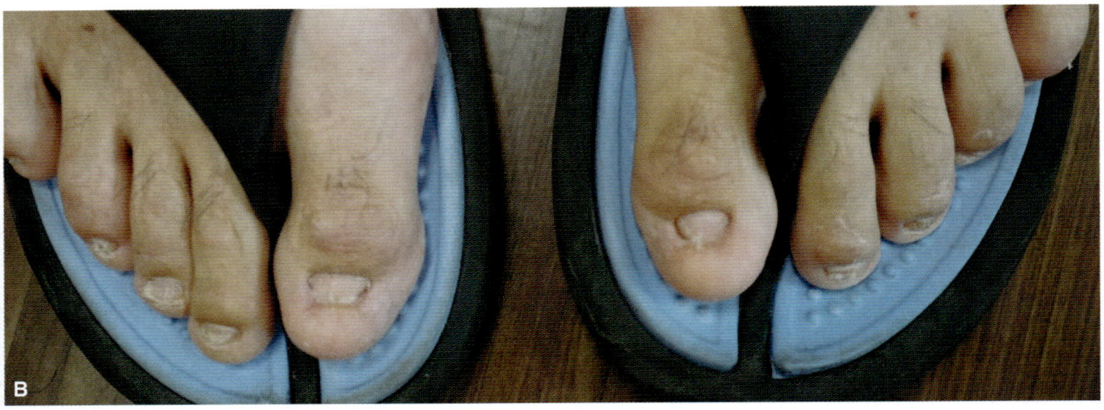

FIGURE 12-10A & 10B. An adult male patient with DEB pruriginosa with recurrent small blisters and erosions that result in persistent, itchy, hyperpigmented-to-erythematous papules, mostly affecting the extensor surfaces of the legs. The patient also has absent great toenails.

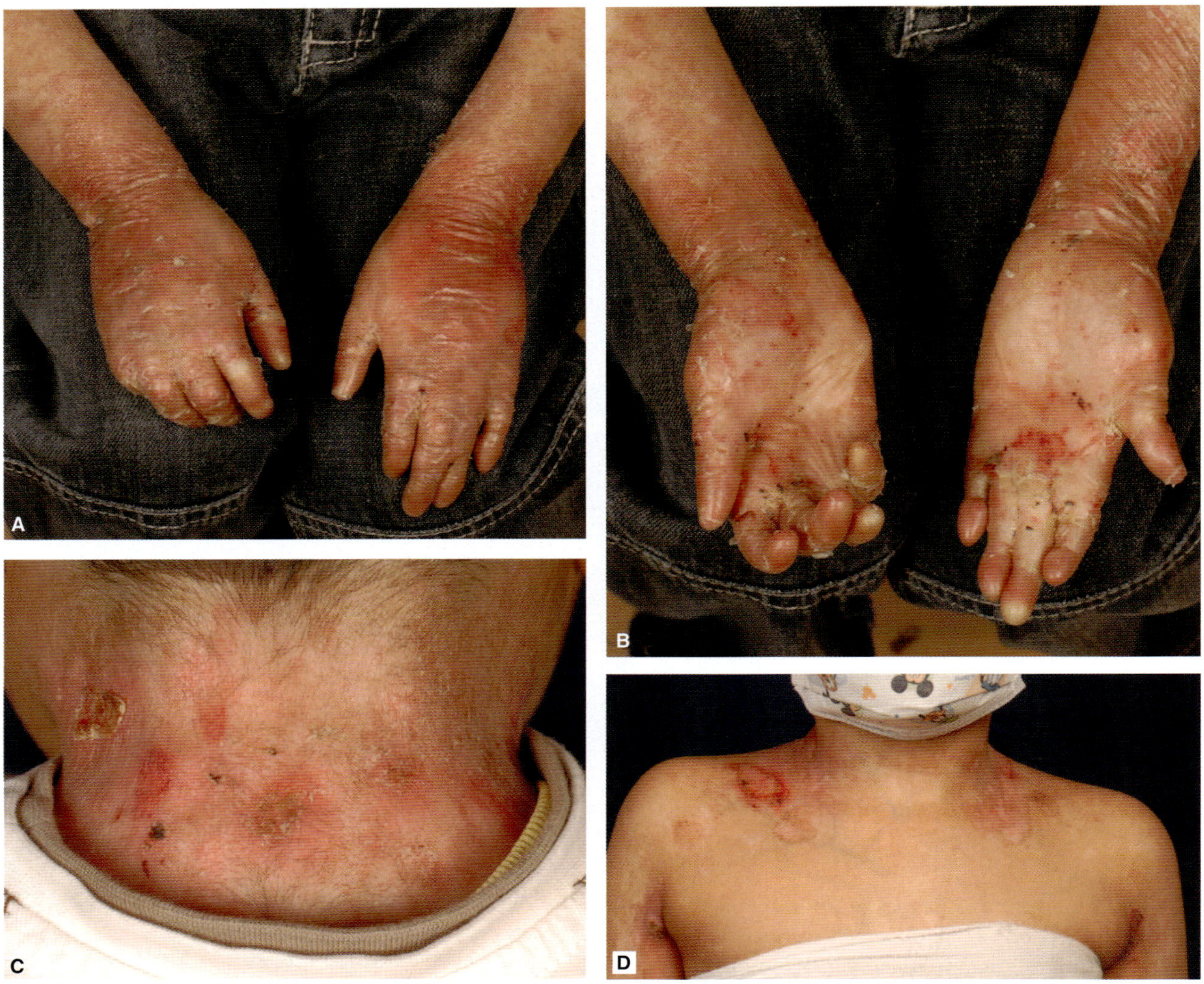

FIGURE 12-11A–11D. Recessive DEB in an Indian boy with severe scarring and pseudosyndactyly of his hands with loss of nails. There are also widespread erosions and scarring on his trunk.

- EB subtypes with mottled pigmentation have been described in pigmented skin. This can be seen in patients with EBS or DEB.
- DEBRA, the support group for EB, now has many branches around the world, although it is not present in all countries in Asia. Clinical guidelines for the management of EB can be downloaded from the EB-Clinet website (www.eb-clinet.org).

Bibliography

1. Has C, Bauer JW, Bodemer C, et al. Consensus reclassification of inherited epidermolysis bullosa and other disorders with skin fragility. Br J Dermatol 2020;183(4):614-27.

INHERITED ICHTHYOSIS

The inherited ichthyoses are a group of disorders characterized by impairment in stratum corneum desquamation, leading to hyperkeratosis and scaling. This results from either abnormal corneocyte shedding (retention hyperkeratosis) or increased epidermal cell proliferation (epidermal hyperplasia). In nonsyndromic ichthyosis, only the skin is affected. In syndromic ichthyosis, other organ systems besides the skin are also affected.[1]

Clinical Features

- Ichthyosis vulgaris (common ichthyosis)
  - This is the most common form of inherited ichthyosis and is associated with pathogenic variants in the *FLG* gene, which encodes the filaggrin protein, responsible for maintenance of the epidermal barrier. It is an autosomal dominant disorder with variable expression.
  - It is characterized by scaling and generalized xerosis, with onset during late childhood or adolescence.
  - It most commonly affects the lower limbs, especially the calves and shins.
  - Patients with ichthyosis vulgaris may have other features of atopy, including atopic dermatitis, allergic rhinitis, and asthma. Other cutaneous features include keratosis pilaris and hyperlinear palms.
- X-linked ichthyosis
  - This is an X-linked recessive condition with an incidence of 1 in 6000 males, caused by a mutation in the *STS* gene on chromosome Xp22, resulting in a deficiency of steroid sulfatase.
  - Onset is usually in infancy or early childhood. Affected boys present with large light-brown scales resembling fish scales over the extensor extremities, posterior neck, and upper trunk, with a symmetrical distribution. In most cases, the antecubital and popliteal fossa, palms, and soles are unaffected. The hair and nails are normal.
  - The scales become thicker and grayish yellow-brown in color as the child ages, leading to a "dirty" appearance. Scales on the scalp, neck, and preauricular areas may improve in childhood.
  - Associated features include cryptorchidism (undescended testis) in the affected male and corneal opacities in both the affected male and the carrier female.
  - Placental steroid sulfatase deficiency in the mother may result in low estrogen levels and a failure of initiation or prolonged labor.
  - It can be associated with Kallmann syndrome, as the *KAL1* and *STS* genes are contiguous on the Xp22 chromosome.
- Autosomal recessive congenital ichthyosis (ARCI)
  - ARCI encompasses a group of nonsyndromic congenital ichthyoses that present at birth either as a harlequin or collodion baby.
  - The harlequin baby represents the most phenotypically severe form of ARCI and is caused by pathogenic variants in the *ABCA12* gene. Babies are often born prematurely, with a thick plate-like covering with deep cracks and fissures. There is marked ectropion (outturning of the eyelids), eclabium (fish-mouth deformity) and flattening of the ears.[2] Most harlequin babies are stillborn or have poor survival in the early neonatal period, and have a complicated clinical course, with poor feeding, temperature and electrolyte dysregulation, and dehydration, which may be life-threatening. Movement and respiration maybe impaired by the rigidity of the skin. They are at risk of infection and sepsis.
  - The collodion baby is a descriptive term for babies born with a cellophane-like covering. Pathogenic variants in several genes are associated: *ABCA12*, *ALOX12B*, *ALOXE3*, *CERS3*, *CYP4F22*, *lipase (LIPN)*, *NIPAL4/ICHTHYIN*, *PNPLA1*, and *TGM1*.[2] At birth, there is variable thickness of the membrane, which may distort facial features and extremities, leading to digital constriction, flattened ears, ectropion, and eclabium. After a few weeks, the collodion membrane is shed and replaced by large scales. During the neonatal period, some babies may have complications such as reduced ability to suck, respiratory difficulty, aspiration pneumonia, fluid and electrolyte imbalances, temperature instability, increased metabolic requirements, and cutaneous and systemic infections. Hyperkeratosis in the older child can result in obstruction of eccrine sweat glands, resulting in hypohidrosis and risk of overheating. Over time, the clinical features evolve to either a lamellar ichthyosis (LI) phenotype with thick, brown, dirty scales or a congenital ichthyosiform erythroderma (CIE) phenotype with generalized redness and thinner scaling.

Differential Diagnoses

- Acquired forms of ichthyosis
  - Ichthyosis may be induced by drugs such as retinoids, chemotherapy, and targeted cancer drugs. A detailed past medical history and drug history is useful in eliciting a temporal sequence of the inciting drug and onset of ichthyosis.

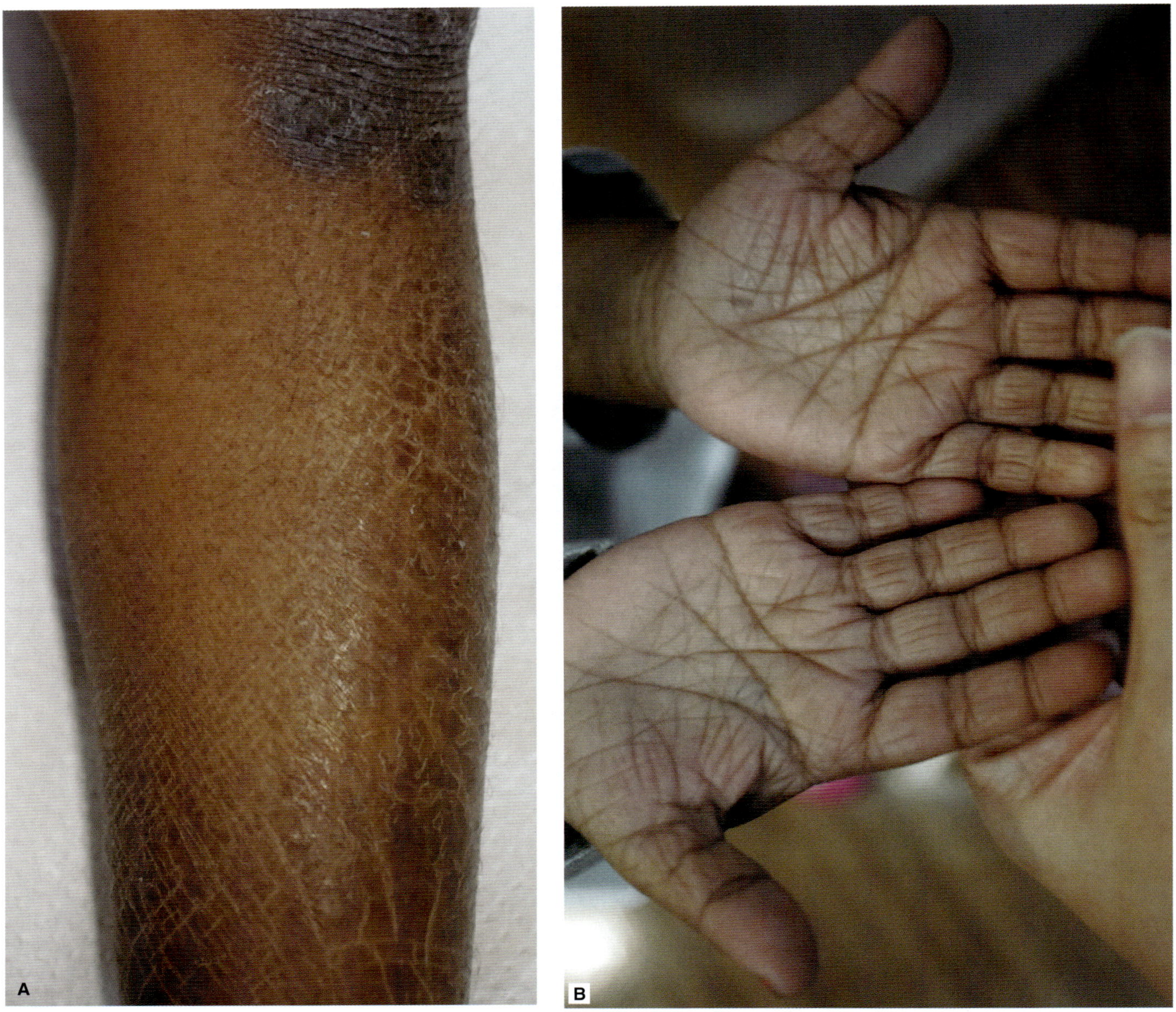

FIGURE 12-12A & 12B. Ichthyosis vulgaris occurring on the shins of this Indian girl. She also has hyperlinearity of the palms and patches of eczema.

- Other rarer causes of acquired ichthyosis include infections (e.g., HIV, leprosy), systemic disease (e.g., renal failure, malnutrition, hypothyroidism, hypopituitarism, diabetes), malignancy (e.g., mycosis fungoides and other cutaneous T-cell lymphomas, Hodgkin's disease).

Investigations & Treatment

- Ichthyosis vulgaris
  - Ichthyosis vulgaris is diagnosed clinically. Treatment involves frequent application of topical moisturizers.
- X-linked ichthyosis
  - Diagnosis can usually be made from family history and clinical findings. Mutation analysis for *STS* gene may be performed to confirm the diagnosis. Skin biopsy is usually not useful, with nonspecific findings of hyperkeratosis and hypergranulosis.
  - Treatment involves the use of keratolytics (e.g., urea, lactic acid, glycolic acid, and salicylic acid) and frequent application of topical moisturizers.
  - Topical retinoids may be useful in some patients. Severe cases may require oral acitretin, but its use is limited due to adverse effects.
- Autosomal recessive congenital ichthyosis
  - Genetic studies can be performed to detect the causative gene mutation. This is now performed with next-generation sequencing.

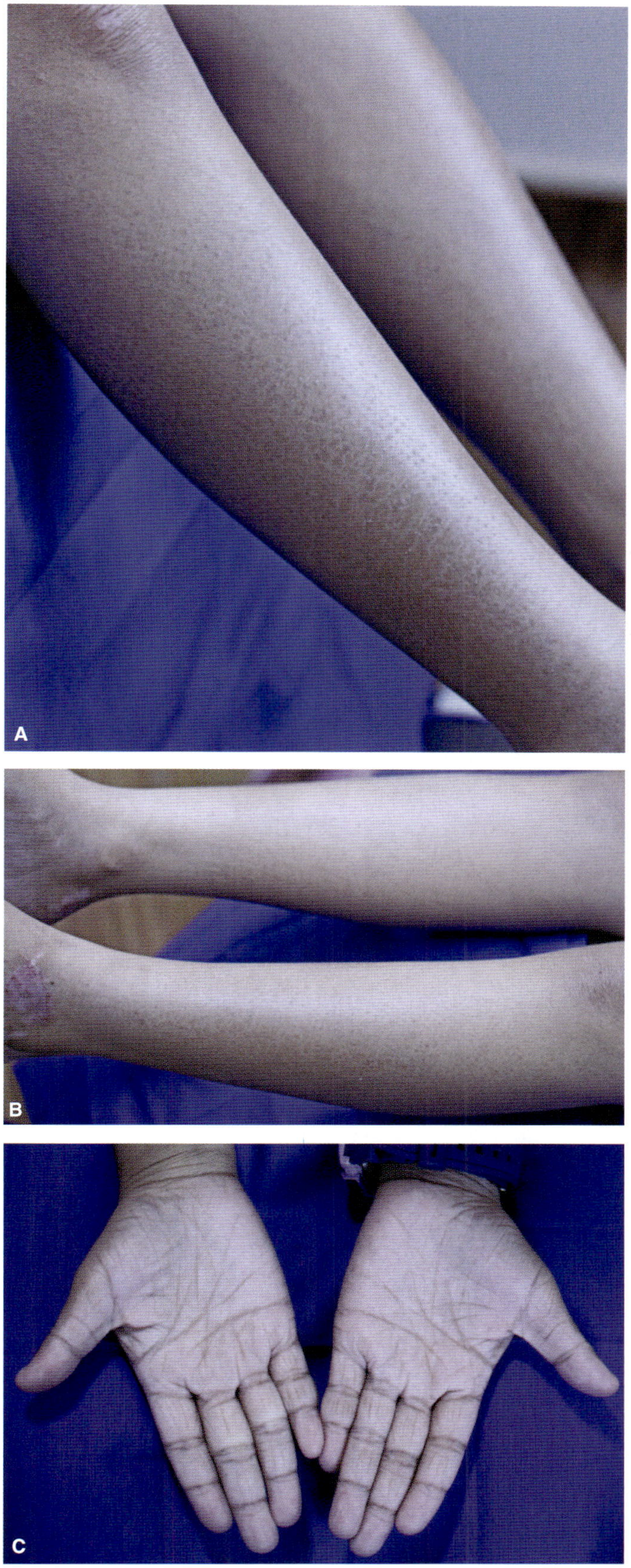

FIGURE 12-13A–13C. Ichthyosis vulgaris in a 10-year-old Chinese girl with mild scaling on the lower legs, in addition to hyperlinear palms. She also has mild eczema over the ankle area.

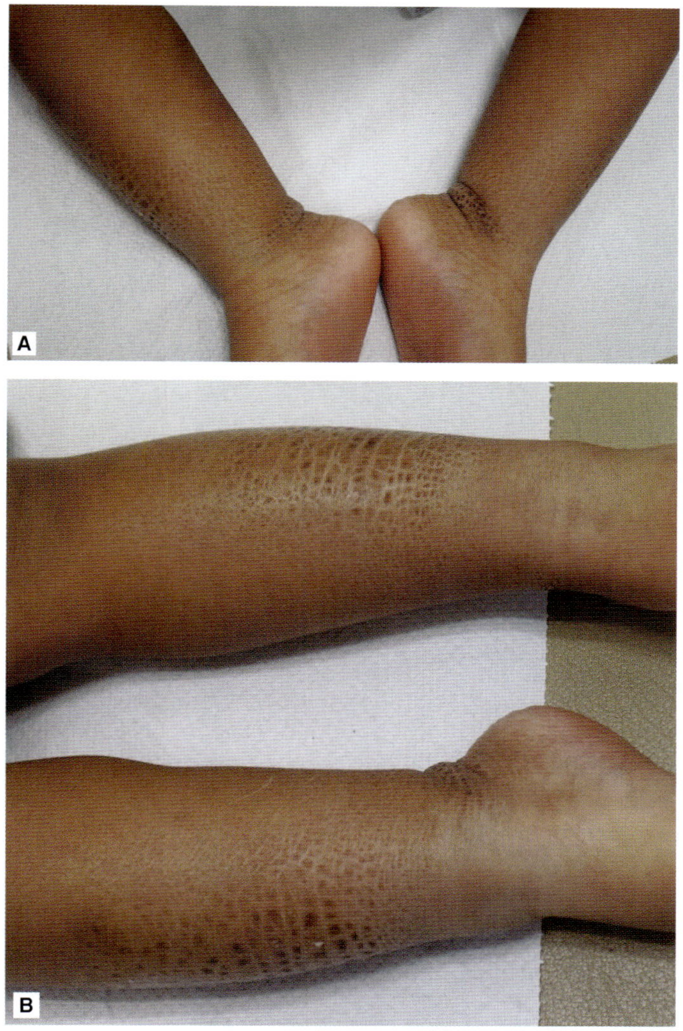

FIGURE 12-14A & 14B. Three-year-old Malay boy, with X-linked ichthyosis, presenting with hyperpigmented scales on the extensor surfaces from a few months of age.

- Skin biopsies for routine histology are nondiagnostic, as there will be variable hyperkeratosis, parakeratosis, and acanthosis. Immunohistochemical staining, such as transglutaminase-1, can be performed to detect loss of affected protein.
- Treatment involves regular application of moisturizers to alleviate symptoms of dryness, thickening, and fissuring. An exfoliating soft sponge can be used to remove scales. Non-soap cleansers should be used.
- Topical and systemic retinoids can be effective in reducing scaling and improving both function and appearance.[3]
- If there is antenatal suspicion of a harlequin ichthyosis, a neonatal team should be on standby at birth for resuscitation. Subtle signs on antenatal ultrasound include polyhydramnios, echogenic amniotic fluid, fetal growth restriction, ectropion and eclabium, flat

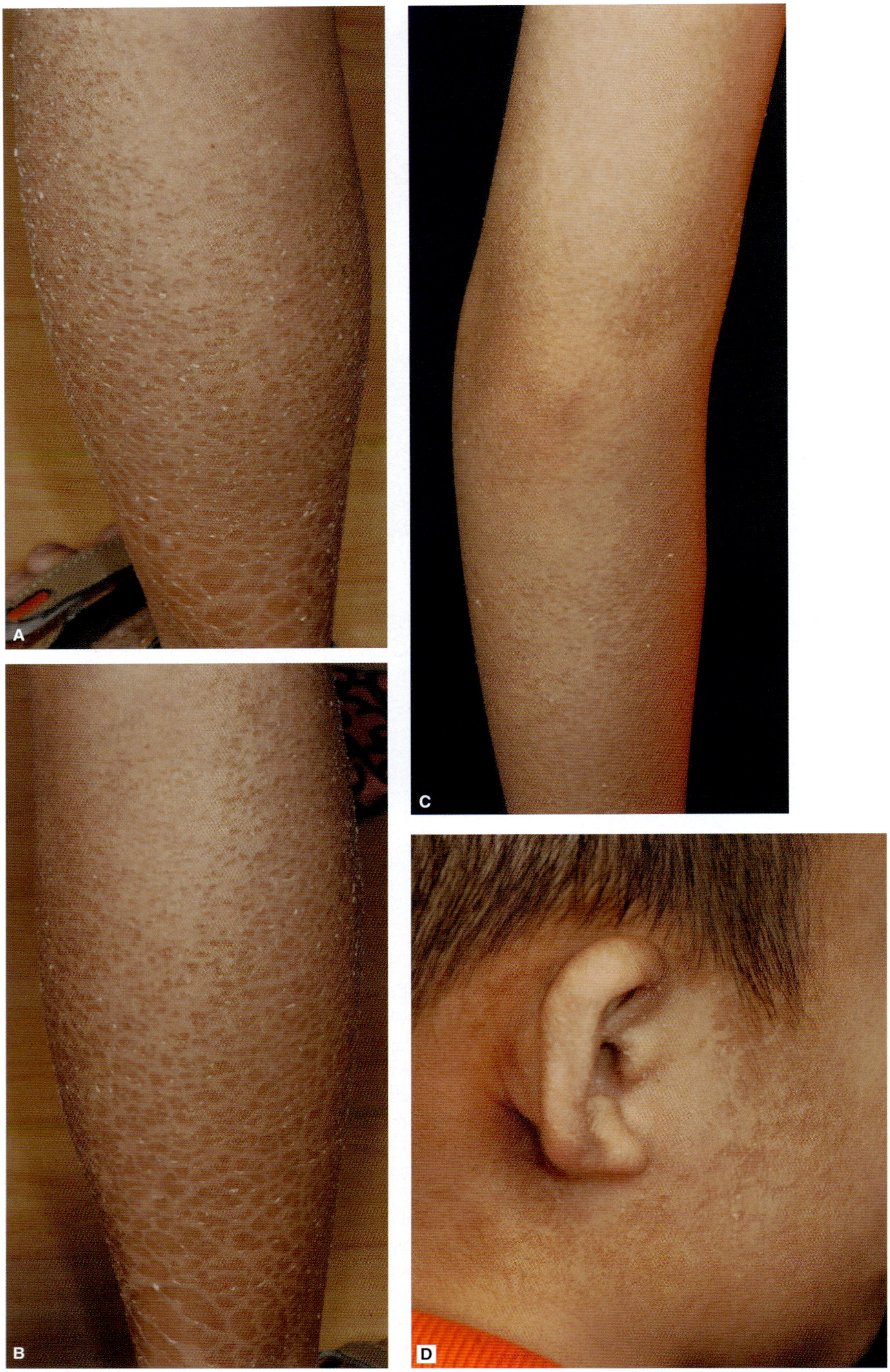

FIGURE 12-15A–15D. X-linked ichthyosis in a Chinese boy presenting with "dirty" scaling on the extensor surfaces of the legs, with less severe involvement of the arms and face.

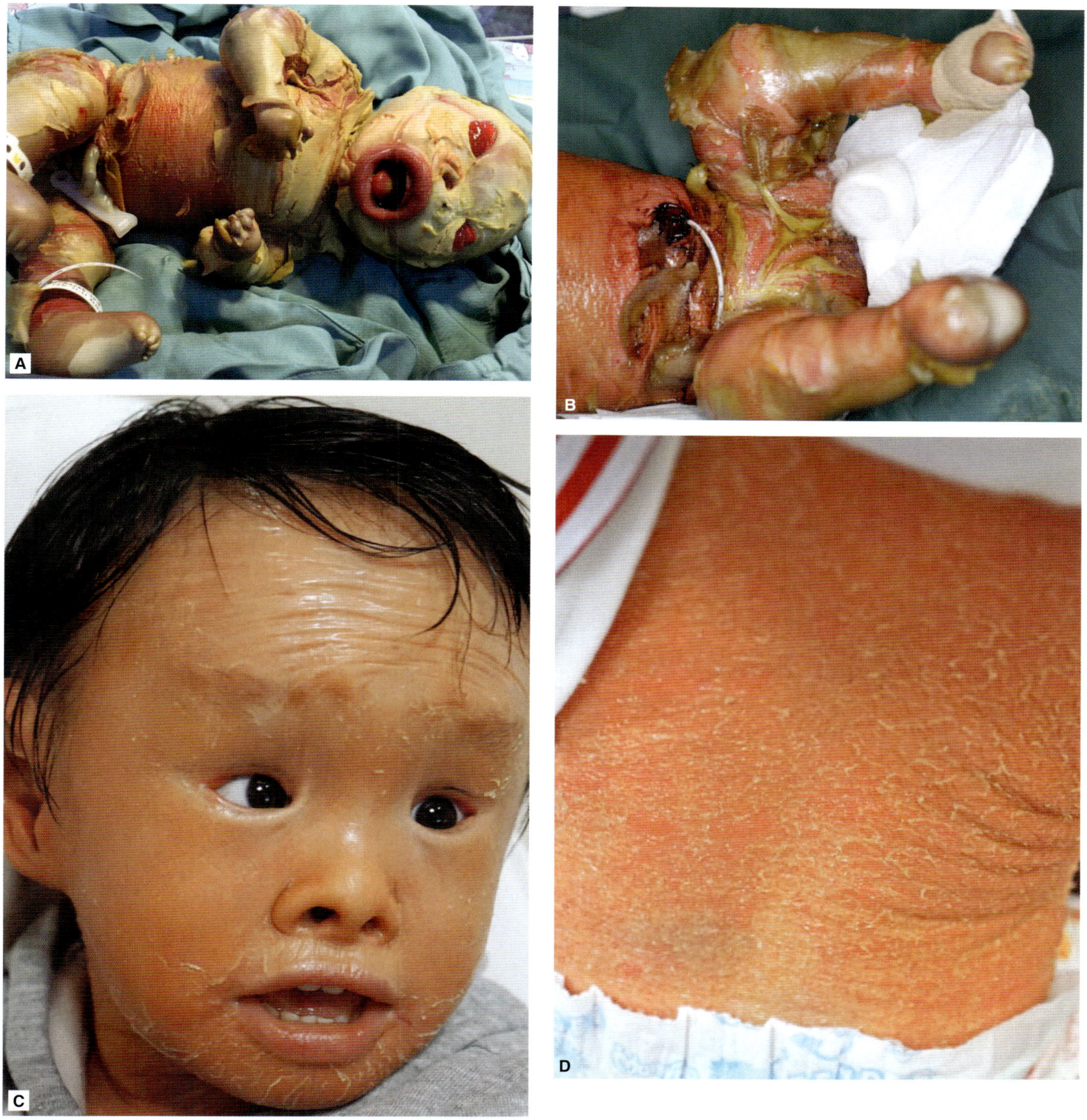

FIGURE 12-16A–16D. Harlequin ichthyosis presenting in a newborn Chinese girl with *ABCA12* mutation. There are thick plate-like scales covering the entire skin surface with ectropion and eclabium. The fingers and toes are underdeveloped. Figures 12-16C & 16D show the same child at 4 years of age after treatment with high-dose oral acitretin, with residual generalized erythema and scaling. There is still mild ectropion.

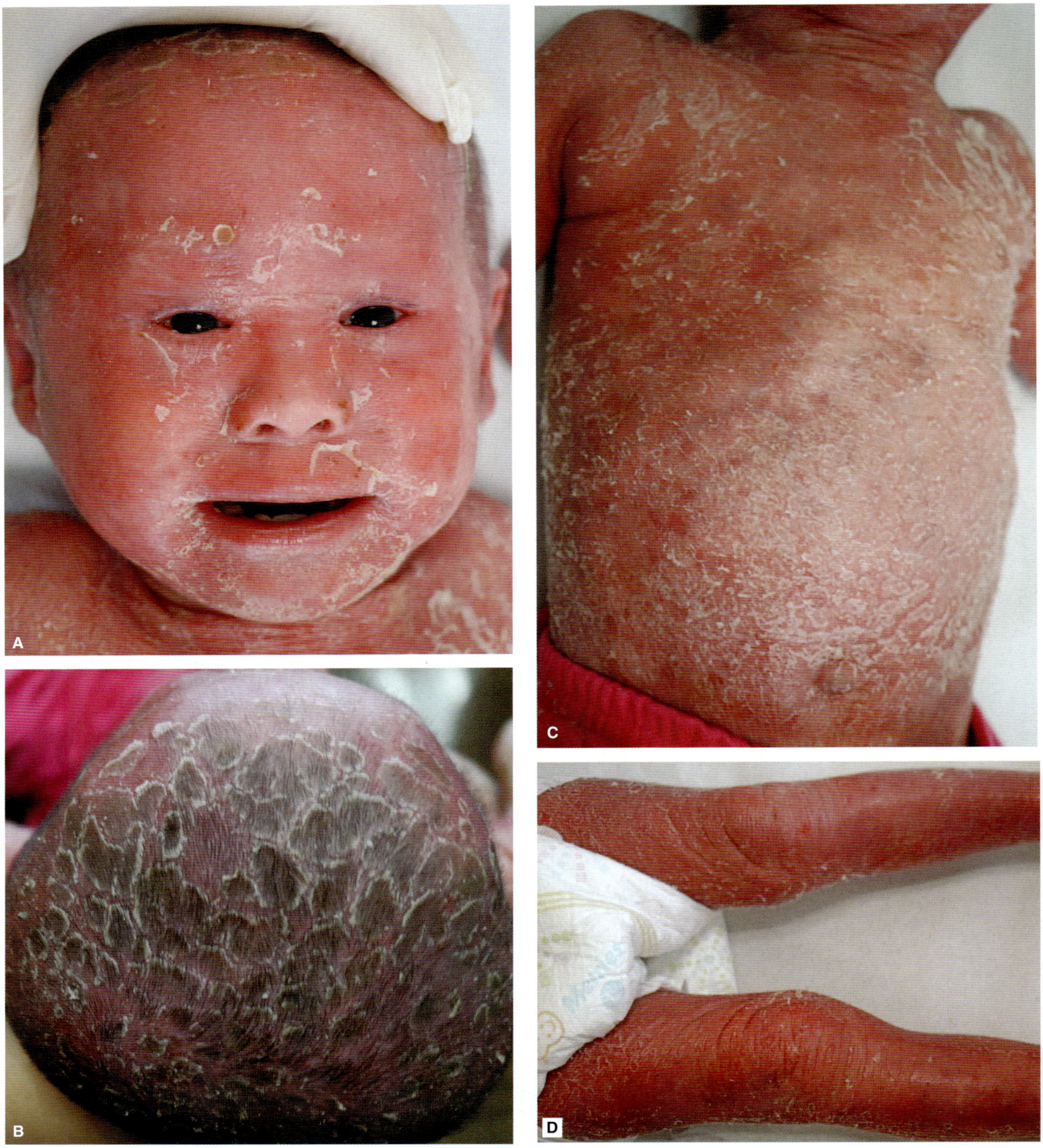

FIGURE 12-17A–17F. Autosomal recessive congenital ichthyosis associated with mutation in *ABCA12* gene presenting with generalized erythema and scaling from birth in a Vietnamese toddler.

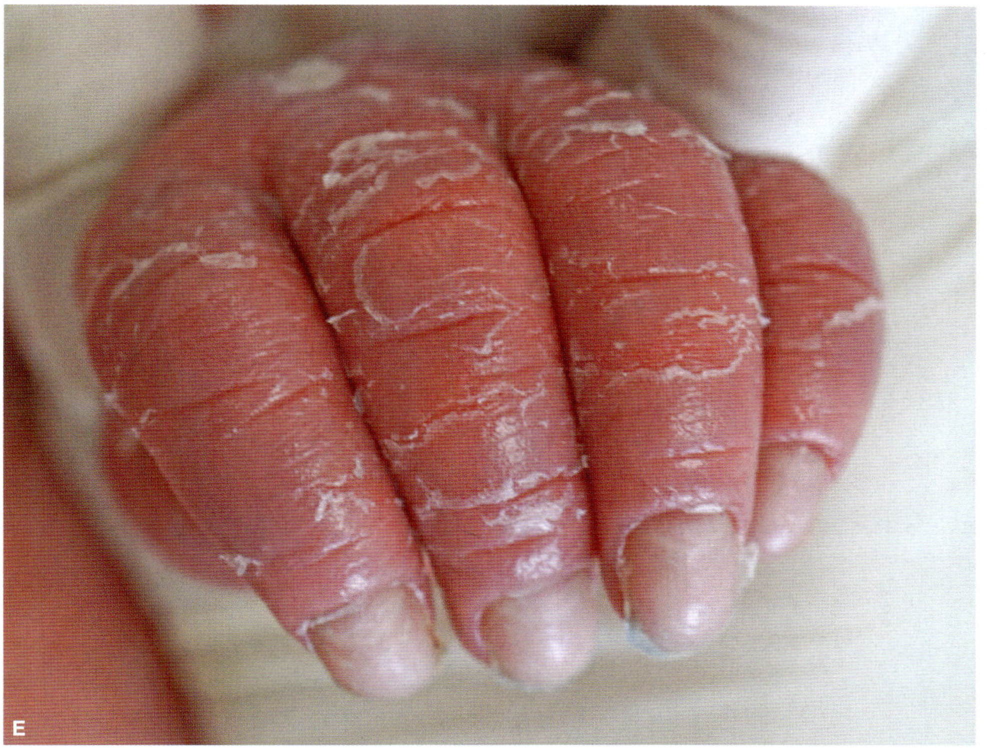

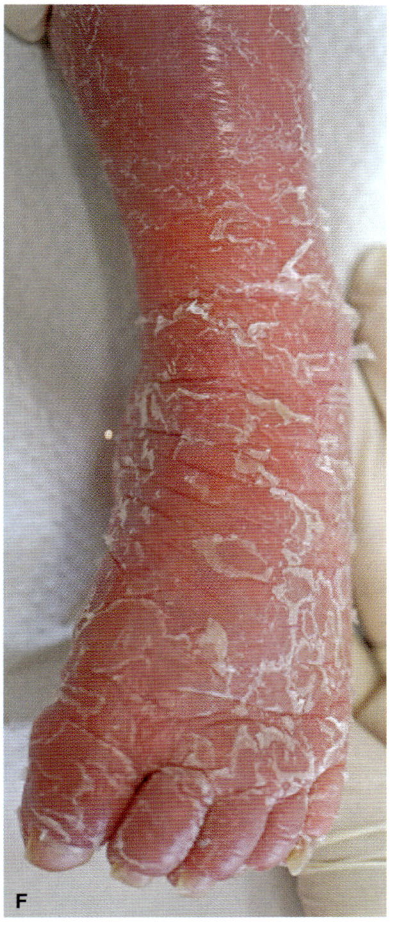

FIGURE 12-17A–17F. (Continued)

nose, wide-open mouth, poorly formed ears, flexion of extremities, hyperflexion of fingers and toes, and absence of opening movements of fingers. At birth, treatment includes intensive care nursing in a humidified incubator for management of body temperature, and fluid and electrolyte status. Regular application of moisturizers should be immediately initiated. Non-soap cleansers should be used. Systemic retinoids such as isotretinoin and acitretin are useful in increasing the survival and improving the quality of life.[3]

Pearls & Practical Tips

- It may be difficult to differentiate ichthyosis vulgaris from X-linked ichthyosis, especially in the younger male child. In general, X-linked ichthyosis occurs much earlier, in the first few months of life, compared to ichthyosis vulgaris, which usually occurs after a few years. Children with ichthyosis vulgaris may have other signs of atopy. The extent of involvement of X-linked ichthyosis is more widespread than ichthyosis vulgaris and also affects the upper limbs, trunk, and face, compared to only the lower limbs in ichthyosis vulgaris.
- Newborns with harlequin ichthyosis and severe collodion membranes should be nursed in a humidified incubator. However, the humidity should be reduced after the first few days of life to prevent overgrowth of pathogenic bacteria, especially *Pseudomonas aeruginosa.*
- Newborns with severe harlequin ichthyosis may require higher doses of retinoids for treatment, such as acitretin >1 mg/kg/day.
- Recent studies have shown clinical improvements with the use of monoclonal antibodies targeting the Th17 immune pathway.[4]

References

1. Oji V, Tadini G, Akiyama M, et al. Revised nomenclature and classification of inherited ichthyoses: results of the first ichthyoses consensus conference in Sorèze 2009. J Am Acad Dermatol 2010;63(4):607-41.
2. Takeichi T, Akiyama M. Inherited ichthyosis: non-syndromic forms. J Dermatol 2016 Mar;43(3):242-51.
3. Zaenglein AL, Levy ML, Stefanko NS, et al. Consensus recommendations for the use of retinoids in ichthyosis and other disorders of cornification in children and adolescents. Pediatr Dermatol 2021 Jan;38(1):164-80.
4. Paller AS, Renert-Yuval Y, Suprun M, et al. An IL-17-dominant immune profile is shared across the major orphan forms of ichthyosis. J Allergy Clin Immunol 2017 Jan;139(1):152-65.

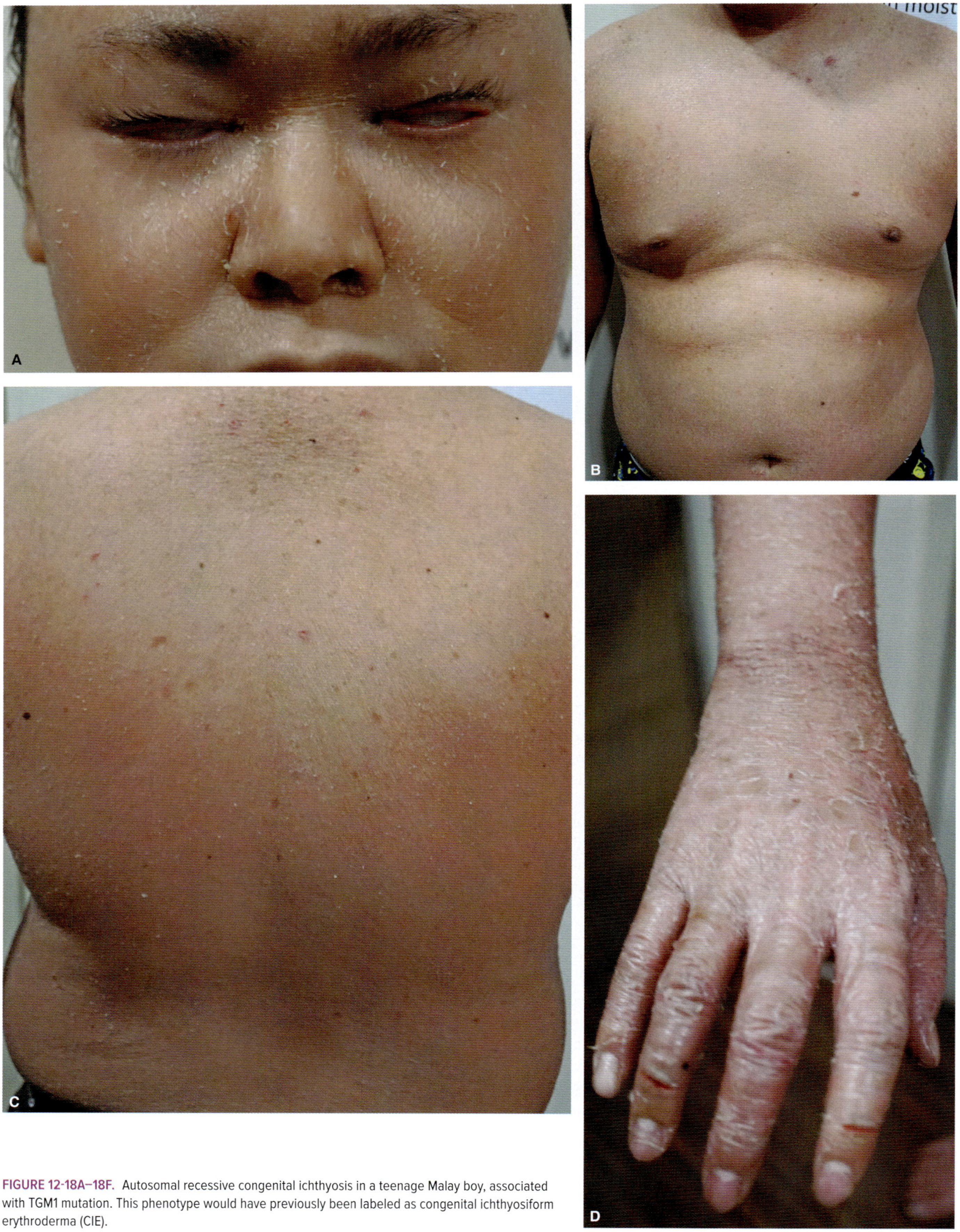

FIGURE 12-18A–18F. Autosomal recessive congenital ichthyosis in a teenage Malay boy, associated with TGM1 mutation. This phenotype would have previously been labeled as congenital ichthyosiform erythroderma (CIE).

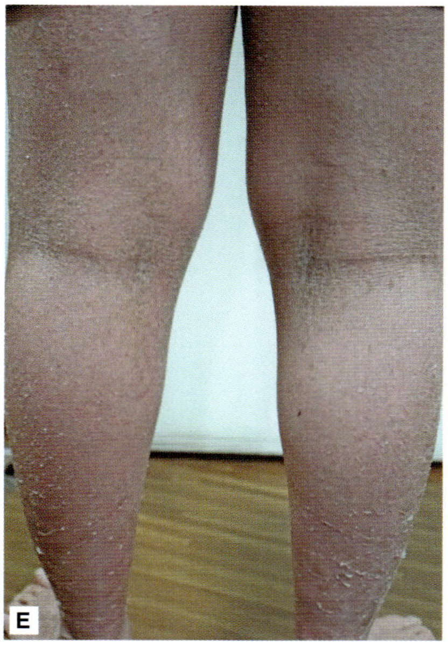

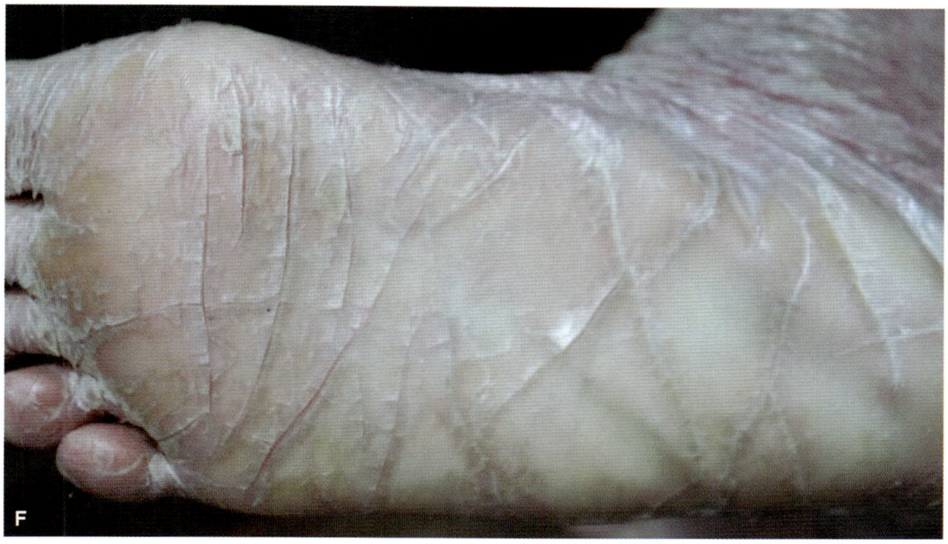

FIGURE 12-18A–18F. (Continued)

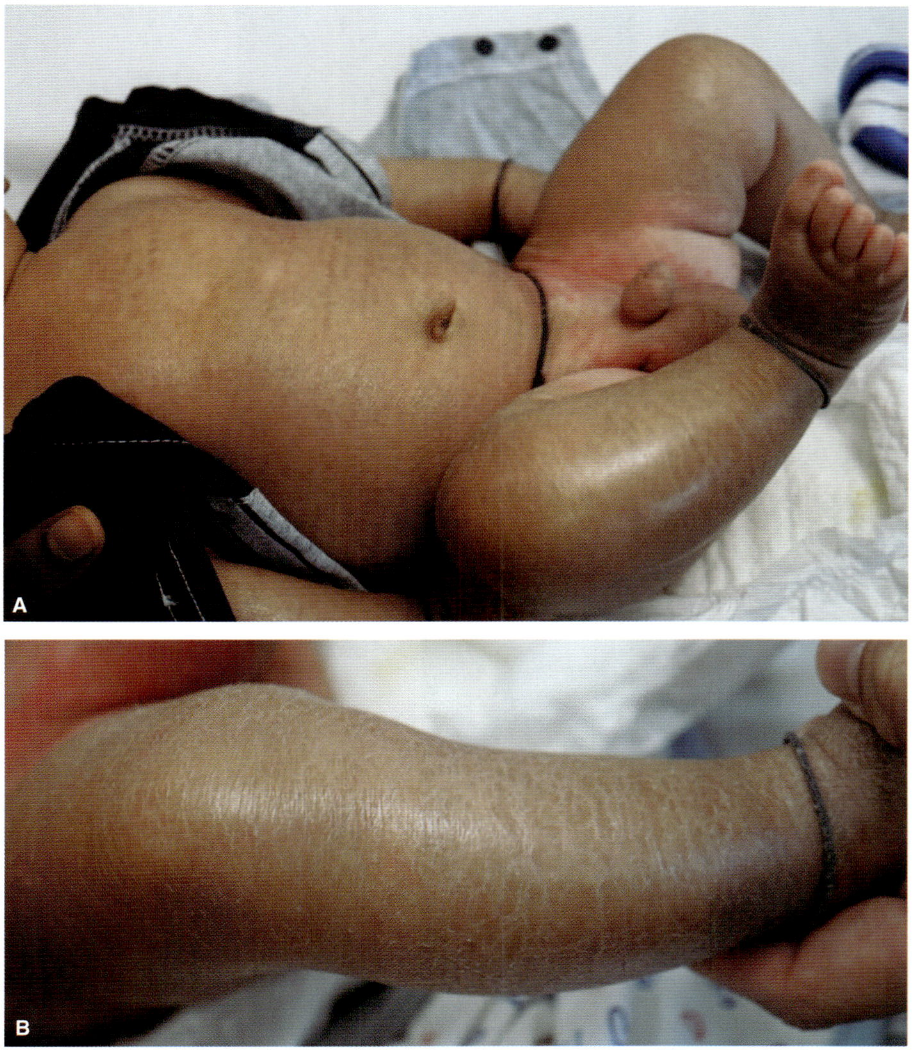

FIGURE 12-19A & 19B. Autosomal recessive congenital ichthyosis presenting with a mild phenotype in a neonate born to consanguineous parents, associated with *ALOXE3* mutation.

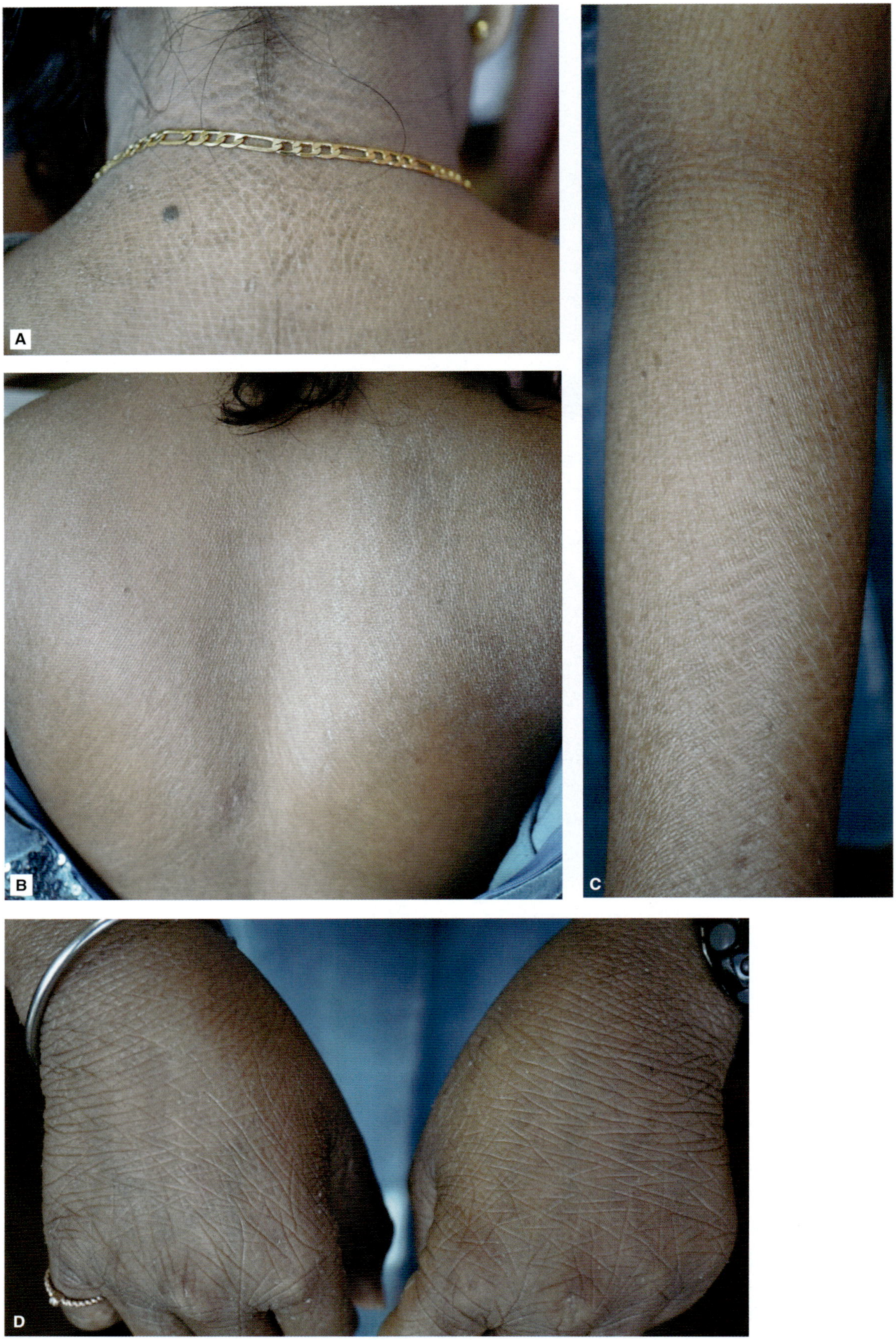

FIGURE 12-20A–20D. Autosomal recessive congenital ichthyosis in an adolescent Indian girl, presenting with generalized, thickened, "dirty" scales. This phenotype would have previously been labeled "lamellar ichthyosis."

KERATINOPATHIC ICHTHYOSIS

The keratinopathic ichthyoses are a group of rare inherited disorders of cornification, associated with pathogenic variants in various keratin genes, resulting in a poorly functioning keratin network in the superficial epidermis. Epidermolytic ichthyosis, formerly known as bullous congenital ichthyosiform erythroderma (BCIE), Broq type, is due to variants in *KRT1* or *KRT10* genes. Superficial epidermolytic ichthyosis, formerly known as ichthyosis bullosa of Siemens, is due to variants in *KRT2*, found more superficially in the epidermis.[1] All the keratinopathic ichthyoses are inherited in an autosomal dominant fashion.

Clinical Features

- Epidermolytic ichthyosis
  - At birth and during the first weeks to months of life, the affected neonate presents with very superficial bullae that break easily, with background erythema, leading to superficial desquamation, erosions, and denuded areas.
  - From a few months of life, there is gradual skin thickening, evolving eventually into ichthyosiform grayish-brown scales with variable erythema. Palms and soles may have varying degrees of thickness and scaling.

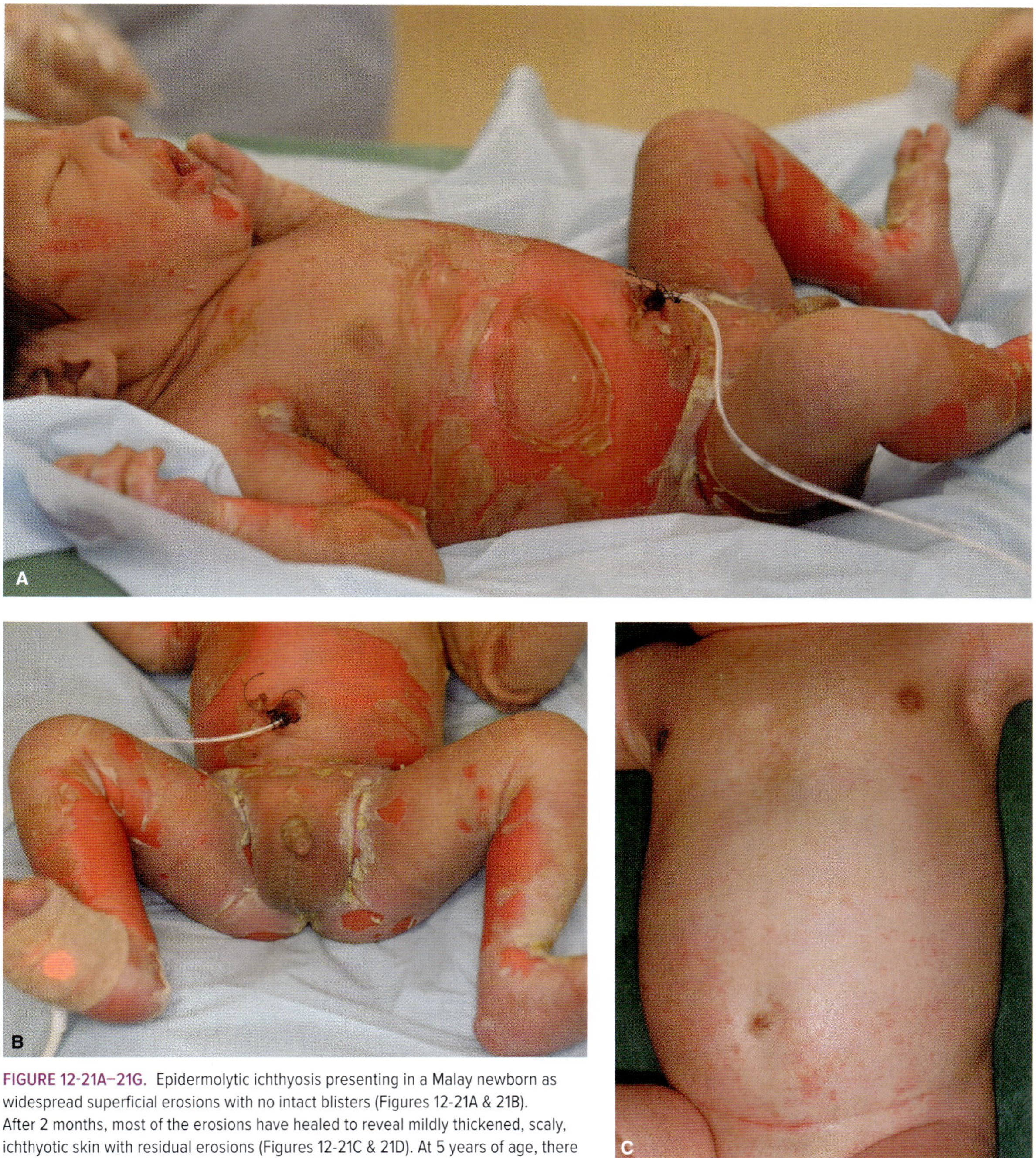

FIGURE 12-21A–21G. Epidermolytic ichthyosis presenting in a Malay newborn as widespread superficial erosions with no intact blisters (Figures 12-21A & 21B). After 2 months, most of the erosions have healed to reveal mildly thickened, scaly, ichthyotic skin with residual erosions (Figures 12-21C & 21D). At 5 years of age, there is persistent generalized erythema and scaling, with hyperkeratosis of the palms and soles (Figures 12-21E–21G).

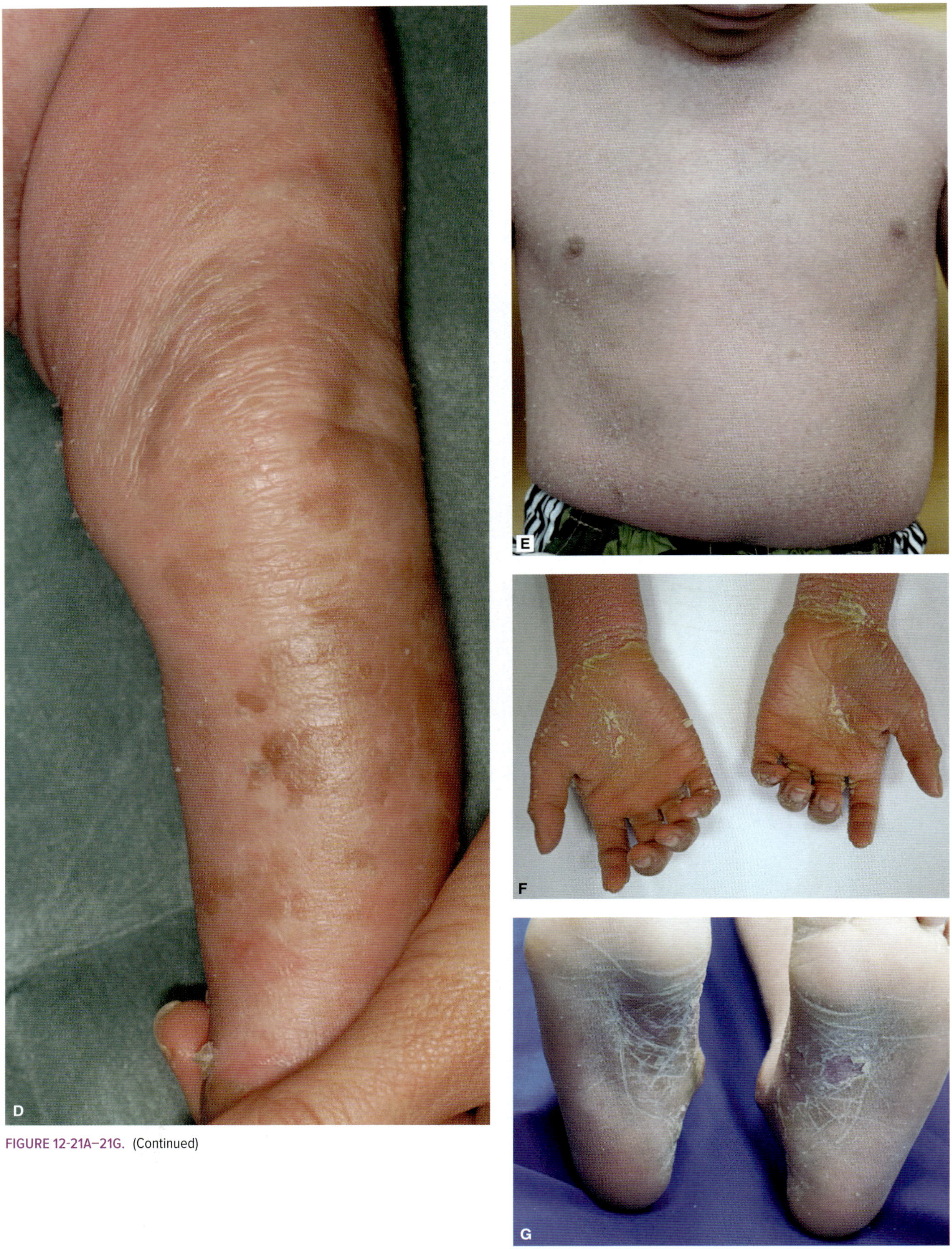

FIGURE 12-21A–21G. (Continued)

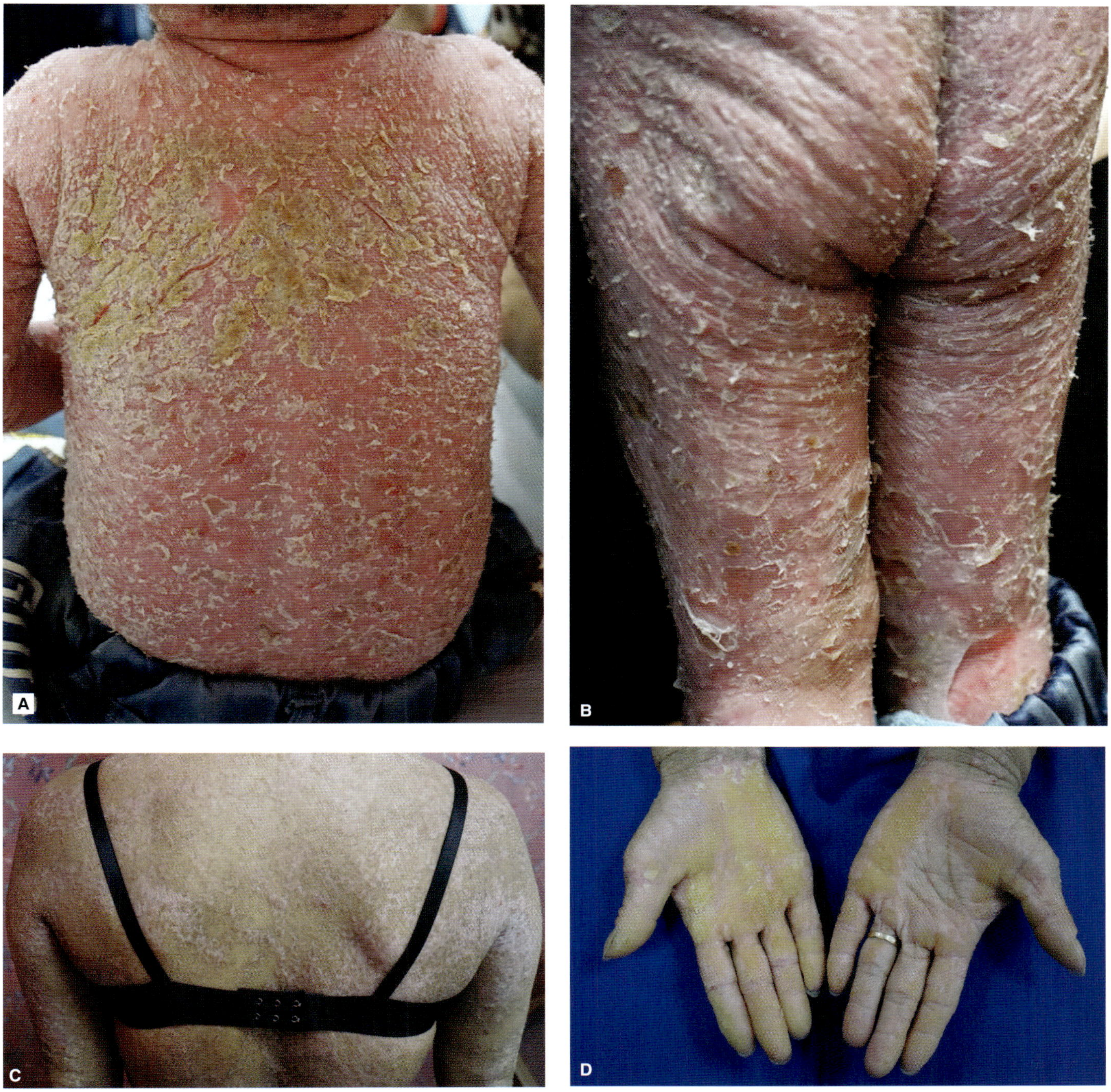

FIGURE 12-22A–22D. Epidermolytic ichthyosis in a young Vietnamese child with generalized erythema, superficial erosions, and scaling (Figures 12-22A & 22B). His mother has systematized epidermal nevus with features of epidermolytic hyperkeratosis on histology (Figures 12-22C & 22D). The child carries a germline *KRT1* mutation, inherited from the mother with gonosomal mosaicism for the same mutation.

- Superficial epidermolytic ichthyosis
    - There is milder thickening and more superficial blistering compared to epidermolytic ichthyosis. The superficial blisters and scaling have been described as "Mauserung phenomenon," in which the skin appears to be molting. Thickening of the palms and soles is not seen.

Differential Diagnoses

- Epidermolysis bullosa simplex (EBS)
    - EBS is a rare genetic disorder of skin fragility, which also manifests as superficial, chronic blistering with erosions. With time, EBS patients may also develop hyperkeratosis at the sites of friction, such as palms and soles. However, the thickening is not as marked

as seen in epidermolytic ichthyosis. Intact blisters are usually also not seen in epidermolytic ichthyosis.
  - The classical histological pattern of epidermolytic hyperkeratosis seen in epidermolytic ichthyosis is not seen in EBS.
- Bullous impetigo/staphylococcal scalded skin syndrome (SSSS)
  - Bullous impetigo and SSSS can also present in the neonatal period with superficial bullae and erosions. The classical honey-yellow crusting and pus discharge may provide a clue to the diagnosis. Babies may be febrile and unwell.
- Stevens-Johnson syndrome/toxic epidermal necrolysis
  - This is extremely rare in the neonatal period, as the neonatal immune system is too immature to mount the immunological response.
- Autosomal recessive congenital ichthyosis (ARCI)
  - ARCI can present with thickened skin and scaling at birth, but blisters and erosions are not a feature.

Investigations & Treatment

- Skin biopsies can be performed, which show the classical feature of epidermolytic hyperkeratosis, which is a characteristic vacuolar degeneration with hypergranulosis of the stratum granulosum and stratum spinosum.
- Genetic studies can be performed to detect the causative gene variants in *KRT1*, *KRT2*, and *KRT10*.
- In the early blistering stage of the disease, supportive care of the young infant is important to prevent infection, dehydration, fluid/electrolyte imbalances, and temperature fluctuations.
- Judicious application of emollients, careful handling, and application of nonadherent dressings over eroded areas is helpful in the early period.
- In the later hyperkeratotic, verrucous stage, keratolytic agents with urea, salicylic acid, and alpha-hydroxy acids can be used to assist with exfoliation of the scales. This should be avoided in young children due to the possible irritation and stinging.

Pearls & Practical Tips

- Epidermolytic ichthyosis may occur in the offspring of a parent with systematized epidermal nevi, where the inheritance pattern would be from mosaic to germline. It is important to examine the parents. Genetic counseling is important for future family planning.
- Advice to reduce dehydration and overheating should be given to the patient and the family.
- Systemic retinoids are usually not helpful in patients with keratinopathic ichthyosis.

Reference

1. Paller AS, Syder AJ, Chan YM, et al. Genetic and clinical mosaicism in a type of epidermal nevus. N Engl J Med 1994; 331:1408-15.

NETHERTON SYNDROME

Netherton syndrome is one of the most common of the syndromic ichthyoses. The syndromic ichthyoses encompass a wide range of inherited disorders of cornification that presents with variable spectrum of ichthyosis associated with manifestations in other organ systems such as neurological, hearing, gastrointestinal, and so forth. Netherton syndrome is a rare genodermatosis presenting with the classical triad of congenital ichthyosiform erythroderma, trichorrhexis invaginate, and atopic diathesis.

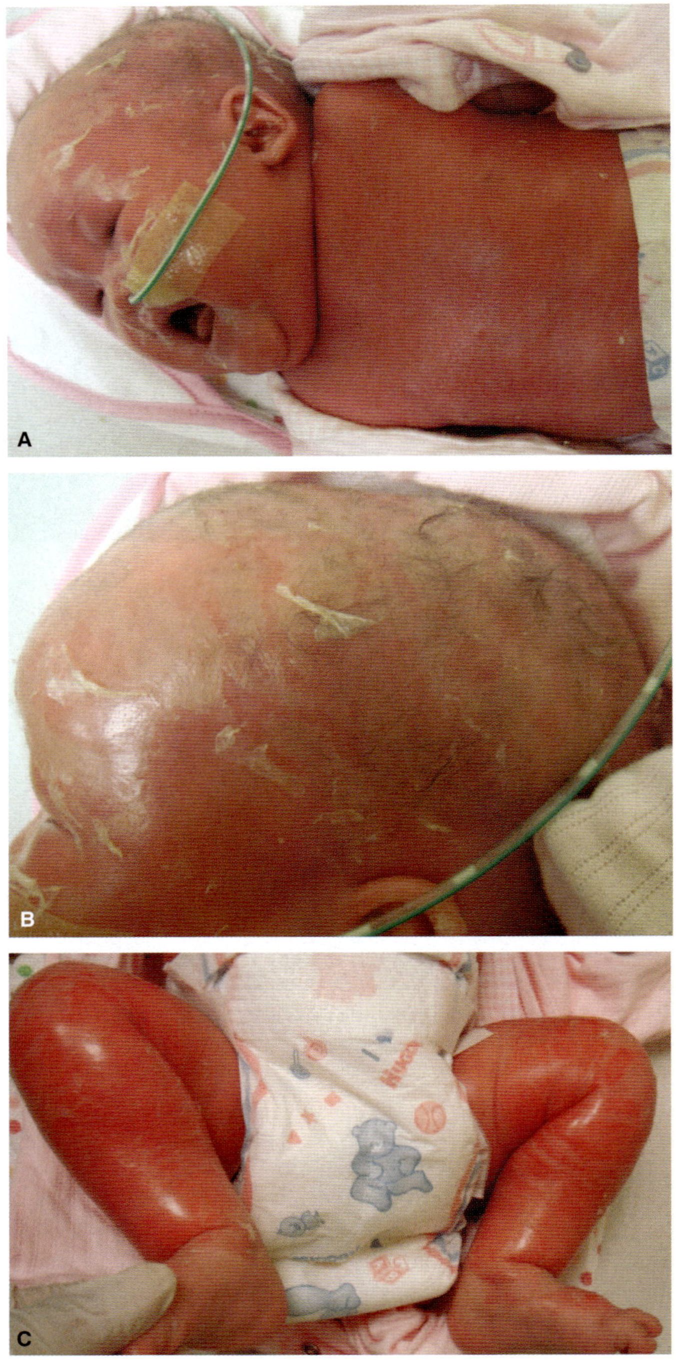

FIGURE 12-23A–23C. Netherton syndrome presenting as neonatal erythroderma associated with alopecia in this Nepalese neonate.

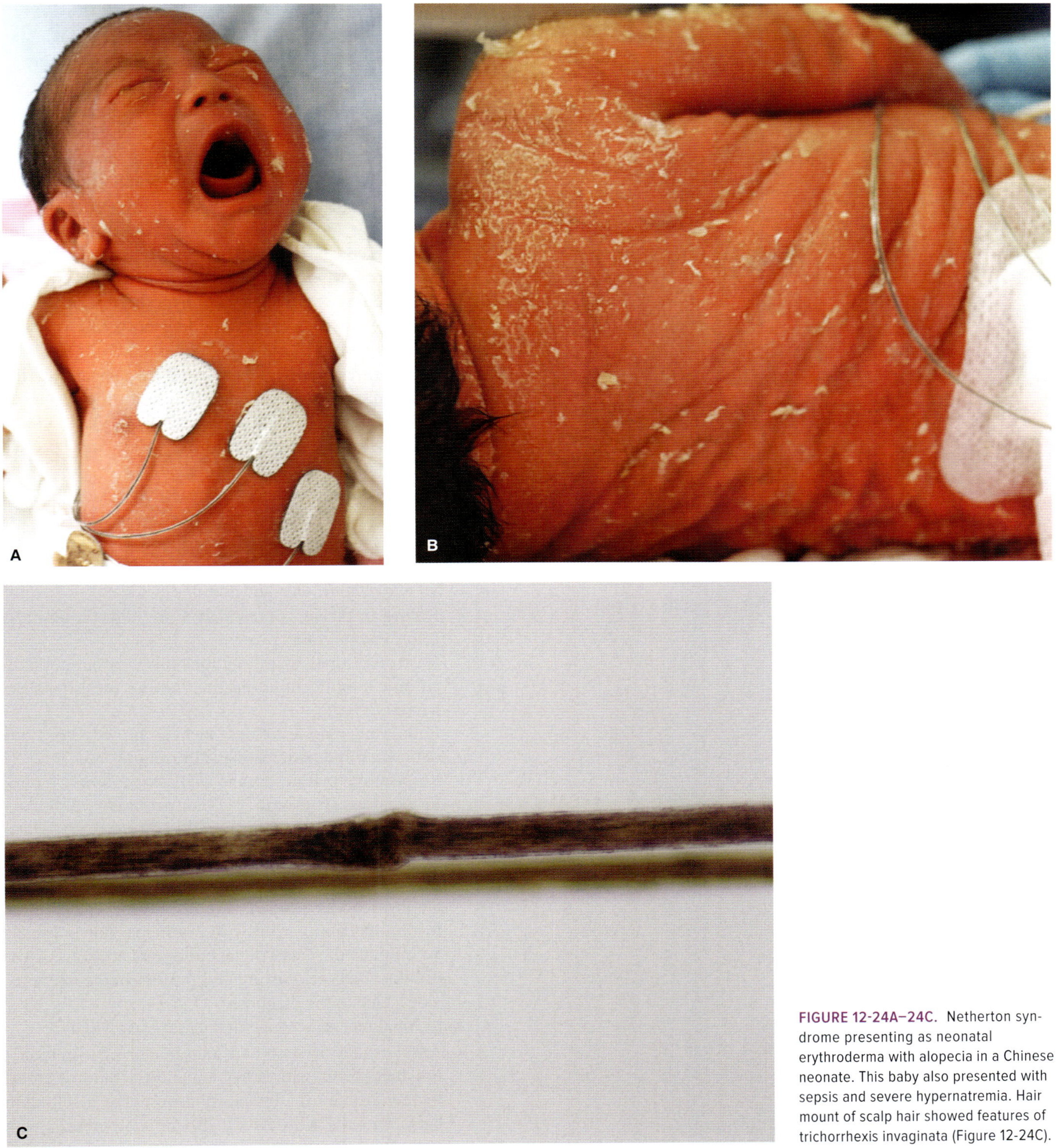

FIGURE 12-24A–24C. Netherton syndrome presenting as neonatal erythroderma with alopecia in a Chinese neonate. This baby also presented with sepsis and severe hypernatremia. Hair mount of scalp hair showed features of trichorrhexis invaginata (Figure 12-24C).

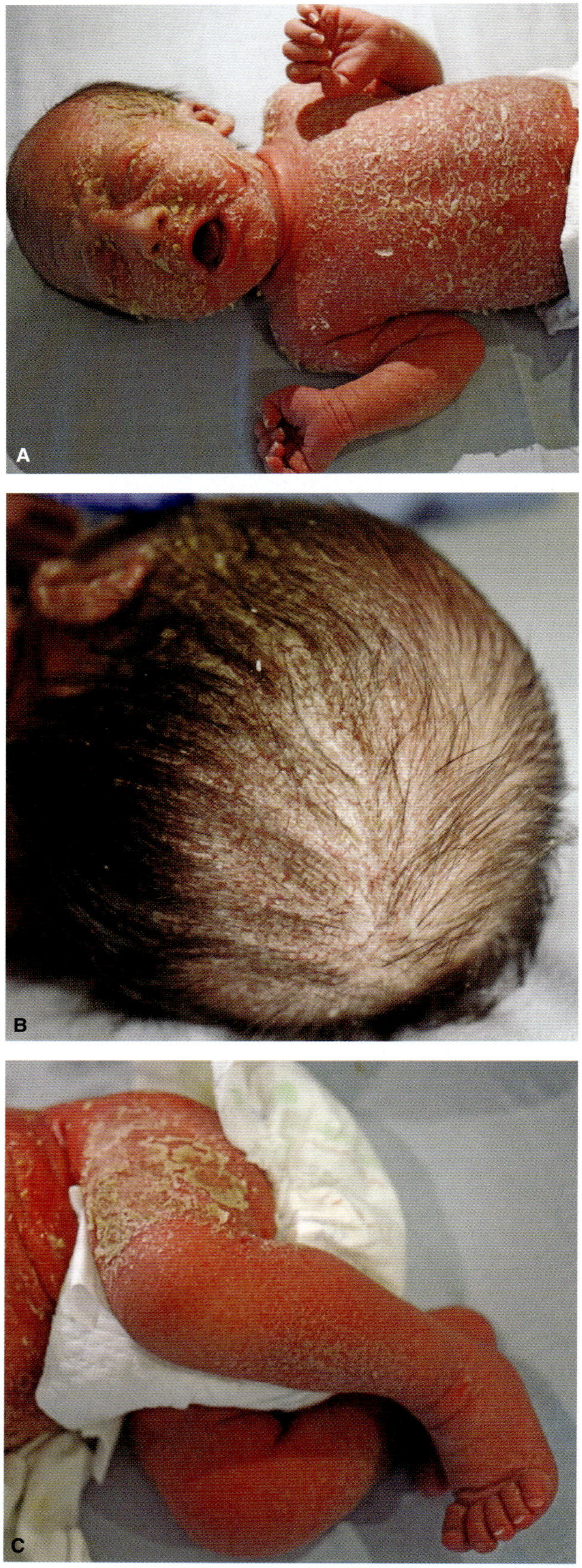

FIGURE 12-25A–25C Chinese neonate with Netherton syndrome, presenting as neonatal erythroderma. Alopecia is subtle in this child, who also presented with hypernatremia and feed intolerance.

Clinical Features

- Netherton syndrome affects 1 in 200,000 individuals, and the phenotype can vary from mild desquamative dermatitis to lethal forms.
- It is caused by loss-of-function mutations in the *SPINK5* gene on chromosome 5q32 encoding for lymphoepithelial Kazal-type-related inhibitor (LEKTI), a serine protease inhibitor that is usually expressed in stratified epithelia.
- Affected neonates present with ichthyosiform erythroderma at birth. Sparse hair or congenital alopecia may be present. They are often born premature and medically labile in the first few weeks of life, with potential life-threatening complications of hypothermia, infection, and sepsis secondary to immunodeficiency, and hypernatremic dehydration.
- Atopic features, which may start in the neonatal period and worsen with age, are associated with high levels of IgE. These patients may have increased likelihood of eczema, asthma, allergic rhinitis, cow's milk protein allergy, or other food allergies.
- Another classical cutaneous feature that begins to manifest after a few years is ichthyosis linearis circumflexa (ILC). This presents as a circular or arcuate erythema and scaling of the skin with a "double-edged" scale.
- Other extracutaneous manifestations include the following:
  - Failure to thrive, contributed to by high protein and caloric requirements.
  - Gastrointestinal manifestations such as enteropathy, chronic noninfectious diarrhea, and severe esophageal barrier defect.
  - Endocrine manifestations such as growth hormone deficiency and pancreatic insufficiency.
  - Respiratory manifestations such as neonatal respiratory distress syndrome (RDS) or persistent pulmonary hypertension of the newborn (PPHN).

Differential Diagnoses

- Staphylococcal scalded skin syndrome
  - Staphylococcal scalded skin syndrome can present in the neonatal period with erythema, but is usually accompanied by superficial bullae and erosions. Areas of honey-yellow crusting and pus discharge may provide a clue to the diagnosis.
- Autosomal recessive congenital ichthyosis (ARCI)
  - ARCI usually presents as a collodion or harlequin phenotype at birth, with ectropion and eclabium. Netherton syndrome usually does not present as a collodion baby. Patients with ARCI also do not present with extracutaneous involvement.

Investigations & Treatment

- Trichoscopy can be performed to examine for trichorrhexis invaginata and trichorrhexis nodosa. This is most common on the eyebrows or eyelashes during early infancy.
- Hair mounts of cut hairs can also be performed to look for the hair features.

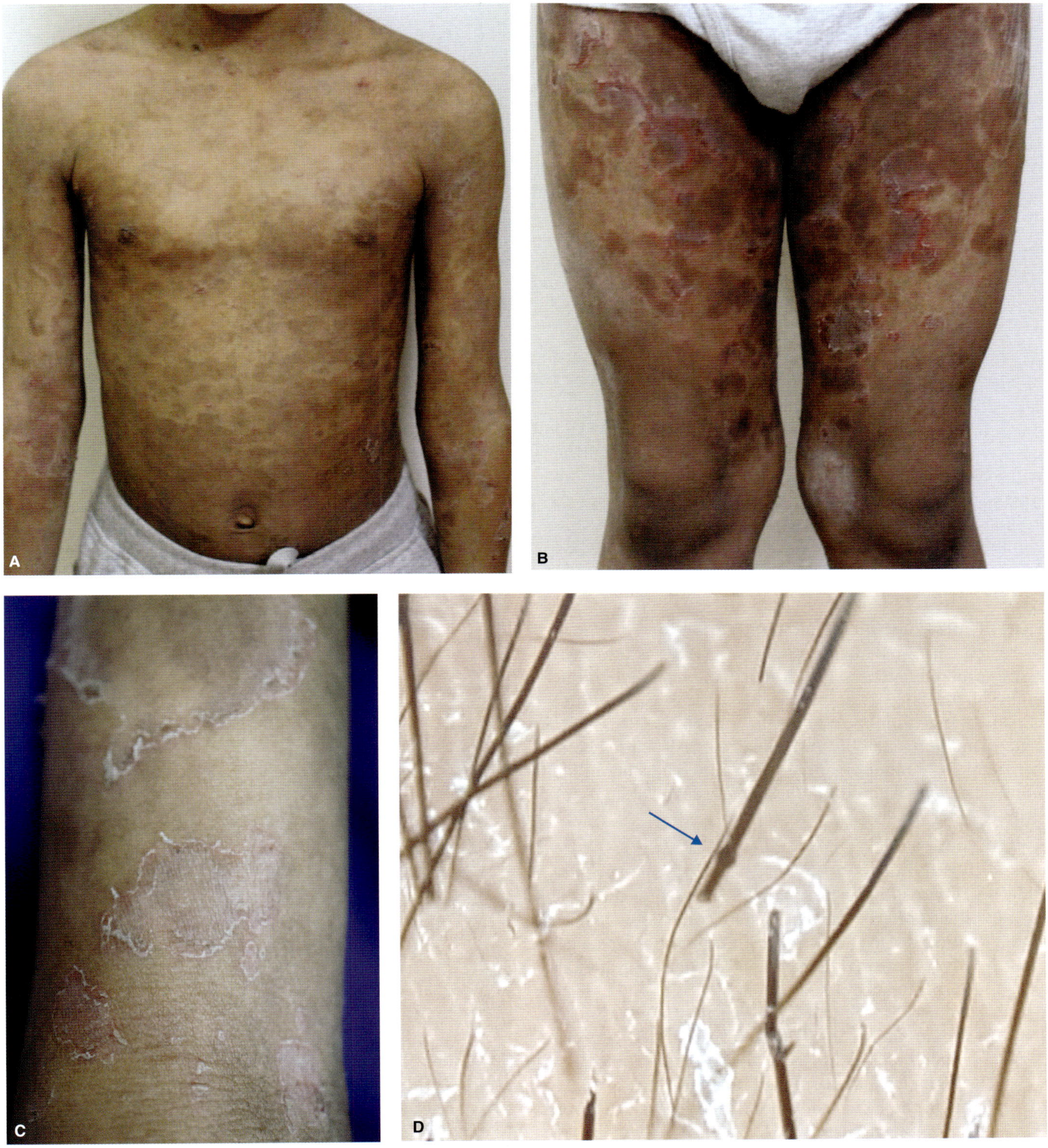

FIGURE 12-26A–26D. Netherton syndrome in an older Indonesian boy who presents with features of ichthyosis linearis circumflexa. He also has features of atopic dermatitis. Dermoscopy of scalp hairs reveals features of trichorrhexis invaginata (Figure 12-26D).

- Genetic studies can be performed to detect the causative gene mutation in *SPINK5*.
- Management is multidisciplinary, requiring supportive therapy of the neonate in a humidified incubator.
- Special attention should be paid to prevention and treatment of temperature instability, sepsis, and fluid and electrolyte imbalance, with prompt management of hypernatremic dehydration.

- Frequent application of moisturizers is useful to alleviate the dryness and scaling of the skin.
- The use of keratolytic agents should be avoided.
- Some patients may benefit from systemic retinoids such as acitretin or isotretinoin.

Pearls & Practical Tips

- Monitor the neonate closely for hypernatremic dehydration with regular serum electrolyte levels. This may last for the first few months of life.
- Due to the impaired epidermal barrier, the risk of transcutaneous absorption is extremely high. Topical medications, such as potent topical corticosteroids and calcineurin inhibitors, should be avoided or used with great caution.
- The classical hair changes are more prominent on the eyebrows and eyelashes early in life. It can be seen less frequently on scalp hair.
- The use of new monoclonal antibodies against IL-17 and IL-4/-13 have recently been used for the treatment of Netherton syndrome.

Bibliography

1. Bellon N, Hadj-Rabia S, Moulin F, et al. The challenging management of a series of 43 infants with Netherton syndrome: unexpected complications and novel mutations. Br J Dermatol 2021 Mar;184(3): 532-7.

HEREDITARY PALMOPLANTAR KERATODERMA

Hereditary palmoplantar keratoderma (PPK) is a heterogenous group of genetic skin disorders characterized by thickening of the skin of the palms and soles. It can be further classified into four morphological subtypes: diffuse, focal, striate, and punctate PPK. PPK can occur in isolation without involvement of other organ systems (non-syndrome PPK) or be associated with abnormalities in other organ systems (syndromic PPK).

Clinical Features

- Diffuse PPK
  - Diffuse PPK can be subclassified into those that exhibit transgrediens, where the keratoderma beyond the volar surfaces of the hands and feet, and non-transgrediens, in which the keratoderma is limited to the volar surfaces of the palms and soles.
  - Diffuse PPK without transgrediens has been associated with mutations in *KRT1*, *KRT9*, and *DSG1* genes, and is inherited in autosomal dominant fashion. Patients present from infancy with progressive diffuse thickening of the palms and soles that does not extend onto the dorsal surfaces.
  - Diffuse PPK with transgrediens includes several phenotypes and is caused by mutations in different genes, namely *SERPINB7* (Nagashima, AR), *SLURP1* (Mal-de-Maleda, AR), *AQP5* (Bothnian, AD), and *KRT1* (Greither, AD). In addition to PPK, other manifestations include hyperhidrosis and whitish change upon contact with water.

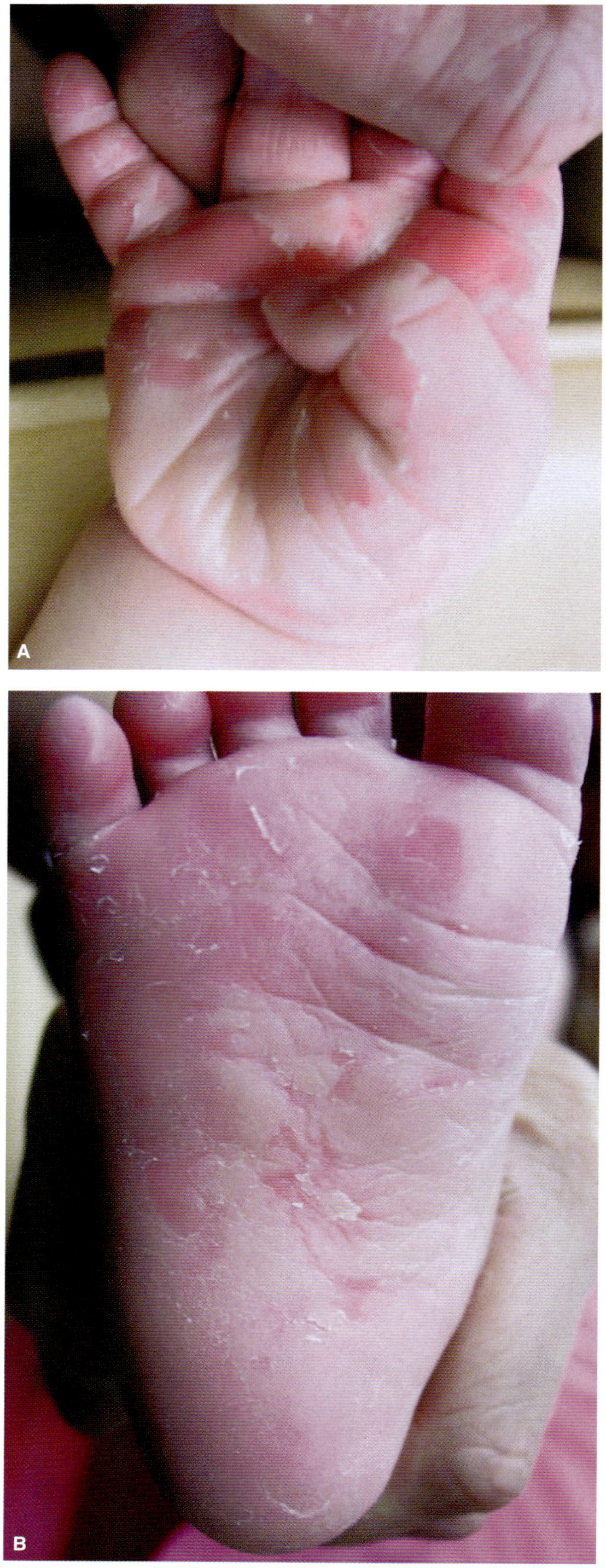

A

B

FIGURE 12-27A & 27B. Diffuse PPK with superficial erosions are seen in this Chinese infant with a family history of diffuse PPK.

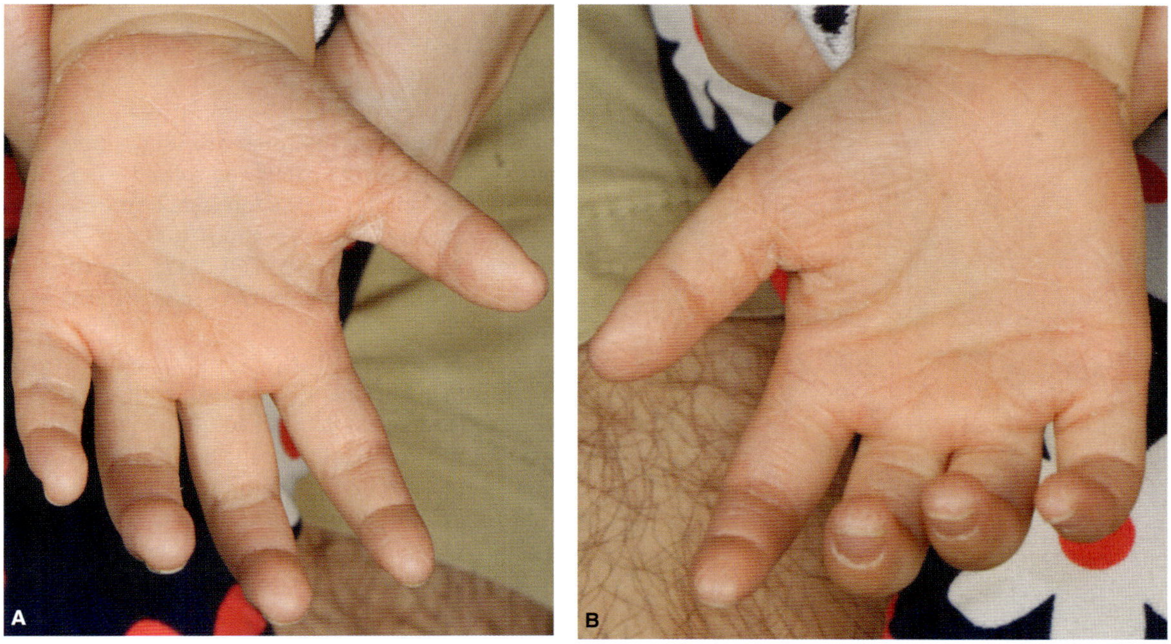

FIGURE 12-28A & 28B. Diffuse PPK in a 3-year-old Chinese girl, first noticed when she was a few months old.

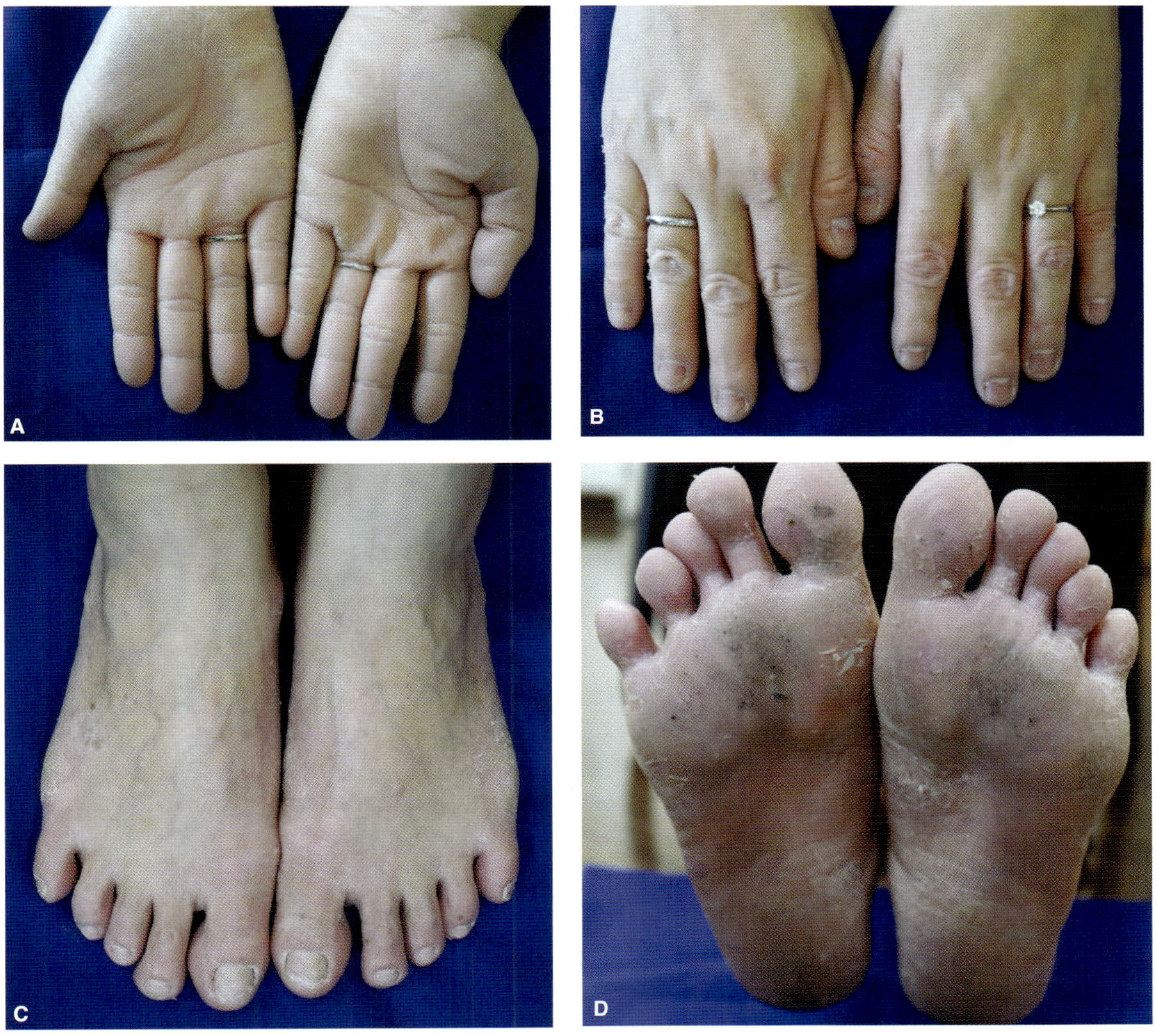

FIGURE 12-29A–29D. Diffuse PPK seen in a young adult female since early childhood, presenting as diffuse thickened of bilateral palms and soles.

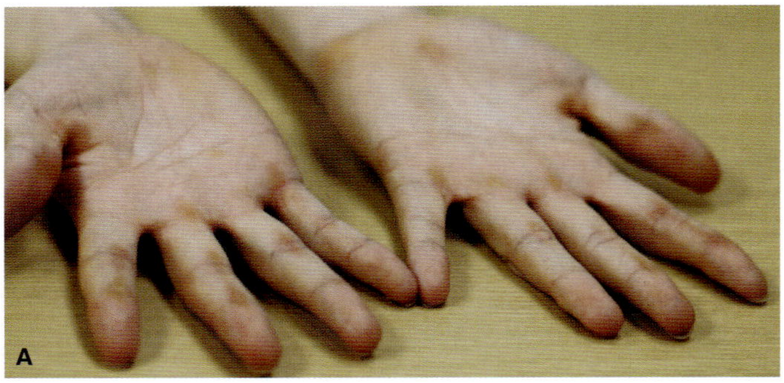

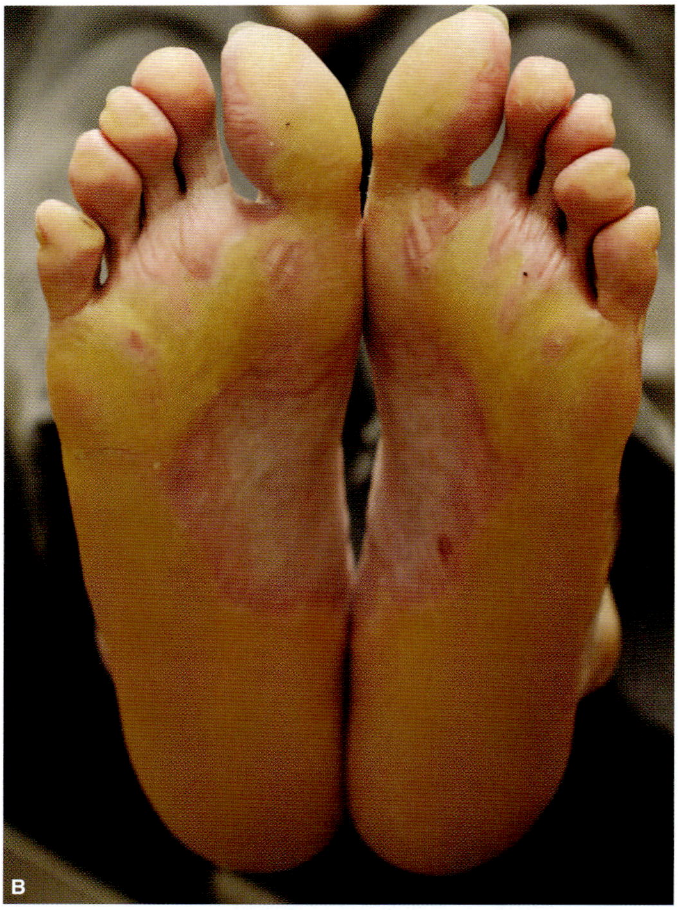

FIGURE 12-30A & 30B. Striate PPK occurring in an adolescent male since early childhood. This appears as striate thickening on the palms and thickening at pressure points on the soles. The patient's father was similarly affected.

- Focal PPK
  - Focal PPK presents with painful hyperkeratosis involving the weight-bearing areas of the soles.
  - Focal PPK is seen in pachyonychia congenita, an autosomal dominant condition, associated with mutations in *KRT6A*, *KRT6B*, *KRT16*, or *KRT17*. These patients also present with thickened nails and other cutaneous manifestations. Mutations in *KRT6C*, *DSG1*, and *TRPV3* are also associated with focal PPK.
- Striate PPK
  - Striate PPK is characterized by thickened skin in a linear configuration along the palmar surface of the fingers and pressure points of the soles.
  - It has been associated with mutations in *DSG1*, *DSP*, and *KRT1*, and is inherited in an autosomal dominant fashion.
- Punctate PPK
  - Patients with punctate PPK present with multiple, tiny keratotic papules on the palms and soles. Lesions usually appear in childhood or adolescence and can progressively increase in number and size.
  - Mutations in *AAGAB* and *COL14A1*, inherited as autosomal dominant traits, have been associated with punctate PPK.
- Syndromic PPK
  - Patients with syndromic PPK present with manifestations in other organ systems in addition to the PPK.
  - Important systems to examine include hearing (*GJB2*), hair and nails (*GJB6*), dentition (*CTSC*, *TRPV3*, *WNT10A*, *RHBDF2*), and cardiovascular (*DSP*, *JUP*).
  - Patients with epidermolysis bullosa simplex (*KRT5*, *KRT14*) can also develop PPK during late childhood or adolescence.

Differential Diagnosis

- Acquired palmoplantar keratoderma (PPK)
  - Acquired PPK occurs later in life and may be secondary to various causes, such as eczema, psoriasis, contact dermatitis, infections, medications, and systemic diseases.
- Viral warts/verrucae and calluses
  - Viral warts and calluses are common conditions that can present in childhood with thickened keratotic lesions of the palms and soles. Paring of warts will reveal thrombosed capillaries. Calluses occur more commonly in adolescents and adults and are related to poorly fitting footwear.

Investigations & Treatment

- Skin biopsies are not routinely performed for diagnosis of the various types of PPK. Clinical history and examination will aid in diagnosis, confirmed by targeted mutation analysis.
- Treatment of PPK will require multimodality therapy.
- General measures include the use of comfortable footwear, insoles, or orthotics, and the use of wicking socks to absorb sweat.
- Topical therapies include keratolytics (salicylic acid 5%–10%, urea 10%–30%, propylene glycol 20%–60%, lactic acid), moisturizers, topical corticosteroids, topical retinoids, and topical vitamin D analogues (calcipotriol).
- Oral retinoids (isotretinoin, etretinate, acitretin, alitretinoin) may be useful for some PPK patients who have suboptimal improvements with topical therapies. Botulinum toxin injections and iontophoresis have also been used for PPK.

Pearls & Practical Tips

- A full skin examination and targeted systemic examination is important to differentiate non-syndromic with syndromic PPK. Molecular diagnosis can then be performed using targeted sequencing panels for PPK.

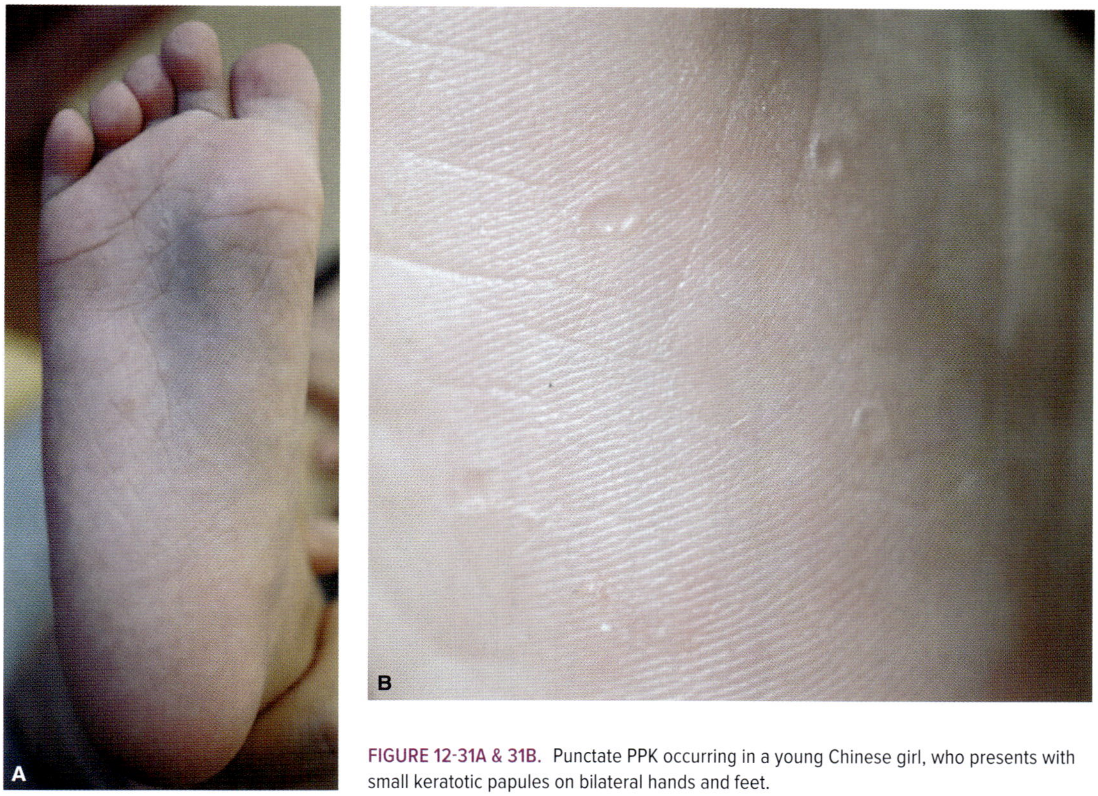

FIGURE 12-31A & 31B. Punctate PPK occurring in a young Chinese girl, who presents with small keratotic papules on bilateral hands and feet.

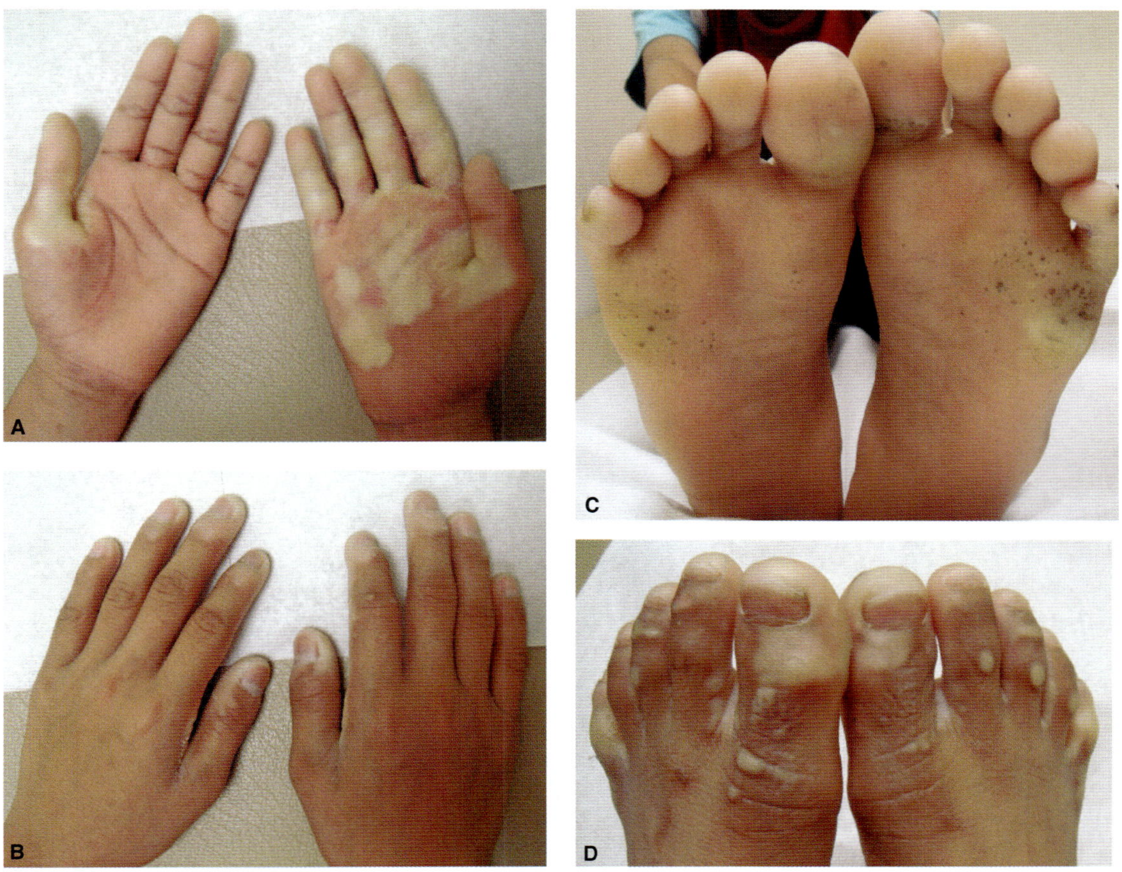

FIGURE 12-32A–32D. Diffuse PPK secondary to mutations in *SLURP1* gene in this Cambodian boy with Mal-de-Maleda syndrome. His parents are consanguineous.

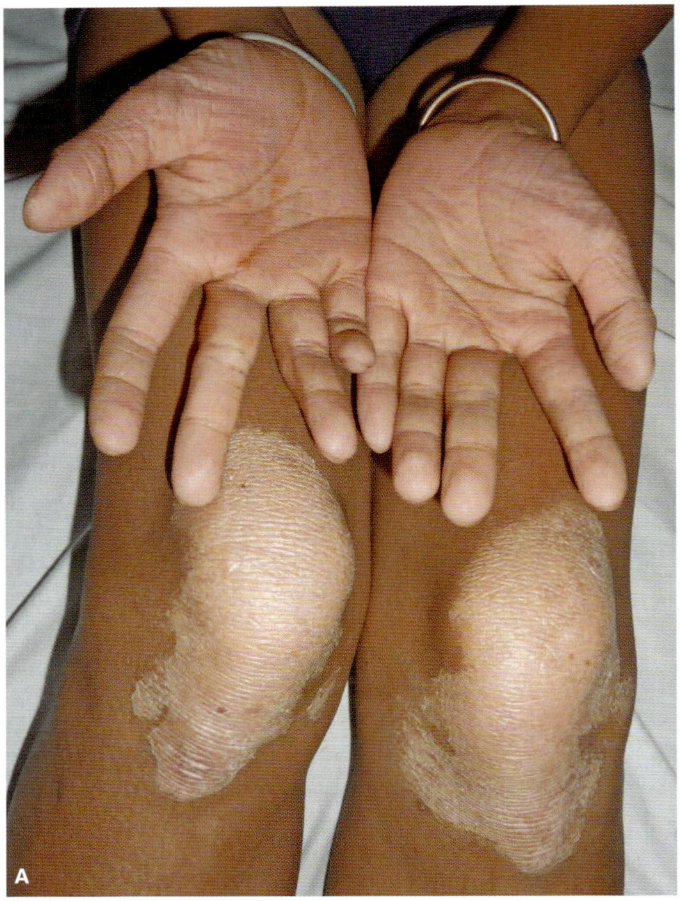

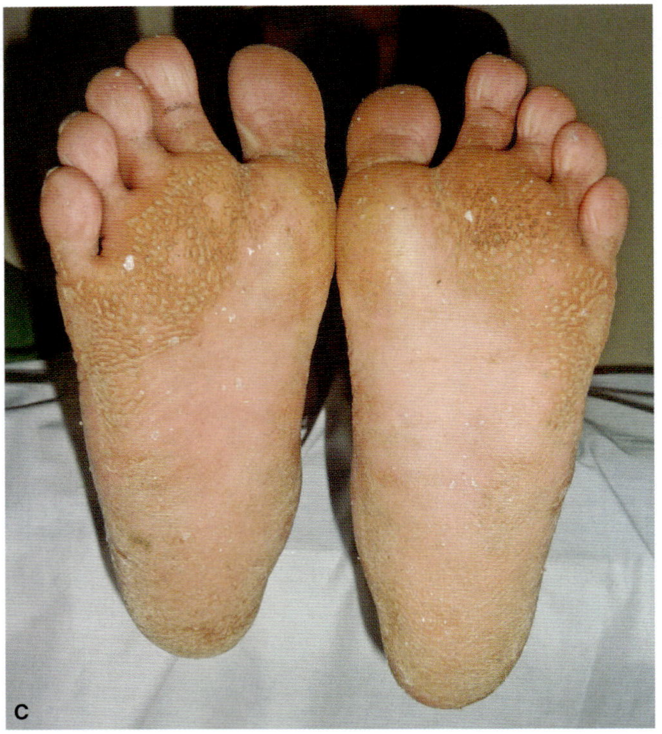

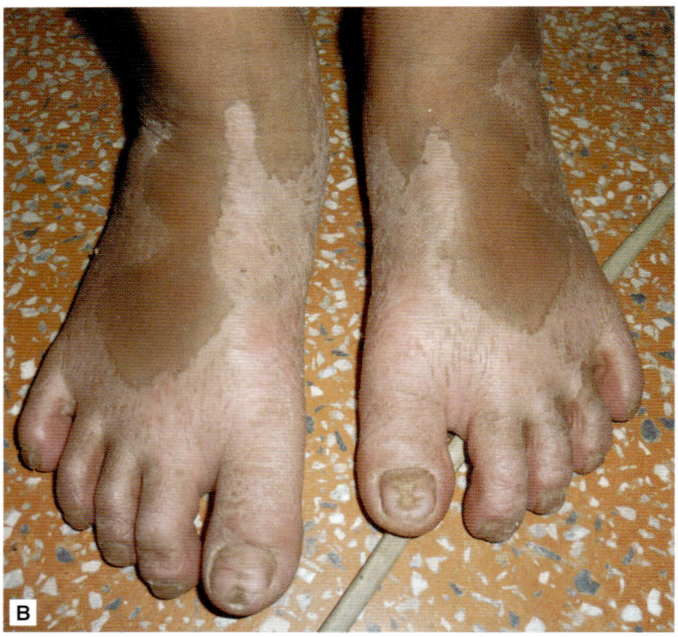

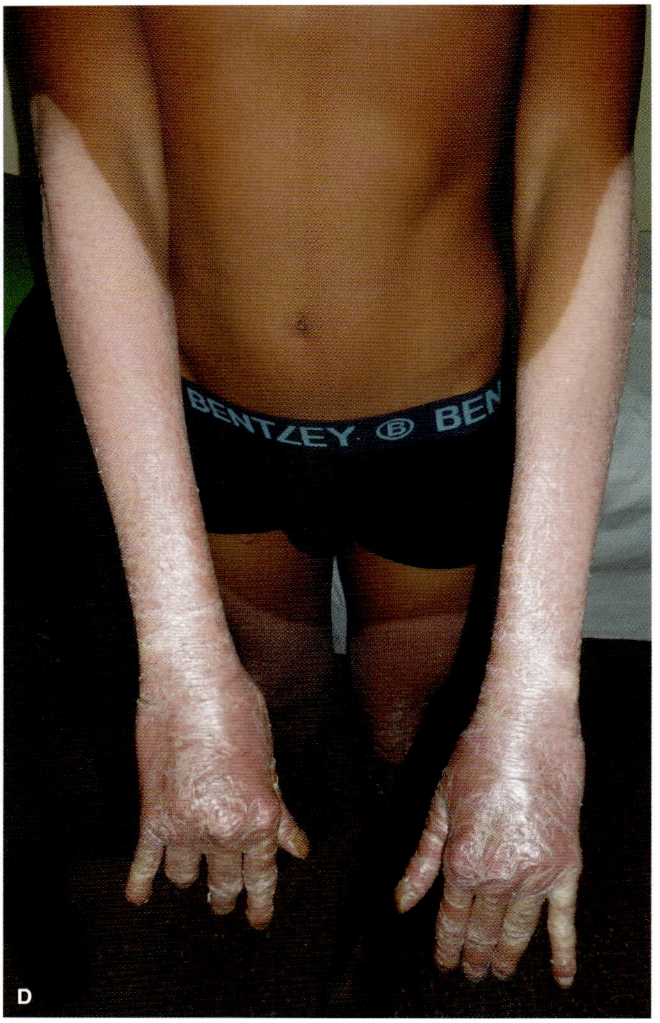

FIGURE 12-33A–33G. Diffuse PPK secondary to mutations in *CTSC* in two Cambodian brothers with Papillon-Lefevre syndrome, also known as Haim-Monk syndrome. Figures 12-33A–33C show the younger brother with less severe and extensive involvement, while Figures 12-33D–33G show the older brother with more severe and extensive involvement, with secondary contractures of the fingers. Both brothers also showed features of periodontitis. (Photographs courtesy of Dr. Sithach Mey, Preah Kossamak Hospital, Phnom Penh, Cambodia.)

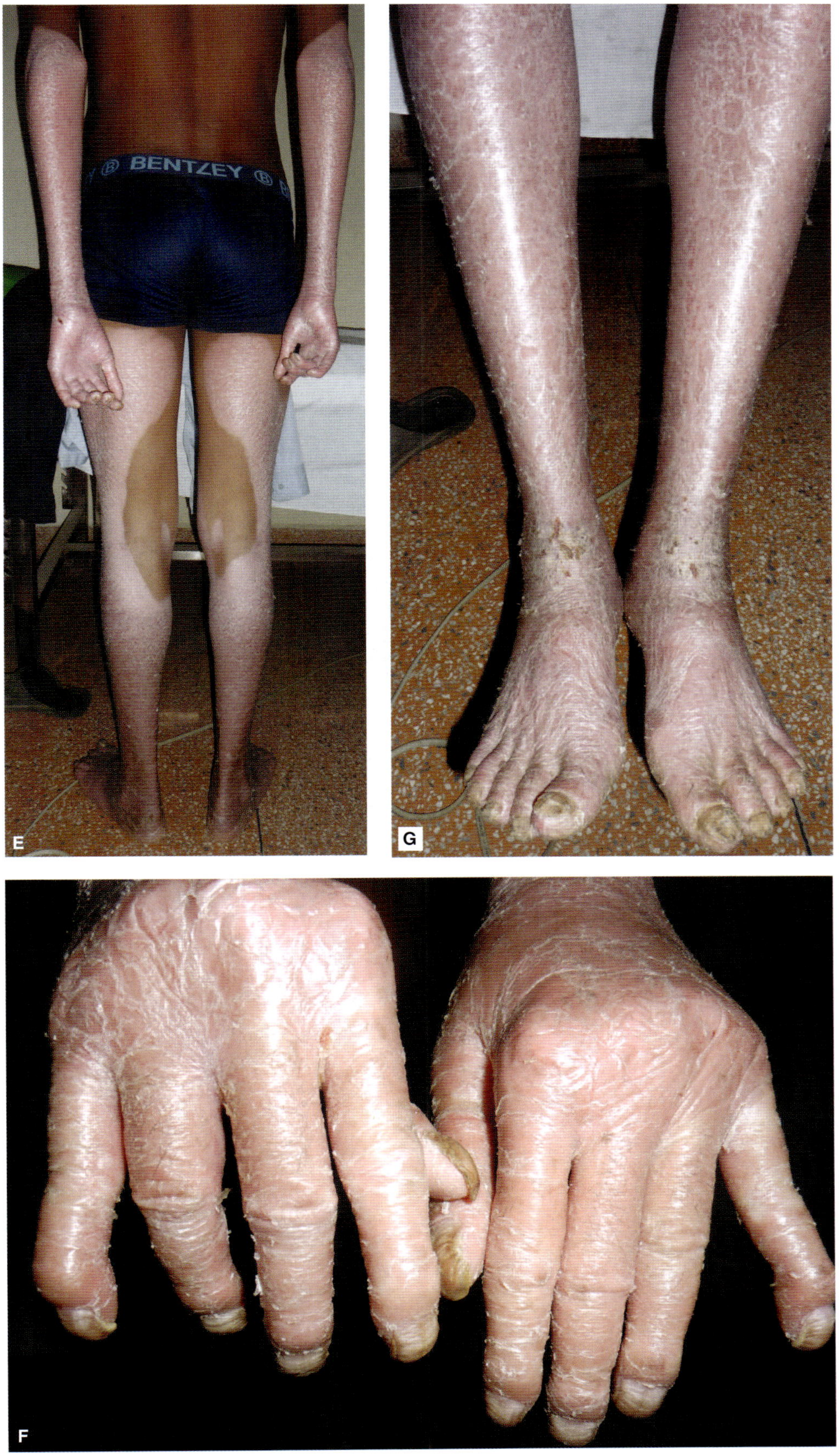

FIGURE 12-33A–33G. (Continued)

- Treatment of PPK is aimed at relieving symptoms and will frequently require multimodality treatment.

Bibliography

1. Sakiyama T, Kubo A. Hereditary palmoplantar keratoderma "clinical and genetic differential diagnosis". J Dermatol 2016;43(3):264-74.
2. Dev T, Mahajan VK, Sethuraman G. Hereditary palmoplantar keratoderma: a practical approach to the diagnosis. Indian Dermatol Online J 2019;10(4):365-79.
3. Bodemer C, Steijlen P, Mazereeuw-Hautier J, O'Toole EA. Treatment of hereditary palmoplantar keratoderma: a review by analysis of the literature. Br J Dermatol 2021;184(3):393-400.

PACHYONYCHIA CONGENITA

Pachyonychia congenita is a rare genetic skin condition caused by mutations in five keratin genes: *KRT6A*, *KRT6B*, *KRT6C*, *KRT16*, and *KRT17*. The inheritance pattern in autosomal dominant.

Clinical Features

- The most prominent clinical manifestations are nail abnormalities and painful palmoplantar keratoderma.
- Nail changes often occur early but sometimes appear only during adolescence. The nails become progressively thicker, tented, and discolored. There is associated paronychia (inflammation of the nail folds) and recurrent nail shedding.
- Painful focal hyperkeratosis of the soles can be progressive and cause significant functional morbidity. There may be associated blister formation and hyperhidrosis.
- Other clinical manifestations include small follicular papules on sites of trauma (e.g., elbows, knees, and buttocks), oral lesions (leukokeratosis or white plaques on the tongue or buccal mucosa), steatocysts, and neonatal teeth.

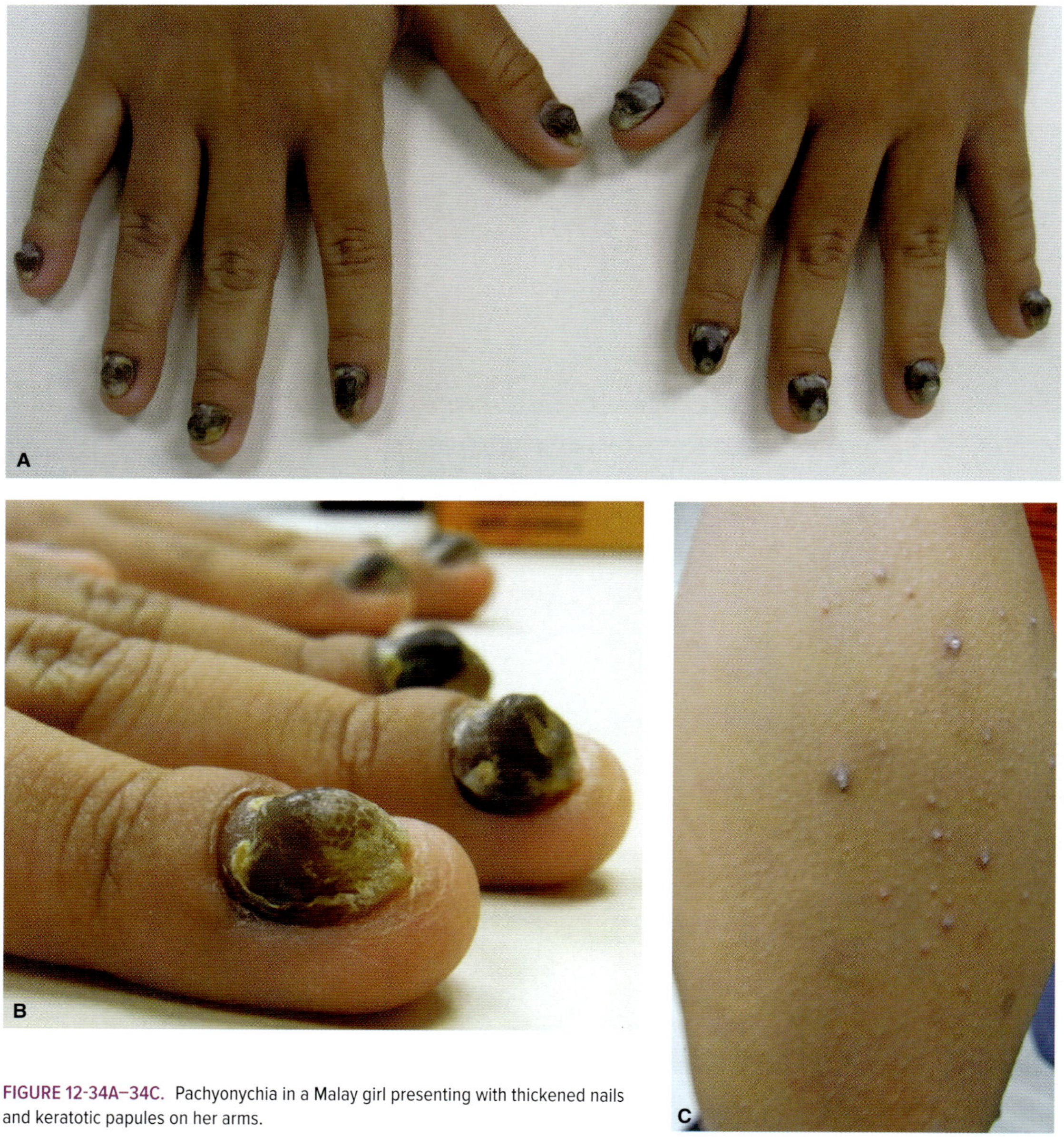

FIGURE 12-34A–34C. Pachyonychia in a Malay girl presenting with thickened nails and keratotic papules on her arms.

Differential Diagnoses

- Other causes of palmoplantar keratoderma (PPK)
  - There are many other causes of hereditary or acquired PPK. A thorough history and examination should be performed in all pediatric patients presenting with PPK to exclude these other causes.
  - Refer to section on inherited PPK.
- Other nail abnormalities
  - Other nail abnormalities that may present with thickened nails include pincer nails, familial onychogryphosis, dyskeratosis congenita, twenty-nail dystrophy, and onychomycosis. Careful history, physical examination, and microbiological investigations will help to exclude these diagnoses.
  - Refer to section on nail disorders.

Investigations & Treatment

- Diagnosis of pachyonychia congenita is suspected clinically and confirmed by genetic testing.
- Treatment of nail thickening is with regular filing and trimming of nails. Application of topical keratolytics to the affected nails and areas of hyperkeratotic skin will help to decrease the thickening and reduce pain. These include urea, propylene glycol, and salicylic acid in various concentrations and vehicles.
- Surgical nail avulsion with matrix destruction may be performed in more severe cases to prevent regrowth of the abnormal nails.
- Botulinum toxin injections may be useful to control hyperhidrosis and reduce blistering.
- Systemic retinoids and rapamycin have been used, but with variable results and significant potential side effects.

Pearls & Practical Tips

- Leukokeratosis can present during infancy and is often mistaken for candidiasis. Poor response to antifungal treatments should prompt investigation of other causes, including pachyonychia congenita.

Bibliography

1. Zieman AG, Coulombe PA. Pathophysiology of pachyonychia congenita-associated palmoplantar keratoderma: new insights into skin epithelial homeostasis and avenues for treatment. Br J Dermatol 2020;182(3):564-73.

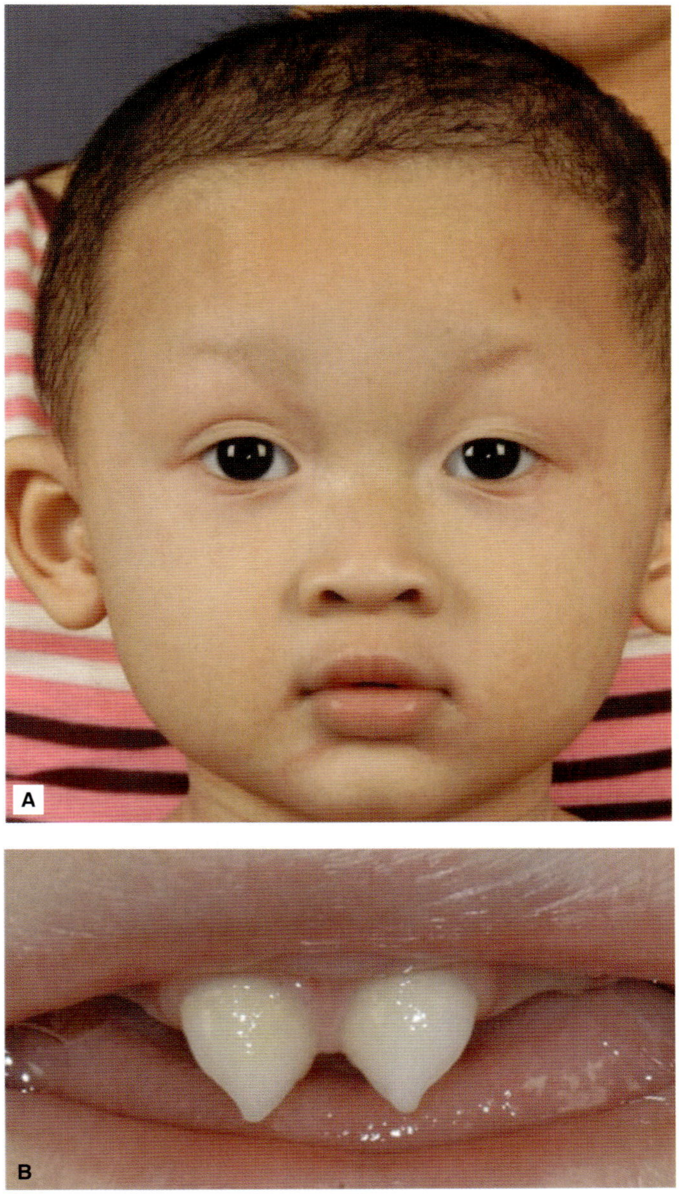

FIGURE 12-35A &35B. A Chinese boy with hypohidrotic ectodermal dysplasia with classical facies and conical teeth.

ECTODERMAL DYSPLASIAS

Ectodermal dysplasias (ED) are a rare group of genodermatoses characterized by abnormalities in the development or functioning of two or more ectodermal derivatives, including hair, teeth, nails, and certain glands such as eccrine glands. ED can be caused by mutations in a number of genes, with different modes of inheritance, and affecting several different developmental pathways. Some ED conditions also affect non-ectodermal-derived tissues.

Clinical Features

- Hypohidrotic ectodermal dysplasia (HED)
  - Mutations in several genes (*ED1*, *EDAR*, *EDARADD*, *IKBKG*) can lead to HED. Different inheritance patterns are seen, including X-link recessive (*ED1*) affecting males and autosomal dominant or autosomal recessive (*EDAR*, *EDARADD*). Patients with mutations in *IKBKG* also have features of immunodeficiency.
  - Patients with HED present with a triad of reduced sweating, hypotrichosis, and abnormal dentition. Reduced sweating can result in intermitted fevers and hyperthermia. Hair is sparse and short, with reduced pigmentation. Teeth eruption is delayed, and abnormalities range from absence of teeth to peg-shaped or conical teeth.
  - Classical facial features include a large forehead with frontal bossing, periorbital pigmentation, prominent nostrils, and flat malar ridges.
  - Atopic dermatitis and other atopic conditions occur more commonly.

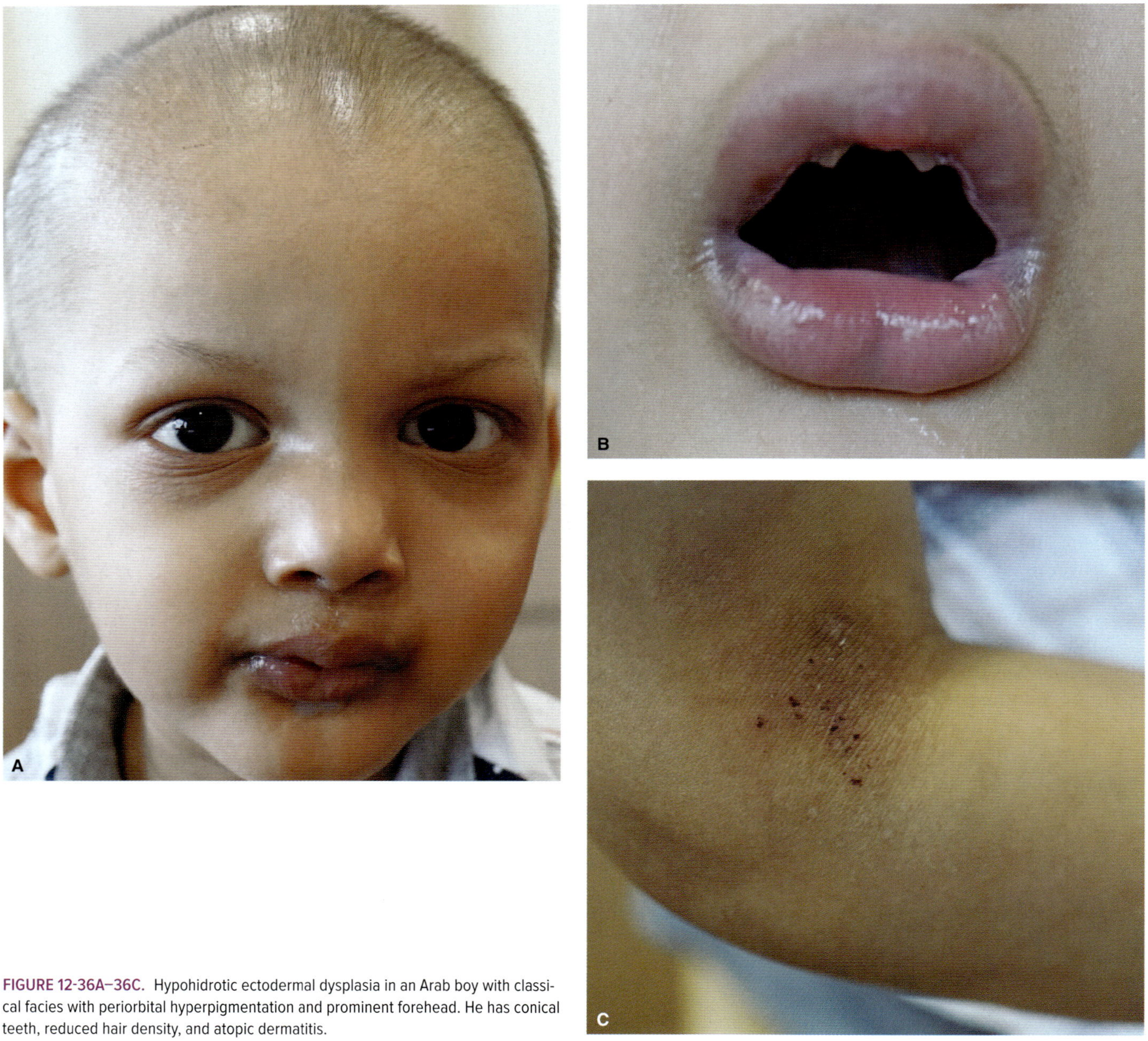

FIGURE 12-36A–36C. Hypohidrotic ectodermal dysplasia in an Arab boy with classical facies with periorbital hyperpigmentation and prominent forehead. He has conical teeth, reduced hair density, and atopic dermatitis.

- Hidrotic ectodermal dysplasia (Clouston syndrome)
  - Mutations in the *GJB6* gene that encodes connexin 30 have been associated. The inheritance pattern is autosomal dominant.
  - Patients with Clouston syndrome present mostly with nail dystrophy. The nails grow slowly and can appear thickened or thinned and discolored. Chronic paronychia may be a problem.
  - Patients are able to sweat but hair may appear sparse, fine, and brittle. Dental caries are common, and eye involvement has been reported.

Differential Diagnoses

- Other rarer forms of ectodermal dysplasias may be explained by mutations affecting the EDA/NFκB pathway (e.g., incontinentia pigmenti), WNT pathway (e.g., focal dermal hypoplasia/Golz syndrome), TP63 pathway (e.g., AEC/Hay-Wells syndrome, Rapp-Hodgkin syndrome, EEC syndrome) and may present with variable features affecting the ectodermal-derived tissues, with associated involvement of other organ systems. Clinical correlation with genetic testing will often aid in a final diagnosis.

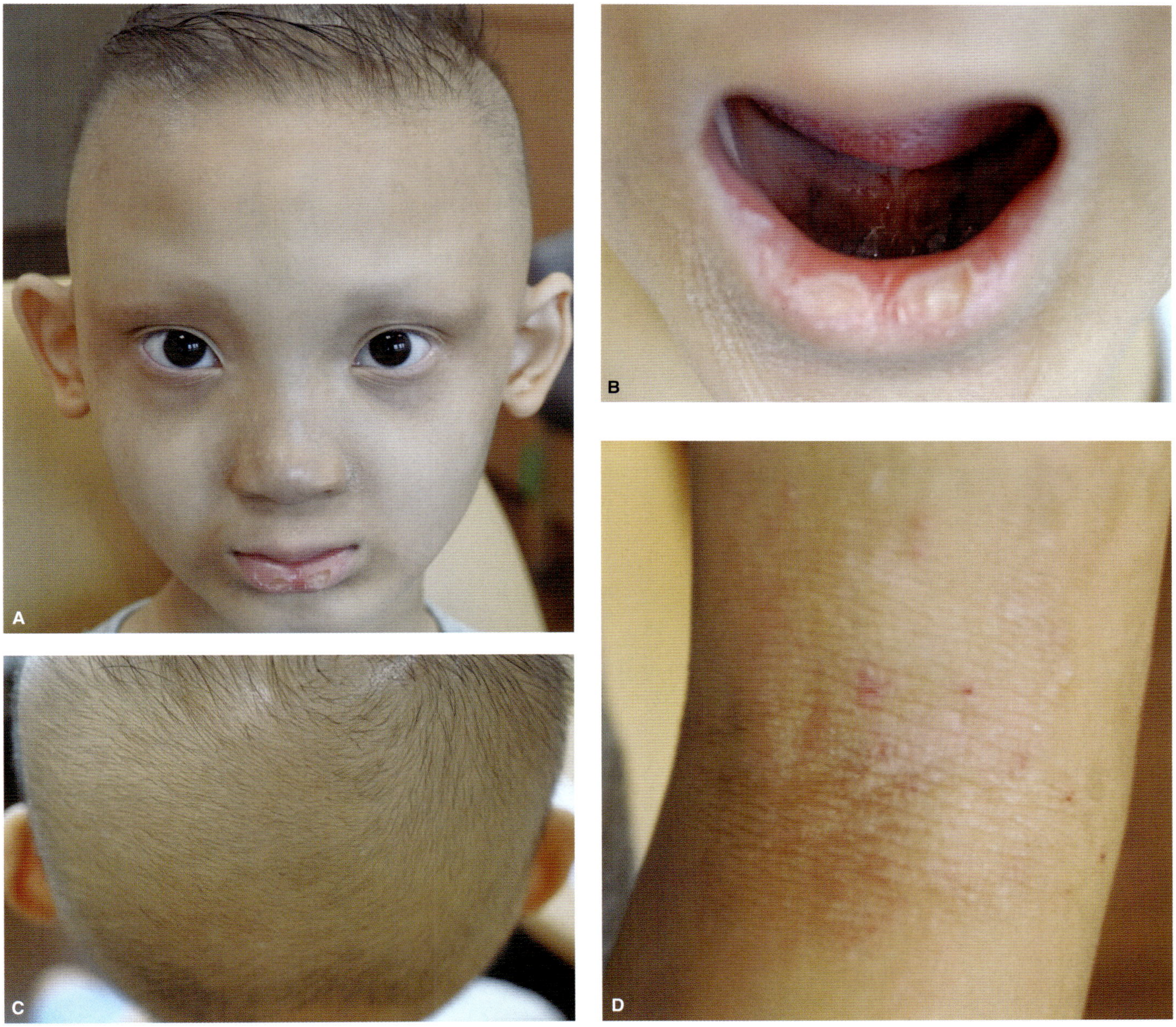

FIGURE 12-37A–37D. Hypohidrotic ectodermal dysplasia in a Chinese boy with classical facies, periorbital hyperpigmentation, anodontia, sparse, short hair, and atopic dermatitis affecting the flexural areas. His nails are normal.

Investigations & Treatment

- Diagnosis of ectodermal dysplasia is clinical and confirmed by genetic testing.
- There is no specific treatment for ectodermal dysplasia. Parents should be advised to prevent and observe for signs of hyperthermia, and learn how to manage these with body cooling measures.
- Dental restoration in the form of dentures, crowns and bridges, and implants should be discussed early with the pediatric dentist or orthodontist.
- Atopic diathesis should be treated as with other patients with atopy.

Pearls & Practical Tips

- Infants and young children with hypohidrotic ectodermal dysplasia may present with fevers of unknown origin and may undergo extensive workup to exclude infections, malignancy, and autoimmune disease. Examine these patients for subtle features of ectodermal dysplasia.
- Although hypohidrotic ectodermal dysplasia is X-linked recessive and affects males, female relatives may present with less severe manifestations of the condition.

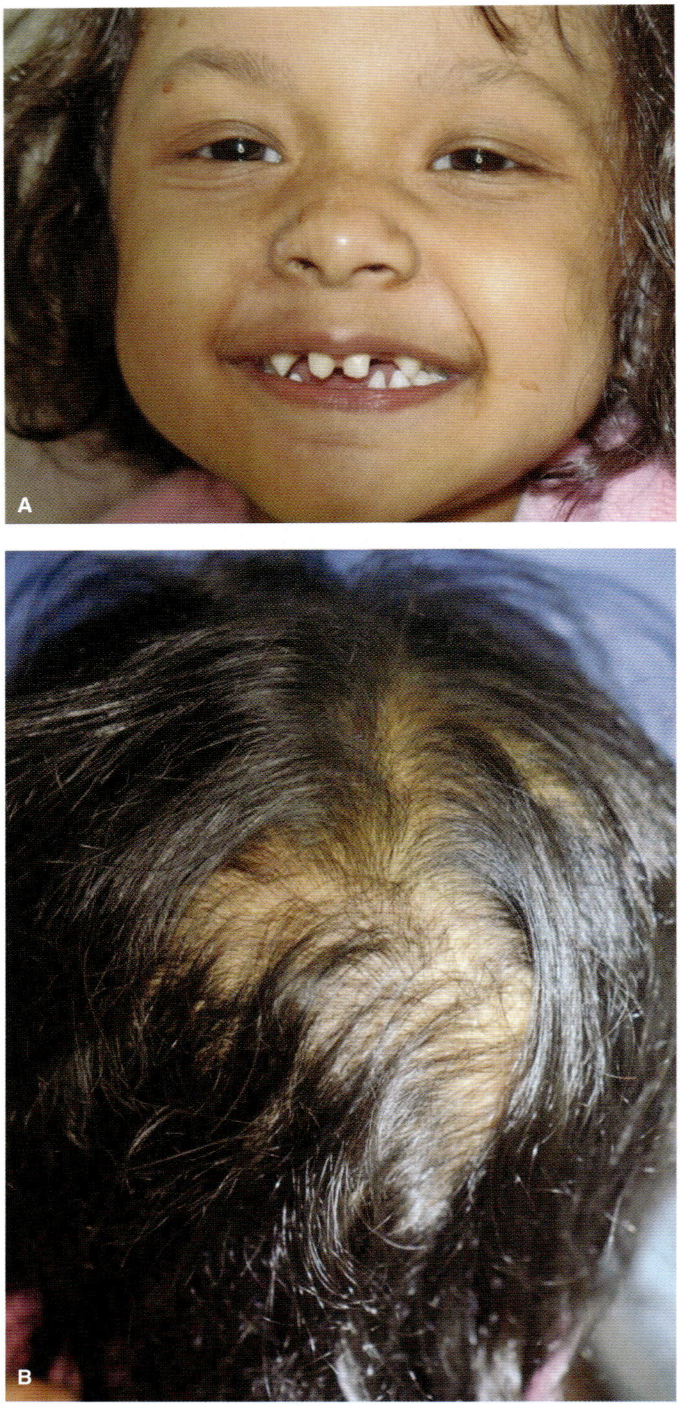

FIGURE 12-38A & 38B. A Malay girl with subtle features of ectodermal dysplasia, with periorbital hyperpigmentation, conical teeth, and thinning of scalp hair. Her father has similar but more severe features.

Bibliography

1. Wright JT, Fete M, Schneider H, et al. Ectodermal dysplasias: classification and organization by phenotype, genotype and molecular pathway. Am J Med Genet A 2019 Mar;179(3):442-7.
2. Spitz JL. Genodermatoses: A Clinical Guide to Genetic Skin Disorders. 2nd ed. Lippincott Williams & Wilkins; 2005.

BASAL CELL NEVUS SYNDROME/GORLIN SYNDROME

Basal cell nevus syndrome (BCNS), or Gorlin syndrome, is a rare autosomal dominant cancer-predisposition syndrome with variable expression. The most characteristic feature is the early development of multiple basal cell carcinomas (BCC). The syndrome is caused by mutations in *PTCH1* or *SUFU* genes.

Clinical Features

- Mutations in the *PTCH1* and *SUFU* genes leads to deregulation of the hedgehog signaling pathway, which plays a vital role in organ development and tumor formation, leading to various developmental abnormalities and tumors.

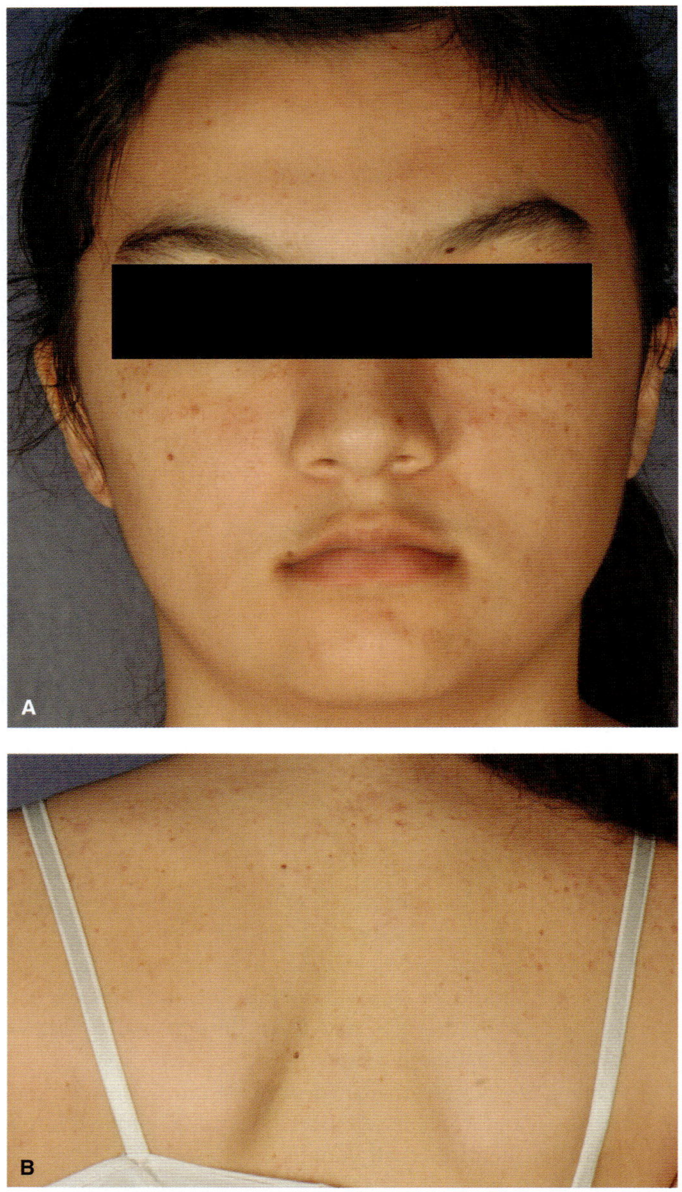

FIGURE 12-39A & 39B. An older adolescent girl with Gorlin syndrome presenting with multiple small basal cell carcinomas on her face, trunk, and limbs.

- Criteria for diagnosis of BCNS: If an individual has two major and one minor criteria OR one major and three minor criteria.
  - Major criteria: Multiple BCC (greater than five in a lifetime, or a BCC before 30 years), lamellar calcification of the falx cerebri, jaw keratocyst, greater than two palmar or plantar pits, and a first-degree relative with BCNS.
  - Minor criteria: Macrocephaly, childhood medulloblastoma, cleft lip/palate, rib or vertebral anomalies (bifid, splayed, missing, or extra ribs; bifid, wedged, or fused vertebrae), preaxial or postaxial polydactyly, cardiac or ovarian fibroma, lymphomesenteric or pleural cysts, and ocular anomalies (cataract, coloboma, microphthalmia).
- BCC can appear within the first year of life but are most common around early adulthood. They appear as skin-colored or brown, dome-shaped papules, measuring 1 to 10 mm in size. There may be central umbilication. Erosions, crusting, and bleeding can occur. The lesions can occur anywhere on the skin but are more common on the head, neck, and trunk.
- Other characteristic features include café-au-lait spots, coarse facies, frontal bossing, broad nasal root, hypertelorism, milia, and epidermal cysts, lipomas, and fibromas.

Differential Diagnoses

- Bazex and Rombo syndrome
  - These are rare genetic syndromes that also present with increased risk of early BCC. Other similar features to BCNS include multiple milia and epidermal cysts.
- Multiple melanocytic nevi
  - Some children or adolescents can develop multiple melanocytic nevi, even in darker-skinned races. They are more common on the face, neck, and trunk.
  - Dermoscopic and histological features will enable differentiation between melanocytic nevi and BCC.

Investigations & Treatment

- Skin biopsy will reveal classical histological features of BCC, with nodules of basaloid cells extending from the epidermis, with peripheral palisading, artefactual retraction, and mucin deposition.
- Regular skin screening for new lesions should be offered to all patients with BCNS.
- Skeletal surveys should be done of the skull, maxilla, mandible, ribs, and vertebrae.
- Genetic testing should be offered to patients with suspected BCNS. If a mutation in *PTCH1* or *SUFU* is confirmed, genetic counseling should be performed, and other family members should be offered genetic testing.
- Treatment of BCC in BCNS is similar to treatment of other BCC. Treatment options include surgery (e.g., simple excision or Moh's surgery), electrocautery, curettage, cryotherapy, photodynamic therapy, topical imiquimod, and topical 5-fluorouracil.
- Oral retinoids may be offered to suppress formation of new BCC.

Pearls & Practical Tips

- Medulloblastoma in BCNS can occur early, before 5 years of age, and usually precedes the development of the multiple BCC.
- Odontogenic keratocysts of the jaw can be destructive and can lead to eating and speech difficulties. Patients should be regularly reviewed by a dentist or oral surgeon.
- Newer treatment options include inhibitors of the hedgehog signaling pathway, such as vismodegib, PIK3-mTOR inhibitors, and the PKC inhibitor. However, their efficacy and long-term safety in children and adolescents is unknown.

Bibliography

1. Spitz JL. Genodermatoses: A Clinical Guide to Genetic Skin Disorders. 2nd ed. Lippincott Williams & Wilkins; 2005.
2. Fujii K, Miyashita T. Gorlin syndrome (nevoid basal cell carcinoma syndrome): update and literature review. Pediatr Int 2014 Oct;56(5):667-74.

NEUROFIBROMATOSIS

Neurofibromatosis type 1 (NF1) is the most common neurocutaneous disorder, with an incidence of 1 in 3000 individuals. Neurofibromatosis type 2 (NF2) is rarer, with an incidence of 1 in 40,000 individuals. Both conditions manifest with various skin lesions associated with involvement of other organs, especially the neurological system and eyes.

Clinical Features

- NF1 is an autosomal dominant (AD) disorder caused by a mutation in the *NF1* gene on chromosome 17q11.2, which encodes the protein neurofibromin, a tumor suppressor gene in the RAS-MAPK pathway.[1]
- NF2 is also inherited in an AD fashion and is caused by a mutation in the *NF2* gene on chromosome 22, which encodes the protein merlin and which also functions as a tumor suppressor.
- NF1 predominantly affects the skin, eyes, central nervous system, peripheral nervous system, and musculoskeletal system, but other organs may rarely also be involved. The following are significant systemic features:
  - Skin: Café au lait macules (CALMs) are usually present from birth, and increase in number and size over several years. Axillary or inguinal freckling may also appear in early childhood.
  - Peripheral nervous system: Neurofibromas are benign nerve sheath tumors typically arising in adolescence. Plexiform neurofibromas are more complex and extensive nerve sheath tumors that arise from bundles of nerve fascicles or nerve plexuses and may be associated with significant morbidity, depending on the site of involvement.
  - CNS: Benign T2-hyperintense lesions may be detected in 60% to 80% of pediatric patients with NF1.[1] Macrocephaly, seizures, hydrocephalus, neurocognitive and behavioral deficits, and learning disorders are also known associations with NF1.

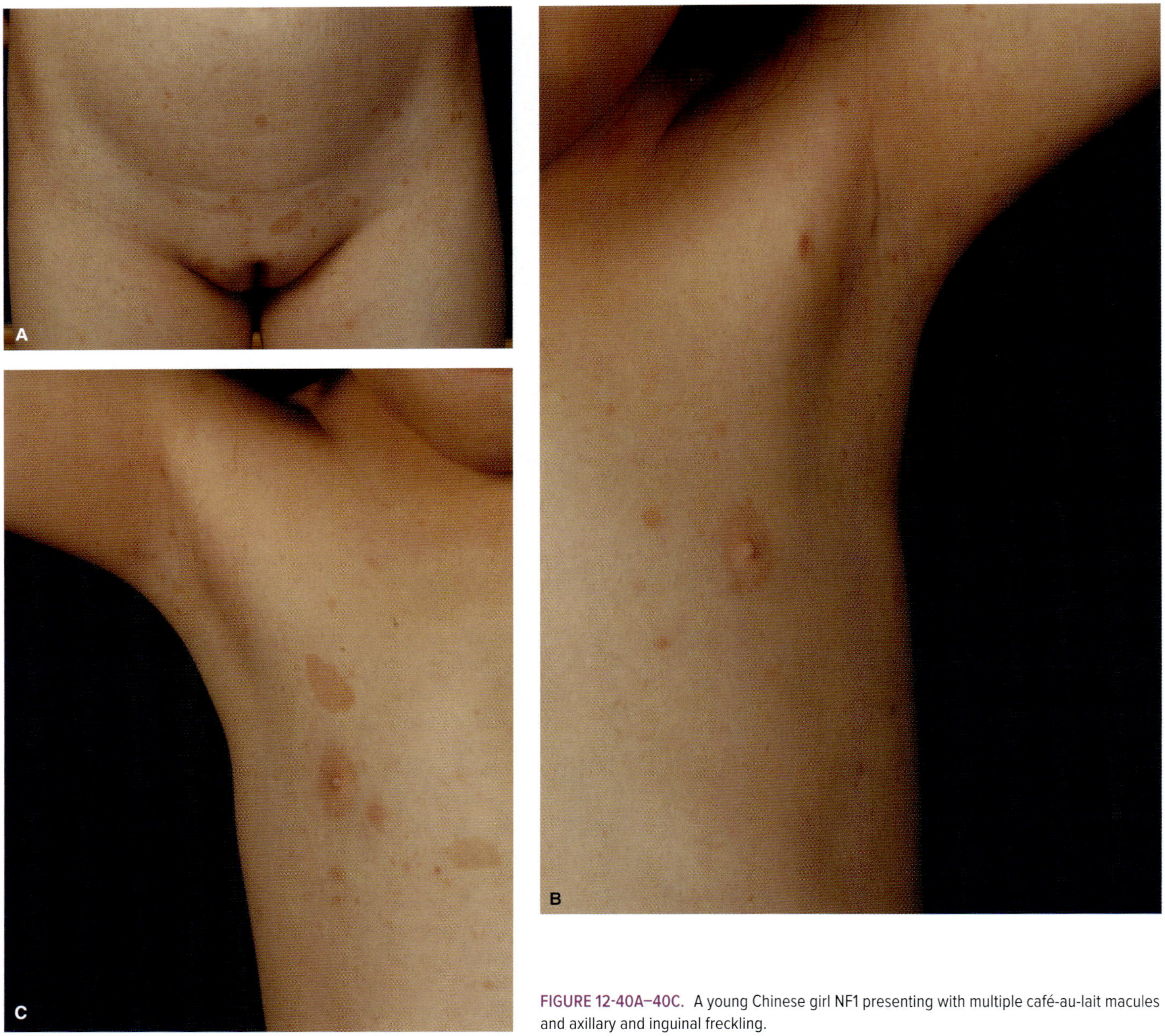

FIGURE 12-40A–40C. A young Chinese girl NF1 presenting with multiple café-au-lait macules and axillary and inguinal freckling.

- Eye: Lisch nodules are hamartomatous lesions of the iris that may be detected from early childhood. Approximately 15% of pediatric patients may have optic gliomas.
- Musculoskeletal system: Sphenoid wing dysplasia, anterior chest wall deformities, and bowing of tibia/fibula are common findings. Pseudoarthrosis may require surgical intervention.
- Vasculopathy: 30% of patients with NF1 have hypertension, which may be secondary to renal artery stenosis, and a small population may have pulmonary stenosis or other vascular abnormalities such as moyamoya syndrome, cerebral aneurysms, and stenotic or tortuous cerebral vessels.

Differential Diagnoses

- Tuberous sclerosis (TS)
  - TS can also present with CALMs during early childhood.
  - Other early clinical features of TS include hypopigmented lesions, shagreen patch, early seizures, developmental delay, cortical tubers in the brain, and myocardial rhabdomyoma.
- McCune-Albright syndrome
  - Also known as polyostotic fibrous dysplasia, and caused by mutations in *GNAS1*, this condition can also present with CALMs, but lesions are usually larger and have a jagged "coast of Maine" border appearance.

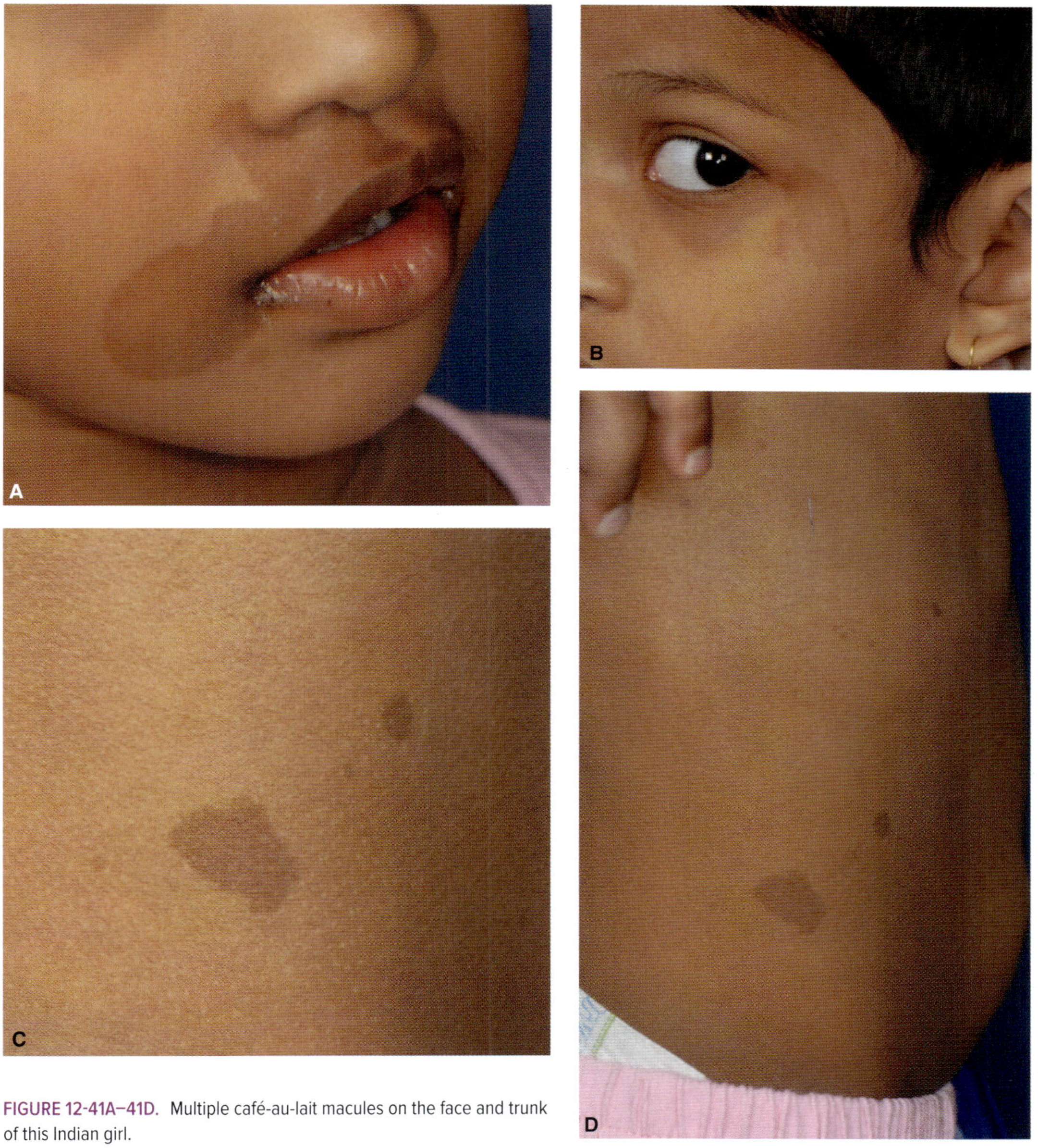

FIGURE 12-41A–41D. Multiple café-au-lait macules on the face and trunk of this Indian girl.

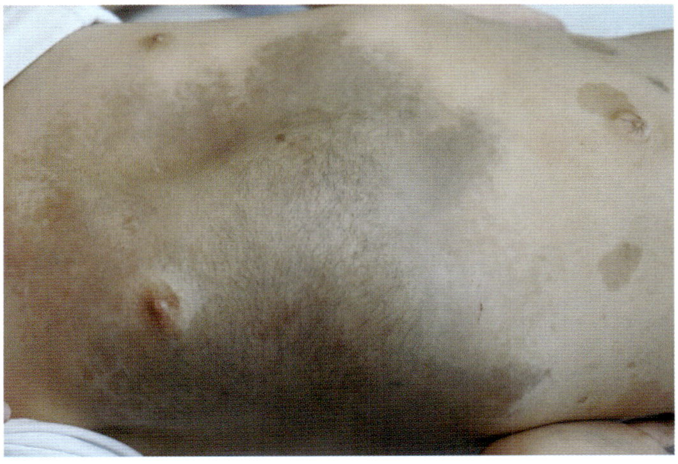

FIGURE 12-42. Large plexiform neurofibroma on the right chest of this Chinese girl with NF1, with overlying grayish-brown, irregular hyperpigmentation, and hypertrichosis.

- Legius syndrome
  - Caused by an autosomal dominant mutation in the *SPRED1* gene, Legius syndrome can also present with multiple CALMs from a young age. However, these patients do not present with other cutaneous or systemic manifestations of NF1.

Investigations & Treatment

- Clinical examination and history will aid in diagnosis, confirmed by targeted mutation analysis.
- Longitudinal monitoring is necessary, as signs and symptoms of NF1 develop over time.
- Multidisciplinary management is essential. Throughout childhood, annual examination of skin, vision, skeletal growth, blood pressure, and neurocognitive development will facilitate early detection of comorbidities.

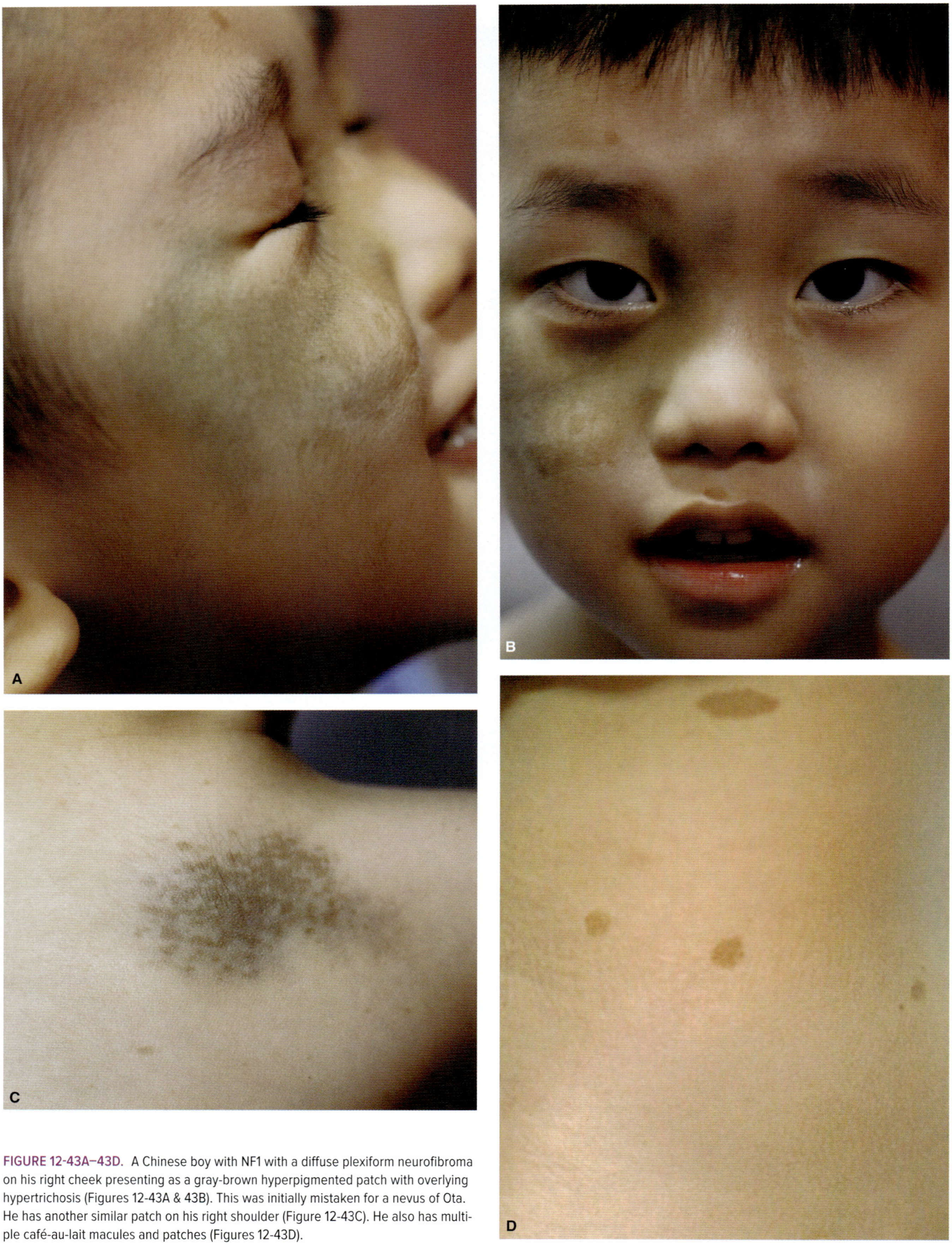

FIGURE 12-43A–43D. A Chinese boy with NF1 with a diffuse plexiform neurofibroma on his right cheek presenting as a gray-brown hyperpigmented patch with overlying hypertrichosis (Figures 12-43A & 43B). This was initially mistaken for a nevus of Ota. He has another similar patch on his right shoulder (Figure 12-43C). He also has multiple café-au-lait macules and patches (Figures 12-43D).

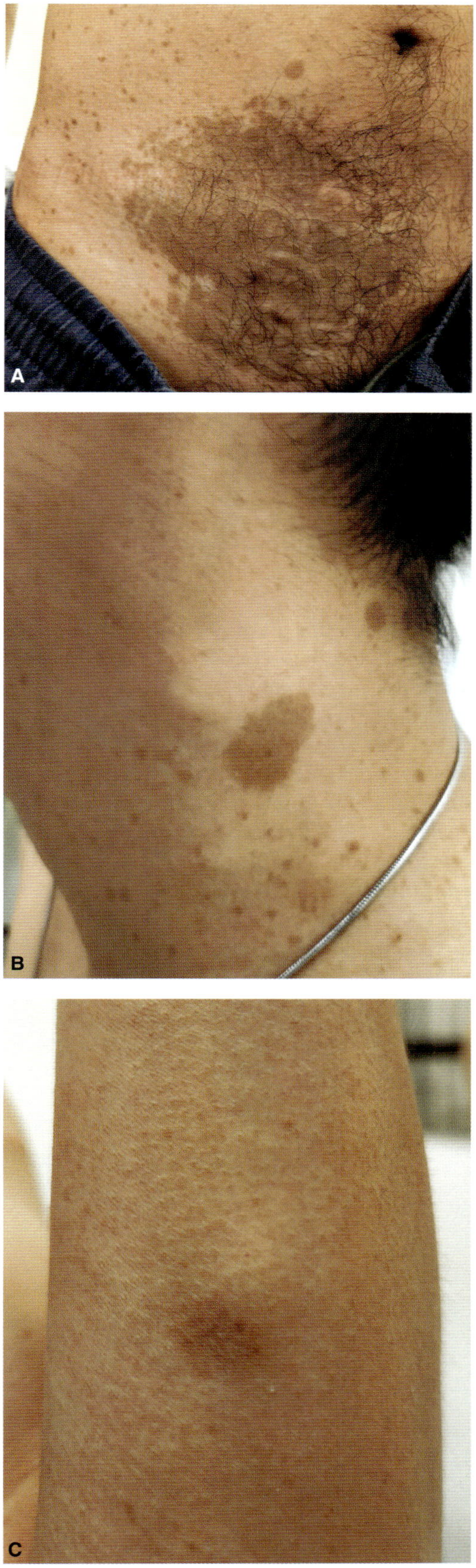

FIGURE 12-44A–44C. An older adolescent Chinese male with NF1 with a large plexiform neurofibroma on his abdomen with smaller, deeper nodules on his neck and arm. There are multiple café-au-lait macules.

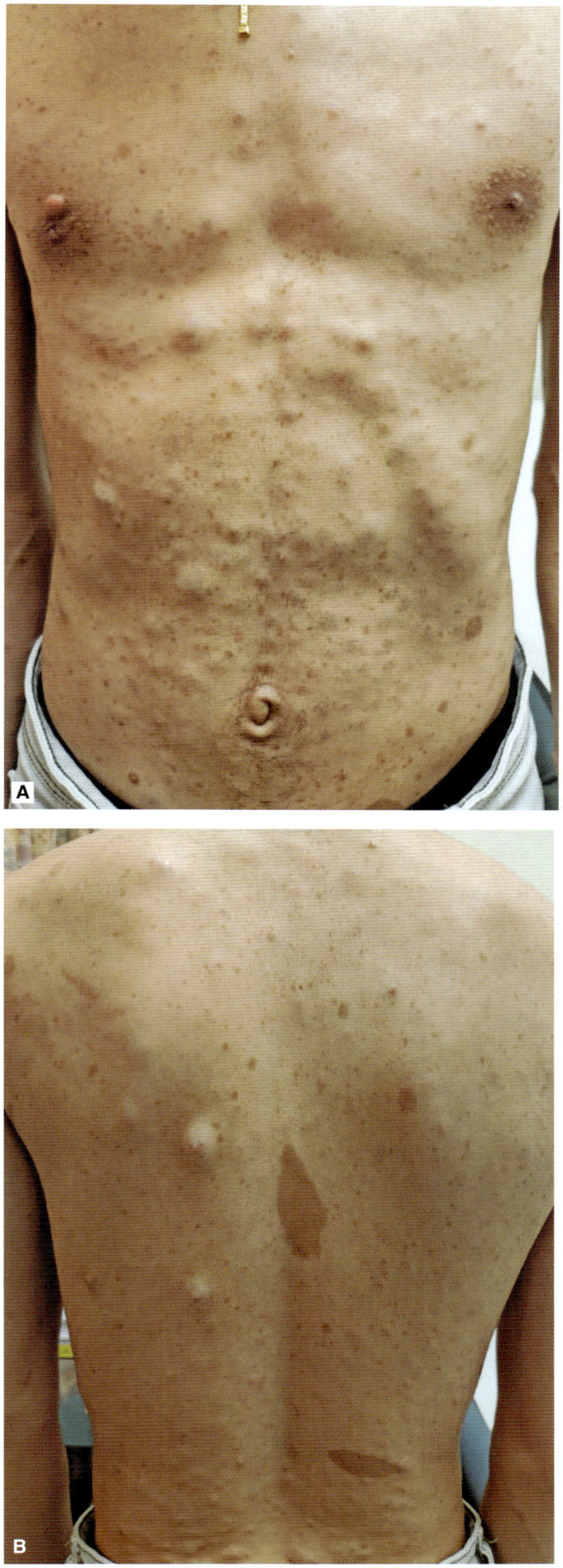

FIGURE 12-45A & 45B. An older adolescent Chinese male with NF1 with multiple café-au-lait macules and patches, and multiple neurofibromas over his trunk and back.

TABLE 12-1. NF1 diagnostic criteria[2] (requires the presence of two of seven clinical features).

Organ	Clinical Features
Skin	• Six or more café au lait macules > 5 mm in diameter in prepubertal children and >15 mm in post-pubertal children • Two or more neurofibromas or one plexiform neurofibroma • Axillary or inguinal freckling
Eyes	• Two or more Lisch nodules • Optic pathway glioma
Bone	• A distinctive osseus lesion (long bone thinning, sphenoid wing dysplasia)
Family history	• First-degree relative with NF1 meeting above criteria
Genetic testing	• A germline *NF1* pathogenic variant

- Genetic counseling is an integral part of patient care at the time of diagnosis and for discussions on family planning.
- MEK inhibitors, such as selumetinib and trametinib, have recently been used to treat the various manifestations of NF-1, with variable results.

Pearls & Practical Tips

- Plexiform neurofibromas are often present from birth but may not be recognized. Clues to early presentation include a large, irregular overlying CALM or other abnormal overlying pigmentation, and increased hair growth.

References

1. Rosser T. Neurocutaneous disorders. Continuum (Minneap Minn). 2018 Feb;24(1, Child Neurology):96-129. doi: 10.1212/CON.0000000000000562. PMID: 29432239.
2. National Institutes of Health Consensus Development Conference. Neurofibromatosis conference statement. Arch Neurol 1988;45(5):575-8. doi:10.1001/archneur.1988.00520290115023.

TUBEROUS SCLEROSIS

Tuberous sclerosis (TS) is a fairly common neurocutaneous disorder, with an incidence of 1 in 10,000 births. It is characterized by a triad of skin findings, seizures, and mental disability. Multiple other organ systems may also be involved, including the eyes, heart, lungs, kidneys, liver, and bone.

Clinical Features

- TS is inherited in an autosomal dominant fashion and is caused by mutations in *TSC1* and *TSC2* genes, found on chromosome 9 and 16, respectively. *TSC1* encodes hamartin and *TSC2* encodes tuberin proteins.
- Most white macules appear at birth to 2 years, followed by a shagreen patch between 2 and 5 years of age, and facial angiofibromas at puberty. Systemic symptoms may follow skin manifestations, such as seizures or infantile spasms, with an association between early onset of seizures and mental disability.
- Clinical manifestations of TS
  - Skin (present in 96% of patients with TS):
    - Hypomelanocytic macules (three or more) are usually present from birth and increase in number with age.
    - Facial papules/nodules (facial angiofibromas, or "adenoma sebaceum") present usually from puberty.
    - Truncal connective tissue nevi (shagreen patch) may appear in early childhood.
    - Peri-/subungual fibromas occur usually from puberty or early adulthood.
    - Forehead fibrous plaque (hamartomas).
    - Café-au-lait macules are less commonly seen compared to neurofibromatosis type 1.
  - Eye: Retinal hamartomas, retinal astrocytomas, achromic retinal patches
  - CNS: Seizures, infantile spasms, subependymal nodules, cortical tubers, intracranial calcification, giant cell astrocytoma, mental retardation
  - Dental: Pitted enamel, gingival fibromas
  - Musculoskeletal: Cystic bone refraction
  - Pulmonary: Lymphangioleiomyomatosis
  - Renal: Bilateral angiolipomas, renal cysts, carcinoma
  - Endocrine: Precocious puberty, hypothyroidism
  - Cardiac: Myocardial rhabdomyoma, Wolff-Parkinson-White syndrome

Differential Diagnoses

- Nevus depigmentosus
  - Nevus depigmentosus is a common birthmark presenting with a hypopigmented patch. Lesions are usually solitary and not associated with other systemic or cutaneous manifestations.

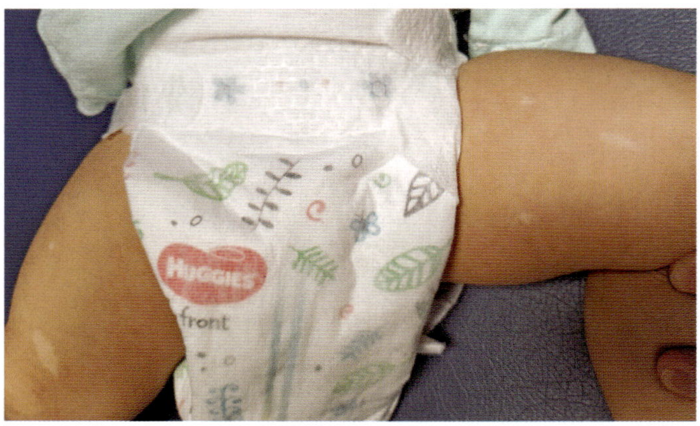

FIGURE 12-46. Multiple ash-leaf hypopigmented patches on the legs of this Chinese infant with tuberous sclerosis. The patient also presented with infantile seizures.

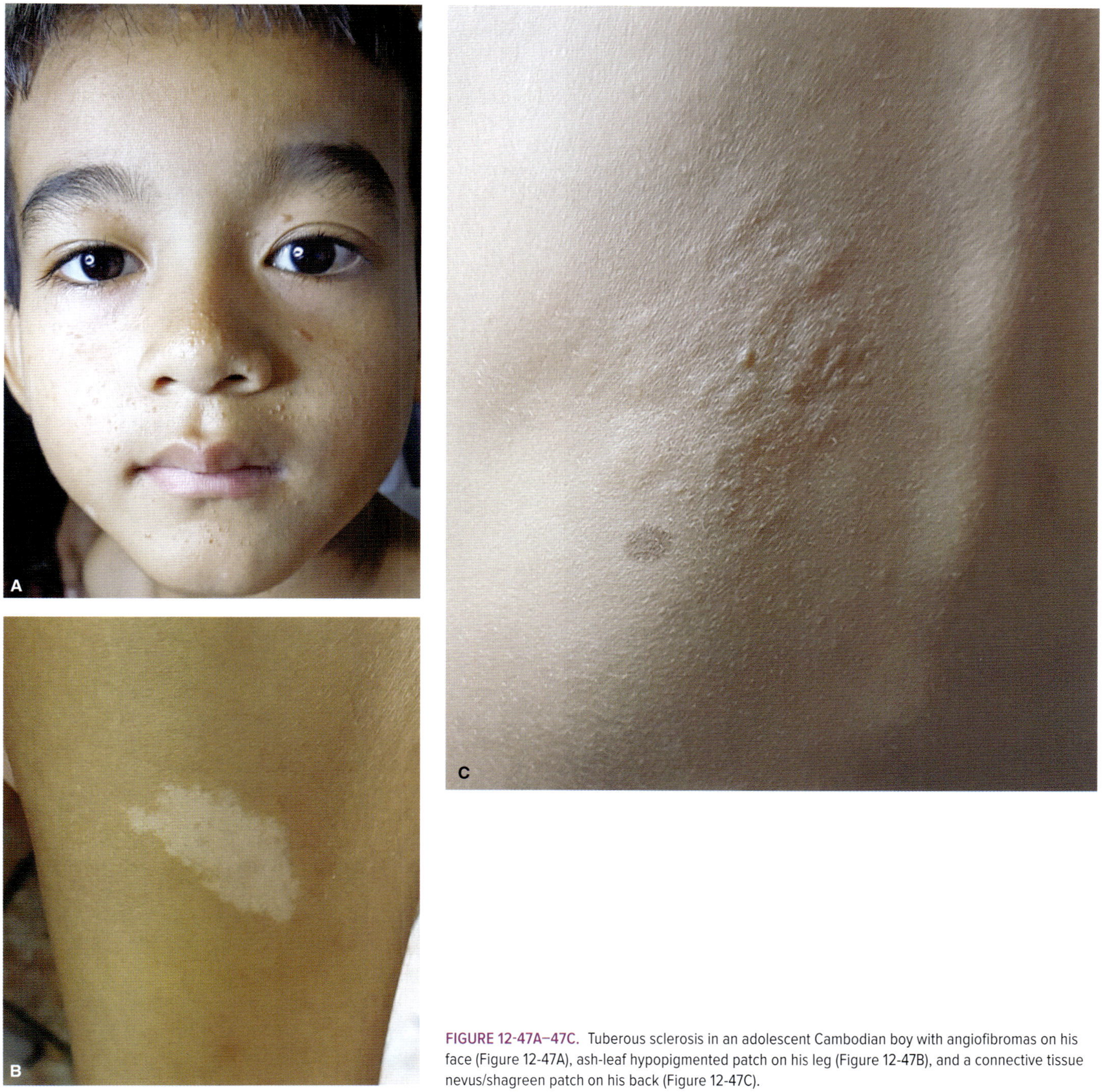

FIGURE 12-47A–47C. Tuberous sclerosis in an adolescent Cambodian boy with angiofibromas on his face (Figure 12-47A), ash-leaf hypopigmented patch on his leg (Figure 12-47B), and a connective tissue nevus/shagreen patch on his back (Figure 12-47C).

- Vitiligo
  - Vitiligo is an acquired disorder and is not present from birth. There are no associated systemic manifestations.
- Piebaldism and Waardenburg syndrome
  - These two conditions present with hypopigmented or depigmented lesions from birth or early childhood. A white forelock is usually also present.

Investigations & Treatment

- Clinical history and examination will aid in diagnosis, confirmed by targeted mutation analysis.
- Regular ultrasound of the kidneys will facilitate detection of any renal angiolipoma or polycystic kidney disease.
- Neuroimaging such as CT brain or MRI brain will be useful in a child with recurrent seizures and may detect subependymal nodules, cortical tubers, calcifications, or ventricular dilatation.

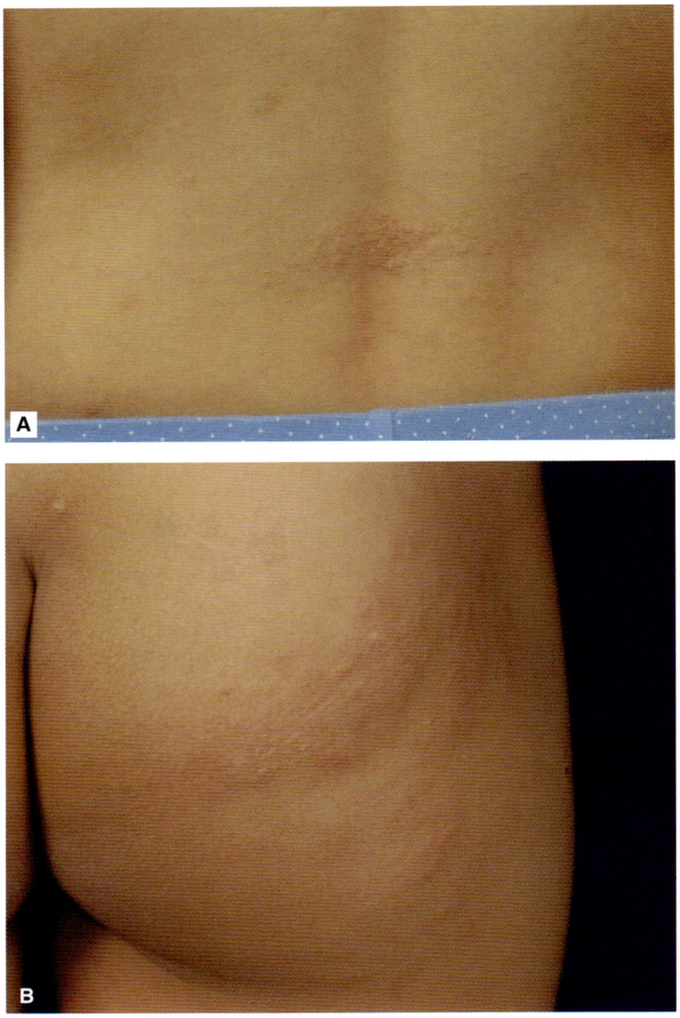

FIGURE 12-48A & 48B. Connective tissue nevi on the back and buttock of a young Chinese girl with tuberous sclerosis.

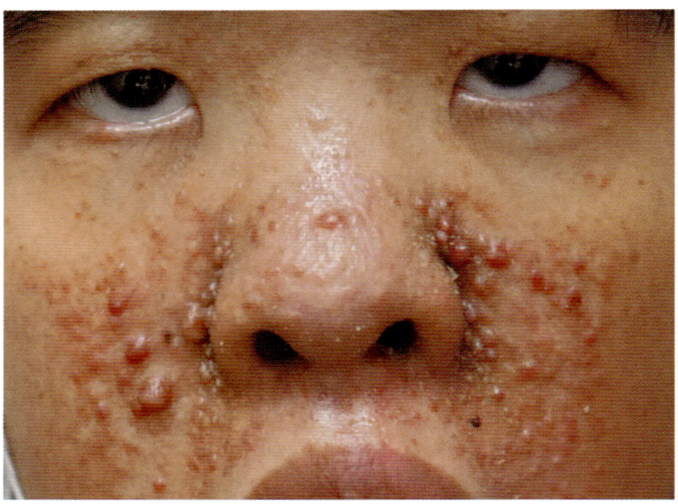

FIGURE 12-49. Multiple angiofibromas (adenoma sebaceum) in a young adult female with tuberous sclerosis. She has epilepsy, developmental delay, and renal angiomyolipomas.

TABLE 12-2. Tuberous sclerosis diagnostic criteria.[2]

• Definite tuberous sclerosis complex: either two major features or one major feature with two minor features. • Probable tuberous sclerosis complex: one major plus one minor feature. • Possible tuberous sclerosis complex: either one major feature or two or more minor features.	
Major features	• Facial angiofibromas or forehead plaque • Nontraumatic ungula or periungual fibroma • Hypomelanotic macules (three or more) • Shagreen patch (connective-tissue nevus) • Multiple retinal nodular hamartomas • Cortical tuber • Subependymal nodule • Subependymal giant-cell astrocytoma • Cardiac rhabdomyoma, single or multiple • Lymphangiomyomatosis • Renal angiomyolipoma
Minor features	• Multiple, randomly distributed pits in dental enamel • Hamartomatous rectal polyps • Bone cysts • Cerebral white-matter radial migration lines • Gingival fibromas • Nonrenal hamartoma • Retinal achromic patch • Confetti-like skin lesions • Multiple renal cysts

- Anticonvulsant therapy should be commenced for a child with infantile spasms or seizures.
- ECG can be performed to detect arrhythmias, and a 2D-echocardiogram will detect cardiac rhabdomyoma. Rhabdomyomas are usually present congenitally or in early infancy.
- Multidisciplinary management with eye examination, neurodevelopmental assessment, genetic counseling, and support groups are essential.
- mTOR inhibitors, such as sirolimus, has recently been used for the treatment of TS, with variable results.

Pearls & Practical Tips

- Patients should be followed up longitudinally and detailed physical examination performed to detect evolving systemic involvement and comorbidities.
- Wood's lamp examination is useful in identifying hypopigmented lesions, especially in infants and young children with fairer skin.
- Ash-leaf lesions are the most classical type of hypopigmented lesions seen in TS. Other hypopigmented lesions seen in TS include "thumbprint"-like macules and confetti hypopigmentation.

References

1. Kurlemann G. Neurocutaneous syndromes. Handb Clin Neurol 2012;108:513-33. doi: 10.1016/B978-0-444-52899-5.00046-0. PMID: 22939051.
2. Roach ES, Gomez MR, Northrup H. Tuberous sclerosis complex consensus conference: revised clinical diagnostic criteria. J Child Neurol 1998;13(12):624-8. doi:10.1177/088307389801301206.

INCONTINENTIA PIGMENTI

Incontinentia pigmenti (IP) is an X-linked dominant genodermatosis that affects the integument (skin, hair, and nails), central nervous system, eyes, and skeletal system. Patients usually present to the pediatric dermatologist for skin lesions at birth or shortly after birth. It is usually lethal in male fetuses.

Clinical Features

- IP is caused by a mutation in *IKBKG* gene (previously known as *NEMO* gene or NF-kB essential modulator) found on chromosome Xq28.
- Affected females present with four distinct stages, with lesions following a Blaschkoid distribution on the skin:
  - Inflammatory/vesicular or bullous stage: Newborn to a few months of age

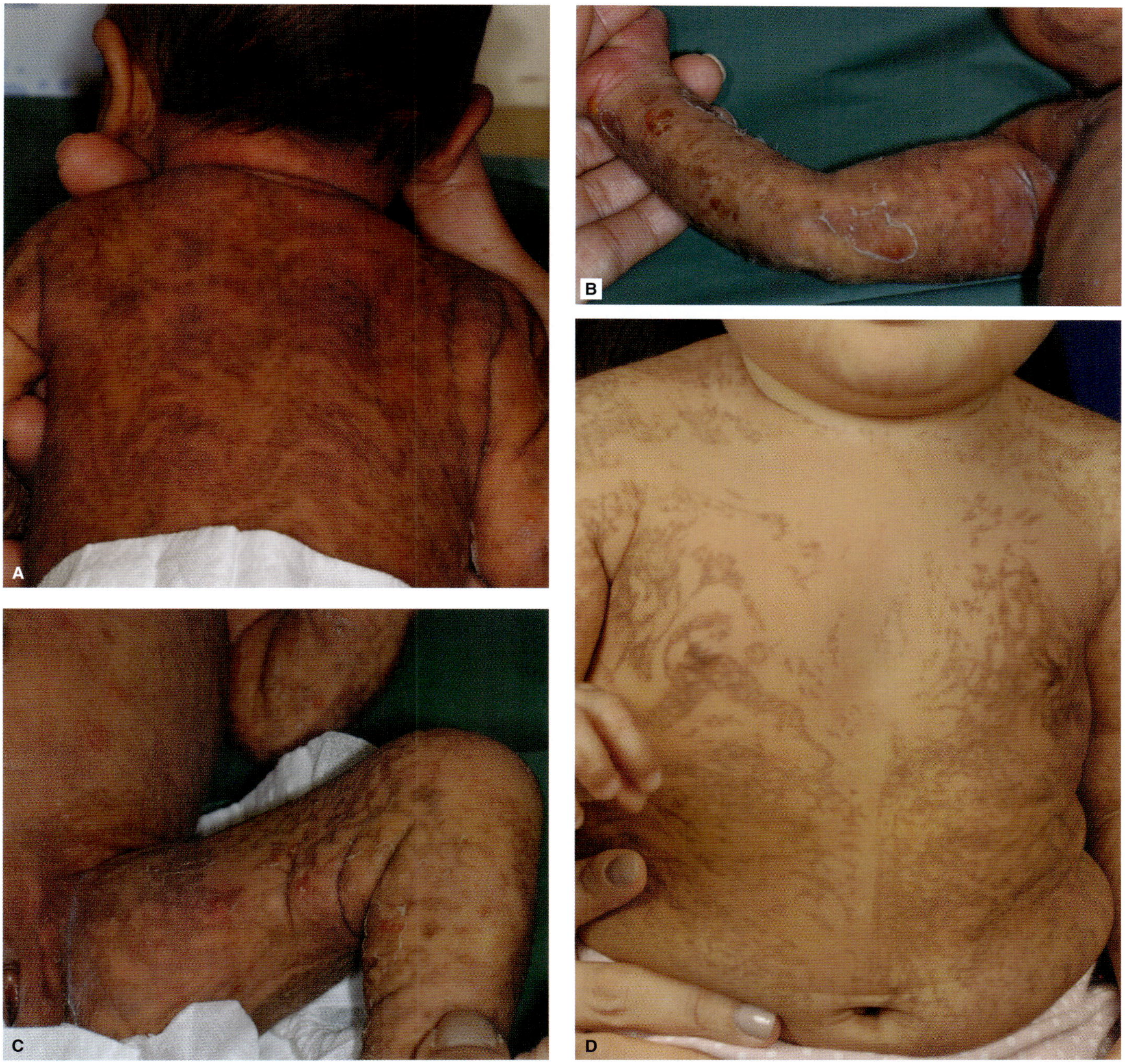

FIGURE 12-50A–50H. A newborn Chinese girl with IP, presenting at birth with extensive hyperpigmented streaks following lines of Blaschko, with blisters and keratotic lesions in linear configuration (Figures 12-50A–50C). Figures 12-50D & 50E show the same child at 9 months of age. The blisters and keratotic lesions have resolved to leave hyperpigmented streaks following lines of Blaschko. Figures 12-50F–50H shows the same child at 7 years of age. She has abnormal dentition and scarring alopecia. The hyperpigmented streaks have lightened considerably by this age.

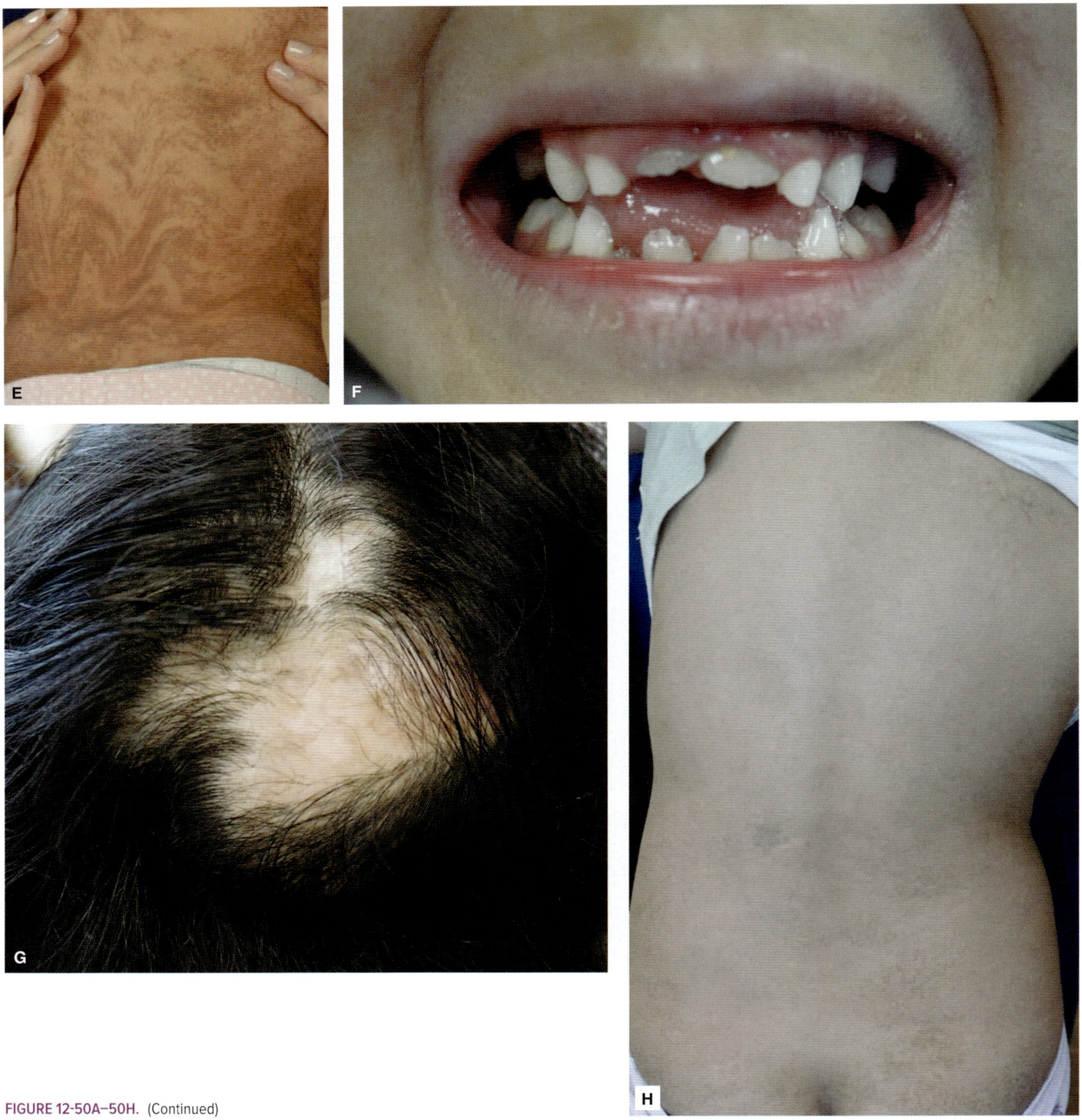

FIGURE 12-50A–50H. (Continued)

- Verrucous stage: A few months to 1 year of age
- Hyperpigmented stage: 1 year to adolescence
- Hypopigmented stages: Adulthood

- Involvement of other systems include:
  - Eye: Microphthalmia, retinal vascular abnormalities, strabismus, nystagmus, cataracts, retinal detachment, optic atrophy
  - CNS: Seizures, mental retardation, spastic paralysis, slow motor development
  - Dental: Conical or missing teeth
  - Nail: Nail dystrophy, nail tumors
  - Other: Pulmonary hypertension, asymmetric breast development, supernumerary nipples, peripheral eosinophilia during the inflammatory phase

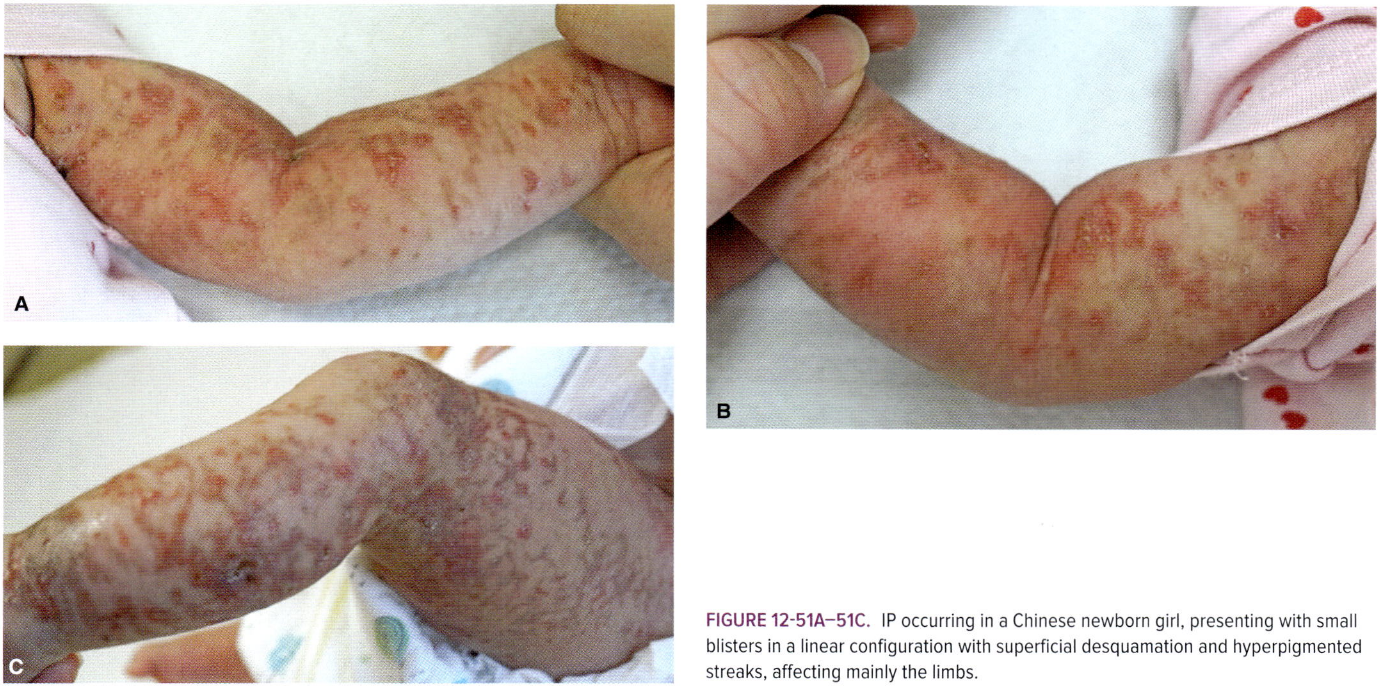

FIGURE 12-51A–51C. IP occurring in a Chinese newborn girl, presenting with small blisters in a linear configuration with superficial desquamation and hyperpigmented streaks, affecting mainly the limbs.

Differential Diagnoses

- Differentials will differ between the various stages
  - Inflammatory/vesicular stage
    - » Infective causes of vesicles and bullae, such as herpes simplex infection, varicella, and impetigo
    - » Epidermolysis bullosa
    - » Autoimmune bullous disorders due to transplacental transmission of maternal autoantibodies in an affected mother
  - Verrucous stage
    - » Epidermal nevus, inflammatory linear verrucous epidermal nevus (ILVEN)
  - Hyperpigmented stage
    - » Pigmentary mosaicism
    - » Lichen planus
  - Hypopigmented stage
    - » Pigmentary mosaicism
    - » Vitiligo

Investigations & Treatment

- Skin biopsy in the inflammatory and verrucous stage will show intraepidermal vesicles with eosinophils and focal dyskeratosis.
- Genetic studies to confirm the mutation in the *IKBKG* (*NEMO*) gene.
- Multidisciplinary management with eye examination, dental, neurological, and neurodevelopmental assessment, genetic counseling, and support groups are essential.

Pearls & Practical Tips

- Rare occurrence of IP in males have been reported and can occur as a result of mosaicism or as part of Klinefelter syndrome with an XXY karyotype.
- It is common for the initial three stages of skin lesions (bullous, verrucous, and hyperpigmented) to occur simultaneously at birth or early infancy. Rarely, the first two stages (bullous and verrucous) can occur in utero, and babies only present with the hyperpigmented stage. This occurrence can lead to misdiagnosis of pigmentary mosaicism until other systemic manifestations occur, such as seizures.
- Although usually more severe in the first few weeks of life, blisters can recur over the initial few months or years of life, especially during times of intercurrent illness.
- Prompt referral to a pediatric ophthalmologist is essential to detect early retinal abnormalities which may require treatment, such as lasers. Further eye complications, even blindness, can occur if not detected and treated early.

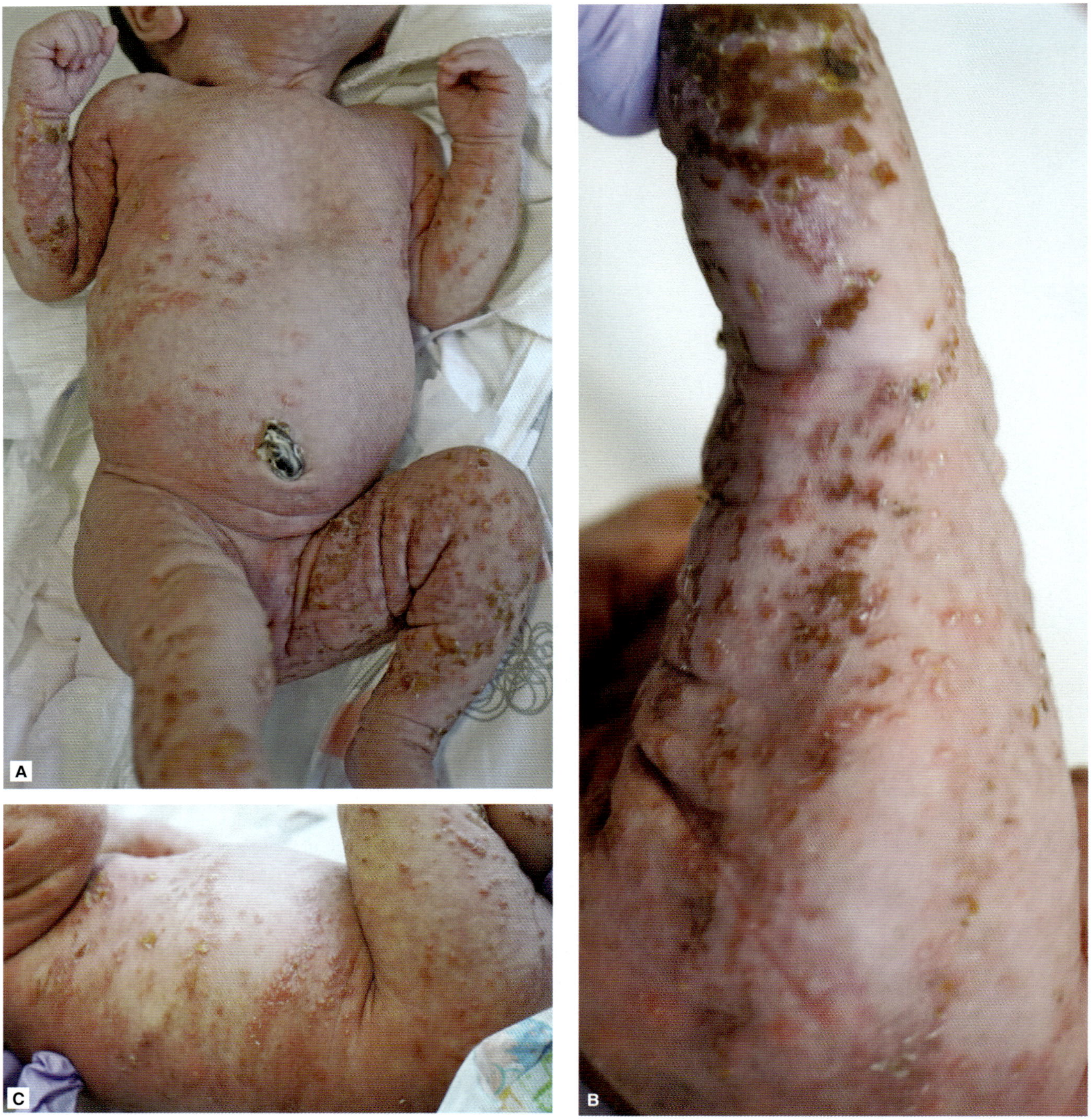

FIGURE 12-52A–52C. Extensive lesions in a newborn Chinese baby girl with IP, with blisters, erosions, and crusted keratotic lesions in a Blaschkoid and liner distribution over the trunk and limbs.

INHERITED DISORDERS OF CONNECTIVE TISSUE

Inherited disorders of connective tissue are caused by mutations in genes encoding proteins that provide cohesion and support for various structures like skin, tendons, ligaments, and vessels. Collagen and elastin are the proteins most commonly affected.

Clinical Features

- Ehlers-Danlos syndrome (EDS)
  - EDS is a group of inherited connective tissue disorders currently classified into 13 subtypes, with substantial overlap between the various phenotypes. Inheritance can be autosomal dominant or autosomal recessive.
  - Skin hyperextensibility is the most characteristic feature. The skin is also soft, doughy to touch, and extremely fragile, which results in easy bruising.
  - Wound healing is poor and delayed, leaving thin atrophic scars. Wound dehiscence is common.
  - Joint hypermobility manifests as chronic joint pains, joint dislocations, and instability.

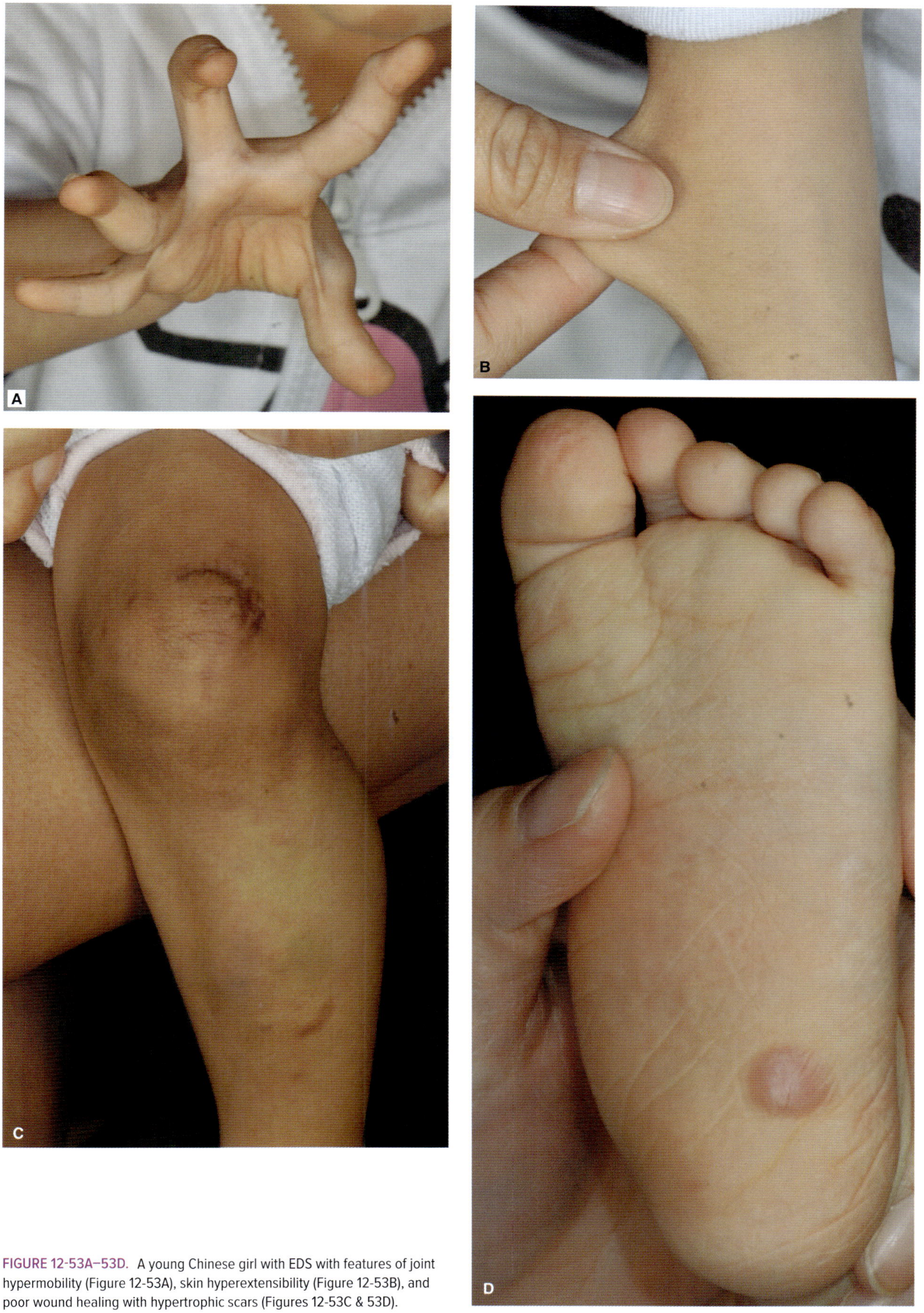

FIGURE 12-53A–53D. A young Chinese girl with EDS with features of joint hypermobility (Figure 12-53A), skin hyperextensibility (Figure 12-53B), and poor wound healing with hypertrophic scars (Figures 12-53C & 53D).

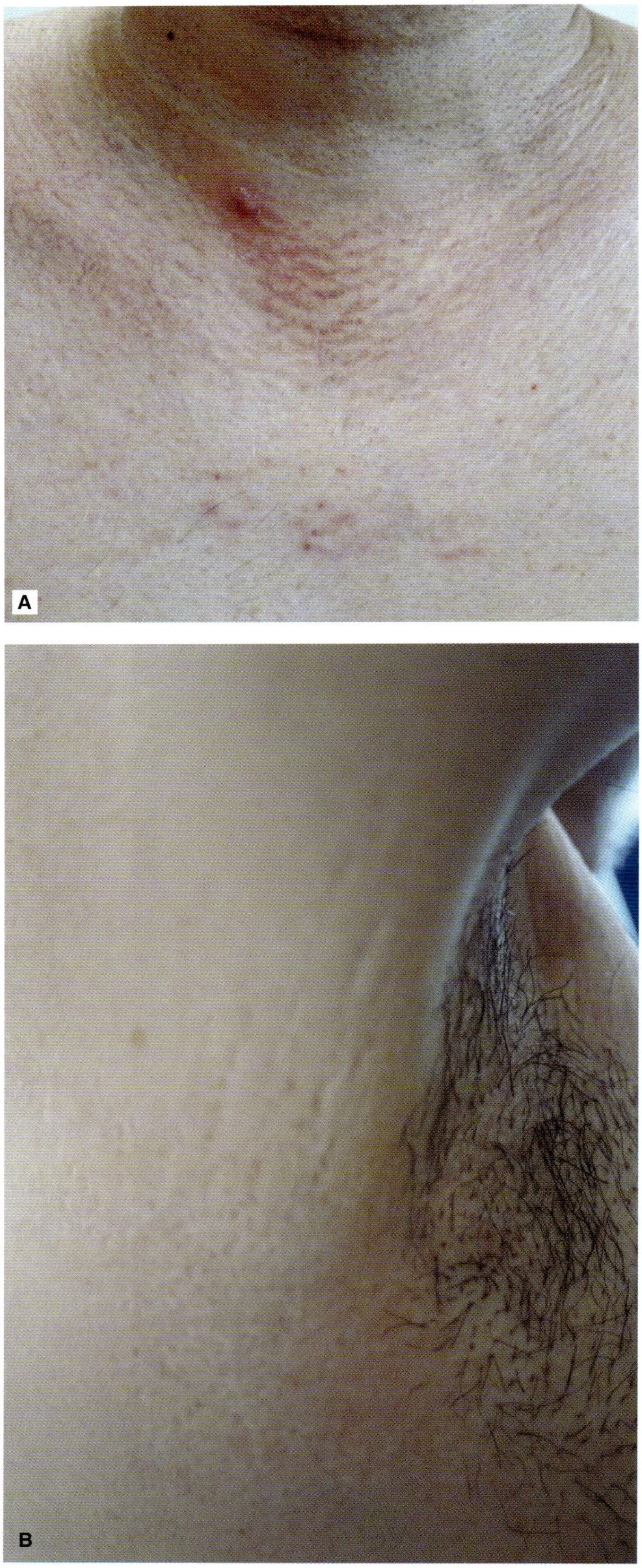

FIGURE 12-54A & 54B. PXE occurring in an adult Chinese male who presented with massive gastrointestinal bleeding but was also found to have angioid streaks on retinal examination, and cardiovascular problems. Examination of his skin shows linear and papular streaks over his upper chest and axillae, resembling plucked chicken skin.

- Pseudoxanthoma elasticum (PXE)
  - PXE is a recessively inherited genetic disorder with mutations in *ABCC6* gene. It is characterized by deposition of calcium in connective tissues, mainly in elastic fibers present in the skin, eyes, and blood vessels.
  - Skin manifestations are some of the earliest manifestations of PXE and can appear from late childhood or adolescence. Characteristic skin lesions are asymptomatic soft, small, yellowish papules and plaques that resemble "plucked chicken skin." They most commonly affect the neck and intertriginous areas. The affected skin can become progressively loose and wrinkled.
  - Ocular involvement in the form of retinal neovascularization and hemorrhage can appear from the first decade of life. Angioid streaks are characteristic and are seen as irregular, brown lines radiating from the optic disk.
  - Mineralization of vessels presents as premature atherosclerosis and myocardial infarction. Other manifestations include gastrointestinal bleeding, claudication, hypertension, and stroke.

Investigations & Treatment

- Ehlers-Danlos syndrome
  - EDS is a clinical diagnosis supported by genetic testing wherever possible. Genetic testing helps with prognostication and monitoring for systemic complications.
  - Echocardiogram is required to assess for cardiac involvement such as mitral valve prolapse and aortic dilatation.
  - There is no specific treatment for EDS, and management is mainly supportive, including avoidance of trauma and wearing of protective pads over trauma-prone sites, regular physiotherapy, and non-weight-bearing exercises such as swimming.
  - Wounds should be closed without tension in two layers, and suture removal should be delayed to reduce the risk of dehiscence.
- Pseudoxanthoma elasticum
  - Skin biopsy for histological evaluation is required for definitive diagnosis. Classical histological features are fragmented elastic fibers with deposition of calcium in the dermis.
  - There is no definitive treatment available for PXE. Active surveillance and treatment of systemic complications is essential, with regular reviews by ophthalmologists, vascular surgeons, and gastroenterologists.
  - Contact sports should be avoided as they increase the risk for ocular and head trauma that may result in retinal hemorrhage.

Bibliography

1. Malfait F, Francomano C, Byers P, et al. The 2017 international classification of the Ehlers-Danlos syndromes. Am J Med Genet C Semin Med Genet 2017;175(1):8-26.
2. Germain DP. Pseudoxanthoma elasticum. Orphanet J Rare Dis 2017;12(1):85.

Vascular Anomalies

INFANTILE HEMANGIOMA

Infantile hemangiomas (IH) are one of the most common vascular tumors of infancy, occurring in 2% to 4% of infants. They are most commonly found on the skin, but rarely may occur in visceral organs, such as the liver. They have a characteristic growth pattern, with spontaneous involution thereafter. Most IH do not require treatment, but those with potential to cause complications require urgent diagnosis and treatment.

Clinical Features

- Usually not present at birth, or appearing as a gray, pink, or hypopigmented, flat, stain, IH grows fairly rapidly in the first 5 to 6 months of life ("proliferation phase") before the growth rate slows down over the next 4 to 6 months.
- Superficial IH present as bright red, raised papules, nodules, or plaques, while deep IH present as soft bluish swellings. Mixed IH combine both a superficial, reddish component and a deeper, bluish component. All IH are soft on palpation and feel warmer than the surrounding skin.
- After the initial 10 to 12 months of growth, most IH undergo slow involution to become flatter and paler. They regress at about 10% a year, with smaller IH involuting more quickly than larger and thicker IH.
- Residual skin changes such as telangiectasias, uneven skin texture and color, and scarring may remain even after complete involution. This is more common with larger and/or more protruding IH.
- Spontaneous ulceration can complicate IH occurring on the lips or at intertriginous sites, such as the groin, axillae, neck, and behind the ears. This usually occurs at 2 to 3 months of age. Ulcerated IH is painful and is at risk for secondary infections.
- IH affecting the eyes or eyelids can lead to ocular complications such as amblyopia and astigmatism. IH affecting the nose can lead to distorted nasal anatomy.

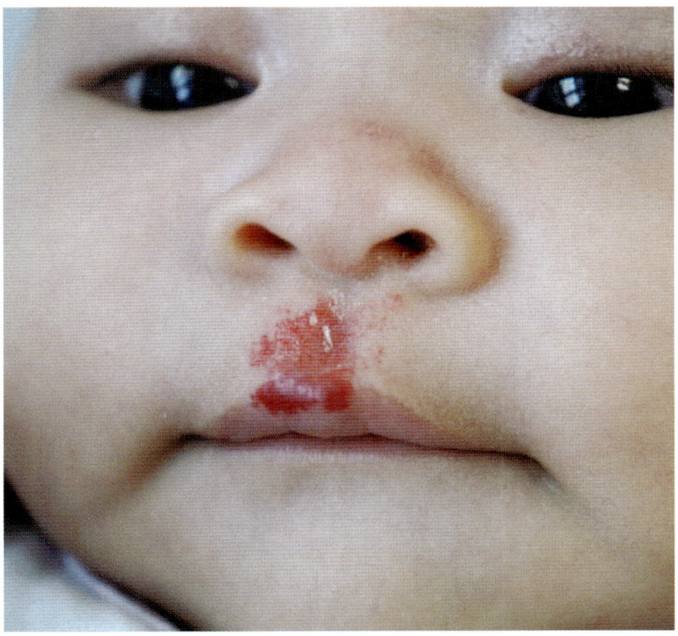

FIGURE 13-1. Superficial IH on the upper lip of a 2-month-old Chinese infant.

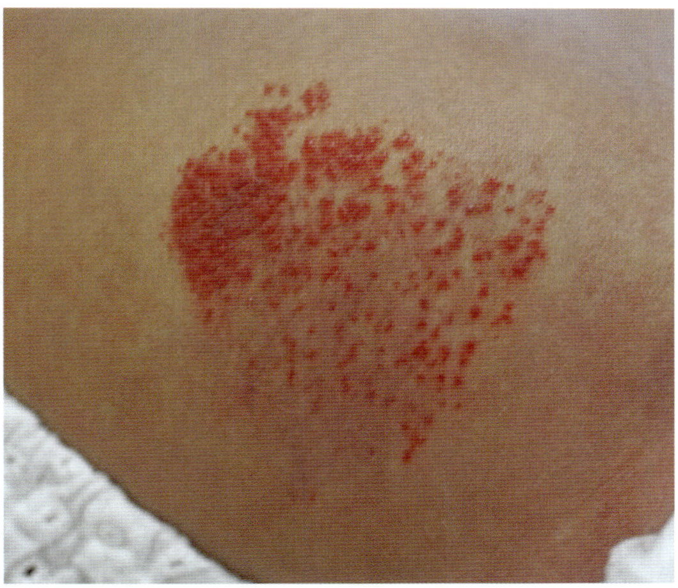

FIGURE 13-2. Superficial IH on the back of a 3-month-old infant.

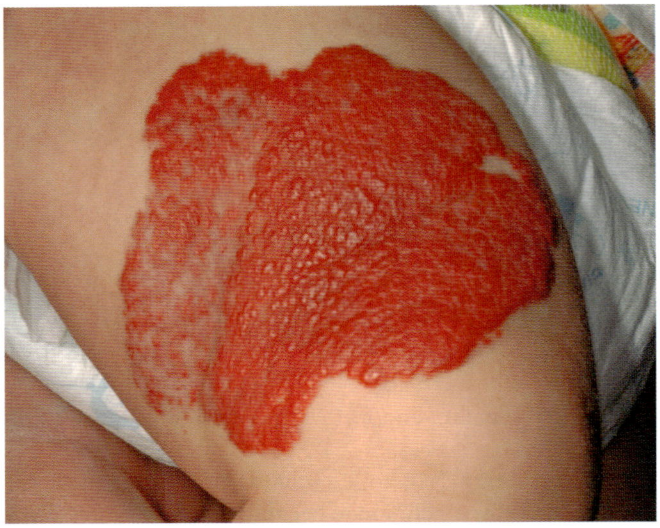

FIGURE 13-3. Large, segmental superficial IH on the thigh of a 3-month-old Chinese infant.

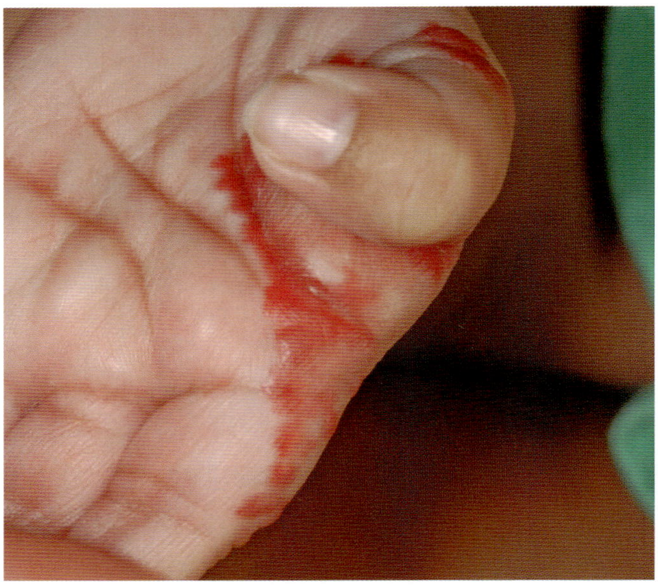

FIGURE 13-4. Superficial IH on the palm of a 2-month-old child.

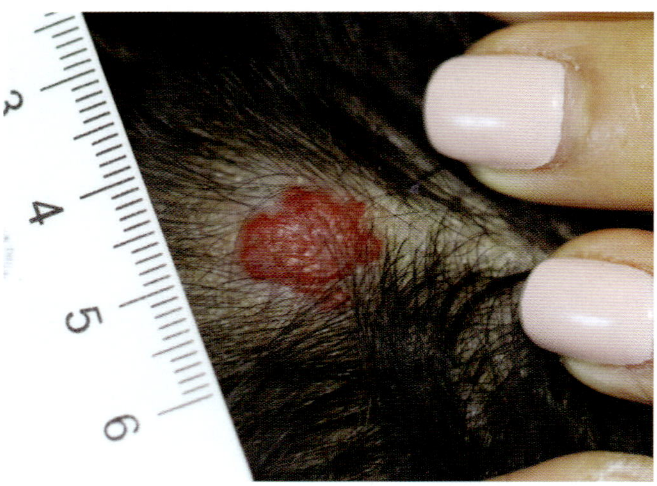

FIGURE 13-5. Scalp IH in a 2-month-old child with accompanying alopecia.

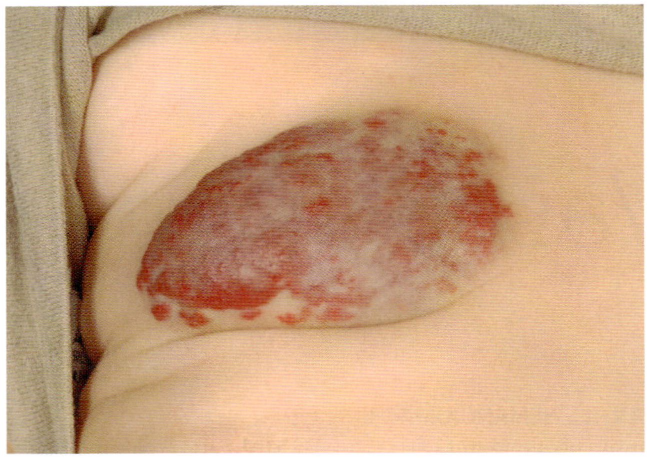

FIGURE 13-6. Mixed IH with both superficial and deep components on the chest of a Chinese infant.

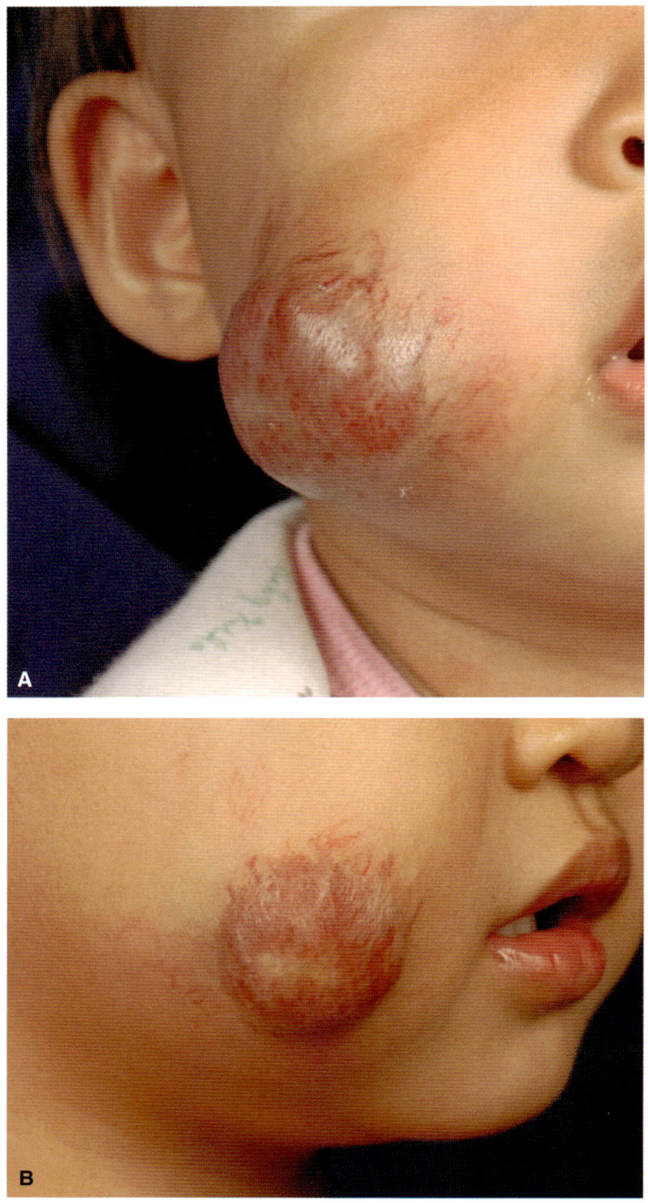

FIGURE 13-7A & 7B. Mixed IH on the cheek of a 4-month-old child. This lesion did not respond optimally to treatment with oral propranolol for 6 months (Figure 13-7B).

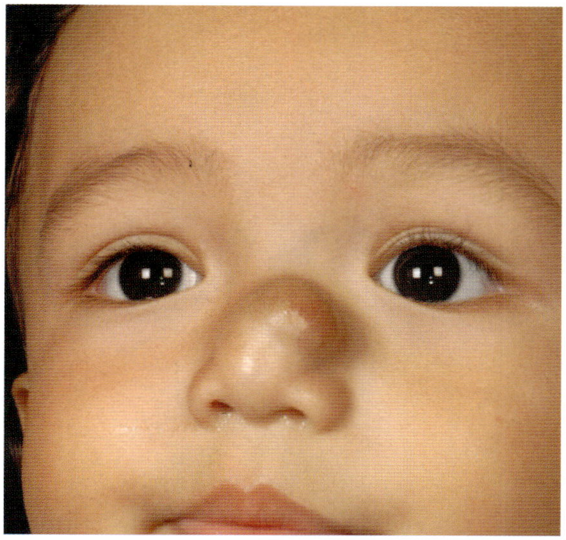

FIGURE 13-8. Deep IH on the nose of a 3-month-old child.

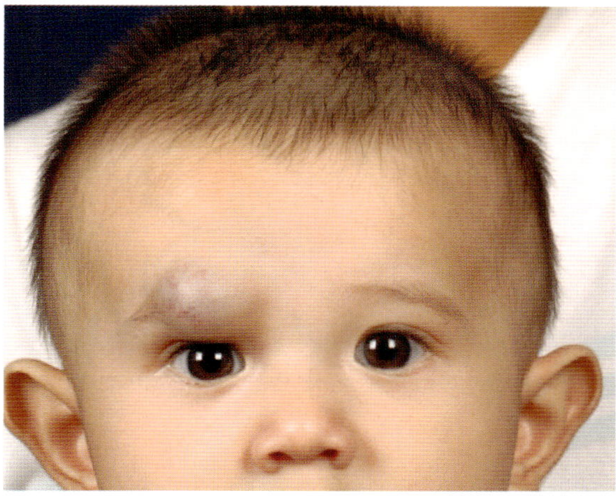

FIGURE 13-9. Deep IH over the right brow in a 3-month-old causing partial ptosis of the upper eyelid.

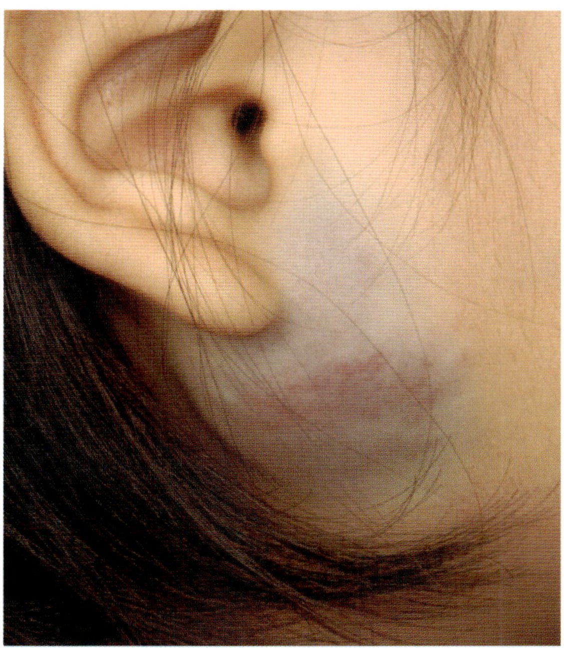

FIGURE 13-10. Deep IH on the right cheek and jaw of a Malay infant.

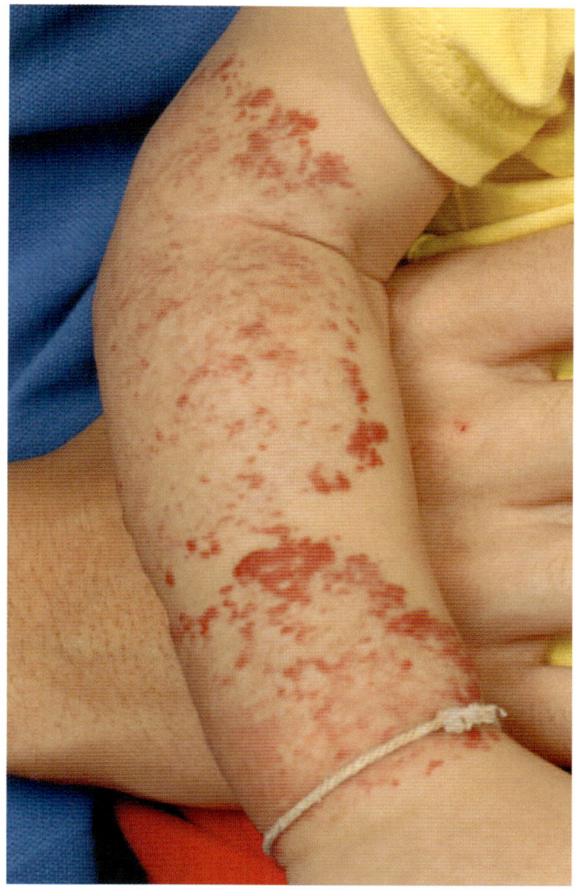

FIGURE 13-11. Abortive IH or IH with minimal or arrested growth (IH-MAG) on the arm of a Chinese infant, with proliferation of only the peripheral areas of the lesion.

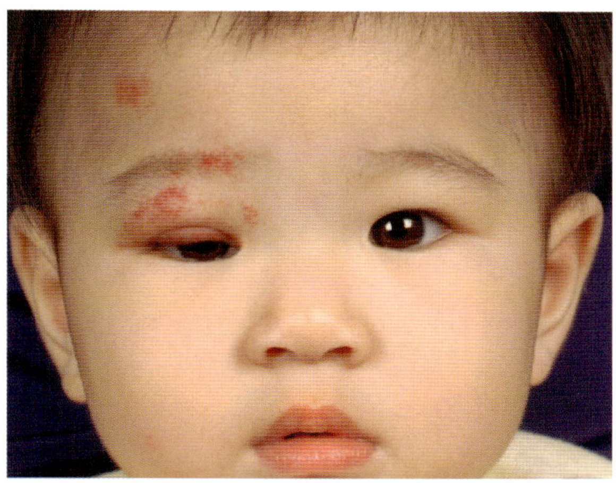

FIGURE 13-12. Segmental IH affecting the forehead and upper eyelid of this 4-month-old girl, causing obstruction of the visual axis. Associated manifestations of PHACES need to be excluded in this patient.

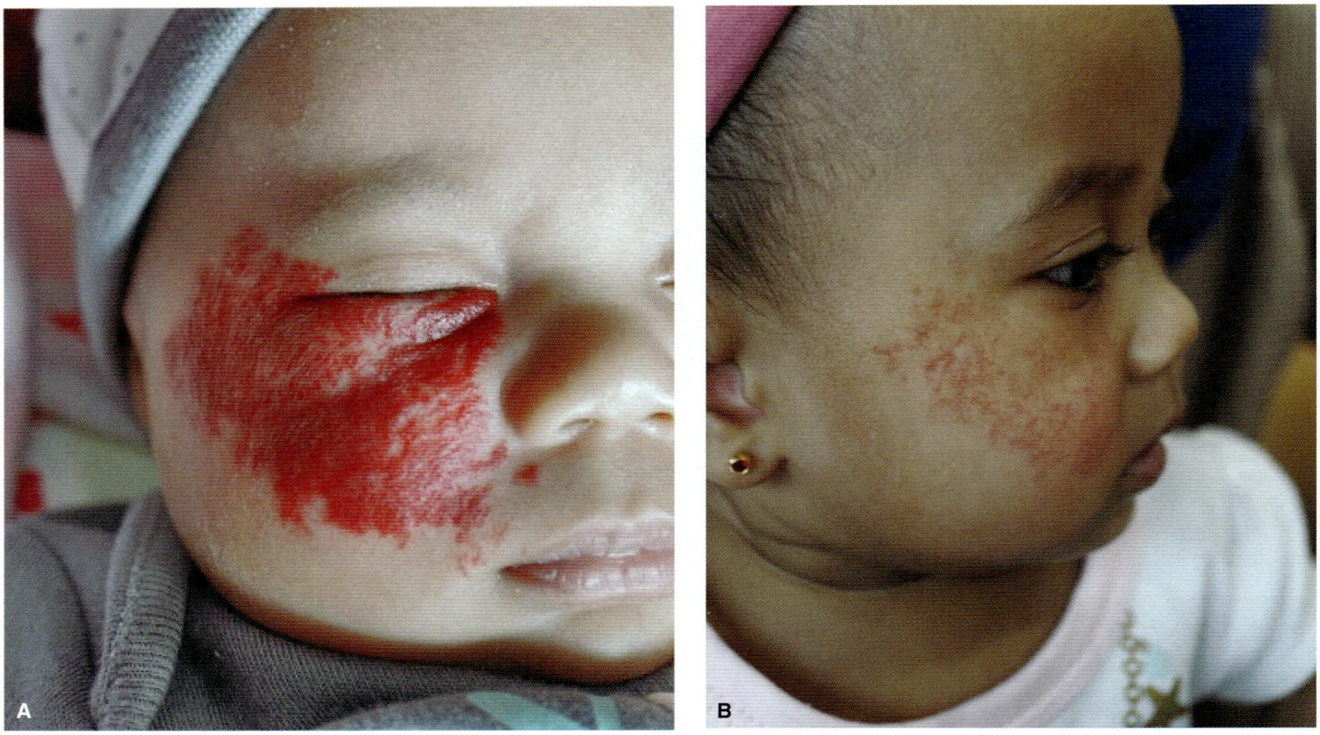

FIGURE 13-13A & 13B. Segmental IH affecting the right cheek of a 2-month-old Malay girl. PHACES was excluded in this patient. Figure 13-13B shows the same child after 6 months of treatment with oral propranolol.

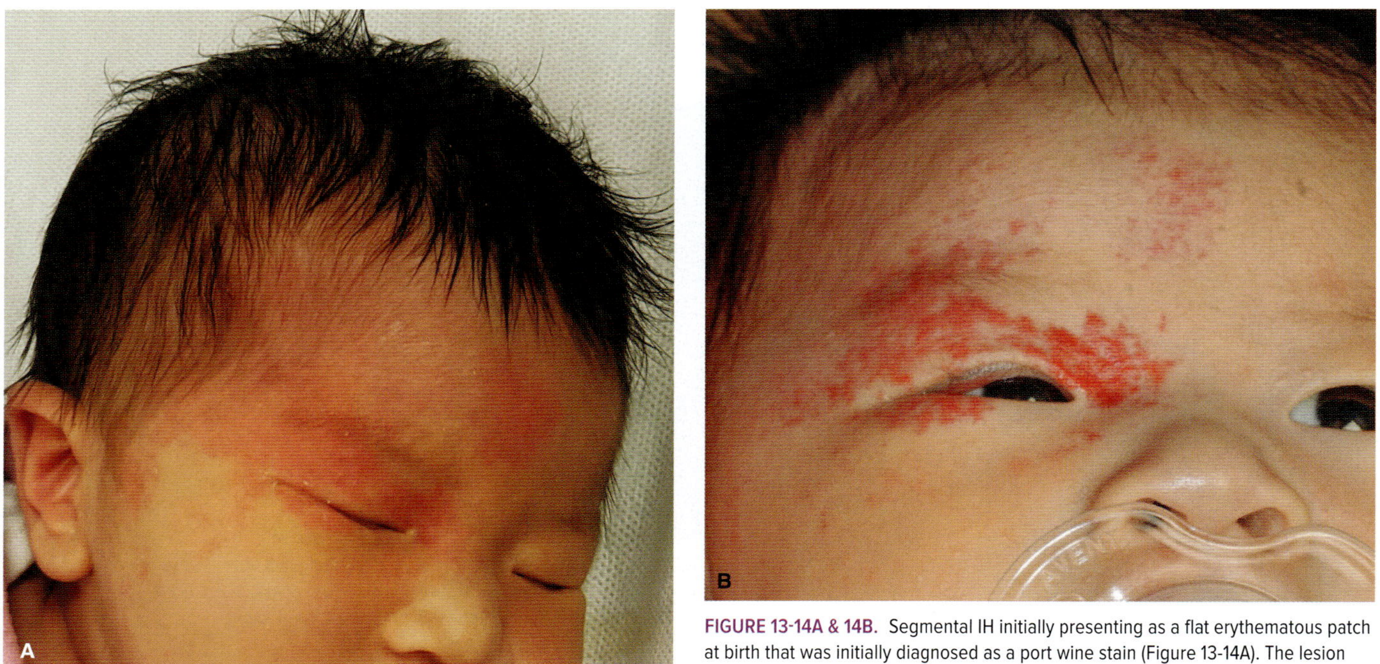

FIGURE 13-14A & 14B. Segmental IH initially presenting as a flat erythematous patch at birth that was initially diagnosed as a port wine stain (Figure 13-14A). The lesion proliferated over the next weeks (Figure 13-14B).

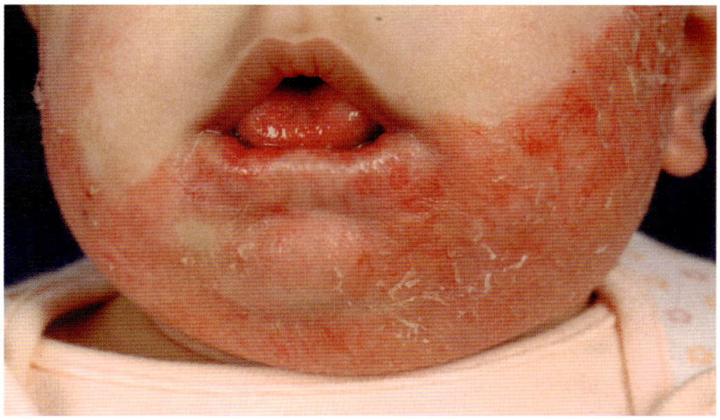

FIGURE 13-15. Segmental IH affecting the "beard" area of a 4-month-old Arab female with overlying eczematous changes (Meyerson phenomenon). Airway involvement and PHACES syndrome were excluded.

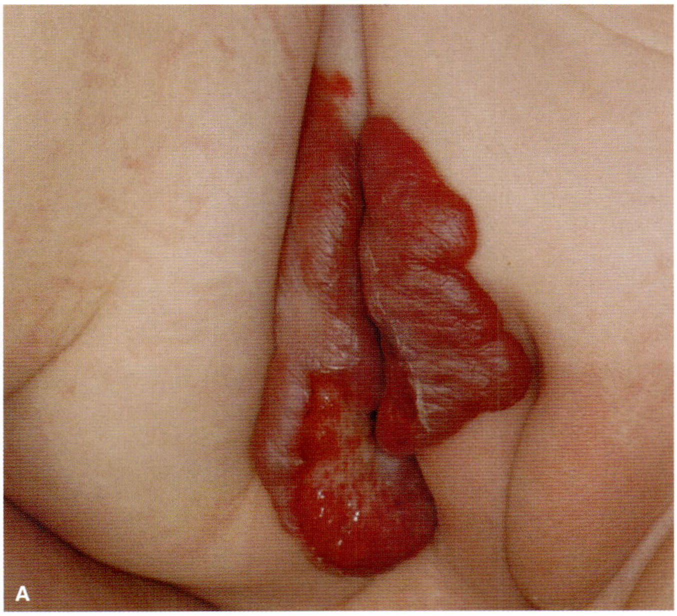

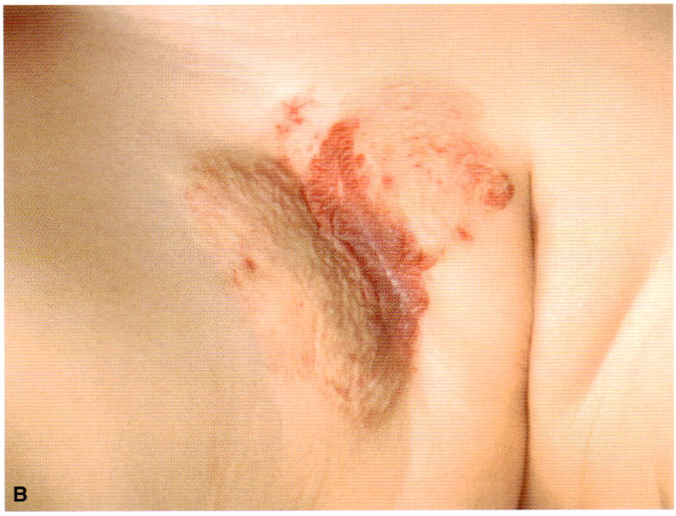

FIGURE 13-16A & 16B. Segmental IH affecting the groin and thigh in a 3-month-old Chinese girl. PELVIS syndrome needs to be excluded. Figure 13-16B shows the same child at 10 months of age after treatment with oral propranolol. There are residual redness and textural changes.

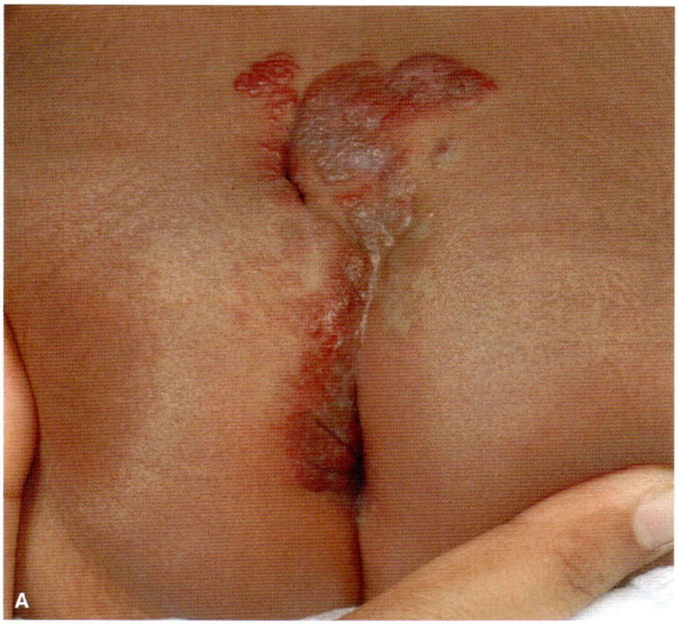

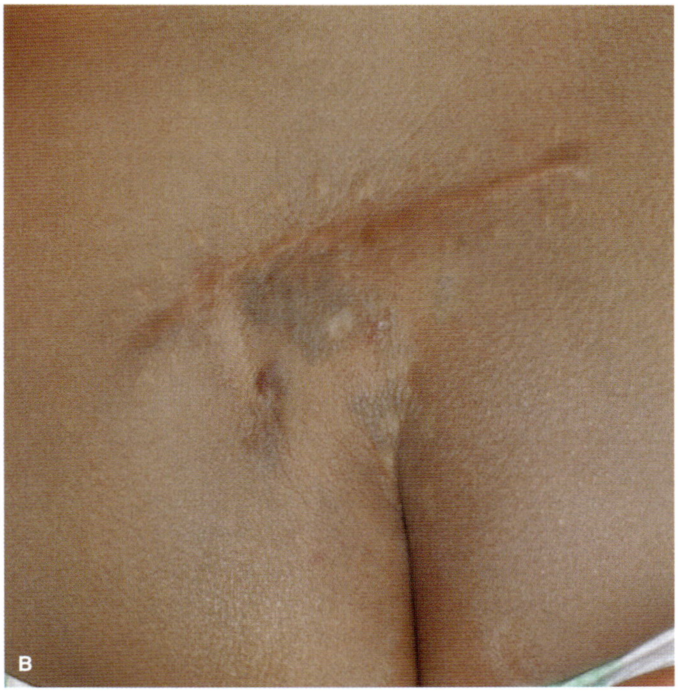

FIGURE 13-17A & 17B. Segmental IH affecting the lumbosacral region of a 2-month-old Malay girl with associated PELVIS syndrome. Figure 13-17B shows the child at 1 year of age after treatment of oral propranolol. The scar is from surgery to correct lipomyelomeningocele and spinal dysraphism.

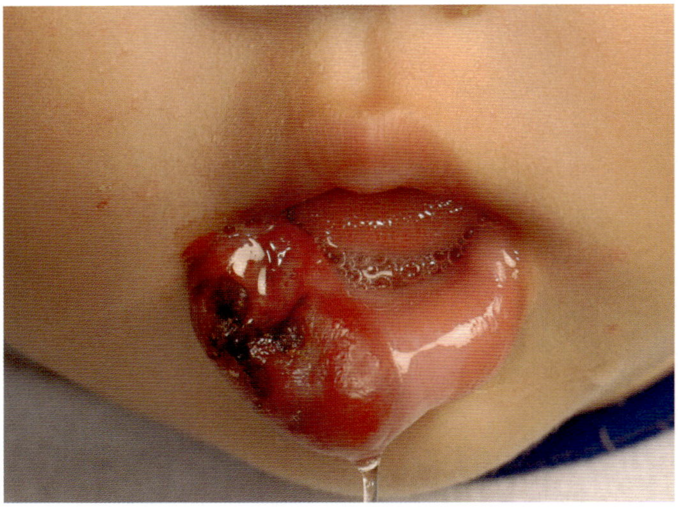

FIGURE 13-18. Ulcerated IH on the lip of a 3-month-old Vietnamese girl.

- IH affecting the preauricular region may be associated with parotid gland IH.
- PHACES syndrome is a combination of **P**osterior fossa malformations, **H**emangiomas (segmental), **A**rterial abnormalities, **C**ardiac abnormalities, **E**ye abnormalities, and **S**ternal cleft/**S**upraumbilical raphe. It can occur in infants with large, segmental IH affecting the head and neck region, and rarely the chest and upper limbs.
- Segmental IH affecting the "beard region" of the lower lip, chin, neck, and mandibular region may have associated airway IH.
- PELVIS syndrome is a combination of **P**erineal hemangiomas, **E**xternal genital malformations, **L**ipomyelomeningoceles, **V**esicorenal abnormalities, **I**mperforate anus, and **S**kin tags. It can occur in infants with large, segmental IH affecting the groin, perianal, or lumbosacral area.
- Multiple IH (more than five discreet lesions) may be associated with visceral involvement, such as liver IH. Liver IH may be associated with consumptive hypothyroidism.

Differential Diagnoses

- Congenital hemangiomas
  - Congenital hemangiomas are fully or almost fully grown at birth, and present with soft, erythematous and/or bluish nodules or plaques, usually surrounded by a pale halo. Unlike IH, there is no proliferative phase.
- Capillary malformation or port wine stain
  - Capillary malformations present as flat, pink-to-erythematous patches that do not proliferate or involute.
- Kaposiform hemangioendothelioma or tufted angioma
  - These are rare vascular tumors which can also present in infancy. They can be associated with the Kasabach-Merritt phenomenon, which does not occur in IH. They present with firm, indurated, violaceous plaques.

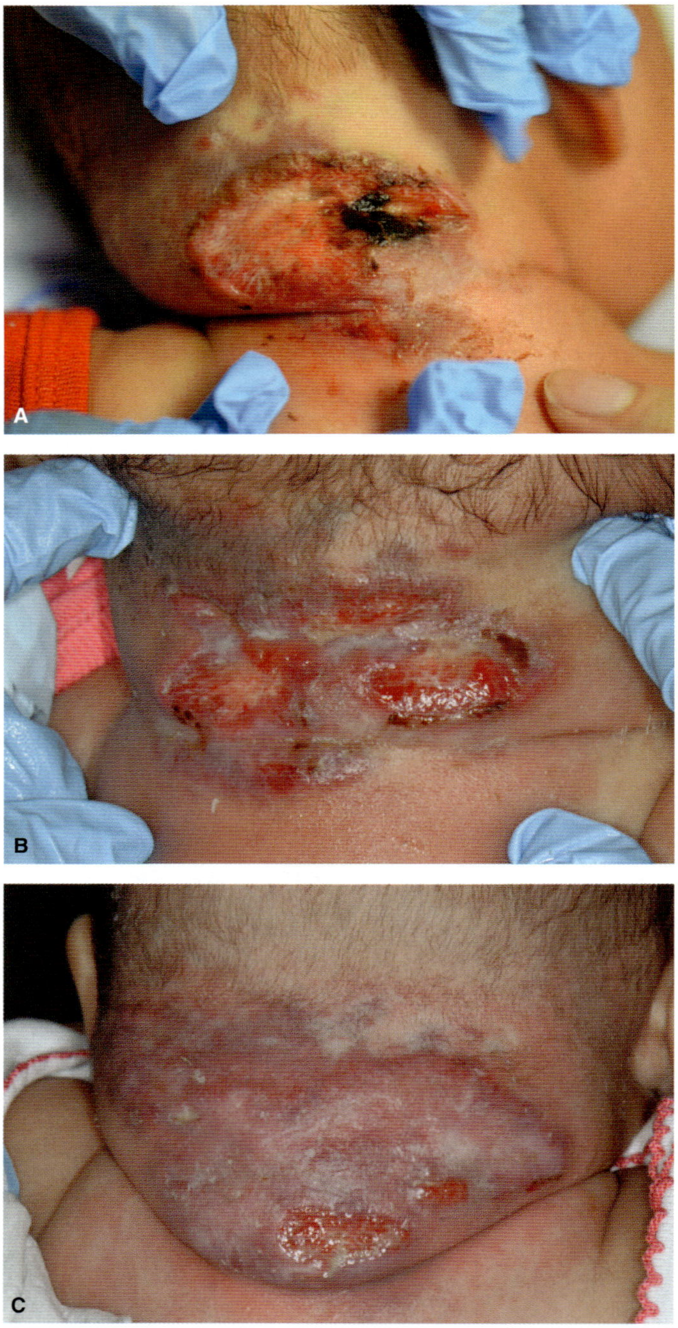

FIGURE 13-19A–19C. Ulcerated IH over the posterior neck in a 2-month-old Chinese twin girl with partial response to treatment with oral propranolol. Figures 13-19B and 13-19C show the same child after 3 weeks (b) and 3 months (c) of treatment, respectively.

- Dermoid cyst
  - These can mimic deep IH, presenting as slightly bluish, deep nodules. They occur along lines of skin fusion such as upper outer eyelids. Unlike IH, they do not feel warmer than surrounding skin.
  - A Doppler or ultrasound may be required to differentiate.

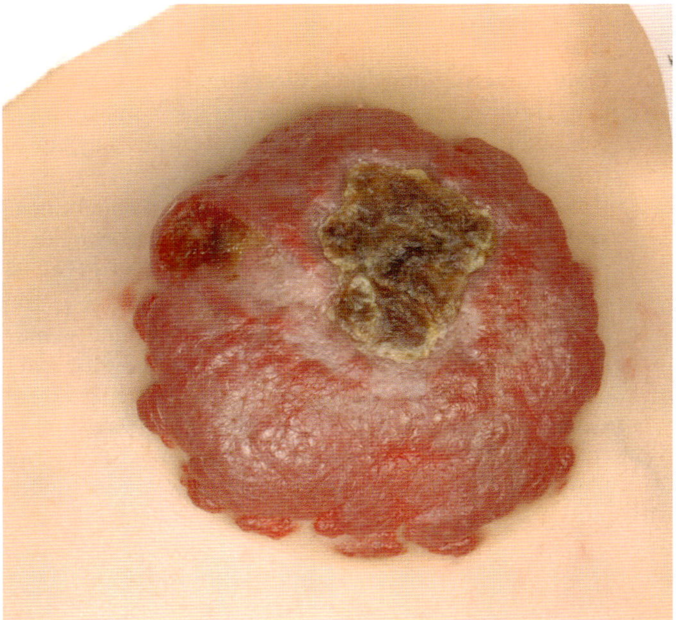

FIGURE 13-20. Ulcerated IH on the back of a 6-month-old Chinese boy with superficial scabbing.

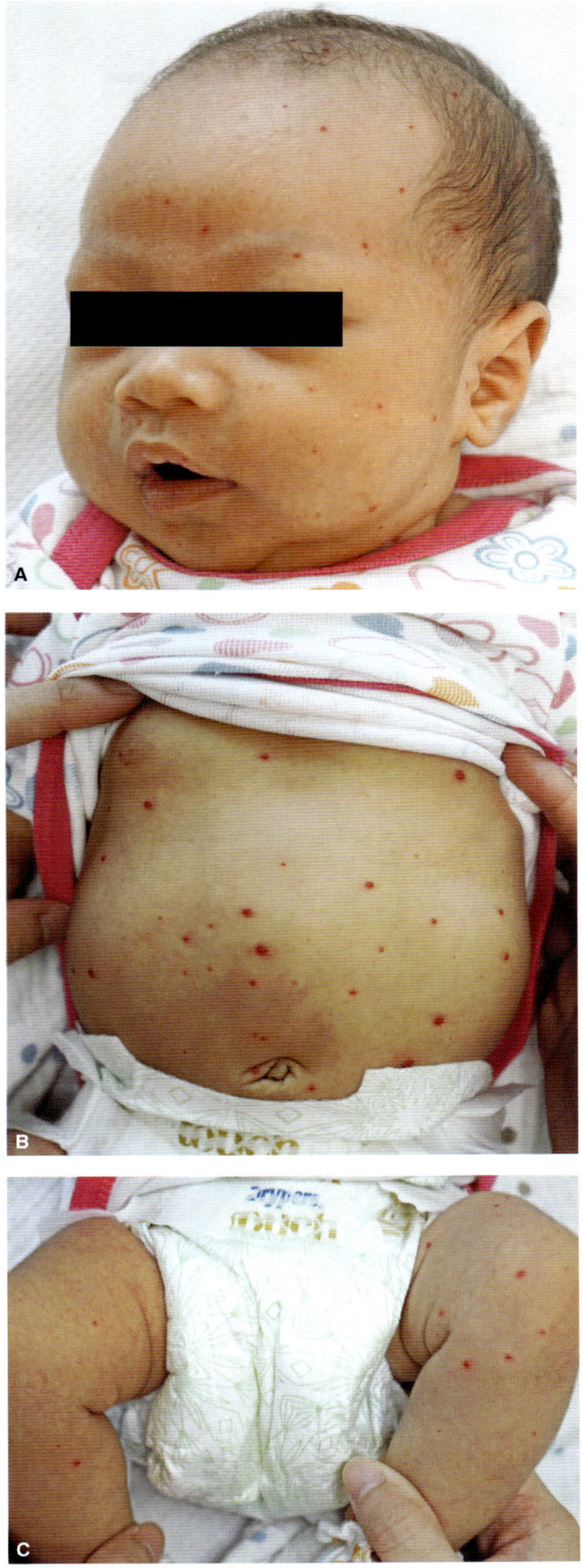

FIGURE 13-21A–21C. Multiple "miliary" IH affecting the face, trunk, and limbs of a 1-month-old Chinese girl. There was concomitant liver IH.

Investigations & Treatment

- Diagnosis of IH is usually made clinically. Pulsatile flow can be demonstrated using a bedside Doppler.
- If biopsied, classical histological findings show lobules of plump endothelial cells that line thin vascular channels with small or inconspicuous lumens. The endothelial cells stain positively for GLUT1 immunohistochemical stain.
- Most isolated, small and nonsegmental IHs do not warrant further investigation.
- If PHACES syndrome is suspected, an eye evaluation, MRI, and MRA of the head and neck, and echocardiogram should be performed.
- Periorbital IH with suspected retro-orbital extension will require MRI of the orbit and a detailed ophthalmological evaluation.
- Segmental IH involving the "beard distribution" will require referral to a pediatric otolaryngologist (ENT) for further evaluation.
- If PELVIS syndrome is suspected, ultrasound or MRI of the kidneys and MRI of the lumbosacral spine should be performed.
- Infants presenting with multiple (more than five) cutaneous IH will require abdominal ultrasound and thyroid function test.
- Most IH do not require treatment. However, IH with complications or with potential to cause complications require urgent evaluation and treatment.
- Treatment options include topical and systemic β-blockers, such as topical timolol and oral propranolol, oral corticosteroids, lasers (such as the pulsed-dye laser or Nd:YAG laser), and surgical excision.

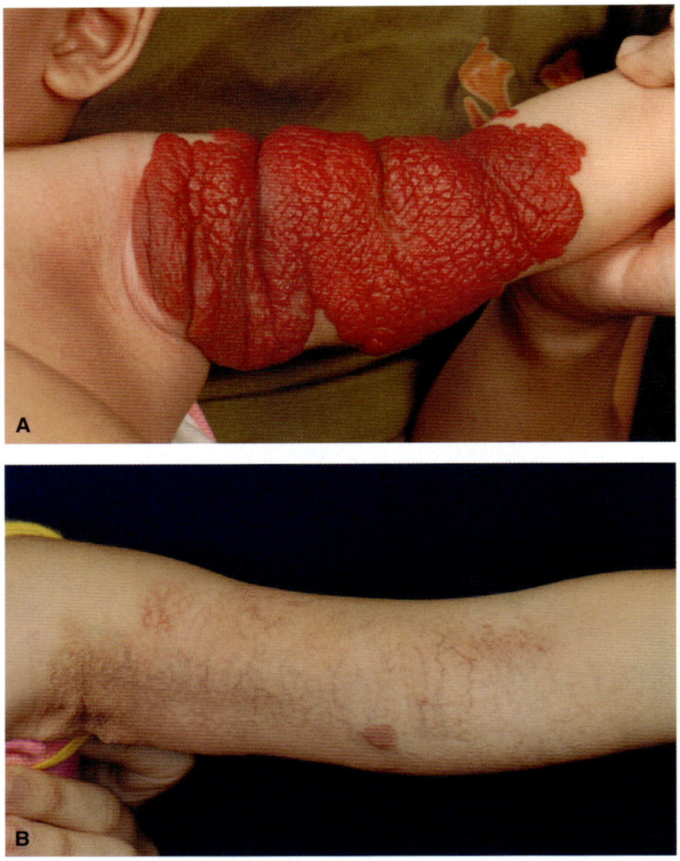

FIGURE 13-22A & 22B. Large, segmental IH on the arm of a 3-month-old Chinese girl who was treated with oral propranolol. Figure 13-22B shows the same child at 3 years of age with residual skin atrophy and telangiectasias.

- The use of β-blockers has revolutionized the treatment of IH in the past decade.
- Flatter lesions will respond well to topical timolol. This should be started early and continued until the child is about 1 year of age. Minimal monitoring is required unless large areas are treated.
- Oral propranolol is useful for larger and more protruding lesions. It works the best if started in the first 6 months of life, but is still useful if started before 1 year of age. It is given as either a twice or three times daily dose of 1.5–3 mg/kg/day. Common side effects include sleep disturbance and cool hands and feet. Rare side effects include hypoglycemia, bradycardia, hypotension, and wheezing. It should be continued until 1 year of age.

Pearls & Practical Tips

- A detailed history on the growth pattern of the lesion is important to differentiate IH from congenital hemangiomas and port wine stains. Early segmental IH can mimic port wine stains. Parents should be told to observe for thickening of the stain within the first few weeks or months of life.
- In premature infants, the growth of IH follows chronological age and not corrected age; that is, it appears after the first few weeks after birth, and not a few weeks after the infant reaches term.
- Besides intertriginous sites, ulceration can also occur in large, protruding IH located on the back and limbs in older infants at about 4 to 6 months of age, usually due to friction as the infant becomes more active.
- IH involving the eye region may have retro-orbital extension and require further evaluation by a pediatric ophthalmologist. These patients may have associated PHACES syndrome.
- The residual skin changes of larger IH can lead to significant psychosocial impairment in patients and their caregivers, especially if located on the face. Early treatment reduces the risk of these residual skin changes.
- Ulcerated IH respond more quickly to treatment with both oral propranolol and a tailing course of oral prednisolone. Other adjunctive treatments include optimal wound care and pulsed-dye laser treatment. Pain control is essential.

BIBLIOGRAPHY

1. Tan JMC, Lim HW, Koh MJA. Oral propranolol for the treatment of infantile haemangiomas in Singapore. Singapore Med J 2021;62(3):139-42.
2. Ng MSY, Tay YK, Ng SSY, Foong AYW, Koh MJA. Comparison of two formulations of topical timolol for the treatment of infantile hemangiomas. Pediatr Dermatol 2017;34:492-3.

CONGENITAL HEMANGIOMA

Congenital hemangiomas are uncommon vascular tumors that are fully formed at birth. Unlike infantile hemangiomas, they do not proliferate after birth. Most involute spontaneously, although the rate of involution varies. A small proportion do not involute.

Clinical Features

- Congenital hemangiomas present at birth as erythematous-to-bluish, soft, compressible nodules or plaques with overlying telangiectasia and a pale halo at the base. Sometimes there may be slightly firmer nodules felt within the hemangioma.
- They are fully formed at birth and generally do not proliferate.
- Three subtypes have been described based on clinical behavior:
  - Rapidly involuting congenital hemangiomas (RICH) tend to involute by 12 to 15 months of age or sometimes a few years, but may leave residual dermal and subcutaneous atrophy.
  - Non-involuting congenital hemangioma (NICH) do not undergo involution.
  - Partially involuting congenital hemangioma (PICH) lie along the spectrum between RICH and NICH.

Differential Diagnoses

- Infantile hemangioma (IH)
  - Unlike congenital hemangiomas that are fully formed at birth, IH are not present at birth and undergo

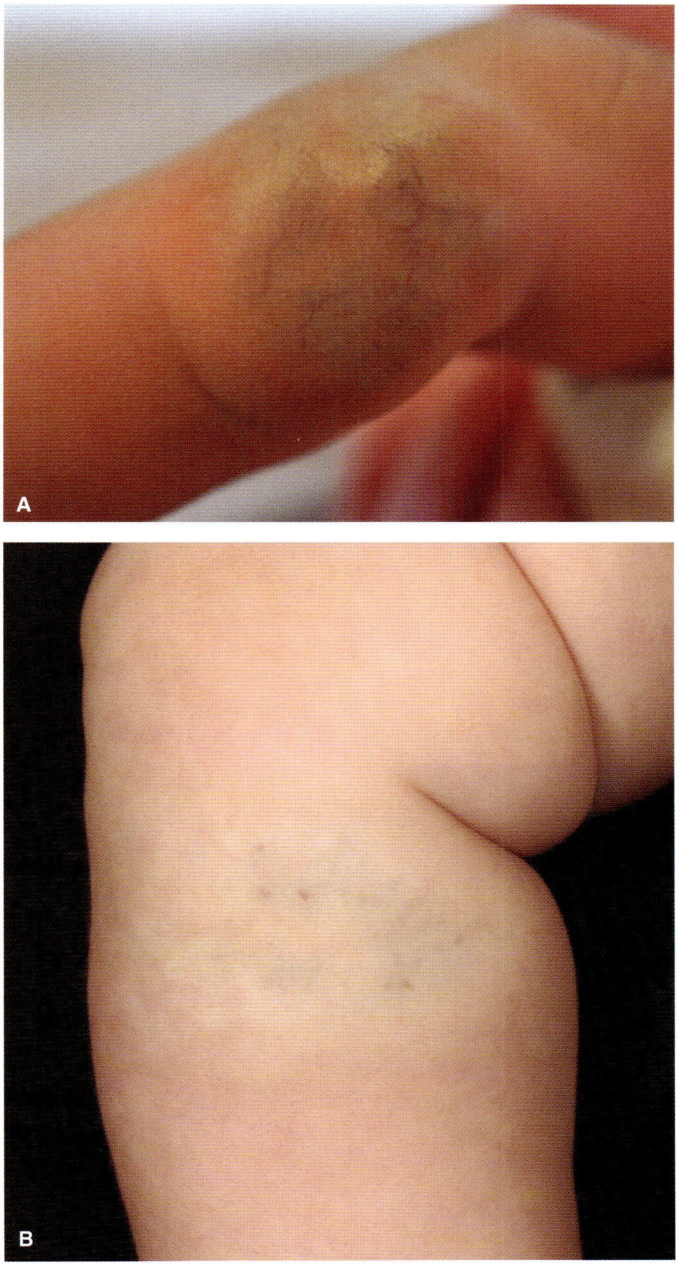

FIGURE 13-23A & 23B. RICH on the leg of a newborn. Note the central telangiectasias and peripheral pallor of the lesion at birth. Figure 13-23B shows the same lesion at 8 months of age.

proliferation over the first year of life, followed by slow involution over years.

- Kaposiform hemangioendothelioma or tufted angioma
  - These may be present from birth but can also proliferate thereafter. Clinically, they are firmer and more indurated than congenital hemangiomas and may be associated with the Kasabach-Merritt phenomenon.
- Malignant tumors, such as fibrosarcoma or rhabdomyosarcoma
  - Unlike congenital hemangiomas, malignant tumors are firmer and may appear more violaceous than

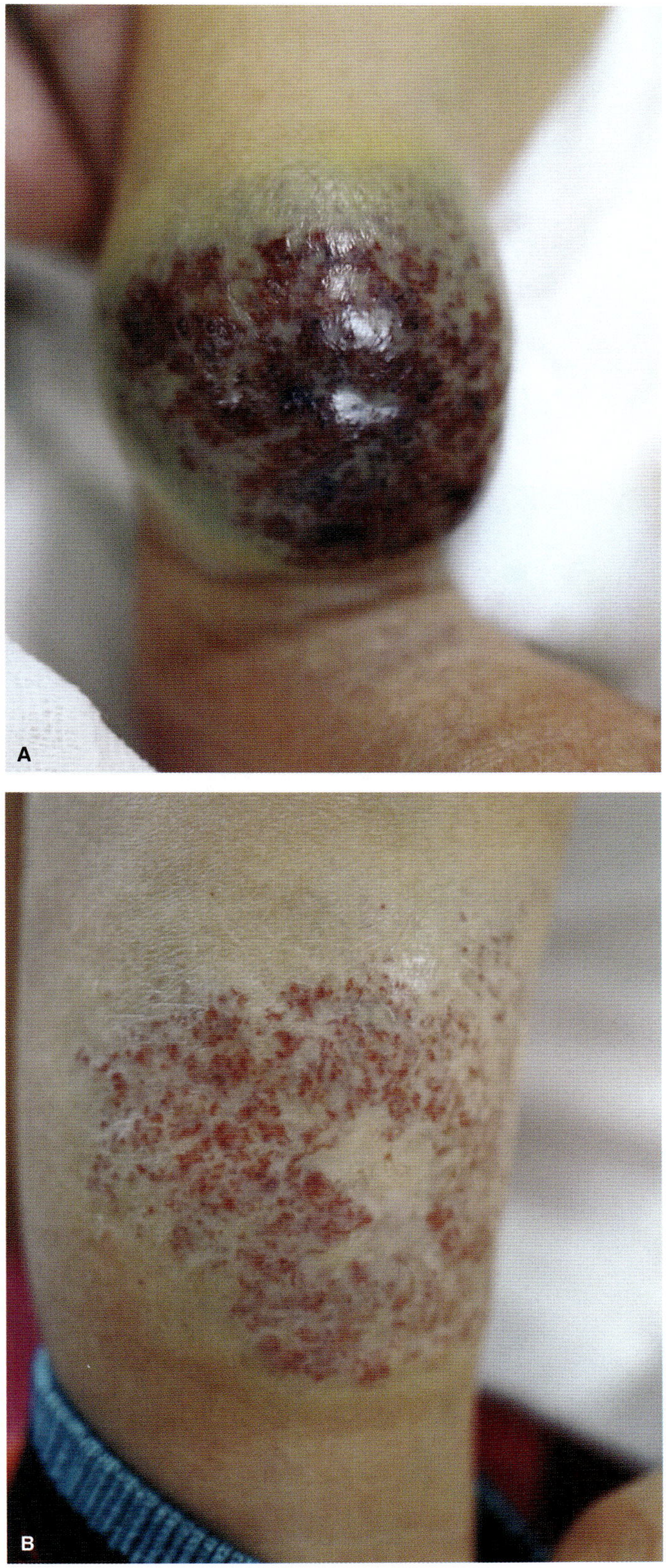

FIGURE 13-24A & 24B. A RICH on the leg of a newborn presenting with a fairly large, protruding but soft nodule. Figure 13-24B shows the same lesion at 18 months of age with gradual involution.

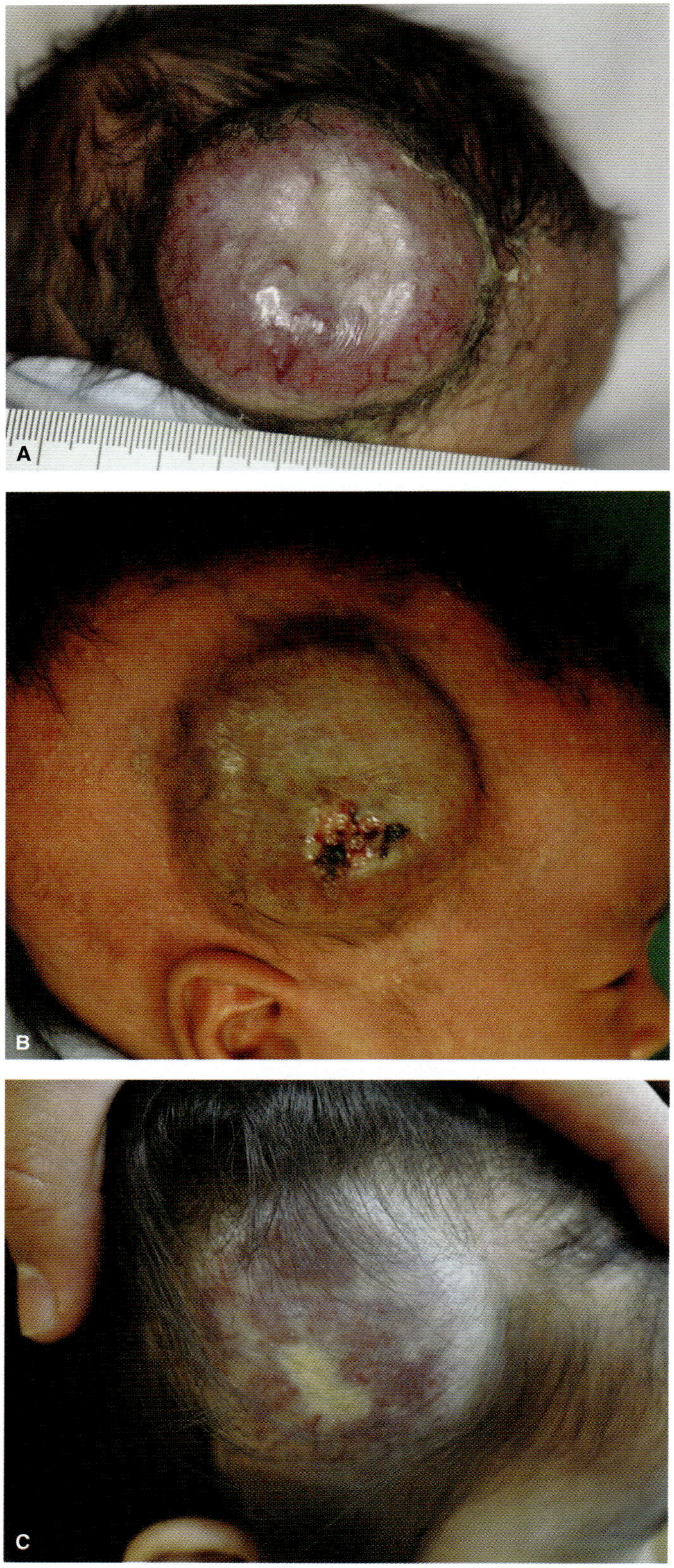

FIGURE 13-25A–25C. Large congenital hemangioma on the right scalp of a newborn Malay boy (Figure 13-25A), complicated by ulceration and bleeding at 3 weeks (Figure 13-25B). Figure 13-25C shows the same lesion at 3 years of age with some regression. These lesions may be classified as a PICH.

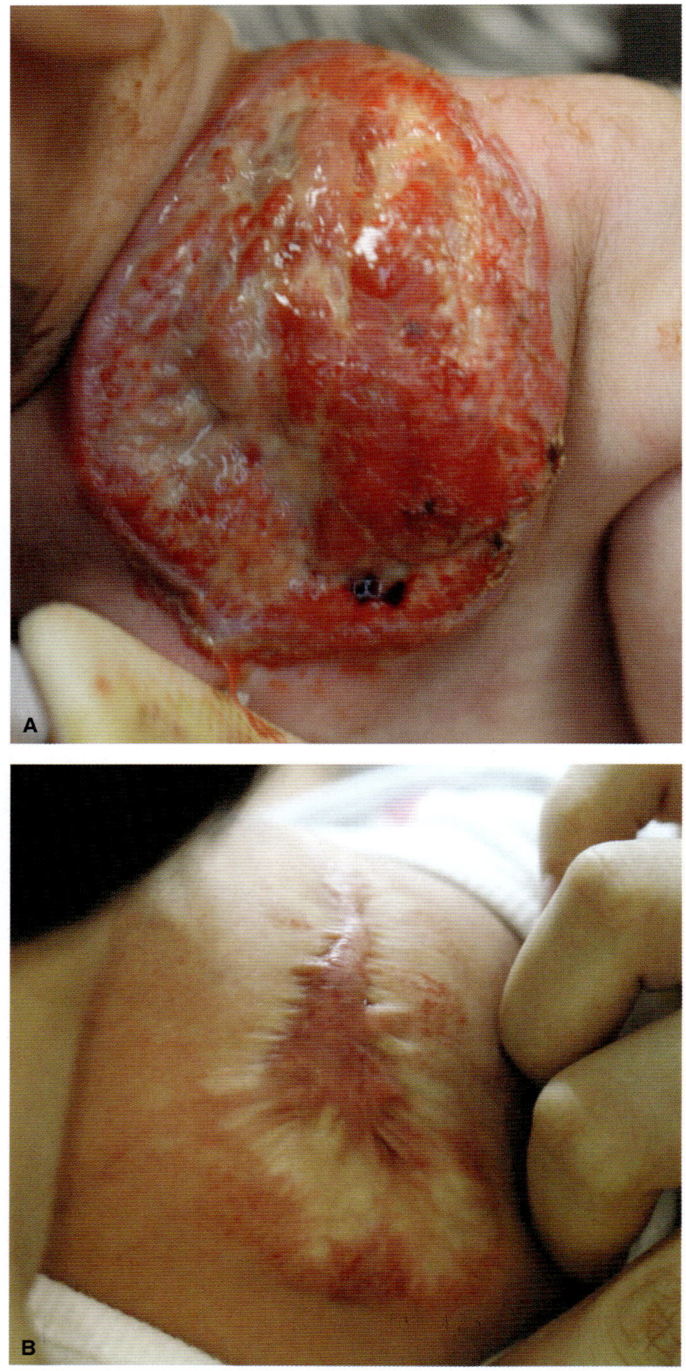

FIGURE 13-26A & 26B. A large congenital hemangioma with severe ulceration that occurred at 3 weeks of age (Figure 13-26A). The ulceration healed slowly, with residual keloid scarring (Figure 13-26B).

congenital hemangiomas. They also continue to proliferate over weeks or months. A biopsy is required to confirm the diagnosis.

Investigations & Treatment

- Diagnosis is usually made clinically based on history and physical examination findings.

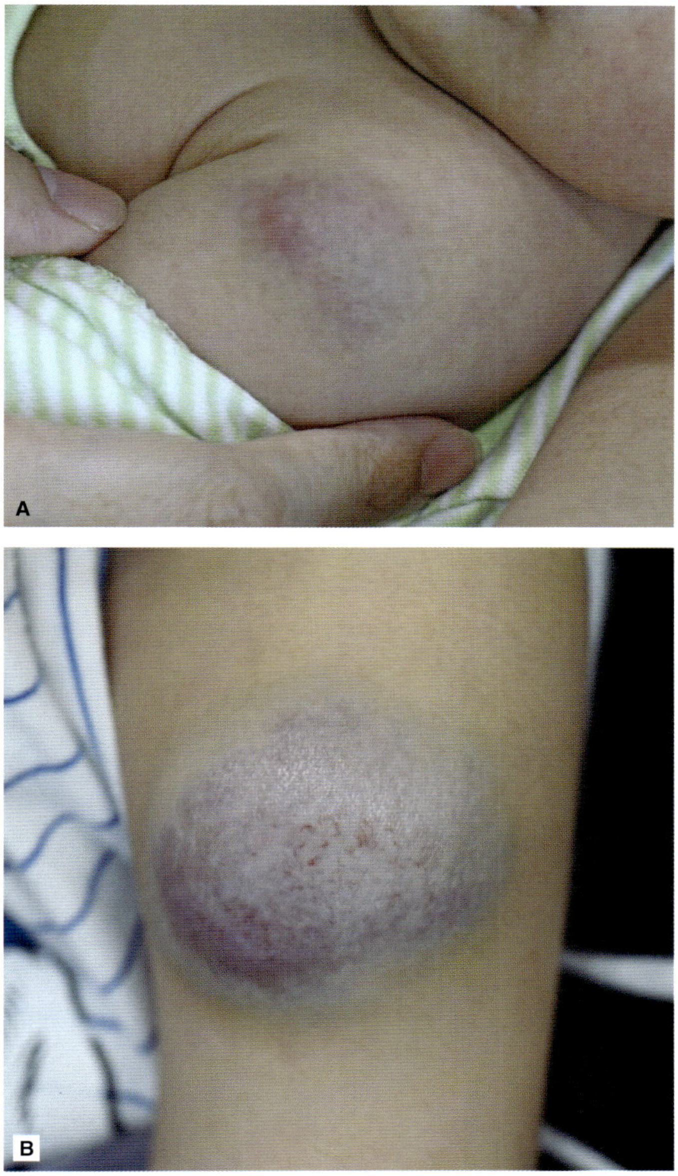

FIGURE 13-27A & 27B. A NICH on the upper arm of a Chinese boy. Figure 13-27A shows the lesion at a few days of life, and Figure 13-27B shows the lesion at 5 years of age with no signs of involution.

- Pulsatile flow can be demonstrated using a bedside Doppler.
- An MRI is usually required prior to planning for surgical excision to delineate the planes of involvement by the congenital hemangioma.
- A skin biopsy may be needed in atypical cases. Classical histological findings are that of packed lobules of capillaries with thrombus formation. The endothelial cells are negative for GLUT1 immunohistochemical stain.
- Depending on the size and site, most congenital hemangiomas can be treated conservatively. If required, surgical excision or interventional embolization may be considered, especially for NICH.

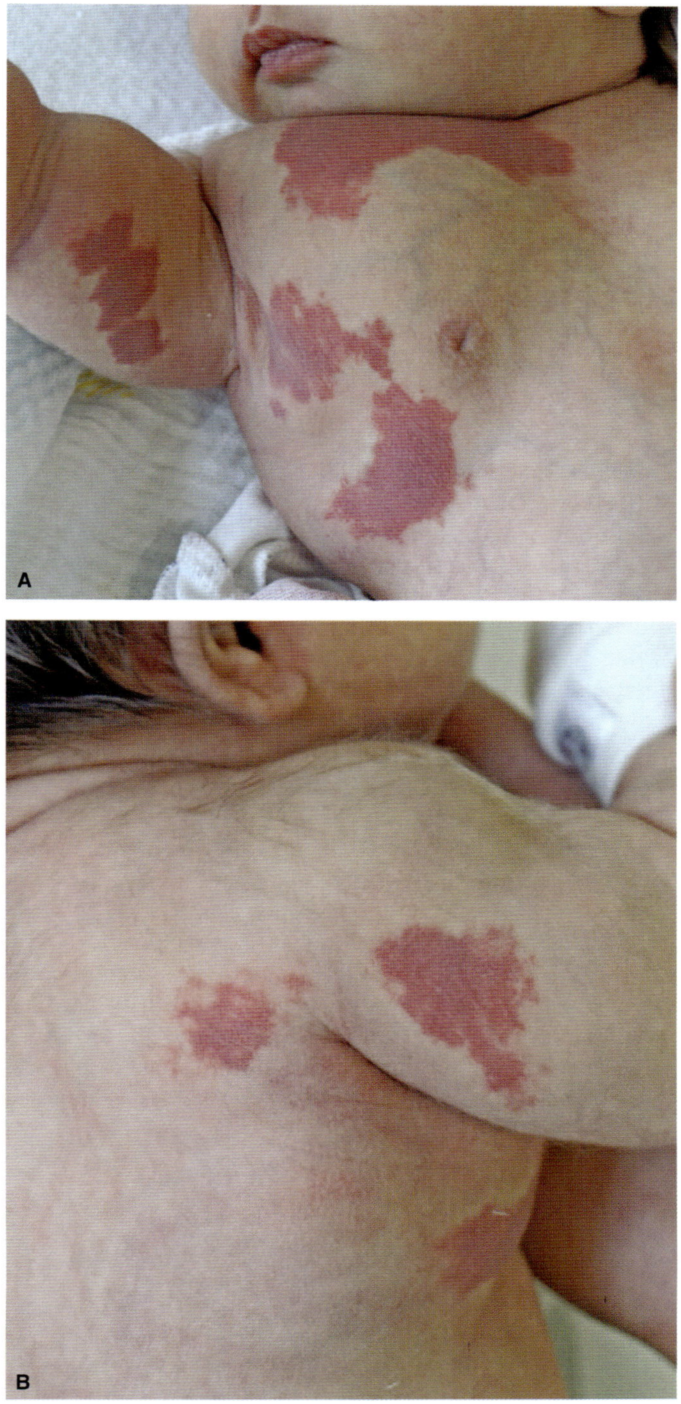

FIGURE 13-28A & 28B. A large congenital hemangioma affecting the right upper back, chest, shoulder, and arm of a Chinese baby, with overlying vascular stain. This presentation is unusual, and diagnosis was confirmed on radiological imaging and biopsy.

Pearls & Practical Tips

- Pulsatile flows can be demonstrated using a Doppler for both congenital hemangiomas and IH. The clinical history and course are used to differentiate the two entities, as well as the clinical appearance.

- Rarely, some congenital hemangiomas may increase in size after birth, although the rate and volume of growth are much less compared to IH.
- Ulceration and bleeding, which can be torrential, can occur in congenital hemangiomas, especially in the first few weeks of life, in lesions that are located over areas with "tighter" skin, such as the scalp. Advice should be provided to caregivers.
- Some lesions of RICH may be complicated by mild thrombocytopenia and hypofibrinogenemia, but not to the level of Kasabach-Merritt phenomenon.
- Congenital hemangiomas do not show good response to treatment with β-blockers.

KAPOSIFORM HEMANGIOENDOTHELIOMA & TUFTED ANGIOMA

Kaposiform hemangioendothelioma (KHE) and tufted angioma (TA) are rare vascular tumors that commonly present in infancy or early childhood. They are now considered on a spectrum, with KHE having more locally aggressive behavior and TA having a more benign course. Both can be associated with the Kasabach-Merritt phenomenon (KMP), a condition characterized by thrombocytopenia, consumptive coagulopathy, and anemia. Both KHE and TA can spontaneously regress over years, although most tend to persist or gradually increase in size.

Clinical Features

- Both KHE and TE present at birth or early infancy, and less commonly in later childhood, or rarely in adolescence or adulthood. Both lesions can present with pain and tenderness, although most are asymptomatic.
- KHE usually presents as a single firm, indurated, erythematous-to-violaceous nodule or plaque with irregular borders. It most commonly affects the extremities but can also occur on the trunk. There is gradual increase in size for most lesions but they can also remain stable for years.

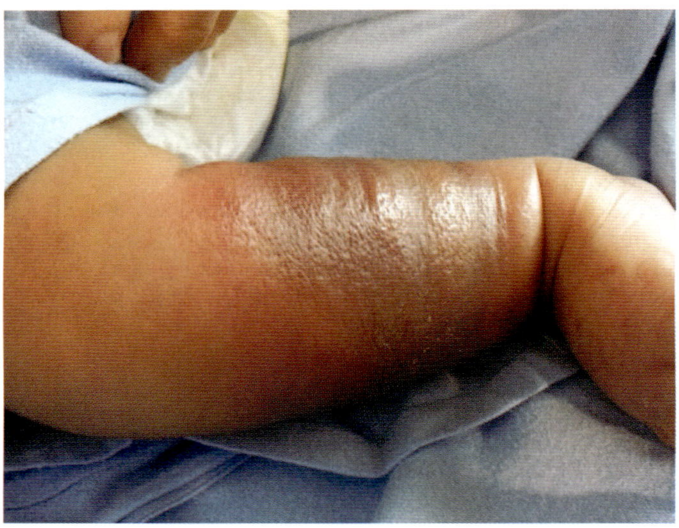

FIGURE 13-29. KHE on the right leg of a Malay infant, presenting as an indurated, bruise-like plaque with overlying puckering of skin. There was concomitant KMP.

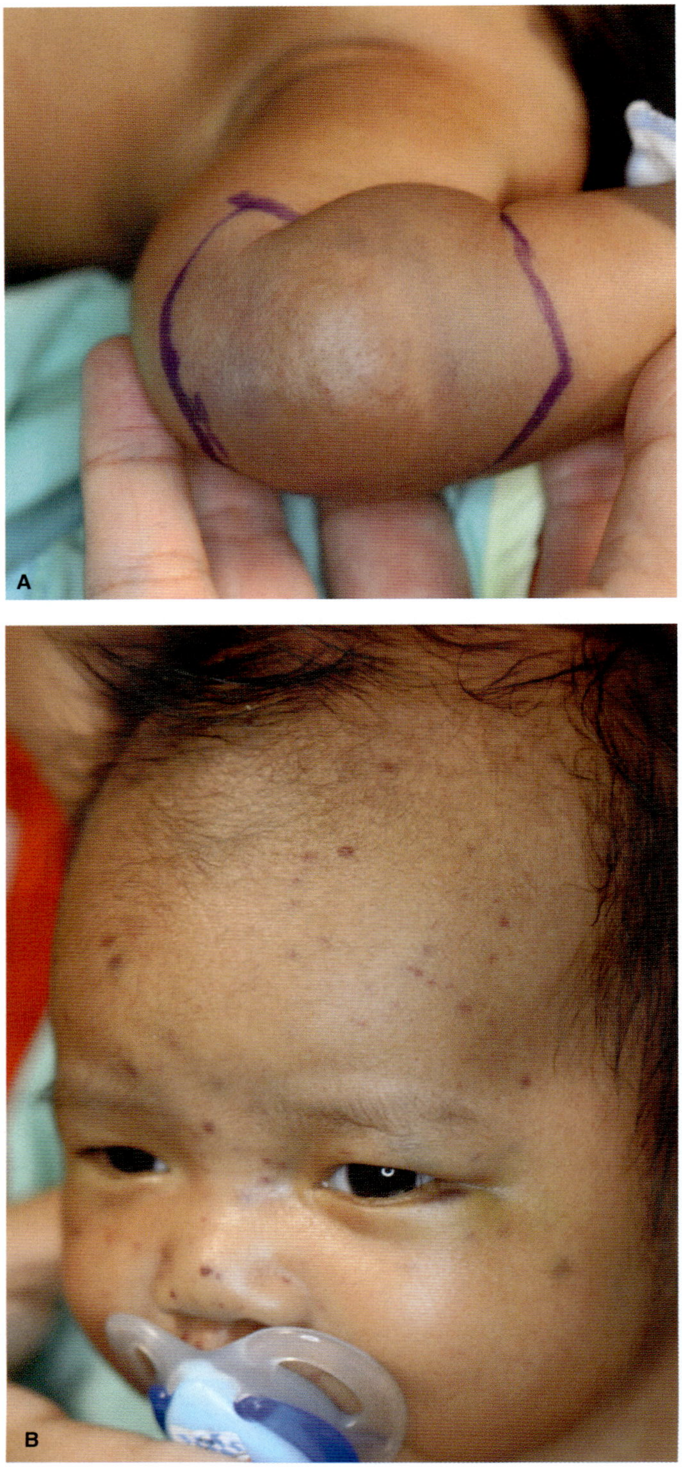

FIGURE 13-30A & 30B. KHE on the arm of a Malay infant, presenting as an indurated, hyperpigmented plaque. He presented with swelling of the lesion associated with multiple petechiae secondary to KMP (Figure 13-30B).

- TA usually presents with erythematous-to-brownish, indurated plaques with ill-defined borders. It is more common over the trunk, neck, and limbs. If present at birth, it may be perceptible as a faint pink or brown discoloration. There can be overlying hyperhidrosis and hypertrichosis.

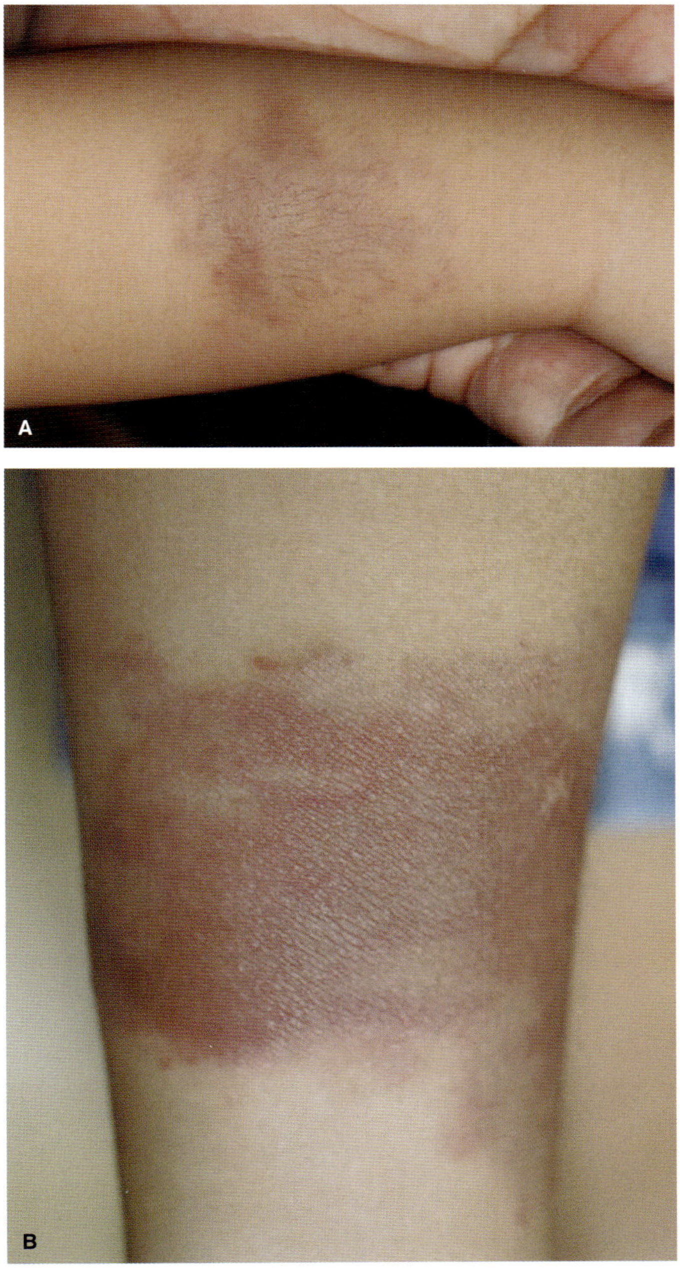

FIGURE 13-31A & 31B. TA on the left forearm of a Chinese boy that presented at 6 months of age with a brown hyperpigmented plaque with overlying hypertrichosis. It gradually progressed to become more confluent and violaceous, as shown in Figure 13-31B, when the child was 4 years of age.

- Both KHE and TA can be associated with KMP, although this is more common in KHE. It usually occurs in the first few weeks or months of life, presenting as induration and rapid expansion of the existing lesion, with purpura, swelling, and tenderness. There can be associated signs of bleeding, such as hematochezia.
- Other complications of KHE include compression of surrounding tissues and musculoskeletal issues.
- Both KHE and TA can rarely regress spontaneously, although this is more common for lesions of TA.

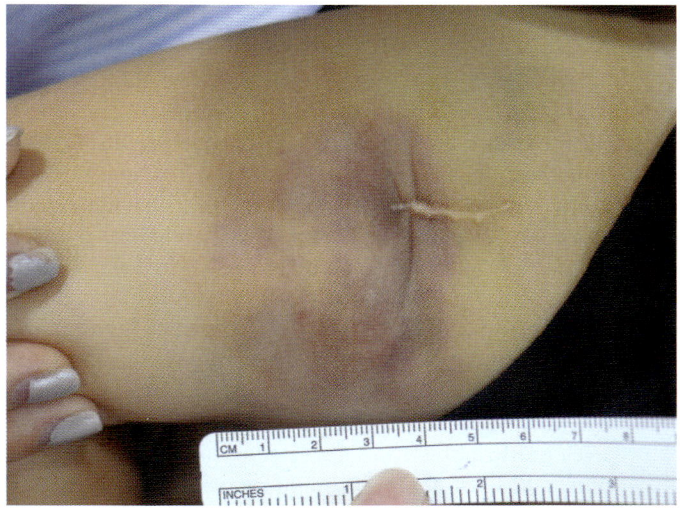

FIGURE 13-32. TA on the right thigh of a Chinese boy with a scar after a previous resection. On palpation, the lesion feels indurated.

Differential Diagnoses

- Congenital hemangioma
  - Congenital hemangiomas have more well-defined borders, often with a pale halo around the lesion. They do not increase in size or thickness after birth.
  - Although some rapidly involuting congenital hemangiomas may have mild thrombocytopenia and hypofibrinogenemia, they do not fulfil the criteria of KMP.
- Malignant tumors, such as fibrosarcoma or rhabdomyosarcoma
  - These are even more rare than KHE and TA in childhood, and are less likely to be associated with KMP. If in doubt, a biopsy is required to confirm the diagnosis.

Investigations & Treatment

- Although they can be diagnosed clinically, especially if associated with KMP, radiological imaging such as

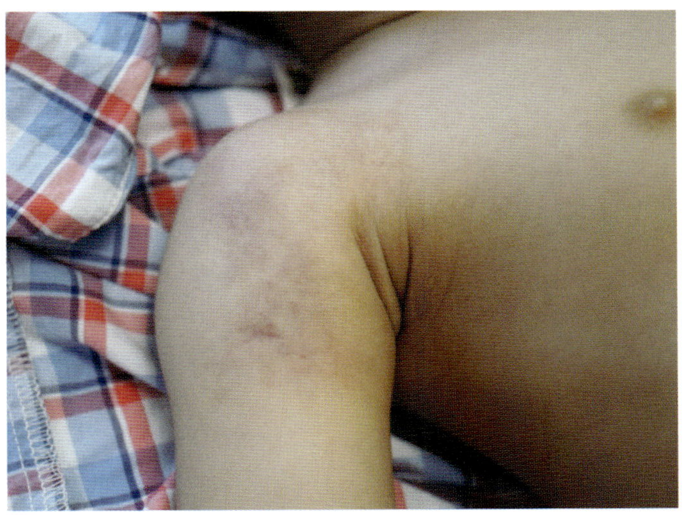

FIGURE 13-33. TA on the right shoulder of a Chinese boy presenting with a diffuse, faint vascular stain with mild induration.

ultrasound and MRI can aid in diagnosis. These also help to delineate the extent of the tumor and monitor response to treatment.

- Skin biopsies can be performed to confirm diagnosis and exclude other conditions. There is considerable overlap in the histological features of KHE and TA, with nodular proliferations of endothelial cells with slit-like lumen and cytoplasmic vacuoles in lesions of KHE, and tufts of capillaries in a "cannonball" or lobular pattern in lesions of TA. There is no significant nuclear atypia or mitotic activity. Often, features of both KHE and TA may be found in the same specimen or in separate specimens from the same lesion.
- If KMP is suspected, complete blood count, fibrinogen level, prothrombin time, activated partial thromboplastin time, and D-dimer level should be performed. This may be repeated to monitor for response to treatment.
- Consideration for treatment depends on severity of symptoms, size and site of lesion, and complications such as the KMP and the degree of functional impairment.
- Treatment options include active non-intervention with regular surveillance, oral corticosteroids, oral mTOR inhibitors (e.g,. sirolimus or everolimus), surgical excision, or vincristine. Arterial embolization may also be considered in symptomatic patients if a feeding vessel can be identified.

Pearls & Practical Tips

- Large KHEs have the highest risk of KMP, especially if located in the retroperitoneum or mediastinum.
- Regression may be more common in congenital or early-onset TA.

PYOGENIC GRANULOMA

Pyogenic granuloma (PG), also known as lobular capillary hemangioma, is a benign, acquired vascular tumor, characterized by proliferation of capillaries of the skin and oral cavity.

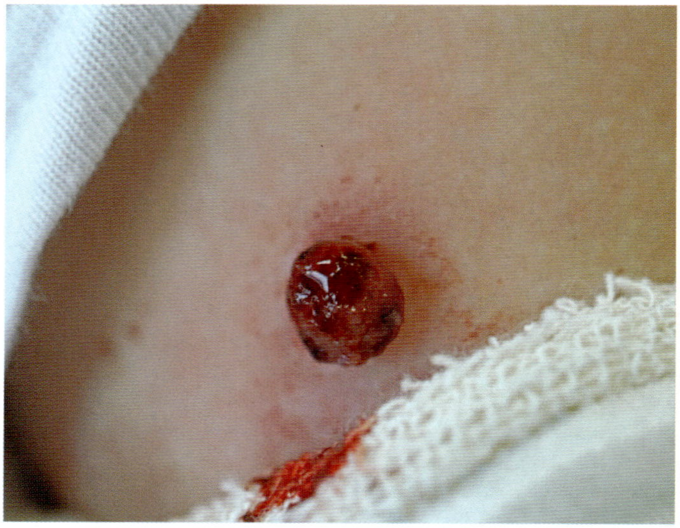

FIGURE 13-34. Bleeding PG on the lower back of a Chinese child.

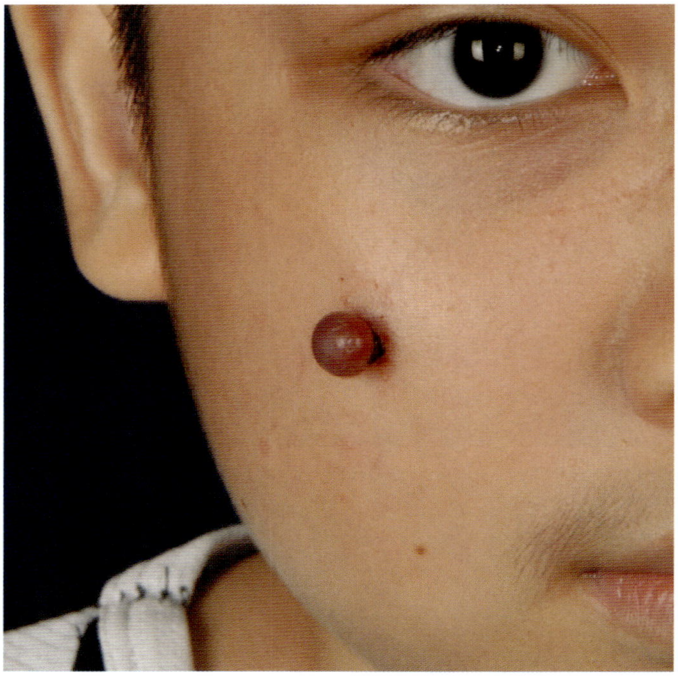

FIGURE 13-35. Pedunculated PG on the right cheek of a Malay boy.

They occur more commonly over areas prone to trauma, such as the face or upper limbs. Superficial ulceration and recurrent bleeding can occur as a complication.

Clinical Features

- PGs can present at any age but are not congenital. They rarely involute spontaneously.
- They present as discrete, erythematous-to-violaceous papules that grow rapidly over weeks, before stabilizing in size.

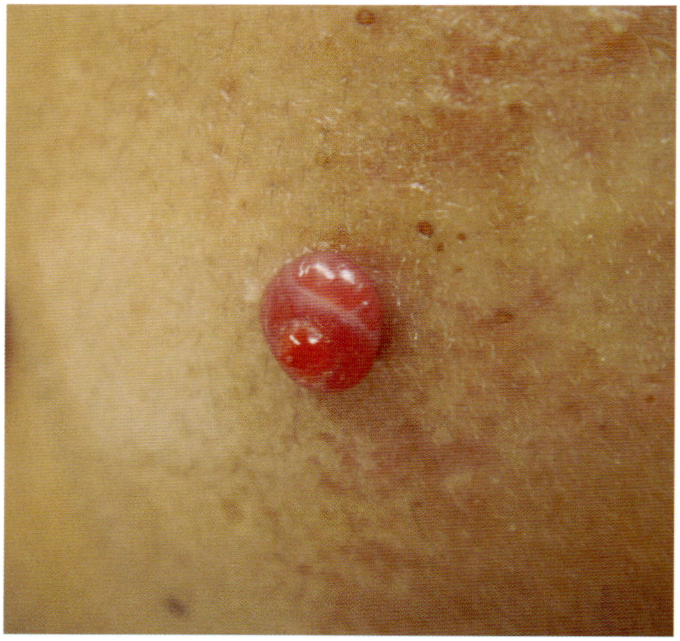

FIGURE 13-36. PG on the cheek of a teenage Chinese male, with surface erosion and bleeding.

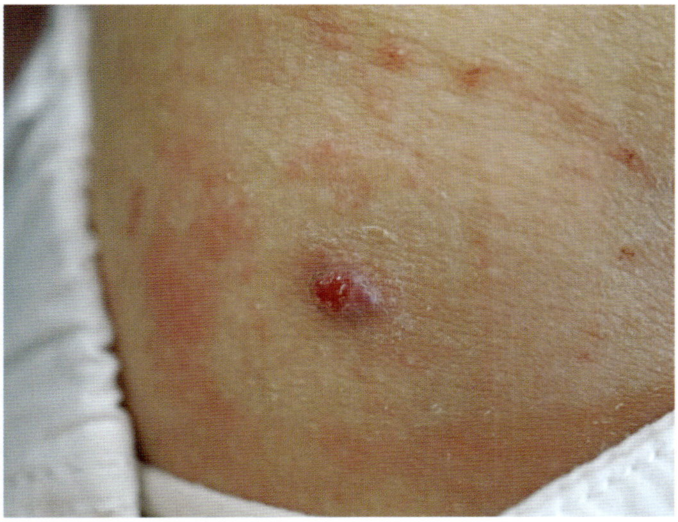

FIGURE 13-37. A more sessile, slightly keratotic PG with surface erosion. There is surrounding contact dermatitis.

- There may be superficial erosions or recurrent contact bleeding.
- They most commonly occur on the face, hands, fingers, and forearms.

Differential Diagnoses

- Spitz nevus
  - Spitz nevi can also present as dome-shaped, pink-red papules on the face or lower extremities. Bleeding is less common compared to PG.
- Viral wart
  - Viral warts, especially over the face, can also present with contact bleeding but have a more verrucous surface compared to PG.

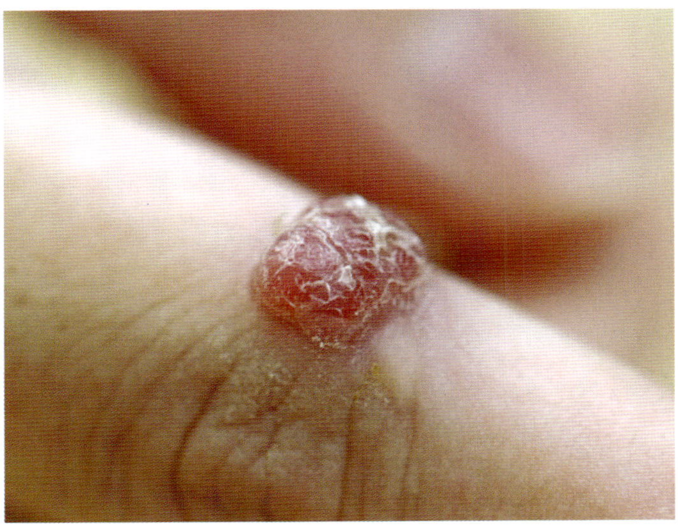

FIGURE 13-38. Keratotic PG on the finger of a Chinese adolescent female.

- Juvenile xanthogranuloma (JXG)
  - JXG are also commonly seen on the face and arms, commonly with a violaceous color. Bleeding and surface erosion is seen less frequently compared to PG.

Investigations & Treatment

- Diagnosis is usually made clinically.
- Typical histological features include a lobular proliferation of capillaries and endothelial cells set in a loose, myxoid stroma with surrounding inflammatory cells.
- Treatment options include shave excision and electrocautery, cryotherapy, and silver nitrate cauterization.
- In younger children, medical treatment options include imiquimod cream or topical timolol, although these need to be applied for weeks or months and may not lead to involution.
- There have been increasing number of reports of successful treatment of PG with table salt daily for 1 to 3 weeks.

Pearls & Practical Tips

- PG should be treated, as they risk ulceration and recurrent bleeding and rarely involute spontaneously.
- There is a relatively high risk of recurrence. This is reduced with complete excision and cauterization of the feeding blood vessel at the base.

CAPILLARY MALFORMATION

Capillary malformations (CM), also commonly known as port wine stains (PWS), are slow-flow vascular malformations. They are fairly common, and occur in about 0.3% of newborns. Although the majority are isolated lesions, extensive lesions can be associated with various malformation syndromes, such as Sturge-Weber syndrome and Klippel-Trenaunay syndrome.

Clinical Features

- CM present at birth or shortly after birth as sharply demarcated, homogeneous, erythematous macules or patches.
- They are usually unilateral and are most commonly located on the face and neck but can also affect the trunk and upper and lower limbs.
- They persist throughout life, growing in proportion to the growth of the child.
- Some CM can darken with age to become more purplish with a cyanotic hue, and develop an irregular, thickened, nodular surface ("cobblestone effect"). This usually occurs in late adolescence or adulthood. Pyogenic granuloma-like nodules can also develop, which can bleed with minor trauma.
- Segmental PWS affecting the forehead and upper eyelids can be associated with Sturge-Weber syndrome, while Klippel-Trenaunay syndrome is associated with PWS on the limbs.
- Nevus simplex, also known as salmon patch, stork-bite, or nevus flammeus, are common forms of capillary malformations that occur as light pink stains on the glabella,

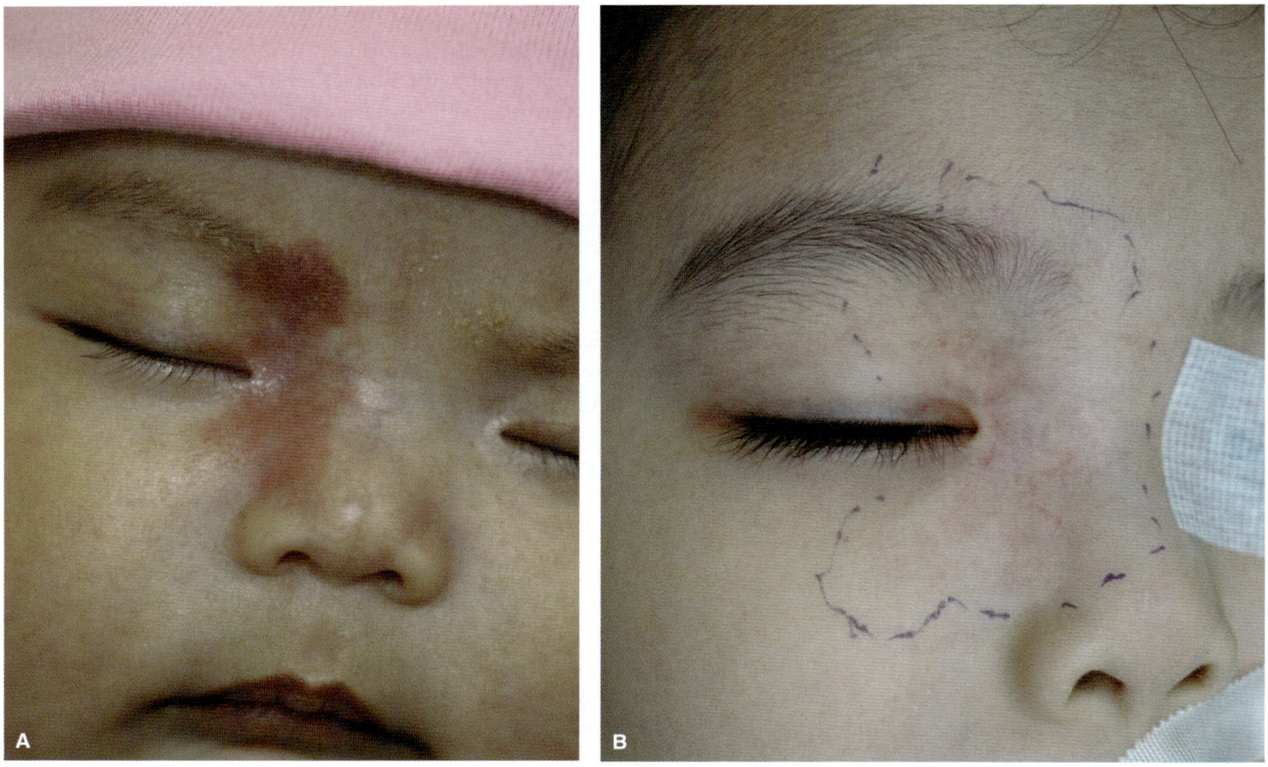

FIGURE 13-39A & 39B. PWS on the right inner canthus and nasal bridge of a Chinese newborn. Figure 13-39B shows the same lesion after multiple treatments of pulsed-dye laser over 3 years.

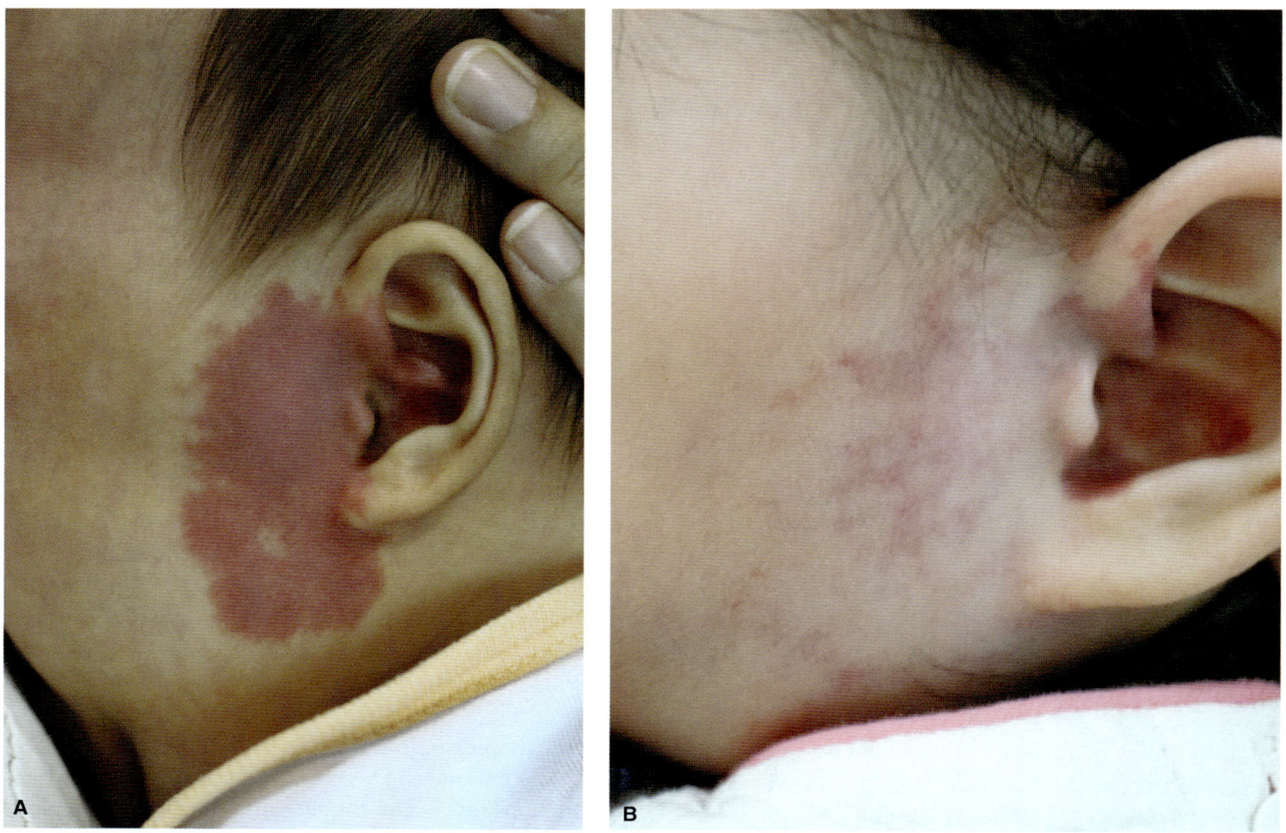

FIGURE 13-40A & 40B. Dark PWS on the left parotid region of a Chinese infant. Figure 13-40B shows the same child at 3 years of age after multiple treatments with the pulsed-dye laser.

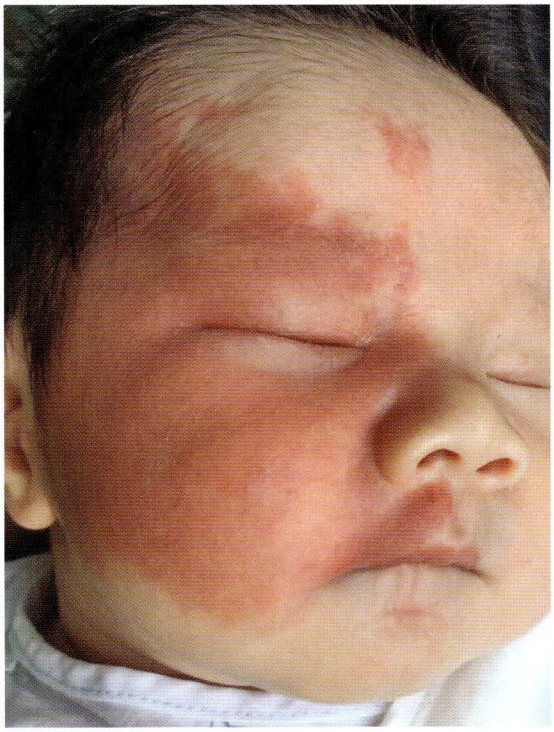

FIGURE 13-41. Large PWS on the right side of the face of a Chinese male infant.

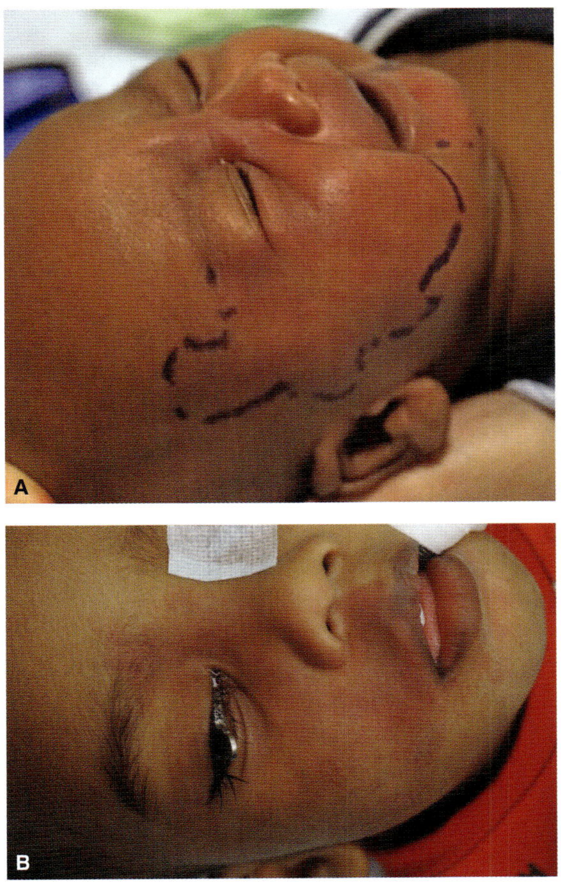

FIGURE 13-42A & 42B. Large PWS on the right face of an Indian male infant. Figure 13-42B shows the same child at 3 years of age after treatment with pulsed-dye laser.

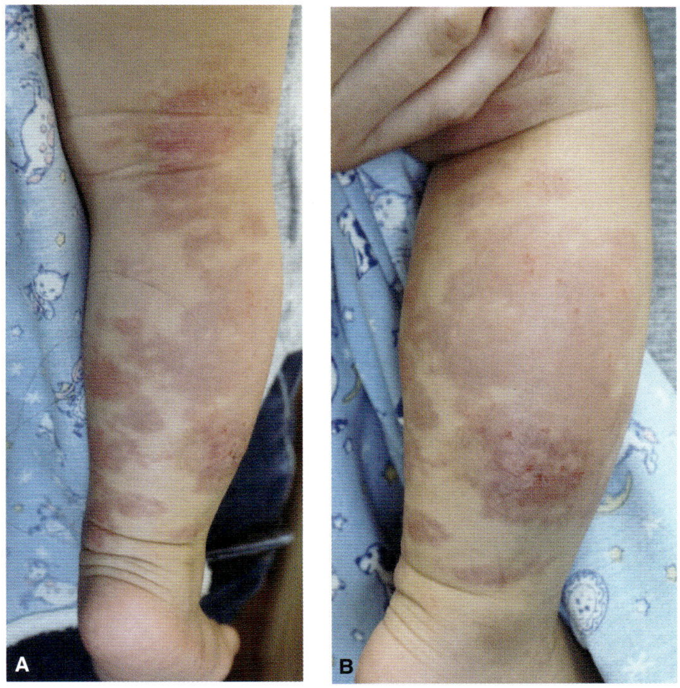

FIGURE 13-43A & 43B. Patchy PWS on the right leg of a Chinese infant with atopic dermatitis. Lesions of AD may frequently be seen over PWS.

eyelids, or central occipital/posterior neck region. These lesions may become more obvious when the child cries or strains, and in warmer weather. Lesions on the face tend to fade over a few years, while lesions on the occipital and neck region do not fade.

Differential Diagnoses

- Early infantile hemangioma (IH)
  - IH may present as a light pink stain at birth, which may be confused with a PWS. Unlike PWS, which remain flat, IH lesions will proliferate over the next few weeks and months to increase in color and depth.
- Capillary malformation-arteriovenous malformation (CM-AVM) syndrome
  - The CM lesions of CM-AVM progressively increase in number and size over time. A pulsatile flow may be demonstrated using a bedside Doppler.

Investigations & Treatment

- Most CM do not require further investigation.
- If Sturge-Weber syndrome is suspected, a detailed eye examination and imaging of the brain should be performed. If Klippel-Trenaunay syndrome is suspected, imaging of the affected limbs should be performed.
- CM can be treated with lasers and light devices that target vascular lesions. These include the pulsed-dye laser (PDL), the long-pulsed Nd:YAG laser, alexandrite laser, and intense pulsed light (IPL). Treatment requires multiple sessions and can be painful.
- Camouflage makeup may be recommended for the older child or adolescent if required for cosmetic concealment.

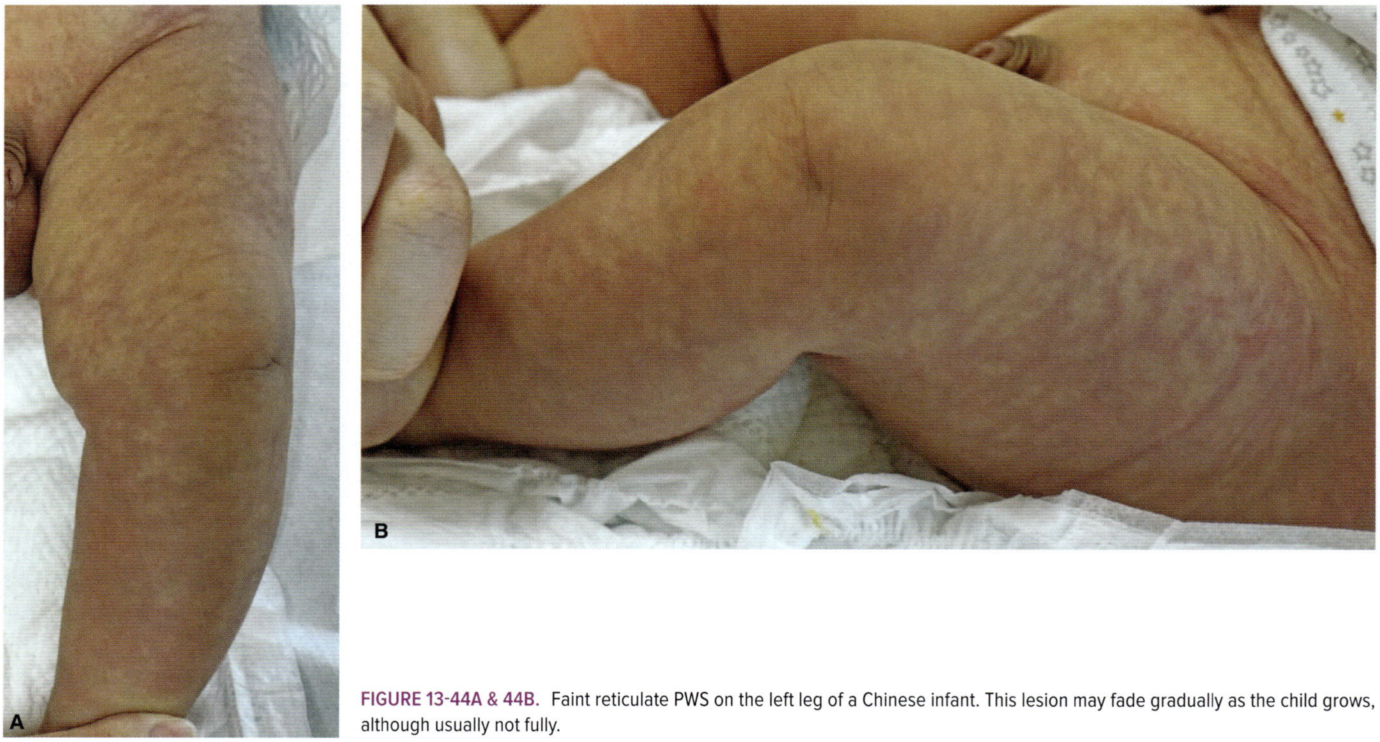

FIGURE 13-44A & 44B. Faint reticulate PWS on the left leg of a Chinese infant. This lesion may fade gradually as the child grows, although usually not fully.

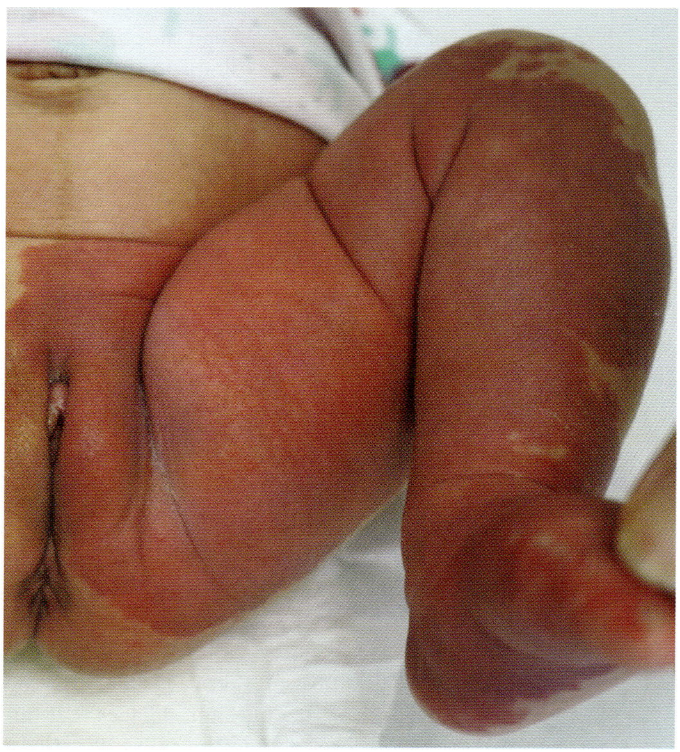

FIGURE 13-45. Extensive PWS on the left lower limb and genitalia of a Chinese infant. These lesions generally do not respond as well to pulsed-dye laser therapy.

Pearls & Practical Tips

- CM often lighten in the first 6 months due to the drop in hemoglobin levels in early infancy.
- Early laser treatment is now recommended, as results may be better when the stains are lighter. Use of general anesthesia may be avoided in younger infants where swaddling and holding the baby is sufficiently calming.
- Intra-ocular metal eye shields should be used if lasers are performed near the eyes.
- Early laser treatment may help to reduce the "cobblestone" effect later in life.

CUTIS MARMORATA TELANGIECTATICA CONGENITA

Cutis marmorata telangiectatica congenita (CMTC) are rare capillary malformations characterized by persistent reticulated marbled erythema, sometimes associated with skin atrophy or ulceration. They are usually isolated findings but can be associated with underlying involvement of other organs.

Clinical Features

- CMTC presents at birth or in the neonatal period.
- CMTC is characterized by bluish to deep purple vascular stains with reticulate or marbling patterns. It becomes more pronounced in lower temperatures and when the child is crying.
- The lesions are most often unilateral, localized, and limited, but segmental or generalized involvement can occur. The most common sites of involvement are the trunk and lower extremities.

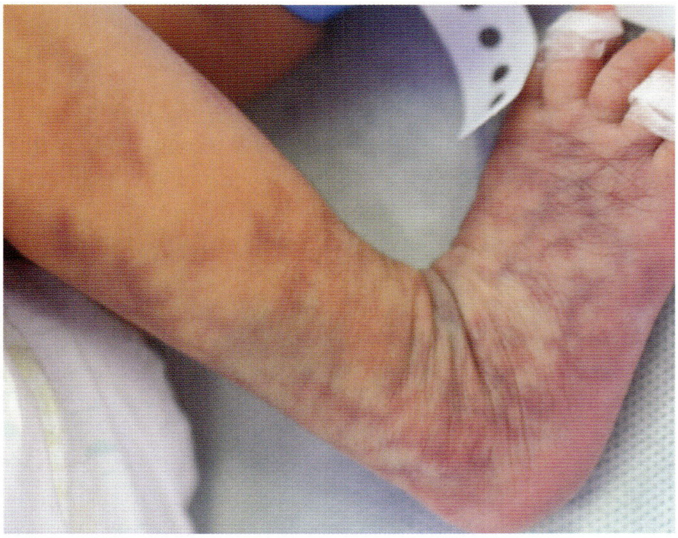

FIGURE 13-46. CMTC affecting the right lower leg of a Malay newborn, presenting with reticulate, violaceous patches.

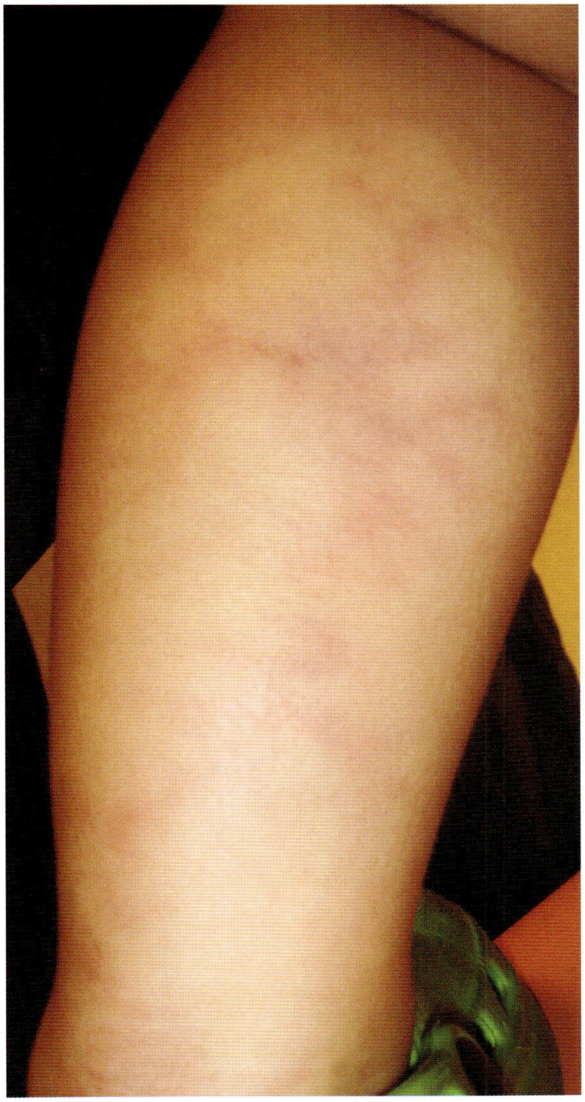

FIGURE 13-47. CMTC affecting the calf of a Chinese infant.

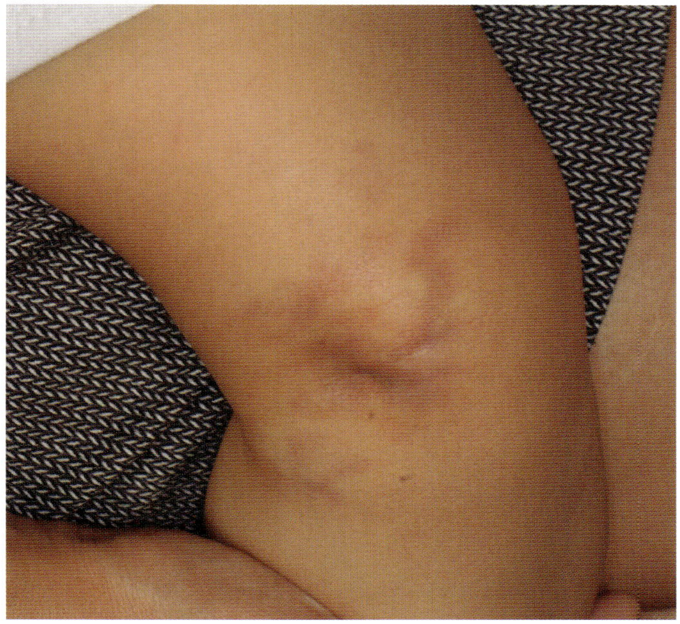

FIGURE 13-48. CMTC affecting the knee of a Chinese infant.

- The affected skin may be atrophic and can ulcerate.
- There may be associated hypotrophy or hypertrophy of the affected limb. If occurring over the face, there may be associated neurological or ophthalmological abnormalities.
- The lesions usually fade within a few years, although they usually do not disappear completely.

Differential Diagnoses

- Physiological cutis marmorata
  - Physiological cutis marmorata also presents with a reticulate pattern over the trunk and extremities. However, it occurs bilaterally and disappears when the ambient temperature is warmer.
- Klippel-Trenaunay syndrome (KTS)
  - Patients with KTS have a combination of port wine stains, venous and/or lymphatic malformations, and soft-tissue hypertrophy.
- Neonatal lupus erythematosus
  - Neonatal lupus erythematosus that occurs during fetal life can result in extensive livedo, telangiectasias, and atrophic scarring resembling CMTC. Lupus antibodies will be present in mother and child.

Investigations & Treatment

- The diagnosis of CMTC is made clinically. Imaging studies are indicated when an associated congenital anomaly is suspected.
- Evaluation by an ophthalmologist, neurologist, and orthopedic surgeon may be necessary if there is a possibility of involvement of the eye, brain, bones, or joints.
- Limb girth and limb length measurements should be monitored regularly.
- Treatment for most cases of CMTC is expectant, as there is spontaneous improvement over a few years.

- Ulcer management should be instituted if present, including regular dressings and treatment of secondary infection and pain.

Pearls & Practical Tips

- The persistence of skin mottling even after warming is a diagnostic pearl of CMTC.
- Unlike port wine stains, CMTC responds poorly to treatment with pulsed dye lasers and may have a higher risk of scarring.

BIBLIOGRAPHY

1. Haidari W, Light JG, Castellanos B, Jorizzo JL. Cutis marmorata telangiectasia congenita with painful ulcerations. Dermatol Online J 2020;26(6):13030.
2. Bui TNPT, Corap A, Bygum A. Cutis marmorata telangiectatica congenita: a literature review. Orphanet J Rare Dis 2019;14(1):283.

VENOUS MALFORMATION

Venous malformations (VM) are fairly common slow-flow vascular malformations that often present at birth or early childhood. Large lesions can be associated with pain and discomfort. Most VM are isolated lesions but may also be found in malformation syndromes such as PIK3CA-related overgrowth syndromes (PROS). Somatic mutations in the PI3K-AKT-mTOR pathways have been associated with VM.

Clinical Features

- VM commonly present at birth, during infancy, or in early childhood. Rare lesions can present later in life. They grow proportionately with the child but can increase more significantly during puberty.
- VM present as bluish, soft, compressible, warm nodules or plaques that can be well defined or diffuse and infiltrative. There may be an erythematous or purplish stain.
- Phleboliths can form as a result of venous stasis and inflammation and can cause pain, which can be significant. They are felt as rubbery-to-firm pellets or nodules within the VM.
- Complications include rapid enlargement and pain after trauma, venous thrombosis, chronic pain from phleboliths, overlying skin changes, and limb overgrowth resulting in functional impairment.

Differential Diagnoses

- Deep infantile hemangioma (IH)
  - VM can be confused with deep IH. The latter will proliferate in the first few months of life, and a pulsatile flow can be demonstrated on bedside Doppler, which is not heard over VM.

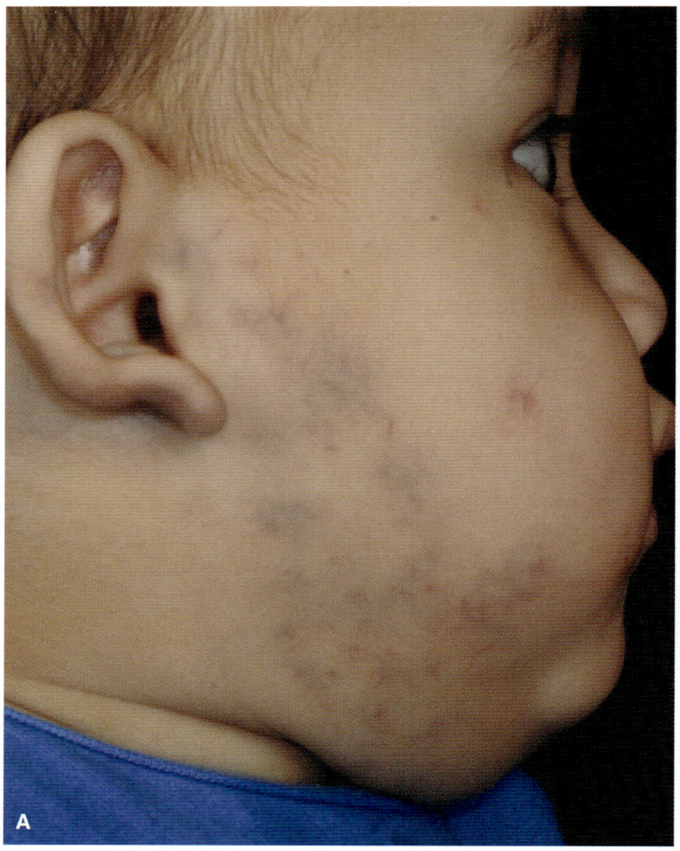

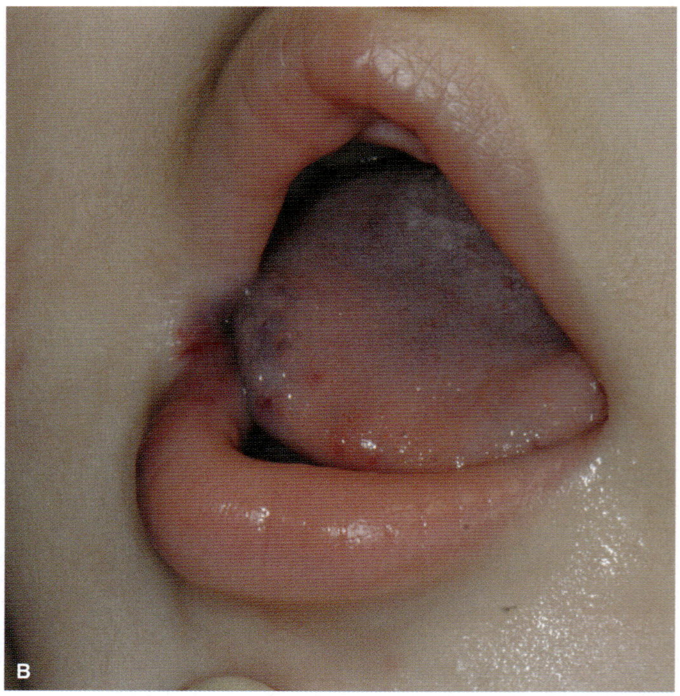

FIGURE 13-49A & 49B. Venous malformation affecting the right cheek, jaw, and neck of a Malay infant, extending onto the lip, tongue, and buccal mucosa

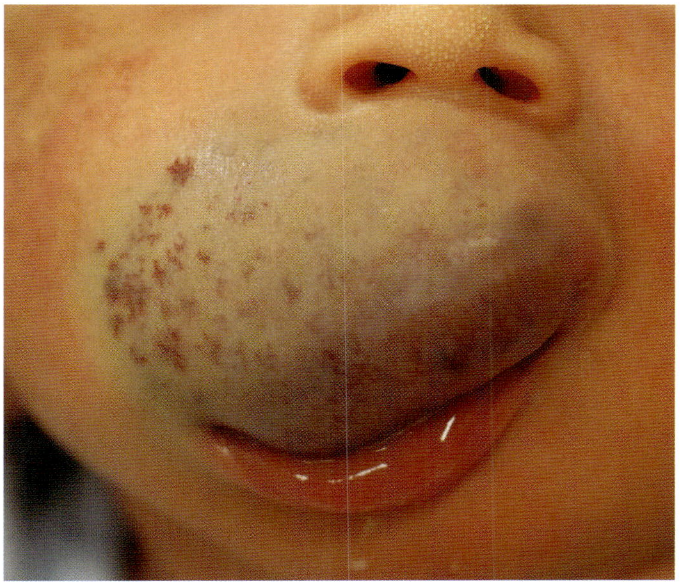

FIGURE 13-50. Large venous malformation affecting the upper lip of a newborn.

- Congenital hemangioma
  - Congenital hemangiomas often have more overlying skin changes, including telangiectasias, and often have a ring of pallor at the base. A pulsatile flow can also be demonstrated on bedside Doppler.
- Kaposiform hemangioendothelioma (KHE)
  - Clinically, KHE are firmer and more indurated and may be associated Kasabach-Merritt phenomenon.
- Lymphatic malformation (LM)
  - LM can appear similar to VM and they often occur together. VM are usually warmer than the surrounding skin, and may contain phleboliths. LM are the same temperature as the surrounding skin and do not contain phleboliths.

Investigations & Treatment

- The diagnosis is often made on history and clinical examination, although radiological investigations are useful to confirm the diagnosis.
- Ultrasound typically shows dilated venous channels, which are compressible, often with presence of phleboliths.
- MRI and MRA are able to show the extent of the lesion, especially if planning for treatment.
- Most small cutaneous VM are asymptomatic and do not usually require treatment.
- Symptomatic and larger VM can be treated with oral mTOR inhibitors (e.g., sirolimus and everolimus), sclerotherapy, and surgical excision.
- Serial compression of VM of the extremities may help to relieve swelling and alleviate symptoms.

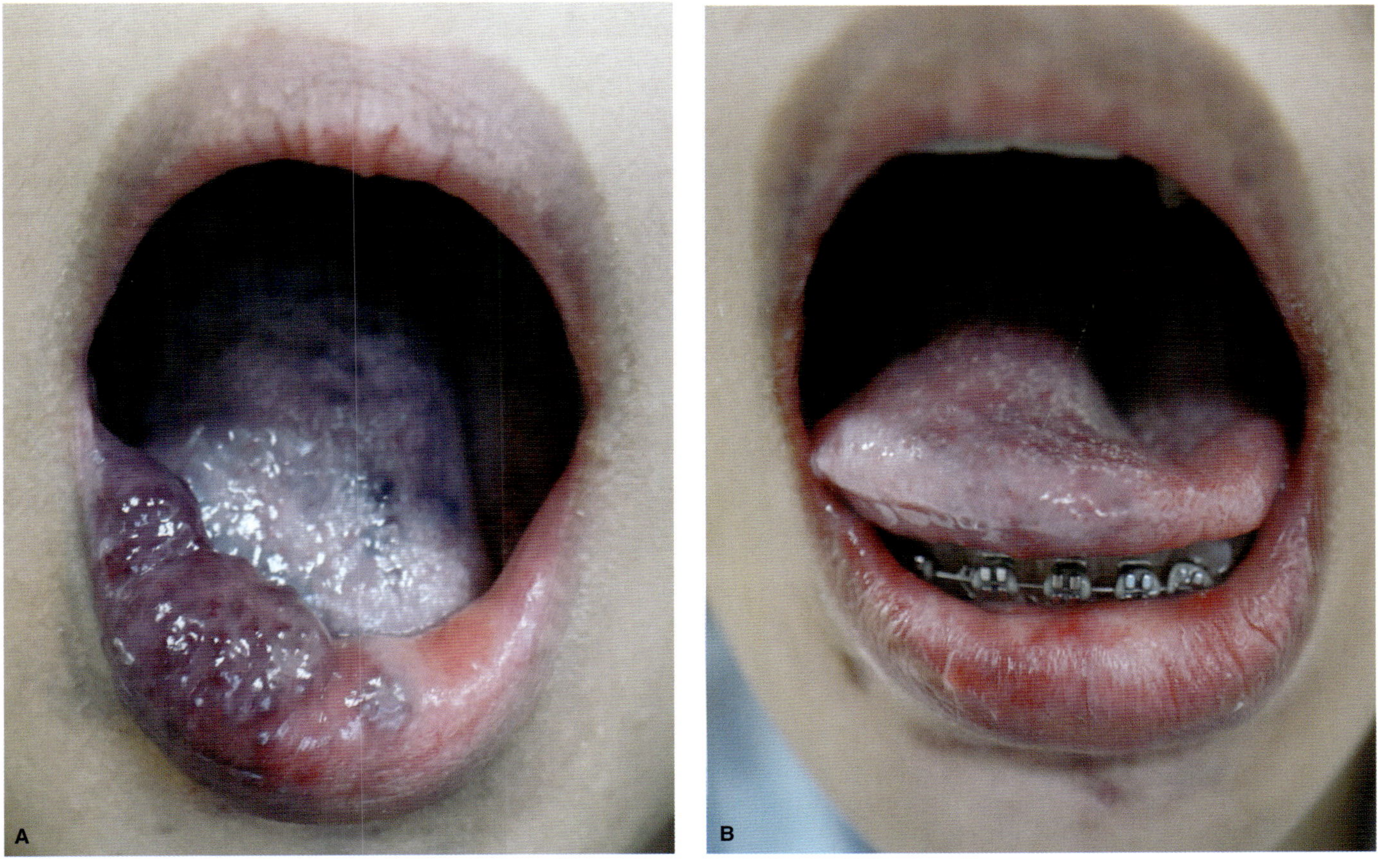

FIGURE 13-51A & 51B. Venous malformation affecting the lip and tongue of this adolescent Malay female. Figure 13-51B shows the same patient after multimodality treatment with oral sirolimus, sclerotherapy, and lasers.

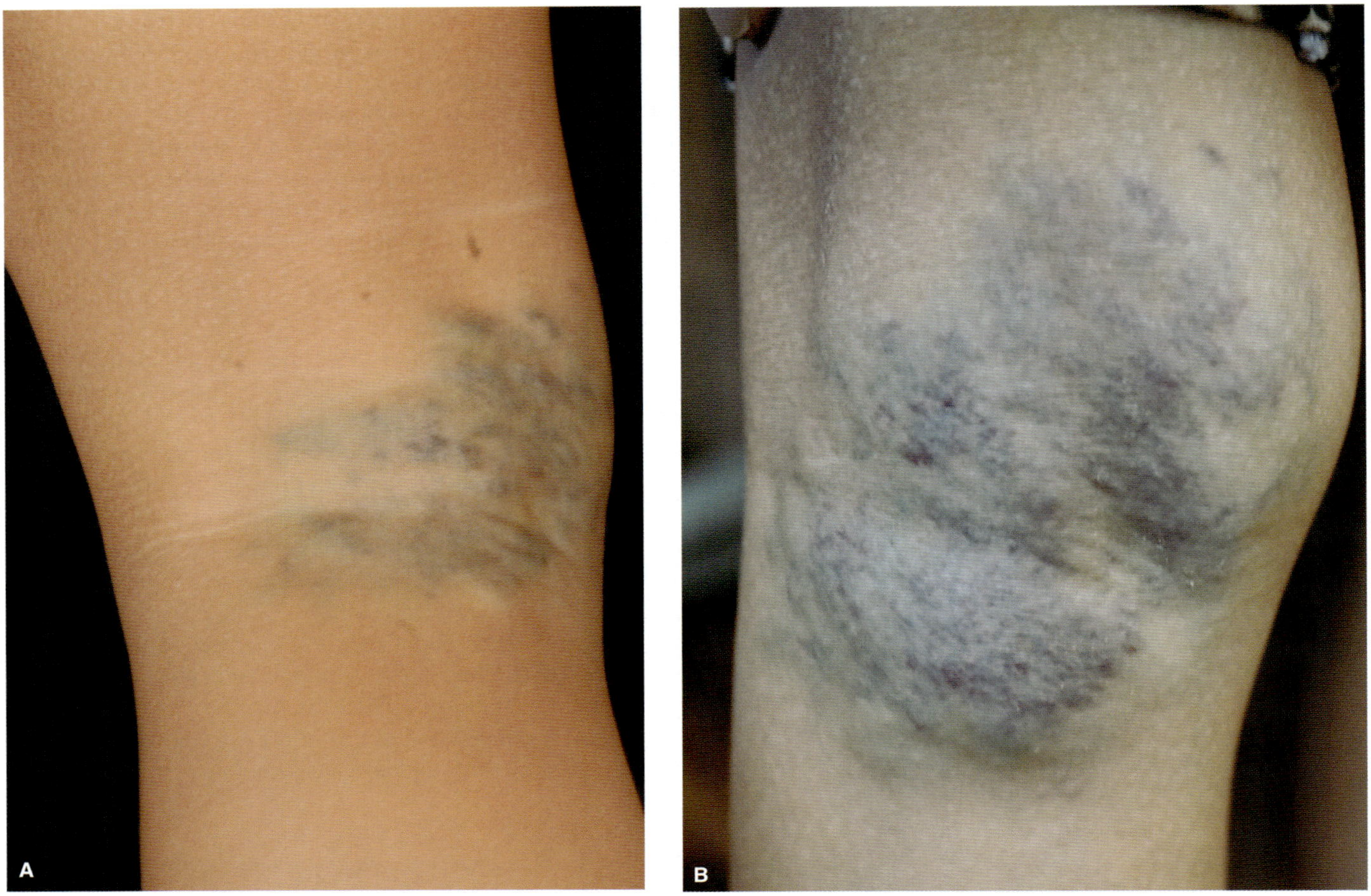

FIGURE 13-52A & 52B. Venous malformation on the popliteal fossa of a 2-year-old Chinese boy. There is gradual enlargement of the lesion, with Figure 13-52B showing the child at 7 years of age.

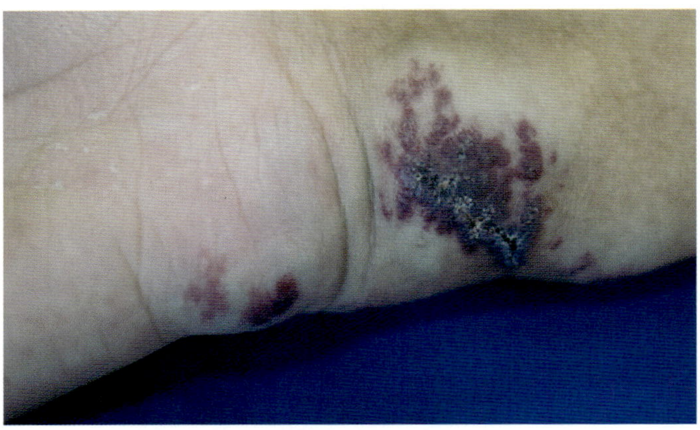

FIGURE 13-53. "Verrucous venous malformation" on the wrist and hand of a 7-year-old Nepalese boy. Note the more keratotic surface.

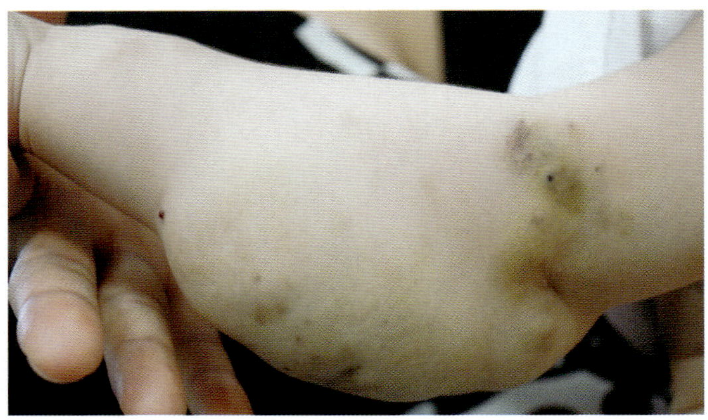

FIGURE 13-54. Veno-lymphatic malformation on the arm of a Vietnamese boy, presenting with soft swelling over the entire arm with a few surface blebs.

Pearls & Practical Tips

- Phleboliths may not be present in young children with VM.
- Patients with larger and more complex VM should be managed in a multidisciplinary team which includes pediatric dermatologists, oncologists, interventional radiologists, surgeons, and physiotherapists.

BIBLIOGRAPHY

1. Behravesh S, Yakes W, Gupta N, et al. Venous malformations: clinical diagnosis and treatment. Cardiovasc Diagn Ther 2016 Dec;6(6):557-69.
2. Cooke-Barber J, Kreimer S, Patel M, Dasgupta R, Jeng M. Venous malformations. Semin Pediatr Surg 2020;29:150976.

LYMPHATIC MALFORMATIONS

Lymphatic malformations (LM) are uncommon slow-flow vascular malformations of the lymphatic system. They can be macrocystic, microcystic, or a combination of both. Most LM are isolated lesions, but they may also occur with other malformations or in malformation syndromes, such as PIK-3CA-related overgrowth syndromes (PROS). Similar to venous malformations, somatic mutations in the PI3K-AKT-mTOR pathway have been associated with LM.

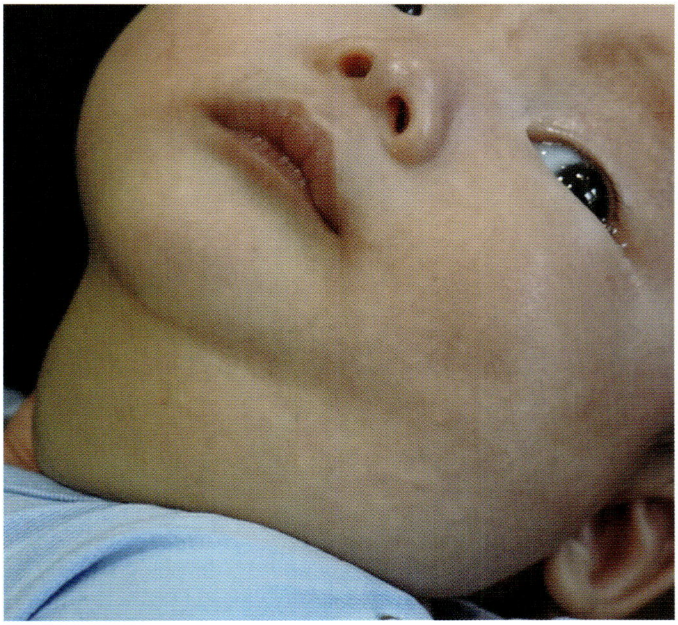

FIGURE 13-55. Macrocystic lymphatic malformation on the left neck of a Chinese infant.

Clinical Features

- LM are usually evident at birth or early childhood. Large LM may be visualized on antenatal imaging. LM may rarely present later in life.
- The lesions most frequently affect the head and neck region but can also affect other sites such as the trunk and limbs.
- LM can be classified as macrocystic, microcystic, or a combination of both.
- Macrocystic LM consist of large interconnected lymphatic channels and cysts (>2 cm) that often distort the anatomy. They present as soft, normothermic, subcutaneous swellings, usually with a light bluish hue.
- Microcystic LM presents as flesh-colored erythematous or hemorrhagic papules (<2 cm) that can coalesce into plaques. The lesions resemble frog spawn and may discharge clear, slightly cloudy, or blood-tinged fluid.
- Combined LM present with both macrocystic and microcystic components.
- Common complications include infection and intracystic bleeding, which can result in pain, rapid enlargement, fever, and anemia. LM around the neck region can cause respiratory distress. LM can enlarge with intercurrent illness or after vaccinations.

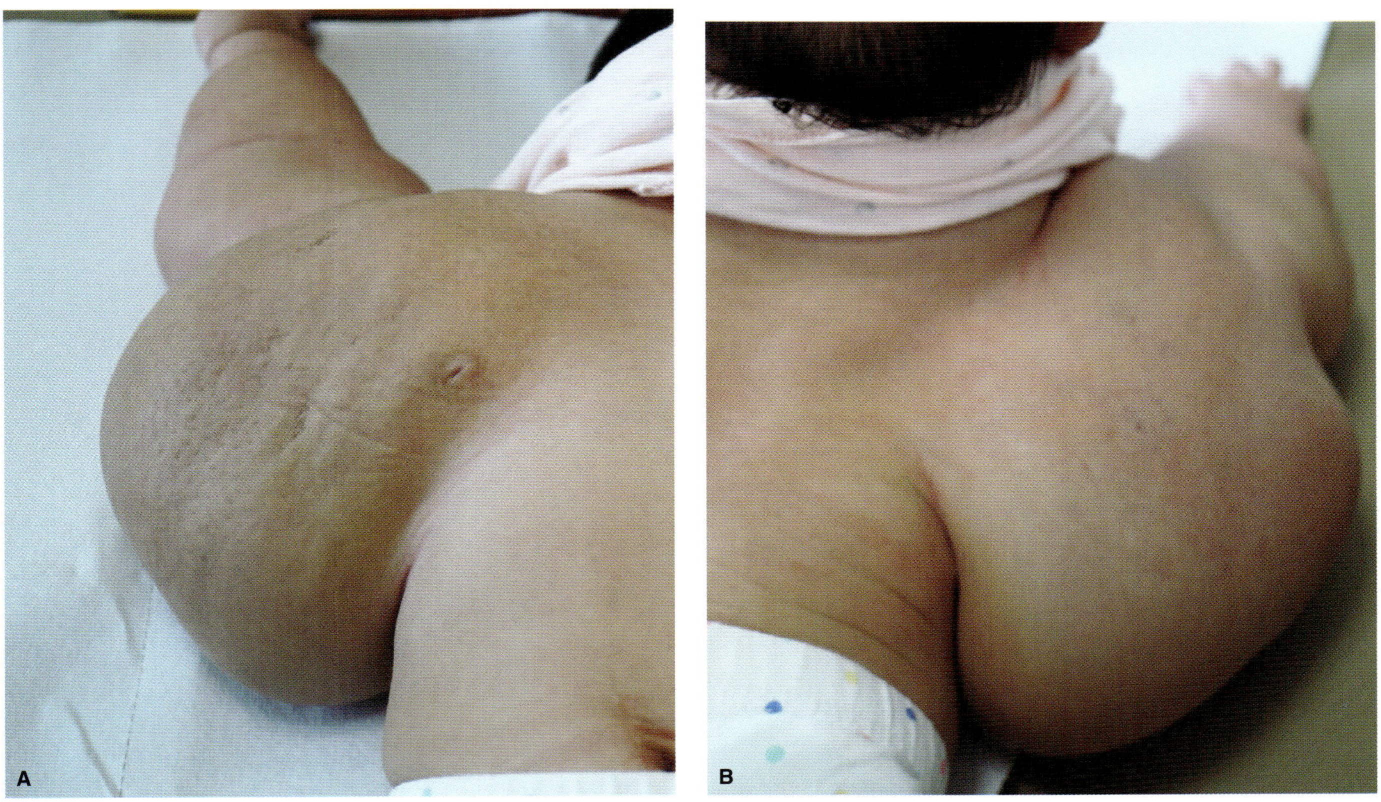

FIGURE 13-56A & 56B. Large lymphatic malformation on the right arm and chest of a Chinese infant girl, with overlying skin changes. The patient underwent sclerotherapy within weeks of life due to recurrent intralesional bleeding.

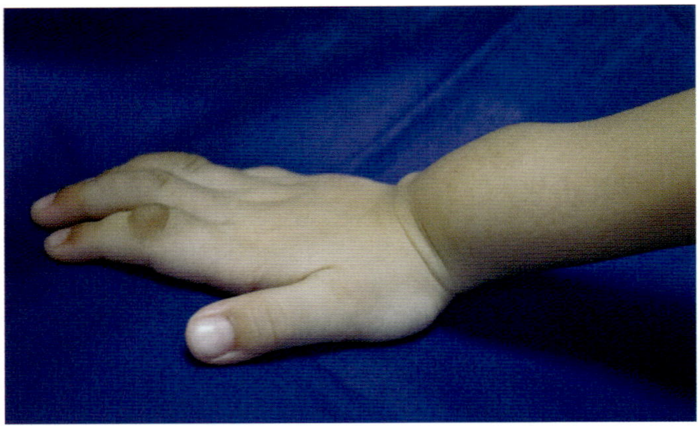

FIGURE 13-57. Lymphatic malformation on the forearm of a child.

Differential Diagnoses

- Deep infantile hemangioma (IH)
  - LM can be confused with deep IH, especially if the latter does not have a superficial component. IH will proliferate in the first few months of life and a pulsatile flow can be demonstrated on bedside Doppler, which is not heard over LM.
- Venous malformation
  - Venous malformation usually feels warmer than LM and may contain phleboliths. Imaging with ultrasound and MRI will help to differentiate the two entities. Both components are often seen in the same lesion.
- Dermoid cyst
  - LM can mimic dermoid cysts if they occur at sites of skin fusion such as eyebrows. Imaging will help to differentiate the two entities.

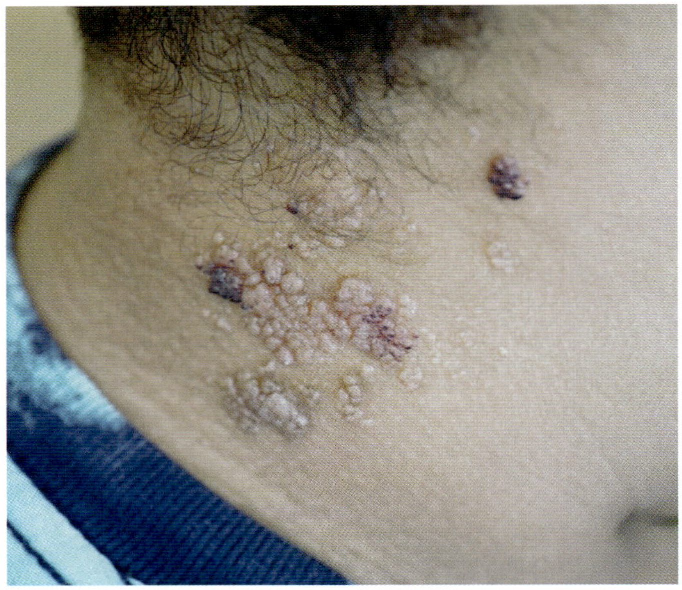

FIGURE 13-59. Microcystic lymphatic malformation on the neck of a Filipino boy, presenting as skin-colored hemorrhagic papules appearing like “frog-spawn.”

Investigations & Treatment

- LM are usually suspected clinically, but imaging studies including ultrasound and MRI will help to confirm the diagnosis and better define the extent and relationship to vital structures. Ultrasound typically shows dilated lymphatic sacs that lack connections with the lymphatic system. There will be no flow seen on Doppler.

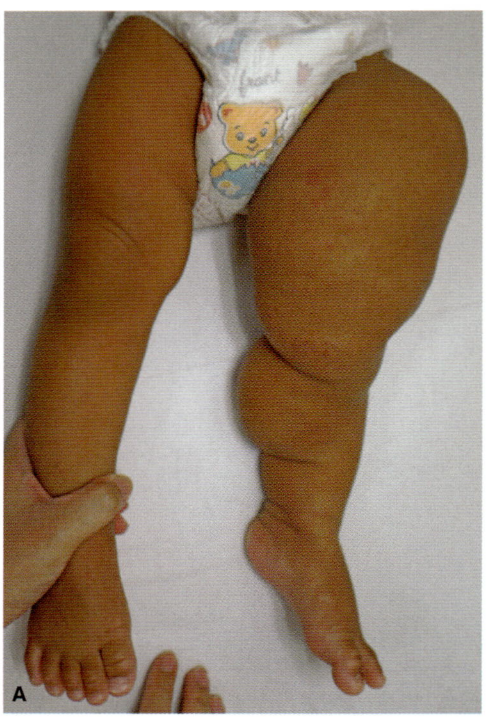

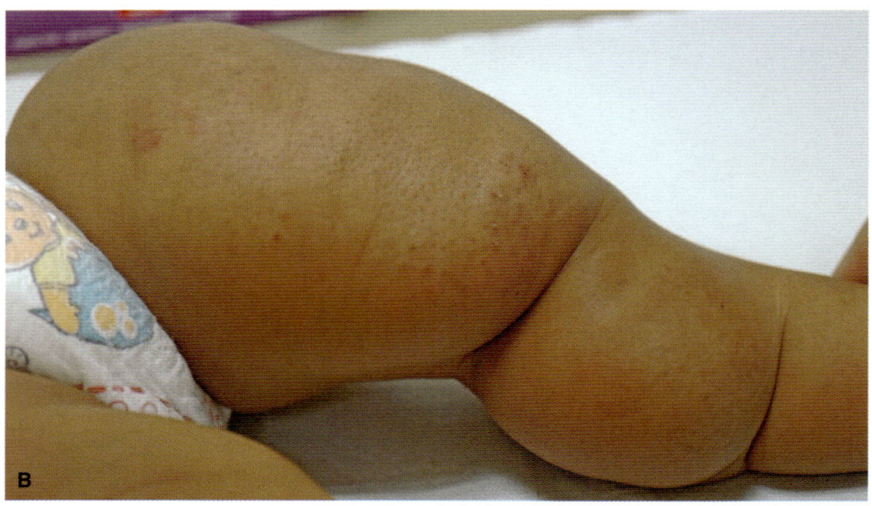

FIGURE 13-58A & 58B. Extensive lymphatic malformation affecting the left thigh and calf of a young Malay child.

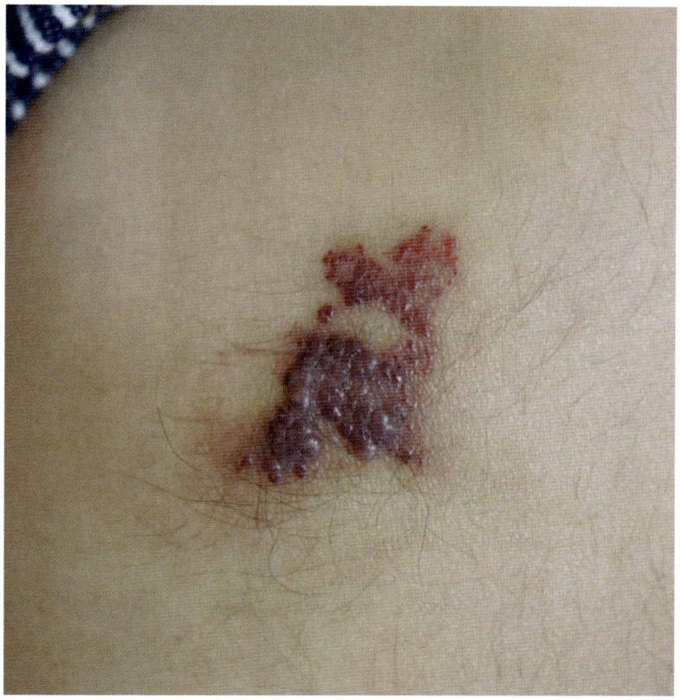

FIGURE 13-60. Microcystic lymphatic malformation on the thigh of a Japanese boy presenting as hemorrhagic papules.

- Treatment of LM depends on various factors, including the size, site, degree of functional impairment, symptoms, complications, and aesthetic impairment. Early intervention should be instituted for cases with life- or function-threatening complications, such as airway compromise.
- For macrocystic lesions, treatment can involve a combination of oral mTOR inhibitors such as sirolimus or everolimus, sclerotherapy, and surgery.
- Microcystic lesions may be treated with ablative techniques such as electrocautery, and ablative lasers such as the carbon dioxide laser or erbium-YAG laser.
- Systemic antibiotics will be required for LM that present with secondary infection. Intralesional antibiotics may also be useful.
- Serial compression bandaging may be useful for LM of the extremities to relieve swelling and alleviate symptoms.

Pearls & Practical Tips

- The recurrence risk of extensive LM after surgery is high. Treatment should be combined with medical and interventional therapies.
- Patients with large and complicated LM should be managed in a multidisciplinary team which includes pediatric dermatologists, oncologists, interventional radiologists, surgeons, and physiotherapists.

BIBLIOGRAPHY

1. Theiler M, Wälchli R, Weibel L. Vascular anomalies—a practical approach. J Dtsch Dermatol Ges 2013;11:397-405.
2. Kulungowski AM, Patel M. Lymphatic malformations. Semin Pediatr Surg 2020;29:150971.

ARTERIOVENOUS MALFORMATION

Arteriovenous malformations (AVM) are rare high-flow vascular malformations comprised of an abnormal tangle of blood vessels that lack capillary beds, resulting in direct connections between the arterial and venous circulations. Most AVM are isolated lesions, but may also be part of malformation syndromes, such as Parkes-Weber syndrome and hereditary hemorrhagic telangiectasia. Somatic or germline mutations in the RAS-MAPK-ERK pathway have been found to be associated with AVM.

Clinical Features

- AVM are very rare in children but can present at any age, including adulthood.
- AVM most commonly occur in the brain and spine, although they can occur in any part of the body. Most cutaneous AVM occur on the head and neck region, although they can also occur on the limbs and trunk.
- The presentation of AVM varies from faint erythematous macules or patches, thin purplish plaques, to larger pulsating nodules or masses with audible bruit. There is a palpable thrill, and a murmur may be heard on auscultation.
- Some AVM may display aggressive growth patterns and result in functional or cosmetic deformity and, in some patients, cardiovascular compromise. Other complications include bleeding, ulceration, and cardiac failure.

Differential Diagnoses

- Slow-flow vascular malformations
  - Venous and lymphatic malformations are usually soft and compressible with a bluish tinge. Thrills and bruits are never present.
- Infantile hemangioma and congenital hemangioma
  - These are much more common than AVM, and there is a characteristic pattern of growth and involution. AVM do not involute spontaneously.

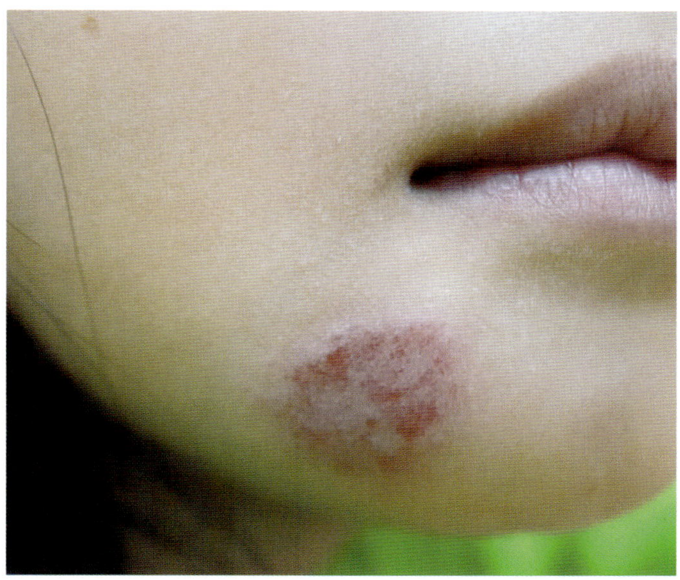

FIGURE 13-61. AVM on the chin of a 7-year-old Chinese girl, presenting with a demarcated red-maroon plaque with a palpable thrill.

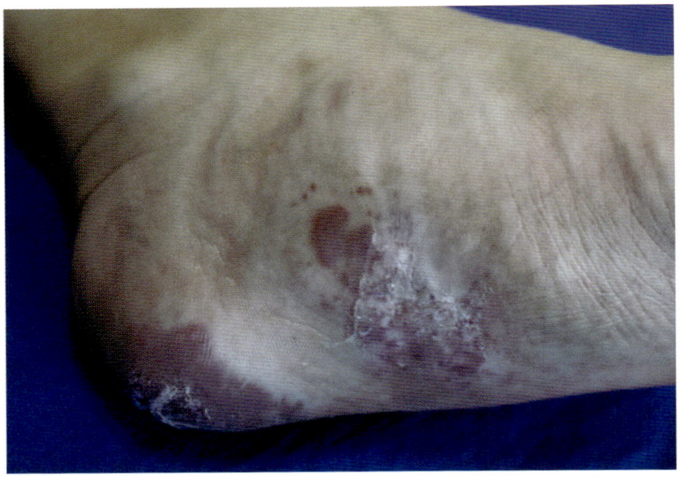

FIGURE 13-62. AVM on the foot of a Filipino boy presenting with a painful, indurated, violaceous plaque with recurrent surface ulceration.

Investigations & Treatment

- The diagnosis can be suspected clinical and confirmed with various imaging modalities, including ultrasound with Doppler and MRI/MRA. The extent of the lesion can also be visualized.
- Angiography will demonstrate the flow characteristics, feeding vessels, and anastomoses. This is useful if there is consideration for embolization or surgery.
- Small and asymptomatic AVM may not require treatment.
- Transcatheter embolization is the mainstay of treatment for most congenital peripheral AVMs, with surgical excision as an adjunctive modality.

Pearls & Practical Tips

- AVM has been known to occur after trauma, especially over the scalp.

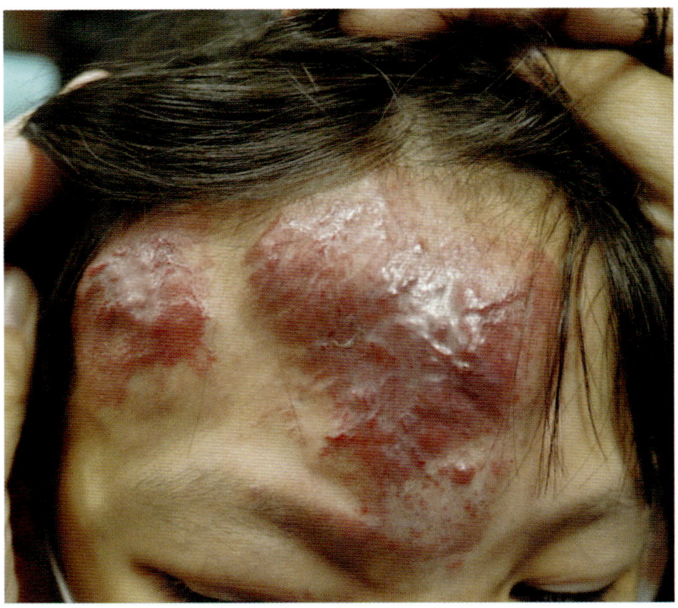

FIGURE 13-63. AVM on the forehead and scalp of a 9-year-old Chinese girl. She had concomitant intracranial AVM.

- Patients with AVM should be managed in a multidisciplinary team which includes pediatric dermatologists, oncologists, interventional radiologists, and surgeons.
- Systemic MEK inhibitors, such as trametinib, have recently been used for the treatment of AVM.

BIBLIOGRAPHY

1. Whitehead KJ, Smith MC, Li DY. Arteriovenous malformations and other vascular malformation syndromes. Cold Spring Harb Perspect Med 2013 Feb 1;3(2):a006635.
2. Manjunath SM, Shetty S, Moon NJ, et al. Arteriovenous malformation of the oral cavity. Case Rep Dent 2014;2014:353580.

STURGE-WEBER SYNDROME

Sturge-Weber syndrome (SWS) is a rare vascular malformation syndrome involving the skin, eye, and brain. It is characterized by facial segmental capillary malformation, or port wine stain (PWS), affecting the forehead and upper eyelids. It has been associated with activating somatic mutations in the *GNAQ* and *GNA11* genes, which encode a G-protein subunit, in the affected tissues.

Clinical Features

- SWS presents at birth with a sharply demarcated, segmental, pink-to-erythematous patch involving the V1 dermatome of the trigeminal nerve, which grows in proportion to the growth of the child.
- The stain may lighten over the first 6 months as the hemoglobin level undergoes a physiological decrease. Subsequently, it remains static but can darken to a dull erythro-cyanotic hue, sometimes with accompanying irregular nodular thickening of the surface over years.
- Brain involvement presents with epilepsy, developmental delay, focal neurological deficits, early handedness, and visual gaze preference. These findings usually present within the first 2 years of life.
- The most common eye manifestation in SWS is glaucoma, which most commonly occurs in the first 2 years of life but can occur later in life. Other eye manifestations include choroidal angiomas, retinal detachment, and visual loss.

Differential Diagnoses

- Segmental infantile hemangioma (IH) and PHACES syndrome
  - Segmental facial IH can appear as a flat, pink stain at birth, mimicking a PWS. However, IH lesions will proliferate over the next few weeks to become a brighter red and thicker in consistency.
  - Segmental facial IH may be associated with PHACES syndrome, also associated with neurological and ophthalmological manifestations.

Investigations & Treatment

- SWS can be clinically suspected in a patient presenting with a segmental PWS affecting the forehead and/or upper eyelids.

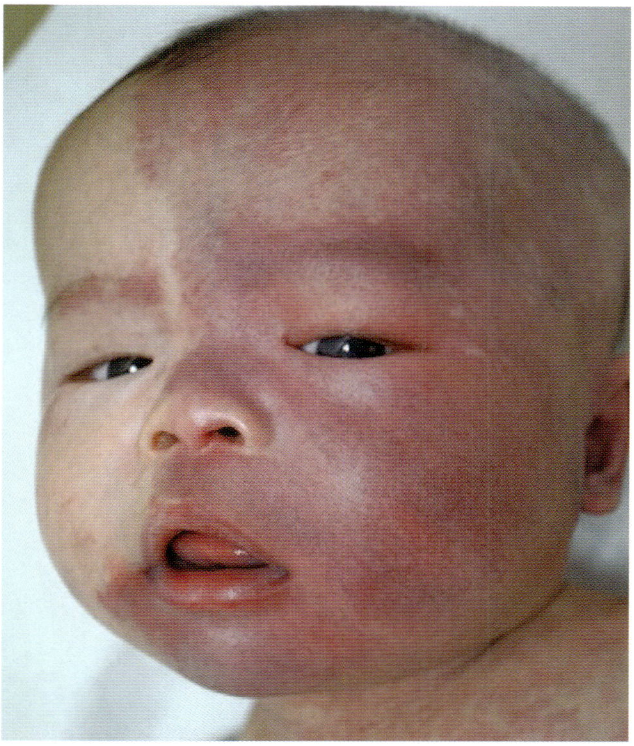

FIGURE 13-64. Sturge-Weber syndrome in a young Chinese infant presenting with extensive PWS bilaterally and affecting several segments, including the forehead.

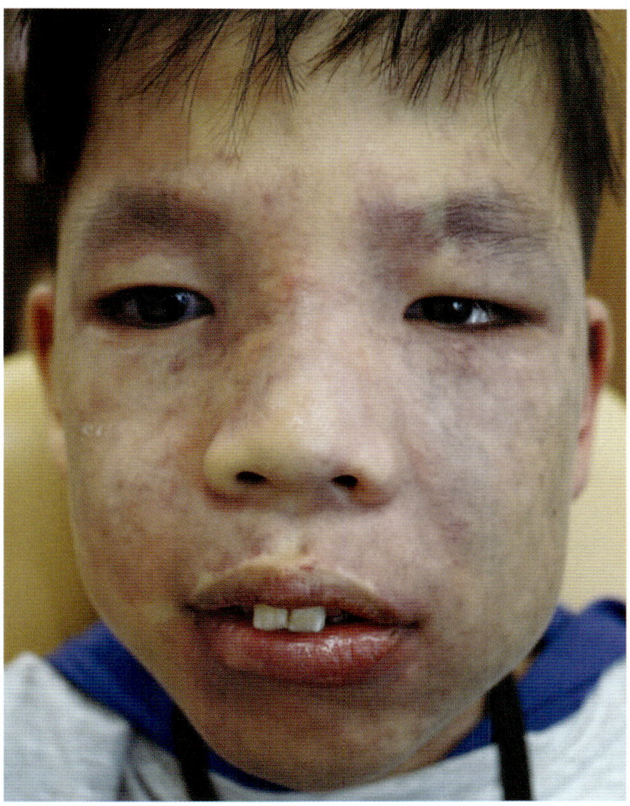

FIGURE 13-65. A Chinese boy with Sturge-Weber syndrome and extensive bilateral facial PWS, for which he has undergone pulsed-dye laser treatment. He has neurological and ophthalmological involvement.

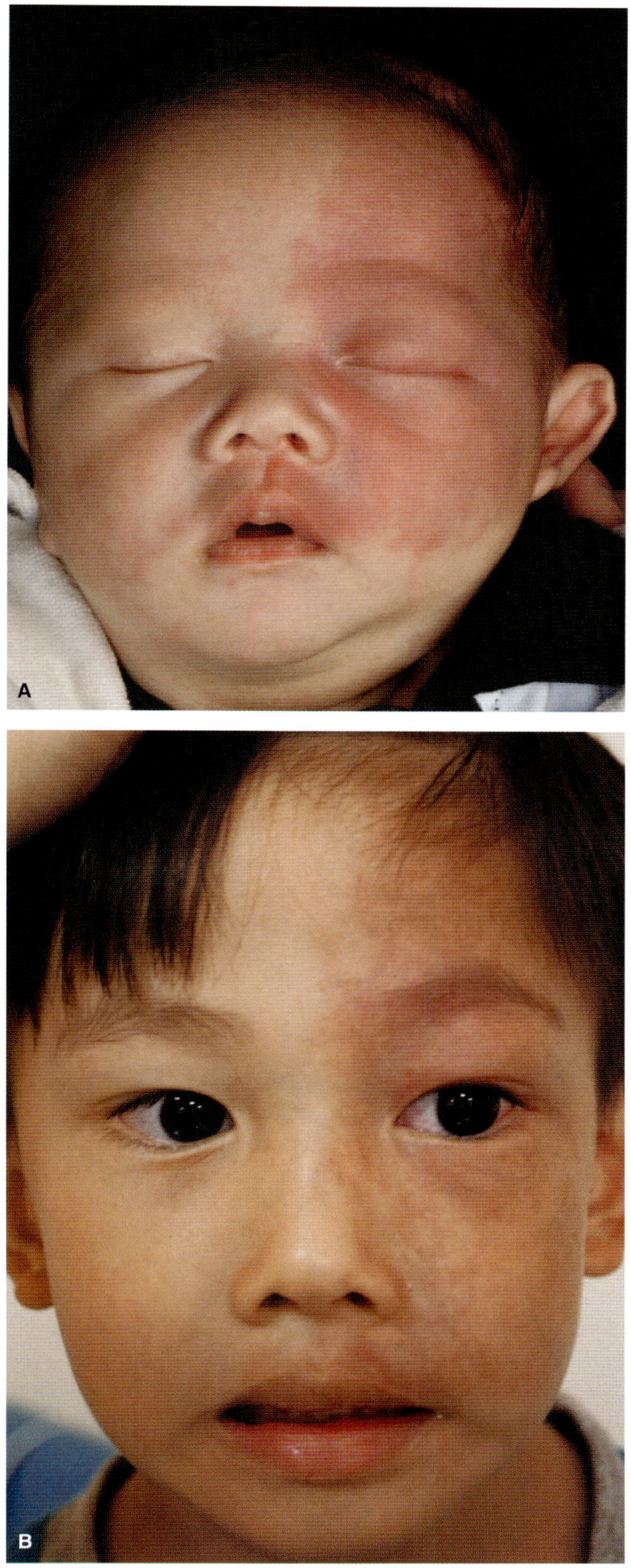

FIGURE 13-66A & 66B. A Chinese boy with Sturge-Weber syndrome, recurrent seizures, and left-sided PWS affecting the forehead, eyelids, and cheeks for which he has undergone several treatments with pulsed-dye laser.

- These patients should be referred for formal eye examination by an ophthalmologist.
- Patients should also undergo cranial MRI, with early findings of transient hyperperfusion with accelerated myelin maturation, leptomeningeal enhancement, and restricted diffusion if there is an associated acute ischemic event. Later findings include gyriform calcifications as well as cortical atrophy.
- Treatment requires a multidisciplinary team approach which should include neurologists, ophthalmologists, dermatologists, developmental pediatricians, physiotherapists, and occupational therapists.
- Regular screening for glaucoma is required for years, as eye involvement may occur later in life.
- The PWS can be treated with vascular lasers, including the pulsed-dye laser (PDL), long-pulsed Nd:YAG laser, and intense pulsed light (see Capillary Malformation section in this chapter).

Pearls & Practical Tips

- Initially thought to follow the V1 distribution of the trigeminal nerve, the PWS in SWS is now known to follow the vascular distribution of the upper face. All babies with PWS affecting the forehead and upper eyelids should be evaluated for SWS.
- There is a relatively high recurrence rate after laser treatment of PWS in SWS.

BIBLIOGRAPHY

1. Comi A. Current therapeutic options in Sturge-Weber syndrome. Semin Pediatr Neurol 2015;22(4):295-301.
2. Marques L, Nunez-Cordoba JM, Aguado L, et al. Topical rapamycin combined with pulsed dye laser in the treatment of capillary vascular malformations in Sturge-Weber syndrome. Phase II, randomized, double-blind, intraindividual placebo-controlled clinical trial. J Am Acad Dermatol 2015;72:151-8.

PIK3CA-RELATED OVERGROWTH SPECTRUM

PIK3CA-related overgrowth spectrum (PROS) refers to a group of vascular anomaly syndromes associated with somatic gain-of-function mutations in *PIK3CA* gene, and with overlapping clinical features. Common features include asymmetric limb overgrowth and various slow-flow vascular malformations. Mutations in *PIK3CA* gene result in constitutional activation of the PI3K-AKT-mTOR pathway, involved in cellular proliferation, survival, and growth as well as vascular development during embryogenesis. The two most common syndromes within the spectrum of PROS are Klippel-Trenaunay syndrome (KTS) and congenital lipomatous overgrowth, vascular malformations, epidermal nevi, and skeletal abnormalities (CLOVES) syndrome. Less common conditions include megalencephaly-capillary malformation (MCAP) syndrome, hemimegalencephaly, fibroadipose hyperplasia, and hemihyperplasia-multiple lipomatosis (HHML) syndrome.

Clinical Features

- PROS usually presents at birth, although diagnosis may be delayed in patients with less obvious features.
- KTS is characterized by a combination of various slow-flow vascular malformations, including capillary, venous,

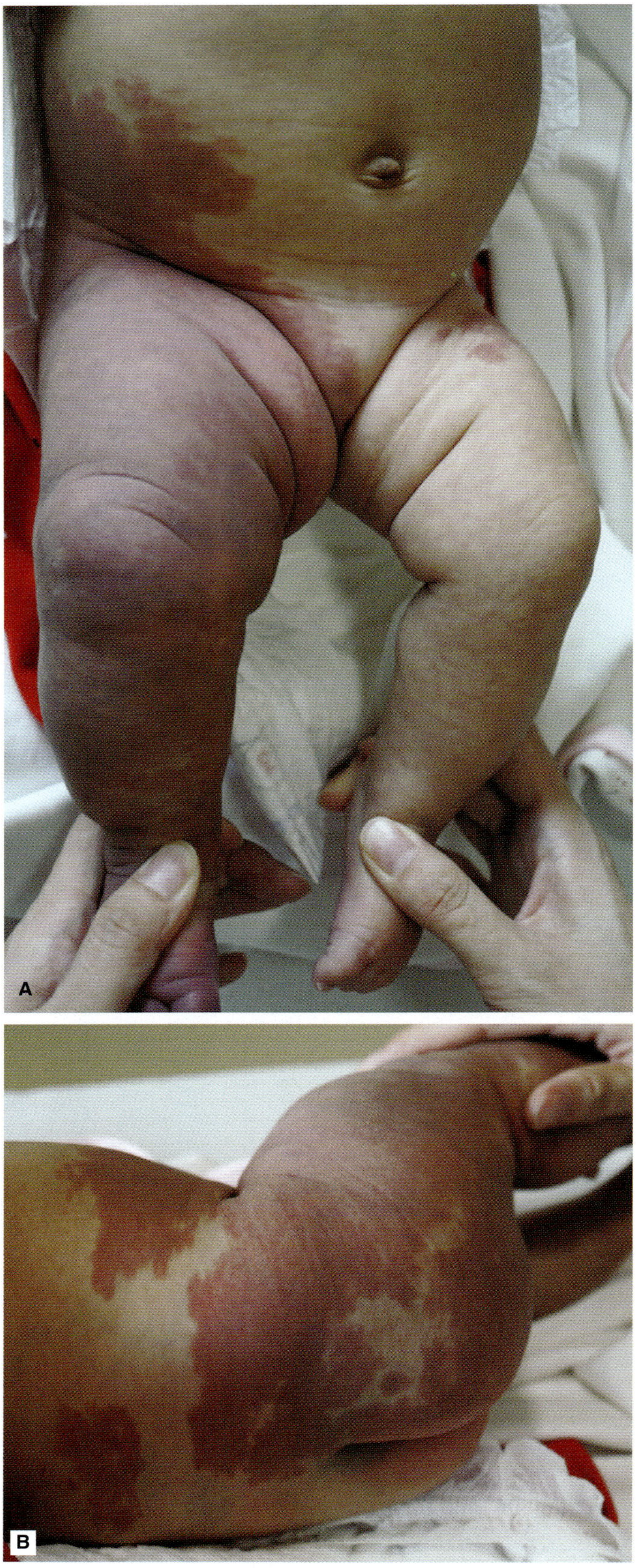

FIGURE 13-67A & 67B. A newborn Chinese girl presenting with KTS affecting the right leg, extending to the genitalia, buttocks, and back.

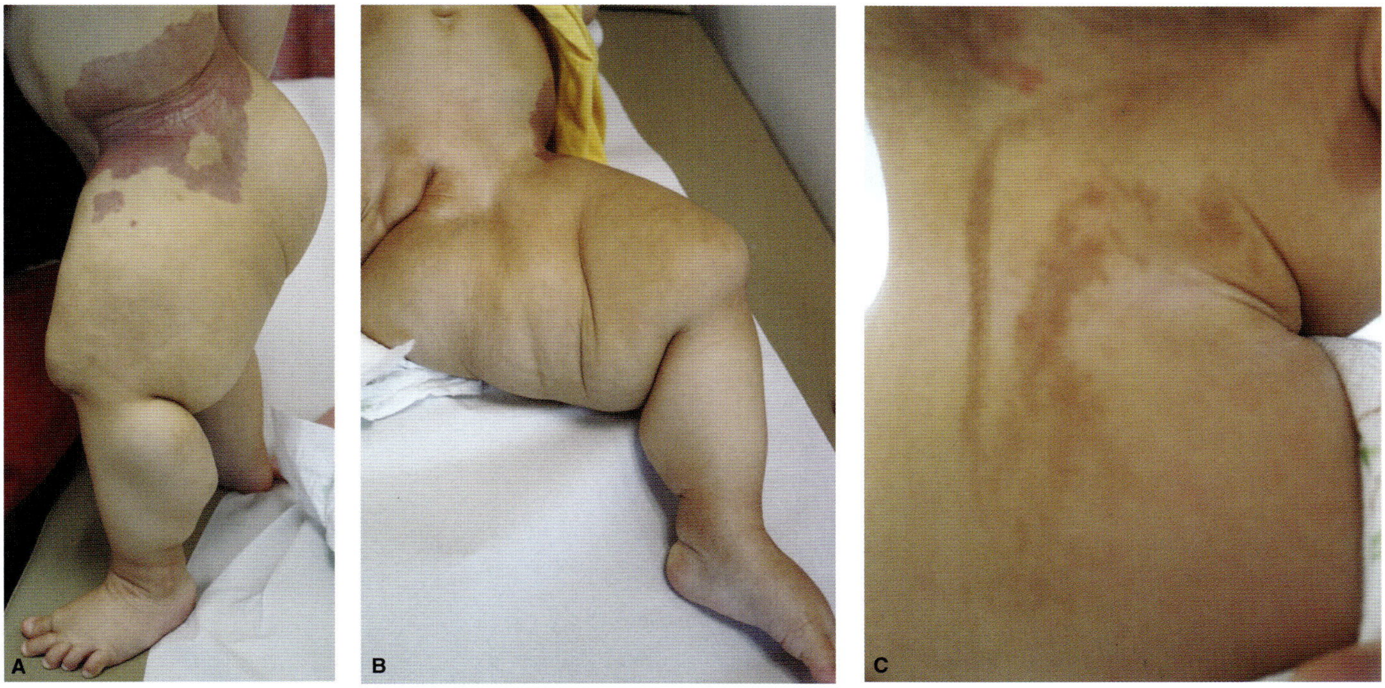

FIGURE 13-68A–68C. A Chinese infant girl presenting with CLOVES syndrome with vascular malformations affecting her left leg with prominent embryonic veins. She has an epidermal nevus on her posterior neck (Figure 13-68C).

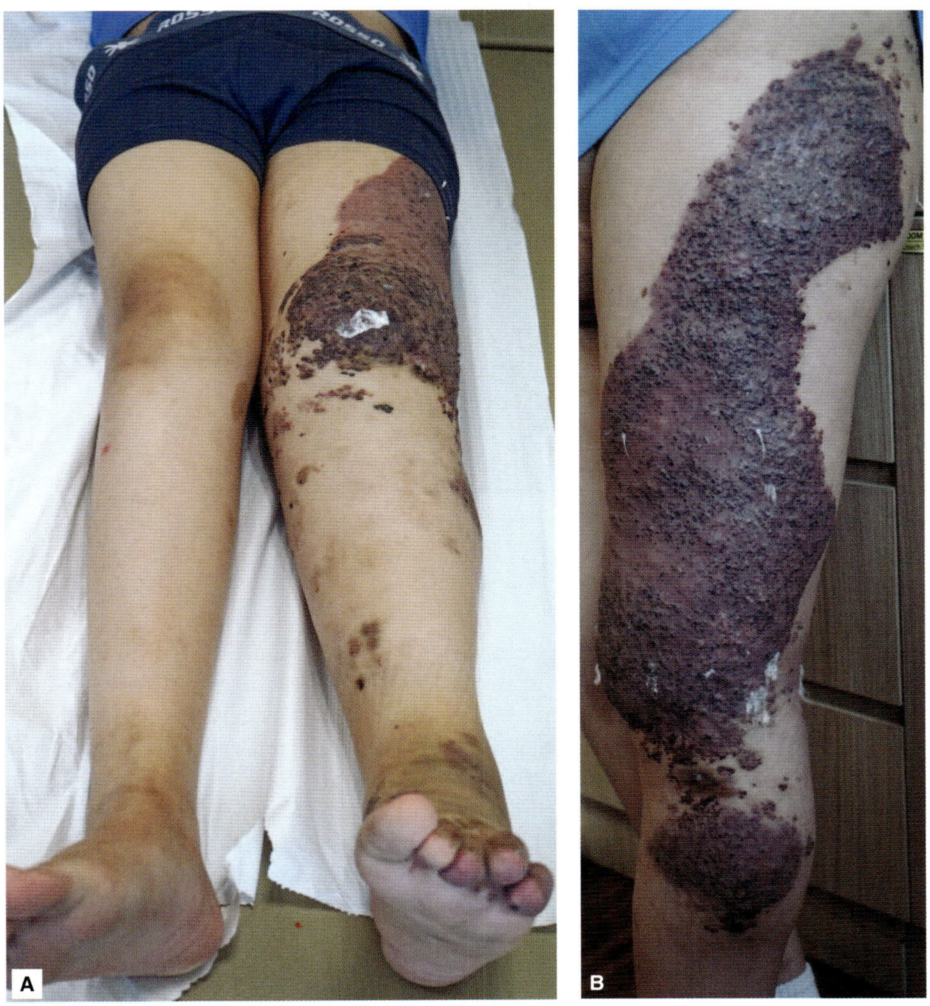

FIGURE 13-69A & 69B. A Malay boy with KTS presenting with vascular stains and blebs on his left leg associated with deeper venous and lymphatic malformations, embryonic veins, and asymmetric limb hypertrophy.

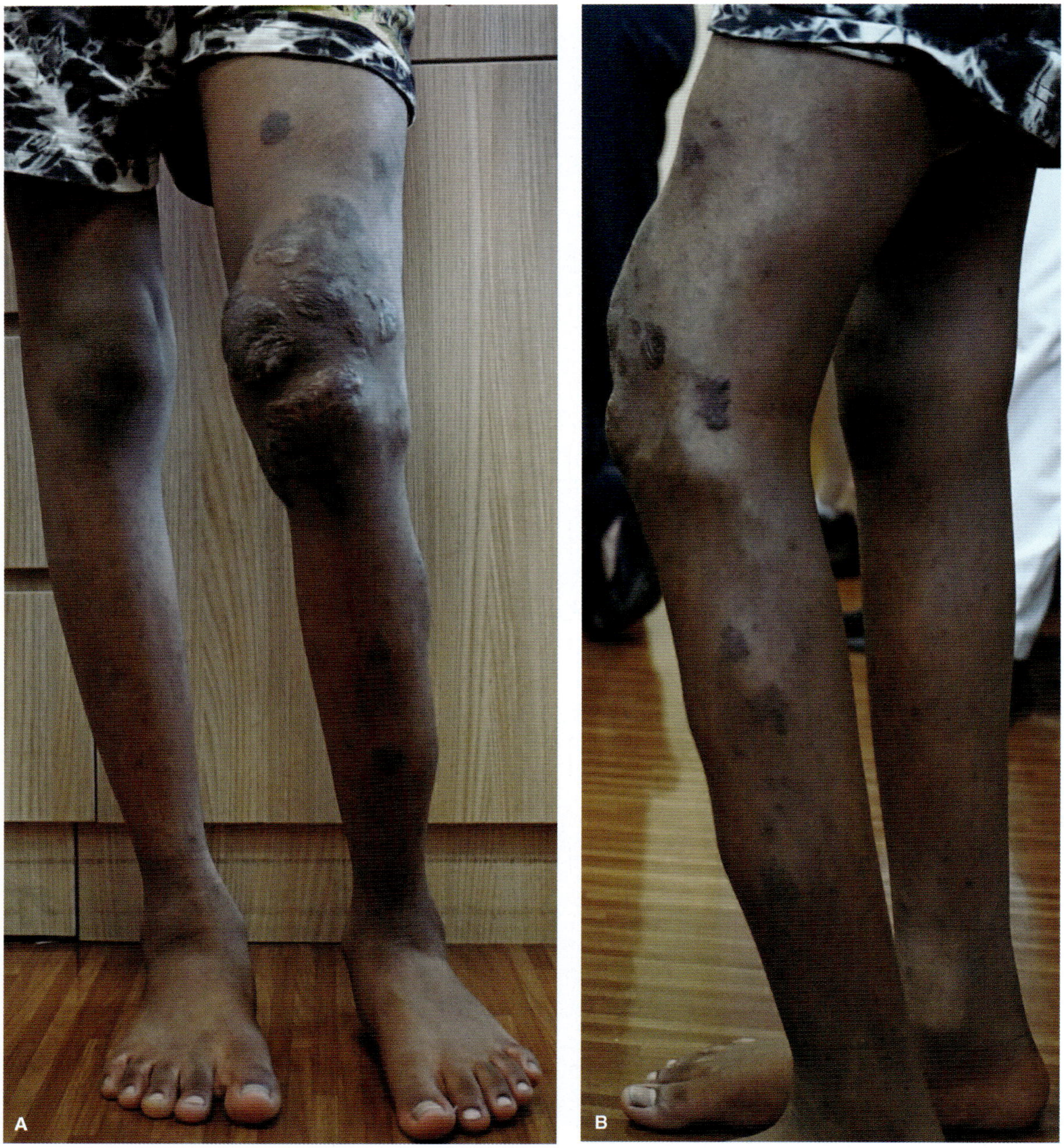

FIGURE 13-70A & 70B. An Indian boy with KTS with irregular leg hypertrophy with severe leg-length discrepancy, vascular blebs, and prominent varicosities.

and lymphatic malformations, and variable degrees of tissue and bony hypertrophy.

- It most commonly affects the lower limbs, but also affects the upper limbs, head, and neck. The majority of cases are unilateral.
- A persistent anomalous embryonic or "marginal" vein is often found in the affected limb of KTS patients. These veins are usually found on the lateral side of the limb.
- Venous and lymphatic malformations can also involve the lower gastrointestinal and genitourinary system, resulting in hematochezia and hematuria.
- Complications include deep vein thrombosis, especially of the dilated marginal vein, leading to pulmonary embolism, musculoskeletal problems such as limb length discrepancy leading to scoliosis and gait disturbances, and chronic lymphedema.
- The clinical features of CLOVES are similar to KTS patients, but also include large lipomatous tumors, epidermal nevi, and skeletal abnormalities most commonly affecting the spine. There are reports of increased risk of Wilms tumor.

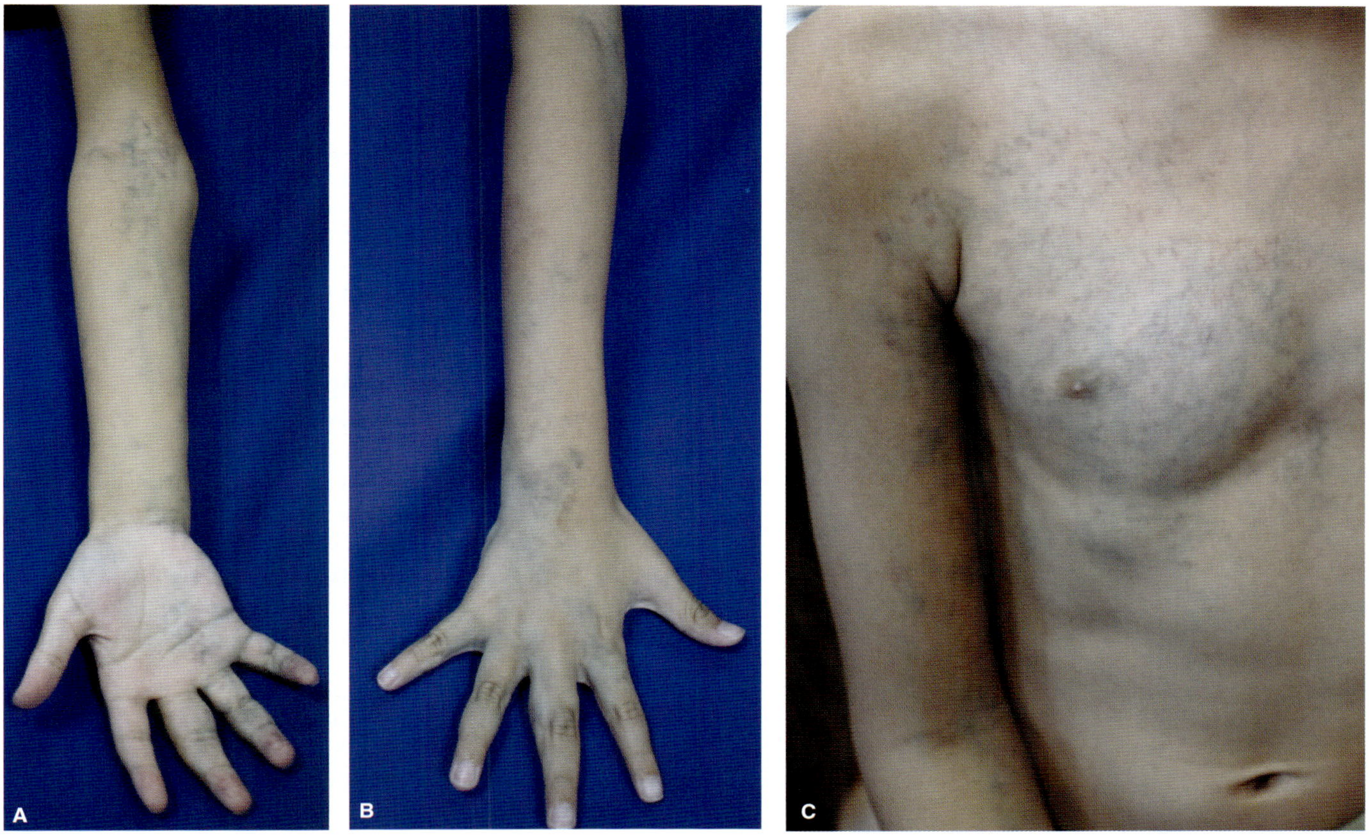

FIGURE 13-71A–71C. PROS affecting the right arm of a Thai Chinese boy. Upper limb involvement is less common than lower limb involvement. There are extensive venous malformations and tissue hypertrophy.

Differential Diagnoses

- Proteus syndrome
  - Proteus syndrome is an extremely rare disorder characterized by disproportionate asymmetric overgrowth caused by somatic activating mutation in *AKT1* gene, also part of the PI3K-AKT-mTOR pathway.
  - Patients present with hemihypertrophy, vascular malformations, progressive skeletal malformations, and tumors, which may be malignant.
  - Unlike KTS, lesions appear in a mosaic or random distribution, with a "patchy" pattern of affected and unaffected areas.
- Parkes-Weber syndrome
  - Parkes-Weber syndrome presents with fast-flow arteriovenous malformations and fistulas, associated with somatic activating mutations in the RAS-MAPK-ERK pathway.
  - Clinically, the hypertrophy seen in Parkes-Weber syndrome is more uniform throughout the limb compared to the non-uniform hypertrophy seen in KTS.
  - The vascular stain of Parkes-Weber syndrome is lighter than the more violaceous stain of KTS.
- Hemihypertrophy
  - Hemihypertrophy is a condition with excessive unilateral overgrowth. It can be isolated or be part of a genetic

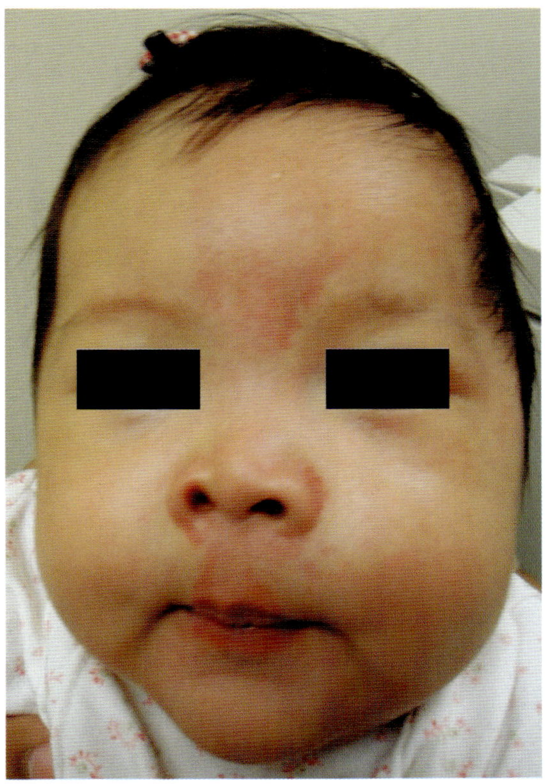

FIGURE 13-72. A rare case of MCAP occurring in a Chinese infant. She has a faint facial PWS associated with hemihypertrophy of her face. Brain imaging revealed megalencephaly.

syndrome, such as Beckwith-Wiedemann syndrome. Unlike the latter two conditions, isolated hemihypertrophy is not associated with vascular malformations.

Investigations & Treatment

- Lesions of PROS are diagnosed clinically and may even be suspected on antenatal imaging.
- Baseline and serial imaging studies, such as ultrasound and MRI, are used to confirm the extent of involvement and monitor for complications and treatment outcome.
- Multidisciplinary and multimodality management is required for patients with PROS, including pain management, rehabilitation, compression bandages, sclerotherapy, embolization, systemic medications such as mTOR inhibitors (e.g., sirolimus and everolimus) and anticoagulants, laser therapy, and surgery.

Pearls & Practical Tips

- Children with CLOVES syndrome should be monitored up to 8 years of age with regular ultrasound surveillance for development of Wilms tumor.
- Patients with PROS should be managed in a multidisciplinary team which includes pediatric dermatologists, hemato-oncologists, interventional radiologists, surgeons, and therapists.
- Molecular genetic testing for somatic *PIK3CA* mutations can be performed on biopsies of affected tissue. However, this requires deep sequencing techniques due to the low level of affected cells, even in lesional tissue.
- Alpelisib, a specific inhibitor of PI3K, is a relatively new systemic medication that has shown some promise in the treatment of *PIK3CA*-related vascular conditions.

BIBLIOGRAPHY

1. Asghar F, Aqeel R, Farooque U, Haq A, Taimur M. Presentation and management of Klippel-Trenaunay syndrome: a review of available data. Cureus 2020 May 8;12(5):e8023.
2. Keppler-Noreuil KM, Rios JJ, Parker VE, et al. PIK3CA-related overgrowth spectrum (PROS): diagnostic and testing eligibility criteria, differential diagnosis, and evaluation. Am J Med Genet A 2015;167A(2):287-95.

CAPILLARY MALFORMATION-ARTERIOVENOUS MALFORMATION SYNDROME/PARKES-WEBER SYNDROME

Capillary malformation-arteriovenous malformation (CM-AVM) syndrome and Parkes-Weber syndrome are rare, and are characterized by fast-flow vascular malformations, arteriovenous malformation or fistulae, with overlying capillary stains. Parkes-Weber syndrome is now recognized as a subset of CM-AVM syndrome. Germline or somatic mutations in *RASA1* and *EPHB4* genes are associated with CM-AVM and Parkes-Weber syndrome.

Clinical Features

- Patients with Parkes-Weber syndrome present at birth or in early childhood with a faint pink-to-hyperpigmented macular stain on one or more limbs, more commonly the lower limb. There is uniform hypertrophy of the affected limb compared to the normal side, and the affected limb

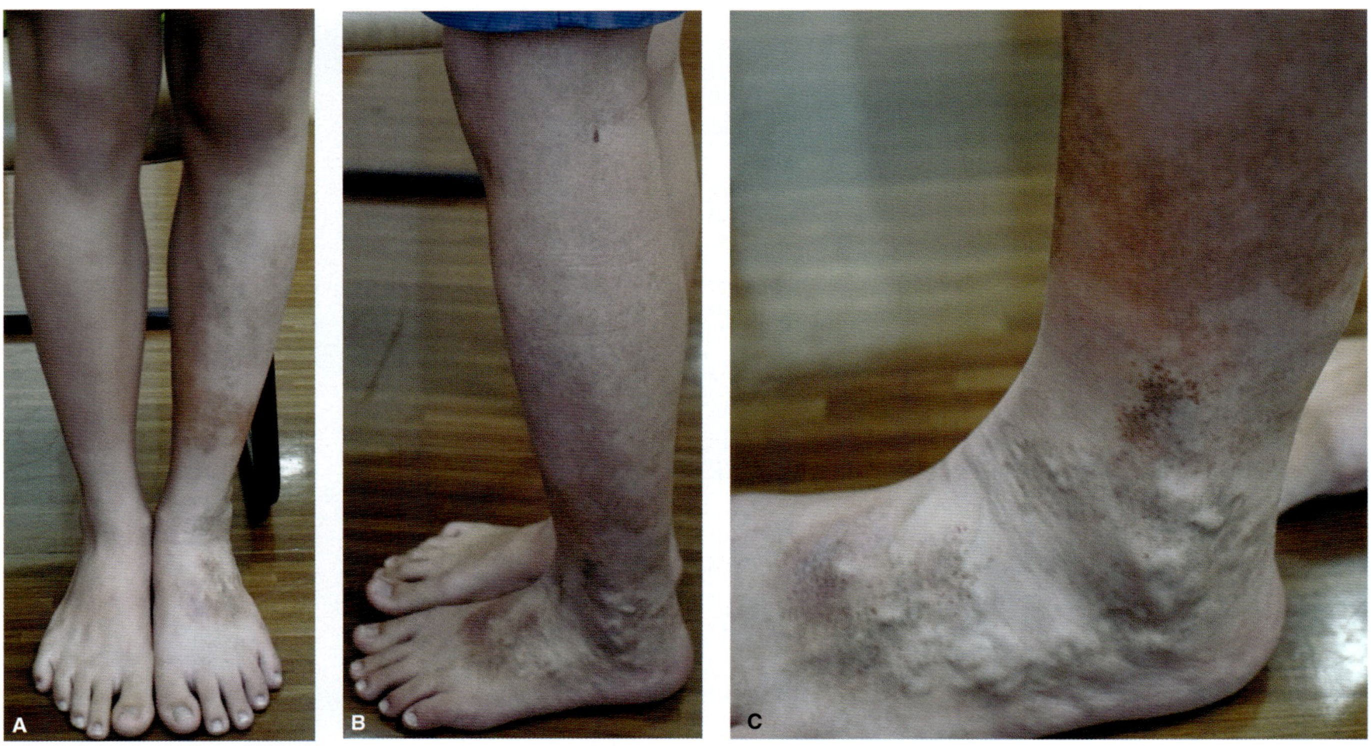

FIGURE 13-73A–73C. Parkes-Weber syndrome in a Chinese boy presenting with a faint hyperpigmented stain on his left leg. There is mild, diffuse hypertrophy of the limb with several enlarged vessels around the ankle area.

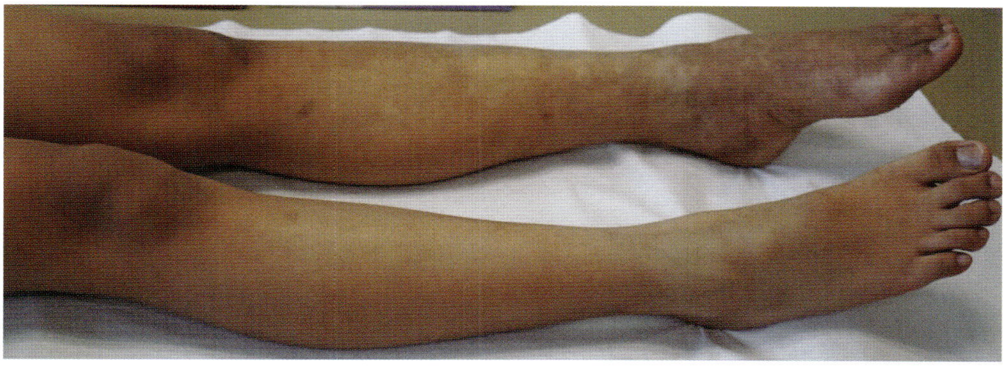

FIGURE 13-74. Parkes-Weber syndrome in a Malay boy presenting with a faint hyperpigmented stain on his left leg associated with diffuse hypertrophy.

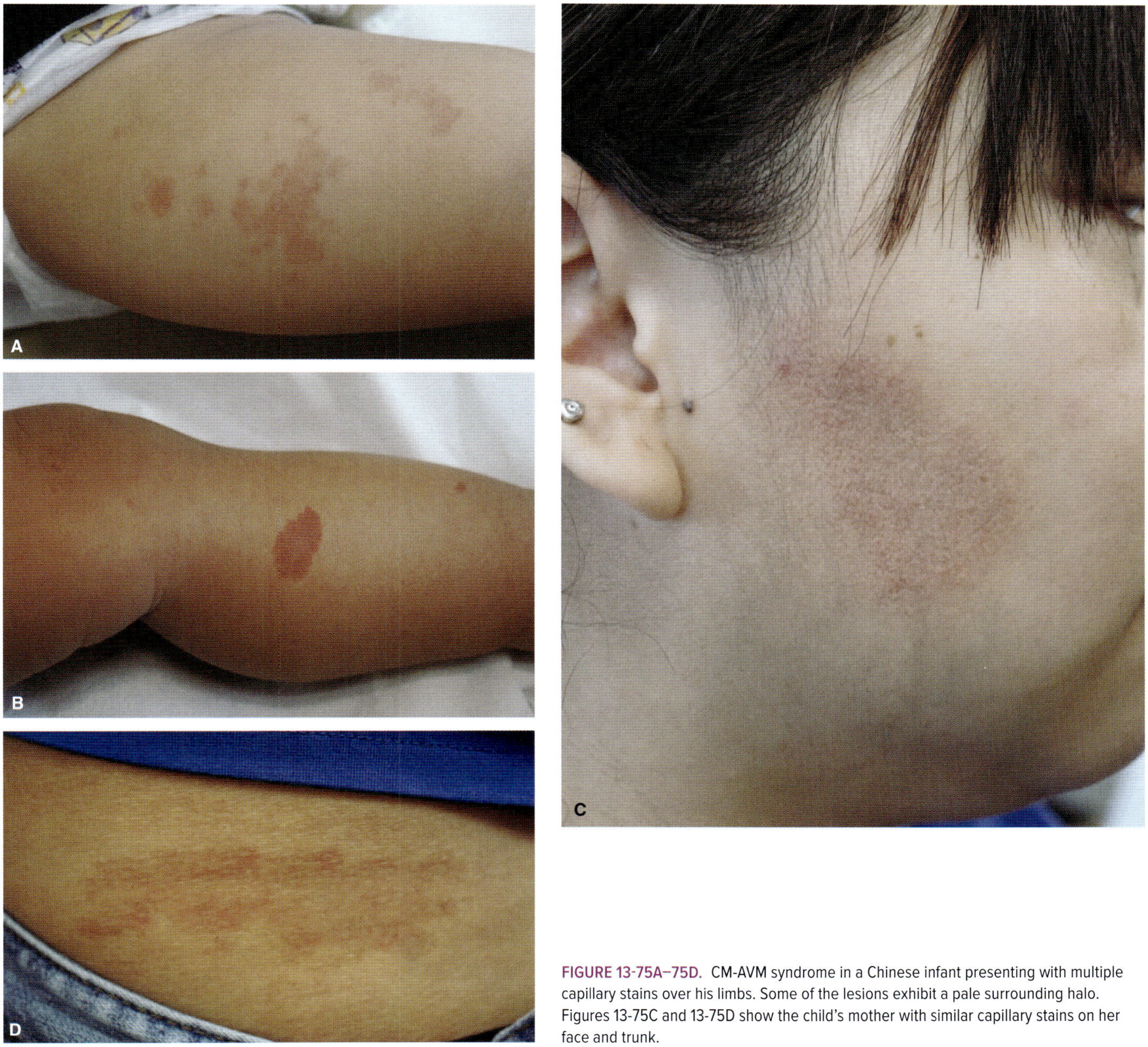

FIGURE 13-75A–75D. CM-AVM syndrome in a Chinese infant presenting with multiple capillary stains over his limbs. Some of the lesions exhibit a pale surrounding halo. Figures 13-75C and 13-75D show the child's mother with similar capillary stains on her face and trunk.

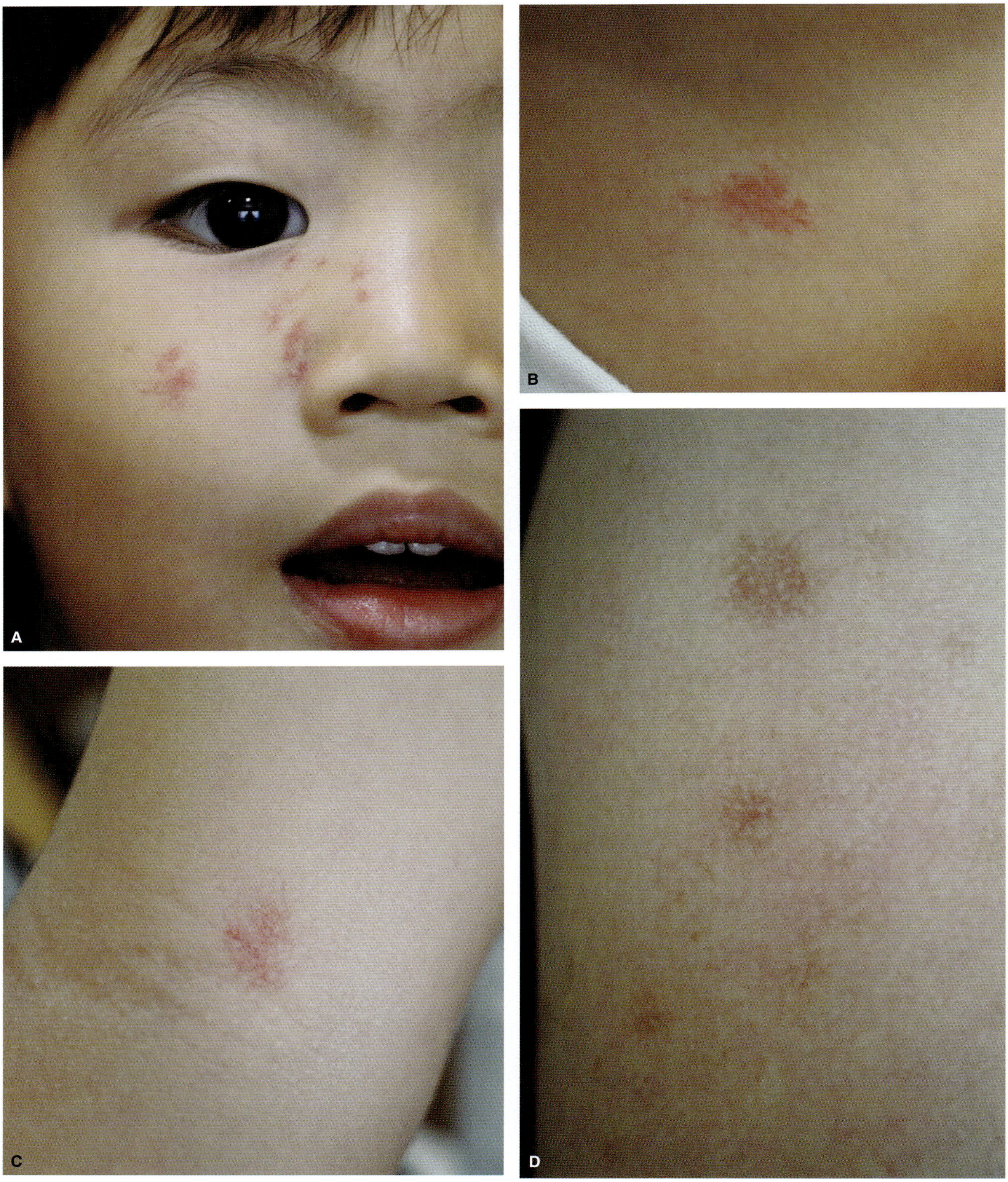

FIGURE 13-76A–76D. CM-AVM syndrome in a Chinese boy with multiple irregular vascular stains with a pale surrounding halo. Figure 13-76D shows similar lesions on his mother's arm.

feels warmer. A bruit from the underlying AVM may be heard on auscultation.

- In CM-AVM syndrome, there are tiny to large pink-orange stains scattered over the body. Some of the stains may show the classical surrounding halo of hypopigmentation. The lesions may be present from birth and can increase in number as the child grows. Bier's spots, which appear as hypopigmented macules on the limbs, may be seen in some patients.
- Patients with Parkes-Weber syndrome may experience pain or heaviness of the affected limb. Cardiac failure is an uncommon complication if the arteriovenous shunting is massive. Limb hypertrophy may lead to limb-length discrepancy with its associated orthopedic problems such as scoliosis.

Differential Diagnoses

- Capillary malformation/port wine stain
  - Simple capillary malformations can also present as light pink-to-purplish stains. They are usually obvious at birth and do not increase in number. Limb hypertrophy is uncommon, and Doppler studies will be negative.
- Klippel-Trenaunay syndrome (KTS)
  - KTS can present with a violaceous capillary stain on a limb, often associated with limb hypertrophy. However, the hypertrophy seen in KTS is usually not uniform, and the overlying stain is darker than that seen in Parkes-Weber syndrome. The limb hypertrophy in the latter is uniform over the entire limb.
  - There are no fast-flow vascular malformations in KTS.

Investigations & Treatment

- A Doppler placed over the stains may reveal an arterial signal or "whoosh."
- Ultrasound, MRI/MRA and angiography of the affected limb will be able to demonstrate the fast-flow arteriovenous malformations or fistulas.
- Management of CM-AVM and Parkes-Weber syndrome can be complex, and ideally should be managed by a multidisciplinary vascular team. Asymptomatic patients can be managed conservatively. If treatment is indicated, options include interventional embolization and surgery. More recently, systemic medications such as mTOR inhibitors, MEK inhibitors, and thalidomide have shown mixed results in treating fast-flow malformations.

Pearls & Practical Tips

- The vascular stain in Parkes-Weber syndrome can appear more "hyperpigmented" in Asian patients.
- Parkes-Weber syndrome is often misdiagnosed as KTS. Fast-flow malformations are not seen in KTS patients.
- Bedside Doppler is useful to detect the fast-flow malformations of Parkes-Weber syndrome and KTS. Patients should be placed in different positions to illicit the pulsatile flow.

BIBLIOGRAPHY

1. Banzic I, Brankovic M, Maksimović Ž, Davidović L, Marković M, Rančić Z. Parkes Weber syndrome-diagnostic and management paradigms: a systematic review. Phlebology 2017 Jul;32(6): 371-83.
2. Mulliken JB, Burrows PE, Fishman SJ. Mulliken & Young's Vascular Anomalies: Hemangiomas and Malformations. 2nd ed. Oxford University Press; 2013.

BLUE RUBBER BLEB NEVUS SYNDROME

Blue rubber bleb nevus syndrome (BRBNS) is a rare vascular anomaly syndrome characterized by multifocal venous malformation that mainly affects the skin and gastrointestinal tract. It can also affect other organs, including liver, spleen, heart, eye, and central nervous system. BRBNS is caused by double somatic activating mutations in the *TIE2* gene, encoding the TEK receptor tyrosine kinase, leading to unregulated angiogenesis.

Clinical Features

- BRBNS usually presents at birth or in early childhood with a large, dominant venous malformation and several, soft, compressible, rubbery, blue-to-purple papules or nodules that represent smaller venous malformations. These smaller lesions increase in size and number over time.
- The lesions are usually asymptomatic but may be painful or tender, hyperhidrotic, and may bleed with trauma. They tend to swell in gravity-dependent positions.
- Venous malformations in the gastrointestinal tract most commonly involve the small bowel but can occur anywhere from the mouth to the anus.
- The most serious complication is severe gastrointestinal hemorrhage resulting in hemodynamic instability, severe anemia, and disseminated intravascular coagulopathy. Intestinal intussusception can also occur.

Differential Diagnoses

- Diffuse neonatal hemangiomatosis/multiple infantile hemangiomas (IH)
  - Diffuse neonatal hemangiomatosis is characterized by multiple IH that rapidly increase in size and number within the first few weeks of life. The evolution is much faster than BRBNS, which evolve over months or years.
  - A pulsatile flow can be demonstrated on bedside Doppler.
- Klippel-Trenaunay syndrome (KTS)
  - KTS can also present with gastrointestinal bleeding caused by venous malformations. However, it usually affects only one limb and is associated with other malformations, such as capillary and lymphatic malformations, and limb hypertrophy.
- Maffucci syndrome
  - This is an extremely rare disorder characterized by multiple enchondromas, skeletal deformities, and cutaneous venous malformations. BRBNS does not typically have skeletal involvement.

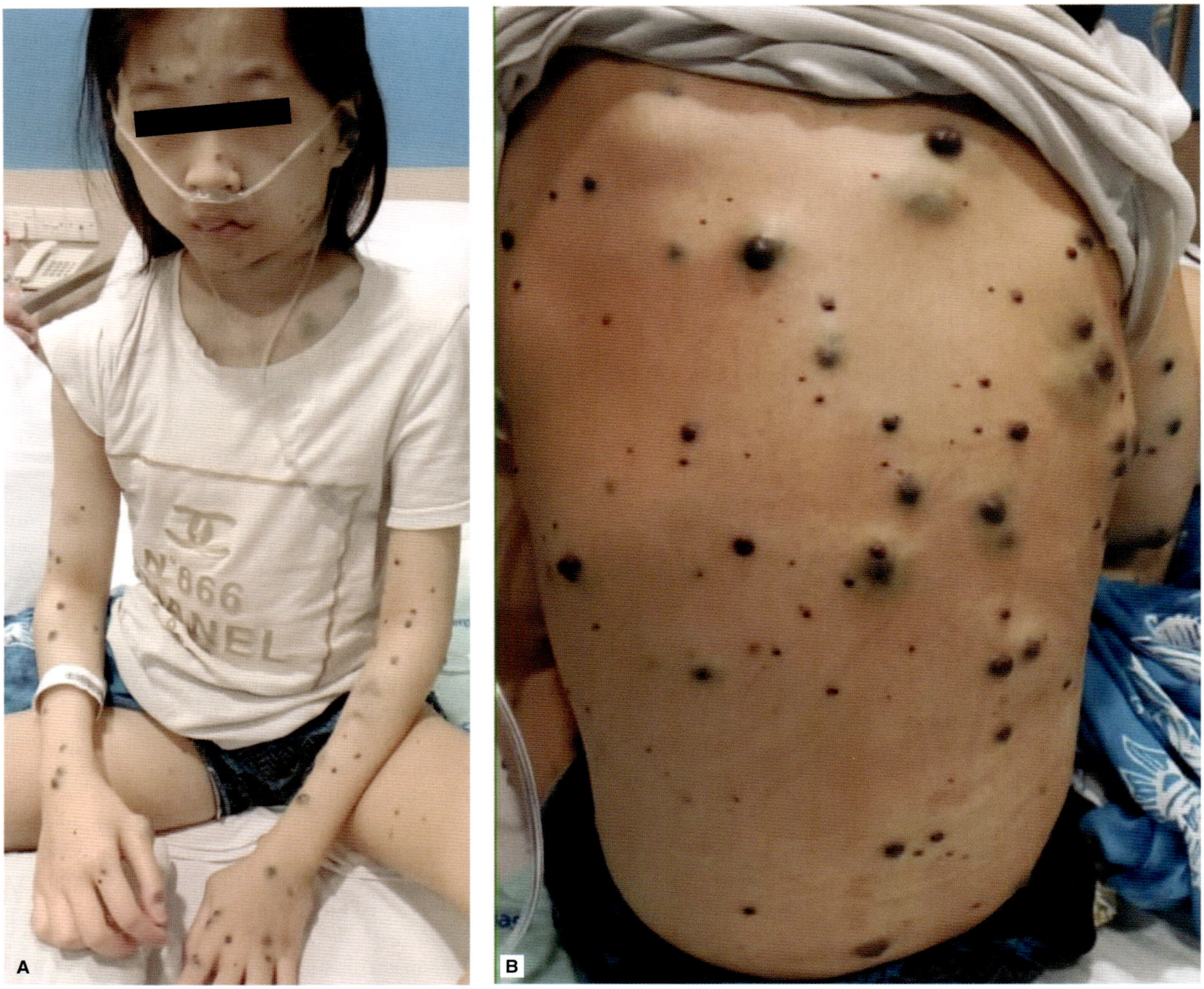

FIGURE 13-77A & 77B. BRBNS in an Indonesian girl presenting with progressively increasing numbers of venous malformations over her entire skin surface. She has multiple gastrointestinal venous malformations causing severe anemia from chronic blood loss. (Photograph courtesy of Dr. Djohan Kho, Medan, Indonesia.)

Investigations & Treatment

- BRBNS is usually clinically suspected, with the diagnosis supported by imaging, histology, and endoscopy.
- Biopsies of the skin or gastrointestinal lesions will reveal increased dilated and tortuous venous channels with dystrophic calcification.
- Endoscopy will aid in diagnosis of gastrointestinal involvement. However, visualization of the small bowel may be difficult with regular esophagoduodenoscopy and colonoscopy, and may require capsule endoscopy.
- MRI may be required to assess for other organ involvement, depending on the clinical presentation.
- Multidisciplinary and multimodality management is required, and varies depending on the severity and location of disease. Treatment of gastrointestinal involvement includes regular blood transfusions and iron supplementation for anemia, sclerotherapy, systemic medications such as mTOR inhibitors (e.g., sirolimus and everolimus), and surgical excision. Patients with life-threatening gastrointestinal bleeding may require partial bowel resection.
- The cutaneous venous malformations may be treated with vascular or ablative lasers, sclerotherapy, or surgical resection.

Pearls & Practical Tips

- Genetic testing for *TIE2* mutations can be performed on lesional tissue, as the mutation is somatic.
- Rarely, patients may present with only gastrointestinal involvement, without cutaneous involvement.

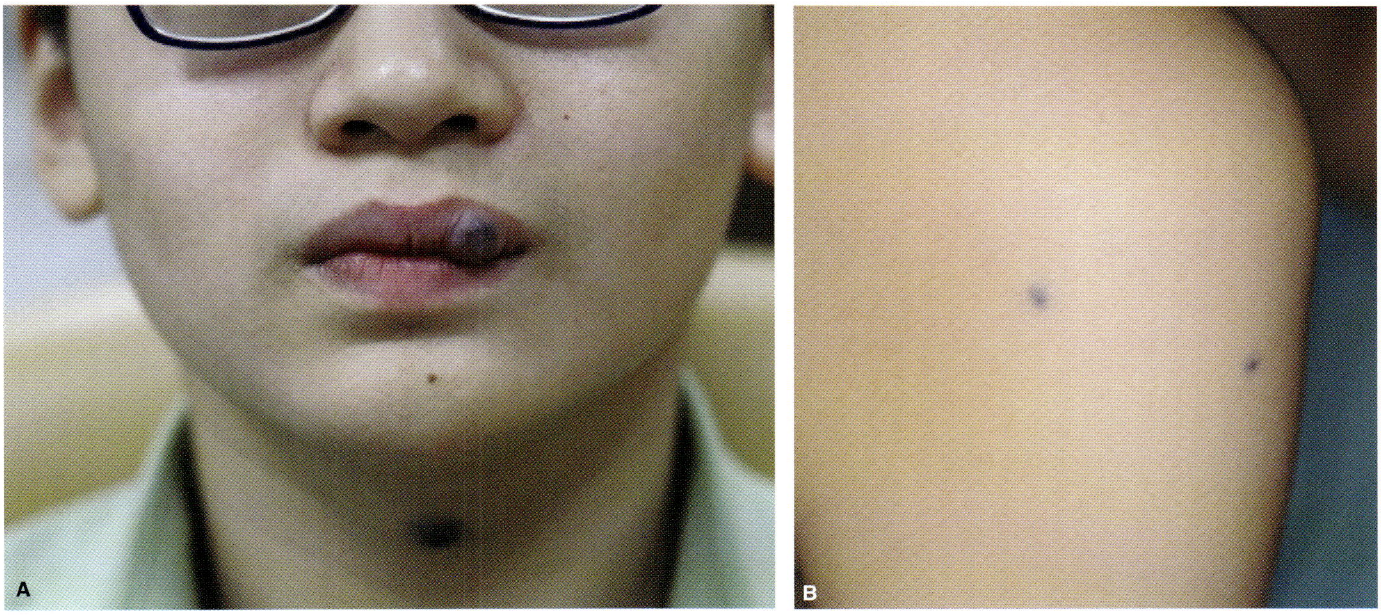

FIGURE 13-78A & 78B. BRBNS in a Chinese boy presenting initially with recurrent anemia secondary to gastrointestinal bleeding. He has several small venous malformations on his face, limbs, and trunk.

- Patients and caregivers should be counseled on the high risk of severe gastrointestinal bleeding and intussusception.

BIBLIOGRAPHY

1. Yuksekkaya H, Ozbek O, Keser M, Toy H. Blue rubber bleb nevus syndrome: successful treatment with sirolimus. Pediatrics. 2012 Apr;129(4):e1080-4.
2. Moser CM, Hamsch C. Successful treatment of cutaneous venous malformations in a patient with blue rubber bleb naevus syndrome by Nd:YAG laser. Br J Dermatol 2012;166(5):1143-5.

14

Skin Tumors and Tumor Syndromes

EPIDERMAL NEVUS

Epidermal nevi are common, benign congenital tumors resulting from proliferation of epidermal keratinocytes. Most commonly an isolated cutaneous finding, extensive epidermal nevi may be associated with other systemic abnormalities (epidermal nevus syndrome).

Clinical Features

- Epidermal nevi are typically present from birth but can develop in early childhood.
- They appear as skin-colored or brown and can be flat or raised at presentation.

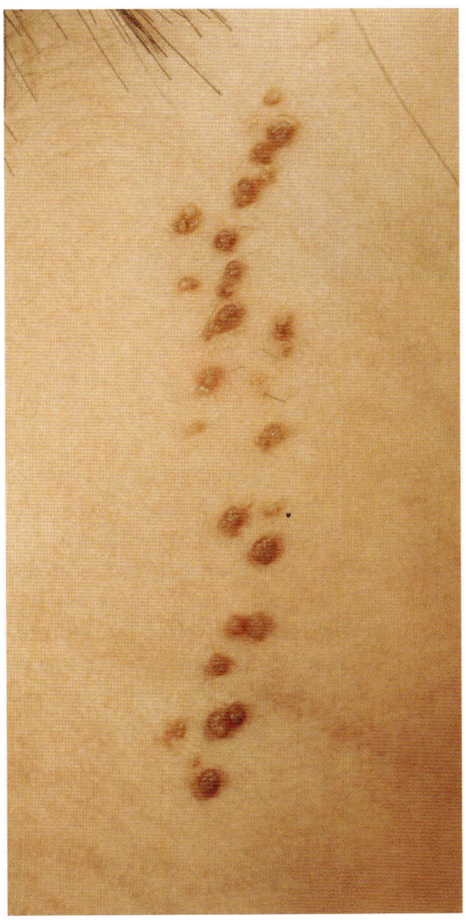

FIGURE 14-1. Epidermal nevus in a linear distribution on the neck of a 5-year-old Chinese girl.

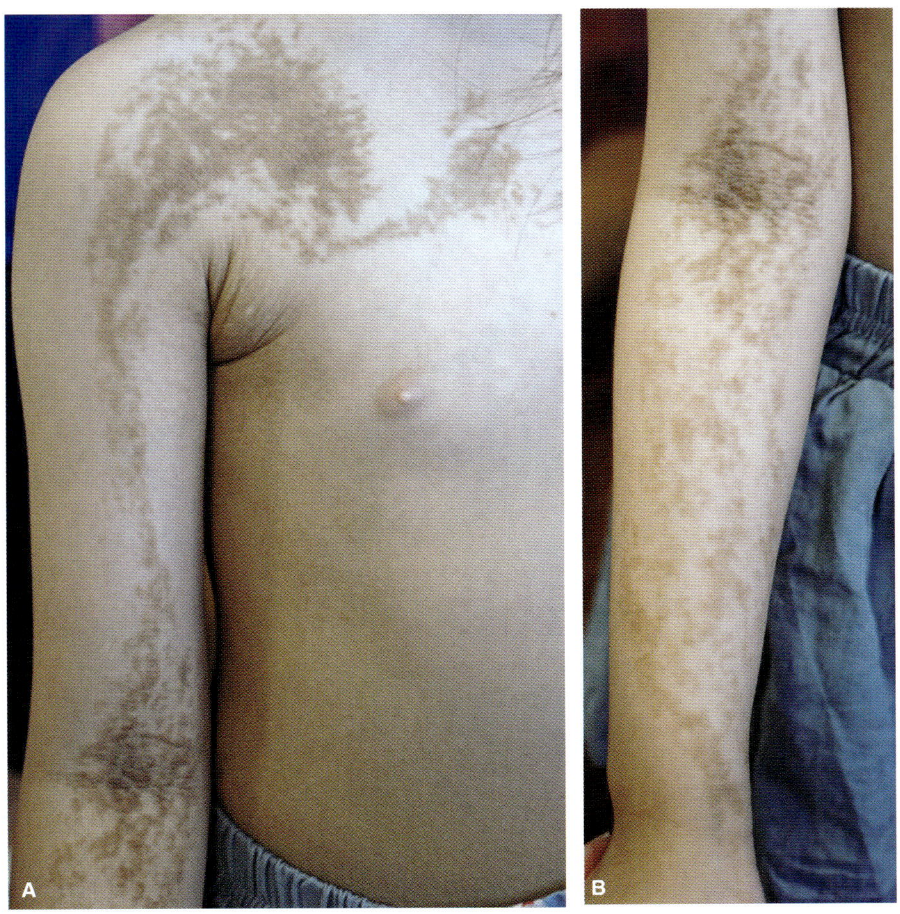

FIGURE 14-2A & 2B. Epidermal nevus on the arm of a Chinese girl. In younger children, the lesions can appear rather flat and be mistaken for pigmentary mosaicism. Closer inspection will reveal the irregular surface.

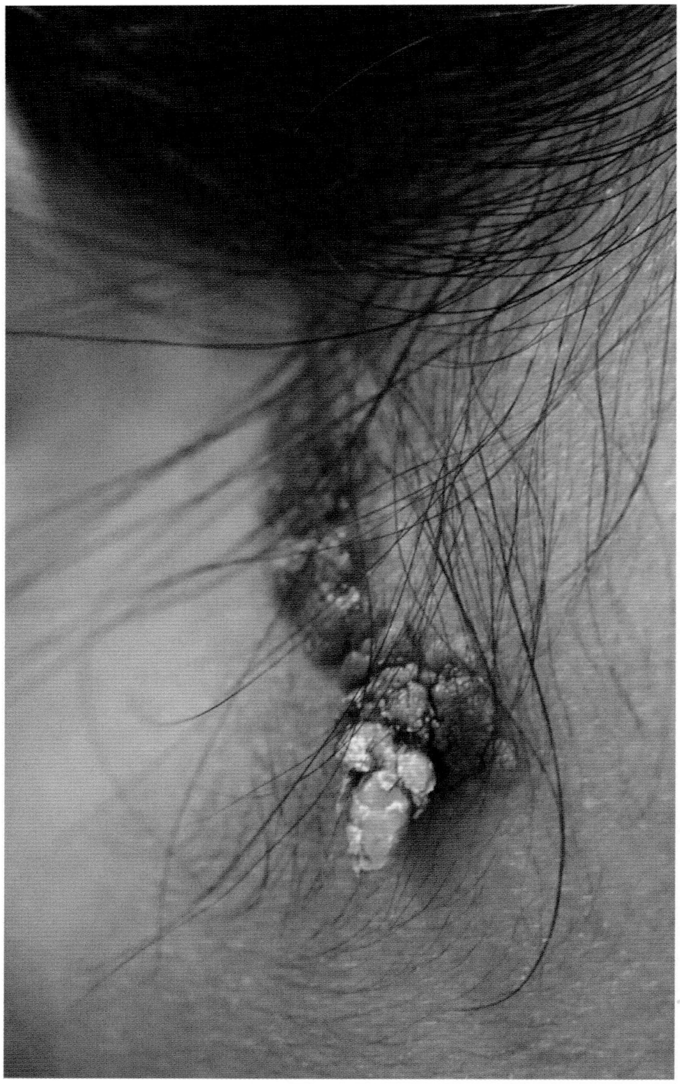

FIGURE 14-3. Epidermal nevus on the cheek of a Malay adolescent, which has become more verrucous and hyperpigmented since puberty.

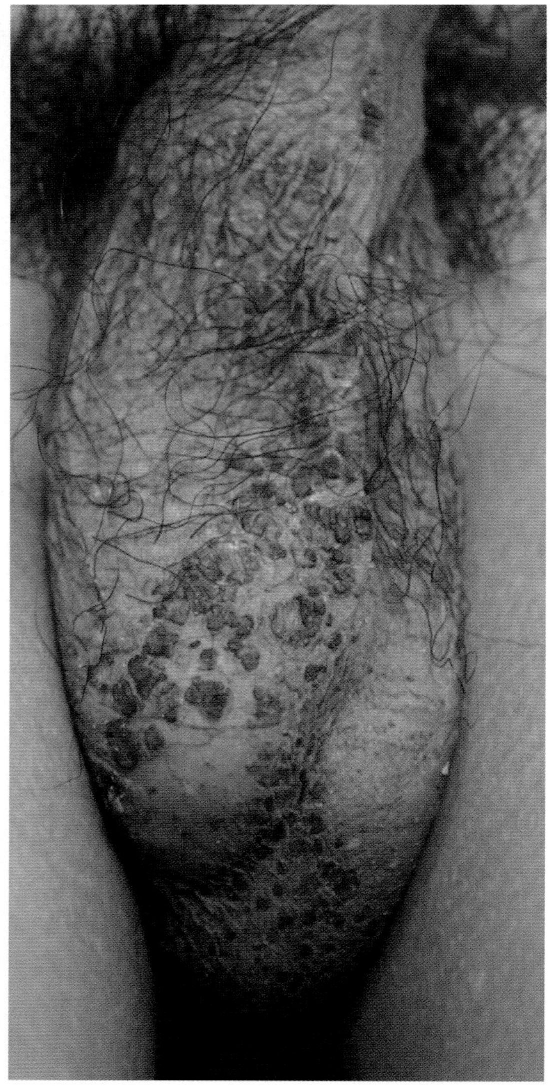

FIGURE 14-4. Epidermal nevus on the scrotum of an adolescent Chinese male. Biopsy showed features of epidermolytic hyperkeratosis, signifying a possible mutation in *KRT1* or *KRT10* genes.

- They are distributed along the lines of Blaschko, and often appear in a linear configuration.
- With time, the lesions can become darker and more raised, developing a verrucous appearance.
- Several subtypes of epidermal nevi have been described:
  - **Epidermolytic nevi** show features of "epidermolytic hyperkeratosis" on histology, with vacuolar degeneration of the granular cell layer with increased numbers of irregularly shaped keratohyaline granules. Somatic mosaic mutations in *KRT1* or *KRT10* have been described in these nevi. In patients with extensive epidermolytic nevi, if the mutation affects gonadal cells, epidermolytic ichthyosis (bullous congenita ichthyosiform erythroderma [BCIE]) can occur in their offspring (see section on genodermatoses).
  - **Acantholytic nevi** have a histological appearance reminiscent of Darier's disease, with loss of adhesion between suprabasal keratinocytes, dyskeratosis, and presence of corps ronds and grains, hyperkeratosis, and parakeratosis.
- Epidermal nevus syndrome is characterized by the presence of epidermal nevi associated with extracutaneous abnormalities, most often affecting the brain, eye, and skeletal systems. In these cases, the epidermal nevi are usually fairly extensive.

Differential Diagnoses

- Viral warts
  - These are benign verrucous growths caused by the human papilloma virus.

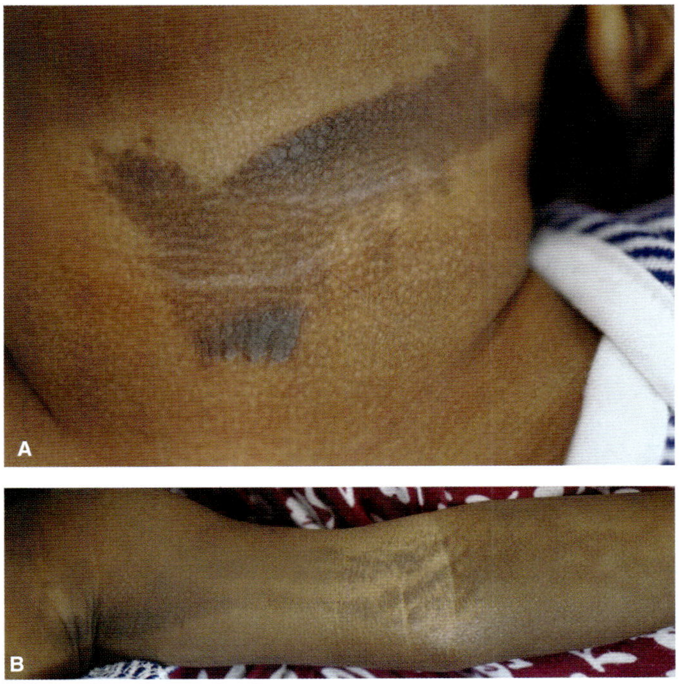

FIGURE 14-5A & 5B. Rather extensive epidermal nevus in an Indian girl affecting the neck, chest, and left arm in a Blaschkoid distribution.

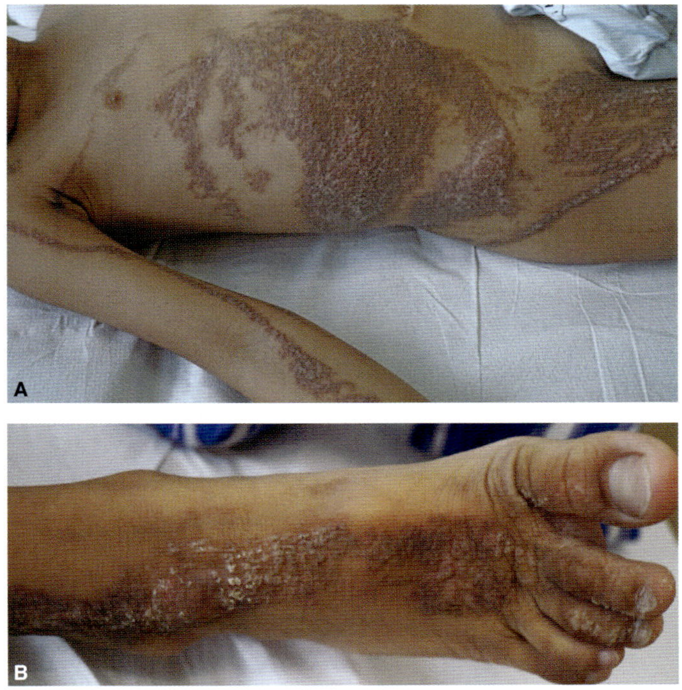

FIGURE 14-6A & 6B. "Systematized" epidermal nevus affecting large areas of one side of the body in a Malay boy. He did not have any associated organ involvement.

  - Lesions are rarely in a linear configuration.
  - Microthrombi may be seen on dermoscopic examination.
- Lichen striatus
  - This is an uncommon, idiopathic papular eruption of childhood characterized by skin-colored or hyperpigmented papules arranged in a linear configuration along the lines of Blaschko.
  - It usually resolves after months, with temporary hypopigmentation.

Investigations & Treatment

- Although not usually required, a biopsy will help to establish the diagnosis.
- Typical histologic features of hyperkeratosis, acanthosis, and papillomatosis may be seen.
- Small lesions may be treated conservatively, especially if not cosmetically significant.
- Dermabrasion, cryosurgery, electrosurgery, and ablative laser surgery can be used to treat epidermal nevi if indicated. Surgical excision can be performed for smaller lesions.

Pearls & Practical Tips

- Children with isolated, small epidermal nevi and no other cutaneous or systemic findings do not need further investigations.
- A systemic review should be performed to rule out neurologic, ocular, skeletal, and cardiovascular manifestations if the epidermal nevus is extensive, to exclude the epidermal nevus syndrome.
- Unlike nevus sebaceous, epidermal nevi do not undergo malignant transformation.

INFLAMMATORY LINEAR VERRUCOUS EPIDERMAL NEVUS

Inflammatory linear verrucous epidermal nevus (ILVEN) is an uncommon condition characterized by inflamed warty lesions that group together in a linear pattern along the lines of Blaschko.

Clinical Features

- Arises usually during the first 5 years of life, and affects females more than males.
- Lesions are usually unilateral and more commonly affect the lower half of the body. They appear as red or pink, inflamed, with overlying scaling or hyperkeratosis. Lesions can be painful.
- The lesions progress gradually over a few months.

Differential Diagnoses

- Lichen striatus
  - More common condition in children and also presents as pinkish-to-erythematous papules or plaques in a linear configuration. Usually less hyperkeratotic than ILVEN.

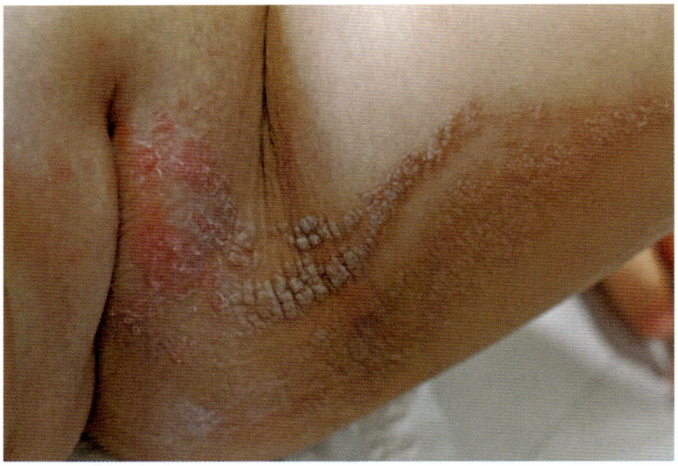

FIGURE 14-7. ILVEN on the perineum and thigh of a Chinese infant girl.

- Tends to resolve faster than ILVEN, to leave a hypopigmented linear streak.
- Linear psoriasis
  - Rare variant of psoriasis characterized by linear distribution of psoriatic lesions along lines of Blaschko.
  - Responds more favorably to topical treatments such as topical corticosteroids and vitamin D derivatives.
- Linear lichen planus
  - Rare variant of lichen planus characterized by violaceous papules distributed along the lines of Blaschko. Usually appears more violaceous and scaly compared to ILVEN.

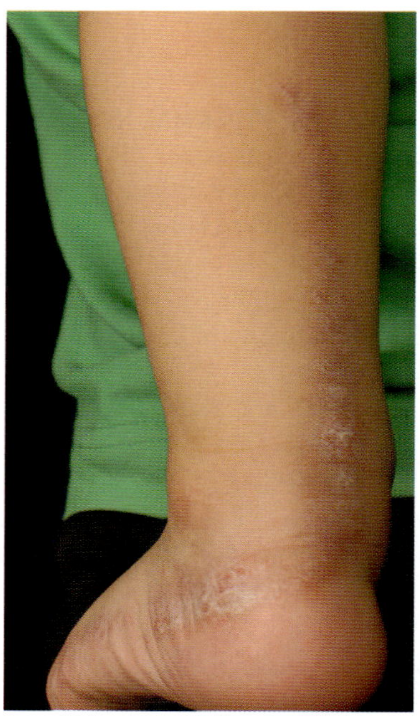

FIGURE 14-8. ILVEN on the posterior calf extending down to the lateral sole of this infant. There is clinical overlap with lichen striatus in this case.

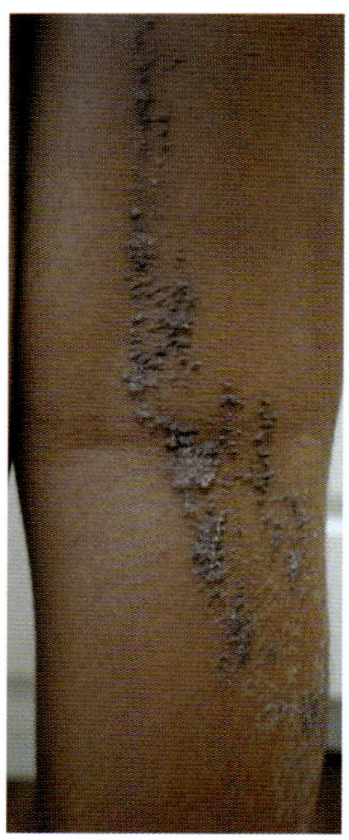

FIGURE 14-9. ILVEN on the posterior thigh of an Indian girl.

Investigations & Treatment

- A skin biopsy can be helpful in making the diagnosis of ILVEN and differentiating it from the other differential diagnoses.
- Histologically, there is psoriasiform epidermal hyperplasia with alternating orthokeratosis and parakeratosis. Areas of orthokeratosis overlie areas of hypergranulosis, while areas of parakeratosis overlie areas of hypogranulosis. A dense mixed inflammatory infiltrate in the superficial dermis is usually seen.
- Emollients and topical corticosteroids may help to alleviate itch. However, treatment can be disappointing.
- Other topical treatments that can be considered include topical calcineurin inhibitors, topical vitamin D analogs, and topical retinoids.
- Surgical modalities such as excision, cryosurgery, and CO_2 laser therapy can also be used.

Pearls & Practical Tips

- ILVEN can clinically and histologically mimic linear psoriasis and may sometimes respond to topical treatments that are commonly used in psoriasis.

NEVUS SEBACEOUS

Nevus sebaceous, also referred to as organoid nevus, is a congenital hamartoma of the pilosebaceous follicular unit. Although benign in nature, secondary tumors, which are infrequently malignant, can occur in later years.

Clinical Features

- Nevus sebaceous most commonly presents at birth as a well-defined, thin, yellow-orange hairless patch or plaque that is usually oval or linear. Lesions are sometimes not noticed until later in childhood or rarely, after puberty.
- After the first 5 to 6 months of life, the lesion may become thinner due to reduction in maternal hormonal stimulation.

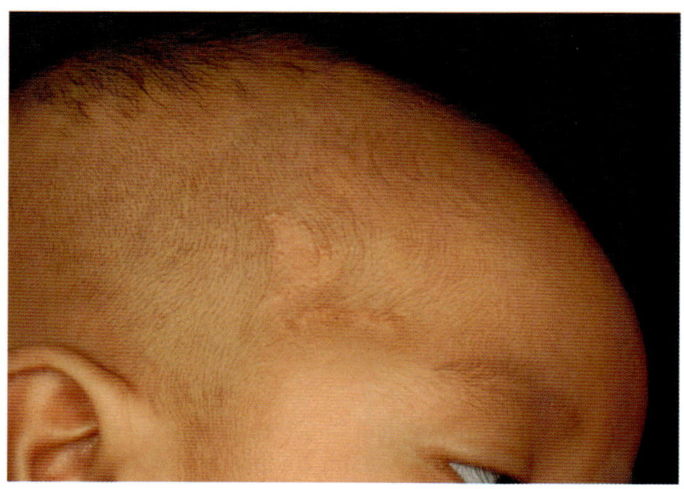

FIGURE 14-10. Nevus sebaceous on the temporal scalp and forehead of an infant Malay boy.

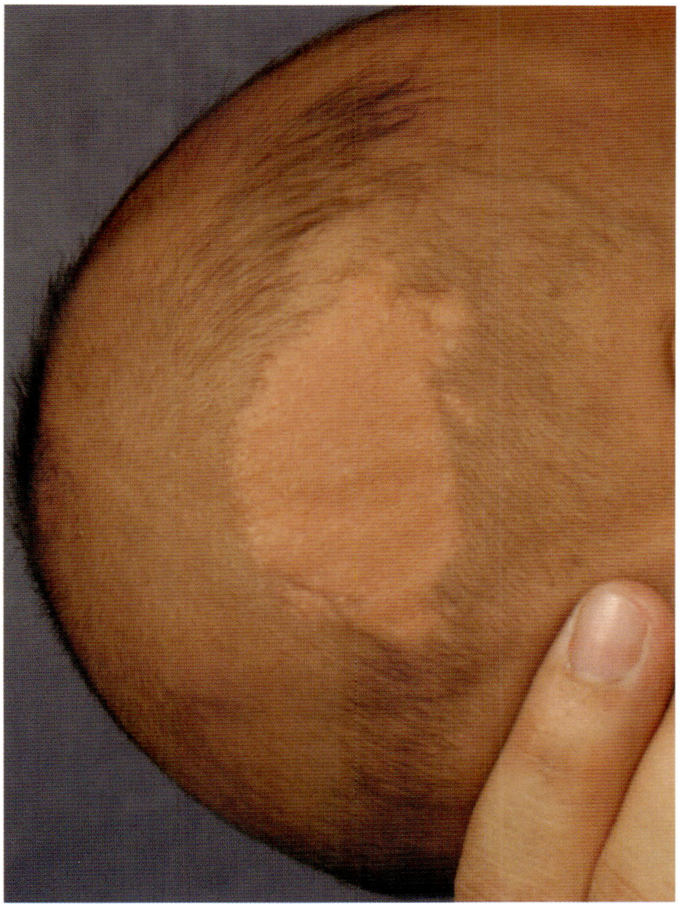

FIGURE 14-11. Large but flat nevus sebaceous on the parietotemporal scalp of an infant Malay boy.

- During puberty and adulthood, lesions tend to become more elevated, verrucous, or nodular.
- The size can range from one to several centimeters. Rarely, lesions can be more extensive.
- Secondary benign and malignant tumors may arise within a nevus sebaceous.
- Common benign tumors include trichoblastoma, syringocystadenoma papilliferum, and trichilemmoma. These tumors can develop at any time, including from birth.
- Malignant neoplasms, which usually occur in adulthood, include basal cell carcinoma, squamous cell carcinoma, apocrine carcinoma, trichilemmal carcinoma, sebaceous carcinoma, and porocarcinoma.
- Extensive nevus sebaceous may be associated with abnormalities affecting the brain, eyes, and bones (Schimmelpenning syndrome). Mosaic mutations in HRAS or KRAS have been identified in some patients. Patients may have neurological abnormalities including seizures, developmental delays, intellectual impairment, and hemimegalencephaly. Skeletal defects include craniofacial defects, hypoplastic bones, short stature, and vitamin D-resistant hypophosphatemic rickets.

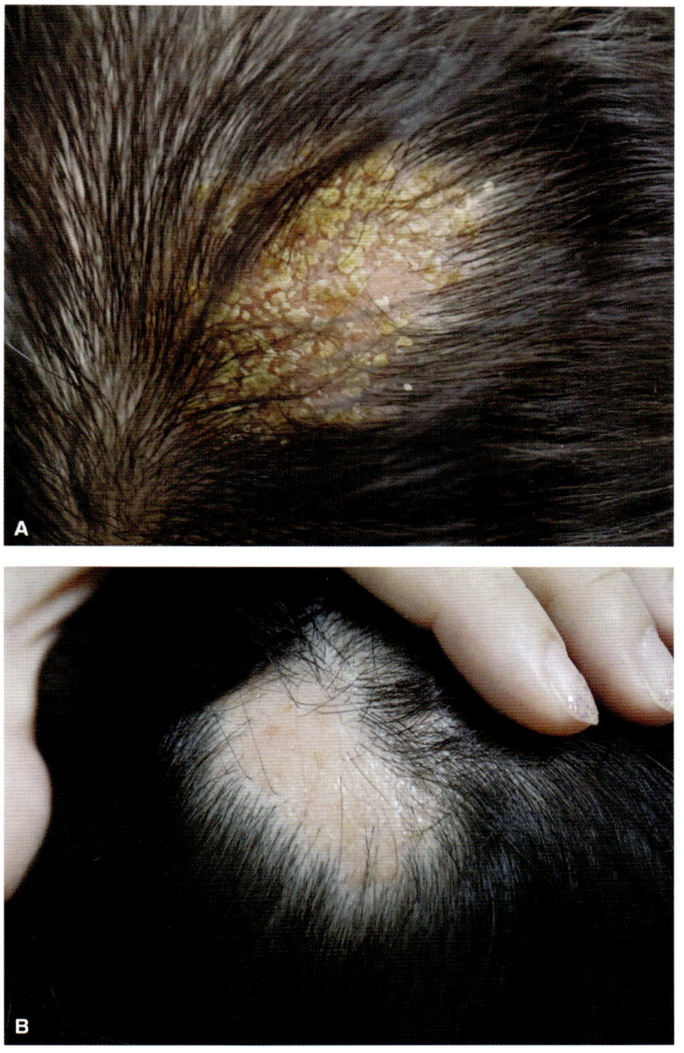

FIGURE 14-12A & 12B. Nevus sebaceous in a 3-month-old infant with overlying seborrheic dermatitis (Figure 14-12A). The same child at 3 years of age when the nevus sebaceous appears flatter (Figure 14-12B).

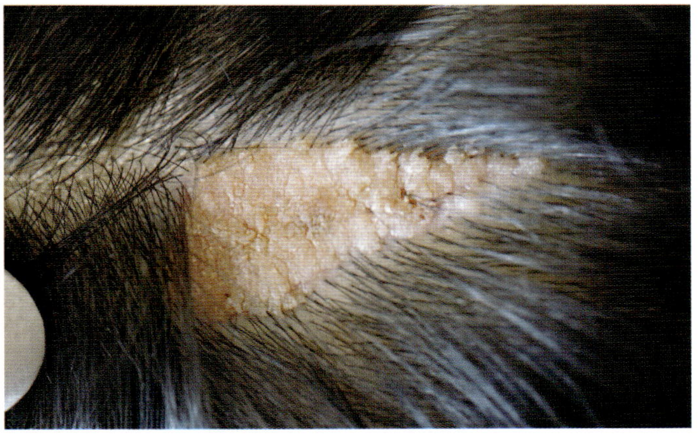

FIGURE 14-13. Nevus sebaceous in a 12-year-old boy which has become more verrucous during puberty.

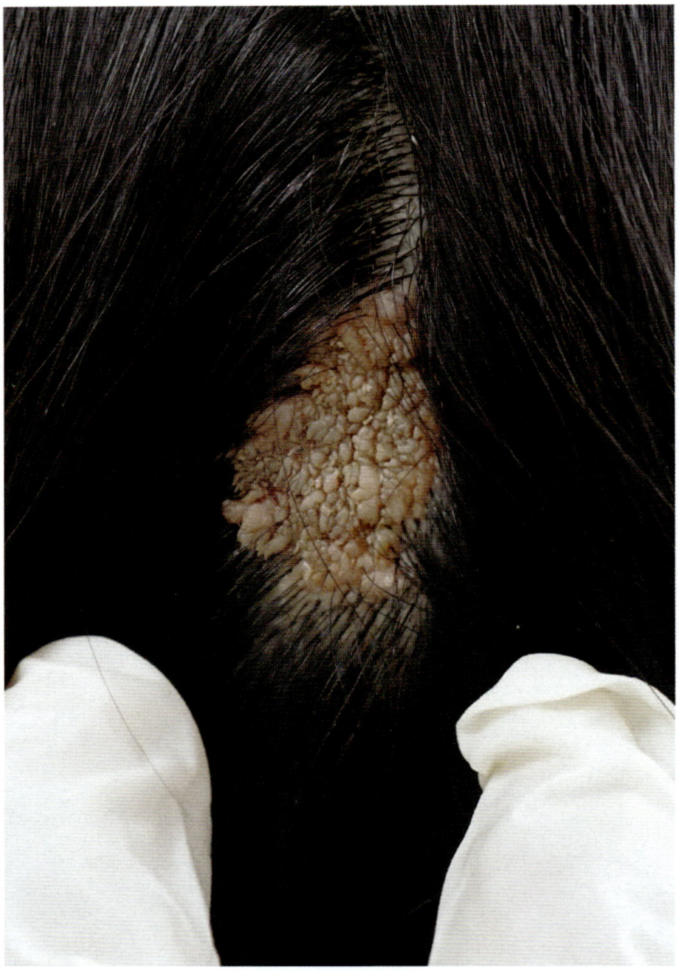

FIGURE 14-14. Hypertrophic nevus sebaceous in a 14-year-old Nepalese female. The lesion was eventually excised.

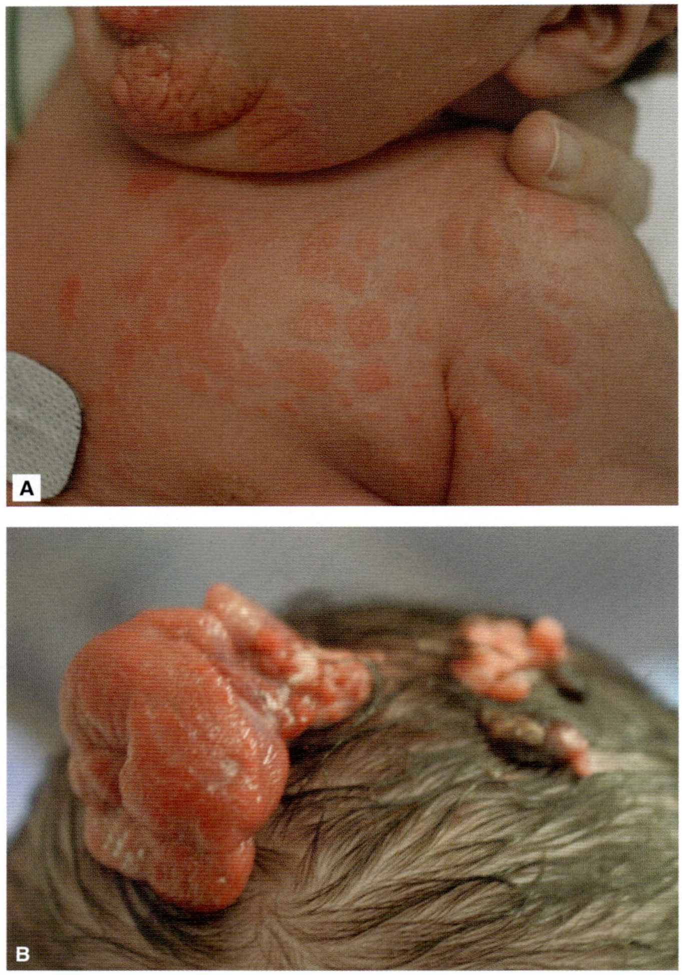

FIGURE 14-16A & 16B. Extensive "systematized" nevus sebaceous affecting the scalp, face, trunk, and upper limbs. Secondary tumors arising from the scalp lesions, representing trichoblastoma and syringocystadenoma papilliferum, were present from birth (Figure 14-16B).

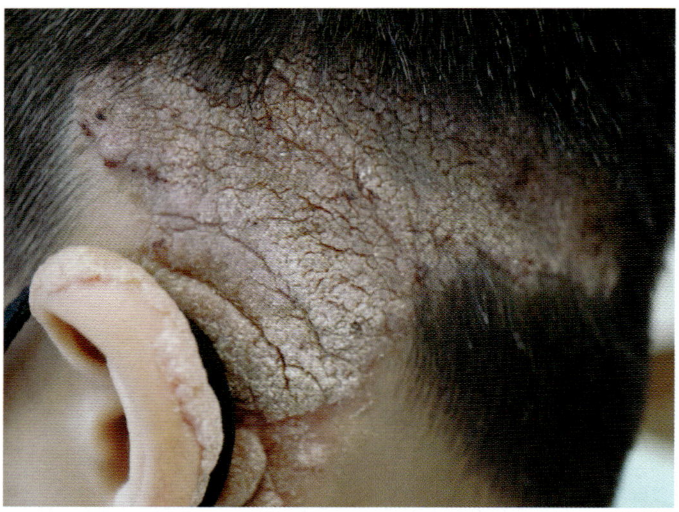

FIGURE 14-15. Hypertrophic nevus sebaceous in a 13-year-old Chinese male. The lesions became thicker with age, especially during puberty.

Differential Diagnoses

- Juvenile xanthogranuloma
  - Usually presents in infants or young children as reddish-to-yellow papules, plaques, or nodules. Rarely occurs congenitally.
- Aplasia cutis congenita
  - Presents at birth as an atrophic or scarred alopecic defect, most commonly on the scalp. They are sharply demarcated, non-inflammatory, and may have surface ulcerations.
  - The lesion usually re-epithelializes over several months and forms a smooth atrophic or fibrotic scar.
- Cutaneous mastocytoma
  - Presents as a yellow to reddish-brown macule, patch, or plaque, usually with a "peau d'orange" surface. Lesions may urticate upon rubbing (Darier sign).
  - Rarely presents at birth but can occur within the first few months of life.
  - Usually resolves within a few years.

Investigations & Treatment

- The diagnosis of nevus sebaceous is usually made clinically.
- A punch biopsy may be performed for histologic confirmation. Typical histopathologic findings include epidermal papillomatosis and acanthosis, high-lying hyperplastic sebaceous glands, decreased or primitive hair follicles, and ectopic apocrine glands.
- Treatment is with full-thickness excision.
- There is a high risk of recurrence after laser resurfacing.

Pearls & Practical Tips

- Most secondary tumors arising in a nevus sebaceous occur in adulthood. However, they can occur congenitally, in childhood, or during adolescence. Malignant tumors occur mostly in adulthood. Multiple secondary tumors can occur simultaneously.
- The most common skin malignancy is basal cell carcinoma.
- As the risk for developing secondary carcinomas is low, excision under local anesthesia can be deferred to late childhood or adolescence. As lesions can become thick and verrucous, they can become traumatized during hair combing or styling. Cosmesis is another indication for excision.
- Seborrheic dermatitis or eczema can occur over a patch of nevus sebaceous during infancy, a phenomenon also known as the "Meyerson phenomenon."

PILOMATRICOMA

Pilomatricoma, or pilomatrixoma, is a benign proliferation derived from hair matrix cells. It most commonly presents in infants and young children.

Clinical Features

- Pilomatricomas are typically found on the head and neck region but can also be found on the trunk or limbs.
- Lesions are usually asymptomatic and grow relatively slowly. They may remain stable for years or grow slowly up to several centimeters in diameter.
- They may be skin-colored, erythematous, or have a bluish hue.
- They characteristically feel firm or hard due to calcification or even ossification within the lesion. This also results in an angulated shape, also known as the "tent" sign.
- If multiple, they can be rarely associated with inherited conditions such as Rubinstein-Taybi syndrome, Gardner syndrome, or myotonic dystrophy.

Differential Diagnoses

- Epidermal cyst
  - Skin-colored or grayish papule or nodule, usually with a central punctum, and does not feel as firm as pilomatricomas.
  - Contains keratinous material that can be expressed through the central punctum

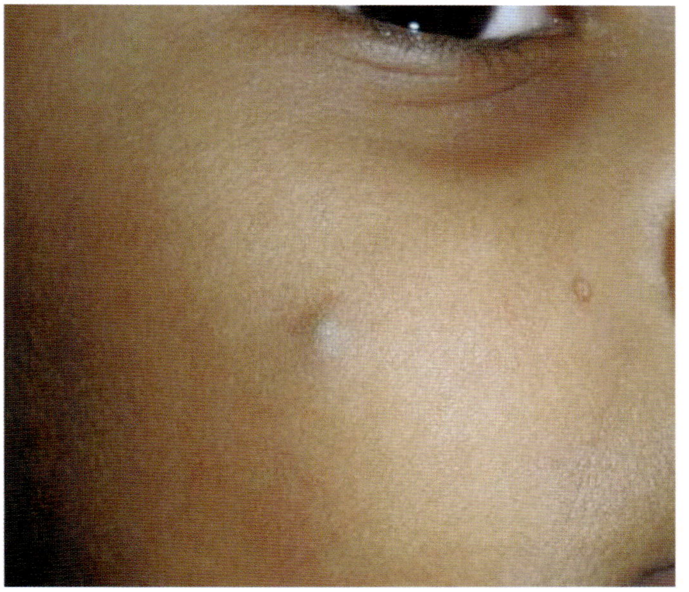

FIGURE 14-17. Pilomatricoma on the cheek of an Indian girl presenting as a firm, bluish, deep papule. (Courtesy of Professor Sandipan Dhar, FRCP.)

- Dermoid cyst
  - Harmless, cystic growth that is present at birth or within the first few years of life.
  - Softer, cystic lesion compared to pilomatricoma, which is usually firmer.
- Dermatofibroma
  - Usually deeper and more rubbery than a pilomatricoma.
  - Color is more hyperpigmented in the center, usually with a depression.

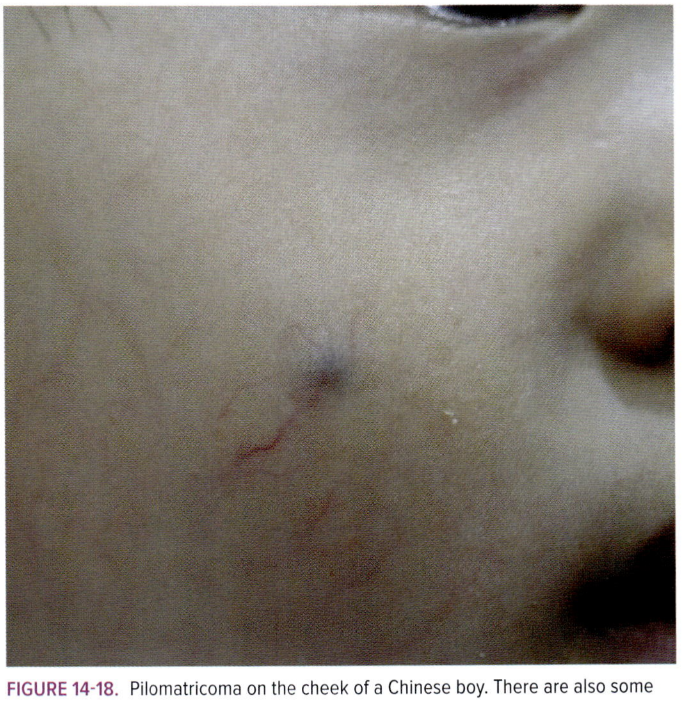

FIGURE 14-18. Pilomatricoma on the cheek of a Chinese boy. There are also some surrounding telangiectasias, which are unrelated to the pilomatricoma.

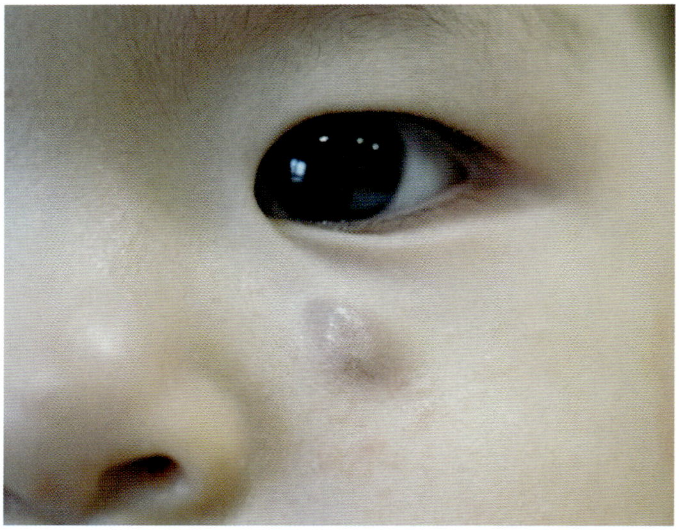

FIGURE 14-19. A large pilomatricoma on the cheek of a Chinese toddler. There is some surrounding eczema in this child, with concomitant atopic dermatitis.

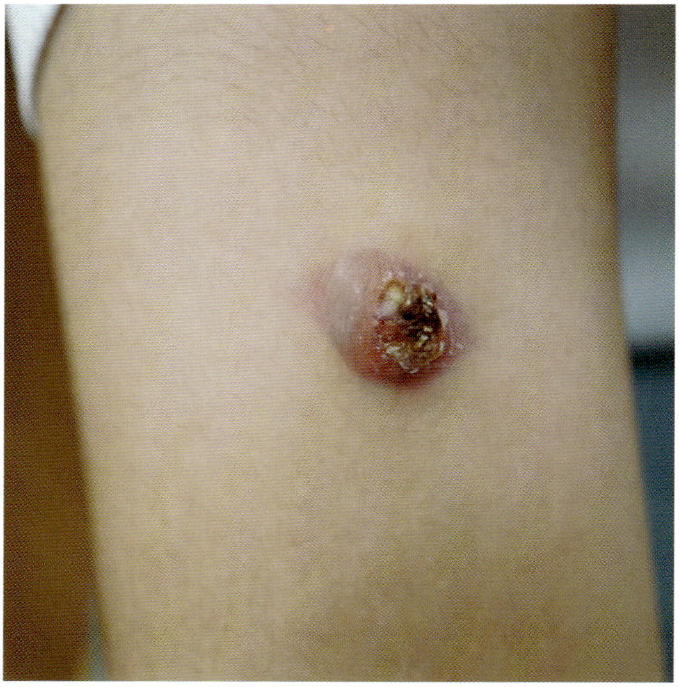

FIGURE 14-21. "Perforating" pilomatricoma on the arm of a Chinese girl, presenting as a ulcerated nodule.

   - Occurs more commonly in adolescents and adults, but can also be seen less commonly in children.

Investigations & Treatment

- Although pilomatricomas may be diagnosed clinically, doubtful cases can be biopsied for confirmation by histology, which is characteristic. There is a well-circumscribed tumor in the dermis consisting of basophilic matrical cells that transition into eosinophilic "shadow" cells with missing nuclei. Calcium deposits and multinucleated cells can also be seen.
- Treatment involves limited excision of the lesion. Recurrences are uncommon.

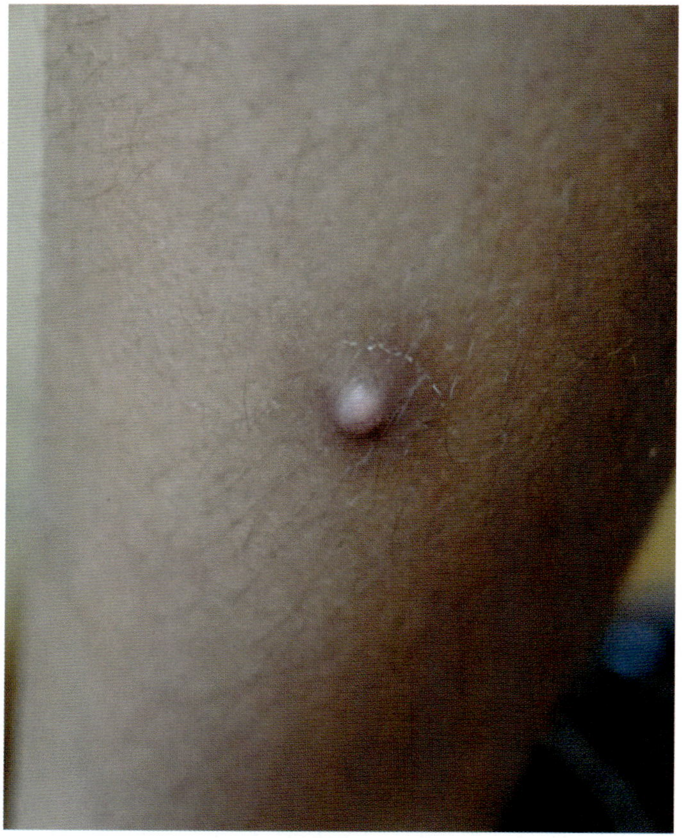

FIGURE 14-20. Pilomatricoma on the calf of an Indian boy, presenting as a firm, pink, sessile papule.

Pearls & Practical Tips

- The "see-saw" or "teeter-totter" sign is a characteristic clinical feature of pilomatricomas—pushing down on one end of the lesion causes the other end to "pop" upward.
- As pilomatricomas are very well circumscribed; they may be removed quite easily with an incision over the surface and delivering the nodule/tumor through the incision, akin to pushing a button through a buttonhole.

DERMOID CYST

Dermoid cysts are fairly common developmental cysts that are lined by epithelium and extend inward from the skin surface. Although they may not be obvious at birth, they usually present in the first few years of life.

Clinical Features

- Usually present at birth but may not be noticeable until a few months, or by 5 years of age.
- Present as soft, round, and rubbery subcutaneous nodules with normal overlying skin.

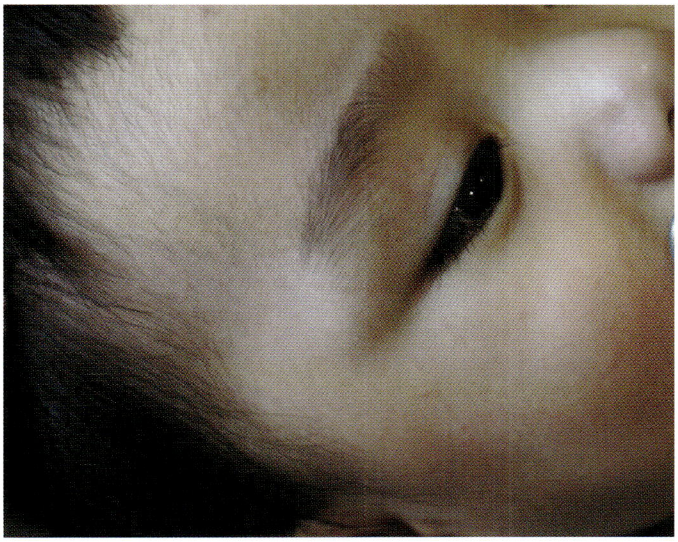

FIGURE 14-22. A Malay infant with dermoid cyst over the lateral third of the eyebrow.

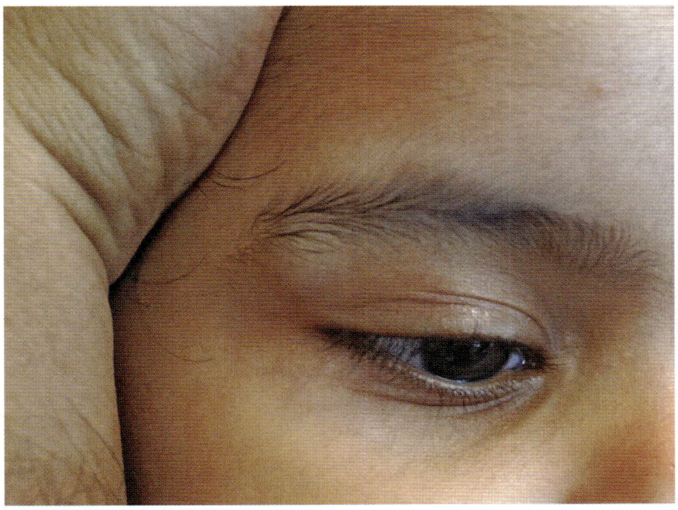

FIGURE 14-23. A young Indian child with dermoid cyst over the lateral third of the eyebrow.

- Most commonly found at the temporal forehead, lateral eyebrow, or lateral canthus, especially the last third of the eyebrow and midline nasal bridge. They can also be found on the scalp.

Differential Diagnoses

- Epidermal cyst
  - Epidermal cysts may have a central punctum.
  - Usually does not occur along embryonic cleft closure sites.
- Trichilemmal cyst
  - Trichilemmal cysts usually occur over the scalp.
- Deep infantile hemangioma
  - The overlying skin may feel warmer than the surrounding skin, and an arterial signal will be elicited on Doppler ultrasound.

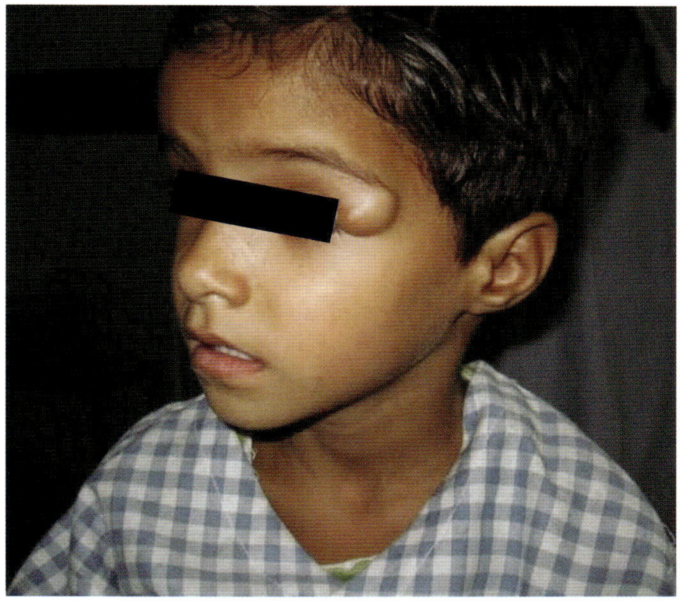

FIGURE 14-24. Dermoid cyst over the lateral third of the eyebrow and lateral canthus. (Courtesy of Professor Sandipan Dhar, FRCP.)

Investigations & Treatment

- Histology shows a cyst lined by stratified squamous epithelium with the presence of pilosebaceous structures within the cyst.
- Midline lesions should have MRI or axial CT prior to excision to exclude any intracranial extension to avoid ascending infection.
- Midline lesions should be managed by a team which may include neurosurgeon, plastic surgeon, and otolaryngologist.
- Lateral lesions usually have no intracranial extension and as such, imaging may not be necessary. These lesions can be removed by primary excision.

Pearls & Practical Tips

- As deep infantile hemangioma is a differential diagnosis, Doppler ultrasound is useful to differentiate the two conditions.
- Small lesions may be treated conservatively.

SYRINGOMA

Syringomas are benign tumors derived from eccrine sweat glands, occur more commonly in adolescents and young adults, and are uncommon in children. They are usually isolated to the face but more eruptive, generalized forms have been described.

Clinical Features

- Syringomas appear as skin-colored papules that may be solitary or in clusters.
- They most commonly occur around the eyes and nose, but can also occur on the chest, abdomen, extremities, axillae, and vulva.
- Patients are usually otherwise healthy.

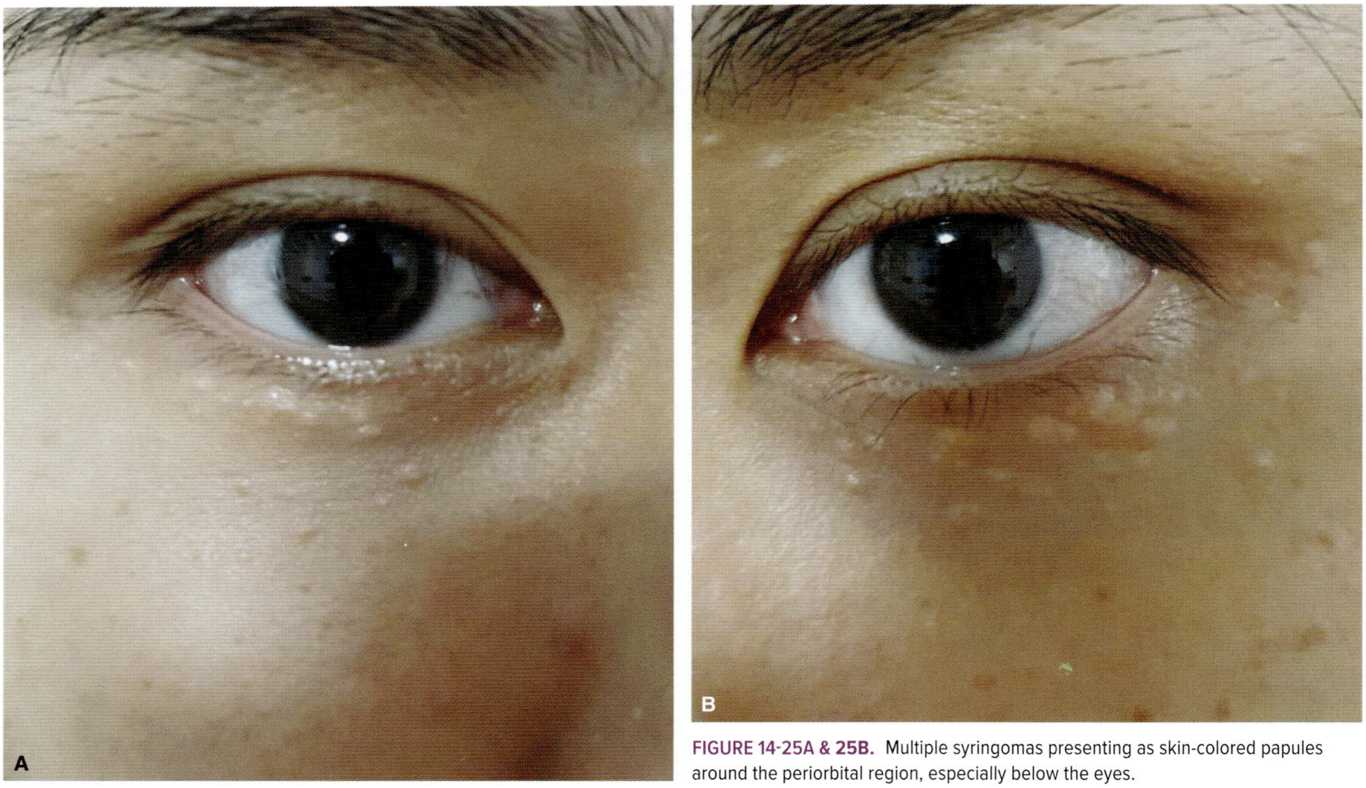

FIGURE 14-25A & 25B. Multiple syringomas presenting as skin-colored papules around the periorbital region, especially below the eyes.

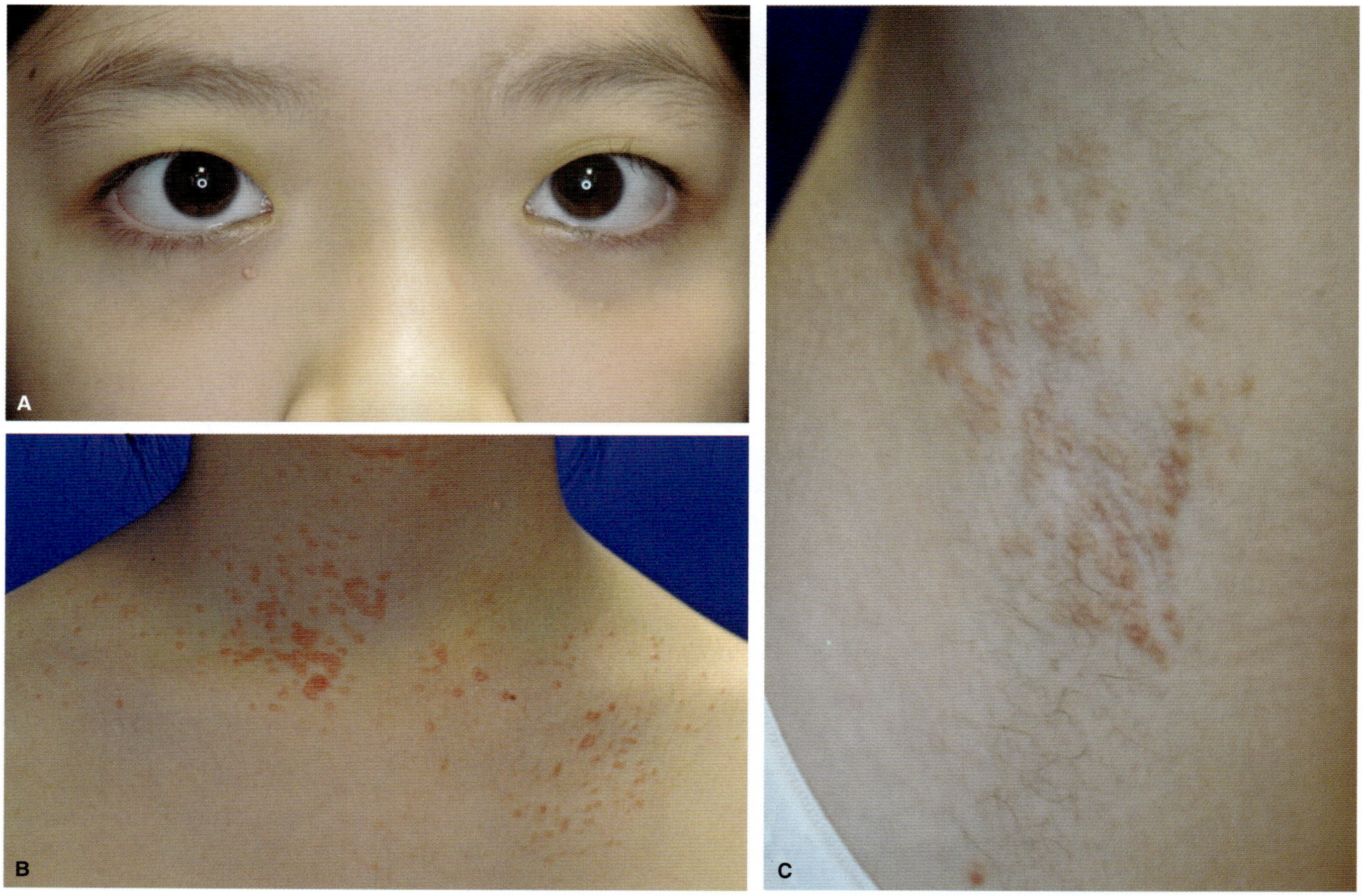

FIGURE 14-26A–26C. Eruptive syringomas in a Chinese adolescent girl, presenting as multiple pink-orange papules over the face, neck, chest, and axillae.

Differential Diagnoses

- Milia
  - Firm, pearly white, well-circumscribed dome-shaped papules that are also commonly seen around the eyes. May also be multiple.
- Trichoepithelioma
  - Firm papules which may appear as yellow, pink, brown, bluish, or skin-colored and have predilection for the nose and nasolabial folds.
  - May require biopsy to differentiate from syringomas, especially in children.
- Angiofibroma/fibrous papule
  - Presents as a solitary, flesh- to tan-colored papule, most often on the nose.
  - Multiple lesions may be seen in patients with tuberous sclerosis.

Investigations & Treatment

- Histology shows small ducts with dilated lumen lined by two-layered epithelium, often with comma-shaped extensions with a "tadpole" pattern.
- Can be treated conservatively.
- If required, treatment options include topical retinoids, electrocautery, ablative lasers (e.g., carbon dioxide laser), and excision.

Pearls & Practical Tips

- The risk of recurrence is common after treatment, and patients and caregivers should be advised accordingly.

TRICHOEPITHELIOMA

Trichoepitheliomas are fairly common, benign tumors derived from hair follicles. They can be inherited in an autosomal dominant fashion. Although more common in late adolescence and adulthood, they can occur in children.

Clinical Features

- Trichoepitheliomas present as small, firm, skin-colored papules. They occasionally can also appear yellow, pink, or brown. They measure between 2 and 5 mm in size.
- The distribution is usually on the central face, especially around the nose and nasolabial folds. Rarely, they can occur on the scalp, neck, trunk, and genitalia.
- Mutations in *CYLD* gene have been found in patients with syndromes characterized by multiple trichoepitheliomas, such as multiple familial trichoepithelioma and Brooke-Spiegler syndrome. The latter is an autosomal dominant condition, with multiple trichoepitheliomas, spiradenomas, and cylindromas.

Differential Diagnoses

- Milia
  - Firm, pearly white, well-circumscribed dome-shaped papules that are also commonly seen around the eyes. May also be multiple.
- Syringomas
  - Skin-colored papules usually symmetrically over the eyelids, cheeks.

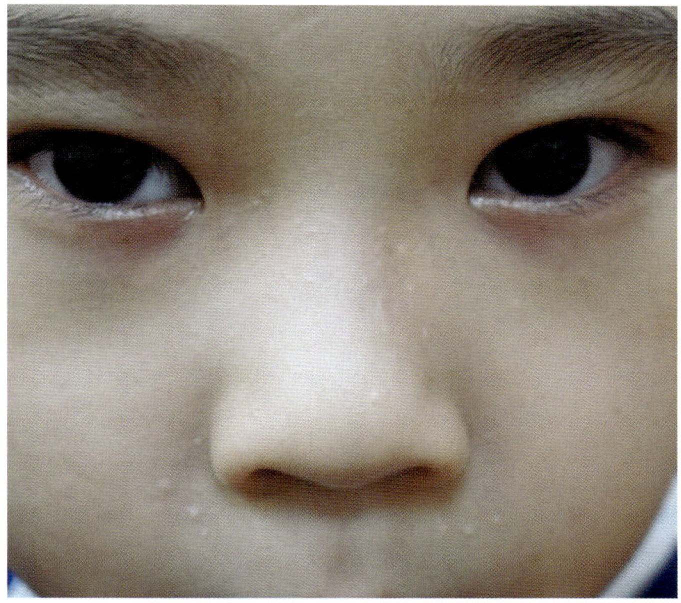

FIGURE 14-27. Multiple trichoepitheliomas presenting on the face of a Chinese boy.

  - May be difficult to differentiate from trichoepitheliomas if solitary, and require histology for confirmation.
- Angiofibroma/fibrous papule
  - Presents as a solitary, flesh- to tan-colored papule, most often on the nose.
  - Multiple lesions may be seen in patients with tuberous sclerosis.

Investigations & Treatment

- Histology is confirmatory and shows a circumscribed tumor comprising of nests of basaloid cells with horn cysts in the dermis. There is associated peripheral palisading with stromal clefting, a fibrotic stroma, and papillary mesenchymal bodies.

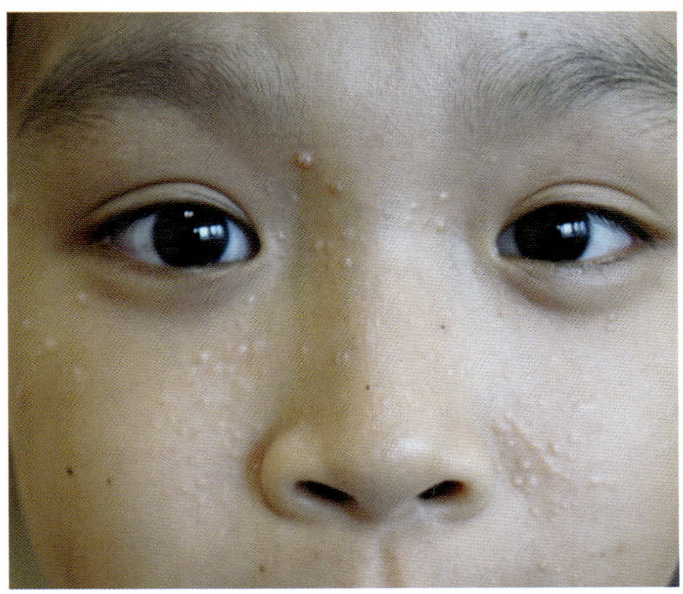

FIGURE 14-28. Multiple trichoepitheliomas on the face of an older Chinese boy presenting with multiple white or skin-colored papules.

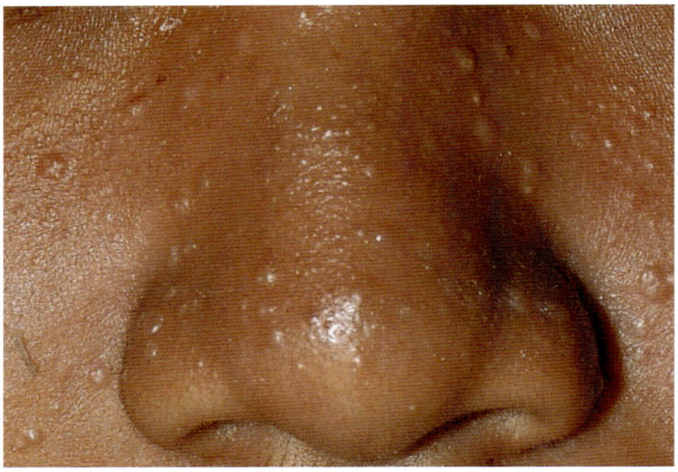

FIGURE 14-29. Multiple trichoepitheliomas presenting as firm, skin-colored papules on the nose and nasolabial fold area. (Courtesy of Dr. Leong Kin Fon, MRCPCH.)

- Excision is usually the treatment of choice if cosmetically indicated. Other treatment options include electrocautery, cryotherapy, and laser ablation.

Pearls & Practical Tips

- Apart from excision, risk of recurrence after other forms of ablative treatment (e.g., electrocautery) is high.

EPIDERMAL CYSTS

Epidermal cysts are more common in adults but can occur in adolescents, and less commonly in children. They represent true cysts with an epithelial lining. They are most common on the scalp, head, neck, and trunk, but may be found anywhere on the skin.

Clinical Features

- Epidermal cysts present as slow-growing, firm or sometimes doughy deep nodules, measuring from a few millimeters to a few centimeters in size. They are attached to the skin surface, and a punctum may be sometimes be seen.

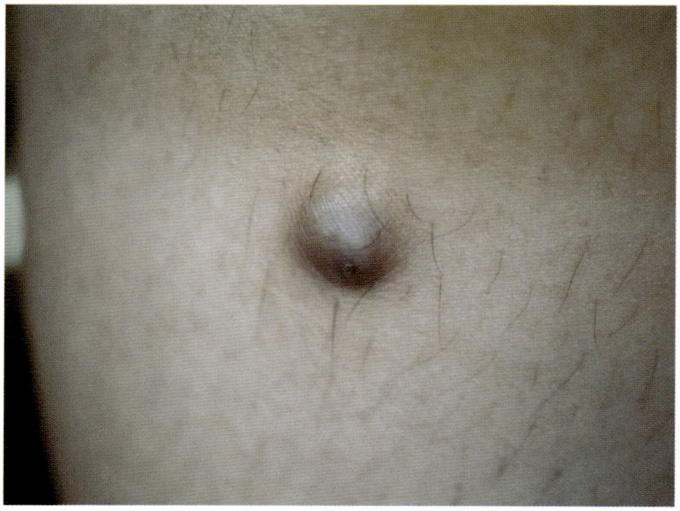

FIGURE 14-30. Small epidermal cyst on the shin of an Indian girl, presenting as a bluish, rubbery papule. A punctum is seen at the inferior pole.

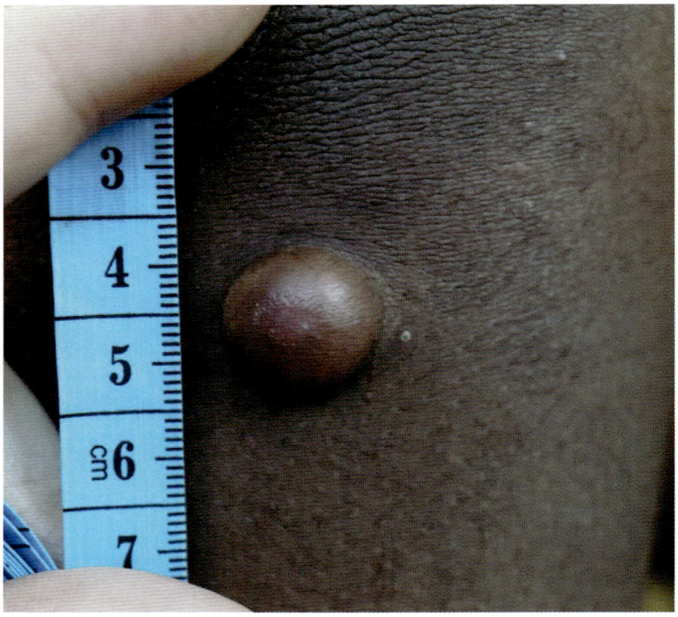

FIGURE 14-31. Epidermal cyst on the elbow of an Indian adolescent presenting as a large, rubbery, skin-colored nodule.

- If punctured, they produce a foul-smelling whitish substance.
- Lesions can become erythematous, swollen, and painful if inflamed or infected.

Differential Diagnoses

- Dermoid cyst
  - Usually occur along embryonic cleft closure sites and do not have a central punctum.

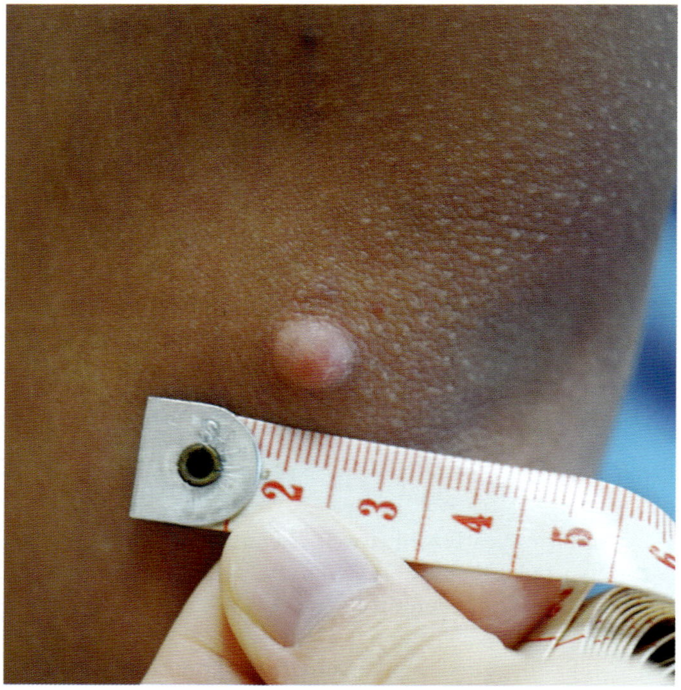

FIGURE 14-32. Epidermal cyst on the elbow of a Chinese adolescent.

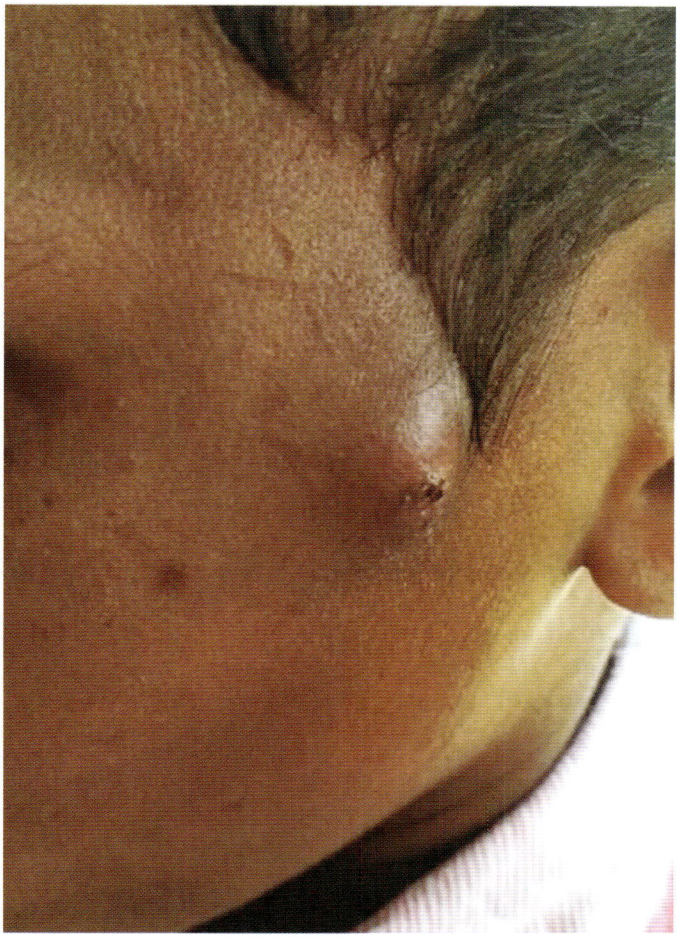

FIGURE 14-33. Inflamed epidermal cyst on the face of an Indian boy. A central punctum can be seen. (Courtesy of Professor Sandipan Dhar, FRCP.)

- Trichilemmal cyst/Pilar cyst
  - Trichilemmal cyst usually occurs over the scalp and can be difficult to differentiate from epidermal cysts unless examined histologically.
- Pilomatrixoma
  - These are more common in children and are firmer in nature, with a positive "see-saw" or "teeter-totter" sign.

Investigations & Treatment

- Histology shows a cyst lined by stratified squamous epithelium with a granular layer. Within the cyst, there is laminated keratin.
- It can be left alone or removed by excision, incision, and expression of its contents.

Pearls & Practical Tips

- Multiple epidermal cysts may occur in Gardner syndrome (familiar adenomatous polyposis) and in Gorlin syndrome (nevoid basal cell carcinoma syndrome).

TRICHILEMMAL CYST/PILAR CYST

Trichilemmal cysts are uncommon in childhood. They are derived from the outer root sheath of the hair follicle.

Clinical Features

- Trichilemmal cysts present as firm skin-colored to yellow-tan subcutaneous nodules. A central punctum is usually not seen.
- They are found most commonly on the scalp, and less commonly over the scrotum.
- Similar to epidermal cysts, they can be painful if inflamed or infected.
- There may be an autosomal dominant inheritance pattern.

Differential Diagnoses

- Epidermal cyst
  - Epidermal cyst may have a central punctum.
  - Histology shows a granular layer in the wall of the cyst, which is absent in a trichilemmal cyst.

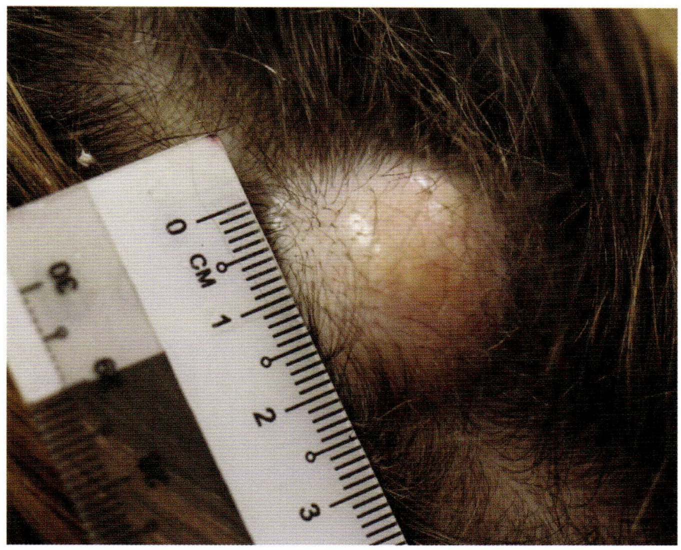

FIGURE 14-34. Trichilemmal cyst on the scalp of an adolescent girl, presenting as a rubbery skin-colored tumor. The diagnosis was confirmed on biopsy.

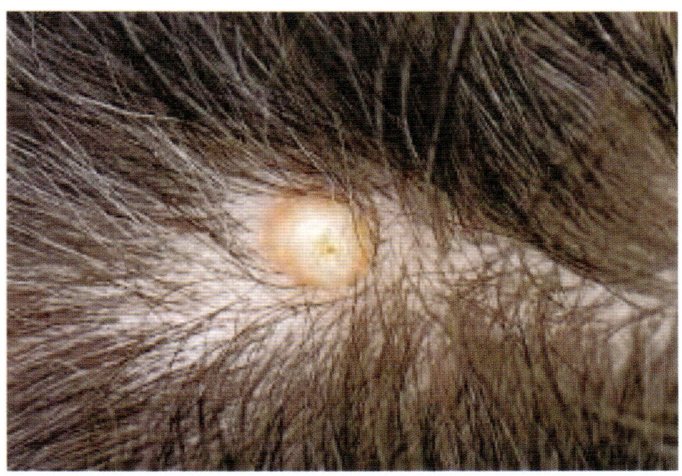

FIGURE 14-35. Trichilemmal cyst on the scalp. (Courtesy of Professor Sandipan Dhar, FRCP.)

Investigations & Treatment

- Histology shows a cyst lined by stratified squamous epithelium with abrupt keratinization with no granular layer. Within the cyst is eosinophilic compact keratin, sometimes with foci of calcification or cholesterol clefts.
- It can be left alone or surgically excised.

Pearls & Practical Tips

- Most often clinically diagnosed as epidermal cysts, and are only confirmed on histological examination.

VELLUS HAIR CYSTS

Vellus hairs are fine hairs with decreased pigmentation that are found on the face, trunk, and limbs. Vellus hair cysts are small cysts that contain vellus hairs and occur due to occlusion at the level of the infundibulum, with subsequent dilatation of the hair follicle. They are fairly uncommon but occur more commonly in children and adolescents than adults.

Clinical Features

- Although mostly sporadic, eruptive vellus hair cysts that occur in childhood can be familial. Both genders are equally affected.
- Vellus hair cysts are usually an isolated finding, but eruptive forms may occur in ectodermal dysplasia or pachyonychia congenita.
- They present as asymptomatic, small, hyperpigmented, dome-shaped papules but can also appear slightly inflamed.
- They most commonly occur over the chest, back, or knees. There are usually multiple, grouped lesions.

Differential Diagnoses

- Epidermal cyst
  - Epidermal cysts usually occur as single or only a few lesions. There is usually a central punctum.
- Steatocystoma multiplex
  - These are "true" sebaceous cysts and usually occur in late adolescence or early adulthood. Lesions are usually multiple and present as soft, skin-colored papules.

Investigations & Treatment

- Vellus hair cysts may be diagnosed clinically, but diagnosis can be confirmed with a biopsy.
- Histology shows a small cyst containing small vellus hairs and lined by stratified squamous epithelium.
- Vellus hair cysts may be left alone or surgically excised.

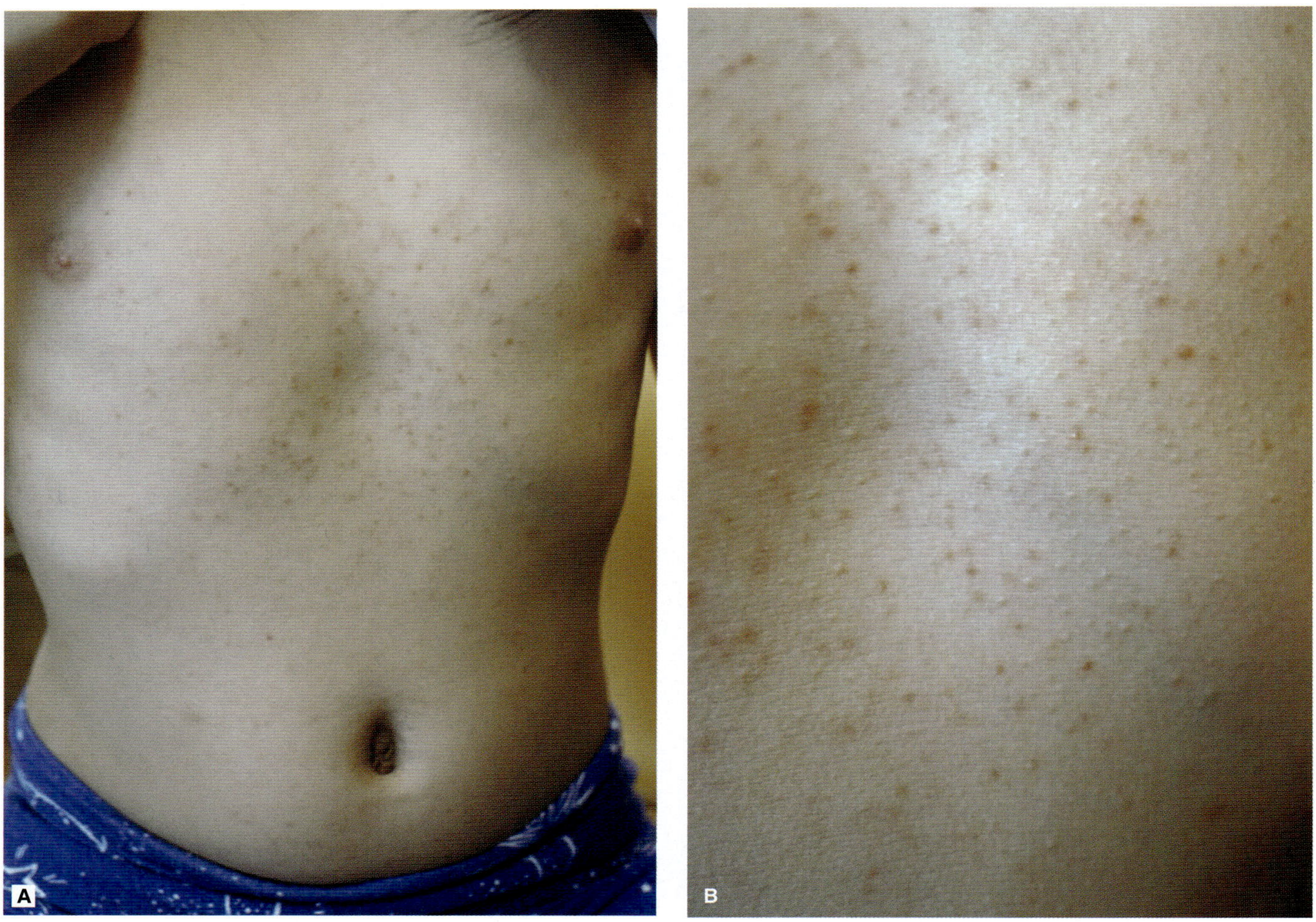

FIGURE 14-36A & 36B. Eruptive vellus hair cysts on the chest and upper abdomen of a Chinese girl presenting as multiple small, hyperpigmented papules.

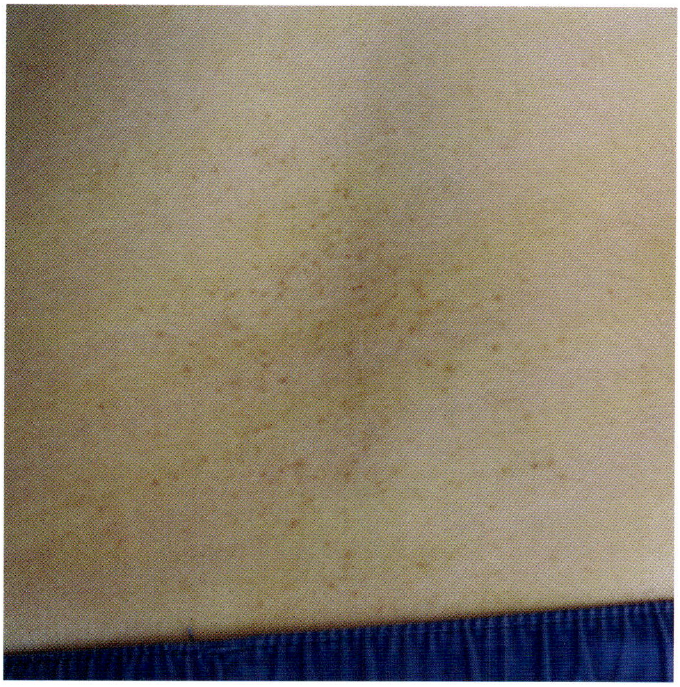

FIGURE 14-37. Vellus hair cysts on the back of a Chinese adolescent boy.

BECKER'S NEVUS

Becker's nevus is a hamartoma or developmental anomaly consisting of changes in pigmentation and increased numbers of hair follicles, sebaceous glands, and smooth muscle. It is distinctive in that the anomaly does not appear at birth, but usually presents during puberty. It is more common in males compared to females.

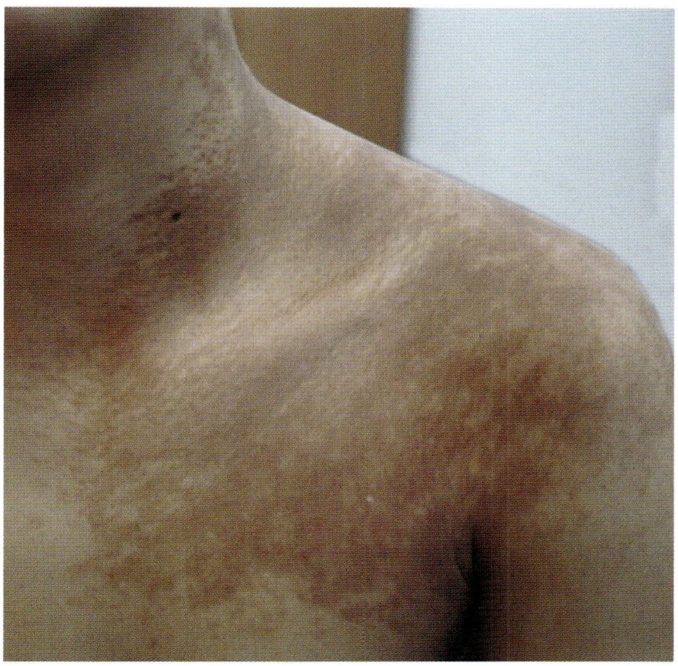

FIGURE 14-38. Classical presentation of a Becker's nevus on the left neck, chest, and shoulder of a Malay adolescent boy, as a medium-brown patch with irregular borders.

Clinical Features

- Becker's nevus presents as an asymptomatic, unilateral, large, hyperpigmented patch with increased hair. It most commonly occurs on the upper back or chest, usually on the scapular area of adolescent males.
- It has been described in all races.
- It may be light or dark brown in color, with a geographic pattern, sharply demarcated but irregular borders. The surface is usually smooth, but some areas may have a slightly elevated verrucous surface.
- Hyperpigmentation precedes development of hypertrichosis, which may be subtle or pronounced, and generally limited to the hyperpigmented area. Some lesions do not develop hypertrichosis ("melanotic" type of Becker's nevus).
- The characteristic onset during puberty is due to hormonal changes and the fact that the lesion shows an increased number of testosterone receptors. Acne may develop over the nevus during puberty due to the increased numbers of sebaceous glands.
- The lesion enlarges for a few years during puberty and then remains stable. It usually does not fade.
- Becker's nevus is most commonly an isolated skin finding; however, it can rarely be associated with an underlying musculoskeletal abnormality (Becker's nevus syndrome), such as ipsilateral limb hypoplasia, reduced breast development in areas under the lesion, or supernumerary nipple.

Differential Diagnoses

- Smooth muscle hamartoma
  - Becker's nevus is considered on a spectrum with smooth muscle hamartoma. The latter usually occurs as an asymptomatic, skin-colored or pigmented plaque

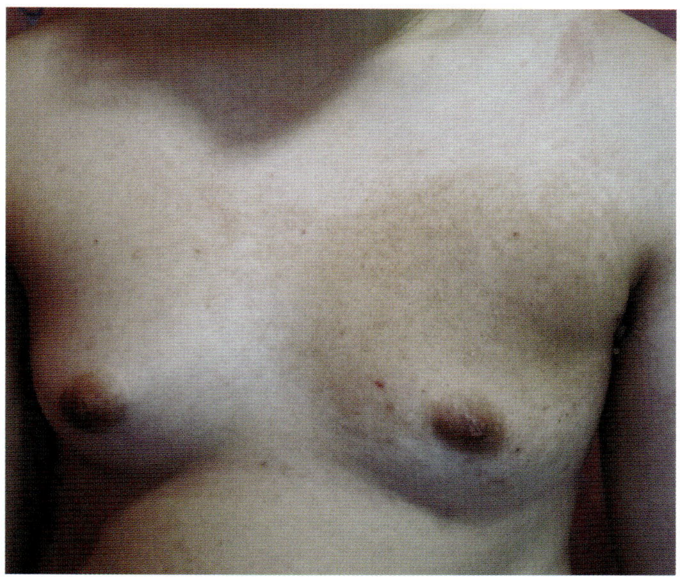

FIGURE 14-39. Becker's nevus on the left chest of an adolescent Chinese female presenting as a hyperpigmented, medium-brown patch with increased hair.

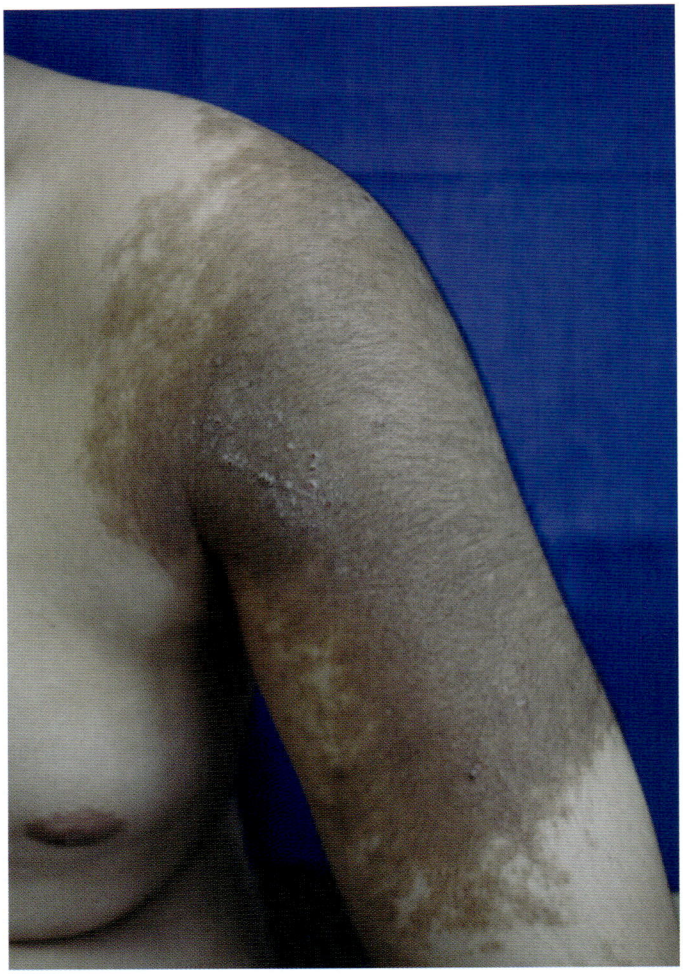

FIGURE 14-40. Becker's nevus on the arm and shoulder of a Chinese adolescent male presenting as a large deep-brown patch with hypertrichosis. Eczema is seen over an area of the nevus.

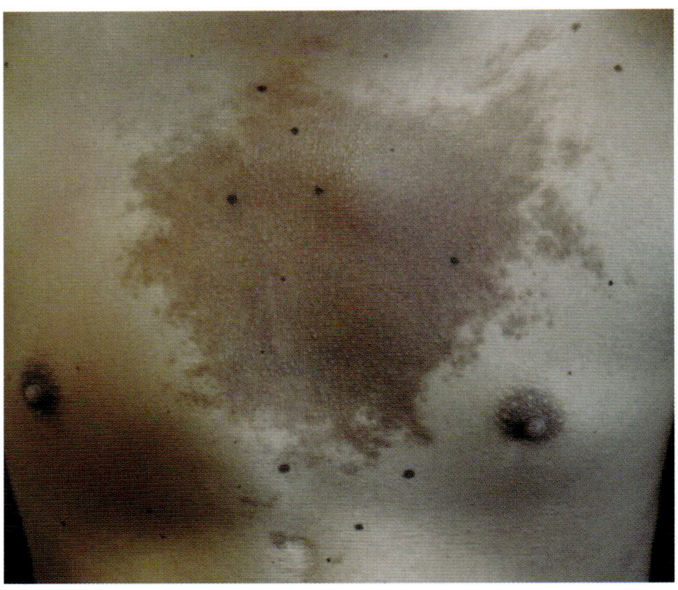

FIGURE 14-41. Becker's nevus on the central chest of a Chinese adolescent boy with background of cardiofaciocutaneous (CFC) syndrome, a type of RASopathy, which also manifests with multiple lentigines and junctional melanocytic nevi.

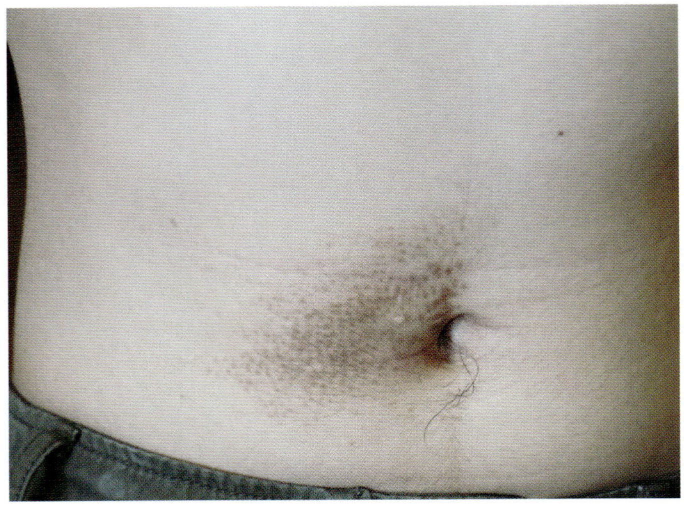

FIGURE 14-42. Am uncommon form of Becker's nevus on the abdomen of a Chinese teenager presenting as follicular pigmentation and hypertrichosis.

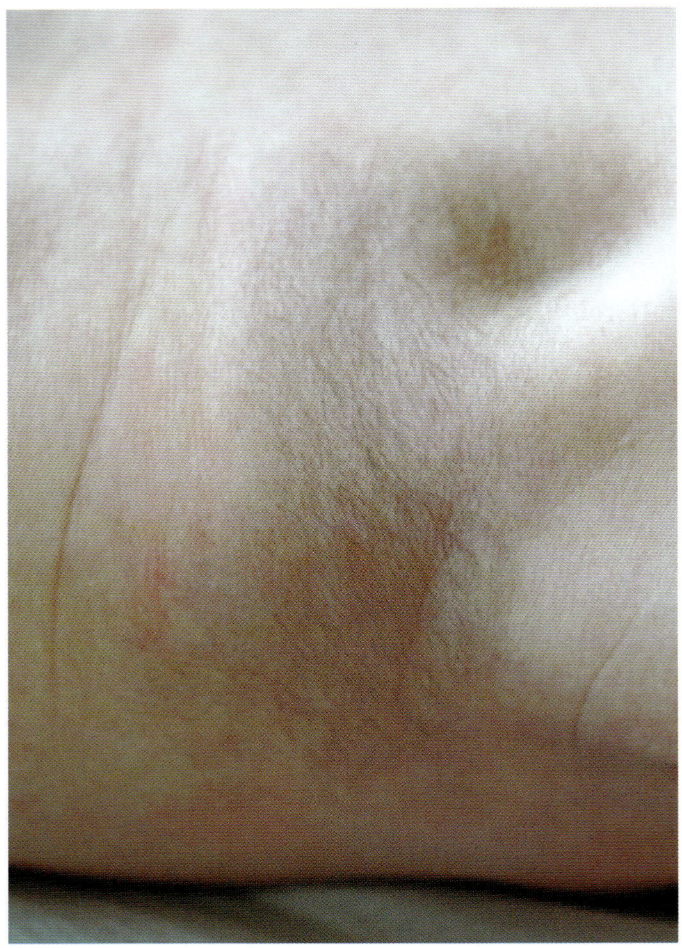

FIGURE 14-43. Smooth muscle hamartoma on the back of a Chinese infant presenting with hypertrichosis and mild hyperpigmentation.

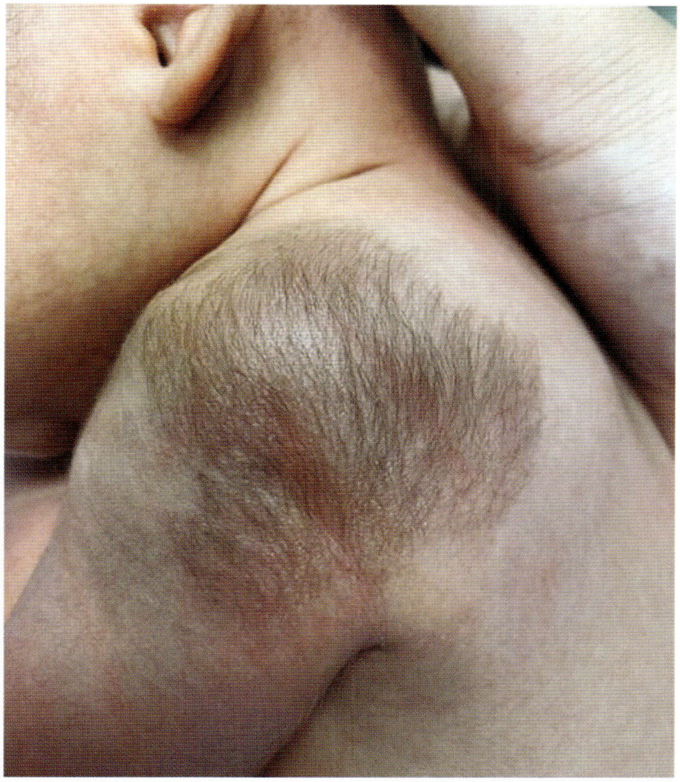

FIGURE 14-44. Smooth muscle hamartoma on the deltoid region of a newborn.

with hypertrichosis. It usually presents earlier than Becker's nevus and is more commonly located on the lumbosacral area, trunk, and proximal extremities. Pseudo-Darier sign may be positive, whereby rubbing of the overlying skin results in transient piloerection.

- Café-au-lait macule (CALM)
  - CALMs also present as brown, hyperpigmented patches. However, there is no increased overlying hair growth. They can also occur in areas that are unusual for Becker's nevus, such as the lower limbs and face.
- Congenital melanocytic nevus
  - A hairy congenital melanocytic nevus is present at birth, in contrast to a Becker's nevus, which usually appears during adolescence. Melanocytic nevi are also more deeply pigmented, with a more irregular surface.
- Plexiform neurofibroma
  - Plexiform neurofibromas often occur in patients with neurofibromatosis type I. They can also have increased overlying hairs. Other signs of neurofibromatosis may also be present, such as café-au-lait macules, axillary or inguinal freckling, and Lisch nodules.

Investigations & Treatment

- The diagnosis can usually be made clinically. Skin biopsy may be performed if the presentation is atypical and exclusion of other differential diagnoses needs to be made.
- Histological examination shows a normal number of basal melanocytes with increased melanin pigmentation in the basal layer of the epidermis. Increased hair follicles and smooth muscle bundles are often present in the dermis.
- It can be left alone if patients are not concerned by the cosmetic appearance. The lesion is often too large for surgical excision and can result in excessive scarring.
- Hypertrichosis is often the most disturbing characteristic, and this can be managed with different hair removal treatments such as waxing, hair electrolysis, or laser hair removal.
- Partial lightening of the hyperpigmentation can be achieved with lasers such as the Q-switched Nd:Yag laser, but results are variable, and recurrence of pigmentation is high.

Pearls & Practical Tips

- It is important to reassure the patient that a Becker's nevus is not associated with an increased risk of development of melanoma or other cancers within the lesion.
- It is useful to reassure parents and patients that the lesion will not continue to grow or get darker once it has stabilized after a few years.
- Patients may report its occurrence after intense sunbathing. This is due to its ability to tan more easily than the surrounding areas and so become more apparent.

CONNECTIVE TISSUE NEVUS

Connective tissue nevi are hamartomas of the dermis and they, result from an increase or change in the amount and distribution of the components of the extracellular matrix of the dermis. One of the three main components is usually affected, namely collagen, elastic tissue, or proteoglycans. They may represent isolated findings or be part of a more complex syndrome or systemic disease.

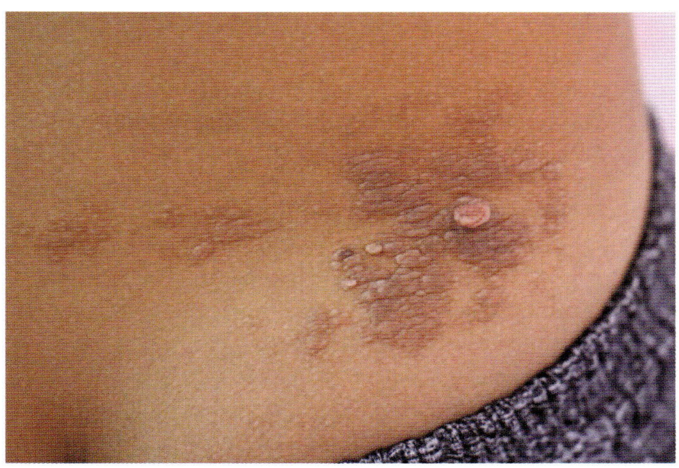

FIGURE 14-45. An unusual case of combined epidermal nevus and connective tissue nevus presenting with hyperpigmented, spongy papules with an irregular surface. Biopsy showed both epidermal hyperplasia and accumulation of mucin in the dermis.

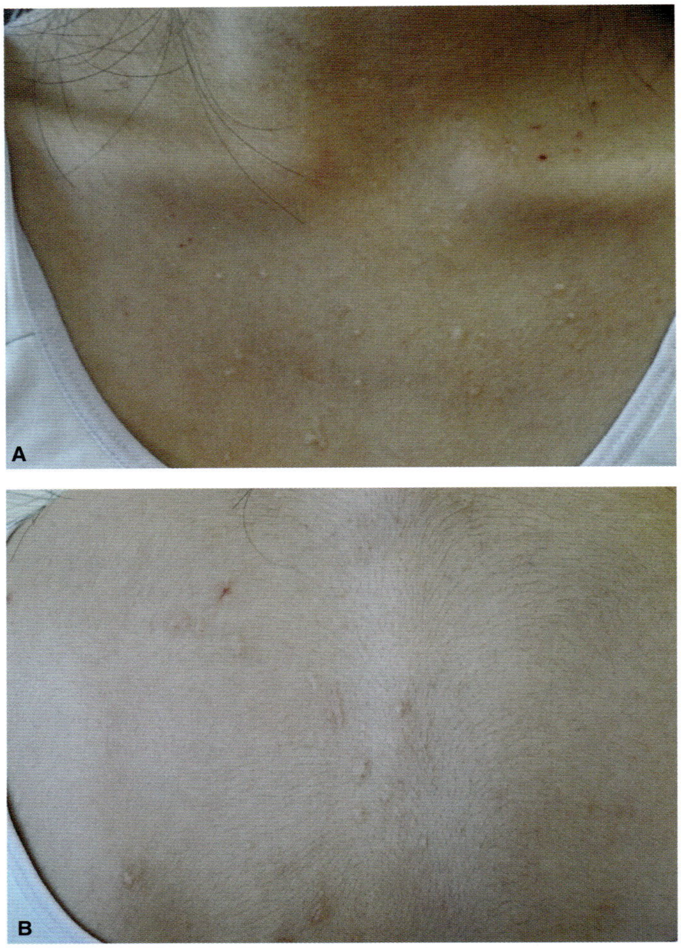

FIGURE 14-46A & 46B. Multiple collagenomas affecting the trunk and limbs of a Chinese adolescent girl, presenting as skin-colored to hypopigmented, rubbery papules. Diagnosis was confirmed on histology.

Clinical Features

- Connective tissue nevi are usually present from birth or in childhood. They may be solitary, multiple, or eruptive.
- Connective tissue nevi can present as asymptomatic papules, nodules, or plaques that are firm or rubbery, skin-colored or yellowish, with a lobulated surface. Lesions on the plantar surface have a cerebriform appearance.
- Although mostly an isolated finding, collagenomas may be associated with other conditions, such as shagreen patch in tuberous sclerosis, familial cutaneous collagenoma, Buschke-Ollendorf syndrome, and multiple endocrine neoplasia type 1.
- Shagreen patch is one of the diagnostic criteria for tuberous sclerosis and describes a "pebbly" plaque with a cobblestone appearance, typically on the lower back or nape of neck.
- Elastomas may be isolated, familial, or part of Buschke-Ollendorf syndrome.
- Connective tissue nevi comprising proteoglycans are rare, and include inherited or acquired localized mucinous nevi.

Differential Diagnoses

- Epidermal nevus
  - Epidermal nevi appear as soft, dome-shaped, skin-colored or hyperpigmented papules, nodules, or plaques, in a linear or blaschkoid configuration. They are also present from birth or in early childhood.
  - Epidermal nevi appear more superficial compared to connective tissue nevi.
- Smooth muscle hamartoma
  - These are benign, asymptomatic, skin-colored or pigmented plaques, usually with overlying hypertrichosis. They may also be present from birth or early childhood. Rubbing of the overlying skin can result in transient piloerection (pseudo-Darier sign).
- Fibrous hamartoma of infancy
  - This is a benign, typically solitary, skin-colored subcutaneous nodule which may have overlying hypertrichosis. Most appear within the first year of life but may be congenital.
- Infantile myofibromatosis
  - Presents with single or multiple firm to rubbery, skin-colored to purple dermal or subcutaneous nodules, commonly on the head and neck region or on the trunk. Most are present at birth and up to the first 2 years of life, and may involve the skeleton and multiple internal organs.
- Dermatofibroma
  - This usually occurs in older children or adolescents and presents as a firm, hyperpigmented papule or nodule.

Investigations & Treatment

- Skin biopsy and histopathological examination can help in confirming the diagnosis and excluding the differential diagnoses.
- Special immunohistochemical stains are required to highlight the various components of the connective tissue nevi.
- Excision of individual lesions is generally effective, although not always feasible, especially in large lesions. Removal of the lesion(s) does not change the course of the systemic disease or genetic syndrome.

Pearls & Practical Tips

- When performing biopsies for diagnosis of connective tissue nevi, a separate biopsy from normal-appearing skin at the same anatomical site should also be done for comparison.
- In a child with a connective tissue nevus, especially if large or multiple, exclusion of an underlying syndrome is important. Personal or family history of similar cutaneous lesions, systemic review, and physical examination for other cutaneous lesions will provide clues.

HYPERTROPHIC SCAR/KELOID

Hypertrophic scars and keloids are excessive proliferations of connective tissue in response to skin trauma. A hypertrophic scar is a thick, elevated scar that does not extend beyond the boundaries of the initiating injury, whereas a keloid extends beyond the boundaries of the initial injury.

Clinical Features

- Hypertrophic scars and keloids can occur in children, adolescents, and adults, although they are less common in younger children. They usually occur after trauma to the skin, although sometimes a history of trauma may not be apparent.
- There may be a family history of similar scarring or keloid formation in other family members. They are also more common in darker-skinned individuals.
- Hypertrophic scars present as elevated pink or erythematous papules or nodules confined to the area of cutaneous injury, often in a linear configuration.
- Keloids present as protuberant, firm or rubbery, erythematous to brown papules, nodules, or plaques, which extend beyond the area of original cutaneous injury or trauma. The surface is usually smooth.
- Both hypertrophic scars and keloids are usually asymptomatic but can be itchy or, less commonly, painful. They can lead to contractures if occurring over the flexural aspects of joints.
- Both occur predominantly over the chest, shoulders, upper back, face (jawline and earlobes), and neck.
- In Asian patients, facial and truncal keloids often develop during adolescence, with acne vulgaris being a common trigger for their development.
- Ear piercing is by far the most common etiology underlying the development of keloids on the earlobe and helix.

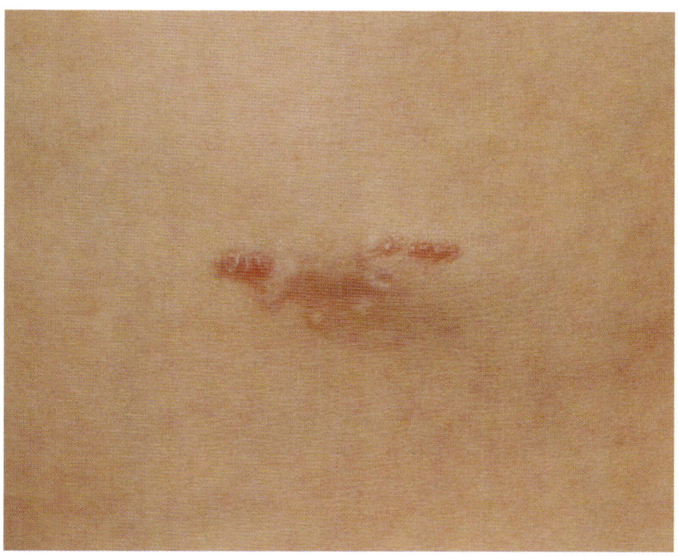

FIGURE 14-47. Hypertrophic scar on the abdomen of a young Chinese girl post-surgery. Note the increased pigmentation at the periphery and decreased pigmentation in the central areas of the scar.

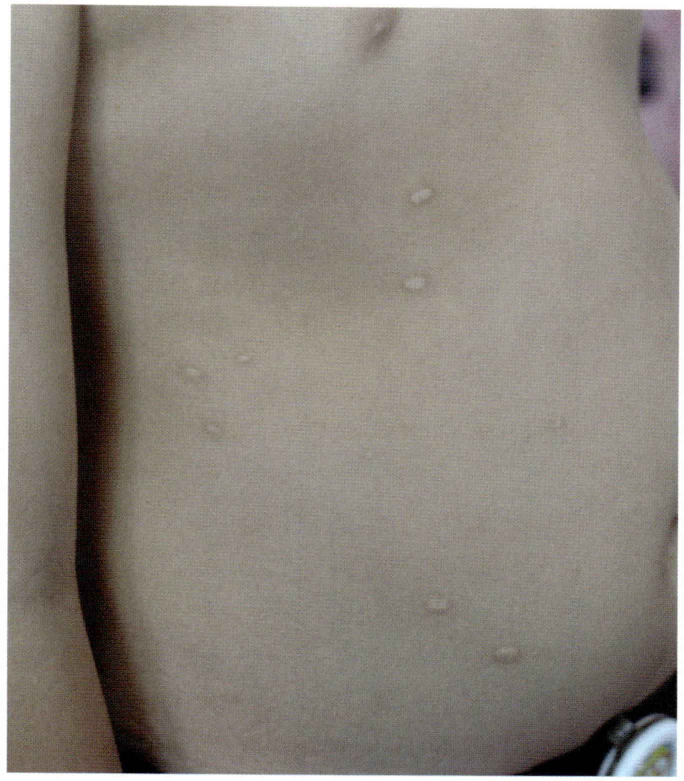

FIGURE 14-48. Multiple varicella induced hypertrophic scars on the trunk of a Malay boy presenting as hypopigmented, firm papules.

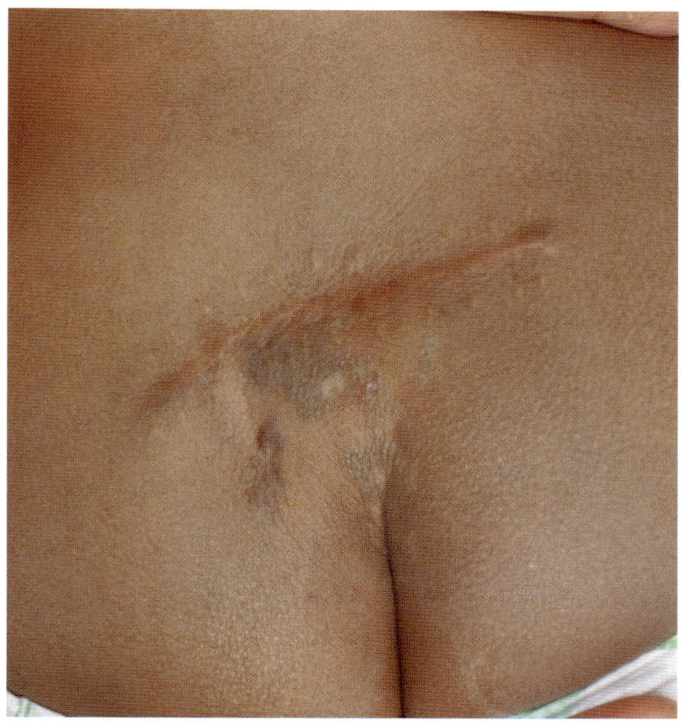

FIGURE 14-49. Hypertrophic scar on the lower back of a Malay infant who underwent spinal surgery.

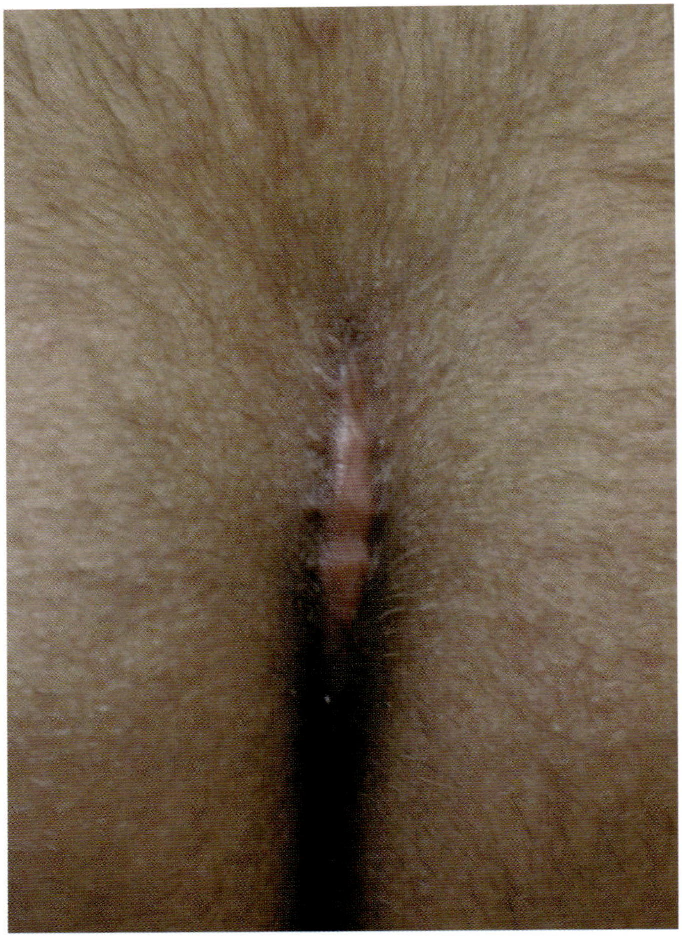

FIGURE 14-50. Keloid on the natal cleft of an Indian teenager after surgery for pilonidal sinus.

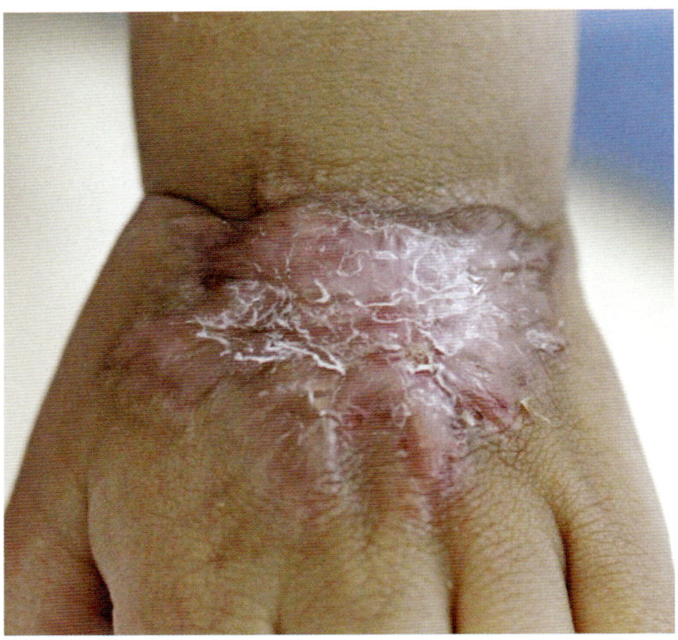

FIGURE 14-51. Keloid on the hand of a 2-year-old Malay toddler after a burn injury, presenting as a large, pink, firm plaque with surface scaling.

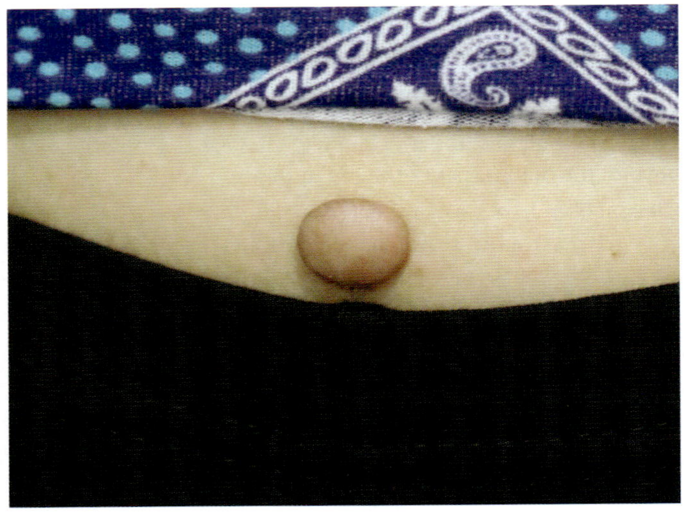

FIGURE 14-52. Keloid on the abdomen of a Malay teenager after ornamental piercing.

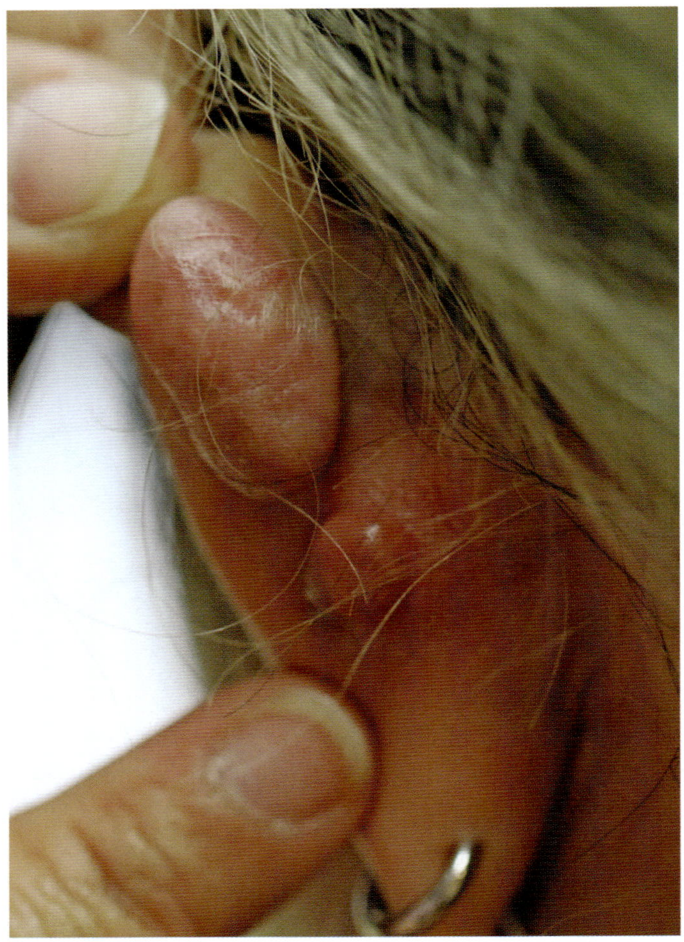

FIGURE 14-53. Two keloids on the posterior surface of the ear of a Malay adolescent after ornamental piercing.

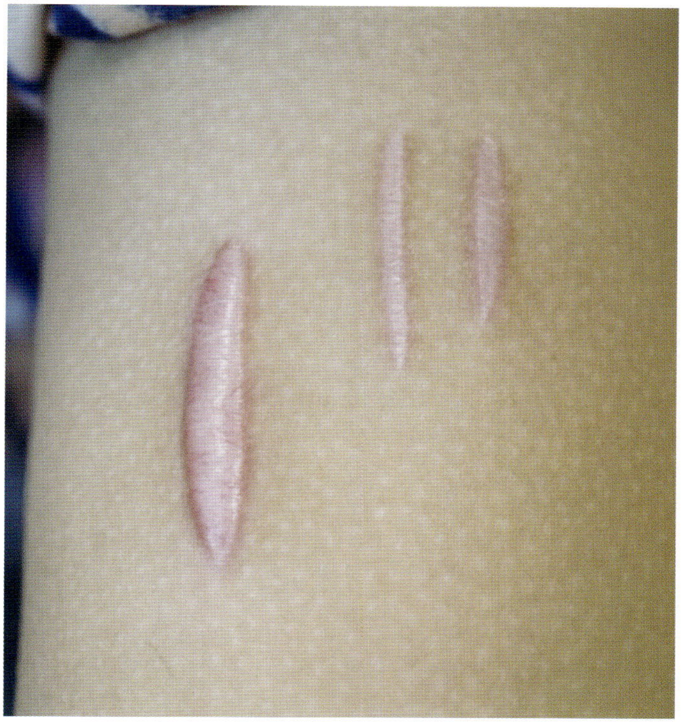

FIGURE 14-54. Linear hypertrophic scars on the arm of a Chinese adolescent after intentional traumatic injury.

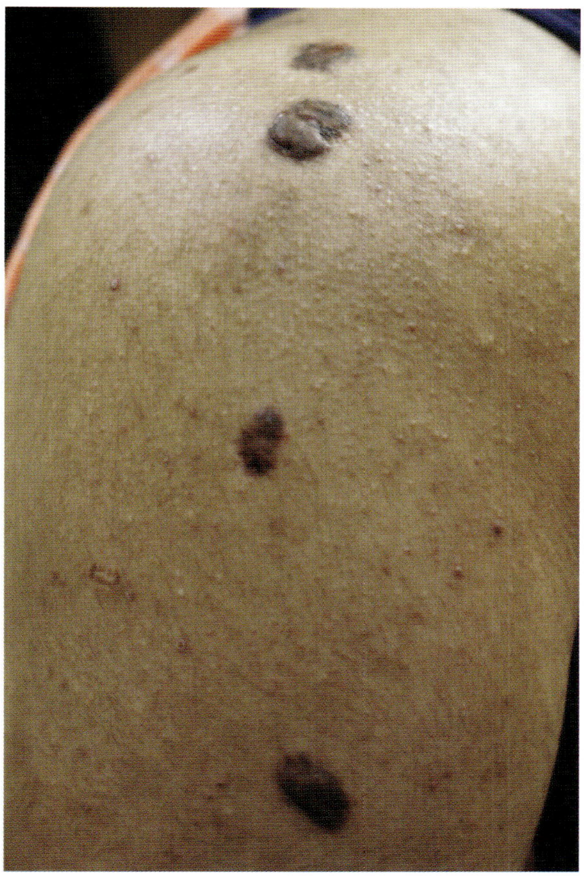

FIGURE 14-55. Keloids on the shoulder of an Indian adolescent from acne. Note the intense hyperpigmentation of the scars.

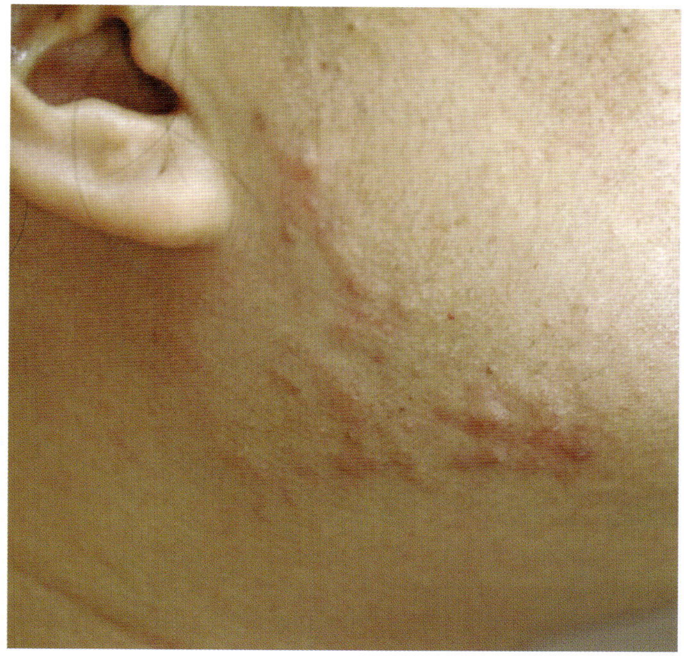

FIGURE 14-56. Hypertrophic scars on the jawline of a 20-year-old woman with severe facial acne.

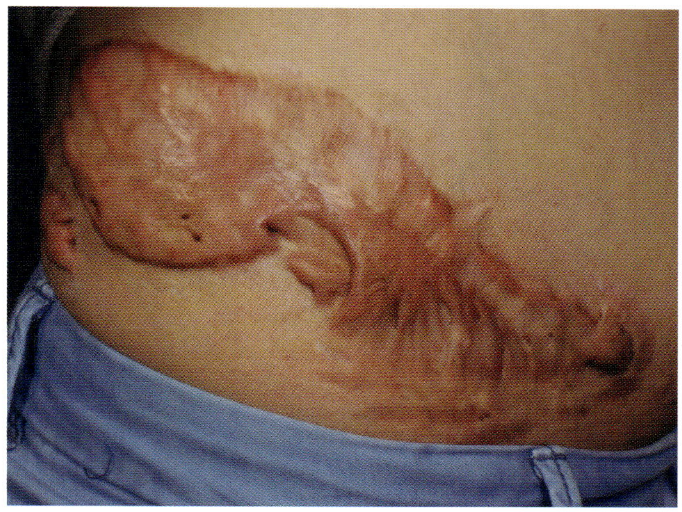

FIGURE 14-57. Extensive keloid scarring on the abdomen of an 8-year-old Nepalese girl post-trauma.

- In children, hypertrophic scars are common following severe burn injuries.

Differential Diagnoses

- Dermatofibroma
  - This presents as a hyperpigmented, firm papule, usually over the legs, especially in adolescents. The "dimple sign" may be present, where squeezing the lesion produces a dimple or wrinkling at the center of the lesion.
- Juvenile xanthogranulomas
  - Often seen in infants and young children, juvenile xanthogranulomas appear as orange-yellow to hyperpigmented papules with a smooth surface. They tend to self-resolve over a few years.

- Dermatofibrosarcoma protuberans
  - This is an extremely rare, locally aggressive fibrohistiocytic tumor that is much more common in adults than children or adolescents. It also presents as a painless, erythematous to skin-colored, firm and fleshy plaque, nodule, or tumor, usually over the trunk, shoulder, and chest area. Diagnosis is by skin biopsy.

Investigations & Treatment

- Hypertrophic scars and keloids are diagnosed clinically. Biopsy is not recommended as further trauma may worsen the scar. It is usually performed when diagnosis is not clear, with a role to exclude other more dangerous diagnoses.
- Histologically, thick homogenous collagen bundles are seen haphazardly throughout the dermis. Hypertrophic scars show an increased number of fibroblasts compared to keloids.
- Treatment can be frustrating, and managing patients' and caregivers' expectations is important.
- Multiple treatment options are available, and there is no universally accepted treatment protocol.
- Treatment with silicone gel or sheets has the advantage of being painless but only works for relatively newer scars. Silicone sheets should be applied for at least 12 hours per day to be effective.
- Intralesional corticosteroids, most commonly with triamcinolone (10–40 mg/mL), can be considered but may be too painful for children. Treatment can be repeated every few weeks until the scar flattens. Side effects include surrounding skin atrophy and telangiectasias. In children afraid of injections, a trial of potent steroids with occlusion can be tried.
- Cryotherapy can be attempted for small keloids (especially earlobe keloids). Laser therapy has also been used with variable results. These include the pulsed-dye laser, Nd:YAG laser, and carbon dioxide lasers.
- Pressure garments can be advised after future surgery to reduce the risk of hypertrophic scar/keloid formation, for a minimum period of 6 months.
- After scar maturation, surgical scar revision can be discussed with a plastic surgeon, but is often challenging.
- Intralesional triamcinolone can be given prophylactically to new surgical wounds to reduce the occurrence of keloid/hypertrophic scars.

Pearls & Practical Tips

- Patients with a history of keloids or hypertrophic scars should be informed that they are prone to develop more lesions and should inform future healthcare professionals or tattoo/piercing artists about their history, as healing after procedures (laser, piercings, surgery) is associated with an increased risk of abnormal scarring.
- Itch can be a sign that the process of scarring is still evolving. The pruritus and erythema subside with scar maturation.
- Treatments are more effective in more recent lesions.
- All healed burn wounds should be treated with pressure garments to prevent abnormal scar formation.
- Combination treatments may work better than monotherapy, such as combining intralesional corticosteroids with lasers.

DERMATOFIBROMA

Dermatofibroma, also known as benign fibrous histiocytoma, represents a benign reactive proliferation of fibroblasts in the skin. Although more common in adults, they can also occur in children and adolescents. They may represent a reaction pattern to an insect bite or other form of trauma, although often no such history is obtained.

Clinical Features

- A dermatofibroma presents as an asymptomatic, firm, well-defined dermal papule or nodule, 5 to 10 mm in diameter (occasionally up to 2 cm), and favors the lower extremities.
- In Asian patients, it is commonly hyperpigmented compared to patients with skin types I–II, where they may appear pink.
- It may enlarge slowly and may partially regress with time.
- Pinching the lesion usually results in a downward movement of the lesion, known as the "dimple sign."
- Occasionally, multiple dermatofibromas are seen in children who are immunocompromised and with conditions such as leukemia, human immunodeficiency virus, systemic lupus erythematosus, and atopic dermatitis.
- Rarely, multiple dermatofibromas run in families, and an autosomal dominant missense mutation in the factor XIII A-subunit has been described.

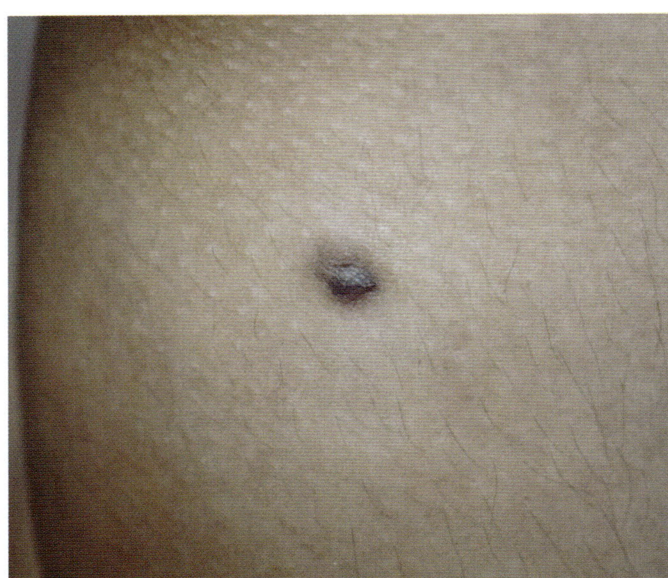

FIGURE 14-58. Dermatofibroma on the calf of a 12-year-old Chinese girl presenting as a deeply pigmented firm nodule.

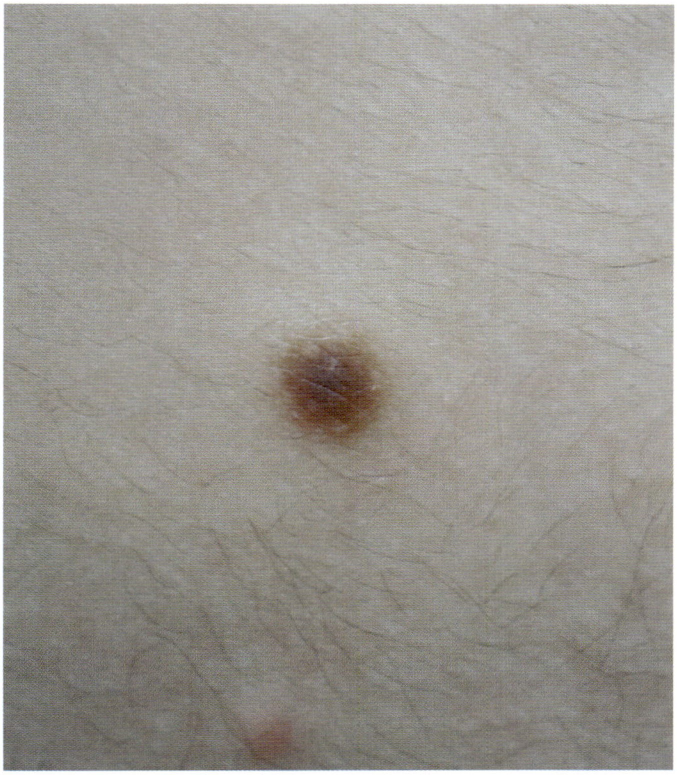

FIGURE 14-59. Dermatofibroma on the thigh of a 13-year-old Chinese girl presenting as a firm hyperpigmented papule.

Differential Diagnoses

- Epidermal cysts
  - These are benign cystic lesions derived from hair follicles. They are attached to the overlying skin and have a rubbery to firm consistency. They tend to be skin-colored or slightly bluish in color. There is often a central punctum.
- Melanocytic nevus
  - Pigmented dermatofibromas may be confused with melanocytic nevi. However, nevi are usually soft, compared to the firmer nature of dermatofibromas.
  - Dermoscopy of dermatofibroma commonly reveals a central white area with surrounding faint pigment network. Suggestive dermatoscopic features for melanocytic nevi include presence of a pigment network and aggregated brown or black globules.
- Hypertrophic scar or keloid
  - A history of preceding trauma, surgery, or inflammatory conditions such as acne vulgaris in keloid-prone areas including jawline, shoulders, and upper chest, should raise suspicion for keloid/hypertrophic scar.
- Juvenile xanthogranuloma
  - Often seen in infants and young children, juvenile xanthogranulomas appear as orange-yellow to hyperpigmented papules with a smooth surface. They tend to self-resolve over a few years.

Investigations & Treatment

- Although most often diagnosed clinically, histological examination may be required if clinical and/or dermoscopic features are not classical.
- Skin biopsy shows a fibrohistiocytic proliferation surrounded by excessive eosinophilic bundles of collagen and an overlying hyperplastic epidermis. Immunohistochemical staining reveals positive staining for CD68, factor XIIIA, and negative staining for CD34.
- Excision is the only treatment and can be considered for diagnostic or cosmetic reasons.

Pearls & Practical Tips

- The dimple sign is useful to differentiate dermatofibromas from other skin lumps.
- In skin of color, dermatofibromas tend to be hyperpigmented.
- Multiple dermatofibromas may be seen in children with compromised immunity or in those with a positive family history.

SKIN TAGS/FIBROEPITHELIAL POLYPS

Skin tags, or fibroepithelial polyps, are less common in children compared to adults. They may be present from birth or are acquired. In older children and adolescents, they are often associated with obesity.

Clinical Features

- Skin tags are skin-colored or hyperpigmented, soft, pedunculated or less commonly sessile, papules, which can be found on any part of the face, body, or limbs, although the most common sites are the neck, axillae, groin, and inframammary area.
- Skin tags are generally not common in babies and children. If present, they may be clues to more complex abnormalities or syndromes; for instance, skin tags in the sacral area may be associated with spinal dysraphism, especially if other cutaneous signs are present in the area.

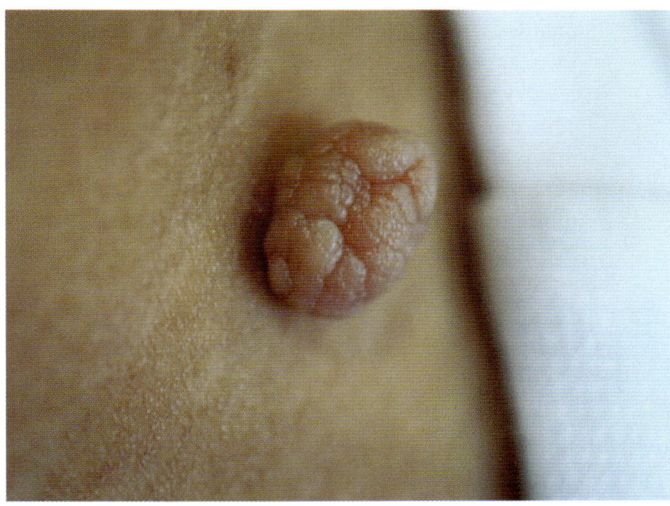

FIGURE 14-60. Fibroepithelial polyp on the axilla of a Chinese adolescent presenting as a pedunculated, skin-colored nodule with an irregular surface.

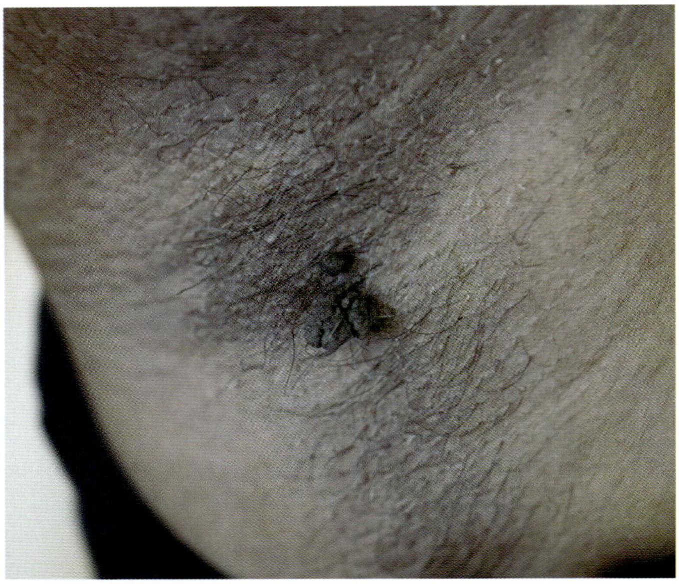

FIGURE 14-61. Skin tag on the axilla of a 13-year-old Indian male, presenting as a soft, deeply pigmented nodule. There is concomitant acanthosis nigricans.

- Solitary skin tags around the nipple have been reported in neonates, and these detach spontaneously.
- Preauricular skin tags (or accessory tragi) are minor developmental abnormalities of the first branchial arch.
- Skin tags on the neck, axillae, and inguinal region of older children and adolescents are often associated with obesity, insulin resistance, and diabetes mellitus.

Differential Diagnoses

- Intradermal melanocytic nevus
  - Presents as a brown hyperpigmented papule and is often sessile. Dermoscopy may reveal a pigment network, brown or black globules in melanocytic nevi.
- Viral wart
  - May present as a soft and skin-colored papule as well. Differentiating characteristics include clustering of papules from auto-inoculation or a verrucous or filiform appearance with surface thrombosed capillaries.
- Accessory nipple
  - This represents a remnant of the embryological milk line which runs from the anterior axillary fold to the anterior thigh. It presents as a small brown, pink, umbilicated papule which may be surrounded by a pigmented areola.
- Seborrheic keratosis
  - These are more common in adults than in children and adolescents. However, small lesions on the neck or cheeks may resemble skin tags. Dermoscopy reveals milia-like cysts, irregular crypts, fissures, and ridges.

Investigations & Treatment

- No investigations are usually required for diagnosis.
- Skin tags may be removed via shave or snip excision.

Pearls & Practical Tips

- Skin tags are not common in the pediatric population.

NEUROFIBROMA

Neurofibromas are common benign dermal tumors that consist of neuromesenchymal tissue, including Schwann cells, endoneurial cells, and perineural cells. They are more commonly seen in adults but can occasionally be seen in children and adolescents. Most neurofibromas occur in isolation, but multiple neurofibromas or plexiform neurofibromas may be seen in type 1 neurofibromatosis. (See Chapter 12 section on neurofibromatosis for photographs of neurofibromas and plexiform neurofibromas.)

Clinical Features

- Neurofibromas present as asymptomatic, soft, flesh-colored to pink or brown, sessile or pedunculated papules or nodules, usually with a smooth surface.
- They can occur anywhere on the skin.
- There is a classical “buttonhole” sign, in which pressure on the surface leads to invagination of the nodule into the dermis.
- Plexiform neurofibromas are rare tumors seen in neurofibromatosis type 1. They often present early in life as a hyperpigmented, brown patch with indistinct borders. There may be overlying hypertrichosis. With time, the surface can become more lobulated and feel like a “bag of worms.” There is a risk of malignant change in plexiform neurofibromas.

Differential Diagnoses

- Intradermal melanocytic nevus
  - Most intradermal melanocytic nevi are pigmented, especially in Asian races. However, they may also appear flesh-colored and mimic neurofibromas.
- Juvenile xanthogranulomas
  - Juvenile xanthogranulomas are far more common in childhood than neurofibromas. They often appear as a rubbery to firm, yellow-orange or brown papules or nodules, with a smooth surface.

Investigations & Treatment

- Although not usually required, a biopsy will help to establish the diagnosis.
- Histologically, neurofibromas appear as well-demarcated, non-encapsulated nodules within the superficial to deep dermis, made up of small, “comma-shaped” spindled cells set in a pinkish-myxoid stroma. Mast cells are prominent.
- Small lesions may be treated conservatively, especially if not cosmetically significant.
- If required, surgical excision is the treatment of choice.

Pearls & Practical Tips

- A diagnosis of plexiform neurofibroma should prompt a search for other features of neurofibromatosis, including café-au-lait macules, axillary or inguinal freckling, neurofibromas and Lisch nodules.
- Plexiform neurofibromas have been misdiagnosed as infantile hemangiomas, smooth muscle hamartomas, nevus of Ota, and melanocytic nevi.

LIPOMA

Lipomas represent collections of increased mature adipose tissue. They are more common in adults compared to children and adolescents. They most commonly present as solitary lesions but can occur as part of lipomatous overgrowth in certain syndromes such as PIK3CA-related overgrowth syndromes.

Clinical Features

- Lipomas present as soft, mobile, skin-colored, painless lumps in the subcutaneous layer.
- They may occur on any part of the body and limbs, and may be solitary or multiple.
- Lipomas occurring on the lower back may be an occult sign of spinal dysraphism, especially if associated with other cutaneous signs, such as a port wine stain or dimpling.
- Certain overgrowth syndromes are associated with lipomas, such as *PIK3CA*-related overgrowth spectrum, which includes CLOVES syndrome (congenital lipomatous overgrowth, vascular malformations, epidermal nevi, and skeletal anomalies) and Proteus syndrome.

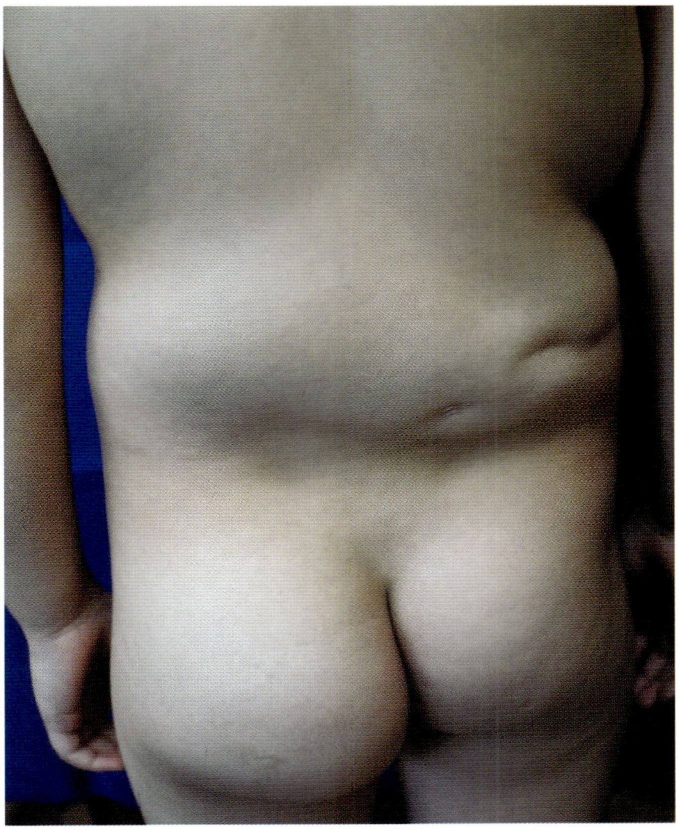

FIGURE 14-62. Multiple large lipomas in a child with suspected PIK3CA-related overgrowth spectrum.

Differential Diagnoses

- Neurofibroma
  - These present as soft, dome-shaped, skin-colored, or pinkish papules or nodules.
- Branchial cyst
  - This presents as a painless, mobile lump on the lateral neck, without a cutaneous or mucosal opening. It presents at birth or shortly after birth.
- Vascular tumor or malformation
  - Deep infantile hemangiomas can present as skin-colored or lightly bluish lumps that can be mistaken for lipomas. The classical growth trajectory and natural history help to differentiate. Placing a Doppler over the hemangioma will produce a pulsatile "whoosh" sound, which is not heard over a lipoma.
  - Deep lymphatic malformations can also present as skin-colored, soft lumps. There may be a light bluish hue. Imaging such as ultrasound or MRI can help to differentiate from a lipoma.
- Cephalocele
  - This is congenital herniation of intracranial structures through a scalp defect. It is a differential for lipomas on the scalp. The "hair collar sign," a ring of coarse, dark hair encircling the cephalocele, may be a clue to this diagnosis. Palpate for an underlying skull defect, which is found in meningoceles and encephaloceles.
- Dermoid cyst
  - This is congenital and results from entrapment of skin along the lines of embryonic fusion. It presents at birth or early in life as an asymptomatic, firm, subcutaneous papule or nodule, most commonly over the periorbital area, especially the lateral eyebrow and/nasal root.
- Epidermal inclusion cyst
  - This is attached to the overlying skin and has a firm consistency, and there is usually a central punctum.

Investigations & Treatment

- An ultrasound with Doppler may assist in differentiating this from vascular lesions. MRI scan can also detect fat.
- Lipomas, if small and solitary, may be left alone.
- If necessary, surgical excision is effective.

Pearls & Practical Tips

- Exclude associated syndromes in children who present with unusual lipomas (e.g, size, number) or lipomatous overgrowth.
- Lipomas can be left alone and are excised mainly for cosmetic reasons.
- If a patient presents with multiple painful lipomas and a positive family history, Dercum's disease should be considered.

Skin Manifestations of Systemic Conditions

SKIN MANIFESTATIONS OF NUTRITIONAL DEFICIENCIES

Nutritional deficiency remains common worldwide, especially in infants and children from lower socioeconomic communities, and includes protein deficiency as well as vitamin and mineral deficiencies. Although less common in more developed countries, it can occur in children who are picky eaters, have impaired absorption, or if caregivers impose restrictive feeding practices due to various reasons. Nutritional deficiencies can remain unrecognized if not suspected by healthcare providers, leading to detrimental health effects. In this chapter, we discuss protein and vitamin deficiencies that present with skin manifestations.

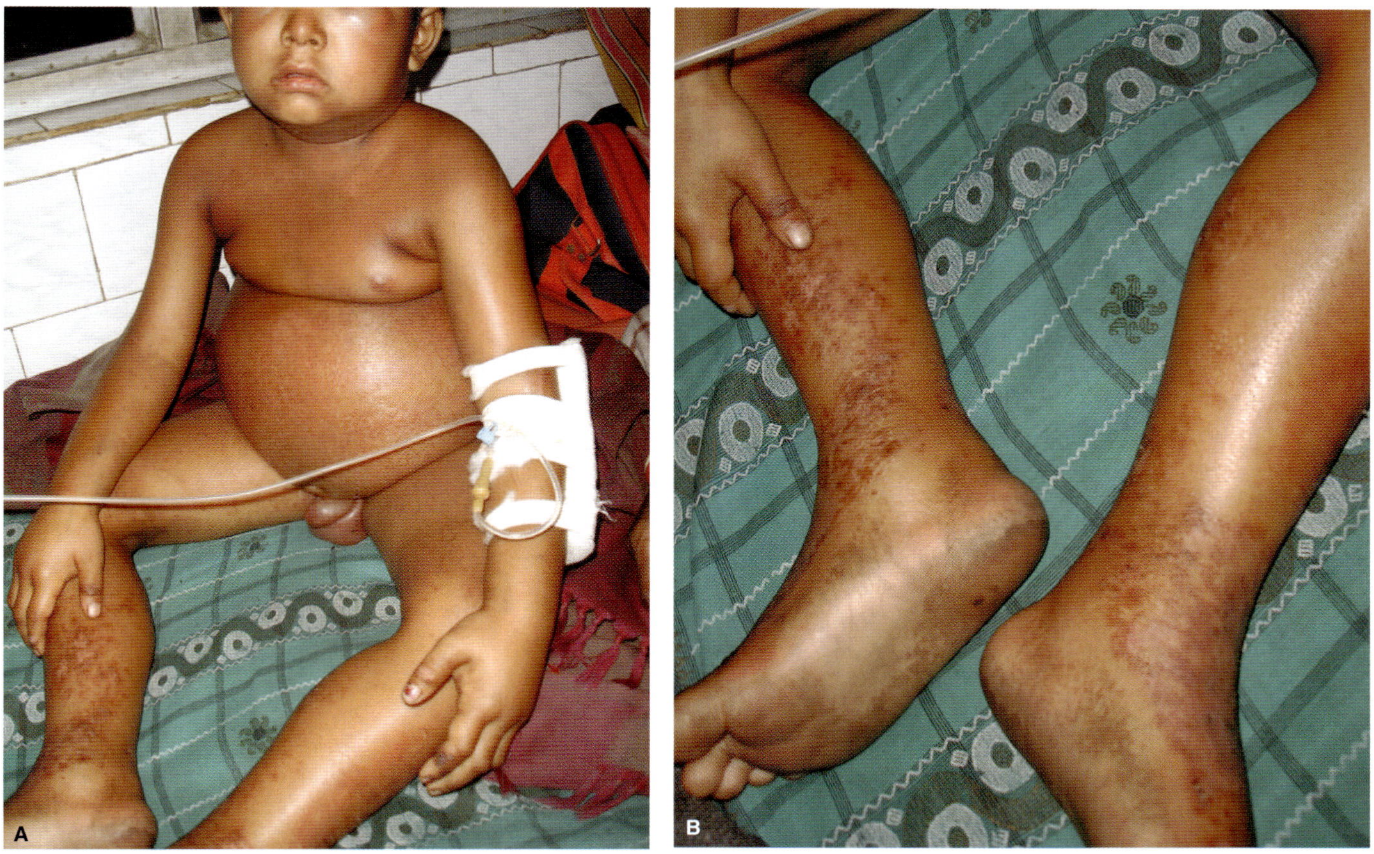

FIGURE 15-1A & 1B. Kwashiorkor in an Indian boy presenting as severe generalized edema associated with flaky, hyperpigmented plaques on his lower limbs. (Photograph courtesy of Dr. Sandipan Dhar, Kolkata, India.)

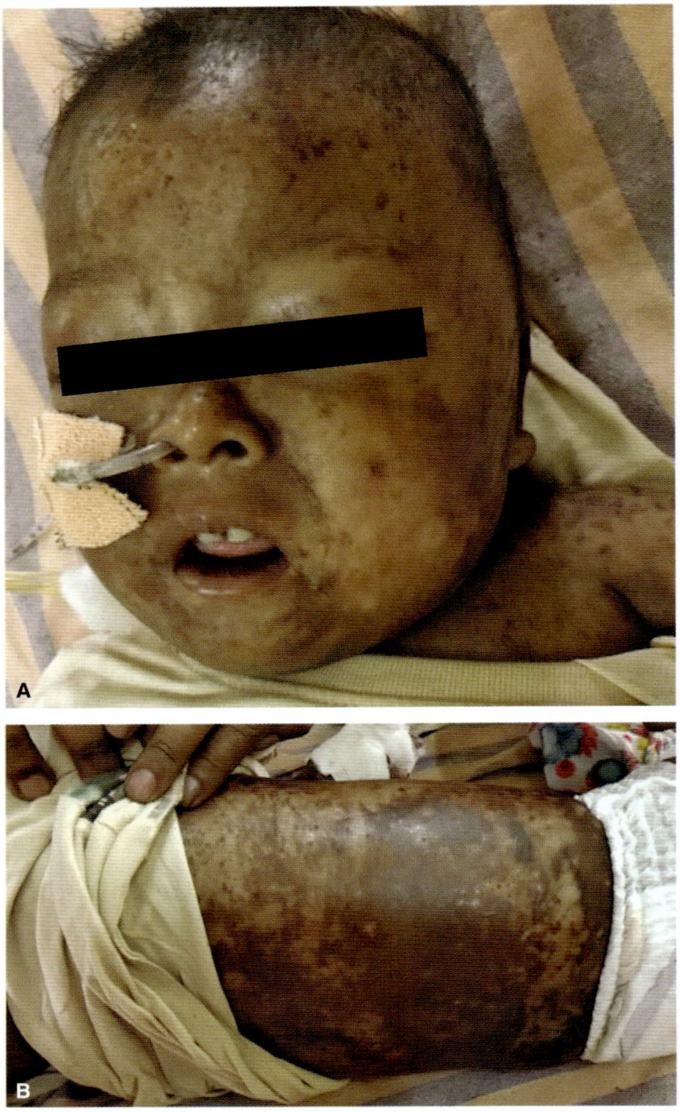

FIGURE 15-2A & 2B. Kwashiorkor in a young Indian boy presenting as edema with generalized hyperpigmented, flaky patches and plaques. (Photograph courtesy of Dr. Sandipan Dhar, Kolkata, India.)

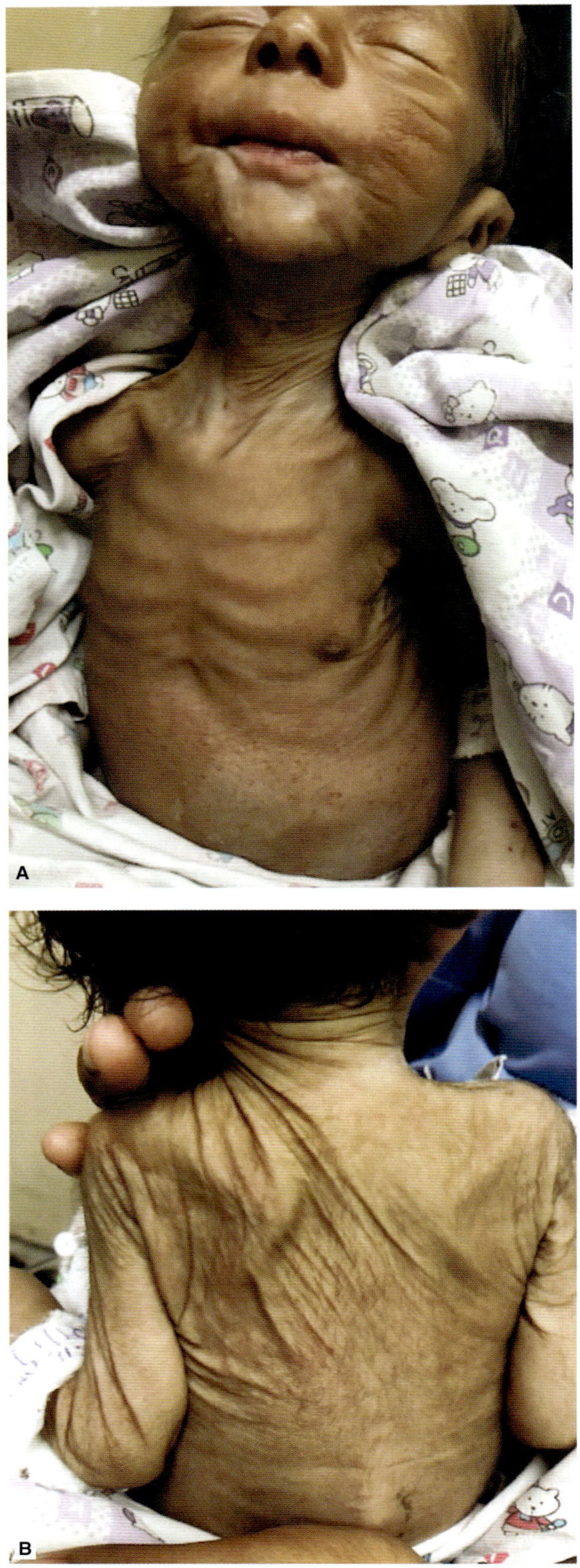

FIGURE 15-3A & 3B. Marasmus in an Indian infant presenting as generalized wasting. (Photograph courtesy of Dr. Sandipan Dhar, Kolkata, India.)

SKIN MANIFESTATIONS OF PROTEIN DEFICIENCY

Protein-energy malnutrition results from insufficient intake of protein and/or calories and includes kwashiorkor and marasmus. Kwashiorkor occurs from a diet high in carbohydrates but low in protein content. Marasmus occurs from both insufficient protein and total calorie intake.

Clinical Features

- Kwashiorkor presents clinically with an erythematous eruption with red-brown overlying flaky scaling, primarily over the sun-covered sites. Other cutaneous manifestations include photosensitivity, purpura, and bruising. There may also be edema of the face, abdomen, and lower limbs. Other associated systemic features include irritability, lethargy, and poor growth.

- Marasmus usually does not present with cutaneous features unless associated with other mineral or vitamin deficiencies. Marasmus usually presents with failure to thrive, irritability, and apathy, with a general appearance of wasting due to loss of subcutaneous tissue.

Differential Diagnoses

- Acrodermatitis enteropathica
  - The cutaneous eruption of kwashiorkor can be fairly similar, although edema is usually not present in acrodermatitis enteropathica.
- Atopic dermatitis
  - The eruption of kwashiorkor can resemble atopic dermatitis, although there is usually a family history of atopy and more prominent flexural involvement in atopic dermatitis.

Investigations & Treatment

- Kwashiorkor and marasmus are usually diagnosed clinically, but investigations to exclude other deficiencies should be undertaken such as complete blood counts, liver function tests, renal function tests, and so forth.
- Treatment of protein malnutrition includes treating dehydration, electrolyte imbalance, hypothermia, micronutrient deficiencies, and infections. Feeding should be started cautiously to achieve adequate catch-up growth.

SKIN MANIFESTATIONS OF VITAMIN DEFICIENCIES

Vitamin deficiencies are common worldwide, but are more common in lower socioeconomic communities. In higher socioeconomic communities, they are often under-recognized, which can lead to detrimental effects for the child. Table 15-1 summarizes the vitamin deficiencies that manifest with cutaneous symptoms and signs.

TABLE 15-1. Vitamin deficiencies with cutaneous manifestations.

	Function	Food Sources	Presentation	Differential Diagnoses	Treatment
A	Fat-soluble vitamin, plays role in cellular differentiation, embryonic and fetal development, immunity, mucosal and skin function	Yellow foods and vegetables, cheese, eggs, offal	• Ocular features: Night blindness, xerophthalmia (dry eyes), Bitot spots (triangular, perilimbal, gray plaques of keratinized conjunctival debris) • Skin: Phrynoderma (follicular hyperkeratosis with small, red-brown follicular papules with central keratotic spinous plug) • Dry lips, thickened tongue	Keratosis pilaris	50,000 IU for <6 months, 100,000 IU for 6–12 months of age, 200,000 IU for 12 months through adulthood
B2 (riboflavin)	Involved in reduction-oxidation reactions; essential for oxidation of fatty acids	Milk, dairy products, cereals, liver, meat, eggs, vegetables	• Skin: Dermatitis on scrotum and labia, nasolabial area, angular stomatitis, glossitis, cheilosis • Others: Anemia, neurodegeneration, and peripheral neuropathy, corneal vascularization, muscular/skeletal/gastrointestinal abnormalities (if deficiency occurs during development)	Other vitamin deficiencies, atopic dermatitis, contact dermatitis	Oral vitamin B2 1.1 mg/kg (women) or 1.3 mg/kg (men)
B3 (niacin)	Cofactor for coenzyme I and II, role in ATP synthesis, glycolysis, and fatty acid and amino acid metabolism	Red meat, liver, lean pork, poultry, salmon, eggs, legumes	• Pellagra: Dermatitis, diarrhea, dementia ("3Ds") • Skin: Hyperpigmented, scaly, eroded patches and plaques over photo-exposed sites, neck ("Casal necklace"), intertriginous areas	Atopic dermatitis, contact dermatitis, collagen vascular disease, autoimmune bullous disease (e.g., pemphigus)	Oral nicotinamide 300 mg in divided doses for 3–4 weeks

(Continued)

TABLE 15-1. Vitamin deficiencies with cutaneous manifestations. (Continued)

	Function	Food Sources	Presentation	Differential Diagnoses	Treatment
B6 (pyridoxine)	Required for tryptophan metabolism and synthesis of nicotinic acid, cofactor to more than 140 enzymes	Plant and animal products	• Skin: Pellagra-like rash, periorificial rash, glossitis, cheilitis, angular stomatitis, oral ulcerations • Neurological: Seizures, peripheral neuropathy • Others: Hypochromic, microcytic anemia, impaired immunity	Atopic dermatitis, contact dermatitis, collagen vascular disease, autoimmune bullous disease (e.g., pemphigus)	Oral vitamin B6 supplementation 30–100 mg/day until resolution of symptoms
B7 (biotin)	Cofactor for carboxylases	Liver, meats, egg yolk, yeast, tomatoes; Avidin in raw egg white can prevent absorption	• Skin: Clinical manifestations similar to zinc deficiency, with crusted, eroded lesions around the mouth and other orifices • Alopecia • Neurological: Lethargy, withdrawn behavior, ataxia, seizures, deafness, developmental delay	Zinc deficiency, atopic dermatitis, contact dermatitis	Oral biotin 10–40 mg/day
B9 (folate)	DNA and RNA synthesis; essential for erythropoiesis	Liver, leafy greens, meat, milk, yeast	• Skin: Hyperpigmentation of oral mucosa, hands, palmar creases, nails, and face; Hunter's glossitis (red, painful tongue with atrophied filiform papillae), angular cheilitis • Others: Macrocytic megaloblastic anemia, fatigue, weakness, neural tube defects (if deficiency occurs during initial weeks of gestation)	Addison's disease	Oral folate 1–5 mg/day
B12 (cyanocobalamine)	Cofactor for homocysteine methyltransferase and methylmalonyl-coA mutase	Animal products such as fish, shellfish, meat, dairy products	• Skin: Hyperpigmentation of palms, soles, flexural areas; vitiligo, angular stomatitis, cheilitis, glossitis, recurrent ulcers, linear streaks on nails, poliosis • Others: Megaloblastic macrocytic anemia, paresthesia, peripheral neuropathy, demyelination of dorsal columns and corticospinal tract, developmental delay, psychiatric manifestations	Addison's disease	Intramuscular vitamin B12 1000 µg/week for 1 month followed by 1000 µg every month
C	Required for growth and repair of tissues, also an antioxidant	Citrus fruits, strawberries, bell peppers, tomatoes, broccoli, cabbage, cauliflower	• Scurvy: Follicular hyperkeratotic papules (upper arms, legs, buttocks) perifollicular hemorrhage, purpura and ecchymoses on the legs, hairs twisted and fragile, poor wound healing and reopening of old scars, splinter hemorrhages, swollen gums • Others: Eye dryness and irritation, subconjunctival, periorbital, or orbital hemorrhage, painful hemarthrosis, subperiosteal hemorrhage (femur, proximal tibia), costochondral junction bleeding, intramuscular bleeding	Vasculitis, thrombocytopenia, pigmented purpuric dermatosis, folliculitis	Oral vitamin C 100 mg TID for at least 1 week, followed by 100 mg daily until symptoms resolve

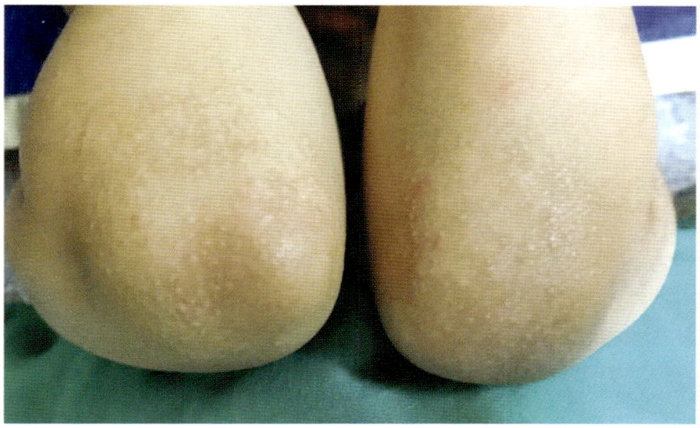

FIGURE 15-4. Phrynoderma in an Indian child presenting as hyperkeratotic, follicular papules on the elbows. (Photograph courtesy of Dr. Sandipan Dhar, Kolkata, India.)

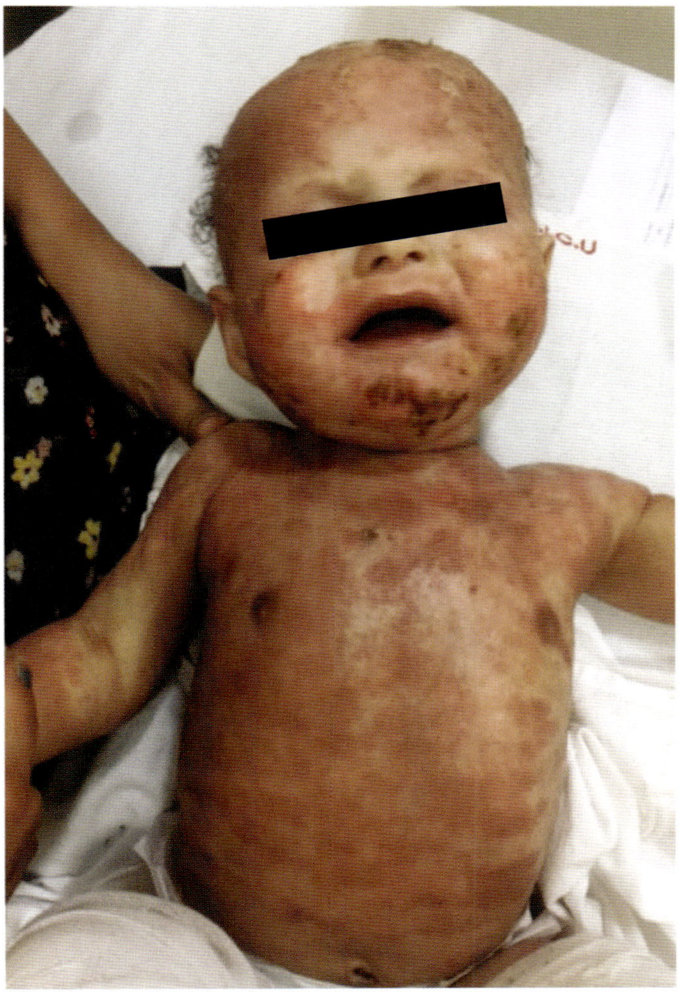

FIGURE 15-5. Biotin deficiency in a young Indian child presenting with widespread crusted, eroded patches and plaques. (Photograph courtesy of Dr. Sandipan Dhar, Kolkata, India.)

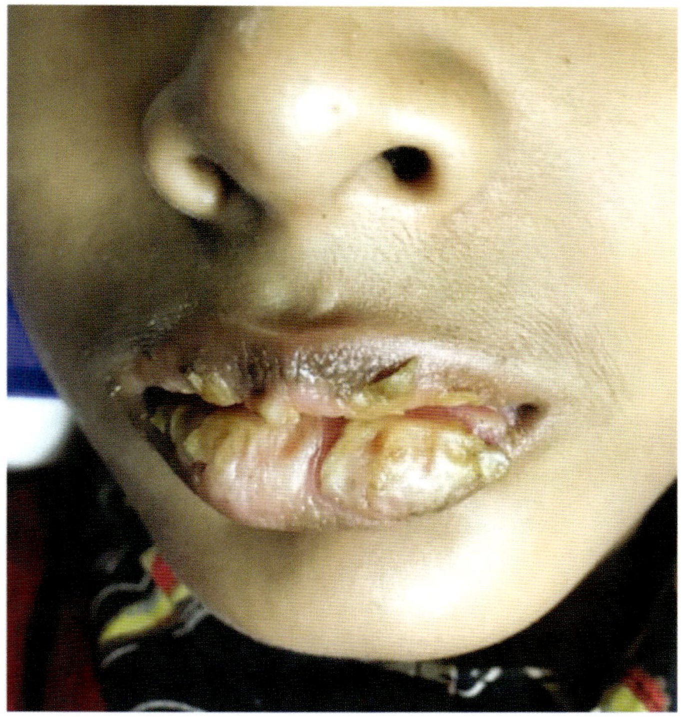

FIGURE 15-6. Vitamin B2 (riboflavin) deficiency in an Indian boy presenting as cheilitis. (Photograph courtesy of Dr. Sandipan Dhar, Kolkata, India.)

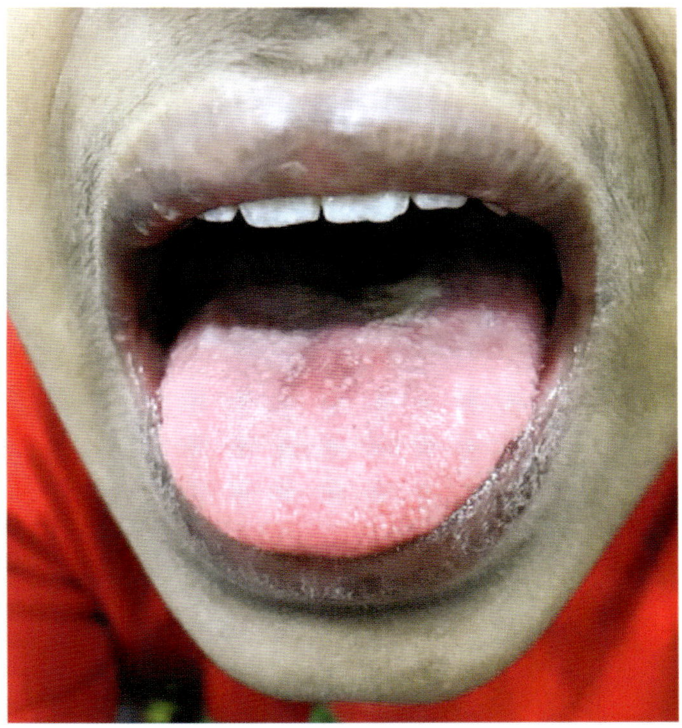

FIGURE 15-7. Vitamin B2 (riboflavin) deficiency in an Indian boy, presenting as glossitis. (Photograph courtesy of Dr. Sandipan Dhar, Kolkata, India.)

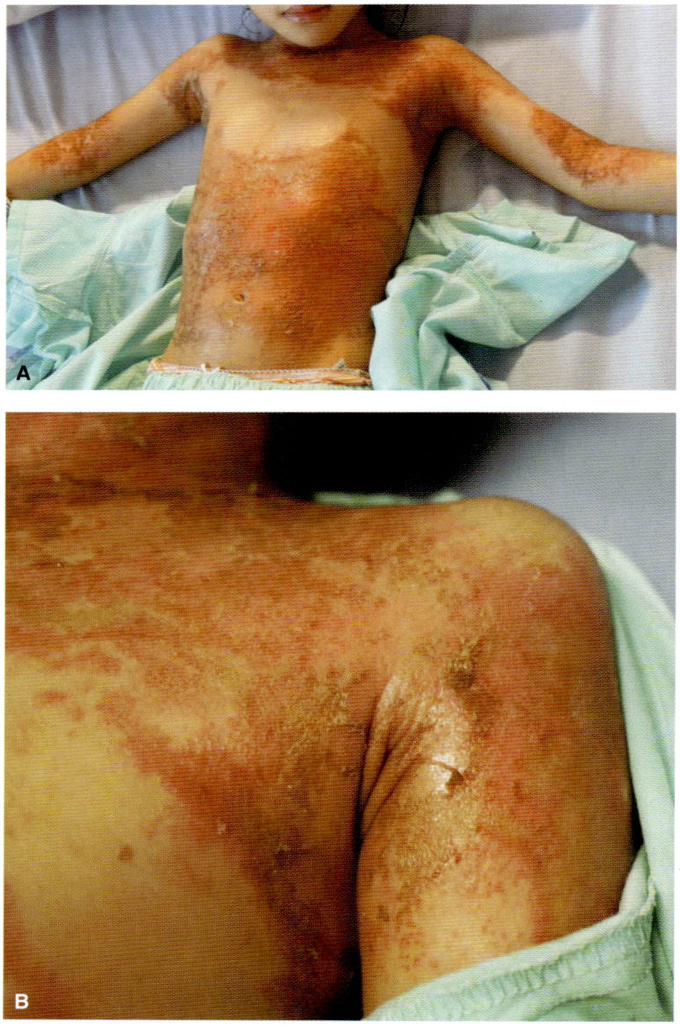

FIGURE 15-8A & 8B. Pellagra caused by niacin deficiency in a 7-year-old Chinese girl presenting with well-demarcated, scaly, eroded plaques over the neck, trunk, and intertriginous areas.

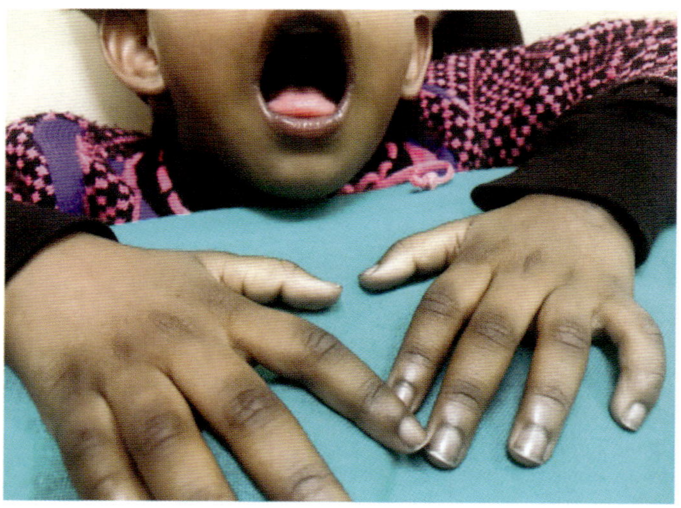

FIGURE 15-9. Vitamin B12 deficiency causing hyperpigmentation of the hands and lips in this Indian child. (Photograph courtesy of Dr. Sandipan Dhar, Kolkata, India.)

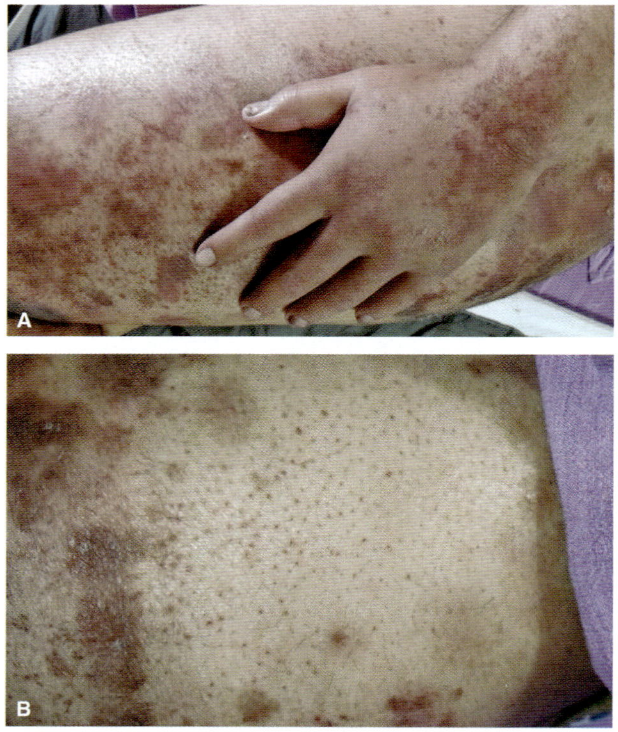

FIGURE 15-10A & 10B. Scurvy caused by vitamin C deficiency presenting as follicular hyperkeratotic papules associated with easy bruising. (Photograph courtesy of Dr. Sandipan Dhar, Kolkata, India.)

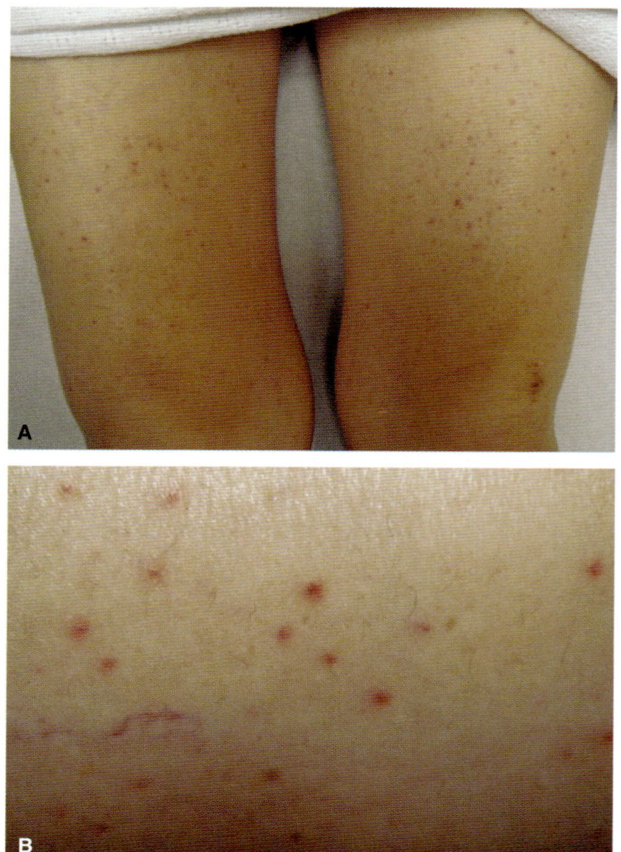

FIGURE 15-11A & 11B. Scurvy presenting as perifollicular hemorrhage associated with twisted hairs.

SKIN MANIFESTATIONS OF IMMUNODEFICIENCY

Immunodeficiency can be primary or acquired. Primary immunodeficiencies or inborn errors of immunity occur from mutations in various genes encoding different components of the immune system. Acquired immunodeficiency in children and adolescents occurs from medications (e.g., prolonged systemic corticosteroids, chemotherapy), hematological malignancies (e.g., lymphomas), or HIV infection. Immunodeficient patients are susceptible to various microbes which usually do not cause invasive disease in immunocompetent individuals. Depending on the immune defect, these patients may have variable susceptibility to viruses, bacteria, and fungi.

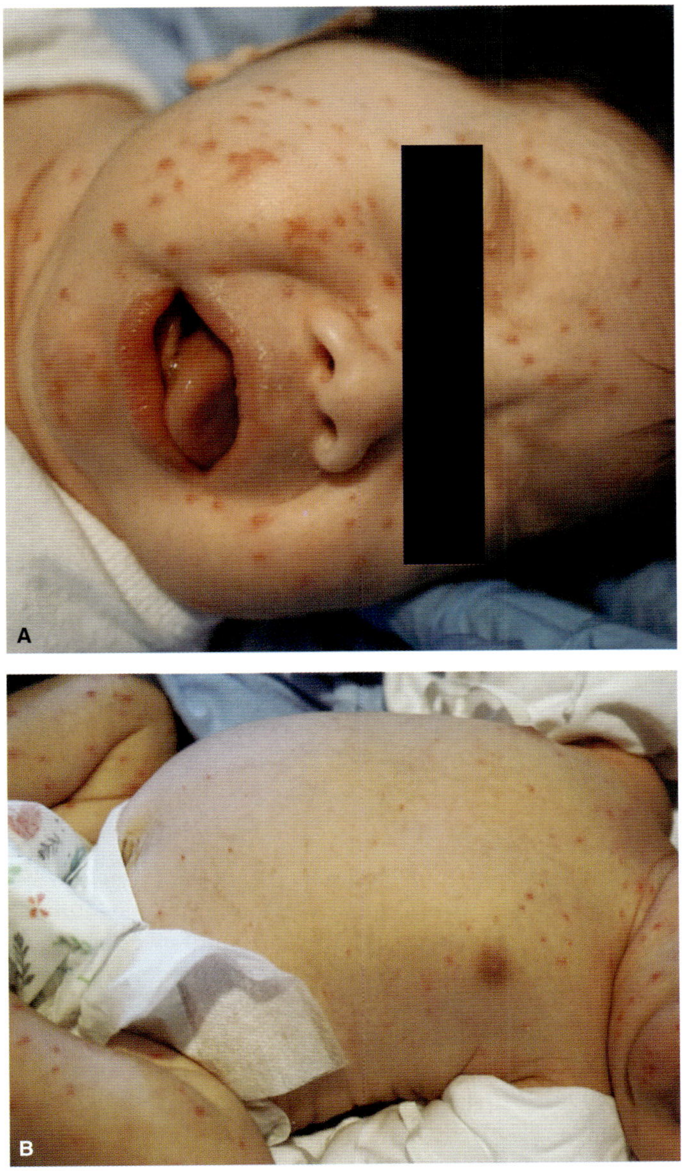

FIGURE 15-12A & 12B. Disseminated fungal infection in a Eurasian infant with chronic granulomatous disease (CGD), presenting as widespread violaceous macules and papules.

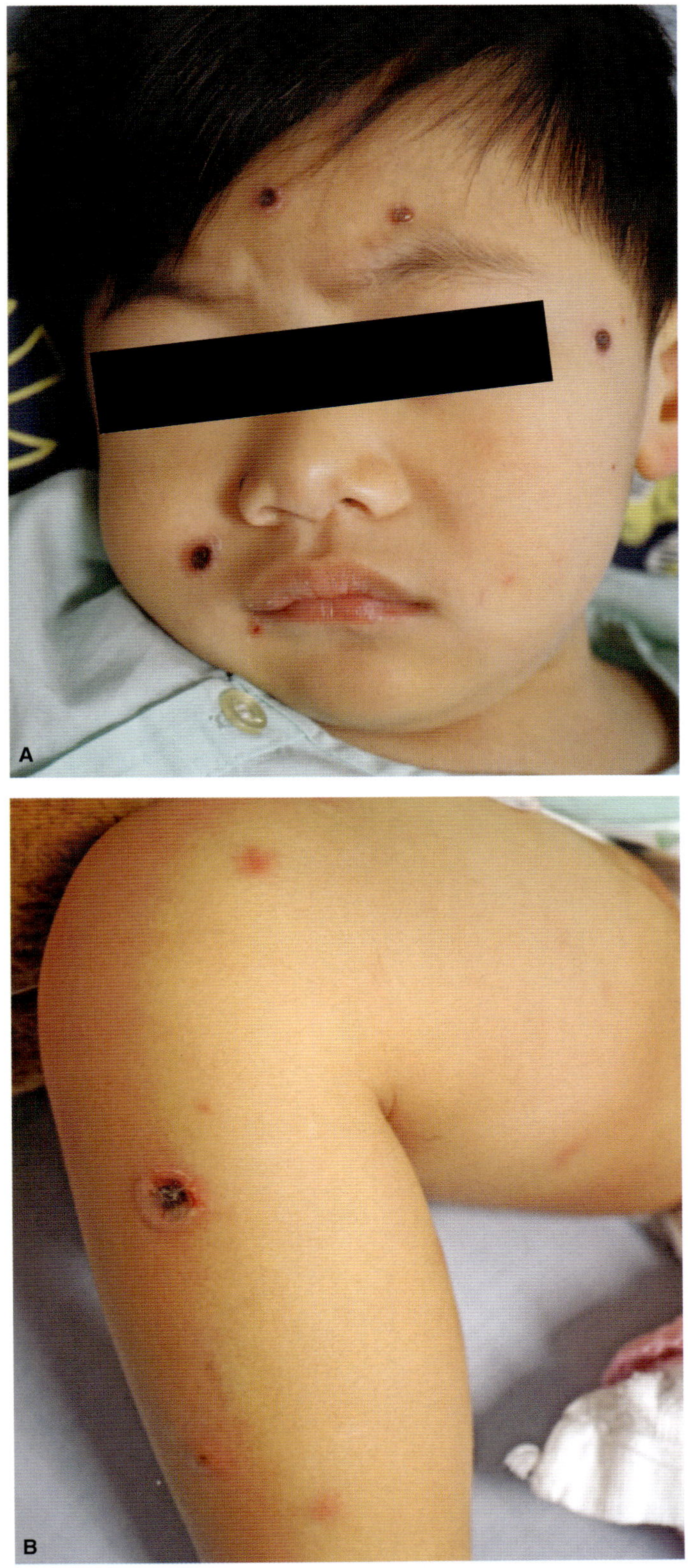

FIGURE 15-13A & 13B. Ecthyma gangrenosum caused by disseminated pseudomonas infection in a Chinese boy with Bruton's agammaglobulinemia, presenting as ulcerated papules with overlying eschar.

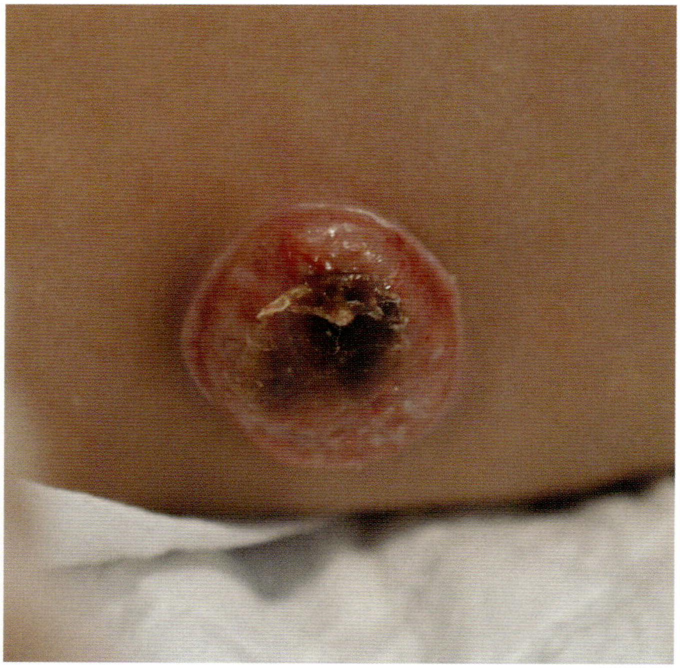

FIGURE 15-14. Non-healing BCG site in an Indonesian infant with primary immunodeficiency presenting as an ulcerated, crusted nodule. Mycobacterial culture was positive for *Mycobacterium bovis*.

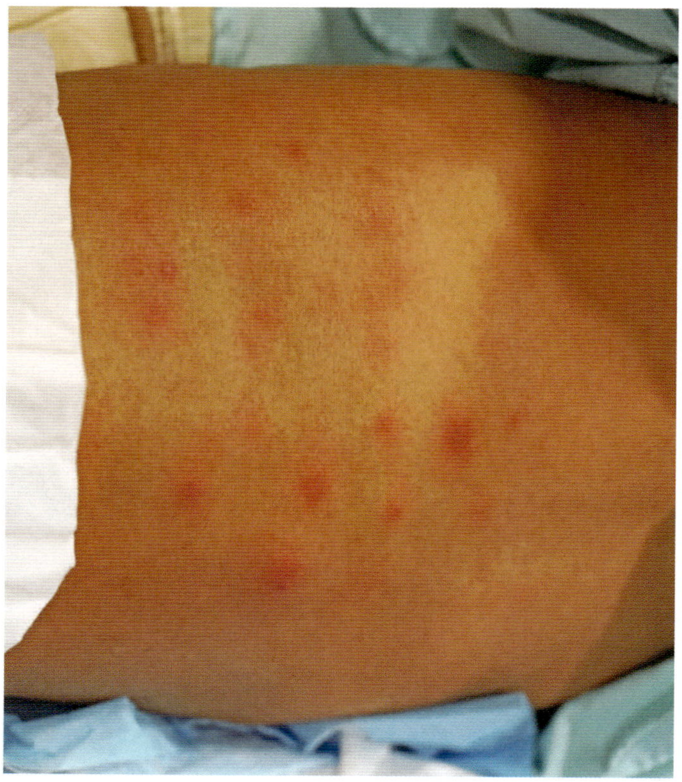

FIGURE 15-15. A Malay toddler with background of immunodeficiency from chemotherapy, presenting with disseminated opportunistic fungal infection, with scattered erythematous-to-violaceous papules and plaques on his trunk.

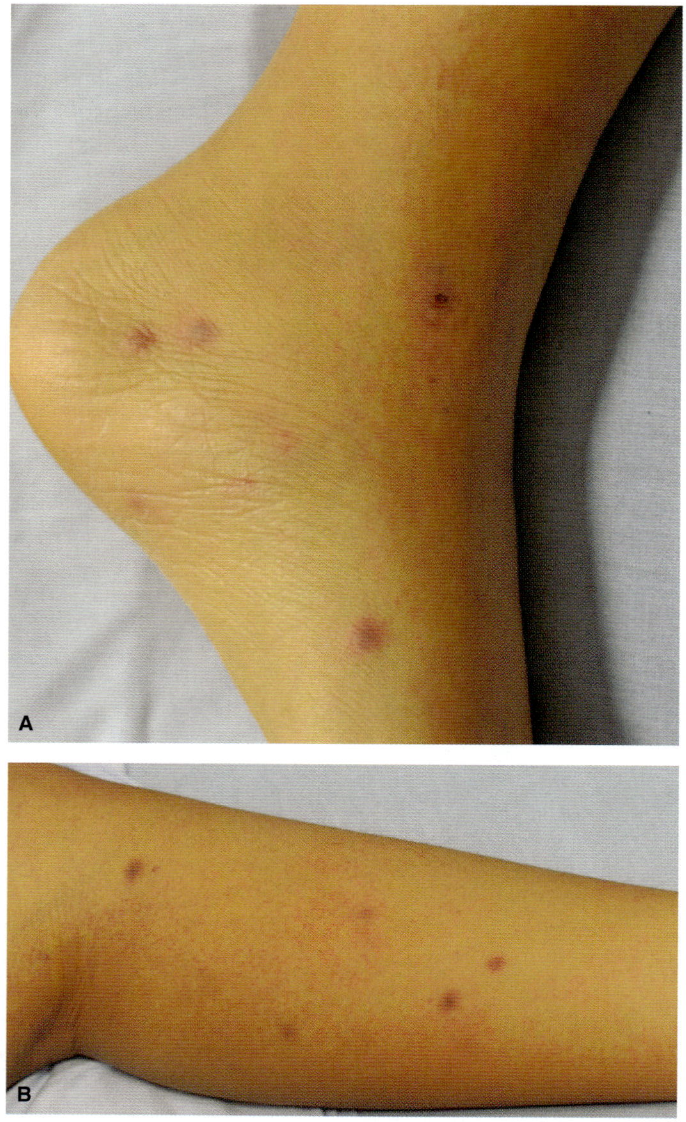

FIGURE 15-16A & 16B. Saprocheate, an opportunistic yeast, infection in a Chinese boy with underlying leukemia undergoing chemotherapy, presenting with scattered purpuric papules.

Clinical Features

- Patients with primary immunodeficiency can present with severe, recalcitrant eczematous eruptions, prompting further immunological evaluation if associated with other features of immunodeficiency. Also known as primary atopic disorders, immunodeficiency syndromes associated with early, severe eczema include hyper-IgE syndrome, Wiskott-Aldrich syndrome, severe combined immunodeficiency (SCID) or Omenn syndrome, and Netherton syndrome.
- Granulomatous skin lesions can occur in chronic granulomatous disease (CGD) and common variable immunodeficiency (CVID).

- Nail, hair, and tooth abnormalities can occur in various immunodeficiency syndromes, such as ectodermal dysplasia with immunodeficiency, dyskeratosis congenita, and autoimmune polyendocrinopathy-candidiasis-ectodermal dysplasia (APECED) syndrome.
- Other features that point to a diagnosis of primary immunodeficiency include infections in multiple locations with increasing frequency and severity with age, recurrent infections with common pathogens, serious infections with unusual pathogens, and failure to thrive.
- Opportunistic skin infections may be seen in both primary and acquired immunodeficiency.
- Bacterial infections (e.g., impetigo, folliculitis, and furunculosis) may occur more frequently in patients with neutrophilic disorders, such as leukocyte adhesion deficiency (LAD). It can also occur more frequently in CGD and hyper-IgE syndrome. Apart from common skin bacteria (e.g., *Staphylococcus aureus*), skin infections with less common bacteria may also occur (e.g., *Klebsiella*, *Pseudomonas*, *Escherichia coli*, *Serratia*, *Salmonella*).
- Mycobacterial infections can present on the skin in immunodeficient patients (e.g., SCID and Mendelian susceptibility to mycobacterial diseases [MSMD]) and can be associated with invasive disease. "BCGosis" can present as localized or disseminated cutaneous or systemic infection after BCG vaccination in these patients, presenting with ulcerated, scabbed, and necrotic papules and nodules.
- The most common fungal infection seen in primary immunodeficient patients is *Candida* species. Persistent and difficult-to-treat candida infections in infancy may be a sign of T-cell immunodeficiency, including SCID and DiGeorge syndrome. Patients with immunodeficiency secondary to iatrogenic causes, such as chemotherapy or stem-cell transplants, are particularly prone to opportunistic invasive fungal infections that can present as deep nodules or plaques on the skin, such as *Aspergillus* spp., *Cryptococcus* spp., *Fusarium* spp., and *Dematiaceous* fungi.

Differential Diagnoses

- Eczematous eruptions
  - Severe atopic dermatitis with concomitant food allergies, seborrheic dermatitis, and infantile psoriasis are differential diagnoses of widespread eczematous eruptions in infancy.
- Neonatal or infantile erythroderma
  - Differential diagnoses, including congenital ichthyoses, epidermolytic ichthyoses, scalded skin syndrome, and cutaneous candidiasis, can also present with early erythroderma.
- Granulomatous skin lesions
  - Differential diagnoses include mycobacterial (tuberculous or atypical mycobacteria) or fungal infections, granuloma annulare, and rheumatoid nodules.

Investigations & Treatment

- If primary immunodeficiency is suspected, patients should be referred to a pediatric immunologist for further evaluation. Initial investigations to screen for underlying immunodeficiency include complete blood count with differential counts, immunoglobulin (IgG, IgA, IgM, and IgE) levels, human immunodeficiency virus (HIV) serology, and complement levels (CH_{50}, AH_{50}, and CH_{100}).
- Skin biopsies are essential to exclude opportunistic infections in suspected immunodeficient patients.
- Definitive treatment of the underlying immunodeficiency is paramount in the management of these patients. Skin manifestations may be treated with the usual treatments for the dermatosis as seen in immunocompetent children such as topical moisturizers, topical corticosteroids, and topical calcineurin inhibitors. However, due to the underlying immunodeficiency or skin barrier defects, side effects from these topical medications may occur more often.

Pearls & Practical Tips

- Suspect an underlying immunodeficiency in patients presenting with severe eczematous eruptions, especially if associated with other manifestations such as failure to thrive.
- The threshold to perform skin biopsies in immunodeficiency should be very low, as these patients are prone to multiple infections, especially to pathogens that usually do not cause disease in normal children. Systemic dissemination can occur, which can lead to mortality or severe morbidity.
- Bacterial, mycobacterial, and fungal cultures should always be sent when a biopsy is performed in a patient with suspected or known immunodeficiency presenting with an unusual rash.

Bibliography

1. Al-Herz W, Nanda A. Skin manifestations in primary immunodeficient children. Pediatr Dermatol 2011 Sep-Oct;28(5):494–501.
2. Reust CE. Evaluation of primary immunodeficiency disease in children. Am Fam Physician 2013 Jun;87(11):773–8.
3. Lehman H. Skin manifestations of primary immune deficiency. Clin Rev Allergy Immunol 2014 Apr;46(2):112–9.

SKIN MANIFESTATIONS OF HEMATOLOGICAL CONDITIONS

Hematological system disorders can present with mucocutaneous symptoms and signs, such as anemia and disorders of hemostasis. Early recognition of these features will prompt further investigations for early determination and management of underlying causes.

SKIN MANIFESTATIONS OF ANEMIA

True anemia is defined as a decrease in the circulating red cell mass, leading to impaired ability to meet the body's oxygen demands. Spurious anemia occurs when there is a dilutional effect of an increase in plasma volume, such as in fluid overload states.

Clinical Features

- Patients present with fatigue, breathlessness, tachypnea, tachycardia, decrease in effort tolerance, dizziness, presyncope, and syncope.
- Skin signs include pallor, which is best seen in the conjunctiva or palmar creases.

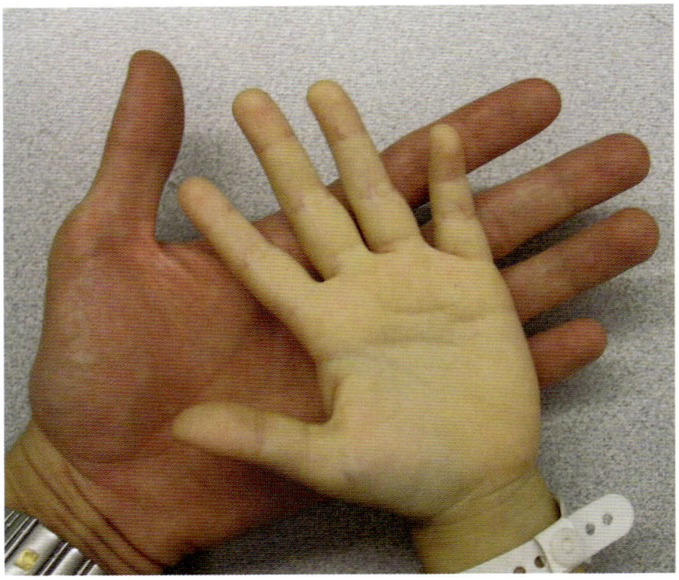

FIGURE 15-17. Palmar pallor in a child with hemolytic anemia, compared to the hands of her normal parent. (Photograph courtesy of Dr. Kumudhini Rajasegaran, Adolescent Medicine, KK Women's & Children's Hospital, Singapore.)

- Other associated signs that should be elicited to determine a cause for the anemia include petechiae, purpura and ecchymoses, and jaundice.
- Koilonychia may be seen with iron deficiency, leukonychia from chronic kidney disease, digital clubbing from chronic liver disease, or congenital heart disease.
- A detailed examination of other organ systems should be performed, including cardiovascular, gastrointestinal, renal, neurological, and endocrinological systems.

Differential Diagnoses

- Differential diagnoses for causes of anemia include:
  - Decreased production of red cells, including nutritional deficiencies (e.g., iron, folate, vitamin B12, and vitamin C), reduction in precursors for red cell production (e.g., hematological malignancies, myelofibrosis, aplastic anemia), ineffective erythropoiesis (e.g., hemoglobinopathies such as thalassemia, myelodysplastic syndrome, anemia of chronic disease), and increased destruction or loss of red cells (e.g., infections, autoimmune hemolytic anemia, blood loss).

Investigations & Treatment

- A complete blood count, peripheral blood film, and reticulocyte count are the most useful initial tests to guide further investigations.
- Further investigations should be guided by the clinical presentation and possible causes, and may include liver function test, renal function tests, thyroid function test, iron studies, lactate dehydrogenase, haptoglobin, hemoglobin electrophoresis, autoimmune markers, vitamin B12 and folate levels, infective screen, and bone marrow examination.
- Treatment of the underlying cause of the anemia will reverse the skin manifestations of the condition.

SKIN MANIFESTATIONS OF DISORDERED HEMOSTASIS

Disordered hemostasis can occur due to conditions that affect platelets, coagulation factors, or the vascular endothelium.

Clinical Features

- The classical skin signs of disordered hemostasis are petechiae, purpura, and ecchymoses (bruising).
- Petechiae are small reddish or purplish pinpoint round spots, less than 2 mm in size, that appear on the skin or mucous membrane as a result of localized hemorrhage. They are caused by platelet disorders.
- Purpura present as non-blanchable, red or violaceous patches that can appear on the skin or mucous membranes and are more than 3 mm in diameter. Ecchymoses are larger than purpura. They occur as a result of disorders of platelets or coagulation factors.
- A thorough history and systematic physical examination is important to determine the cause of disordered hemostasis. Important causes to exclude are inherited causes of coagulation, infections, hematological malignancies, connective tissue diseases, nutritional deficiencies, and chronic liver diseases. Traumatic causes such as injury (accidental or non-accidental), torniquet effect, and local pressure should also be considered.

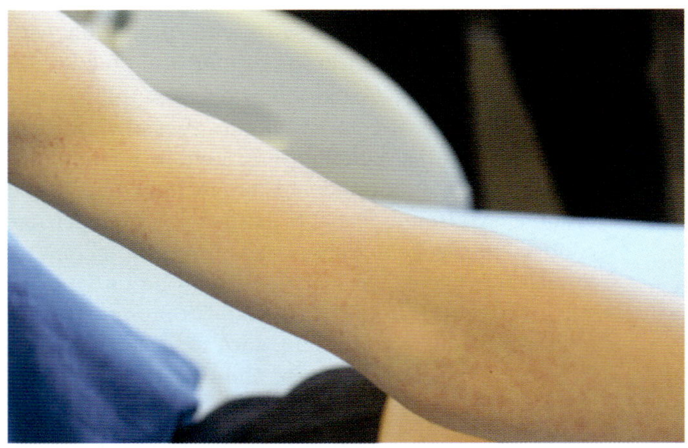

FIGURE 15-18. Petechiae in a Chinese teenager due to underlying thrombocytopenia.

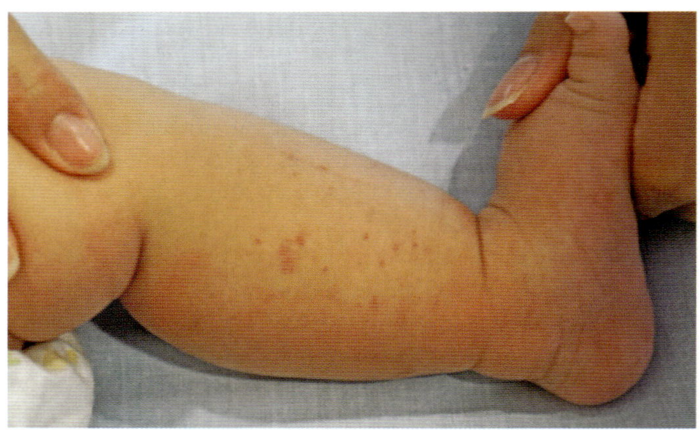

FIGURE 15-19. Petechiae on the legs of an infant associated with prolonged carriage in a baby carrier (Rumpel-Leede phenomenon).

Differential Diagnoses

Differential diagnoses of disordered hemostasis include platelet disorders, coagulopathies, and vascular disorders.

- Platelet disorders
  - Disordered production, which may be inherited (e.g., Wiskott-Aldrich syndrome, Fanconi anemia) or acquired (e.g., hematological malignancy, bone marrow failure, drugs).
  - Increased destruction, including infections (viral, bacterial, or parasitic) and autoimmune conditions (e.g., idiopathic thrombocytopenic purpura or lupus erythematosus).
  - Increased consumption, including sequestration from hypersplenism and Kasabach-Merritt phenomenon.
- Coagulopathies
  - Genetic causes (e.g., von Willebrand disease, factor VII deficiency, hemophilia, fibrinolytic defects).
  - Acquired causes (e.g., severe infection, malignancy, liver disease).
- Vascular endothelium dysfunction
  - Increased vascular fragility (e.g., Ehlers-Danlos syndrome, Marfan syndrome, connective tissue disorders, excessive use of corticosteroids, scurvy).
  - Vasculitis (e.g., Henoch-Schonlein purpura [HSP]).
  - Traumatic (e.g., tourniquet effect, localized pressure, non-accidental injury).

Investigations & Treatment

- Initial investigations include complete blood count, peripheral blood film, prothrombin time (PT), and activated thromboplastin time (aPTT).
- With derangements in PT and/or aPTT, mixing studies and subsequent factor assays can be performed. Other follow-up tests include thrombin time, fibrinogen, and von Willebrand factor antigen test.
- Treatment and resolution of the underlying cause of the disordered hemostasis will correct the skin manifestations.

Reference

1. Yan AC, Jen MV. Skin signs of pediatric nutritional disorders. Curr Probl Pediatr Adolesc Health Care 2012 Sep;42(8):212–7. doi: 10.1016/j.cppeds.2012.02.003. PMID: 22884028.

GRAFT-VERSUS-HOST DISEASE

Graft-versus-host disease (GVHD) is caused by donor leukocytes targeting host organs, causing apoptosis and organ dysfunction. It occurs most frequently in children with malignancy who have undergone hematopoietic stem cell transplantation, especially if the transplant is from a partially matched family member or unrelated donor. It can also occur in immunodeficient patients who have received non-irradiated blood products.

Clinical Features

GVHD can be classified into acute and chronic forms. Acute GVHD usually occurs in the first few months after transplant, whereas chronic GVHD can occur months to years after transplant. The risk of chronic GVHD is higher in patients who have had acute GVHD.

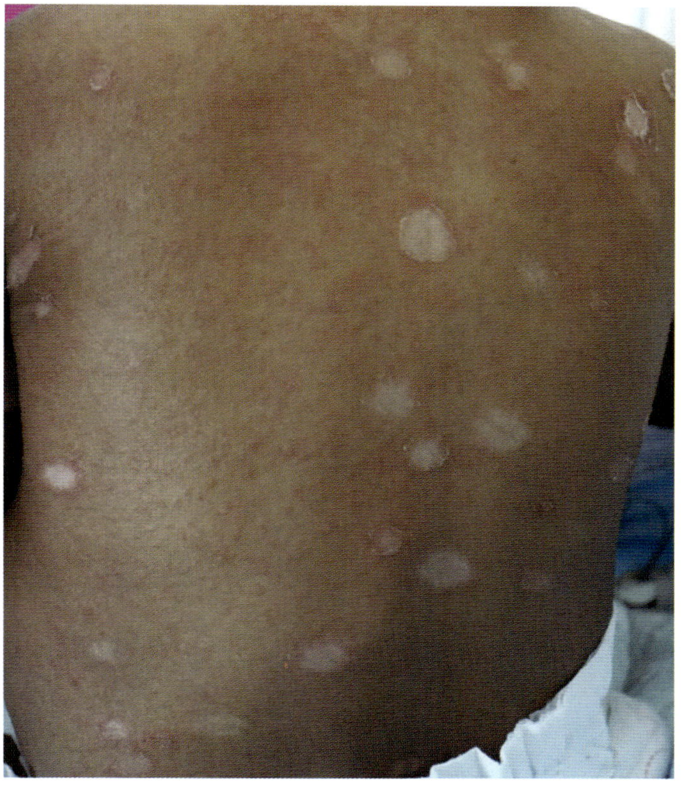

FIGURE 15-20. GVHD in a 2-year-old Malay boy presenting with annular, scaly plaques, affecting the trunk, limbs, and scalp.

- Acute GVHD
  - The condition involves the skin, gastrointestinal tract, and liver.
  - Presents with subacute onset of patchy erythematous macules, papules, patches, and plaques which are only mildly pruritic, becoming more confluent with time. Target or targetoid lesions may sometimes be seen. It usually begins on the face and acral sites before becoming generalized. Scaling and exfoliation can occur, and in severe forms can resemble generalized exfoliative dermatitis or toxic epidermal necrolysis.
  - In people of Asian descent, the rash is often hyperpigmented.
  - There may be accompanying fever, diarrhea (which can be bloody), abdominal pain, nausea, and vomiting. Transaminitis and hepatomegaly may also occur.
- Chronic GVHD
  - This often presents initially as violaceous or pinkish, flat-topped lichenoid papules and plaques. This can be localized, especially over the joints, or more generalized. Mucosal changes resembling lichen planus may also be seen.
  - Other forms of chronic GVHD include acquired ichthyosis and eczematous forms. Late manifestations include sclerodermoid changes, dyspigmentation, poikiloderma, ulcerations, scarring alopecia, and nail dystrophy.

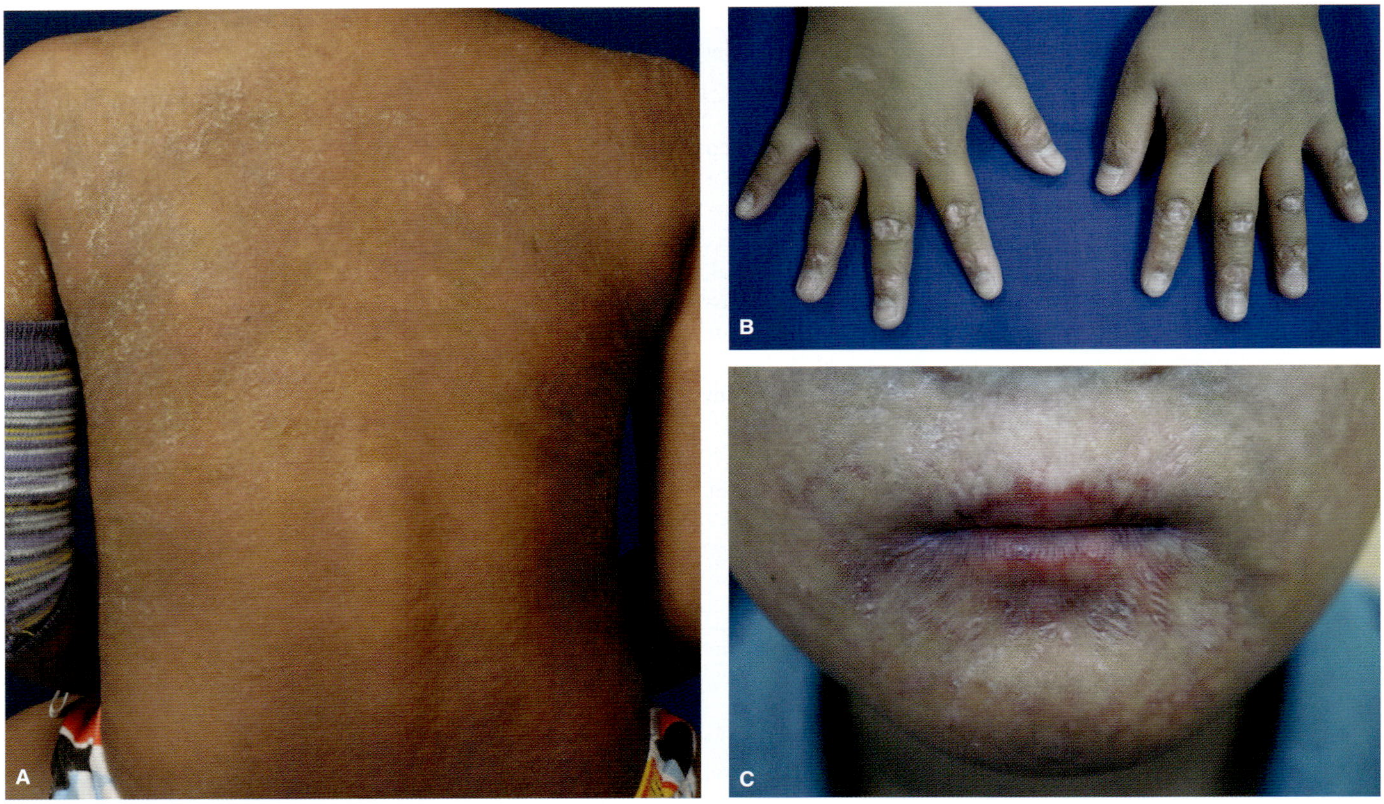

FIGURE 15-21A–21C. Acute GVHD in a 7-year-old Chinese boy with underlying Fanconi anemia, who developed GVHD soon after a bone marrow transplant, presenting as extensive, scaly, hyperpigmented patches and plaques (Figure 15-21A), with more lichenoid features 2 years after the transplant (Figures 15-21B & 15-21C).

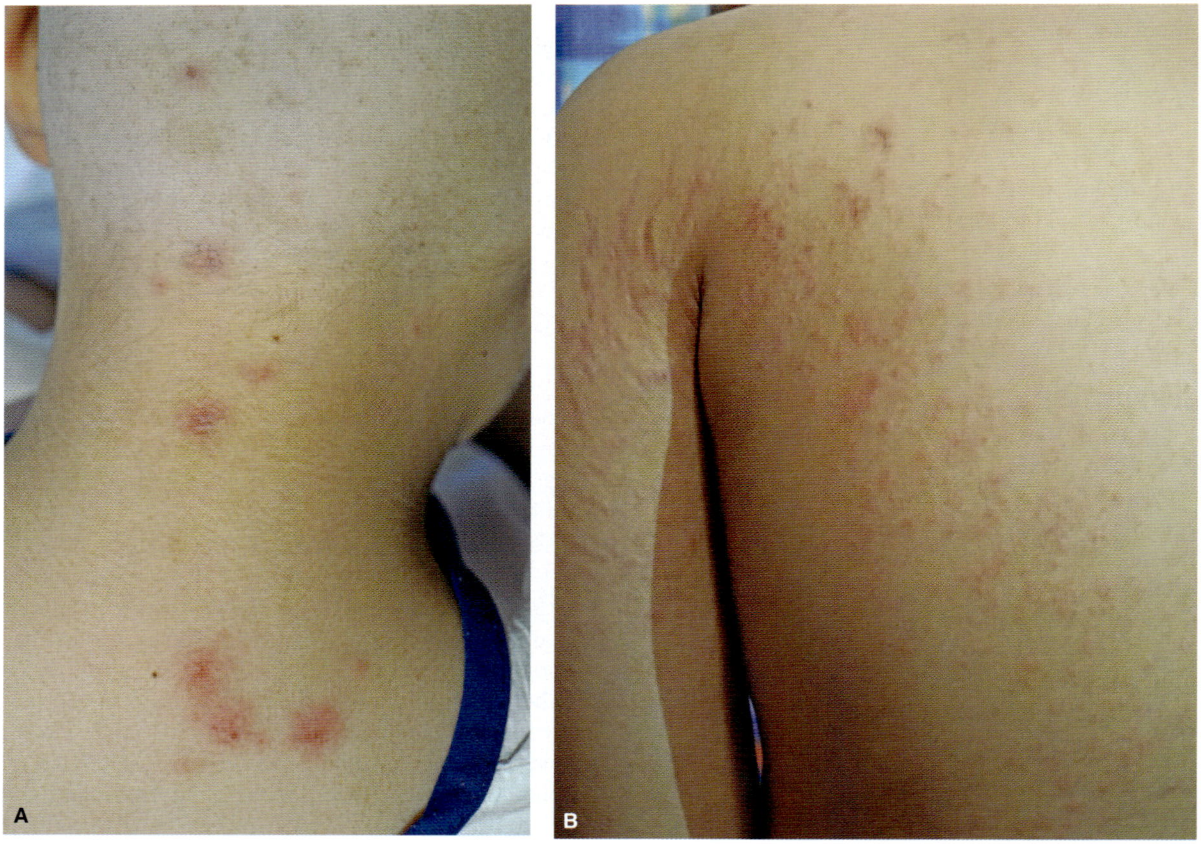

FIGURE 15-22A & 22B. Acute GVHD in a Chinese adolescent boy presenting with urticated and targetoid lesions on his neck and trunk.

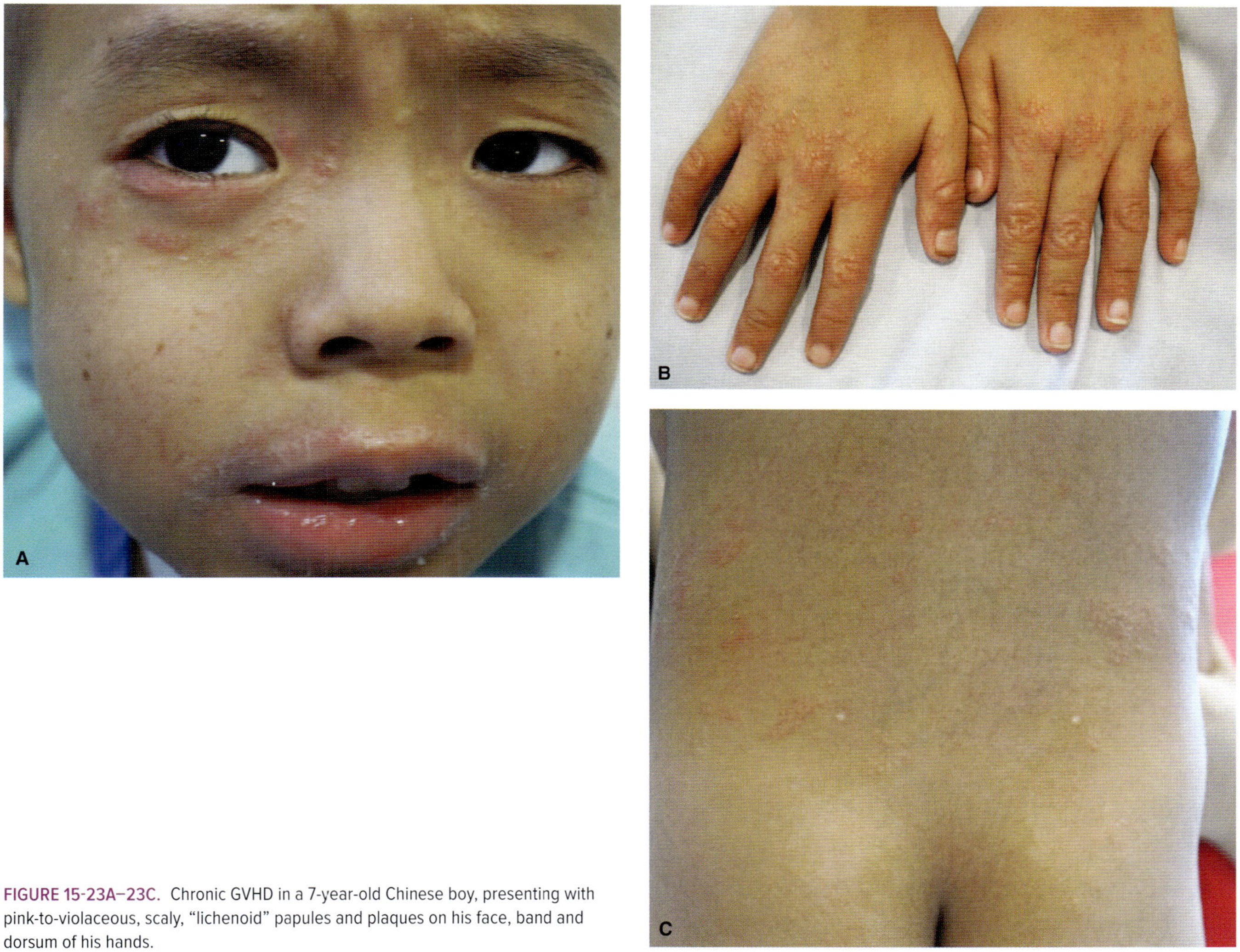

FIGURE 15-23A–23C. Chronic GVHD in a 7-year-old Chinese boy, presenting with pink-to-violaceous, scaly, “lichenoid” papules and plaques on his face, band and dorsum of his hands.

  - Organ involvement is common in chronic GVHD and includes gastrointestinal, hepatic, musculoskeletal, and pulmonary systems.

Differential Diagnoses

- Acute GVHD
  - Differentials from acute GVHD include viral exanthems and drug allergies. Viral exanthems usually resolve in a few days or weeks. Drug allergies, such as erythema multiforme and Stevens-Johnson syndrome, should be excluded by a thorough drug history.
  - Skin biopsies may or may not be useful to differentiate between viral exanthems, drug allergy, and GVHD. Close clinical correlation is important.
- Chronic GVHD
  - Lichenoid presentation can mimic lichen planus and autoimmune disease, such as dermatomyositis and lupus erythematosus. With more sclerodermoid changes, it can mimic morphea and scleroderma. Eczematous forms can mimic atopic dermatitis or other endogenous eczemas.

Investigations & Treatment

- The diagnosis of acute GVHD is made by correlating clinical, hematological, biochemical, and histological features.
- Histological features of acute GVHD include basal vacuolar alteration with exocytosis of lymphocytes and apoptotic keratinocytes. Satellite cell necrosis is classically seen, where a necrotic keratinocyte appears adjacent to a lymphocyte. Severe forms may result in a cleft or blister at the dermal-epidermal junction.
- Histological features of chronic GVHD depend on the clinical presentation. For lichenoid forms, a lichenoid band is seen on histology, sometimes accompanied by satellite cell necrosis. For sclerodermoid forms, sclerosed dermal collagen is seen.
- Treatment of mild acute GVHD, especially in the absence of organ involvement, can be with topical corticosteroids and moisturizers. More severe forms may require treatment with systemic immunosuppression, including corticosteroids. Other treatment options include mycophenolate mofetil, sirolimus, maraviroc (CCR5

antagonist), anti-thymocyte globulins, monoclonal antibodies, and mesenchymal stem cells.

- Similar treatment regimens can be applied to the treatment of chronic GVHD. Topical corticosteroids and calcineurin inhibitors can be used for milder forms. Other treatment options that have been described include systemic retinoids (e.g., acitretin), phototherapy (e.g., narrow-band ultraviolet B, psoralen with ultraviolet A, and UVA1), and thalidomide. Mortality in chronic GVHD can occur.

Pearls & Practical Tips

- With the use of regimens to prevent or reduce GVHD in post-transplant patients, the onset and manifestations of the disease are altered.
- The risk of drug eruptions immediately post-transplantation is extremely low, when the patient's white cell counts have not yet recovered.
- Post-inflammatory dyspigmentation is common in Asian patients with both acute and chronic GVHD, although it is more prominent in the latter.

Bibliography

1. Gatza E, Reddy P, Choi SW. Prevention and treatment of acute graft-versus-host disease in children, adolescents, and young adults. Biol Blood Marrow Transplant 2020 May;26(5): e101–12.

SKIN MANIFESTATIONS OF GASTROINTESTINAL CONDITIONS

SKIN MANIFESTATIONS OF INFLAMMATORY BOWEL DISEASE

Inflammatory bowel disease (IBD) is a chronic inflammatory disorder of the gastrointestinal tract, with two main subtypes, Crohn's disease (CD) and ulcerative colitis (UC). Skin manifestations include erythema nodosum, pyoderma gangrenosum, Sweet syndrome, and recurrent oral ulcers. These are less commonly seen in children compared to adults. Treatment-induced skin lesions may also be seen.

Clinical Features

- Erythema nodosum is the most common skin manifestation in IBD, being more common in CD than UC patients. There is a higher female preponderance.
- Pyoderma gangrenosum is more common in patients with UC compared to CD. There is a high recurrence rate and a female preponderance.
- Sweet syndrome is rare in children with IBD but has a female preponderance.
- Oral ulcers are more common in CD than UC. In 25% of cases, oral ulcers appear before the diagnosis of IBD, and often occur as multiple, painful ulcers over the lips or buccal mucosa. Periodontitis may also be present.
- Orofacial granulomatosis (OFG), also known granulomatous cheilitis, is an uncommon disease characterized by face and lip swelling. The Melkersson-Rosenthal syndrome presents with a triad of recurrent orofacial swelling, relapsing facial paralysis, and fissured tongue.

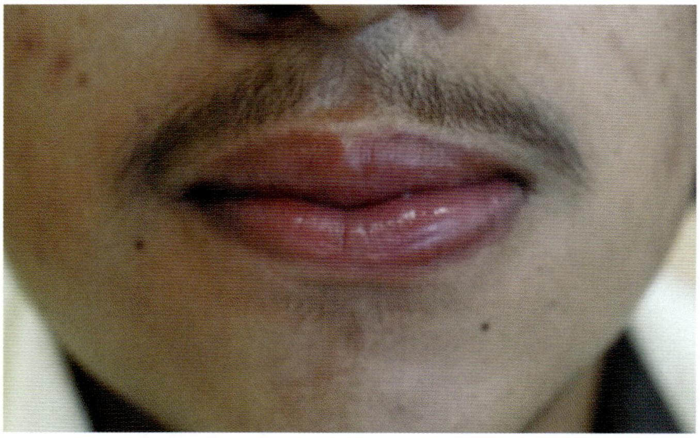

FIGURE 15-24. Granulomatous cheilitis in an Indian adolescent male presenting as thickening of his upper and lower lips.

Investigations & Treatment

- The diagnosis of IBD is based on clinical, endoscopic, histological, and laboratory findings.
- Treatment of dermatoses associated with IBD is similar to patients without IBD (see relevant chapters). Treatment of the underlying IBD may improve the associated dermatoses.
- Similarly, oral lesions can improve with treatment of the IBD. Adjunctive treatment is with antiseptic or anti-inflammatory mouthwashes, while severe cases may require topical or systemic corticosteroids and anti-TNF agents.
- OFG may be treated with intralesional or systemic corticosteroids. Other treatments include minocycline, macrolides, dapsone, azathioprine, clofazimine, thalidomide, and anti-TNF agents.

Pearls & Practical Tips

- The presence of these extra-intestinal manifestations should prompt physicians to screen for underlying IBD, given the significance and potential occurrence even before an IBD diagnosis is established.

Bibliography

1. Greuter T, Navarini A, Vavricka SR. Skin manifestations of inflammatory bowel disease. Clin Rev Allergy Immunol 2017 Dec;53(3):413–27. doi: 10.1007/s12016-017-8617-4. PMID: 28643285.
2. Al-Hamad A, Porter S, Fedele S. Orofacial granulomatosis. Dermatol Clin 2015 Jul;33(3):433–46. doi: 10.1016/j.det.2015.03.008. Epub 2015 May 6. PMID: 26143423.

PEUTZ-JEGHERS SYNDROME

Peutz-Jeghers syndrome (PJS) is a rare autosomal dominant disorder that often presents with mucocutaneous pigmented lesions, and is associated with multiple intestinal hamartomatous polyps and various cancers. The pigmented lesions can present in childhood or adolescence. Causative mutations in the serine-threonine kinase STK11/LKB1 gene have been found in 70% of familial cases.

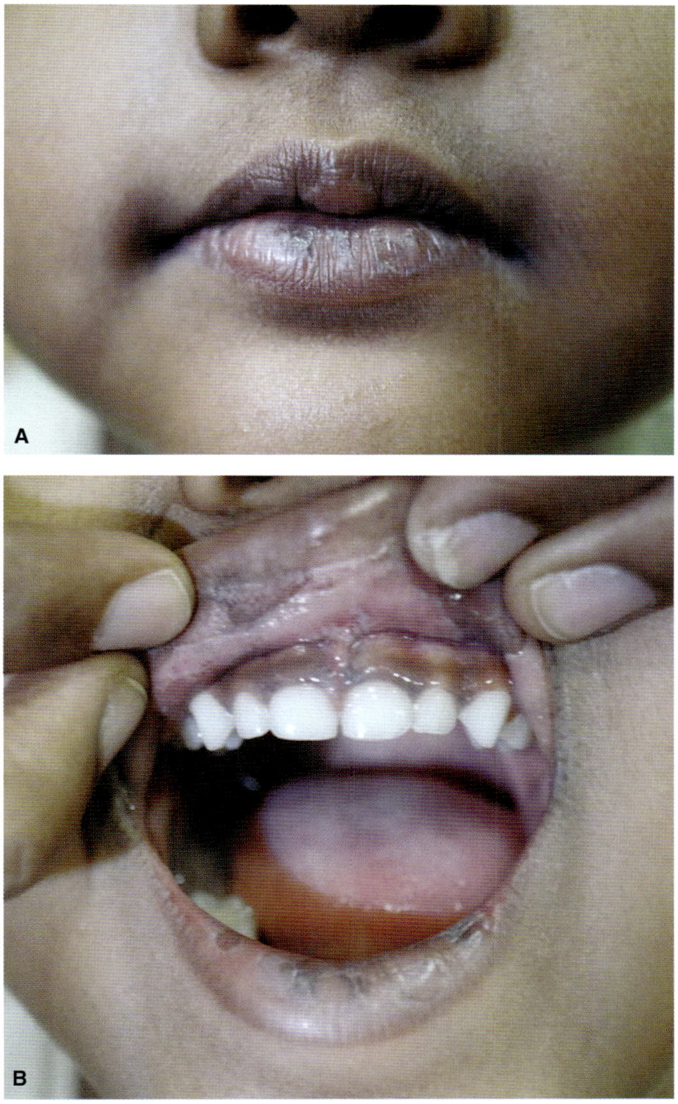

FIGURE 15-25A & 25B. PJS presenting in a young Indian girl with hyperpigmented macules on her lips and oral mucosa.

Clinical Features

- The mucocutaneous lesions of PJS appear as medium-to-dark brown, hyperpigmented macules.
- They are most commonly found on the lips, buccal mucosa, gums, hard palate, and tongue. In addition, they can also occur on the fingers, toes, palms, and periorbital, periumbilical, perianal, and labial areas.
- The pigmented lesions can present in infancy and increase in number with age. The lesions on the skin and lips may fade after puberty, but those on the buccal mucosa, palate, and tongue persist.
- Hamartomatous gastrointestinal polyps are found from the stomach to the anal canal, and may be complicated by gastrointestinal bleeding, intussusception with obstruction, abdominal pain, or rectal prolapse. Approximately 50% of patients may have symptoms in the first 2 decades of life.
- Although most polyps are benign, adenocarcinomas of the gastrointestinal tract, breast and uterine cervical carcinomas, and gonadal sex tumors have been described. Most cancers occur in adulthood.

Differential Diagnosis

- Laugier-Hunziker syndrome
  - This is a benign pigmentary disorder that clinically presents as macular hyperpigmentation of the lips, buccal mucosa, and melanonychia striata, with the absence of visceral manifestations.

Investigations & Treatment

- Genetic studies should be performed to confirm mutations in the *STK11/LKB1* gene.
- Initiation of screening for polyps can be commenced with an esophagogastroduodenoscopy or capsule endoscopy and colonoscopy.
- Yearly screening and evaluation of other organs at risk of malignancy should be performed in adulthood.
- Laser and intense pulsed-light therapy may be attempted for the hyperpigmented lesions if cosmetically disturbing. However, recurrence is common.

Pearls & Practical Tips

- A negative genetic test for *STK11/LKB1* does not entirely exclude PJS, and the patient should still be monitored for development of gastrointestinal symptoms.

Reference

1. Katz SK, Gordon KB, Roenigk HH. The cutaneous manifestations of gastrointestinal disease. Prim Car 1996 Sep;23(3):455–76. doi: 10.1016/s0095-4543(05)70341-9. PMID: 8888338.

CHRONIC LIVER DISEASE

The cutaneous manifestations of chronic liver disease include pruritus, pigmentary changes, vascular changes, and nail changes. Often, these features are present after the diagnosis of chronic liver disease has been made, but in rare cases, the cutaneous manifestations may occur before diagnosis of liver disease.

Clinical Features

- Severe pruritus is one of the most debilitating symptoms of chronic liver disease, and occurs due to cholestasis, with retention of bile acids. Clinically, the patient presents with multiple linear excoriations from chronic scratching, without features of any underlying primary dermatosis.
- Jaundice appears as yellow discoloration of the skin and mucous membranes, secondary to accumulation of bilirubin or its metabolites in the skin. Bilirubin levels greater than 2.5 mg/dL (42.75 µmol/*L*) generally result in clinically apparent jaundice.
- Hypermelanosis may be present in patients with long-standing cirrhosis or hemochromatosis, with a grayish pigmentation caused by an increase in melanin content of the skin in giant melanosomes.
- Vascular changes include spider angiomas (spider nevi), which appear as a telangiectatic network of dilated capillaries radiating from a central arteriole. Compression

of the central punctum results in blanching of the entire lesion. They mostly occur on the face, upper trunk, and distal upper extremities. Palmar erythema presents as increased mottling of the palmar surfaces of the hands, especially the thenar and hypothenar eminences. Bruising or ecchymoses may also be present if coagulopathy occurs as a complication of chronic liver disease.

- Nail changes include Terry-type leukonychia, which appears as an opaque white plate that obscures the lunula and extends to within 1 to 2 mm from the distal nail edge, Muehrcke lines (banded nails), which appear as paired, narrow, and white transverse bands, and digital clubbing.

Investigations & Treatment

- Therapy for pruritus of hepatic failure is directed toward reducing the circulating bile salts. These include oral cholestyramine, colestipol, ursodeoxycholic acid, and rifampicin, or biliary drainage procedures, performed either endoscopically, radiologically, or surgically. Phototherapy has also been used for jaundice-associated pruritus.
- Modifying the central itch signaling by influencing specific receptors in the central nervous system with opioid antagonists, serotonin antagonists, antihistamines, and antidepressants, may also be considered.
- Removing potential pruritogens from the systemic circulation by invasive methods such as molecular adsorbent and recirculating system (MARS), plasmapheresis, and liver transplant.
- Ensuring appropriate skin care with adequate nutrition and fluid intake, emollients, and avoidance of heat.

Bibliography

1. Katz SK, Gordon KB, Roenigk HH. The cutaneous manifestations of gastrointestinal disease. Prim Care 1996 Sep;23(3):455–76. doi: 10.1016/s0095-4543(05)70341-9. PMID: 8888338.
2. Bassari R, Koea JB. Jaundice associated pruritis: a review of pathophysiology and treatment. World J Gastroenterol 2015;21(5):1 404–13. doi:10.3748/wjg.v21.i5.1404.

SKIN MANIFESTATIONS OF ENDOCRINOLOGICAL CONDITIONS

ACANTHOSIS NIGRICANS

Acanthosis nigricans is a fairly common condition that can manifest in childhood or adolescence, especially in individuals who are overweight or obese. It can also occur in children with diabetes mellitus and other endocrine disorders. The skin changes in acanthosis nigricans are postulated to be caused by hormonal overstimulation leading to proliferation of keratinocytes and fibroblasts. In hyperinsulinemia, acanthosis nigricans is caused by excess insulin binding to insulin-like growth factor I receptor and fibroblast growth factor receptor.

Clinical Features

- Acanthosis nigricans appears as symmetric, brown, velvety plaques and hyperpigmentation of the skin. It is usually asymptomatic and has an insidious onset.

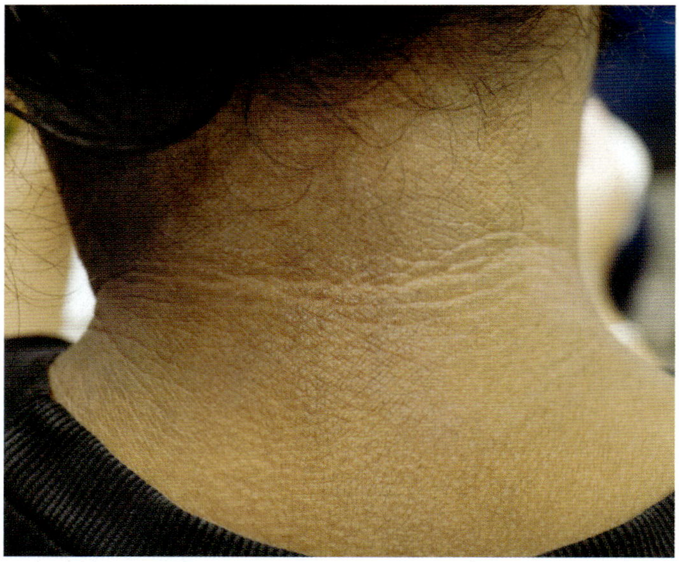

FIGURE 15-26. Acanthosis nigricans affecting the nape of an Indian adolescent girl.

- Typical sites of involvement include the posterior neck, axillae, groin, and other intertriginous sites.
- Acanthosis nigricans can occur in children and adolescents with normal weight and size. However, it is more common in overweight or obese individuals, especially in patients who have concomitant type II diabetes mellitus. Other rare associations include malignancy, genetic syndromes (e.g., Prader-Willi syndrome, Bloom syndrome, and Crouzon syndrome), connective tissue disorders (e.g., lupus erythematosus, dermatomyositis, scleroderma), and medications (e.g., niacin, corticosteroids, oral contraceptives, diethylstilbestrol, growth hormone therapy).

Differential Diagnoses

- Confluent and reticulated papillomatosis of Gougerot and Carteaud
  - Confluent and reticulated papillomatosis is uncommon but often occurs in association with acanthosis nigricans. It appears more reticulated than classical acanthosis nigricans but also affects the intertriginous areas.
- Retention hyperkeratosis
  - This condition can occur at similar sites to acanthosis nigricans but commonly also affects the trunk and limb extensors. Unlike lesions of acanthosis nigricans, the lesions of retention hyperkeratosis may be removed with 70% isopropyl alcohol.
- Epidermal nevus
  - This is usually present from birth or early infancy, and often has a more verrucous surface, and linear or Blaschkoid distribution.
- Addison's disease
  - Acanthosis nigricans can occur in Addison's disease. However, in the latter, the hyperpigmentation is more marked and affects sites beyond the usual sites affected

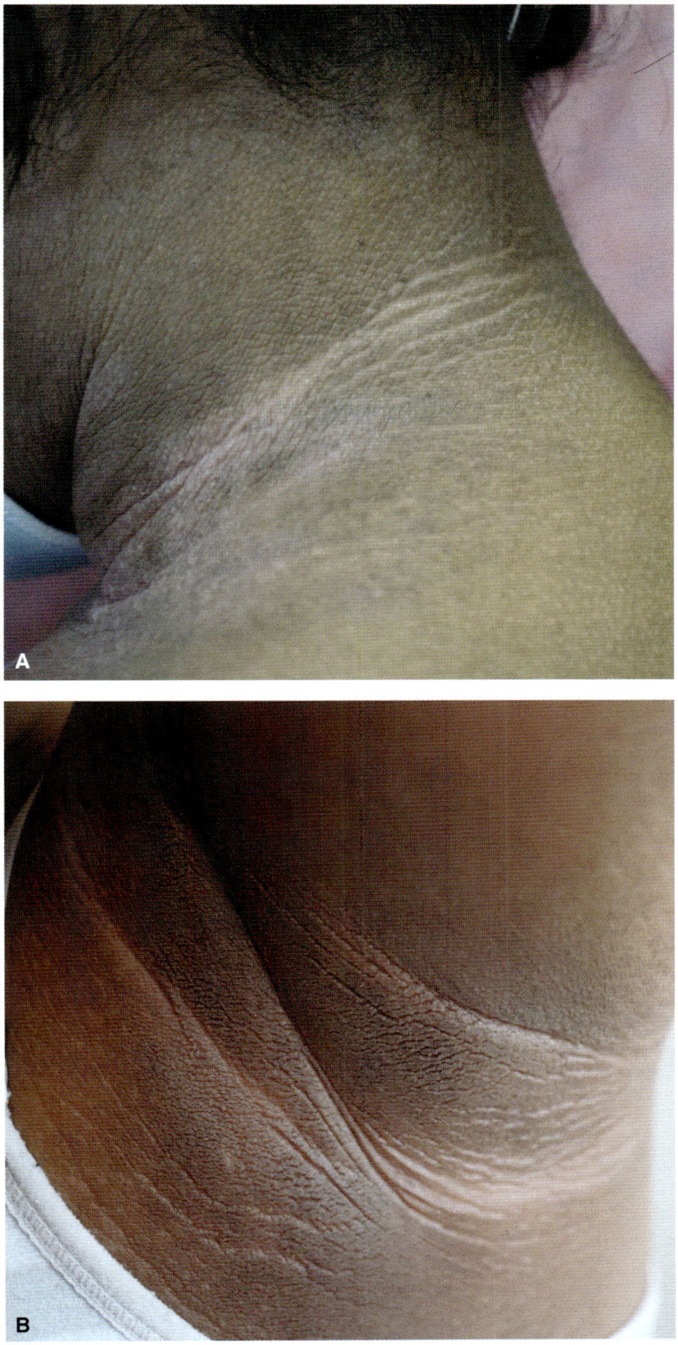

FIGURE 15-27A & 27B. Acanthosis nigricans affecting the neck and axillae of this 14-year-old Indian girl.

by acanthosis nigricans, such as palms, soles, and mucosal surfaces.

Investigations & Treatment

- Investigations should be performed to exclude diabetes mellitus and metabolic syndrome, or an underlying endocrine disorder.
- Treatment and correction of the underlying cause, such as obesity or endocrinological disease, usually results in improvement.

CONFLUENT AND RETICULATED PAPILLOMATOSIS OF GOUGEROT AND CARTEAUD

Confluent and reticulated papillomatosis of Gougerot and Carteaud (CRP) is a benign but chronic dermatosis of unknown etiology, although it is thought to be due to abnormal keratinocyte maturation and differentiation. It has been associated with insulin resistance and acanthosis nigricans.

Clinical Features

- CRP is primarily seen in adolescents and young adults, with females being involved twice as often as males.

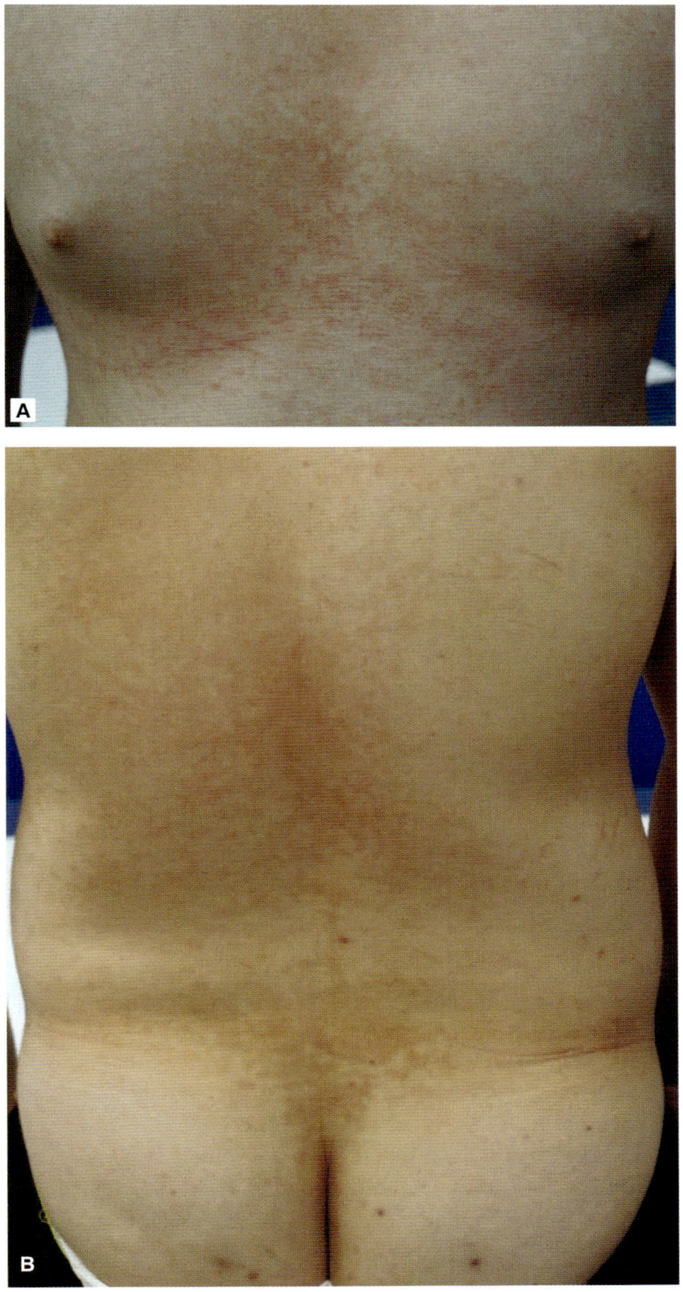

FIGURE 15-28A & 28B. CRP on the chest and back of a 15-year-old Chinese boy, presenting as erythematous-to-hyperpigmented, reticulate patches.

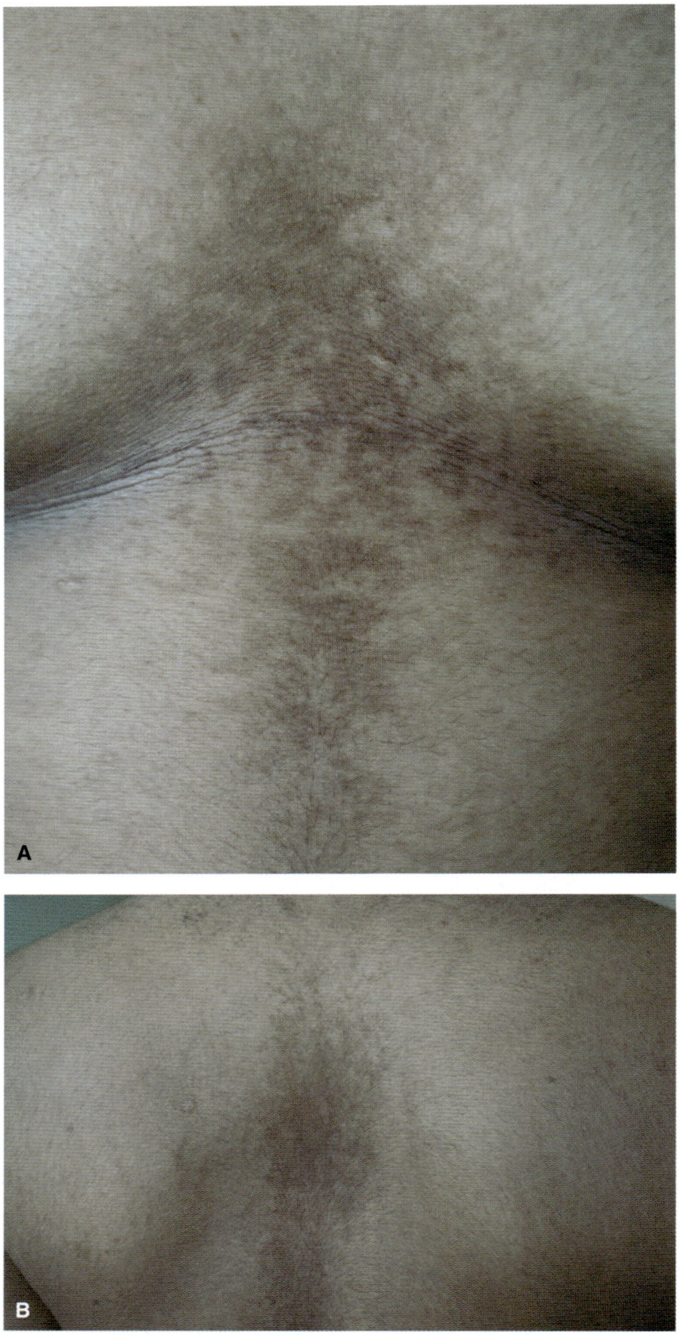

FIGURE 15-29A & 29B. CRP on the central chest and back of a 15-year-old Malay boy presenting as hyperpigmented, reticulate patches.

- It is characterized by elevated, hyperpigmented scaly plaques with a reticulate pattern that spread slowly and insidiously.
- It is usually asymptomatic but can sometimes be pruritic.
- The characteristic distribution involves the axillae, intermammary region, epigastric area, and upper back.

Differential Diagnoses

- Acanthosis nigricans
  - This has a less reticulated pattern compared to CRP. Both conditions can occur concomitantly.

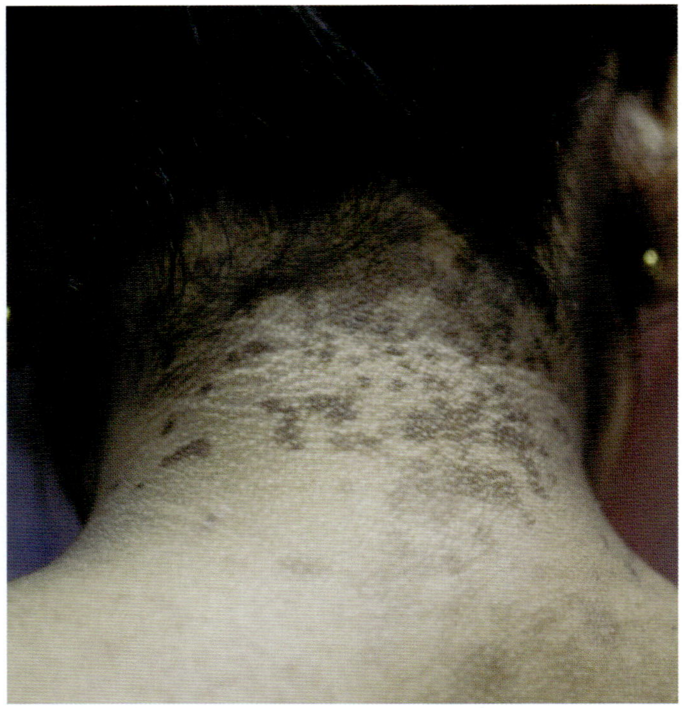

FIGURE 15-30. CRP on the nape of a 13-year-old Indian girl presenting as hyperpigmented, reticulate patches with velvety surface. There is some overlap with acanthosis nigricans in this patient.

- Tinea versicolor
  - This can appear hyperpigmented in darker-skinned individuals. However, the lesions have a circular or oval shape as compared to the reticulated pattern of CRP.

Investigations & Treatment

- Several therapies have been used but may not always be successful.
- Systemic antibiotics such as doxycycline, minocycline, macrolides, or cephalosporine have shown the most improvement.
- Topical antifungal agents, topical calcipotriol, and topical or systemic retinoids may be effective in some patients.
- Weight loss may also be useful.

Pearls & Practical Tips

- Similar to acanthosis nigricans, patients with CRP should be assessed for comorbidities (e.g., diabetes mellitus, hypertension, and hyperlipidemia), especially if overweight or obese.

Bibliography

1. Xiao TL, Duan GY, Stein SL. Retrospective review of confluent and reticulated papillomatosis in pediatric patients. Pediatr Dermatol 2021 Sep 24. doi: 10.1111/pde.14806. Epub ahead of print. PMID: 34561886.

CUSHING SYNDROME

This is a disorder caused by long-term glucocorticoid excess. It is divided into ACTH-dependent types (pituitary-dependent Cushing disease, ectopic ACTH syndrome, and adrenal hyperplasia) and non-ACTH-dependent types (adrenal adenoma, adrenal carcinoma, adrenal hyperplasia). Cushing syndrome may also result from systemic administration of exogenous glucocorticoids.

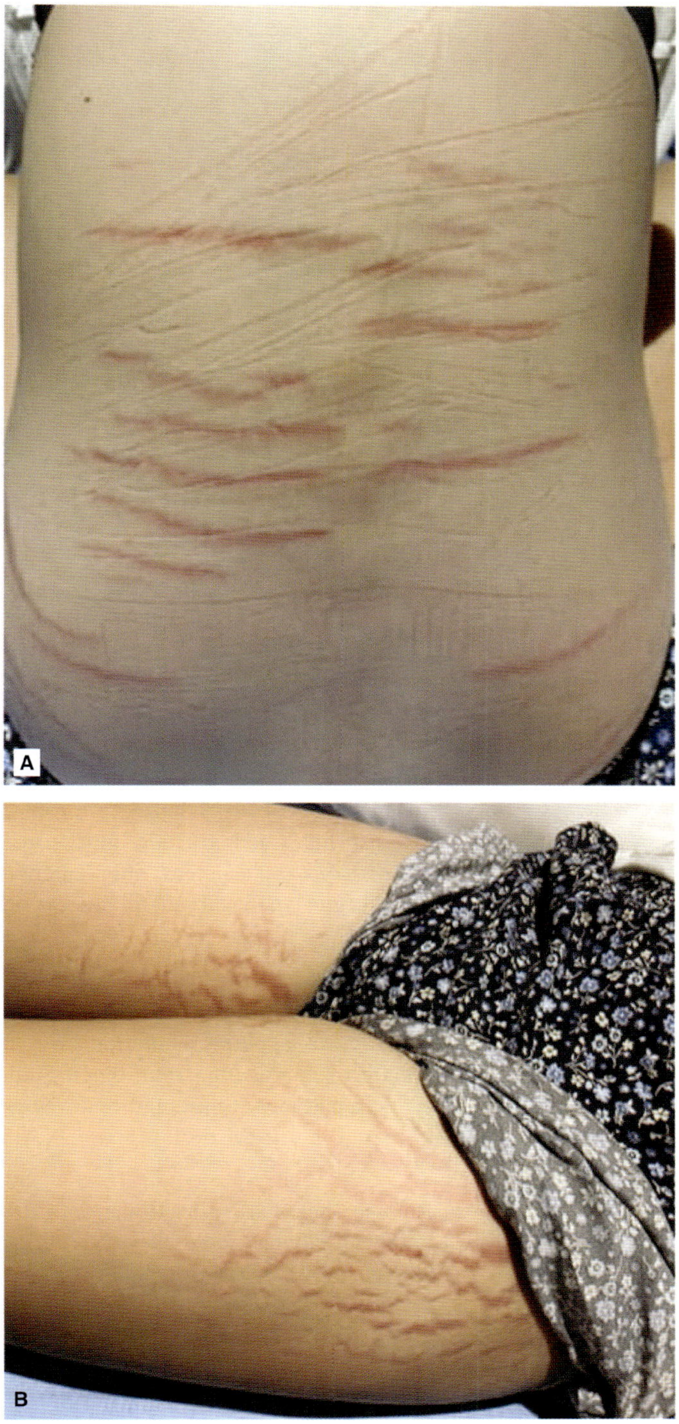

FIGURE 15-31A & 31B. Striae secondary to chronic systemic corticosteroids in a Chinese adolescent girl, presenting as purpuric, atrophic, linear streaks over the back and legs.

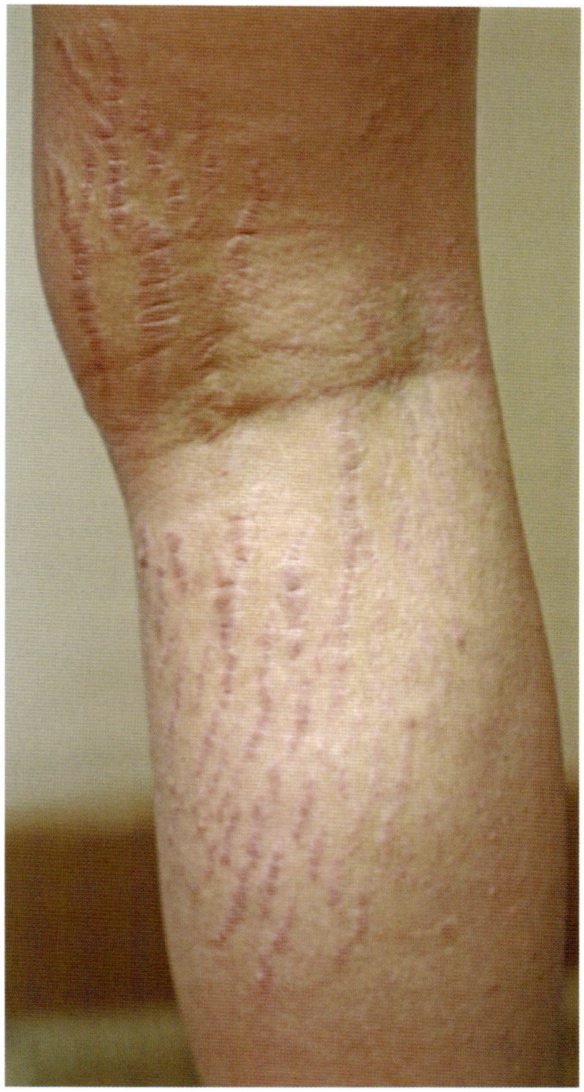

FIGURE 15-32. Steroid-induced striae on the back of the legs of a Chinese adolescent boy, secondary to overuse of potent topical corticosteroids.

Clinical Features

- The cutaneous features of Cushing syndrome include facial plethora and telangiectasias, steroid-induced acne, hirsutism, lanugo hair growth, violaceous striae, striae distensae, easy bruising, poor wound healing, skin atrophy, hyperpigmentation (in ACTH-dependent forms), acanthosis nigricans, frequent fungal infections (e.g., candidiasis, tinea corporis, pityriasis versicolor), androgenetic alopecia (in females), and dorsocervical and supraclavicular fat pad.
- The patient may also exhibit generalized symptoms of fatigue and muscle weakness, hypertension, personality changes, amenorrhea, polyuria, and polydipsia.

Investigations & Treatment

- Investigations to screen for Cushing syndrome include serum blood glucose, serum electrolytes, and 24-hour urinary free cortisol. Confirmatory studies include plasma cortisol levels, dexamethasone suppression test, ACTH and corticotropin-releasing hormone stimulation test.
- Radiographic imaging can be employed for assessment of the pituitary gland and for adrenal tumors.
- Further investigations for complications of Cushing syndrome such as assessment for osteoporosis may be required.
- Management includes elimination of exogenous glucocorticoids or the detection and treatment of the underlying endogenous cause.

Pearls & Practical Tips

- An index of suspicion for Cushing syndrome, supplemented by thorough history taking and physical examination, is pertinent in the assessment of a patient with relevant features. A thorough workup will enable the physician to delineate between the various endogenous or exogenous causes of excess adrenocorticosteroids and institute appropriate treatment.

Bibliography

1. Lause M, Kamboj A, Fernandez Faith E. Dermatologic manifestations of endocrine disorders. Transl Pediat 2017 Oct;6(4): 300–12. doi: 10.21037/tp.2017.09.08. PMID: 29184811; PMCID: PMC5682371.

CONGENITAL ADRENAL HYPERPLASIA

Congenital adrenal hyperplasia (CAH) is caused by impaired steroid metabolism in the adrenal cortex. Due to the defect in cortisol synthesis, the adrenal cortex is stimulated by corticotropin, and overproduction of cortisol precursors occur leading to increased sex hormone synthesis, resulting in hyperandrogenism. The concomitant aldosterone deficiency may result in salt-wasting, failure to thrive, hypovolemia, and shock.

Clinical Features

- The most common cause of CAH is 21-hydroxylase deficiency, with deficiency of 11β-hydroxylase and 3β-hydroxysteroid dehydrogenase less commonly found.
- 21-hydroxylase deficiency classically presents in a female newborn with ambiguous genitalia, with a large clitoris, rugated and partially fused labia majora, and a common urogenital sinus in place of a separate urethra and vagina. The degree of virilization is variable. The absence of testes and presence of normal internal sex organs differentiates a virilized female genitalia from true male genitalia. Hyperpigmentation of the skin creases and genitalia may occur as an early sign of adrenal insufficiency.
- Affected males have no obvious physical signs of the disorder and may present as a medical emergency in hypovolemic shock.

Differential Diagnoses

- Other differentials for ambiguous genitalia and hyperpigmentation may have to be considered.

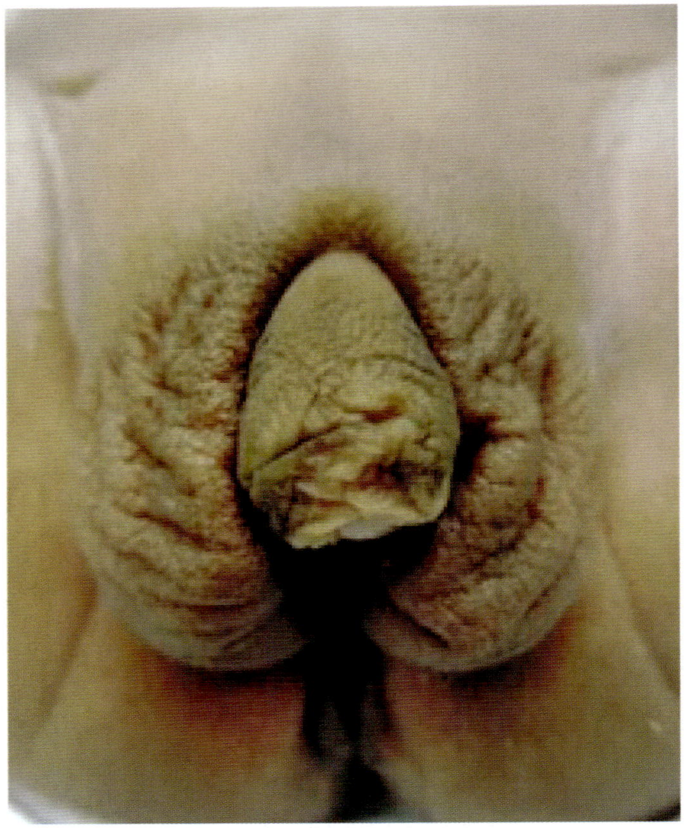

FIGURE 15-33. Ambiguous genitalia in an infant with congenital adrenal hyperplasia.

Investigations & Treatment

- Classic 21-hydroxylase deficiency is confirmed by elevated levels of serum 17-hydroxyprogesterone.
- Genetic testing can be performed for confirmation. Antenatal testing can be performed if suspected.
- Management strategies for CAH include glucocorticoid and mineralocorticoid replacement, supplemental sodium chloride, and surgical management for correction of ambiguous genitalia.

Pearls & Practical Tips

- CAH should be considered in a newborn who presents with ambiguous genitalia, hyperpigmentation, or in hypovolemic shock with salt-wasting. In an older child, it can be considered in a patient with premature development of secondary sexual characteristics.

Bibliography

1. Paller A, Mancini AJ. Hurwitz Clinical Pediatric Dermatology: A Textbook of Skin Disorders of Childhood and Adolescence. 5th ed. Edinburgh: Elsevier; 2016.

XANTHOMAS

Xanthomas represent collections of lipid-containing macrophages in the skin. The mechanism is not completely understood but it is postulated that serum lipids infiltrate the tissues, where they are phagocytized by macrophages. Xanthomas may be a sign of an underlying metabolic or lipid disease.

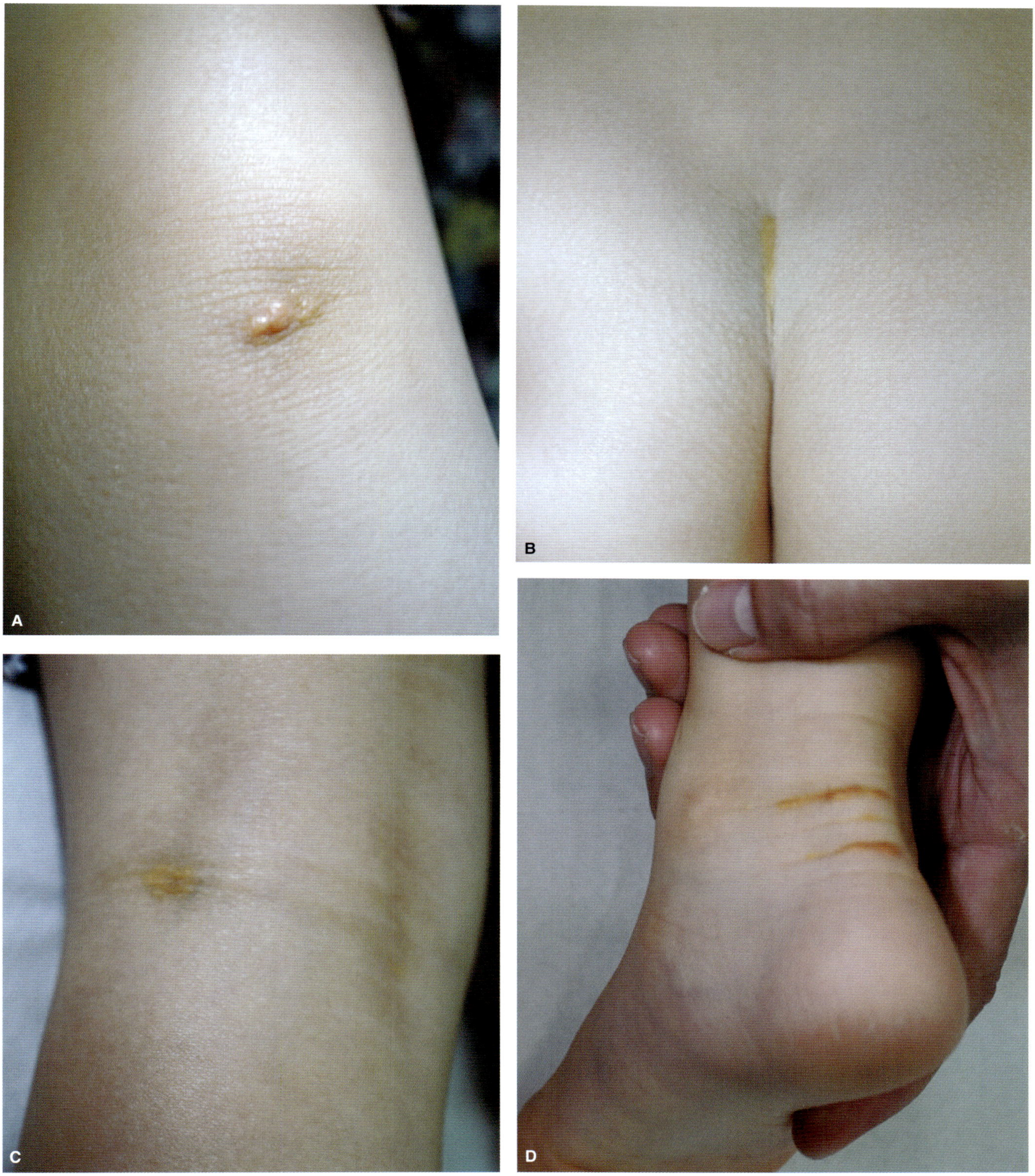

FIGURE 15-34A–34D. Xanthomas in a 4-year-old Chinese girl with underlying familial hypercholesterolemia, presenting as yellow papules and plaques on the extensors and creases.

Clinical Features

- Cutaneous xanthomas present as yellowish-brown, pink, or orange papules, plaques, nodules, or tumors which may occur on the skin or mucous membranes. They commonly occur at sites of pressure or trauma.
- Xanthomas can be classified into several clinical categories:
  - **Plane xanthomas** present as soft, yellow-orange to brown macules to plaques. Examples include xanthelasmas occurring on the eyelids, intertriginous plane xanthomas associated with homozygous familial hypercholesterolemia, and plane xanthomas of the palmar creases associated with dysbetalipoproteinemia.
  - **Eruptive xanthomas** appear in crops of multiple yellow-orange to red papules, commonly on the trunk, oral mucosa, and extensor surfaces of the arms, legs, and buttocks. It is almost always associated with hypertriglyceridemia.
  - **Tendinous xanthomas** present as skin-colored to yellowish, smooth, movable subcutaneous nodules and tumors, commonly on extensor tendons of elbows, knees, heels, hands, and feet. It is most commonly associated with familial hypercholesterolemia.
  - **Tuberous xanthomas** present as large, firm, skin-colored nodules on the palms and extensor surfaces, which can enlarge to over 5 cm. They are found commonly in patients with hypercholesterolemia, especially familial hypercholesterolemia (type II).

Investigations & Treatment

- Although most often diagnosed clinically, a skin biopsy may be required for confirmation, which will show lipid-laden macrophages in various layers of the skin.
- Serum cholesterol and triglyceride levels should be evaluated in all children presenting with xanthomas.
- Co-management with a pediatric endocrinologist and dietician may be necessary.
- Management measures include lifestyle and dietary modification, lipid-lowering medications such as statins, fibrates, ezetimibe, and cholestyramine.

Pearls & Practical Tips

- Cutaneous xanthomas may be the first sign of an underlying serious lipid abnormality in the pediatric patient. Thorough evaluation should be performed.

Bibliography

1. Shah AS, Wilson DP. Primary hypertriglyceridemia in children and adolescents. J Clin Lipidol 2015 Sep-Oct;9(5 Suppl):S20–8. doi: 10.1016/j.jacl.2015.04.004. Epub 2015 Apr 25. PMID: 26343209.
2. Hegele RA. Plasma lipoproteins: genetic influences and clinical implications. Nat Rev Genet 2009 Feb;10(2):109–21. doi: 10.1038/nrg2481. Epub 2009 Jan 13. PMID: 19139765.

CUTANEOUS MANIFESTATIONS OF DIABETES MELLITUS

Cutaneous manifestations of diabetes mellitus (DM) are more commonly seen in the adult population compared to the pediatric population. These include diabetic dermopathy, bullosis diabeticorum, and necrobiosis lipoidica.

Clinical Features

- Diabetic dermopathy most commonly present in adults with long-standing DM. It presents as irregularly shaped, light-brown macules and patches on bilateral anterior shins. Lesions may become atrophic over time.
- Bullosis diabeticorum, or diabetic bullae, present as large, intact bullae which arise spontaneously on the distal extremities, most commonly on the dorsal and lateral surfaces of the lower limbs and feet.
- Necrobiosis lipoidica in a granulomatous skin disorder which is often associated with DM. It may also precede the diagnosis of diabetes by up to several years and present as asymptomatic, slowly enlarging, red to yellow-brown to violaceous plaques in the pretibial areas. Over time, the center may become more atrophic with superficial telangiectasias. Ulceration may occur, and healed ulcers result in depressed scars.

Differential Diagnosis

- A differential for necrobiosis lipoidica is granuloma annulare, especially in the early stages.

Investigations & Treatment

- No therapy is required for diabetic dermopathy.
- Standard wound care is required for diabetic bullae. Good DM control can prevent further lesions.
- Skin biopsy is usually required for diagnosis of necrobiosis lipoidica. Treatment includes topical or intralesional corticosteroids. Pentoxifylline may also be useful.

PSYCHODERMATOLOGICAL CONDITIONS

CHILD ABUSE/NON-ACCIDENTAL INJURIES

Child abuse includes physical abuse, sexual abuse, and neglect, and is one of the most significant causes of childhood morbidity and mortality. Recognition of abuse is vital, as trauma tends to be repeated on the child, increasing future risk of injury or death.

Clinical Features

- Physical abuse, or non-accidental injury (NAI), can present with various cutaneous manifestations, including bruises, patterned injuries, bites, and burns.
- Bruising or ecchymoses in various stages of healing are more suggestive of abuse, with involvement of padded areas (e.g., buttocks, torso, face, genitalia) or uncommonly injured areas (e.g., earlobe, neck, lip, philtrum). Another red flag is bruising in the non-cruising infant less than 9 months of age.
- Patterned injuries typically have a configuration morphologically similar to the objects or methods inflicted on the child. Suspicious features include multiple evenly spaced markings or a patterned imprint (e.g., slap marks, pinch marks, shackle marks on the wrists, ankles, or neck, and ligature marks on the neck or extremities).
- Bite marks should be suspected when lesions such as ecchymoses, abrasions, or lacerations are in an elliptical or ovoid pattern.

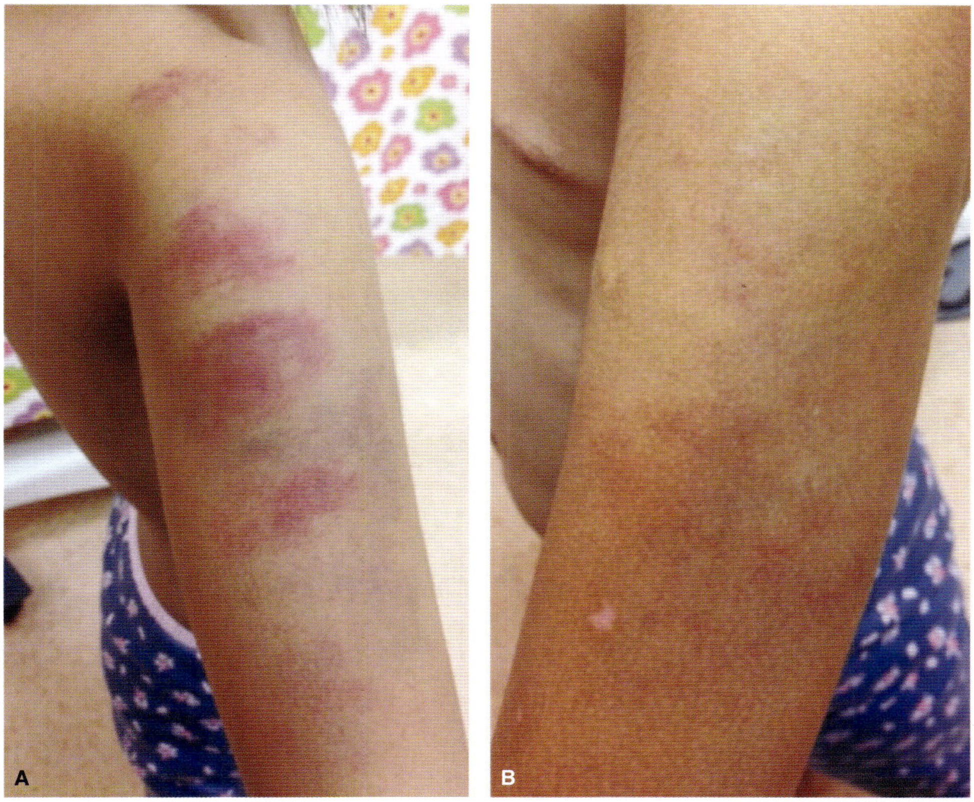

FIGURE 15-35A & 35B. NAI presenting as multiple bruises on the limbs at different stages of evolution, with more recent lesions appearing as red and tender patches with prominent petechiae, and earlier lesions appearing as faint gray patches. (Photograph courtesy of Dr. Peter Wong, Children's Emergency, KK Women's & Children's Hospital, Singapore.)

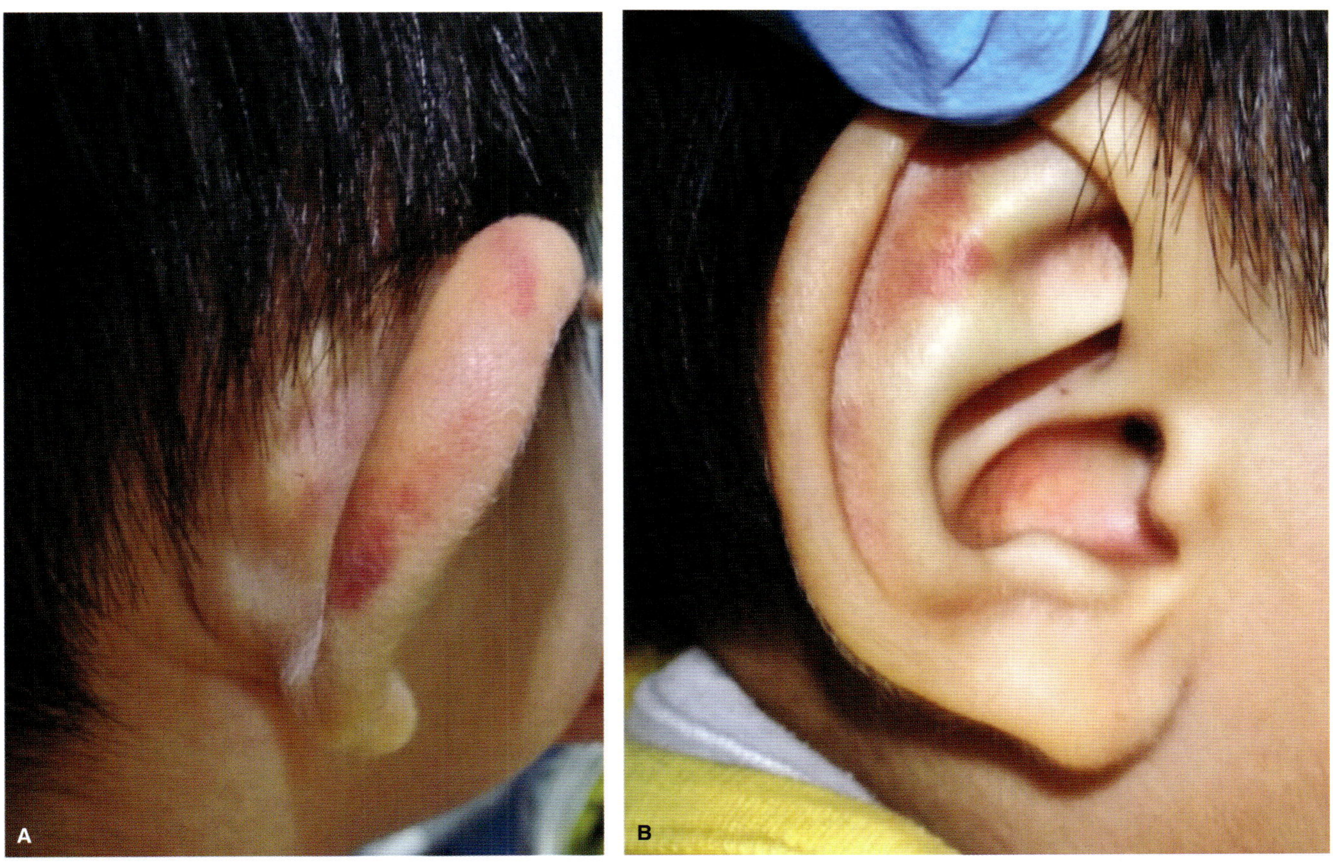

FIGURE 15-36A & 36B. NAI presenting as bruising involving the posterior aspect of the pinna away from the edge or helix (Figure 15-36A). There is also involvement of the base of the pinna, scapha, triangular fossa, and concha on the inside, sites not consistent with an accidental trauma. (Photograph courtesy of Dr. Peter Wong, Children's Emergency, KK Women's & Children's Hospital, Singapore.)

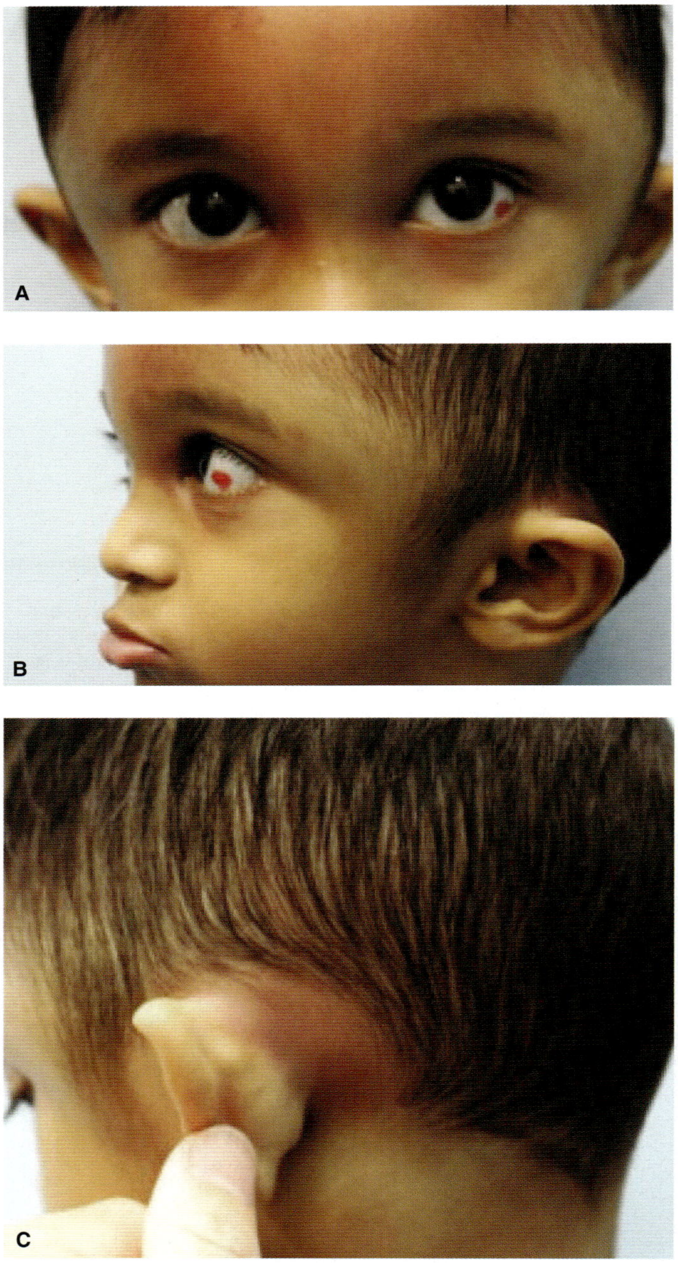

FIGURE 15-37A–37C. NAI in a young Indian boy, presenting with large boggy forehead hematoma, left subconjunctival hemorrhage, and bruising of the base of pinna and mastoid bilaterally. (Photograph courtesy of Dr. Peter Wong, Children's Emergency, KK Women's & Children's Hospital, Singapore.)

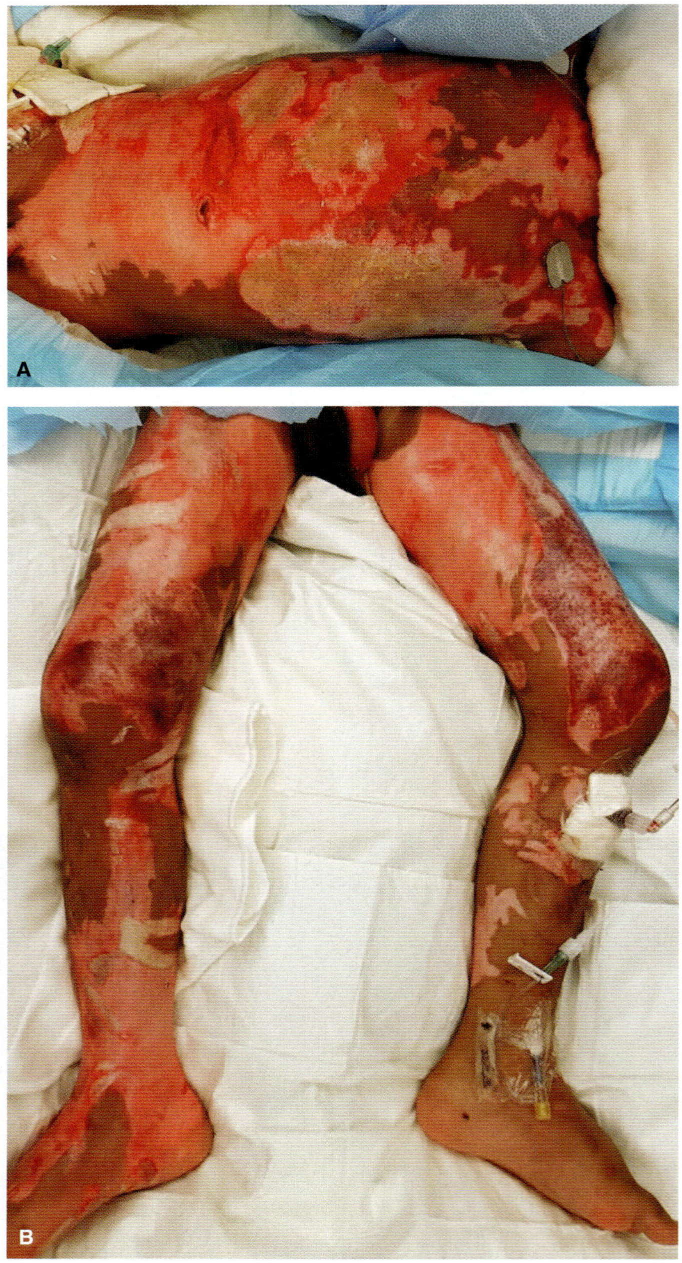

FIGURE 15-38A & 38B. Extensive burns cause by NAI in a young Malay boy, presenting as well-demarcated, fresh erosions and bullae. (Photograph courtesy of Dr. Por Yong Chen, Plastic, Reconstructive & Aesthetic Surgery, KK Women's & Children's Hospital, Singapore.)

- Burns can occur from electrical, chemical, thermal, or radiant heat sources. Abusive burns tend to occur in the age group of 1 to 3 years, where assessment may be difficult due to underdeveloped verbal skills. Red flags include burns that appear older than the history, presence of other injuries, symmetrically distributed lesions, burns to the perineum or buttocks, burns suggestive of immersion (no splash marks, clear tide levels), and demarcated outline of the surface in contact (branding).

- Sexual abuse can occur in both boys and girls. Mucocutaneous findings of sexual abuse include hymenal disruption, laceration, or ecchymoses; anal abrasions, lacerations, scarring, or dilatation; scarring of the posterior fourchette; inner thigh bruising and abrasions; labia minora scars or tears; circumferential injuries to penile shaft or glans penis; oral injuries such as unexplained erythema, bruising, or petechiae of the oral cavity or palate. However, many sexually abused children may have a normal physical examination.

Differential Diagnoses

- Bruising or ecchymoses
  - This should be differentiated from accidental bruising, which occurs over bony prominences such as the shins or forehead, and other non-abuse related causes such as Mongolian spots, Henoch-Schonlein purpura or vasculitis, purpura fulminans of meningococcemia, vascular malformations, chilblains, and bleeding disorders.
- Burns
  - Differential diagnoses for a circular-patterned burn include ecthyma, cellulitis, bullous impetigo, herpes, fixed drug eruption, dermatitis herpetiformis, and pyoderma gangrenosum.
  - Differential diagnoses for other burns include sunburn, contact dermatitis, and non-intentional burns.
- Sexual abuse
  - Differentials include straddle injuries, zipper entrapment, and hair tourniquet, and dermatological conditions, such as lichen sclerosis, vulvovaginitis, seborrheic dermatitis, atopic or contact dermatitis, scabies, lichen simplex chronicus, lichen planus, psoriasis, and hemangiomas.

Investigations & Treatment

- This is guided by the signs and symptoms of the patient. In cases of bruising or ecchymoses, a complete blood count and coagulation profile, looking for any underlying thrombocytopenia or coagulopathy.
- Radiographs are useful in looking for concomitant fractures.
- For suspected sexual abuse, investigations should be done to exclude other sexually transmitted infections such as HIV, syphilis, hepatitis B and C, gonorrhea, chlamydia, trichomonas, and herpes simplex. Pregnancy tests should be performed for pubertal females.

Pearls & Practical Tips

- An index of suspicion for NAI should be high when an injury has suspicious features and is inconsistent with the history or developmental age of the child.

Bibliography

1. Mudd SS, Findlay JS. The cutaneous manifestations and common mimickers of physical child abuse. J Pediatr Health Care 2004 May-Jun;18(3):123–9. doi: 10.1016/j.pedhc.2003.11.004. PMID: 15129212.
2. Andronicus M, Oates RK, Peat J, et al. Non-accidental burns in children. Burns 1998:24;552–8.
3. Swerdlin A, Berkowitz C, Craft N. Cutaneous signs of child abuse. J Am Acad Dermatol 2007 Sep;57(3):371–92. doi: 10.1016/j.jaad.2007.06.001. PMID: 17707148.

FACTITIAL DERMATITIS

Although more common in adults, factitial dermatitis can also occur in children and adolescents, and is often unrecognized. It is caused by conscious or subconscious behaviors driven in response to internal psychologic stressors. These are often not driven by secondary gain, but by the need to satisfy internal psychological needs. Factitial skin diseases include dermatitis artefacta, neurotic excoriations, acne excoriee, and trichotillomania.

Clinical Features

- Dermatitis artefacta
  - This is characterized by the production of self-inflicted skin lesions and occurs predominantly in females, with onset usually during adolescence or young adulthood.

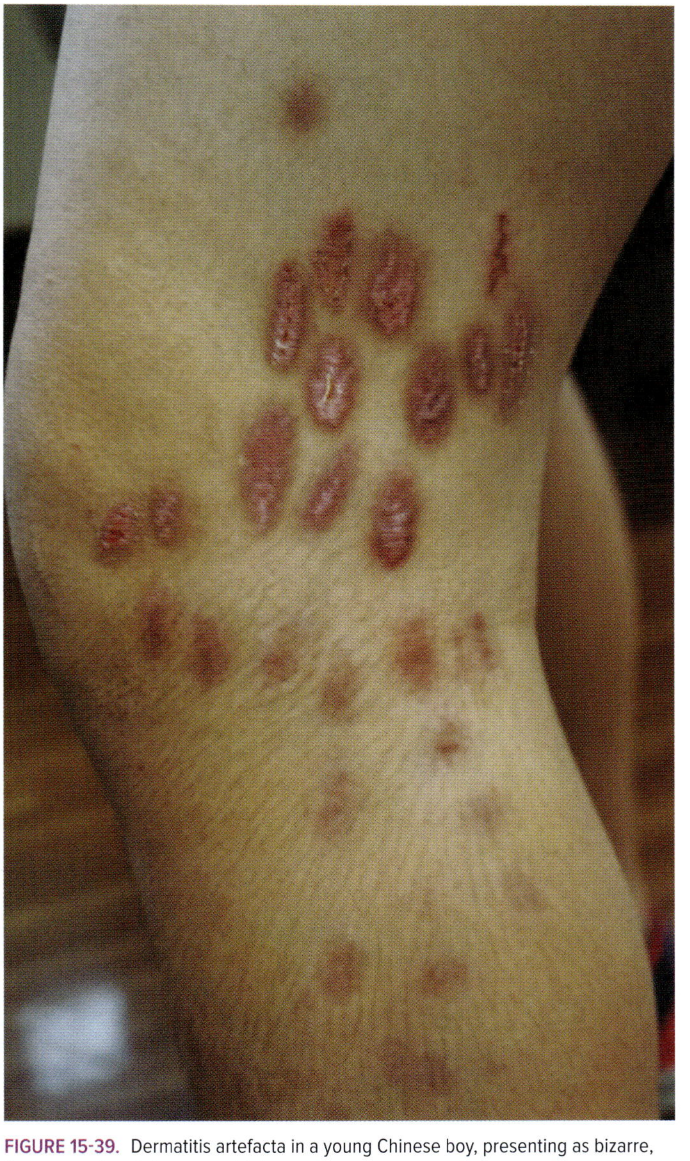

FIGURE 15-39. Dermatitis artefacta in a young Chinese boy, presenting as bizarre, linear, excoriated plaques on his legs.

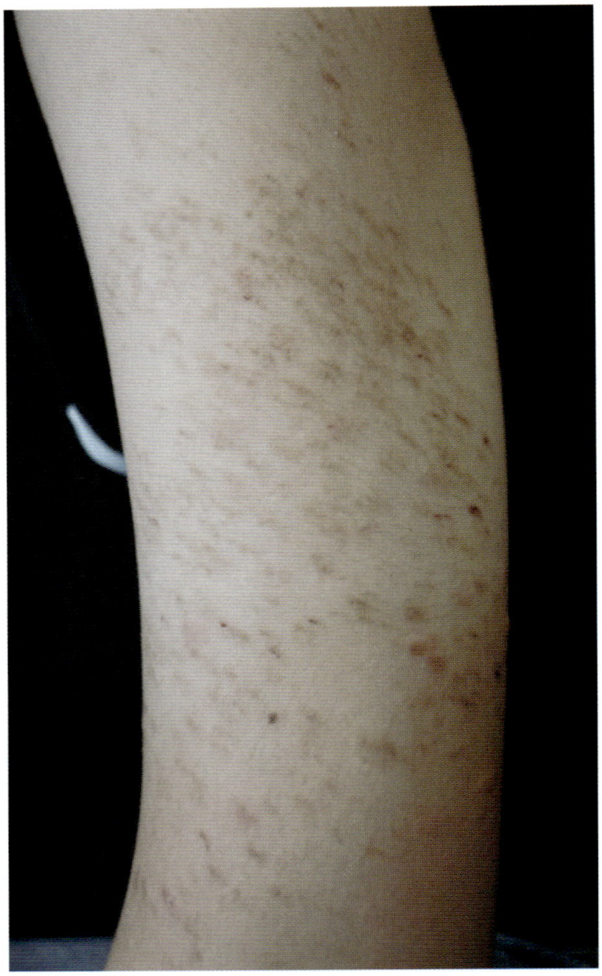

FIGURE 15-40. Dermatitis artefacta in an adolescent Chinese male with underlying behavioral and developmental problems.

- It is often seen in association with comorbid psychiatric conditions such as body dysmorphic disorder, borderline personality, depression, anxiety, obsessive-compulsive disorder, and psychotic disorders.
- Clinically, the skin lesions do not conform to the distribution and morphology of any known skin disease.
- Lesions are concentrated in areas that are easily accessible, displaying a geometric, linear, or bizarre morphology, and may appear as bruising, purpura, excoriations, abrasions, necrosis, ulcerations, burns, erosions, erythema, or scarring. It may also take the form of blisters caused by thermal, electrical, or chemical burns.

- Neurotic excorations
  - These are lesions self-inflicted by patients who have an irresistible urge to manipulate their skin.
  - They are frequently related to psychiatric disorders such as mood disorders, anxiety disorders, or obsessive-compulsive disorders.
  - The cycle of neurotic excoriations may commence with a physical stimulus such as itch or the presence of an irregular skin lesion such as an acne papule.
- Acne excoriee
  - This occurs when acne lesions are picked or excoriated, resulting in scarring, and may be exacerbated by a compulsive need to pick at the skin.
  - Acne lesions appear excoriated or manipulated. Often this leads to hyperpigmentation in darker-skinned patients.

Differential Diagnoses

- Dermatitis artefacta
  - Differential diagnoses include folliculitis, vasculitis, connective tissue disorders, chronic opportunistic

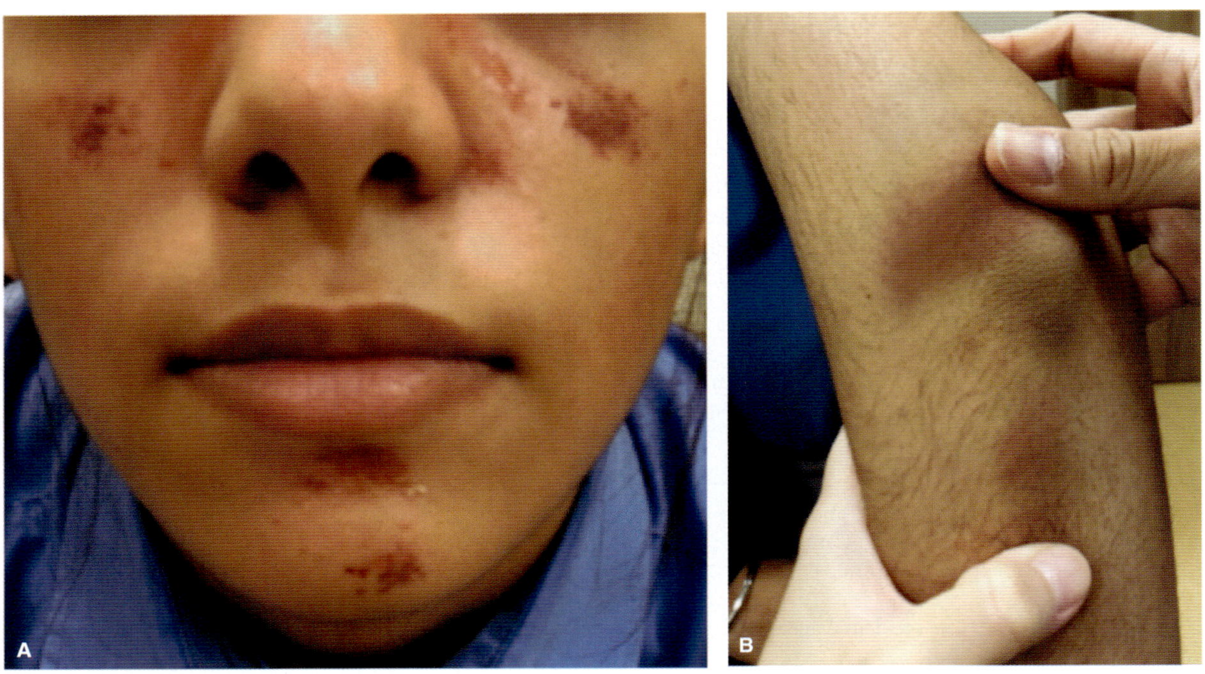

FIGURE 15-41A & 41B. Self-inflected abrasions and bruises in an Indian adolescent girl with underlying psychiatric condition.

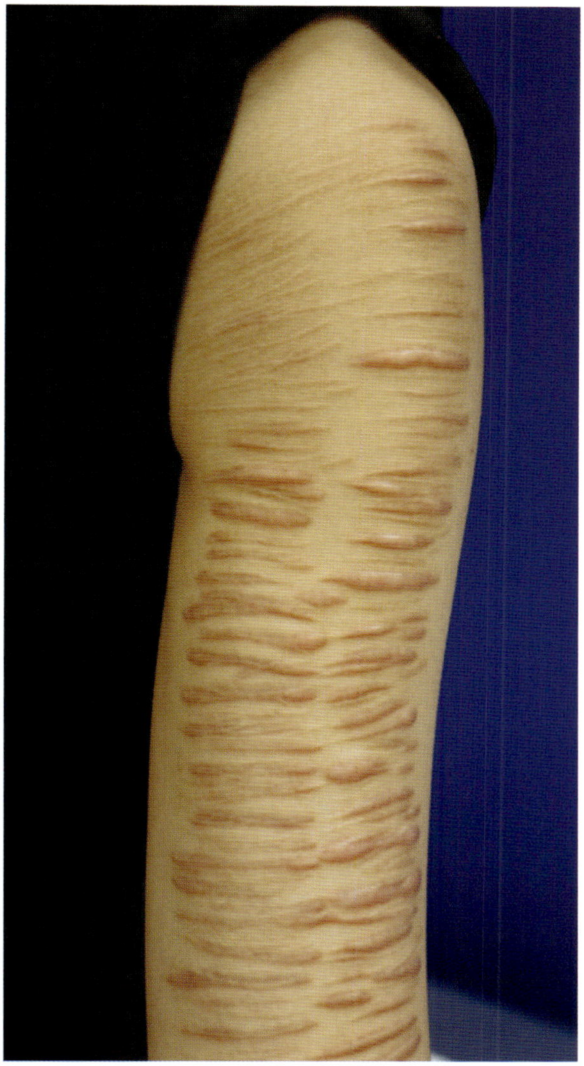

FIGURE 15-42. Self-inflicted injuries in an adolescent Chinese girl, presenting with linear scars.

skin infections, autoimmune bullous disease, and pyoderma gangrenosum.

- Neurotic excoriations
  - Differential diagnoses include arthropod bite reactions, folliculitis, atopic dermatitis or other eczemas, and organic causes of generalized pruritus (e.g., renal disease, liver disease, HIV, lymphoma).

Investigations & Treatment

- Treatment of factitious skin disorders is often challenging. Frequent clinical reassessment and reassurance is key. Patients and caregivers require guidance through a chronic and often recurrent course.
- Younger children without severe psychopathology tend to have better prognosis.
- Adjunctive therapy may be useful, including individual or family psychotherapy, and cognitive behavioral therapy, such as aversion therapy and habit reversal techniques.
- Multidisciplinary management with a psychologist, medical social worker, and psychiatrist enables better administration of adjunctive therapy.
- Pharmacologic treatment (e.g., antidepressants and anxiolytics) may be used in older children or adolescents, especially if associated with an underlying psychiatric disorder.

Pearls & Practical Tips

- An index of suspicion for factitious dermatitis should be present in cases that have a patterned or bizarre configuration.
- Patients often do not openly admit to the self-inflicted trauma, especially during the initial consultations.

Bibliography

1. Shah KN, Fried RG. Factitial dermatoses in children. Curr Opin Pediatr 2006 Aug;18(4):403–9. doi: 10.1097/01.mop.0000236390.41462.39. PMID: 16914995.

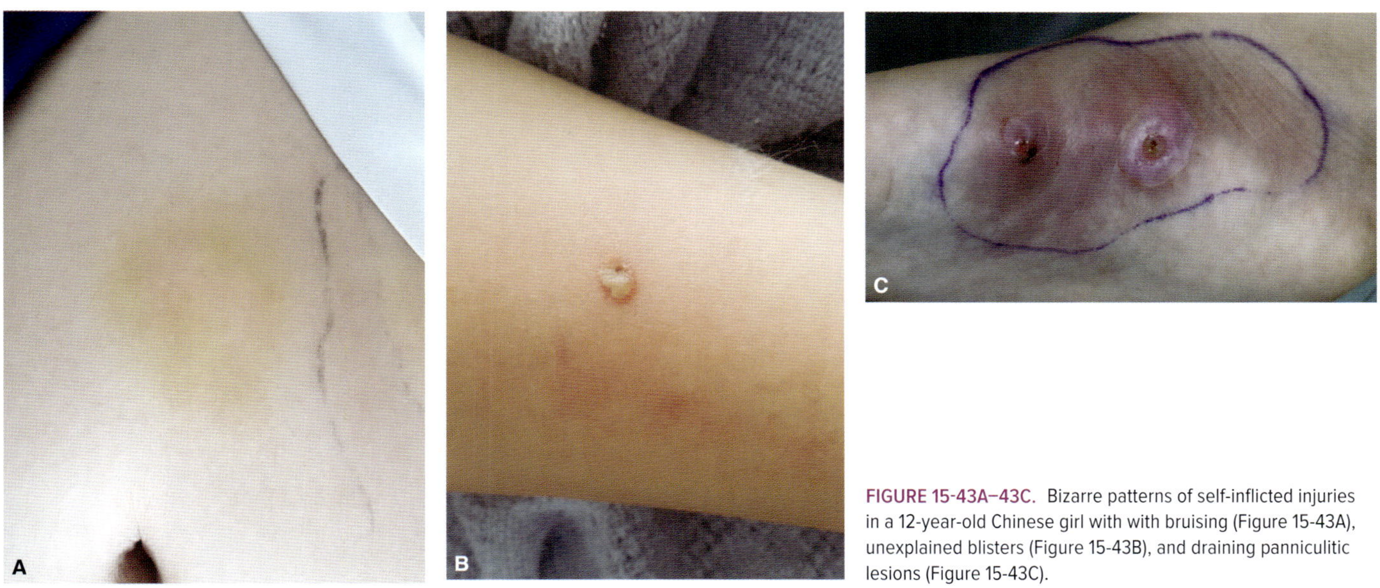

FIGURE 15-43A–43C. Bizarre patterns of self-inflicted injuries in a 12-year-old Chinese girl with with bruising (Figure 15-43A), unexplained blisters (Figure 15-43B), and draining panniculitic lesions (Figure 15-43C).

16

Dermatological Procedures

DERMATOLOGICAL PROCEDURES IN CHILDREN

Although less commonly performed than in adults, dermatological procedures may be required for pediatric patients for diagnostic and/or treatment purposes. Although mostly similar to older patients, younger children may require different approaches and techniques when performing these procedures. This chapter provides a guide, pearls, and practical tips for performing common dermatological procedures in children. Videos of these procedures may be viewed in the online version of this atlas on AccessDermatologyDxRx.com.

CRYOTHERAPY

Cryotherapy is one of the most common dermatological procedures performed for adults and children, for the treatment of various dermatological conditions. Common indications in children include viral warts and molluscum contagiosum.

Procedure

- Liquid nitrogen, at −196°C, is the most commonly used cryogen. It destroys tissues when used to treat benign, premalignant, or malignant skin lesions.
- Repeat freeze–thaw cycles and slowing thaw times creates more tissue injury and is more effective than a single freeze-and-thaw cycle.
- The standard spot-freeze technique is performed using a spray gun nozzle positioned about 1 cm from the skin surface, with the nozzle perpendicular to the skin and aimed at the target lesion.
- The liquid nitrogen is sprayed until an ice ring is created on and around the target lesion. The margin of this ice ring varies according to the nature and thickness of the lesion. Benign lesions require a margin of about 1 to 2 mm, while malignant lesions require margins of 5 mm.
- When the desired margin is attained, maintain the spray to keep the "freeze cycle" for about 5 to 20 seconds, depending on the size and depth of the lesion. After this, allow a complete "thaw cycle" of about 1 to 2 minutes before repeating the next freeze–thaw cycle again.
- For benign lesions, perform at least two to three freeze–thaw cycles, while for malignant lesions, three to four cycles may be required.

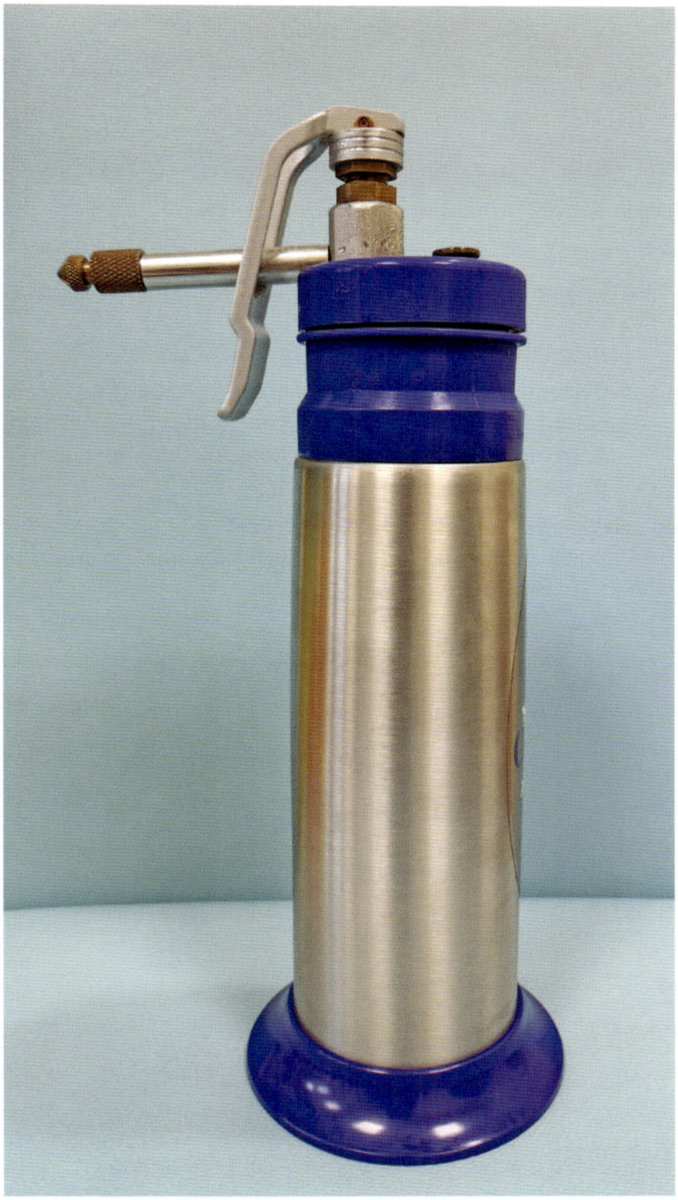

FIGURE 16-1. Cryogen spray gun.

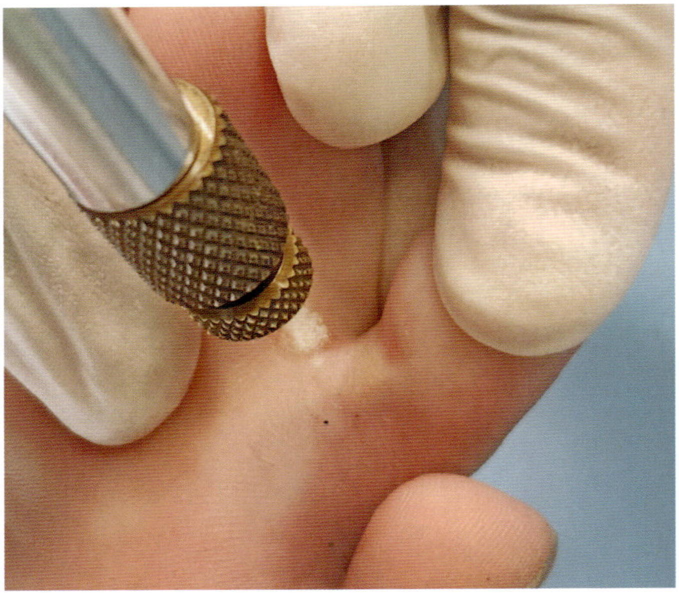

FIGURE 16-2. The cryogen spray is held at about 1 cm away from the skin.

- The procedure may be repeated at one to four week intervals, depending on the type and size of the lesion.

Side Effects

- Common side effects include pain and discomfort, erythema, blistering, post-inflammatory hypo- or hyperpigmentation.
- Scarring is uncommon but can occur if the procedure is performed too aggressively.

Pearls & Practical Tips

- Use a dipstick or cryotip applicator for smaller lesions or lesions on delicate areas such as the face.

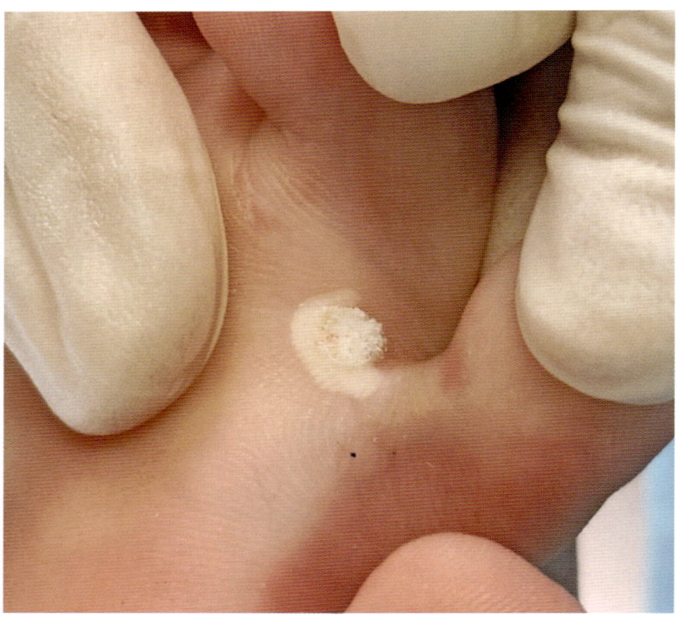

FIGURE 16-3. Cryogen should be applied until the formation of an ice ring around the lesion.

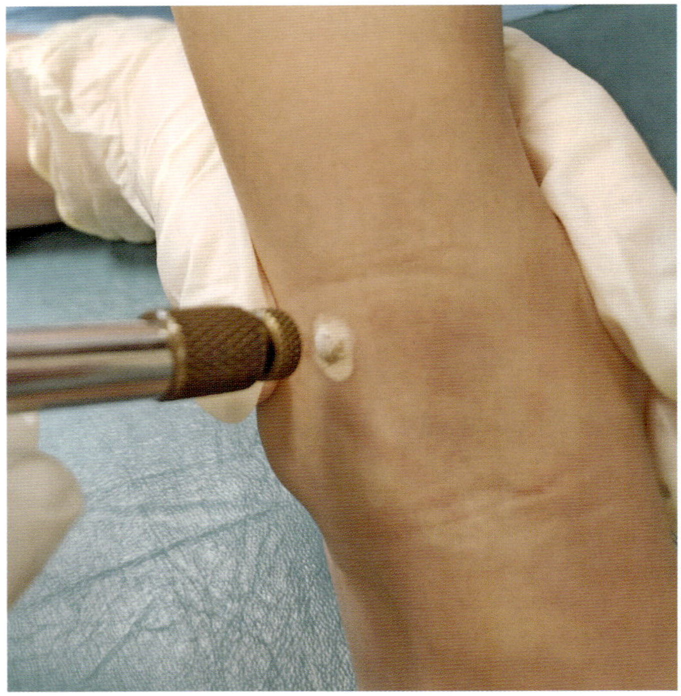

FIGURE 16-4. Another photograph showing the ice ring around the lesion.

- For pediatric patients who have a lower pain threshold, a topical anesthetic such as EMLA (2.5% lignocaine, 2.5% prilocaine) may be applied 30 to 60 minutes before the procedure.
- Avoid performing liquid nitrogen on cosmetically sensitive sites, such as the face, in darker-skinned patients (e.g., Fitzpatrick type V and VI), as depigmentation can occur, which can be permanent.

SAMPLING FOR FUNGAL INVESTIGATIONS

Skin scrapings are commonly performed to diagnose or exclude tinea or other superficial fungal infections of the skin. Hair and nail clippings may also be obtained for suspected tinea capitis or onychomycosis.

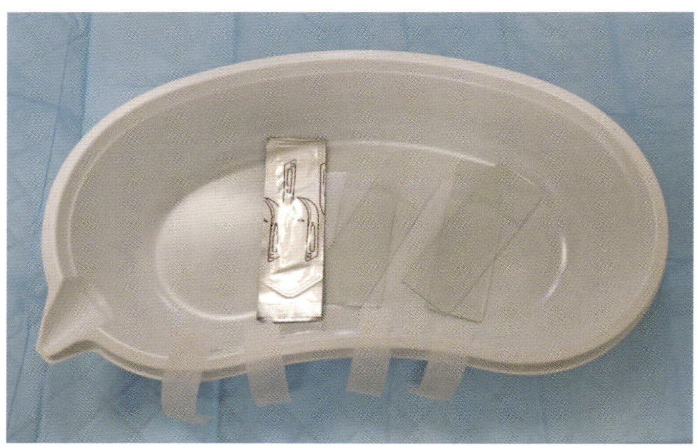

FIGURE 16-5. Equipment required for performing skin scraping for fungal microscopy or culture.

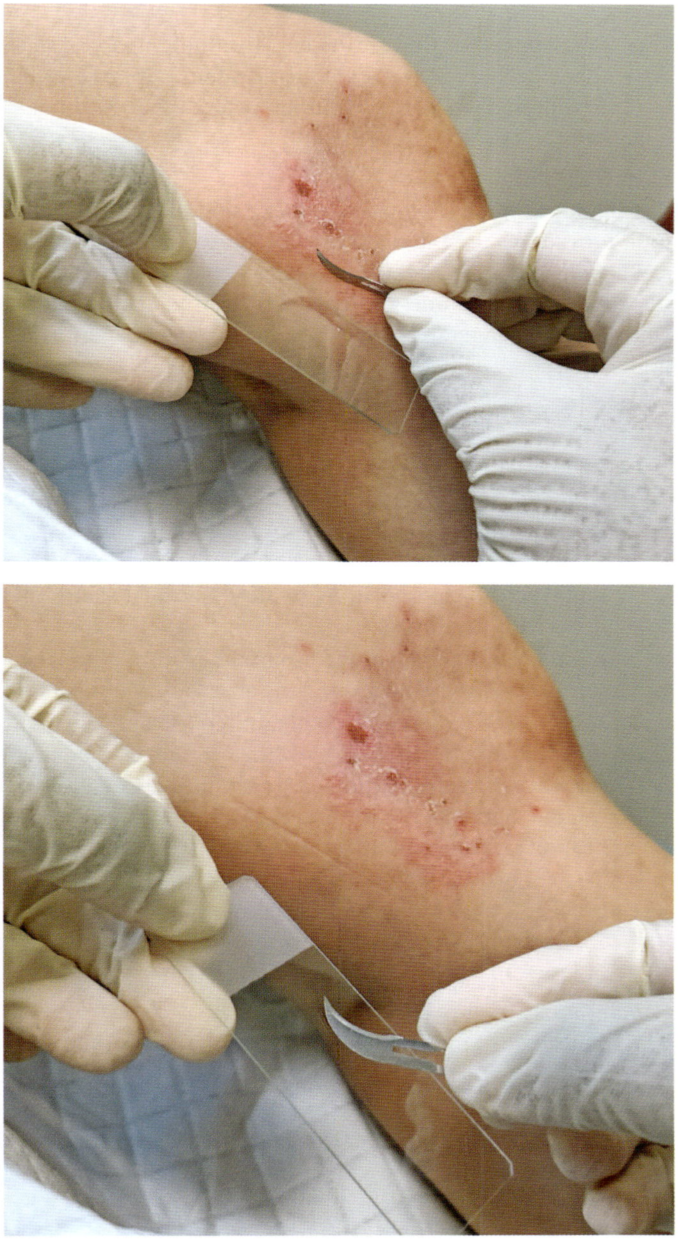

FIGURE 16-6A & 6B. Use of a sterile blade to gently scrape the edge of the skin lesion onto a slide.

Procedure

- Clean the defined area with 70% alcohol before sampling. This is to remove any topical medications that may have been applied prior to sampling, and to minimize contamination.
- For skin samples, use a sterile blade to gently scrape the edge of the skin lesion.
- For nail samples, use a nail clipper to clip a portion of the affected nails, and include the subungual debris if present.
- For hair samples, pluck the hairs from the affected area on the scalp with forceps and scrape the affected part of the scalp gently with a sterile blade. Cut hair is not ideal, as the yield is much lower.

Side Effects

- There are minimal side effects except for mild discomfort and mild and self-limiting bleeding from the scraped area.

Pearls & Practical Tips

- Include as much specimen as possible to increase the yield for both fungal microscopy and fungal culture.
- If a blade is not available, the edge of a microscope glass slide may be used.
- Scraping is performed from the annular edge of the suspected lesions of tinea, and not the central hyperpigmented area.

INTRALESIONAL STEROID INJECTIONS

Intralesional injections are common procedures performed to administer corticosteroids directly into a skin lesion or into the dermis. It is most commonly performed for keloids, hypertrophic scars, prurigo nodularis, or alopecia areata in older children and adolescents. Other less common indications include discoid lupus erythematosus, hypertrophic lichen planus, and granuloma annulare.

Procedure

- The most commonly used steroid is triamcinolone (Kenacort or Kenalog), which is most often available as 40 mg/mL or 10 mg/mL concentrations. These can be further diluted with normal saline. Higher concentrations are usually used for thicker lesions, such as keloids and prurigo nodularis, while lower concentrations are used for thinner lesions and for alopecia areata.

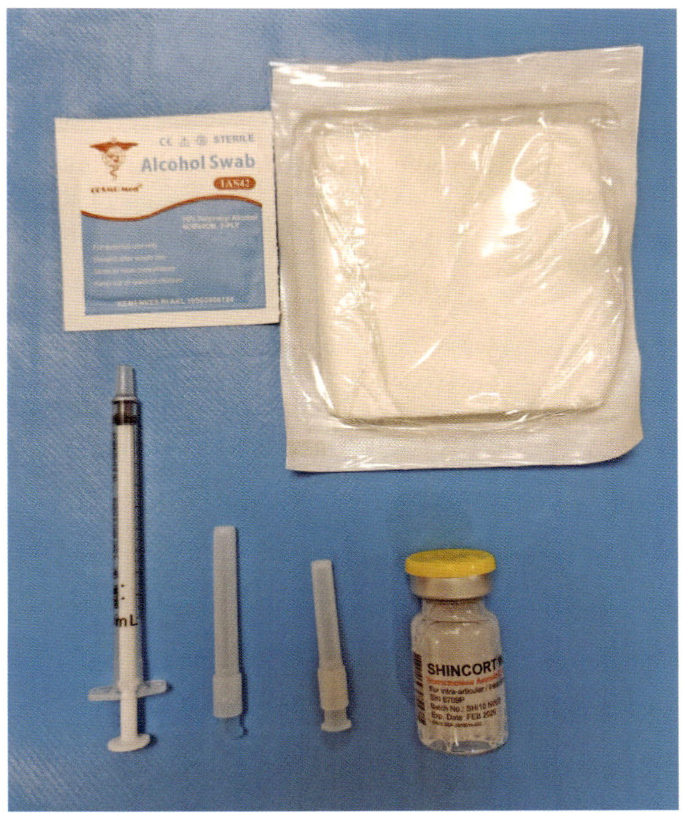

FIGURE 16-7. Equipment required for intralesional corticosteroid injection.

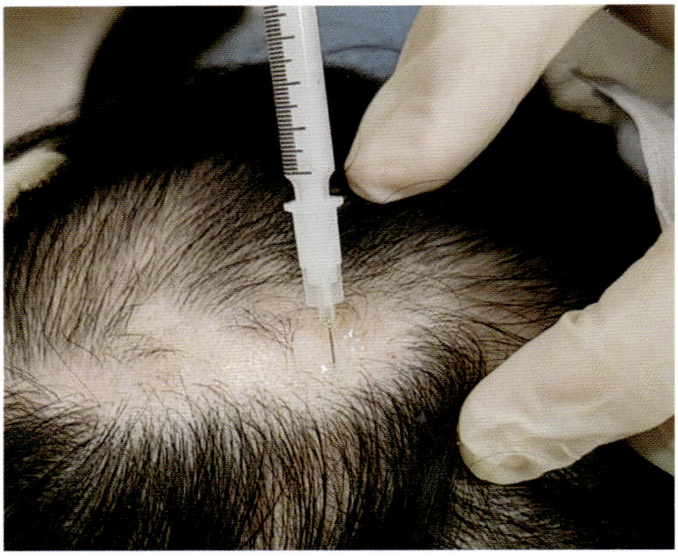

FIGURE 16-8. Intralesional corticosteroid injection for alopecia areata.

- The site for intralesional injection is cleaned with alcohol or other antiseptic solution.
- For keloids, hypertrophic scars, and prurigo nodules, the steroid is injected directly into the lesion, until the overlying skin is blanched.
- For alopecia areata, the steroid is injected into the dermis of the affected areas.
- Repeated injections are performed for each square centimeter, with approximately 0.1 mL of steroid for each injection.
- Light pressure is applied for a few minutes after injection.
- The procedure may be repeated at 4 to 8 weekly intervals.

Side Effects

- Common side effects include pain, bleeding, and bruising. Less common side effects include infection and abscess formation, skin atrophy, hypopigmentation, telangiectasias, and hypertrichosis.

Pearls & Practical Tips

- For patients who have lower pain threshold, a topical anesthetic such as EMLA (2.5% lignocaine, 2.5% prilocaine) may be applied 30 to 60 minutes before the procedure.

SKIN BIOPSIES

Punch biopsies, shave biopsies, and excision biopsies are common procedures used to diagnose or treat various dermatological conditions. Most of these procedures may be performed in the clinic with local anesthetic. However, in younger children who are less cooperative, the procedures may be performed under conscious sedation or general anesthesia.

Procedure

- The site of biopsy is identified and marked.
- The patient is positioned adequately with good lighting, with the bed or couch at an appropriate height for the proceduralist.
- The area to be biopsied is sterilized using a cleansing solution, such as chlorhexidine or sterile normal saline, and dried with sterile gauze.
- Local anesthetic is injected around the biopsy area, and a sterile sheet is placed around the area to be biopsied.
- After the procedure, topical antibiotics and a simple dressing can be applied over the wound. Patients and caregivers should be advised to avoid excessive friction, trauma, and sun exposure to the wound site for optimal healing and to minimize scarring and dyspigmentation.
- The time to suture removal depends on the anatomical site of the biopsy, with facial biopsies requiring 5 to 7 days, truncal biopsies requiring about 10 days, and limb biopsies 10 to 14 days.

Punch Biopsy

- The aim of a punch biopsy is to obtain full thickness skin specimens.
- Punch biopsy tools have circular blades in various diameters (2 to 12 mm) to obtain a cylindrical tissue specimen. The depth of the biopsy is proportional to the diameter of

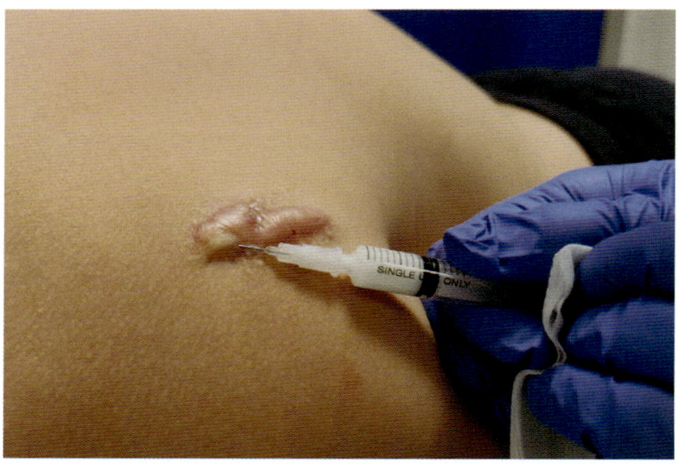

FIGURE 16-9. Intralesional corticosteroid injection for keloid.

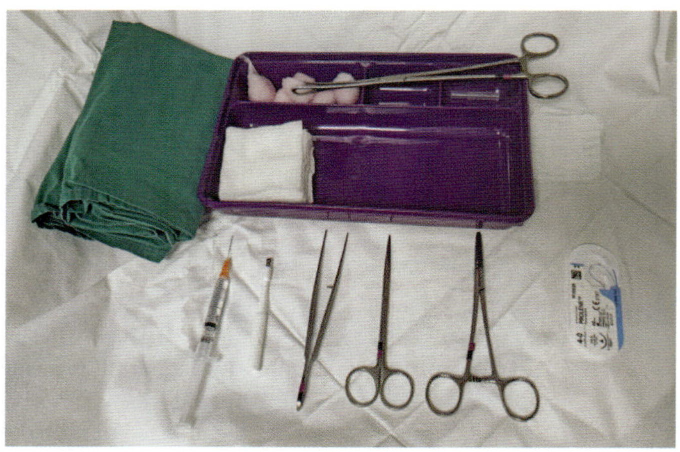

FIGURE 16-10. Instruments required for performing a punch biopsy procedure.

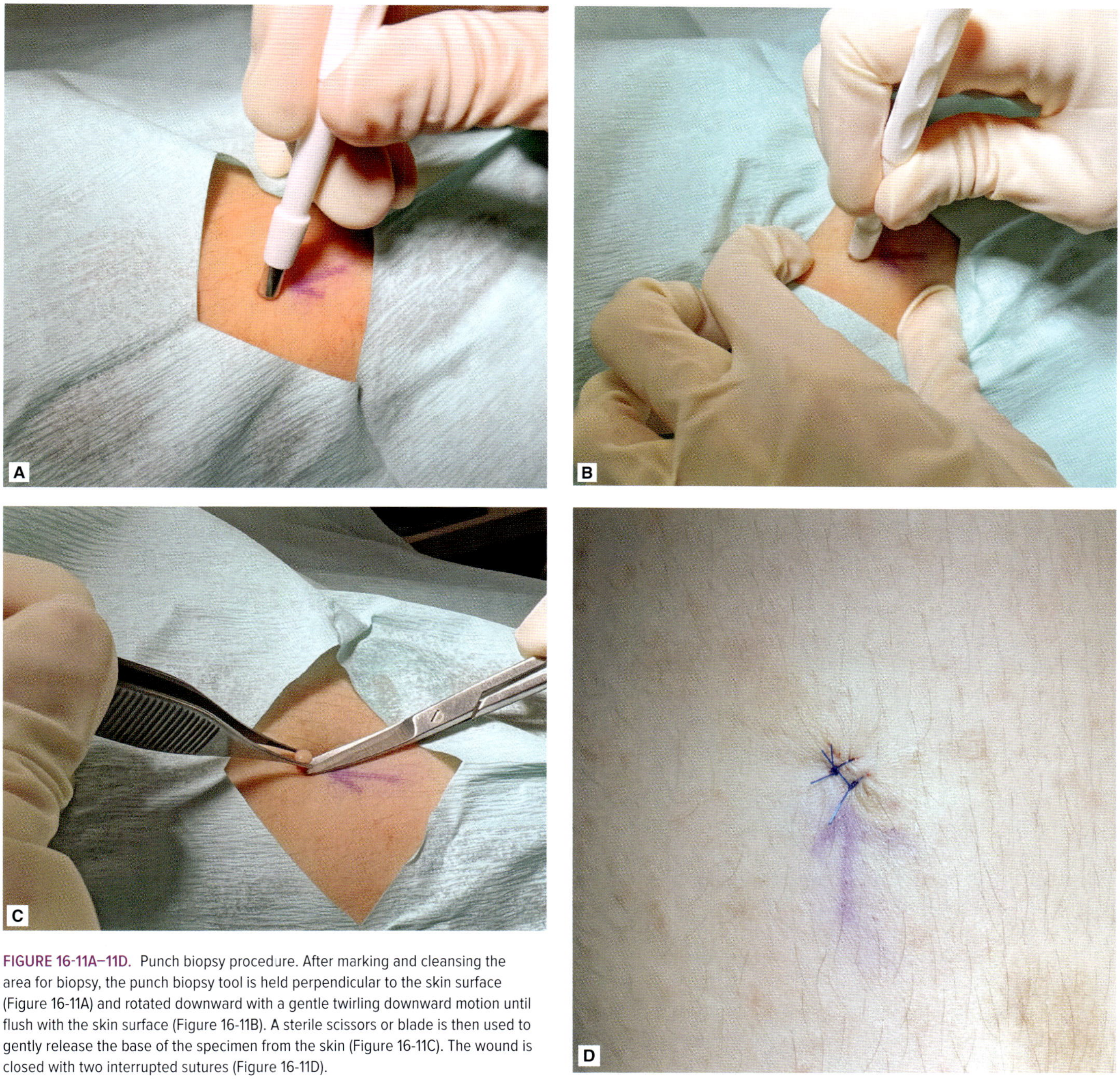

FIGURE 16-11A–11D. Punch biopsy procedure. After marking and cleansing the area for biopsy, the punch biopsy tool is held perpendicular to the skin surface (Figure 16-11A) and rotated downward with a gentle twirling downward motion until flush with the skin surface (Figure 16-11B). A sterile scissors or blade is then used to gently release the base of the specimen from the skin (Figure 16-11C). The wound is closed with two interrupted sutures (Figure 16-11D).

the tool. The most commonly utilized tool size is 4 mm, while 3 mm can be used for facial biopsies. The obtain adequate subcutaneous tissue, a 5- or 6-mm biopsy is required, depending on the age of the patient and site of biopsy.

- The skin is stretched at 90 degrees perpendicular to Langer's lines using the non-dominant hand, while the dominant hand performs the punch biopsy. This is done to obtain an elliptical-shaped wound oriented parallel to Langer's lines.
- The punch biopsy tool is held perpendicular to the skin surface and rotated downward with a gentle twirling downward motion. A sterile scissors or blade is then used to release the base of the specimen from the skin.
- Avoid over-manipulating the specimen with a forceps to avoid crush artifacts, and the specimen is gently transferred into the sterile specimen container.
- The wound can then be closed with one or two interrupted sutures.

Shave Biopsy

- A superficial shave biopsy can be performed for benign epidermal lesions such as viral warts, skin tags, pyogenic granulomas, and epidermal nevi.

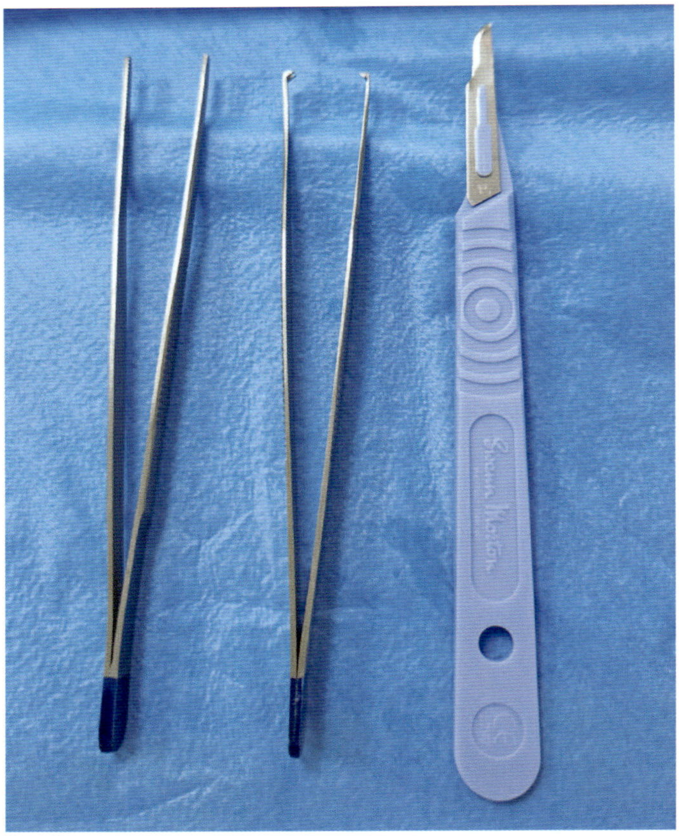

FIGURE 16-12. Instruments required for performing a shave biopsy procedure.

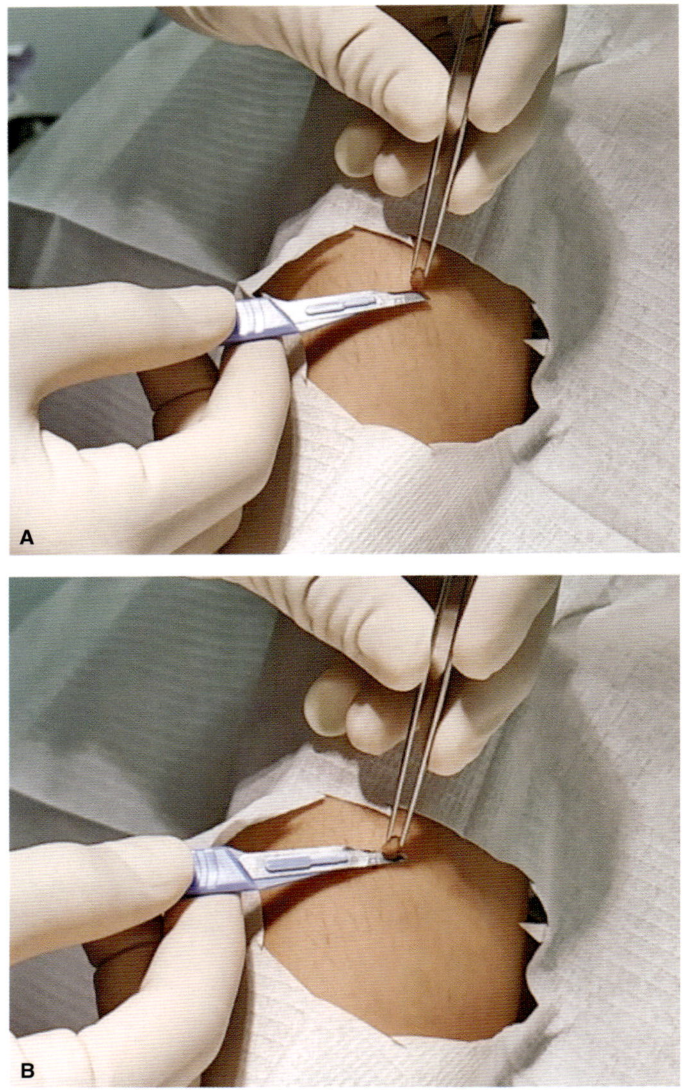

FIGURE 16-13A & 13B. Shave biopsy performed by grasping the lesion with a forceps and gently slicing the base of the lesion with a scalpel.

- A scalpel or Dermablade shave biopsy instrument may be used.
- The scalpel or Dermablade is held parallel to the skin and sliced through the base of the lesion in a side-to-side motion.
- Hemostasis can be achieved with aluminum chloride 20% solution or electrocautery.
- No suturing is required unless performed over an area of excessive tension, such as the sole of the foot.

Excision Biopsy

- Excision biopsies are utilized to remove skin lesions with margins. An incisional biopsy is performed in the same way if a larger or deeper biopsy is required for diagnostic purposes, such as panniculitis.
- The lesion with the appropriate margins is marked out with a surgical marker. The resultant shape should be an ellipse with an ideal length-to-width ratio of 3:1. This is to reduce any "dog-ear" formation upon closure. The eventual scar should be long, thin, and follow the lines of least tension.
- The elliptical incision is made with a sterile surgical blade along the drawn markings. The non-dominant hand is used to maintain traction of the surrounding area.
- A toothed forceps is used to hold the tissue at the apex while gently dissecting the rest of the tissue at the level of the subcutis with a scalpel or scissors. The specimen should be dissected along an even plane to facilitate easy wound closure and for best surgical outcome.
- Hemostasis can be achieved with direct tamponade and/or electrocautery.
- At areas with tighter skin, such as the back, undermining of the surrounding skin is performed using a blade or scissors.
- The defect is closed in layers with absorbable deep sutures and nonabsorbable superficial sutures. Layered closure is essential, as the deep sutures eliminate dead space, decrease wound tension, and facilitate wound eversion.

Side Effects

- Common side effects include bleeding, pain, swelling, erythema, and scarring.
- Less common side effects include postinflammatory hyper- or hypopigmentation, infection, and wound dehiscence (if sutures are used).
- If the biopsy is performed to remove a lesion, recurrence of lesions can occur.

Pearls & Practical Tips

- Always cut the skin under tension, and close any wounds with minimal tension.
- Snip biopsies may be performed for small pedunculated lesions such as skin tags. This is performed in the same way as a shave biopsy except that a curved, small scissors is used to snip the lesion at the stalk.
- If deep pathology is suspected, such as panniculitis, either a 6-mm or incisional biopsy is recommended for optimal tissue sampling. Performing punch biopsies larger than 6 mm is not ideal, as formation of "dog-ears" at the ends of wound sites is common.

ELECTROCAUTERY

This is a commonly performed dermatological procedure to destroy superficial skin lesions, such as viral warts, skin tags, epidermal nevi, and superficial vascular lesions. The device utilizes a direct electric current to generate heat through a cautery probe or electrode. The heated probe is then applied to tissue, resulting in direct heat transference to the tissue leading to local tissue destruction and hemostasis.

Procedure

- As the procedure is painful, topical anesthetic and/or local anesthetic should be used pre-procedure. In younger children, the procedure should be performed under conscious sedation or general anesthesia.
- The area for electrocautery is cleaned using a cleansing solution, such as chlorhexidine or sterile normal saline, and dried with sterile gauze.
- The cautery probe is applied to the lesion for a duration that is determined by the thickness of the lesion. The lesion is destroyed down to the desired level of skin.

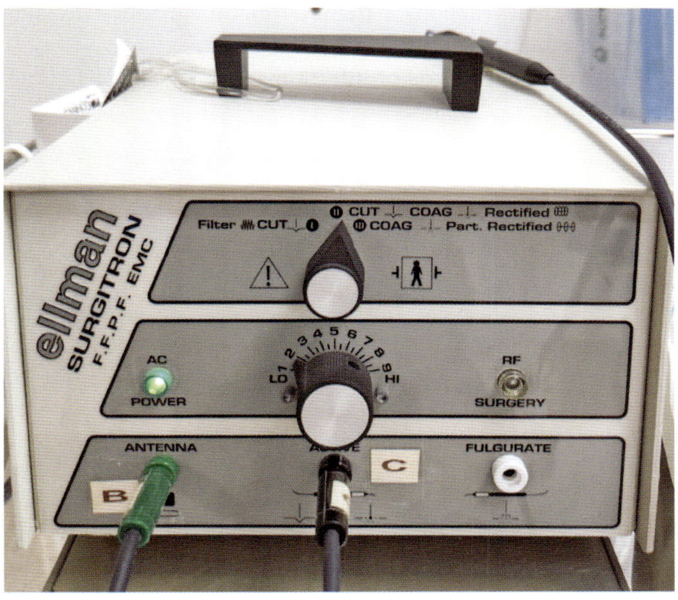

FIGURE 16-14. Electrocautery machine.

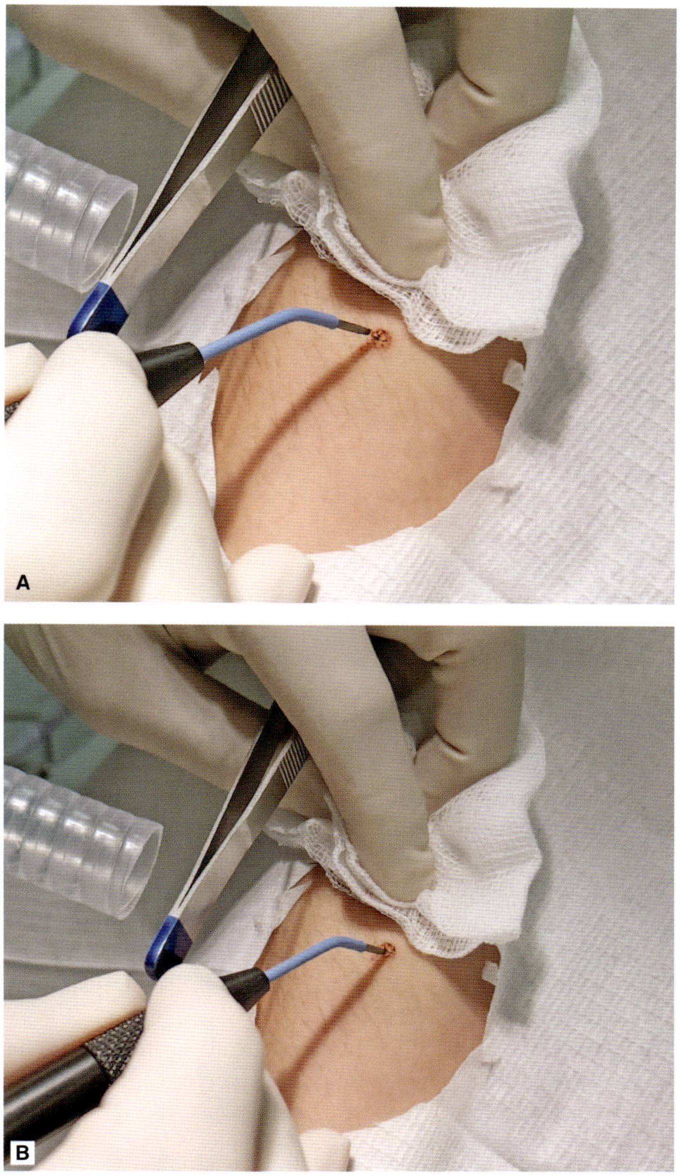

FIGURE 16-15A & 15B. Electrocautery of a lesion on the forearm.

- Hemostasis is usually achieved simultaneously or by application of aluminum chloride 20% solution.
- After the procedure, topical antibiotics and a simple dressing can be applied over the wound. Patients and caregivers should be advised to avoid excessive friction, trauma, and sun exposure to the wound site for optimal healing and to minimize scarring and dyspigmentation.

Side Effects

- Common side effects include pain, swelling, bleeding, and erythema. Both hypertrophic and atrophic scarring may also occur, in addition to post-inflammatory hypo- or hyperpigmentation.

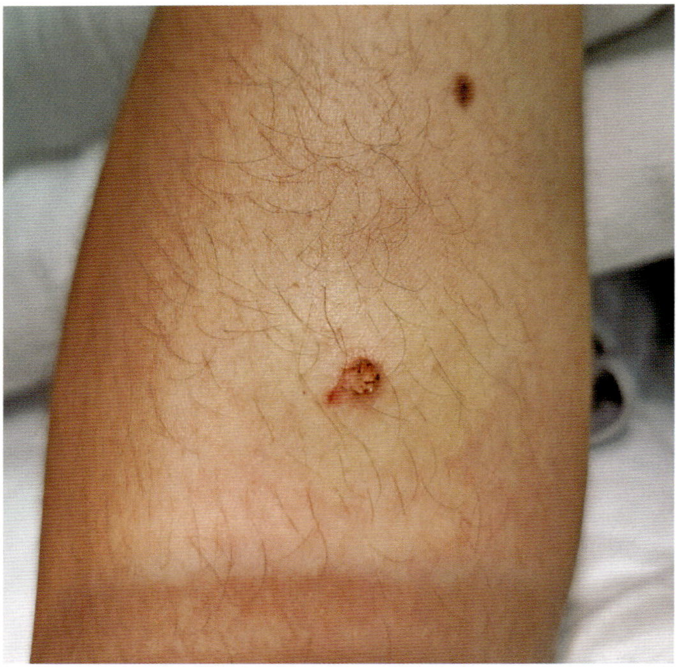

FIGURE 16-16. A scab is seen after the lesion has undergone electrocautery.

Pearls & Practical Tips

- Unlike true electrosurgery, no electric current flows through the patient in electrocautery and therefore it can be safely used in patients with implanted electrical or metallic devices.
- A fume extractor should be utilized to minimize inhalation of the fumes caused by electrocautery. Laryngeal warts have been reported to occur in proceduralists after electrocautery of viral warts.
- For thicker lesions, the superficial portion may be removed by a shave or snip biopsy before application of electrocautery to the base of the lesion.

PATCH TESTING

Patch testing is used to diagnose or exclude allergic contact dermatitis. It can be performed safely in adolescents, children, and even infants. Although most patients undergoing patch testing will be tested against a standard panel, depending on the clinical history and suspicion, additional panels, individual allergens, or patients' own products may also be tested. The results should be interpreted with close clinical correlation.

Procedure

- The allergens are placed in small metal chambers affixed to adhesive patches that are securely taped to the patient's back.
- Markings are drawn with a surgical marker to outline the patches and number the wells.
- The patches are left for 48 hours before removal by parents or caregivers, or in the clinic.
- The skin must remain dry during the period that the patches are in place. Patients should be advised to avoid vigorous physical activity during this period to allow the patches to maintain contact with the skin.

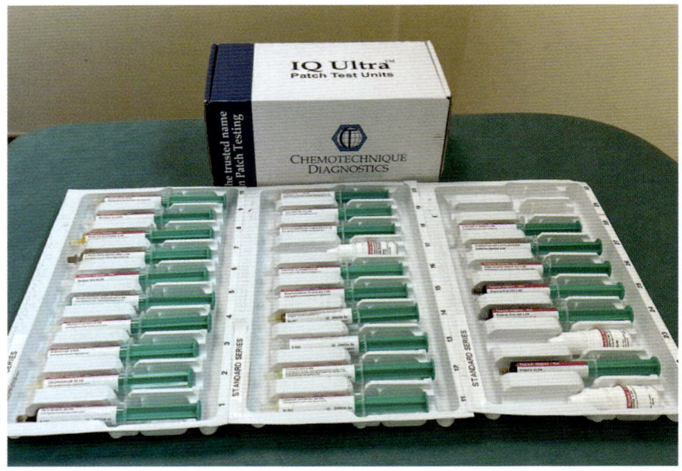

FIGURE 16-17. Trays of patch testing allergens.

- The first reading is performed in the clinic between 48 and 72 hours after placement of the patches. If a delayed reaction is suspected, such as to topical corticosteroids, patients should return between day 5 and 7 after placement of the patches for delayed reading.
- Positive reactions can be labeled as "present relevance" where the allergen is causing the current dermatitis, "past relevance" where the allergen had caused dermatitis in the past but is not a cause of the current dermatitis, "exposed" if the allergen had been previously encountered by the patient but did not develop dermatitis at that time, or "unknown" if there is no known exposure to the allergen.

Side Effects

- Patch testing is a relatively safe procedure. More common side effects include flaring of existing dermatitis, persistent reactions, irritant dermatitis to adhesives, and hyperpigmentation.
- Rarely, anaphylaxis or infection at the patch test site can occur.

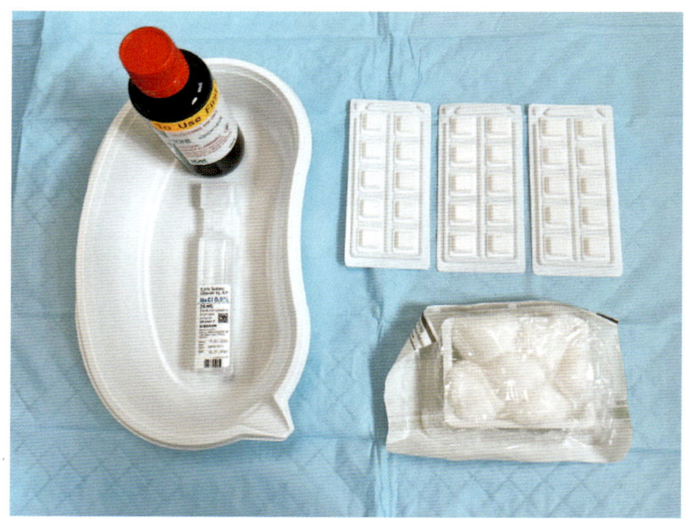

FIGURE 16-18. Other equipment required for performing a patch test.

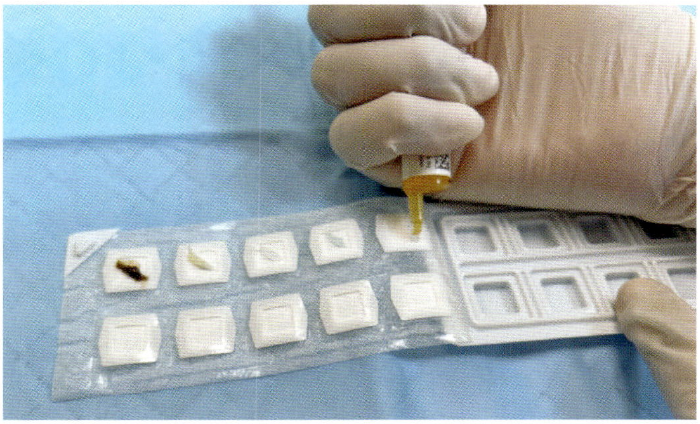

FIGURE 16-19. Allergens are being syringed onto a tray of metal chambers.

Pearls & Practical Tips

- Patients should not be on systemic corticosteroids for 3 to 4 weeks before the patch test, and preferably topical corticosteroids should not be applied to the patch test area 1 to 2 weeks before placement of the patches. Antihistamines are not contraindicated for patch testing.
- Patch testing should not be performed when patients are experiencing a flare of eczema. This is to prevent worsening of the eczema flare and "angry back" syndrome where false positive reactions occur to many of the allergens.
- In infants and younger children who have limited skin area for placement of patch tests, select the most likely allergens to test, or testing can be done sequentially at 2- to 3-week intervals.
- Depending on the clinical history or indications, patients may be patch tested to their own materials or products.
- If an irritant reaction is suspected, patients can return for repeat reading a day later, whereby the reaction would have resolved, unlike a true allergic reaction where it will persist for a few more days.

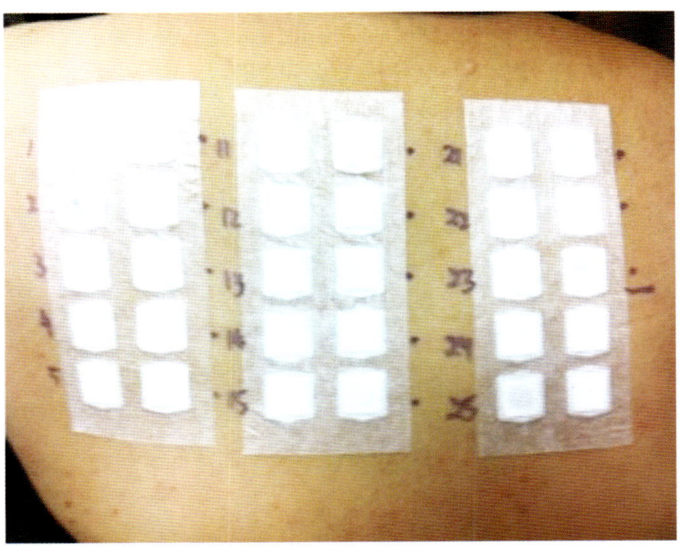

FIGURE 16-20. Patches on the back of a patient undergoing patch testing. These are left in contact with the skin for approximately 48 hours.

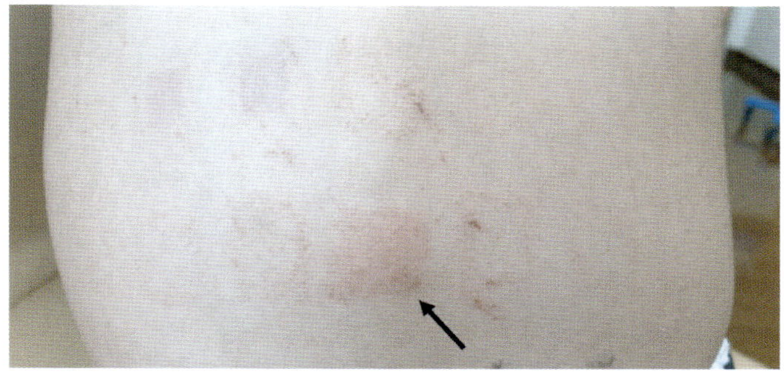

FIGURE 16-21. Example of a positive reaction, read at 72 hours after placement of the patch, with removal at 48 hours.

SKIN PRICK TESTING

Skin prick testing is utilized to identify or exclude drug, food, and aeroallergens, especially in children, although it can also be performed in adolescents and adults. Depending on the clinical history and patient profile, different prick test allergen panels or individual allergens can be selected for the test. Clinical correlation is important to conclude if a positive reaction is relevant and is a cause of the patient's symptoms.

Procedure

- Skin prick tests are usually performed on the inner forearm or the back.

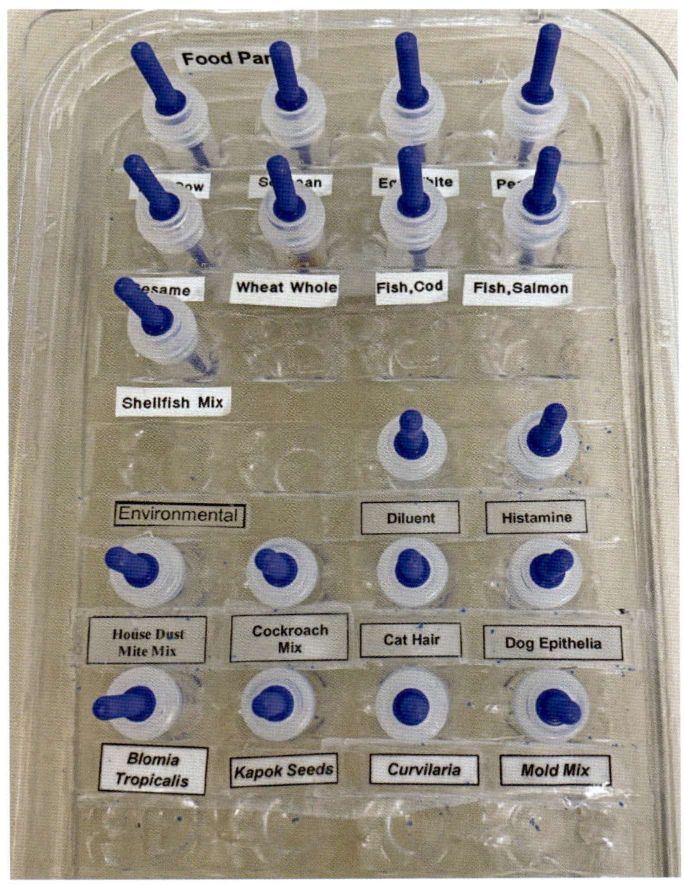

FIGURE 16-22. A tray of skin prick test allergens.

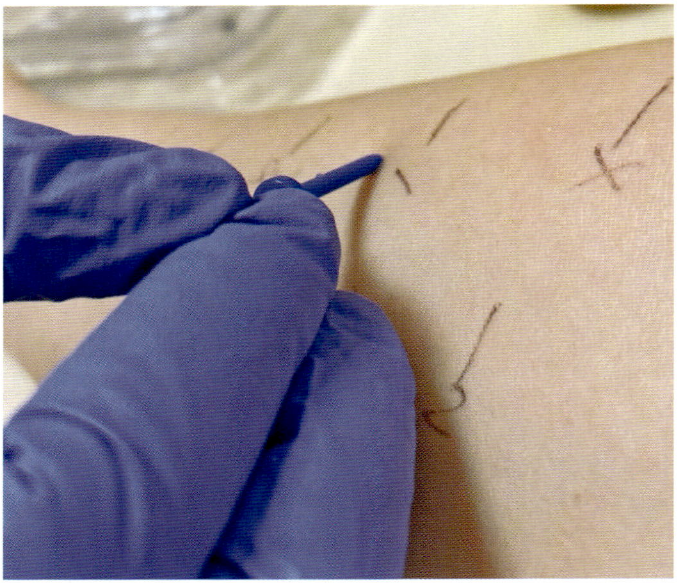

FIGURE 16-23. A small prick is performed using a sterile lancet.

- The area is cleaned with alcohol and markings are made corresponding to the allergens being tested. Each allergen should be pricked at least 2 cm apart.
- A positive and negative control is included. Histamine solution is used for the positive control, while normal saline solution is used as the negative control.
- A drop of each allergen is placed beside the marking and a small prick is performed on the skin beneath the allergen with a sterile lancet or needle.
- A new needle or lancet is used for each allergen being tested.
- Readings are performed after 15 to 30 minutes. A reaction should be observed for the positive control, while the negative control should elicit no response.

Side Effects

- Skin prick testing is relatively safe.
- The most common side effects include itch, urticaria, and flare of underlying dermatosis. Rarely, anaphylaxis can occur.

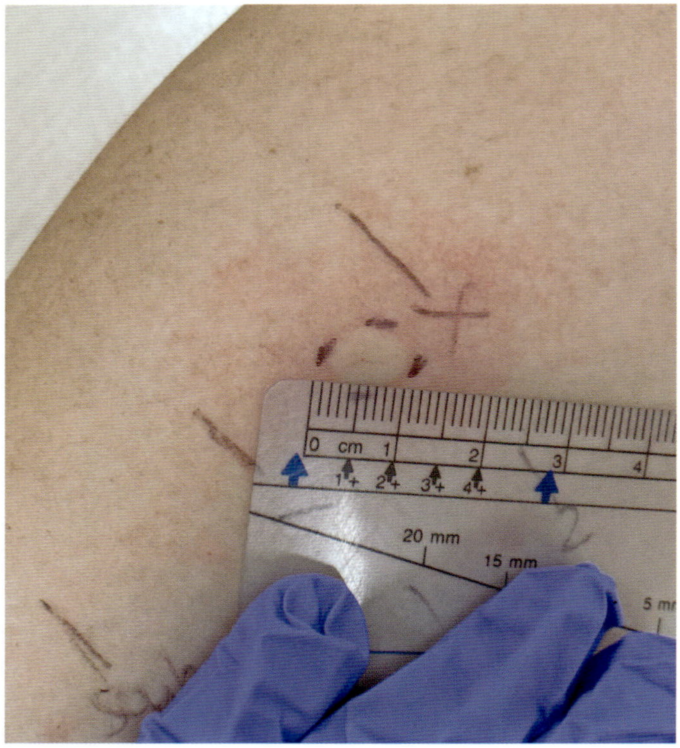

FIGURE 16-24. Wheal and flare indicates a positive skin prick test result.

Pearls & Practical Tips

- Antihistamines should be avoided for approximately a week before the skin prick test. The results will be falsely negative if the patient is on antihistamines.
- Skin prick tests have a high negative predictive value but a lower positive predictive value. The sensitivity and specificity of skin prick tests is approximately the same as specific IgE testing.
- Most children with atopic dermatitis are sensitized to house dust mites from 2 to 3 years of age. Food allergies as a trigger of atopic dermatitis is more common in infants and young children, with milk, eggs, and peanuts being the most common in this age group.

Index

Page numbers followed by *f* indicate figures and *t* indicate tables.

D

O

P